Provocation Testing in Clinical Practice

CLINICAL ALLERGY AND IMMUNOLOGY

Series Editor

MICHAEL A. KALINER, M.D.

Medical Director
Institute for Asthma and Allergy
Washington, D.C.

1. Sinusitis: Pathophysiology and Treatment, *edited by Howard M. Druce*
2. Eosinophils in Allergy and Inflammation, *edited by Gerald J. Gleich and A. Barry Kay*
3. Molecular and Cellular Biology of the Allergic Response, *edited by Arnold I. Levinson and Yvonne Paterson*
4. Neuropeptides in Respiratory Medicine, *edited by Michael A. Kaliner, Peter J. Barnes, Gert H. H. Kunkel, and James N. Baraniuk*
5. Provocation Testing in Clinical Practice, *edited by Sheldon L. Spector*

ADDITIONAL VOLUMES IN PREPARATION

Mast Cell Proteases in Immunological Responses, *edited by George H. Caughey*

Provocation Testing in Clinical Practice

edited by

Sheldon L. Spector
Allergy Medical Clinic and Allergy Research Foundation
Los Angeles, California

Marcel Dekker, Inc. New York • Basel • Hong Kong

Library of Congress Cataloging-in-Publication Data

Provocation testing in clinical practice / edited by Sheldon L. Spector.
p. cm. — (Clinical allergy and immunology; 5)
Includes bibliographical references and index.
ISBN 0-8247-9249-1 (alk. paper)
1. Provocation tests (Medicine) 2. Bronchial provocation tests.
3. Allergy—Diagnosis. I. Spector, Sheldon L. II. Series.
[DNLM: 1. Hypersensitivity. 2. Bronchial Provocation Tests. 3. Nasal Provocation Tests. 4. Immunologic Tests. W1 CL652 v. 5 1995 / QW 900 P968 1995]
RC587.P76P74 1995
616.97'075—dc20
DNLM/DLC
for Library of Congress 94-33912
CIP

The publisher offers discounts on this book when ordered in bulk quantities. For more information, write to Special Sales/Professional Marketing at the address below.

This book is printed on acid-free paper.

Marcel Dekker, Inc.
270 Madison Avenue, New York, New York 10016

Current printing (last digit):
10 9 8 7 6 5 4 3 2 1

PRINTED IN THE UNITED STATES OF AMERICA

Preface

There are a multitude of books dealing with general topics such as asthma, eye conditions, rhinitis, or skin diseases; however, there are very few, if any, dealing with provocative challenges to various organs in the body. My interest in provocative challenges has led me to seek out experts who could provide background information as well as details regarding the challenges themselves. This book will therefore serve as a rather unique reference work.

Many articles have appeared on scientific programs regarding pharmacological challenges such as methacholine and histamine, and the number of such challenges continues to increase. Adenosine and leukotriene challenges were virtually unheard of only a few years ago. Some of the challenges discussed in this volume are induced from natural sources such as air pollution and infectious agents. In vitro studies and animal models that have helped us understand mechanisms are also included in this book.

The main thrust of this work, however, represents details regarding challenges in humans. This means that guidelines must be utilized for the proper performance of such challenges to be done in a scientific and moral way. Humans are not as homogeneous as many of the animals that are studied, so it is not unusual for a paradoxical or unpredictable response to occur. This is an even greater reason for precautions to be taken, since quantification becomes important. The dose of metabisulfite or aspirin administered to someone with asthma must be tailored to the potential disease as well as the heterogeneous patient. As new data emerge, so dose the breadth of the discussion on challenges. Even a few years ago it was not appreciated that certain loop diuretics might protect against provocative challenge. Medications such as adenosine or one of the products of the arachidonic acid pathway were also not mentioned because they had not been isolated or purified to the point of giving a challenge. Many procedures described in this volume are of practical value to the practicing physician since skin tests in both immediate, delayed, and contact sensitivity are discussed.

This book will prove important to clinical researchers, interested in the various aspects of allergy, clinical immunology, and pulmonary medicine. There is an in-depth discussion of the background as well as the practical aspects of performing these challenges for those who are interested in state-of-the-art procedures. In this respect, the volume will be a reference guide for serious investigators as well as a guide to the practicing allergist/immunologist. In addition, there is an international character to this compendium, with authors from such places as England, Australia, France, and Canada. I sincerely wish that the information provided in this book will serve the physician well in understanding the mechanisms, diagnosis, and even treatment when normal physiological mechanisms are challenged.

Sheldon L. Spector

Contents

Contributors

Murray D. Altose UCLA Medical Center, Los Angeles, California

John A. Anderson Henry Ford Hospital, Detroit, Michigan

Sandra D. Anderson Royal Prince Alfred Hospital, Sydney, Australia

Jonathan P. Arm Brigham and Women's Hospital and Harvard Medical School, Boston, Massachusetts

A. K. Bewtra Creighton University School of Medicine, Omaha, Nebraska

James D. Blanchard Harvard School of Public Health, Boston, Massachusetts

Joseph D. Brain Harvard School of Public Health, Boston, Massachusetts

S. Bianco Ospedale S. Raffaele, Milan, Italy

Jean Bousquet Centre Hospitalier Universitaire, Montpellier, France

William W. Busse University of Wisconsin School of Medicine, Madison, Wisconsin

William J. Calhoun University of Pittsburgh, Pittsburgh, Pennsylvania

John E. Connett UCLA Medical Center, Los Angeles, California

Elliot C. Dick University of Wisconsin School of Medicine, Madison, Wisconsin

Jacqueline I. du Toit Royal Prince Alfred Hospital, Sydney, Australia

Peyton A. Eggleston The Johns Hopkins University School of Medicine, Baltimore, Maryland

Philip Fireman University of Pittsburgh School of Medicine and Children's Hospital of Pittsburgh, Pittsburgh, Pennsylvania

Henry Gong, Jr. Rancho Los Amigos Medical Center, Downey, California and University of Southern California, Los Angeles, California

David J. Hendrick University of Newcastle upon Tyne, Newcastle, England

Carol A. Hirshman The Johns Hopkins University, Baltimore, Maryland

Russell J. Hopp Creighton University School of Medicine, Omaha, Nebraska

Nizar N. Jarjour University of Wisconsin School of Medicine, Madison, Wisconsin

Richard E. Kanner UCLA Medical Center, Los Angeles, California

Charles H. Kirkpatrick University of Colorado Health Sciences Center, Denver, Colorado

Antti I. Lauerma University of California School of Medicine, San Francisco, California

Tak H. Lee Guy's Hospital, London, England

Wondra Wong Lee UCLA Medical Center, Los Angeles, California

Robert F. Lemanske, Jr. University of Wisconsin School of Medicine, Madison, Wisconsin

Lawrence M. Lichtenstein The Johns Hopkins University School of Medicine, Baltimore, Maryland

Howard I. Maibach University of California School of Medicine, San Francisco, California

William A. Massey The Johns Hopkins University School of Medicine, Baltimore, Maryland

David A. Mathison Scripps Clinic & Research Foundation, La Jolla, California

François-B. Michel Centre Hospitalier Universitaire, Montpellier, France

Nicki M. Nair Creighton University School of Medicine, Omaha, Nebraska

Harold S. Nelson National Jewish Center for Immunology and Respiratory Medicine, Denver, Colorado

Paul M. O'Byrne McMaster University, Hamilton, Canada

M. G. Pieroni University of Siena, Siena, Italy

Michael B. Raizman Tufts University School of Medicine, Boston, Massachusetts

R. M. Refini University of Siena, Siena, Italy

Josef Riedler Royal Children's Hospital, Melbourne, Australia

Colin F. Robertson Royal Children's Hospital, Melbourne, Australia

M. Robuschi University of Milan, Milan, Italy

Leanne T. Rodwell Royal Prince Alfred Hospital, Sydney, Australia

Richard R. Rosenthal Consultant, Fairfax, Virginia

John E. Salvaggio Tulane University Medical Center, New Orleans, Louisiana

Hugh A. Sampson The Johns Hopkins University School of Medicine, Baltimore, Maryland

P. Sestini University of Siena, Siena, Italy

Gail Shapiro University of Washington School of Medicine, Seattle, Washington

Ronald A. Simon Scripps Clinic & Research Foundation, La Jolla, California

Christine M. Smith Royal Prince Alfred Hospital, Sydney, Australia

William R. Solomon University of Michigan Hospitals, Ann Arbor, Michigan

J. F. Souhrada The John B. Pierce Laboratory and Yale School of Medicine, New Haven, Connecticut

M. Souhrada The John B. Pierce Laboratory and Yale School of Medicine, New Haven, Connecticut

Sheldon L. Spector Allergy Medical Clinic and Allergy Research Foundation, Los Angeles, California

Donald D. Stevenson Scripps Clinic & Research Foundation, La Jolla, California

Donald P. Tashkin UCLA Medical Center, Los Angeles, California

Robert G. Townley Creighton University School of Medicine, Omaha, Nebraska

A. Vaghi Ospedale di Garbagnate, Milan, Italy

Paul V. Williams University of Washington School of Medicine, Seattle, Washington

Robert Wise UCLA Medical Center, Los Angeles, California

Robert A. Wood The Johns Hopkins University School of Medicine, Baltimore, Maryland

John W. Yunginger Mayo Clinic and Foundation, Rochester, Minnesota

Noe Zamel University of Toronto, Toronto, Canada

Provocation Testing in Clinical Practice

1

Allergenic Extracts

John W. Yunginger

Mayo Clinic and Foundation
Rochester, Minnesota

I. INTRODUCTION

Sales of allergenic extracts for diagnostic and therapeutic use in the United States amount to more than $30,000,000 annually. These sales are divided among approximately 12 commercial suppliers, whose catalogs collectively list over 1000 different extracts. In most cases, these extracts are crude complex mixtures of not only allergens but also pigments, enzymes, toxins, nonallergenic proteins, and/or sugars. In only a few cases have the active allergenic materials been isolated and characterized with respect to their physicochemical, biochemical, and immunochemical properties. This review will deal mainly with the preparation, labeling, and regulation of allergenic extracts. Standardization of allergenic extracts is discussed more extensively in Chapter 2.

II. ALLERGENIC EXTRACTS

A. Source Materials

1. Pollens

Anemophilous (wind-pollinated) plants are much more common causes of clinical allergy than are entemophilous (insect-pollinated) plants. Some pollens are collected by the "water set" method, in which cuttings from plants are brought indoors and arranged in water-filled containers; liberated pollen can be collected from waxed paper spread beneath the containers. Other pollens are collected with a portable vacuum in the field or by crushing the thoroughly dried pollen-containing anthers harvested from the heads of the plants. Pollens are cleaned by sieving; additionally, pollens from a few insect-pollinated plants may be cleaned with perchloroethylene. The cleaned pollen is dried to low residual moisture under controlled conditions of time and temperature [1].

The identity and purity of collected pollen can usually be established by microscopic examination, wherein grains are stained with Calberla's solution, a mixture of basic fuchsin, glycerin, ethanol, and water [2]. However, other pollens, such as grass pollens, are indistinguishable microscopically, and identification is verified by comparing the Coomassie blue–stained banding patterns produced by grass pollen extracts separated by thin-layer isoelectrofocusing [3].

2. Animals

For several decades, it was assumed that mammalian allergens were derived only from animal hair or dander. More recently, however, allergenic components have also been identified in animal saliva, serum, and urine. Table 1 lists the principal sources of various animal allergens [4].

Cat. Of all the animal allergens, those from the domestic cat have been studied most extensively. The major cat allergen, *Fel d* I [30], is present in cat salivary glands, pelts, hair follicles, and brains, and in surface washes of living cats [31,32]. Cat serum albumin (*Fel d* II) is also allergenic in a minority of cat-sensitive persons [33]. Although several other minor cat allergens have been

Table 1 Principal Sources of Several Mammalian Allergens

Animal	Allergen sources	Selected references
Cat	Epithelium Saliva Serum	4–11
Dog	Epithelium Serum	10,12–17
Mouse	Urine	18,19
Rat	Urine Serum	20–22
Guinea pig	Urine	23
Rabbit	Saliva	24
Horse	Epithelium Serum	25–27
Cattle	Epithelium Serum	28,29

identified [7], it is not clear whether their presence is essential in cat extracts sold for diagnostic or therapeutic use. Until recently, cat extracts were labeled simply as "cat" and could be prepared from cat dander, cat hair, or pelts from sacrificed animals. Commercial cat extracts are now prepared from either cat hair and dander or from cat pelts, with the source material specifically labeled.

Dog. Less is known about dog allergens. Most clinical studies involving dog allergy have used extracts derived from dog pelts or serum. Although the question of breed-specific allergens is frequently raised in clinical settings, and some reports have purported to show such allergens [14], no convincing evidence of breed-specific allergens has emerged in more recent studies [16,34–36]. Dog extracts used for provocative challenge procedures should probably be mixtures of pelt extracts from several different breeds.

Other Animals. The major source of allergen from laboratory animals, including mice, rats, and guinea pigs, is the urine. Nevertheless, commercial extracts from these animals, as well as rabbits, horses, and cattle, are prepared from the animals' hair, dander, or pelt.

3. Fungi

The most important allergenic fungi belong to the Deuteromycetes form class, or fungi imperfecti. These are asexual stages of a variety of ascomycetes and basidiomycetes [2]. However, the fungi imperfecti classification system is an artificial one, based largely on the macroscopic and microscopic appearance of spores and mycelium [37]. Such morphological classifications may not reflect the immunological and biochemical properties of the fungi that are important in clinical allergy.

The question of whether spores or mycelium should be the source materials for fungal extracts has been debated for decades. Most commercial extracts are prepared from both spores and mycelial mats. Some commercial fungal extracts (for example, MMP® extracts, from Miles/Hollister-Stier) also contain metabolic antigens isolated from dialyzed lyophilized synthetic culture medium [38].

4. Mites

House dust mites, of which *Dermatophagoides pteronyssinus* and *Dermatophagoides farinae* have been studied most extensively, occur in most parts of the world. The mites are grown in culture, and there are two methods of preparing mite extracts [39]. In one method, mites are removed from the culture medium by sieving and then extracted to produced "whole mite" extracts. All mite extracts licensed for sale in the United States are prepared in this manner. The other type of extract is a "whole mite culture" extract, in which the spent medium (including fecal particles and decaying mite carcasses) and living mites are collectively extracted [40]. The physicochemical and immunochemical profiles of these two types of extracts differ, and they may contain different relative concentrations of allergens [41].

Other species of house dust mite, including *Euroglyphus maynei* and *Blomia tropicalis*, are also recovered from homes in selected areas of the United States and are capable of eliciting human immunoglobulin E (IgE) responses [42]. In addition, grain storage mites such as *Lepidoglyphus destructor*, *Tyrophagus putrescentiae*, *Glycophagus domesticus*, and *Acarus siro* are allergenic to humans [43]. Very little is known about the allergenic composition of these mites.

5. Insects

Persons allergic to Hymenoptera stings are tested and treated with Hymenoptera venoms. Bee venom is obtained by electrical stimulation of honeybees [44], whereas vespid venoms are obtained by extracting extirpated venom sacs from yellow jackets, yellow hornets, white-faced hornets, and wasps [45]. Yellow jacket and wasp venom sac extracts are prepared from a mixture of several different insect species. Imported fire ant extracts are currently prepared from crushed whole bodies of the insects; fire ant venom may be available at some future time [46].

Among the biting insects, kissing bugs of the genus *Triatoma* may induce human allergic responses. Here, the major allergen is contained in the insects' salivary glands [47].

Inhalant allergy to insects is being recognized with increasing frequency [48]. When outdoor concentrations of insects reach a high level, a sizable proportion of the local population may become sensitized. Chironomid midges have been reported to cause seasonal outbreaks of rhinitis and asthma in several areas of the world [49,50]; the insects' hemoglobin is a major allergen [51]. Cockroaches produce important indoor aeroallergens [52], and the insects' cast skins, fecal pellets, and egg capsules all contain allergens. Inhalant insect allergy may also be an occupational hazard to persons working with moths, butterflies, crickets, or flies [53]. In all these cases, allergenic extracts are prepared from crushed whole insect bodies.

B. Extract Preparation

1. Extraction

With certain source materials, such as fungi and insect bodies, the raw material is routinely disrupted by grinding. Pollens and other materials are usually defatted with petroleum ether or diethyl ether before extraction. Source materials may be extracted in distilled water, sodium bicarbonate, ammonium bicarbonate, sodium chloride, or 50% glycerin. Ideally, the extraction fluid, its pH and temperature, and the duration of extraction should be optimized for each source material. The final form of the extract (that is, aqueous, glycerinated, or lyophilized) also determines the extraction buffer used. Concentration and/or dialysis steps may be included in the preparation of some extracts.

2. Labeling

For decades, allergenic extracts marketed in the United States have been labeled in weight:volume units or in protein nitrogen units (PNU). The weight:volume system merely tells how the extract was prepared. For example, a 1:10 weight:volume extract is prepared by extracting 1 g of source material in 10 ml of appropriate buffer. Because almost all allergens are proteins, a measurement of the total protein in an allergenic extract might be expected to correlate with its biologic potency. However, both allergenic and nonallergenic proteins are included in this quantitation. Total protein measurements have traditionally been reported as PNU [54] One PNU equals 10^{-5} mg of protein.

Allergenic extracts used in the Scandinavian countries are labeled on the basis of their prick skin test reactivity in sensitive persons, as compared to the subjects' prick skin test reactivity to histamine [55]. These units are called histamine equivalent potency (HEP) units. A smaller unit ("biological unit" [BU]) is used to permit use of whole numbers when dealing with dilute solutions; 1 HEP = 1000 BU.

Another method of measuring the biological activity of an extract is used in the United States [56]. This involves intradermal skin testing of several sensitive persons with serial threefold dilutions of both test and reference allergenic extracts, the latter having been assigned previously a potency in "allergy units" (AU). Although this skin test method is used initially to standardize the extract in question, subsequent commercial lots of the same extract are released following appropriate in vitro tests in which the extract is compared with a reference extract labeled in AU.

However, it is desirable to have one unit of a pollen extract be biologically equivalent to one unit of a mite extract, and so forth. Consequently, the Food and Drug Administration recently introduced the bioequivalent allergy unit (BAU); the intent is to have all allergen extracts with the same BAU labeling produce intradermal skin test reactions of the same size in sensitive persons. At present, only cat extracts are available in the United States with BAU labeling [57]. BAU-labeled standardized cat pelt extracts are not interchangeable with BAU-labeled standardized cat hair/dander extracts or with older AU-labeled cat extracts.

3. Sterility and Safety Testing

Allergenic extracts are usually clarified by centrifugation or coarse-membrane filtration and then sterilized by filtration through 0.2-μm membranes. Extracts packaged in multiple-dose containers contain phenol, at a concentration of 0.4%, and/or 50% glycerin, to inhibit microbial growth. The final product must pass a sterility test as defined by the United States Pharmacopeia. Extracts are also tested for safety by injection into guinea pigs and mice and tested for pyrogens by injection into rabbits. The expiration date shown on the label of the extract depends on the physical state or the diluent used. When shipped by the manufacturer, aqueous extracts are given a 12- to 18-month dating, while glycerinated extracts and lyophilized extracts are given a 3-year dating.

4. Stability

The potency of allergenic extracts decreases gradually during storage. The most important variables affecting loss of potency include temperature [58], the presence of proteases in the crude extract [59], and, particularly with dilute extracts, the adsorption of allergen to the inner wall of the partially filled containers [60]. The stability of allergenic extracts is enhanced by lyophilizing, packaging in 50% glycerin [61], or incorporating human serum albumin into the diluent [62]. It is technically possible to nebulize allergen solutions containing 5% or less glycerin for nasal or bronchial provocation challenges.

III. PURIFIED ALLERGENS

During the past two decades, many purified allergens have been isolated from crude allergenic extracts and have been well characterized with respect to their

Table 2 Nomenclature for Selected Highly Purified Allergens

Allergen source	New	Old	Ref.
Ambrosia artemisiifolia	*Amb a I*	AgE	65
(short ragweed)	*Amb a II*	AgK	65
	Amb a III	Ra3	66
	Amb a IV	Ra4, BPA-R	67
	Amb a V	Ra5	68
Dermatophagoides pteronyssinus (house dust mite)	*Der p I*	P_1, Ag42, Dpt12	69
Dermatophagoides farinae	*Der p II*	AgX	70
(house dust mite)	*Der f I*	Ag11	71
	Der f II	Ag19/20 IIa	72
Felis domesticus (cat)	*Fel d I*	Cat-1	73
	Fel d II	Cat serum albumin	33
Alternaria alternata (fungus)	*Alt a I*	Alt-I	74
Gallus domesticus	*Gal d I*	Ovomucoid	75
(chicken egg white)	*Gal d II*	Ovalbumin	
	Gal d III	Conalbumin	

Source: Abbreviated from Ref. 64.

immunochemical, physicochemical, and biological activities. These allergens, along with polyclonal and monoclonal antibodies thereto, are valuable reagents for studying allergen chemistry and human immune response mechanisms and for standardizing allergenic extracts.

The Subcommittee for Allergen Nomenclature of the International Union of Immunological Societies has established a nomenclature system for these purified allergens [63]; an abbreviated listing is shown in Table 2. Under this system, highly purified allergens are designated by the first three letters of the genus (italicized), space; the first letter of the species name (italicized), space; and a roman numeral. Allergens are numbered either in the order in which they were isolated or with the major allergens having the lower numbers. Several allergens have been assigned biochemical names, e.g., egg white ovomucoid; in these cases, both the assigned allergen nomenclature and the biochemical name are first specified and used interchangeably thereafter.

IV. REGULATION OF ALLERGENIC EXTRACTS

In the United States, commercial allergenic extracts are regulated by the Center for Biologics Evaluation and Research of the Food and Drug Administration. The efficacy and safety of allergenic extracts were extensively studied several years ago by a Food and Drug Administration Expert Panel, whose members were appointed in 1971 and charged with classifying these extracts into three categories. Category I included allergenic extracts that were safe and effective and not mislabeled; these products were to remain licensed. Category II included extracts that were unsafe or ineffective; the license for these products was to be revoked. Category III included extracts for which there were insufficient data to classify them into category I or II. The first report of the panel was published in 1979, but the recommendations were challenged; a final report with recommendations for implementation was issued in 1985. The panel recommended separate safety and efficacy criteria for diagnostic and therapeutic extracts. To receive the category I designation, diagnostic extracts were required to be (1) safe; (2) prepared from well-defined source materials; (3) capable of being standardized; and (4) proved to be diagnostically effective for skin testing in allergic and nonallergic persons, or presumed effective by close analogy to other extracts shown to be effective. Category I immunotherapy extracts were required to meet the above category I criteria for diagnostic extracts and to be proved to be immunotherapeutically effective by a valid clinical study or by analogy with products for which therapeutic effectiveness had been shown.

A summary of the recommendations of the panel has been published [76]. In part because of funding restrictions and organizational realignments at the Food and Drug Administration, the recommendations of the Panel on Review of Allergenic Extracts have not been implemented.

V. STANDARD OR REFERENCE EXTRACTS

Standardization and quality control efforts require that well-characterized standard or reference extracts be available to calibrate the potencies of other extracts of the same allergens.

International standards meet the specifications established by the World Health Organization and are available for extracts of short ragweed [77], birch [78], timothy grass [79], and ryegrass [80] pollens, *D. pteronyssinus* mite [39], and dog [81]. These reference standards may be purchased from the National Institute of Biological Science and Control, Hertfordshire, England. There has been no study of the biological activity of these international standards, and thus they should not be used for provocation challenge testing.

The Center for Biologics Evaluation and Research of the U.S. Food and Drug Administration also makes available a variety of national reference allergenic extracts that can be used by manufacturers or researchers to calibrate in-house secondary standards.

VI. COMPARISON OF ALLERGEN QUANTITIES USED IN CHALLENGE PROCEDURES AND NATURAL EXPOSURE LEVELS

Relatively few studies are available to compare allergen levels encountered by natural exposure and allergen concentrations used for inhalation challenge studies.

In an early study from Johns Hopkins University, ragweed-sensitive patients underwent intradermal skin tests, leukocyte histamine release assays, and quantitative bronchial inhalation challenge [82]. In the bronchial inhalation study, the median cumulative provocation dose causing a 35% decrease in specific airway conductance was approximately 48 μg protein/ml of ragweed extract. As *Amb a* I accounts for 6% of pollen protein [65], the calculated delivered dose of *Amb a* I was 3 μg/ml of extract. In the Baltimore area, the average hourly seasonal *Amb a* I dose is 8×10^{-4} μg [83], while in the Rochester, Minnesota, area, the average hourly seasonal dose of ragweed pollen is 2×10^{-2} μg [84], assuming an average pollen count of 187 grains m^3/day [85]. However, these calculated hourly doses vastly overestimate the actual dosage, because a 24-hour/day exposure to these levels of pollen is very unlikely.

During the past several years, immunochemical assays employing human IgE antibodies have been developed to quantitate aeroallergens [84]. These assays are particularly useful to quantitative amorphous indoor home or occupational allergens, such as cat, dust mite, rodent, guinea pig, or cockroach allergens [86]. Monoclonal or monospecific animal antibody–based immunoassays have also been established for quantitating *Fel d* I [87], *Can f* I (the major dog allergen) [88,89], and *Der p* I and *Der f* I [90] in ambient air or household dust. In each case, these natural exposure levels are much lower than those used in bronchial or nasal inhalation provocation testing.

ACKNOWLEDGMENTS

The author thanks Mr. Charles Clark for helpful discussions and Ms. Marian Bortolon for secretarial assistance. Supported by the Mayo Foundation.

REFERENCES

1. Wodehouse, R. P., *Pollen Grains*, Hafner Publishing Co., New York, 1965.
2. Platts-Mills, T. A. E., and Solomon, W. R., Aerobiology and inhalant allergens, in *Allergy Principles and Practice, 4th ed.* (E. Middleton, Jr, C. E. Reed, E. F. Ellis, et al., eds.), Mosby Year Book, St. Louis, 1993, p. 469–528.
3. Anderson, M. C., The effect of the quality of source materials on reference preparations, in *Regulatory Control and Standardization of Allergenic Extracts* (M. Schaeffer, C. Sisk, and H. D. Brede, eds.), Gustav Fischer Verlag, Stuttgart, 1987, p. 1–6.
4. Schou, C., Defining allergens of mammalian origin. *Clin. Exp. Allergy*, *23*, 7–14 (1993).
5. Ohman, J. L., Jr, Lowell, F. C., Bloch, K. J., et al., Allergens of mammalian origin. V. Properties of extracts derived from the domestic cat, *Clin. Allergy*, *6*, 419–428 (1976).
6. Anderson, M. C., and Baer, H., Allergenically active components of cat allergen extracts, *J. Immunol.*, *127*, 972–975 (1981).
7. Anderson, M. C., Baer, H., and Ohman, J. L., Jr., A comparative study of the allergens of cat urine, serum, saliva, pelt, *J. Allergy Clin. Immunol.*, *76*, 563–569 (1985).
8. Løwenstein, H., Lind, P., and Weeke, B., Identification and clinical significance of allergenic molecules of cat origin, *Allergy*, *40*, 430–441 (1985).
9. Wüthrich, B., and Arrendal, H., RAST in the diagnosis of hypersensitivity to dog and cat allergens. A comparison of different extract preparations with clinical history, skin test, and provocation tests, *Clin. Allergy*, *9*, 191–200 (1979).
10. Hoffman, D. R., Dog and cat allergens: urinary proteins or dander proteins? *Ann. Allergy*, *45*, 205–206 (1980).
11. Didierlaurent, A., Foglietti, M. J., Guérin, B., et al., Comparative study on cat allergens from fur and saliva, *Int. Arch. Allergy Appl. Immunol.*, *73*, 27–31 (1984).
12. Uhlin, T., Reuterby, J., and Einarsson, R., Antigenic/allergenic composition of poodle/Alsatian dandruff extract, *Allergy*, *39*, 125–133 (1984).
13. Yman, L., Brandt, R., and Ponterius, G., Serum albumin: an important allergen in dog epithelia extracts, *Int. Arch. Allergy Appl. Immunol.*, *44*, 358–368 (1973).
14. Varga, J. M., and Ceska, M., Characterization of allergen extracts by polyacrylamide gel isoelectrofocusing and radioimmunosorbent allergen assay. II. Dog and cat allergens, *Int. Arch. Allergy Appl. Immunol.*, *42*, 438–453 (1972).

15. Viander, M., Valovirta, E., Vanto, T., et al., Crossreactivity of cat and dog allergen extracts. RAST inhibition studies with special reference to the allergenic activity in saliva and urine, *Int. Arch. Allergy Appl. Immunol.*, *71*, 252–260 (1983).
16. Blands, J., Løwenstein, H., and Weeke, B., Characterization of extract of dog hair and dandruff from six different dog breeds by quantitative immunoelectrophoresis. Identification of allergens by crossed radioimmunoelectrophoresis (CRIE), *Acta Allergologica*, *32*, 147–169 (1977).
17. Ford, A. W., Alterman, L., and Kemeny, D. M., The allergens of dog. I. Identification using crossed-radioimmunoelectrophoresis, *Clin. Exp. Allergy*, *19*, 183–190 (1989).
18. Schumacher, M. J., Characterization of allergens from urine and pelts of laboratory mice, *Mol. Immunol.*, *17*, 1087–1095 (1980).
19. Price, J. A., and Longbottom, J. L., Allergy to mice. II. Further characterization of two major mice allergens (Ag 1 and Ag 3) and immunohistochemical investigations of their sources, *Clin. Exp. Allergy*, *20*, 71–77 (1990).
20. Lutsky, I., Fink, J. N., Kidd, J., et al., Allergenic properties of rat urine and pelt extracts, *J. Allergy Clin. Immunol.*, *75*, 279–284 (1985).
21. Walls, A. F., and Longbottom, J. L., Comparison of rat fur, urine, saliva, other rat allergen extracts by skin testing, RAST, and RAST inhibition, *J. Allergy Clin. Immunol.*, *75*, 242–251 (1985).
22. Longbottom, J. L., Crossed radio-immunoisoelectric focusing as a method of identifying isoallergens: identification of isoallergens in rat urine extracts, *J. Immunol. Methods*, *68*, 297–304 (1984).
23. Walls, A. F., Taylor, A. J. N., and Longbottom, J. L., Allergy to guinea pigs: I. Allergenic activities of extracts derived from the pelt, saliva, urine, and other sources, *Clin. Allergy*, *15*, 241–251 (1985).
24. Price, J. A., and Longbottom, J. L., Allergy to rabbits. II. Identification and characterization of a major rabbit allergen, *Allergy*, *43*, 39–48 (1988).
25. Løwenstein, H., Markussen, B., and Weeke, B., Identification of allergens in extract of horse hair and dandruff by means of crossed radioimmunoelectrophoresis, *Int. Arch. Allergy Appl. Immunol.*, *51*, 38–47 (1976).
26. Ponterius, G., Brandt, R., Hulten, E., et al., Comparative studies on the allergens of horse dandruff and horse serum, *Int. Arch. Allergy Appl. Immunol.*, *44*, 679–691 (1973).
27. Wahn, U., Herold, U., Danielsen, K., et al., Allergoprints in horse allergic children, *Allergy*, *37*, 335–343 (1982).
28. Prahl, P., Bucher, D., Plesner, T., et al., Isolation and partial characterization of three major allergens in an extract from cow hair and dander, *Int. Arch. Allergy Appl. Immunol.*, *67*, 293–301 (1982).
29. Prahl, P., Weeke, B., and Løwenstein, H., Quantitative immunoelectrophoretic analysis of extract from cow hair and dander, *Allergy*, *33*, 241–253 (1978).
30. Ohman, J. L., Lowell, F. C., and Bloch, K. J., Allergens of mammalian origin. III. Properties of a major feline allergen, *J. Immunol.*, *113*, 1668–1677 (1974).
31. Ohman, J. L., Jr., Baer, H., Anderson, M. C., et al., Surface washings of living cats: an improved method of obtaining clinically relevant allergens, *J. Allergy Clin. Immunol.*, *72*, 288–293 (1983).

32. Brown, P. R., Leitermann, K., and Ohman, J. L., Jr., Distribution of cat allergen 1 in cat tissues and fluids, *Int. Arch. Allergy Appl. Immunol.*, *74*, 67–70 (1984).
33. Ohman, J. L., Jr., Bloch, K. J., Kendall, S., et al., Allergens of mammalian origin. IV. Evidence for common allergens in cat and dog serum, *J. Allergy Clin. Immunol.*, *57*, 560–568 (1976).
34. Brandt, R., and Yman, L., Dog dander allergens. Specificity studies based on the radioallergosorbent technique, *Int. Arch. Allergy Appl. Immunol.*, *61*, 361–370 (1980).
35. Wuthrich, B., Guérin, B., and Hewitt, B. E., Cross-allergenicity between extracts of hair from different dog breeds and cat fur, *Clin. Allergy*, *15*, 87–93 (1985).
36. Lindgren, S., Belin, L., Dreborg, S., et al., Breed-specific dog-dandruff allergens, *J. Allergy Clin. Immunol.*, *82*, 196–204 (1988).
37. Aukrust, L., Selections of source materials for reference preparations of molds, in *Regulatory Control and Standardization of Allergenic Extracts* (M. Schaeffer, C. Sisk, and H. D. Brede, eds.), Gustav Fischer Verlag, Stuttgart, 1987, p. 7–13.
38. Prince, H. E., Molds and bacteria in the etiology of respiratory allergic diseases. XXI. Studies with mold extracts produced from cultures grown in modified synthetic media: a preliminary report, *Ann. Allergy*, *19*, 259–267 (1961).
39. Ford, A., Seagroatt, V., Platts-Mills, T. A. E., et al., A collaborative study on the first international standard of *Dermatophagoides pteronyssinus* (house dust mite) extract, *J. Allergy Clin. Immunol.*, *75*, 676–686 (1985).
40. Lind, P., Standardization of mite extracts: qualitative and quantitative investigations of three kinds of preparations with CRIE and RAST, *Allergy*, *35*, 227–230 (1980).
41. Maasch, H. J., Wahl, R., and Fuchs, T., Application of the first international standard of *Dermatophagoides pteronyssinus* (house dust mite) in the evaluation of allergen extracts produced from two different source materials, *Int. Arch. Allergy Appl. Immunol.*, *84*, 363–372 (1987).
42. Arlian, L. G., Vyszenski-Moher, D. L., and Fernandez-Caldas, E., Allergenicity of the mite, *Blomia tropicalis*, *J. Allergy Clin. Immunol.*, *91*, 1042–1050 (1993).
43. Cuthbert, O. D., Storage mite allergy, *Clin. Rev. Allergy*, *8*, 69–86 (1990).
44. Benton, A. W., Morse, R. A., and Stewart, J. D., Venom collection from honeybees, *Science*, *142*, 228–230 (1963).
45. Hunt, K. J., Valentine, M. D., Sobotka, A. K., et al., Diagnosis of allergy to stinging insects by skin testing with Hymenoptera venoms, *Ann. Intern. Med.*, *85*, 56–59 (1976).
46. Lockey, R. F., Systemic reactions to stinging ants, *J. Allergy Clin. Immunol.*, *54*, 132–146 (1974).
47. Marshall, N. A., and Street, D. H., Allergy to *Triatoma protracta* (Heteroptera: Reduviidae). I. Etiology, antigen preparation, diagnosis and immunotherapy, *J. Med. Entomol.*, *19*, 248–252 (1982).
48. Wirtz, R. A., Allergic and toxic reactions to non-stinging arthropods, *Annu. Rev. Entomol.*, *29*, 47–69 (1984).
49. Kagen, S. L., Inhalant allergy to arthropods. Insects, arachnids, and crustaceans, *Clin. Rev. Allergy*, *8*, 99–125 (1990).
50. Gad El Rab, M. O., and Kay, A. B., Widespread immunoglobulin E–mediated hypersensitivity in the Sudan to the "green nimitti" midge, *Cladotanytarsus lewisi*

(Diptera: Chironomidae). I. Diagnosis by radioallergosorbent test, *J. Allergy Clin. Immunol.*, *66*, 190–197 (1980).

51. Baur, X., and Liebers, V., Insect hemoglobins (*Chi t* I) of the Diptera family Chironomidae are relevant environmental, occupational, and hobby-related allergens, *Int. Arch. Occup. Environ. Health*, *64*, 185–188 (1992).
52. Kang, B., Study on cockroach antigen as a probable causative agent in bronchial asthma, *J. Allergy Clin. Immunol.*, *58*, 357–365 (1976).
53. Mathews, K. P., Inhalant insect-derived allergens, *Immunol. Allergy Clin. North Am.*, *9*, 321–338 (1989).
54. May, J. C., Sih, J. T. C., Miller, J. R., et al., Optimization of parameters in protein nitrogen unit precipitation procedure for allergenic extracts, *J. Allergy Clin. Immunol.*, *63*, 87–97 (1979).
55. Backman, A., Belin, L., Dreborg, S., et al., Standardization of allergenic preparations. Comments with reference to the second edition of the common Nordic guidelines for registration of allergenic preparations, *Allergy*, *46*, 81–84 (1991).
56. Turkeltaub, P. C., Rastogi, S. C., Baer, H., et al., A standardized quantitative skin-test assay of allergen potency and stability: studies on the allergen dose-response curve and effect of wheal, erythema, and patient selection on assay results, *J. Allergy Clin. Immunol.*, *70*, 343–352 (1982).
57. Nightengale, S. L., Alert on changes in standardized cat allergen extract products, *JAMA*, *268*, 2491 (1992).
58. Anderson, M. C., and Baer, H., Antigenic and allergenic changes during storage of a pollen extract, *J. Allergy Clin. Immunol.*, *69*, 3–10 (1982).
59. Blanchard, G. C., and Gardner, R., Characterization of some of the enzymes in ragweed pollen, *Ann. Allergy*, *36*, 410–418 (1976).
60. Foucard, T., Bennich, H., and Johansson, S. G. O., Studies on the stability of diluted allergen extracts using the radioallergosorbent test (RAST), *Clin. Allergy*, *3*, 91–102 (1973).
61. Nelson, H. S., The effect of preservatives and dilution on the deterioration of Russian thistle (*Salsola pestifer*): a pollen extract, *J. Allergy Clin. Immunol.*, *63*, 417–425 (1979).
62. Norman, P. S., and Marsh, D. G., Human serum albumin and Tween 80 as stabilizers of allergen solutions, *J. Allergy Clin. Immunol.*, *62*, 314–319 (1978).
63. Marsh, D. G., Goodfriend, L., King, T. P., et al., Allergen nomenclature, *Bull. W.H.O.*, *64*, 767–774 (1986).
64. Ipsen, H., Klysner, S. S., Larsen, J. N., et al., Allergenic extracts, in *Allergy Principles and Practice, 4th ed.* (E. Middleton, Jr., C. E. Reed, E. F. Ellis, et al., eds.), Mosby Year Book, St. Louis, 1993, p. 529–553.
65. King, T. P., Chemical and biological properties of some atopic allergens, *Adv. Immunol.*, *23*, 77–105 (1976).
66. Underdown, B. J., and Goodfriend, L., Isolation and characterization of an allergen from short ragweed pollen, *Biochemistry*, *8*, 980–989 (1969).
67. Griffiths, B. W., and Brunet, R., Isolation of a basic protein antigen of low ragweed pollen, *Can. J. Biochem.*, *49*, 396–400 (1971).
68. Roebber, M., Klapper, D. G., and Marsh, D. G., Two isoallergens of short ragweed component Ra5, *J. Immunol.*, *129*, 120–125 (1982).

69. Chapman, M. D., and Platts-Mills, T. A. E., Purification and characterization of the major allergen from *Dermatophagoides pteronyssinus*—antigen P_1, *J. Immunol.*, *125*, 587–592 (1980).
70. Lind, P., Purification and partial characterization of two major allergens from the house dust mite *Dermatophagoides pteronyssinus*, *J. Allergy. Clin. Immunol.*, *76*, 753–761 (1985).
71. Dandeu, J. P., Le Mao, J., Lux, M., et al., Antigens and allergens in *Dermatophagoides farinae* mite. II. Purification of Ag11, a major allergen in *Dermatophagoides farinae*, *Immunology*, *46*, 679–687 (1982).
72. Holck, A., Dale, S., and Sletten, K., Purification and characterization of a major allergen from the house dust mite *Dermatophagoides farinae*, *Allergy*, *41*, 408–417 (1986).
73. Leitermann, K., and Ohman, J. L., Cat allergen 1: biochemical, antigenic, and allergenic properties, *J. Allergy Clin. Immunol.*, *74*, 147–153 (1984).
74. Yunginger, J. W., Jones, R. T., Nesheim, M. E., et al., Studies on *Alternaria* allergens. III. Isolation of a major allergenic fraction (Alt-I), *J. Allergy Clin. Immunol.*, *66*, 138–147 (1980).
75. Hoffman, D. R., Immunochemical identification of the allergens in egg white, *J. Allergy Clin. Immunol.*, *71*, 481–486 (1983).
76. Schaeffer, M., and Sisk, L. C., Allergenic extracts: a review of their safety and efficacy, *Ann. Allergy*, *52*, 2–14 (1984).
77. Helm, R. M., Gauerke, M. B., Baer, H., et al., Production and testing of an international reference standard of short ragweed pollen extract, *J. Allergy Clin. Immunol.*, *73*, 790–800 (1984).
78. Arntzen, F. C., Wilhelmsen, T. W., Løwenstein, H., et al., The international collaborative study of the first international standard of birch (*Betula verrucosa*) pollen extract, *J. Allergy Clin. Immunol.*, *83*, 66–82 (1989).
79. Gjesing, B., Jäger, L., Marsh, D. G., et al., The international collaborative study establishing the first international standard for timothy (*Phleum pratense*) grass pollen allergenic extract, *J. Allergy Clin. Immunol.*, *75*, 258–267 (1985).
80. Stewart, G. A., Turner, K. J., Baldo, B. A., et al., Standardization of rye-grass pollen (*Lolium perenne*) extract. An immunochemical and physicochemical assessment of six candidate international reference preparations, *Int. Arch. Allergy Appl. Immunol.*, *86*, 9–18 (1988).
81. Larsen, J. N., Ford, A., Gjesing, B., et al., The collaborative study of the international standard of a dog, *Canis domesticus*, hair/dander extract, *J. Allergy Clin. Immunol.*, *82*, 318–330 (1988).
82. Bruce, C. A., Rosenthal, R. R., Lichtenstein, L. M., et al., Diagnostic tests in ragweed-allergic asthma: a comparison of direct skin tests, leukocyte histamine release, and quantitative bronchial challenge, *J. Allergy Clin. Immunol.*, *53*, 230–239 (1974).
83. Marsh, D. G., Allergens and the genetics of allergy, in *The Antigens*, Vol. 3 (M. Sela, ed.), Academic Press, New York, 1975, p. 271–359.
84. Agarwal, M. K., Yunginger, J. W., Swanson, M. C., et al., An immunochemical method to measure atmospheric allergens, *J. Allergy Clin. Immunol.*, *68*, 194–200 (1981).

85. Welsh, P. W., Butterfield, J. H., Yunginger, J. W., et al., Allergen-controlled study of intranasal immunotherapy for ragweed hay fever, *J. Allergy Clin. Immunol.*, *71*, 454–460 (1983).
86. Swanson, M. C., Agarwal, M. K., and Reed, C. E., An immunochemical approach to indoor aeroallergen quantitation with a new volumetric air sampler: studies with mite, roach, cat, mouse, and guinea pig antigens, *J. Allergy Clin. Immunol.*, *76*, 724–729 (1985).
87. Van Metre, T. E., Marsh, D. G., Adkinson, N. F., et al., Dose of cat (*Felis domesticus*) allergen 1 (*Fel d* I) that induces asthma, *J. Allergy Clin. Immunol.*, *78*, 62–75 (1986).
88. De Groot, H., Goei, K. G. H., van Swieten, P., and Aalberse, R. C., Affinity purification of a major and a minor allergen from dog extract: serologic activity of affinity-purified *Can f* I and of *Can f* I–depleted extract, *J. Allergy Clin. Immunol.*, *87*, 1056–1065 (1991).
89. Schou, C., Hansen, G. N., Lintner, T., et al., Assay for the major dog allergen *Can f* I: investigation of house dust samples and commercial dog extracts, *J. Allergy Clin. Immunol.*, *88*, 847–853 (1991).
90. Luczynska, C. M., Arruda, L. K., Platts-Mills, T. A. E., et al., A two-site monoclonal antibody ELISA for the quantitation of the major *Dermatophagoides* spp. allergens, *Der p* I and *Der f* I, *J. Immunol. Methods*, *118*, 227–235 (1989).

2

Standardization of Allergens

Jean Bousquet and François-B. Michel

Centre Hospitalier Universitaire
Montpellier, France

I. INTRODUCTION

Allergen extracts prepared from biological materials are very complex, heterogeneous, and particularly unstable. They are composed of a mixture of proteins, carbohydrates, enzymes, and other substances, some of them having a biological or a toxic activity. In the majority of extracts, allergens represent only a small fraction of the total mixture. For a given allergen, the quality and shelf-life of the extract vary according to the nature of the raw material, preparation, and storage.

Since the introduction of immunotherapy in 1911, allergen extracts have been used in millions of subjects throughout the world for the diagnosis and treatment of allergy. The production of allergens has been strongly influenced by the fundamental work of pioneers of allergology. Noon and Cantar [1] proposed that extracts be defined in units of weight to volume (w/v), and Stull and Cooke [2] devised protein nitrogen units (PNU). These two units are completely independent of the biological activity of the extract, and when the Panel on Review of Allergenic extracts [3] published its report in 1985 (but the report was submitted to the U.S. Food and Drug Administration [FDA] in 1981), most extracts were labeled in these allergen-independent units and their quality was often not optimal. It is only within the past 20 years that the introduction of in vitro techniques based on immunoglobulin E (IgE) have made it possible, at least for the main allergenic materials, to characterize and quantify the major allergens in the extracts and to quantitate the total allergenic potency. These methods have permitted the definition and preparation, under the aegis of the International Union of Immunological Societies (IUIS), of extracts of reference called "standards," of which six have been accepted by the World Health Organization (WHO). The Bureau of Biologics in the United States has prepared for this country a range of national extracts of reference. Since 1980, new technologies based on monoclonal antibodies and recombinant allergens have been made available. They are increasingly used in the standardization of allergenic extracts, and they are likely to improve significantly the preparation and control of allergen extracts.

In 1994, many allergen extracts are standardized throughout the world, and the overall quality of these extracts has been considerably improved. It is proposed that most if not all allergens should be standardized in order to improve practice for both the diagnosis and the treatment of allergic diseases [4,5]. However, the characterization and quantification of allergens used for provocation tests, including skin tests, is relatively easy by comparison with that of extracts used for treatment, especially if the extract is adsorbed, chemically modified, or both.

II. CONTROL OF ALLERGEN EXTRACTS

The composition of allergen extracts, which is, because of the nature of the raw material, more heterogeneous than that of other biological products, does not make it possible to conceive a system of control based only on a definition of analytical normal values. It requires the definition and production of reference extracts that may be compared, batch to batch, with routine production extracts, using methods that have been well established.

The potency of allergen extracts is defined in CRF 21 600.3 (U.S. Code #) [5] as follows: "The word potency is interpreted to mean the specific ability or capacity of the products, as initiated by appropriate laboratory tests or by adequately controlled clinical data obtained through the administration of the product in the manner intended, to effect a given result." The control of an allergen extract requires several methods to assay its total potency and composition by comparison with reference standards.

It is likely that the new recombinant cDNA technology will considerably modify the standardization of allergens in the future, since it is a potent tool for characterizing allergens and could provide large amounts of identical cloned allergens for diagnosis and standardization purposes. The cDNAs of a number of important human allergens have been isolated and sequenced, including house dust mites [6,7], insect venoms [8], cat [9], various pollens [10–16], and some molds [17]. Some of the recombinant allergens (RAs) are able to react with human IgE in solid-phase assays and to stimulate allergen-specific T cells [15,16]. Recombinant allergens used for in vitro diagnosis should have the same IgE-binding activity as their natural counterparts, but this is rarely obtained. Rafnar et al. [18] compared *Amb a* V and *Amb t* V RAs with native proteins by immunologic assays and nuclear magnetic resonance spectroscopy and found that although RAs may be effective in stimulating T cells, they have different three-dimensional structures. Moreover, the strategy of cDNA cloning requires that IgE epitopes be mainly proteins and that the carbohydrate moiety of the allergen participates only to a minor extent in IgE binding. Moreover, RAs should possess all IgE-binding epitopes relevant to the standardizing of a given native allergen. The production in unlimited amounts of perfectly characterized proteins bearing an identical structure makes their use in standardization very attractive.

A. Allergen Extracts Used for Diagnosis

Allergen extracts used for the diagnosis of allergic disorders include those for skin tests and provocative challenges. To measure allergenic potency and composition, both in vivo and in vitro tests have been proposed (Tables 1 and 2).

1. In vivo Tests

In vivo methods directly carried out in allergic persons are wildly used for the standardization of allergenic extracts. They measure the biological reaction of sensitized persons to allergens, and their results are given in biological units. The only in vivo tests available are based on skin tests, since provocative challenges are not possible for standardization purposes. Moreover, skin tests are the only biological tests that can be used in humans, since the production of histamine-release assays is not feasible for a manufacturer [19].

Methods. Several methods of performing skin tests have been proposed (Table 3), but there is no general agreement on methods of performing quantitative skin tests. Variable parameters include the selection of the allergic patients (from unselected to highly allergic); the method of skin testing (prick test or intradermal reaction); the analysis of the wheal or the flare or both; whether or not the allergen-induced skin test is compared with a reference standard preparation (histamine, codeine phosphate, or compound 48/80); the statistical analysis; and finally the unitage. There are two methods that are more commonly accepted: the U.S. [20,21] and Nordic methods [22–27]. However, other methods are also used [28–30].

The method proposed ($ID_{50}EAL$) as the reference in the United States is based on the study of Turkeltaub et al. [20,21]. It is thoroughly described and published, so that manufacturers can use it easily. Only highly sensitized subjects are selected for the purpose of standardization. Patients receive several intradermal injections of dilutions (threefold increment) of the allergen extract, and the flare is recorded. Both a reference extract and the extract to be tested are injected, and the results of the flare are compared by parallel-line bioassay. This technique is very sensitive, although time-consuming, and results are given in allergy units (AU) or bio-

Table 1 Methods of Analysis of Allergen Extracts Used in Standardization

1. In vivo techniques
    - Skin test titration
2. In vitro techniques
    - Physical methods
        - *Characterization using molecular size*
            - Ultracentrifugal analysis
            - Gel filtration
            - Sodium dodecyl sulfate gel electrophoresis (polyacrylamide gel electrophoresis)
            - Chromatographic methods
        - *Characterization using electrical charge*
            - Isoelectric focusing (IEF)
            - Electrophoresis (starch, gel, agarose gel)
    - Chemical methods
        - Protein analysis (protein nitrogen units, total protein content, amino acids analysis)
        - Carbohydrate analysis
        - Enzyme assays
    - Immunologic methods
        - Inhibition immunoassays including radioallergosorbent test and ELISA-based techniques
        - Monoclonal antibody–based assays
        - Immunodiffusion
        - Quantitative immunoelectrophoresis
            - Crossed immunoelectrophoresis
            - Rocket immunoelectrophoresis
            - Crossed radioimmunoelectrophoresis (CRIE)
        - Immunoprecipitation and laser nephelometry
        - Electroimmunodiffusion
        - Radioimmunoprecipitation
        - Histamine release
        - Complement consumption
    - Combined methods
        - Allergenic profiles of isoelectric focusing
        - Allergenic profiles of chromatographic fractions including CRIE

equivalent allergy units (BAU). The goal is that 1 BAU of all extracts will be biologically equivalent.

The method proposed by the Nordic Authorities is based on the work of Aas et al. [22], published in 1972. The Nordic Authorities recommended the histamine equivalent potency (HEP) unit in their guidelines for registration of allergen preparations published in 1980: The activity of an allergen extract is 1 HEP when

Table 2 Comparison of Techniques Used in Standardization and Control of Allergen Extracts

	Skin tests	PNU and w/v	Inhibition immunoassay	Histamine release	RID	Monoclonal assay	IEF or SDS PAGE	CRIE	Immuno-blotting
Economically feasible	+++	+++	++	+	++	++	+++	+	++
Easy to perform	+++	+++	+++	+	+++	+++	+++	++	+++
In routine standardization									
Total allergenic potency	+	−	+	+	+	+	−	−	−
Components of an extract	−	−	−	−	+[a]	+[a]	+	+	+
Purity of an extract	−	−	−	−	−	−	Proteins	Allergens	Allergens

[a]single component.

PNU = protein nitrogen units; w/v = weight/volume; RID = radial immunodiffusion; IEF = isoelectric focusing; SDS PAGE = polyacrylamide gel electrophoresis; CRIE = crossed radioimmunoelectrophoresis.

Table 3 Comparison Between Skin Test Methods to Standardize Allergens

	U.S. method	Nordic Council method
Skin test method	Intradermal	Prick test
Dosage increment	Threefold	Tenfold
Number of patients tested	15	20
Selection of patients	Highly allergic	No selection
Reaction analyzed	Erythema	Wheal
Histamine reference	No	Yes
Calculation	Means	Geometric means
Units	Allergy unit (AU) and bio-equivalent allergy unit (BAU)	Biological unit (BU)

the extract provokes a specific skin reaction with a wheal of the same median size as a positive reference consisting of histamine 5.43 mmol/L (e.g., histamine dihydrochloride 1 mg/ml), when both solutions are used with the same technique (prick testing) on at least 20 selected subjects who are clinically allergic and cutaneously reactive to the allergen concerned. The selection of patients should be based on their reactivity to the present reference allergen or to another preparation of equivalent quality. The tests must be performed on anatomically corresponding sites. An equivalent designation for the concentration of the preparation is 1000 biological units (BU/ml (1 HEP = 1000 BU/ml). The definition also constitutes the basis for the detailed formulation of a biological method to be used for the calibration of the reference preparation, as well as a corresponding method for the check of the biological activities of subsequent batches in terms of the same reference factors. However, this report did not give the procedure of the test or the statistical analysis, and it has recently been proposed that a histamine reference solution of 54.3 mmol/L be used. Several methods have been proposed and are completely described in the medical dissertation of Dreborg [31]. Although the new guidelines published in 1989 gave a complete description of the test and statistical analysis [32], manufacturers still use their own in-house methods derived from the 1980 recommendations.

On the basis of HEP, it is possible to define other equivalent potencies, but the best positive reference control solution has yet to be discovered. Codeine phosphate [30,33] may be used instead of histamine, since it is a mast cell–degranulating agent.

Brighton et al. have suggested that allergen batches may be assayed by tenfold dilutions of prick tests in sensitive persons [28]. The wheal sizes are recorded for a group of about 30 patients, and the geometric mean wheal size is plotted. It is then possible to define a unit in terms of biological activity in the population tested. This method is currently applied in some European countries [34].

Problems. Skin tests performed for standardization purposes should follow precise guidelines; in particular, the investigator should be aware of drugs possibly taken by the patients, the tests should be done in a given anatomical site, and the time of the day should be identical for all tests, since these factors affect the performance of skin tests. Moreover, there are problems directly related to standardization. In particular, the selection of patients is critical, but there are no definite data indicating that standardization in highly allergic persons is more relevant than that done in unselected allergic subjects. Unitage systems have been modified within the past 15 years because of our evolving knowledge. Finally, the three main units (IU, AU, or BAU and BU) have not yet been compared.

Importance of Skin Testing in Allergen Standardization. Skin testing is of paramount importance, since it represents the only feasible method of obtaining extracts standardized biologically in sensitive subjects. These extracts give skin reactions of a comparable size whatever the allergen species tested (Figure 1), whereas those standardized only by radioallergosorbent test (RAST) inhibition do not. Usually, manufacturers standardize their reference extracts in biological units and then compare their in-house reference preparations with freshly prepared extracts by means of allergen-related in vitro assays.

2. In Vitro Assays Unrelated to Allergens

For decades, allergen extracts have been standardized either by the weight/volume method proposed in 1911 [1] or by their content of proteins, such as the total nitrogen unit proposed in the 1920s by Cooke et al. [2] and the PNU [35], since most allergens are of protein origin. More recently, the analysis of amino acids has also been used. Some allergens are glycoproteins, and the carbohydrate content of allergens may be measured by techniques such as gas-liquid chromatography. Studies examining the correlation between these unitages and allergen-related in vitro assays did not find any significant correlation, even for pollen extracts. It is therefore desirable to avoid labeling extracts in such units only.

3. In Vitro Assays Measuring Total Allergenic Potency

RAST Inhibition and Inhibition Immunoassays. The direct RAST titration [36] has been replaced by inhibition immunoassays such as RAST inhibition (Fig. 2) and derived techniques such as the CAP system, other techniques of solid-phase immunoassay, or ELISA tests [37–45]. Inhibition immunoassays are the most widely used for the control of the total allergenic potency of an extract. These assays should follow precise procedures and require

A solid-phase allergen prepared from a high-quality source material, in which all major and minor allergens are represented. This solid phase can be a paper disk (RAST), magnetic beads (Magic Lite or AlaSTAT), CAP-sponge (CAP System), or plastic well. Allergens are at best covalently coupled.

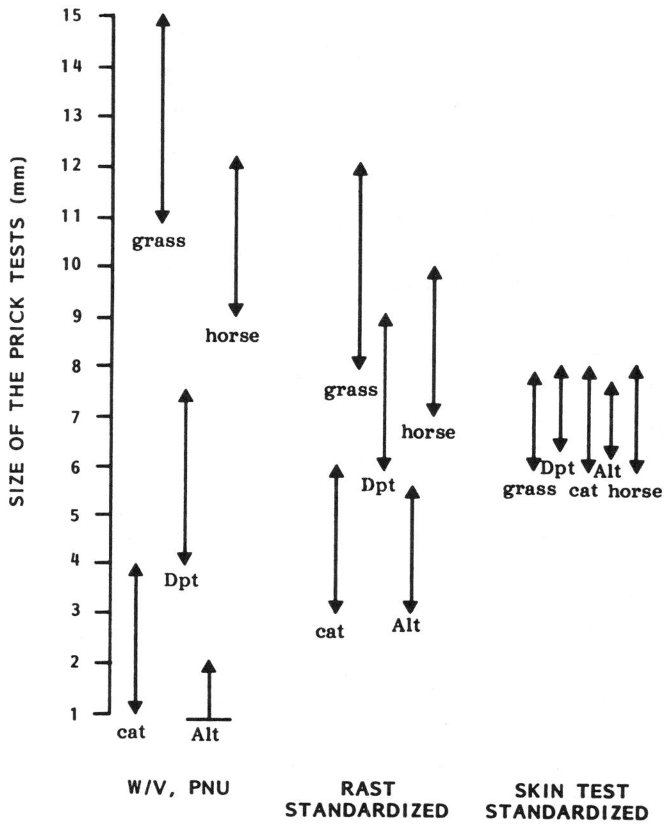

Figure 1 Mean wheal sizes induced by unstandardized and standardized allergen extracts. (From Ref. 26.)

A pool of serum prepared from multiple subjects sensitive to the allergen tested. It has been shown that an individual serum contains only a fraction of these determinants [41,42]. Minor and major allergens should all be recognized in the pool of human sera. It is usually established that a pool of antiserum should contain at least 30 sera. When possible, only patients having a high IgE titer should be included in the pool.

A high-quality reference extract to be used as a standard [43].

These inhibition immunoassays express only the sum of the total allergenic activity and do not give any information on individual allergenic components. Moreover, it has been shown that a single purified major allergen such as *Amb a* I can totally inhibit the RAST (to short-ragweed pollen). The parallelism of the

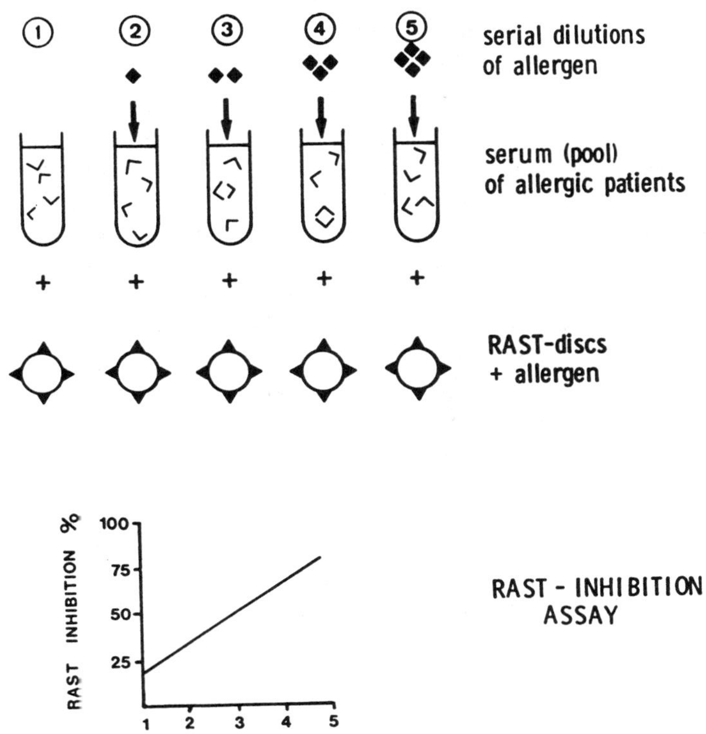

Figure 2 Radioallergosorbent test (RAST)-inhibition assay. (From Ref. 26.)

different curves has to be examined, because extracts that give nonparallel curves may not have the same antigenic composition. The concentration of extract required to induce a 50% inhibition represents a measure of the potency (Fig. 2). The technique has been standardized and is now suitable for allergen standardization.

The inhibition immunoassays offer several advantages [43–45]. The solid-phase supports are remarkably constant; it appears that virtually all allergens can be standardized using this procedure as long as they can be covalently bound to a solid-phase support; it is a test that is independent of the patients; it is convenient; it is standardized in terms of procedure and statistical analysis of the data; and it is usually reproducible within certain limits. This technique has been shown to compare favorably with other in vivo and in vitro standardization techniques for pollens, molds, mites, and venoms.

Histamine Release. Histamine release from blood basophils triggered by serial dilutions of allergen extracts has been used for research purposes and to standardize reference extracts, but it is not a technique that can be routinely performed by manufacturers [19].

Titration of Individual Allergenic Components.

Purified Antigens Without Enzymatic Activity. When pure antigens have been isolated, their concentration in extracts can be determined using either a gel-diffusion technique (radial immunodiffusion [RID]) [46,47] or more sensitive techniques such as two-site immunometric assay using polyclonal or monoclonal antibodies [48–50]. Monoclonal antibodies are now available for many purified allergens of cat (*Fel d* I), house dust mites (*Der p* I, *Der f* I: group I allergens; *Der p* II, *Der f* II: group II allergens), and various pollens and molds [48–52]. Monoclonal antibodies are monospecific, inexhaustible, homogeneous with respect to chemical composition, structure, specificity and combining site, and potentially suitable for absolute quantitation. Moreover, the two-site ELISA assays are simple, rapid, and cost-effective. However, the selection of monoclonal antibodies is difficult, since they are directed against a single epitope of an allergen and should have a high binding activity. Monoclonal antibody affinity chromatography may also be used to purify allergens.

The standardization of allergens using single allergen components has raised questions, since it had to be demonstrated that the measurement of a single component was representative of the total allergenic potency of the extract. Using

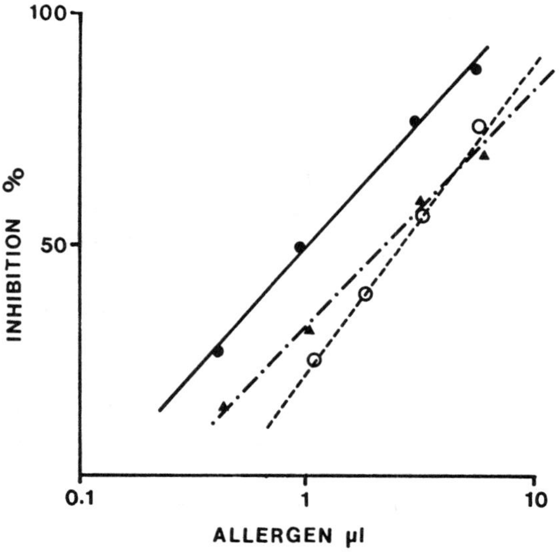

Figure 3 Radioallergosorbent test (RAST)-inhibition assay of four orchard grass pollen extracts. (From Ref. 26.)

RID to measure antigen E (*Amb a* I) and ryegrass group I antigen (*Lol p* I), Baer et al. [46,47] found that the total allergenic potency of short-ragweed extracts was correlated closely with their *Amb a* I content, and that the total allergenic potency of timothy extracts was correlated with *Lol p* I content. Techniques using polyclonal antibodies and RID are in current use for the standardization of short-ragweed (*Amb a* I) and cat (*Fel d* I) extracts. In the case of house dust mites, however, several assays may be required. It has been observed that depending on the source material (mite bodies or mite bodies and spent culture), the ratio between group I and group II allergens varies widely. Moreover, the group II allergens are much more stable than group I, and poor conditions of storage can thus lead to a selective loss of group I allergens [52]. In a recent study, it has been observed that the major allergen content of allergenic preparations reflects their biological activity measured by skin tests, and that for birch, *Dermatophagoides pteronyssinus*, cat, *Alternaria*, and ragweed pollen, 1 BU was equivalent to 1 ng of the major allergen [53]. This observation is of great importance but needs confirmation.

The titration of single components is now largely used in the standardization of allergenic extracts for both potency and composition assays. In particular, the WHO international standard preparations (ISPs) are partly standardized by means of single components. Moreover, the new U.S. regulations will largely use the titration of single allergenic components by means of monoclonal antibody ELISA to standardize allergen extracts. At present, however, only few purified allergens are available to assay allergenic extracts. In the near future, the production in sufficient quantity of RAs of some or all of the important major allergens will be possible without recourse to complex physicochemical procedures and will make the determination of major components easier.

Individual Components with Enzymatic Activity. Phospholipase A [54] and hyaluronidase [55] are allergens of hymenoptera venoms with enzymatic activity. This activity is used for the standardization of the venoms [56]. In the United States, venom extracts are standardized on the basis of their hyaluronidase content.

4. Study of the Composition of Allergen Extracts

Besides the total allergenic potency, it is necessary to measure the composition of the allergen extract.

Physicochemical Techniques. Proteins in an allergenic extract can be separated by isoelectric point or molecular size using isoelectric focusing (IEF) [57–61], polyacrylamide gel electrophoresis (PAGE) [62], gel chromatography [63], isotachophoresis, or high-performance liquid chromatography (HPLC). These are relatively simple techniques that separate proteins without taking into account the antigenic and allergenic composition. However, they are widely used for the batch-to-batch quality control of allergenic extracts.

Immunochemical Techniques. Crossed radioimmunoelectrophoresis (CRIE) [64,65], immunoblotting [66–69], and the titration of purified antigens using monoclonal antibodies [48–52] are preferred, since they give the composition of one or all allergens present in the extract.

Immunoblotting has gained wide acceptance in the standardization of allergens, since it is relatively simple and gives information on the composition of allergen extracts. It is based on a three-step technique. First, allergens are separated either by molecular weight using SDS-PAGE electrophoresis or by isoelectric point using IEF. Then the print of the agarose gel is taken on a nitrocellulose sheet by blotting. Finally, allergens are revealed on nitrocellulose by incubating sera of allergic persons and subsequently revealing IgE bound to allergens, through an immunochemical technique using ^{125}I-labeled IgE or an enzymatic marker (Fig. 4). This elegant technique has been popularized by Peltre et al. [66] and is now widely used to screen the allergens recognized by IgE antibodies, to

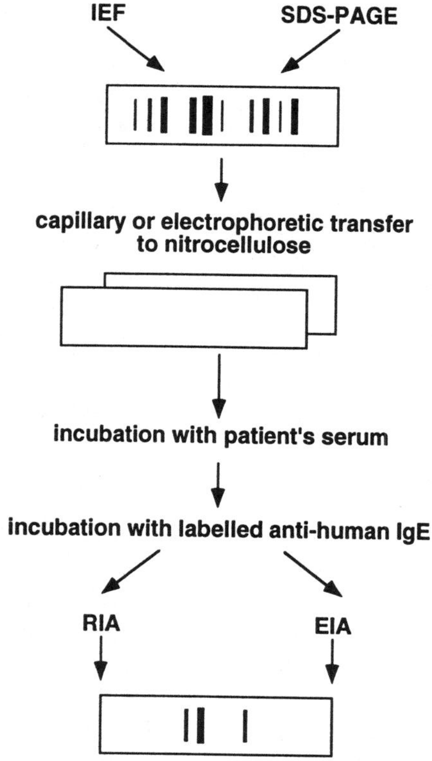

Figure 4 Immunoblotting technique. (From Ref. 26.)

characterize allergens as a research tool, and to standardize allergens in routine use [67,68]. The immunoblotting techniques suffer from limitations of SDS-PAGE or IEF. Only water-soluble allergens can be separated, and all allergens are not equally transferred to nitrocellulose. The binding capacity of allergens should eventually be checked for allergens other than pollens. However, these techniques are simpler than most other immunochemical methods.

Immunochemical techniques using immunoglobulins from animals as a reagent have been used for the characterization and quantification of allergen extracts [64,65,70,71] (Table 4). Single immunodiffusion techniques have been employed for the measurement of concentrations of single individual allergens [46,47], whereas double immunodiffusion methods are able to give either the analysis of the antigen composition in a mixture or the identification of allergens [72,73]. A number of techniques derived from crossed immunoelectrophoresis (CIE) [64,74–76] have been named quantitative immunodiffusion (QIE) techniques [77]. They are all quantitative or semiquantitative and have been widely used for the control and standardization of allergen extracts [90]. They may be used for the control of both the potency of allergen extracts and their allergen composition (Fig. 5).

In the CIE technique [64,65], proteins are separated electrophoretically in an agarose gel and subsequently run perpendicularly into a gel containing antibodies to the proteins. Every protein to which a corresponding antibody exists gives rise to a precipitation peak whose area is correlated to the amount of the protein. This

Table 4 Comparison Between Isoelectric Focusing (IEF), Crossed Radioimmunoelectrophoresis (CRIE), and Immunoblotting

	IEF	CRIE	Immunoblotting
Protein separation	+	+	+[a]
Detection of allergens	No	One precipitate for each allergen	One precipitate for each protein (possibly denaturated)
Sensitivity	200 μg	10–100 μg	200 μg
Reproducibility	+	+	+
Quantification	+	+	+
Performance	Easy	More difficult	Relatively easy
Polyspecific rabbit IgG against all antigenic and allergenic material	No	+	No
Pool of allergic sera	No	+	+
^{125}I–anti–human IgE or enxyme–anti–human IgE	No	+	+

[a]Protein separation by IEF or SDS-PAGE electrophoresis.

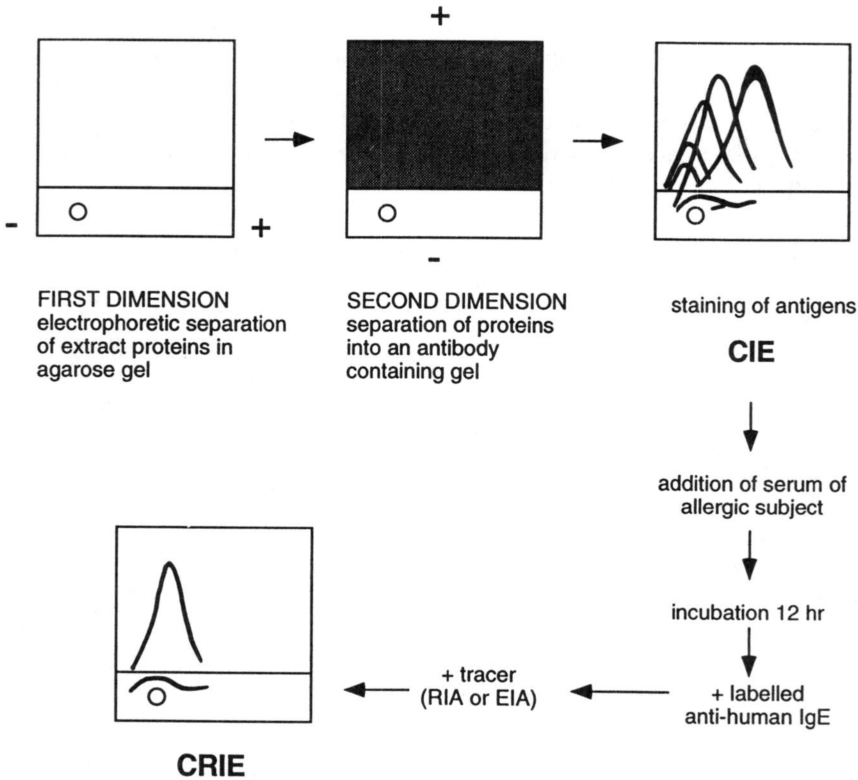

Figure 5 Crossed immunoelectrophoresis (CIE) and crossed radioimmunoelectrophoresis (CRIE). (From Ref. 26.)

double immunodiffusion method is one of the most widely used in allergen standardization and was the basis of several other techniques. Cross radioimmunoelectrophoresis [64,78,79] is one of the methods of choice to detect allergen-specific IgE. It combines the CIE precipitation of an allergen extract by rabbit antiserum, which indicates the antigenic composition of the extract, and the identification of the allergen composition of the extract. This second step is obtained by incubating the cross immunoprecipitates with serum IgE and subsequently adding ^{125}I–anti-IgE. The allergens are then revealed by autoradiography. A semiquantification of specific IgE binding may be obtained using a CRIE reference system [79]. The CRIE technique, like RAST inhibition, was used to identify single allergens in a mixture of allergens and to determine the specificity of human IgE antibodies to a given allergen. The CRIE technique was used to produce "allergograms" of several allergens including grass, ragweed, weed, and tree pollens, several kinds of hair and dandruff, mites, and *Cladosporium* and other molds [80–83]. This technique was also used to control the fractionation and purification of allergens and to study cross-allergenicity among pollens. Overall, CRIE is a very useful tool for allergen standardization, since it is able to identify and quantify the allergens in a complex allergen mixture. However, it has some limitations. The specificity and standardization of the animal antibody reagent is a prerequisite. Furthermore, problems may arise if rabbit IgG is directed against the same antigenic determinants as human IgE, thus inhibiting the binding of the latter to the immunoprecipitates.

B. Allergen Extracts Used for Treatment

It is now recognized that efficacy of specific immunotherapy requires relatively large doses of allergens that are close to the dose that can elicit anaphylactic reactions. Thus, it is important for safety that the amount of allergen be accurately known and be consistent lot to lot [4]. Although assays of potency of therapeutic extracts can be made only by controlled clinical trials in humans, it is absolutely impossible to do so with sequential production batches. It is not possible at present to assay potency in the accepted sense of efficacy, but it is possible to assay the composition of the vaccines. In this respect aqueous extracts present few problems, as they can be directly assayed by the methods described for extracts used in diagnosis. However, skin test titration may not always be possible because of the lower potency of the extracts used for treatment.

For adsorbed vaccines it is necessary either to release the allergen or to use a modified RAST assay [84,85]. When the allergenic components have been chemically modified, it is more difficult to assay the final product except if there is a marker that is easy to titrate, such as *Amb a* I (if not modified). Some of these extracts can be standardized by means of skin test titration [86,87].

In the case of adsorbed or modified extracts, the composition of the finished product cannot be extrapolated from the initial composition of the standardized extracts, for even simple adsorption on gel introduces selection to the molecules that have been insolubilized.

III. UNITS OF STANDARDIZED EXTRACTS

A. Arbitrary Units

Each allergen extract, once standardized, is assigned a potency unit. Several approaches to the choice of potency have been suggested. The "old" allergen-independent units are still in use, but they tend to be replaced by "allergen-related" units. Either these are assigned an arbitrary unitage (e.g., 100,000 AU to the reference), or units are based on the quantity of allergen in the extract (e.g., amount of antigen *Amb a* I) or, finally, on the quantity of protein with defined allergenic activity (e.g., μg of hyaluronidase).

The International Units (IU) labeling the International Reference Preparations and the International Standardized Preparations (ISP) are "an arbitrary measure adopted in the absence of any absolute measurement that can be invariably related to allergic activity [88]. By way of example, the *Dermatophagoides pteronyssinus* ISP of 100,000 IU/ml has been standardized by skin testing, RAST inhibition, and the measurement of *Der p* I and *Der p* II using monoclonal antibody–based assays [89,90]. When an extract is compared by one or several of these techniques to the ISP, a given number of IU will be ascribed to it. They are of relevant importance, since it is hoped that in the future all extracts will be labeled in IU and that this will end much of the confusion that makes communication between physicians and/or researchers using extracts difficult.

B. Biological Units

Several biological units have been proposed since the introduction of the HEP in 1972 by Aas et al. [22]. The HEP (1 HEP = 1,000 BU/ml) is a biological unit based on the skin sensitivity of the patients by comparison with histamine. The skin activity reference unit (SARAH) [29] and the index of reactivity (IR) [30] are close to the HEP and are used by companies in Europe. However, these units are almost completely independent, since the comparison of two similar techniques (SARAH and IR) gave a ratio between both units ranging from 3 (grass pollens) to 60 (olive pollens). Other biological units in current use do not include a reference test with histamine or codeine. The biological activity unit defined by Brighton et al. [26] in 1979 and refined by Carreira et al. [34] is used by a Spanish company. Some of the AUs and all the BAUs (bioequivalent allergy unit) are based on the $ID_{50}EAL$ skin test procedure [20,21,91].

C. Modifications of Unitage

Depending on the evolving knowledge on allergen standardization within the past 15 years, some units have been modified. These modifications have unfortunately caused confusion among clinicians. The HEP was initially based on a histamine dihydrochloride concentration of 5.43 mmol/L. However, the size of the histamine skin test was found to be too small, and later the histamine strength was tenfold increased without any change in the name of the unit.

There have been several changes in labeling in the United States within the past 15 years (Kenimer, Workshop, American Academy of Allergy and Immunology, 1993). The AU nomenclature for potency labeling of allergen extracts was originally an arbitrary system in which units were assigned on the basis of general clinical experience with the various extracts. The initial extracts assigned arbitrary AUs were pollen extracts that were all labeled at 100,000 AU/ml and controlled by

Table 5 Current Status of Allergen Extracts in the United States

Extract	Unstandardized	Current unit label	Current unit method	Future unit
Cat	Removed	BAU/ml	ID_{50} EAL *Fel d* I RID	
Short ragweed	Soon removed	AU/ml	*Amb a* I RID	BAU/ml
Grasses	Licensed	AU/ml	Inhibition[a]	BAU/ml
Weeds	Licensed	AU/ml	Inhibition[a]	BAU/ml
Trees	Licensed	AU/ml	Inhibition[a]	BAU/ml
Mites	No extract	AU/ml	Inhibition[a]	BAU/ml
Venoms	No extract	μg HA	Enzyme activity	

[a]Radioallergosorbent test (RAST) or immunoassay inhibition.
BAU = bioequivalent allergy unit; RID = radial immunodiffusion; AU = allergy unit; HA = hyaluronidase.

in vitro techniques such as RAST inhibition. Following validation of skin test methods for the assessment of extract potency [20,21], AUs have been assigned on the basis of the results of skin testing (ID_{50}EAL skin test procedure). The first extracts evaluated by this method were the house dust mite extracts, and it was shown that they warranted assignment of 10,000 AU/ml (based on the assignment of 100,000 AU to a D_{50} of 14 as determined by the ID_{50}EAL skin test procedure). In 1992 the Center for Biologics Evaluation and Research (CEBR) of the FDA completed an evaluation of the potency of various commercial cat extracts using the ID_{50}EAL Skin Test Procedure [92]. Results for cat extract were not consistent with the arbitrary AU/ml (10 to 19.9 *Fel d* I FDA U/ml = 100,00 AU/ml) that had been originally assigned to these products, and it was observed that cat extracts containing 10–19.9 *Fel d* I FDA U/ml should be labeled 10,000 AU/ml rather than 100,000 AU/ml as originally assigned. This discrepancy between potency as determined by skin testing and the previously assigned potency units created a problem, and the CEBR decided to change the AU to BAU (100,000 AU/ml = 10,000 BAU/ml). A warning from the FDA indicates that products labeled in AU/ml and BAU/ml are not interchangeable [89].

Moreover, extracts within a country may be standardized or not, and the standardized extracts may be labeled in various units (Table 5).

IV. PREPARATION OF ALLERGEN EXTRACTS

The method of manufacture of allergen extracts is complicated by the progressive appearance of techniques of purification and fractionation, but the reference extracts and, more generally, the extracts that are used commercially for diagnosis continue to be obtained by simple extraction. For the commercial products, this is followed by control of the activity obtained by comparison with the internal extract of reference for each drug company; but progressively, comparisons are being made with the international standards.

A. Selection and Control of Raw Materials

The attention given to the final product of the extraction of an allergenic substance often eclipses the importance of the quality of the source material, but this is a prerequisite for any good-quality extract. The selection and control of raw materials are two of the main concerns of the control authorities that regulate allergen extracts. This problem was closely studied by the Allergen Standardization Subcommittee of IUIS, and guidelines have been proposed.

Pollens should be identified, and should be free from contamination by other pollen species or nonpollen contaminants, with limits depending on the practical possibilities of collection. The technique, year [93,94], and place of collection, as well as the conditions of storage and possible chemical modifications of grains (delipidation, use of chemical methods of purification), should be clearly stated [95,96].

For *animal danders, epidermals, and urine* the important data are the identification of the species and breed, the verification of the good health of the animal, the quality and description of the raw materials (epidermal, dermal, pelt, etc.), the presence of blood, and if possible the determination of the bacteria, parasite, mite, and mold load of the specimen [97].

Molds are even more difficult to produce, since there are frequent genetic mutations of the antigenic characters [98]. The strains should be identified by competent mycologists and must be free from contaminants, but some other factors are of importance: the choice of the culture medium (which must be nonallergenic), the method of culture (in continuous phase or stationary), and finally, the method of isolation [99].

Mites also present many problems, not only with respect to their production. Their allergenic content varies according to the culture medium and the fraction used for extraction (whole mite body, excreta, or both) [100,101]. The whole body may contain traces of highly allergenic media such as horse or other animal danders, and their control is very difficult. Finally, some authorities have indicated that mites should not be grown any more on human danders [102].

In some countries, such as Scandinavia, *house dust* extracts have been removed from the market owing to their poor quality and possible side effects.

B. Extraction: Crude Allergen Extracts

Most commercial extracts are crude extracts prepared simply by "subjecting a certain amount of the source material to more or less appropriate liquids in a ratio that has not been scientifically determined." The first allergen extracts were prepared in 1920 by Coca et al. [103], who used a solution as close as possible to biological fluids. It was a mixture of sodium chloride and sodium bicarbonate, with phenol employed as a preservative. In 1927, Stier and Hollister [104] introduced the 50% glycerol solution, which is still commonly used owing to its protective activity against allergen degradation. In fact, the early investigators who prepared allergen extracts tried to come as close as possible to the physiological extraction of allergens that takes place in the nasal and tracheobronchial mucosa, and they used stabilizing agent to best preserve the allergen. These requirements still prevail, but in addition, different research workers and laboratories have scientifically studied the extraction procedures. Among the various aspects studied are the kinetics of release of allergens from a raw material [105–107] and the effect of extractive solutions or temperature on the composition of allergenic extracts [108]. Finally, it is likely that in the future, different raw material will be extracted with different procedures [109,110]. Such extracts should contain all the relevant allergens from a source in the relative proportion found in the raw material. Recently, it has been proposed that the ratio of major allergens present in an extract should be as close as possible to the ratio of these allergens present in the raw material; e.g., the ratio between *Der p* I and *Der p* II should be similar in the allergen extract and in the dust collected [111]. Crude extracts are used for diagnostic and therapeutic purposes.

C. Purification and Fractionation

Allergens constitute only a minor fraction of the crude extracts, so that Scandinavian investigators have suggested that extracts be purified and/or fractionated to discard nonallergenic components and retain the allergens [112].

D. Control of the Freshly Prepared Extract

Since raw materials are of biological origin, they often vary in potency and sometimes in composition, so that when an extract has been freshly prepared it is necessary to control it with in vivo and in vitro tests to assess its potency and composition, using methods described above.

E. Storage and Shelf Life

It has been known for years that diluted allergen extracts preserved in saline lose their activity very rapidly. The first attempt to preserve allergen extracts efficiently was the use of a 50% glycerol solution. More recently, it was observed that the addition of human serum albumin [113,114], Tween 80 [114], or ϵ-aminocaproic acid [115] to the extracting solution diminished the alteration of allergen extracts.

Baer [116] has offered some proposals for maintaining allergenic extracts in an unaltered form:

Freeze-drying or use in a diluent containing 50% glycerol,
Storage of the extract at +4°C,
Addition of stabilizers in diluted extracts to prevent adsorption onto surfaces.

V. STANDARDIZED EXTRACTS

Standardized extracts should contain measured quantities of allergenic activity and are produced with lot-to-lot consistency. Such extracts should at best contain all the relevant allergens from a source in the relative proportion found in the raw material. They should help to improve the reliability of in vivo and in vitro tests as well as that of specific immunotherapy.

A. International Reference Standards

In 1980, allergen extracts were rarely standardized and international standards were not available. The Allergen Standardization Subcommittee of the IUIS decided to prepare international allergen standards. This subcommittee included members of regulatory agencies, scientists in the fields of allergy, chemistry, immunology biology and molecular biology, clinical allergists, and workers from research laboratories of various manufacturers. These members were distributed throughout the world and met regularly several times a year. They first devised the steps to prepare a reliable standard [117]:

1. Review of the published data that make possible the production of a technical dossier for the intended extract.
2. Definition of norms and selection of raw materials.
3. Preparation of a pool of serum from subjects who are clinically allergic and sensitive to the substance under consideration.
4. Preparation of specific reagents that are necessary for the specific techniques (sera from immunized animals, monoclonal antibodies, etc.).
5. An appeal to manufacturing companies or public institutions for production of batches of the future reference material.
6. Analysis of several proposed batches and selection of an ad hoc committee for the product that will be the reference extract.
7. Organization of a multicenter study for validation, using all available methods of control of allergenic extracts.
8. Adoption by the members of the ad hoc committee and then by the members of the Allergen Subcommittee of the IUIS of the preparation and unitage (IU).
9. Conducting of a program of stability studies.

10. Definitive adoption as either an IUIS standard or a WHO standard or reference preparation.
11. Storage of batches on behalf of the IUIS or the WHO.
12. Distribution to laboratories and institutions wishing to define their reference or control their commercial products.

Several allergens have been studied, and reference preparations are available for some of them. To complete the system of standardization, the Subcommittee has started the preparation of a manual of analytical procedures specifying the protocols and reagents that should be used, inspired by the techniques proposed by the Bureau of Biologics in the United States, the National Institute for Biological Standardization and Control in the United Kingdom, and the Nordic Countries guidelines for allergen standardization. These guidelines have thus greatly improved the quality and standardization of the techniques of control [118] and of the allergens used in clinical practice, since the manufacturers have applied their improved knowledge not only to preparing a "good" standard extract that might be accepted as an international standard but also to the preparation of routine extracts.

Each vial distributed by the WHO as a standard (and possibly by other agencies, since some extracts may not be accepted by the WHO as international standard preparations [ISP]) is accompanied by a leaflet defining the major and sometimes the minor allergens, together with reagents required and methods that are appropriate for the measurements. For some allergens there are still unsolved problems. The cat 1 and albumin content of the cat standard allergen is still a matter of discussion. For the *Dermatophagoides pteronyssinus* ISP the problem is even more complicated, since it is made from a spent culture including metabolic and somatic antigens [119], whereas some regulatory agencies specify that extracts should be made from "pure" mites. This is the reason for the preparation of a *Dermatophagoides pteronyssinus* U.S. national standard differing from the ISP.

At present there are five standards that are accepted as being ISPs of WHO: *Dermatophagoides pteronyssinus* [89,90], short ragweed [120], timothy grass [121], birch pollen, and dog hair and dander [122] extracts. One extract is accepted as being an international reference preparation (IRP): Bermuda grass [123]. Cat hair and dander, ryegrass, and *Alternaria* [124,125] extracts may be submitted to the WHO in the future.

The Allergen Standardization Subcommittee of the IUIS, in general recommendations, has emphasized that these international standards should be used as calibrators (i.e., standards for measurement of relative potency) and are not recommended for use as prototypes (i.e., materials to which an extract is to be matched in all respects). The ampoules of standards are available only as reference materials to calibrate national or internal laboratory standards but are not to be used in day-to-day work.

B. National Reference Extracts

National reference extracts have been prepared in the United States by the CEBR (former Bureau of Biologics), in the United Kingdom by the National Institute for Biological Standardization and Control, and in Denmark for several allergens including pollens, mites, molds, foods and venoms [126]. The preparation and control of these extracts usually meet the criteria of the IRPs and the short ragweed ISP is in fact the U.S. national reference extract.

C. Manufacturer Reference Extracts

Since 1980, most manufacturers in the world have prepared "in-house reference preparations" to control the batch-to-batch potency of the major allergens such as mites, many pollen species, some molds such as *Alternaria* and *Cladosporium*, dog and cat dander, venoms, and possibly some foods. Usually, the preparation of these extracts follows the guidelines of the IUIS, but this is not always the case and it is not mandatory. The control of this in-house reference preparation is optimally done by means of skin tests, making it possible to label the extract in biological units; in vitro assay for total allergenic potency, including RAST inhibition in most cases and if possible titration of purified allergen(s); and tests to appreciate the composition of the extract, including IEF, CIE, and if possible CRIE and immunoblotting [127–130]. These reference extracts are labeled in internal units that cannot be directly translated into IU or other units.

In the United States, the labeling of the extracts differs (Table 5). It can be in AU/ml or BAU/ml by comparing the in-house reference preparation with the national standard. In the Nordic countries, extracts are labeled in BU using the method proposed in the Nordic guidelines. In these countries and others, the practice of also comparing the internal standard with the international standards is favored, so that the in-house extract may also be labeled in IU.

D. Preparation and Control of a Commercial Standardized Extract

Manufacturers prepare all new batches of a given allergen exactly as they did for their in-house reference extract, but since the composition of the raw materials may vary, they control the new batch by comparing it with the in-house reference preparation. They use both one or several tests of total allergenic potency (RAST inhibition and/or titration of a purified allergen) and one or several tests assessing the composition of the extract. If the new batch is similar to the reference extract, they store and release the commercial extract. Commercial standardized extracts include venoms, pollens, mites, molds, and foods [131–138]. Comparisons between IRPs and in-house reference preparations are commonly carried out in various companies [139].

E. Clinical Importance of Standardized Extracts with Common Unitage

Standardized allergens of reproducible potency are not prepared for use in laboratories and research institutes but represent a major improvement in allergy clinical practice. Standardized extracts from different manufacturers are less variable in potency, although they are not interchangeable. The batch-to-batch variability of standardized extracts from the same company is now acceptable, and this leads to an increased safety of immunotherapy when vials are changed. However, standardized extracts are more expensive and more potent than older extracts. It is therefore more difficult for nonspecialists to use them.

Hymenoptera venoms were the first standardized and lyophilized extracts. Owing to their remarkable activity, specific immunotherapy with venoms is highly effective. The importance of venoms was emphasized by Yunginger [140], who deemed the availability of standardized hymenoptera venoms one of the major improvements of allergology in the 1970s.

As Dr. P. S. Norman, former chairman of the Subcommittee on Allergen Standardization of the IUIS has stated [141], standardization of allergenic extracts and their labeling in IU allows physicians and investigators to communicate more easily about the sensitivity of their patients as well as about specific immunotherapy protocols. It has been observed that extracts labeled in biological units gave a mean wheal size similar whatever allergen species used when tested by skin tests. Several protocols to study standardized extracts have been proposed [142–145].

1. Diagnosis of Allergic Diseases

Skin Tests. When allergen extracts were not standardized, the positivity of skin tests was largely dependent on their strength. It was common to observe that skin tests with cat, dog, molds, or some pollens difficult to recover (such as *Parietaria* in the Mediterranean area) were negative in patients with a typical history of allergy. On the other hand, some extracts containing large amounts of irritant substances and injected at high concentrations by the intradermal route induced false-positive reactions. When extracts became standardized by RAST inhibition, the sensitivity and specificity of skin tests was increased and most allergic patients were diagnosed. However, the size of the skin tests was highly variable. With allergen extracts standardized by skin tests (biological methods), the sensitivity and specificity of skin tests was slightly increased, and, more important, the mean sizes of the tests are comparable from one allergen species to another and from one batch to another. These considerations strongly support the use of standardized allergens for skin testing [146,147].

Titration of Specific Immunoglobulin E. One of the critical factors for the titration of specific IgE is the quality of allergen extracts. Needless to say, allergen standardization is a prerequisite for any specific IgE test.

Provocative Challenges. The standardization of allergen extracts is also of paramount importance in nasal and bronchial provocative challenges. This is particularly true when challenges are repeated over time to assess the efficacy of an antiallergic treatment. In that case, it is recommended that the same batch of lyophilized standardized extract be reconstituted each test day. It is also recommended that the shelf-life of the lyophilized extract be assayed. Unfortunately, even in 1993, many studies are not properly designed and are overinterpreted because of the decay in activity of unstandardized allergen extracts stored for inappropriate periods of time.

2. Specific Immunotherapy

Safety. The safety of specific immunotherapy is critical. It is now recognized that efficacy of immunotherapy requires relatively large doses of allergen that are close to the dose that may elicit a systemic reaction. Thus, for safety reasons it is important that the amount of allergen be accurately known and consistent from time to time [4]. With unstandardized allergens of variable potency, systemic reactions may occur during the first phase of immunotherapy (since the concentration of a given vial may differ largely from the concentration of another vial, and the starting dose is unknown), as well as when vials are changed, and it has been recommended that the dose of allergen injected be reduced when any new vial is used. It has been proposed that specific immunotherapy may be safer with standardized extracts, but results obtained initially with inhalant allergens were not as satisfactory as expected, since new standardized extracts are far more potent than old ones. Venom immunotherapy has always been considered to be safe, possibly because the first studies were carried out very carefully [148–150]. On the other hand, the first trials using mite, pollen, or mold extracts resulted in a high rate of systemic reactions during the first phase of immunotherapy [151–155]. When these extracts were used more carefully, and eventually with premedication, the rate of systemic reaction with mites, pollens, or molds was low and the severity mild [152,156,157]. On the other hand, with stable extracts or lyophilized extracts reconstituted the day of the injection, maintenance immunotherapy is much safer than when unstandardized extracts are used, and the dose of extract need not be decreased when vials are changed [152,156,157]. When skin tests with standardized extracts are used, it is possible to calculate an optimal dose leading to efficacy and safety [151,157,158].

Efficacy. The efficacy of standardized extracts is now well documented for venoms, pollens, mites, molds, and animal danders.

3. Epidemiological Studies

In epidemiological studies, it is necessary to compare different populations, and for that only standardized extracts can be used.

VI. ALLERGEN NOMENCLATURE

To bring some order into the rather chaotic situation created by the use by different investigators of multiple systems of identification for allergens that have been progressively isolated and described in the main allergenic extracts, a common and unique nomenclature has been proposed [159].

The source of the allergen is clearly defined, including its accepted taxonomic name and any further identification.

Highly purified allergens are designated by the first three letters of the genus (italicized), space, first letter of the species name (italicized), space; and a Roman numeral. For example, *Lol p* I refers to *Lolium perenne* allergen number 1 (perennial rye group I—rye 1). In the rare event that two species have identical designations, they are distinguished by adding one or more letters to each species designation.

The allergens are usually numbered in the order in which they were isolated, or by general agreement of the IUIS Nomenclature Subcommittee. Some exceptions have been proposed to solve, for example, the problems of isoallergens, of chemically defined allergens, or fungal allergens isolated in certain strains.

REFERENCES

1. Noon, L., and Cantar, B. C., Prophylactic inoculation against hay fever, *Lancet*, *i*, 1572 (1911).
2. Stull, A., Cooke, R. A., and Tennant, J., The allergen content of pollen extracts. Its determination and its deterioration, *J. Allergy*, *4*, 455 (1993).
3. Biological products; allergenic extracts; implementation of efficacy review; proposed rule. Department of Health and Human Services, Food and Drug Administration, 21 CRF Parts 6000, 610, and 680
4. Reed, C. E., Yunginger, J. W., and Evans, R., Quality assurance and standardization of allergy extracts in allergy practice, *J. Allergy Clin. Immunol.*, *84*, 4 (1989).
5. Platts-Mills, T. A. E., and Chapman, M. D., Allergen standardization, *J. Allergy Clin. Immunol.*, *87*, 621 (1991).
6. Chua, K. Y., Stewart, G. A., Thomas, W. R., et al., Sequence analysis of cDNA

coding for a major house dust mite allergen, *Der p* 1. Homology with cysteine proteases, *J. Exp. Med.*, *167*, 175 (1988).

7. Baldo, B. A., Structural features of allergens large and small with emphasis on recombinant allergens, *Curr. Opin. Immunol.*, *3*, 841 (1991).
8. Fang, K. S., Vitale, M., Fehlner, P., and King, T. P., cDNA cloning and primary structure of a white-face hornet venom allergen, antigen 5, *Proc. Natl. Acad. Sci. USA*, *85*, 895 (1988).
9. Morgenstern, J. P., Griffith, I. J., Kuo, M. C., et al., Amino acid sequence of *Fel d* I, the major allergen of the domestic cat: protein sequence analysis and cDNA cloning, *Proc. Natl. Acad. Sci. USA*, *88*, 9690 (1991).
10. Rafnar, T., Griffith, I. J., Kuo, M.-C., Bond, J. F., Rogers, B. L., and Klapper, D. G., Cloning of *Amb a* I (antigen E), the major allergen family of short ragweed pollen, *J. Biol. Chem.*, *266*, 1229 (1991).
11. Silvanovich, A., Astwood, J., Zhang, L., et al., Nucleotide sequence analysis of three cDNAs coding for *Poa p* IX isoallergens of Kentucky bluegrass pollen, *J. Biol. Chem.*, *266*, 1204 (1991).
12. Singh, M. H., Hough, T., Theerakulpisut, P., et al., Isolation of cDNA encoding a newly identified major allergenic protein of rye-grass pollen: intracellular targeting to the amyloplast, *Proc. Natl. Acad. Sci. USA*, *88*, 1384 (1991).
13. Breiteneder, H., Petterburger, K., Bito, A., et al., The gene coding for the major birch pollen allergen, *Bet v* 1, is highly homologous to a pea disease resistance response gene, *EMBO J.*, *8*, 1935 (1989).
14. Valenta, R., Duchene, M., Vrtala, S., et al., Recombinant allergens for immunoblot diagnosis of tree-pollen allergy, *J. Allergy Clin. Immunol.*, *88*, 889 (1991).
15. Valenta, R., Vrtala, S., Ebner, C., Kraft, D., and Scheiner, O., Diagnosis of grass pollen allergy with recombinant grass (*Phleum pratense*) pollen allergens, *Int. Arch. Allergy Appl. Immunol.*, *97*, 287 (1992).
16. Yang, M., Olsen, E., Dolovich, J., Sehon, A. H., and Mohapatra, S. S., Immunologic characterization of a recombinant Kentucky blue grass (*Poa pratensis*) allergenic peptide, *J. Allergy Clin. Immunol.*, *87*, 1096 (1991).
17. Moser, M., Crameri, R., Menz, G., et al., Cloning and expression of recombinant *Aspergillus fumigatus* allergen I/a (r*Asp f* I/a) with IgE binding and type I skin test activity, *J. Immunol.*, *149*, 454 (1992).
18. Rafnar, T., Ghost, B., Metzler, W. J., et al., Expression and analysis of recombinant *Amb a* V and *Amb t* V allergens. Comparison with native proteins by immunological assays and NMR spectroscopy, *J. Biol. Chem.*, *267*, 21119 (1992).
19. Maasch, H. J., Fischer, B., Wahl, R., and Wahn, U., Comparison of histamine release assay and RAST inhibition as tools for allergen extract standardization, *Int. Arch. Allergy Appl. Immunol.*, *73*, 314 (1984).
20. Turkeltaub, P. C., Rastogi, S. C., Baer, H., and Norman, P. S., A standardized, quantitative skin test assay of allergen potency, *J. Allergy Clin. Immunol.*, *65*, 213 (1980).
21. Turkeltaub, P. C., Allergenic extracts: In vivo standardization, in *Allergy, Principles and Practice*, 3rd Ed. (E. Middleton, Jr., E. F. Ellis, C. E. Reed, N. F. Adkinson, and J. W. Yunginger, eds.), Mosby Co., St. Louis, 1988, p. 388.

22. Aas, K., and Belin, L., Standardization of diagnostic work in allergy. First report from the standardization committee of the Northern Society of Allergology, *Acta Allergol.*, *27*, 439 (1972).
23. Belin, L., Biologic standardization—the HEP unit, *Proceedings of the Fourth International Paul-Ehrlich-Seminar on Regulatory Control and Standardization of Allergenic Extracts* (M. Schaeffer, C. Sisk, H. D. Brede, eds.), Gustav Fisher Verlag, Stuttgart, 1987, p. 145.
24. Dreborg, S., Basomba, A., Belin, L., Durham, S., Einarsson, R., Eriksson, N. E., Frostad, A. B., Grimmer, O., Halvorsen, R., and Holgersson, M., Biological equilibration of allergen preparations: methodological aspects and reproducibility, *Clin. Allergy*, *17*, 537 (1987).
25. Dreborg, S., Sjogren, I., Eriksson, N. E., and Einarsson, R., Selection of patients for biological standardization as exemplified by standardization of mugwort, goosefoot and English plantain pollen allergen extracts/preparations, *Allergy*, *42*, 485 (1987).
26. Dreborg, S., Belin, L., Eriksson, N. E., Grimmer, O., Kunkel, G., Malling, H. J., Nilsson, G., Sjogren, I., and Zetterstrom, O., Results of biological standardization with standardized allergen preparations, *Allergy*, *42*, 109 (1987).
27. Backman, A., Belin, L., Dreborg, S., Halvorsen, R., Malling, H. J., and Weeke, B., Standardization of allergenic preparations. Comments with reference to the second edition of the common Nordic guidelines for registration of allergenic preparations, *Allergy*, *46*, 81 (1991).
28. Brighton, W. D., Topping, M. D., and Henocq, E., Activity units for allergen extracts, *Clin. Allergy*, *9*, 591 (1977).
29. Watson, H. K., and Rooke, M. B., A proposed unitage system for allergen extracts, *Allergy*, *37* (suppl 1), 24 (1982).
30. Bousquet, J., Djoukhadar, F., Hewitt, B., Guérin, B., and Michel, F. B., Comparison of the stability of a mite extract and a pollen extract stored in normal conditions of use, *Clin. Allergy*, *15*, 29 (1985).
31. Dreborg, S., The skin prick test. Methodological studies and clinical applications, Linköping University Medical Dissertation No. 239, 1987.
32. Nordic Council on Medicines. Registration of allergen preparations, 2nd Ed., Nordiska Läkemedelsnämnden, NLN Publication No 23, Uppsala, 1989.
33. Conroy, M. C., and De Weck, A. L., Codeine: a probe of basophil and mast cell reactivity, *Allergol. Immunopathol.*, *8*, 249 (1980).
34. Carreira, J., Rubio, M., Herrerao, T., et al., Collaborative clinical assay of the biological potency of allergen skin test extracts, *Clin. Allergy*, *14*, 503 (1984).
35. Stull, A., Cooke, R. A., and Chobot, R., The allergenically active substance in pollen. A chemical and biologic study of *Phleum pratense* (timothy) pollen, *J. Allergy*, *3*, 341 (1931).
36. Bousquet, J., Guérin, B., and Michel, F. B., Standardization of allergenic extracts, in *Provocative Challenge Procedures* (S. L. Spector, ed.), Homa Press, Denver, 1989, p. 85. 131.
37. Foucard, T., Johansson, S. G. O., Bennich, H., and Berg, T., In vitro estimation of allergens by a radio-immune antiglobulin using IgE antibodies, *Int. Arch. Allergy*, *43*, 360 (1976).

38. Gleich, G. J., Larson, J. B., Jones, R. T., and Baer, H., Measurement of potency of allergenic extracts by their inhibitory capacities in the ratio-allergo-sorbent tests, *J. Allergy Clin. Immunol.*, *53*, 158 (1974).
39. Yman, L., Allergen assay and extract potency estimation, *Int. Arch. Allergy Appl. Immunol.*, *49*, 55 (1975).
40. Schroder, H., RAST-based techniques for allergen assay, in *Regulatory Control and Standardization of Allergenic Extracts* (H. Brede and H. Going, eds.), Gustav Fisher Verlag, Stuttgart, 1980, p. 139.
41. Maasch, H. J., Wihl, J. A., Schultze-Werninghaus, G., Geissler, W., and Wahl, R., A manufacturer's criteria for in-house reference preparations for RAST inhibition, *Ann. Allergy*, *59*, 29 (1987).
42. Ponterius, G., Brandt, R., Hulten, E., and Yman, L., Comparative studies on the allergens of horse dandruff and horse serum, *Int. Arch. Allergy Appl. Immunol.*, *44*, 679 (1973).
43. Baer, H., and Anderson, M. C., Allergenic extracts. I—Allergenic extracts: sources, preparation, and in vitro standardization, in *Allergy, Principles and Practice*, 3rd Ed. (E. Middleton, Jr., E. F. Ellis, C. E. Reed, N. F. Adkinson, Jr., and J. W. Yunginger, eds.), Mosby Co., St. Louis, 1988, p. 373.
44. Gleich, G. J., Leifermann, K. M., Jones, R. T., Hooton, M. L., and Baer, H., Analysis of the potency of extracts of june grass pollen by their inhibitory capacities in the radio-allergo-sorbent test, *J. Allergy Clin. Immunol.*, *58*, 31 (1976).
45. Yunginger, J. M., Jones, R. T., and Gleich, G. J., Studies on Alternaria allergen. II. Measurement of the relative potency of commercial Alternaria extracts by the direct RAST and by RAST-inhibition, *J. Allergy Clin. Immunol.*, *58*, 405 (1976).
46. Baer, H., Godfrey, H., Maloney, C. J., Norman, P. S., and Lichtenstein, L. M., The potency and antigen E content of commercially prepared ragweed extracts, *J. Allergy*, *45*, 317 (1970).
47. Baer, H., Maloney, C. J., Norman, P. S., and Marsh, D. G., The potency and group I antigen content of six commercially prepared grass pollen extracts, *J. Allergy Clin. Immunol.*, *54*, 157 (1974).
48. Lehrer, S. B., and Salvaggio, J. E., Allergens: standardization and impact of biotechnology—a review, *Allergy Proc.*, *11*, 197 (1990).
49. Platts-Mills, T. A. E., Heyman, P. W., Chapman, M. D., Hayden, M. L., and Wilkins, S. R., Cross reacting and species determinants on a major allergen from *Dermatophagoides pteronyssinus* and *D. farinae*: development of a radioimmunoassay for P1 equivalent in house dust and dust mite extracts, *J. Allergy Clin. Immunol.*, *78*, 398 (1986).
50. Chapman, M. D., Aalberse, R. C., Brown, M. J., and Platts Mills, T. A. E., Monoclonal antibodies to the major feline allergen *Fed d* I. II. Single step affinity purification of *Fel d* I, N-terminal sequence analysis, and development of a sensitive two-site immunoassay to assess *Fed d* I exposure, *J. Immunol.*, *140*, 812 (1988).
51. Chapman, M. D., Allergen-specific monoclonal antibodies: new tools for the management of allergic diseases, *Allergy*, *43*, 7 (1988).
52. Lombardero, M., Heymann, P. W., Platts-Mills, T. A. E., Fox, J. W., Chapman, M.

D., Conformational stability of B cell epitopes on group I and group II *Dermatophagoides* spp. allergens, *J. Immunol.*, *144*, 1353 (1990).

53. Dreborg, S., and Einarsson, R., The major allergen content of allergenic preparations reflects their biological activity, *Allergy*, *47*, 418 (1992).
54. Haberman, E., Bee and wasp venoms, *Science*, *177*, 314 (1972).
55. Baer, H., Hymenoptera venoms: composition, standardization, stability, in *Monograph on Insect Allergy* (M. I. Levine and R. F. Lockey, eds.), Typecraft Press, Pittsburgh, 1981, p. 11.
56. Haberman, E., and Hardt, K. B., Sensitive and specific plate test for the quantification of phospholipases, *Anal. Biochem.*, *50*, 163 (1972).
57. Brighton, W. D., Profiles of allergen extract components by isoelectric focusing and radioimmunoassay, *Dev. Biol. Stand.*, *29*, 367 (1975).
58. Topping, M. D., Brighton, W. D., Stokell, M., and Patterson, J., Fractionation of cocksfoot (*Dactylis glomerata*) pollen by preparative iso electric focusing, *J. Immunol. Methods*, *19*, 61 (1978).
59. Righetti, P.G., Drysdale, J. W., Isoelectric Focusing, Vol. 1, American Elsevier, New York, 1976.
60. Topping, M. D., Brostoff, J., Brighton, W. D., Danks, J., and Minnis, M., Allergenic activity of fractions of cocksfoot (*Dactylis glomerata*) pollen, *Clin. Allergy*, *8*, 33 (1978).
61. Anderson, M. C., Baer, H., and Evans, R., Evaluation of pollen extracts using isoelectric focusing, *J. Allergy Clin. Immunol.*, *61*, 178 (1978).
62. Weber, K., and Osborn, M., The reliability of molecular weight determinations by dodecyl sulfate–polyacrylamide gel electrophoresis, *J. Biol. Chem.*, *244*, 4406 (1969).
63. Fisher, L., An introduction to gel chromatography, in *Laboratory Techniques in Biochemistry and Molecular Biology*, Vol. 1 (T. S. Work and E. Work, eds.), American Elsevier, New York, 1969.
64. Lowenstein, H., Quantitative immunoelectrophoretic methods; a tool for the analysis and isolation of allergens, *Prog. Allergy*, *25*, 1 (1978).
65. Weeke, B., and Lowenstein, H., Quantitative immunoelectrophoresis (QIE) used in analysis of allergen extracts and diagnosis of allergy, *Int. Arch. Allergy Appl. Immunol.*, *49*, 74 (1975).
66. Peltre, G., Lapeyre, J., and David, B., Heterogeneity of grass pollen allergens (*Dactylis glomerata*) recognized by IgE antibodies in human patient's sera by a new nitrocellulose immunoprint technique, *Immunol. Lett.*, *5*, 127–131 (1982).
67. Tovey, E. R., and Baldo, B. A., Standardization of allergens. Qualitative definition of house dust mite extracts following electroblotting and detection of components with antibody and lectin probes, *Int. Arch. Allergy Appl. Immunol.*, *75*, 322 (1984).
68. Bengtsson, A., Rolfsen, W., and Einarsson, R., Characterization of allergens and patient sera by a nitrocellulose immunoprint technique, *Int. Arch. Allergy Appl. Immunol.*, *78*, 139 (1984).
69. Haas, H., Becker, W. M., Maasch, H. J., et al., Analysis of allergen components in grass pollen extracts using immunoblotting, *Int. Arch. Allergy Appl. Immunol.*, *78*, 139 (1986).

70. Laurell, C. B., Quantitative estimation of proteins by electrophoresis in agarose gel containing antibodies, *Acta Biochem.*, *15*, 45 (1966).
71. Weeke, B., Rocket immunoelectrophoresis, *Scand. J. Immunol.*, *2* (suppl. 1), 37 (1973).
72. Ouchterloni, O., Immunodiffusion and immunoelectrophoresis, in *Handbook of Experimental Immunology* (D. M. Weir, ed.), Blackwell Scientific, Oxford, 1967, p. 655.
73. Grabar, P., and Williams, C. A., Methodes permettant l'étude conjuguée des propriétés électrophorétiques et immunochimiques d'un mélange de protéines. Application au sérum sanguin, *Biochim. Biophys. Acta*, *10*, 193 (1953).
74. Weeke, B., Crossed immunoelectrophoresis, *Scand. J. Immunol.*, *2* (suppl. 1), 47 (1973).
75. Kroll, J., Tandem crossed immunoelectrophoresis, *Scand. J. Immunol.*, *2* (suppl. 1), 57 (1973).
76. Sondergaard, I., Standardization of gel-precipitation techniques and their use in allergen standardization, *Allergy*, *35*, 241 (1980).
77. Verbruggen, R., Quantitative immunoelectrophoretic methods. A literature survey, *Clin. Chem.*, *21*, 5 (1975).
78. Lowenstein, H., Physico-chemical and immunological methods for the control of potency and quality of allergenic extracts, in *Regulatory Control and Standardization of Allergenic Extracts* (D. Brede and H. Going, eds.), Gustav Fisher Verlag, Stuttgart, 1980, p. 122.
79. Weeke, B., and Lowenstein, H., Allergens identified in crossed immunoelectrophoresis, *Scand. J. Immunol.*, *2* (suppl. 1), 149 (1973).
80. Lowenstein, H., and Marsh, D. G., Antigens of *Ambrosia eliator* (short ragweed) pollen. I. Cross immunoelectrophoresis analysis, *J. Immunol.*, *126*, 943 (1981).
81. Lowenstein, H., Markussen, B., and Weeke, B., Isolation and partial characterization of three major allergens of horse hair and dandruff, *Int. Arch. Appl. Immunol.*, *51*, 48 (1976).
82. Aukrust, L., Allergens in *Cladosporium herbarum*, in *Advances in Allergology and Applied Immunology* (A. Oehling, I. Glazer, E. Mathov, C. Abresman, eds.), Pergamon Press, Oxford, 1980, p. 475.
83. Lind, P., Korsgaard, J., and Lowenstein, H., Detection and quantitation of *Dermatophagoides* antigens in house dust by immunochemical techniques, *Allergy*, *34*, 319 (1979).
84. Turkeltaub, P. C., Evaluation of modified extracts, in *Proceedings of the Third International Paul Ehrlich Seminar on Regulatory Control and Standardization of Allergen Extracts* (H. D. Brede and E. Stevens, eds.), Stuttgart, Gustav Fisher Verlag, 1984, p. 323.
85. Weeke, B., Aluminum hydroxide absorbed allergens used in a modified RAST (AL-RAST), *Allergol. Immunopathol.*, *5* 321 (1976).
86. Maasch, H. J., and Marsh, D. G., Standardized extracts modified allergens—allergoids, *Clin. Rev. Allergy*, *5*, 89 (1987).
87. Grammer, L. C., Shaughnessy, M. A., and Patterson, R., Standardization of modified allergens using polymerized ragweed as a model, *Clin. Rev. Allergy*, *5*, 89 (1987).

88. Norman, P. S., International Units, in *Proceedings of the Fourth International Paul-Ehrlich-Seminar on Regulatory Control and Standardization of Allergen Extracts* (M. Schaeffer, C. Sisk, and H. D. Brede, eds.), Stuttgart, Gustav Fisher Verlag, 1987, p. 175.
89. Ford, A. W., Rawle, F. C., Lind, P., Spieksma, F. T., Lowenstein, H., and Platts-Mills, T. A., Standardization of *Dermatophagoides pteronyssinus*: assessment of potency and allergen content in ten coded extracts, *Int. Arch. Allergy Appl. Immunol.*, *76*, 58 (1985).
90. Ford, A., Seagroatt, V., Platts-Mills, T. A., and Lowenstein, H., A collaborative study on the first international standard of *Dermatophagoides pteronyssinus* (house dust mite) extract, *J. Allergy Clin. Immunol.*, *75*, 676 (1985).
91. Baer, H., Potency units for allergenic extracts in the USA, in *Proceedings of the Fourth International Paul-Ehrlich-Seminar on Regulatory Control and Standardization of Allergen Extracts* (M. Schaeffer, C. Sisk, and H. D. Brede, eds.), Stuttgart, Gustav Fisher Verlag, 1987, p. 167–168.
92. Center for Biologics Evaluation and Research, Alert on changes in standardized cat allergen extract products. From the Food and Drug Administration, *JAMA*, *268*, 2491 (1992).
93. Maasch, H. J., Hauck, P. R., Oliver, J. D., et al., Allergenic activity of short ragweed pollen (*Ambrosia eliator*) from different years and/or suppliers: criteria for the selection of an in-house allergen reference preparation, *Ann. Allergy*, *58*, 429 (1987).
94. Maasch, H. J., Geissler, W., Winter, H. G., and Wahl, R., Quality of timothy pollen (*Phleum pratense*) from different pollen seasons and different suppliers, *Int. Arch. Allergy Appl. Immunol.*, *81*, 85 (1986).
95. Anderson, M. C., The effect of the quality of source materials on reference preparations, in *Proceedings of the Fourth International Paul-Ehrlich-Seminar on Regulatory Control and Standardization of Allergen Extracts* (M. Schaeffer, C. Sisk, and H. D. Brede, eds.), Stuttgart, Gustav Fisher Verlag, 1987, p. 1.
96. Baer, H., and Anderson, M. C., Preparation and stability of pollen extracts, in *Highlights in Asthmology* (F. B. Michel, J. Bousquet, and P. Godard, eds.), Munich, Springer Verlag, 1987, pp. 291–293.
97. Ohman, J. L., Selection of source materials for preparation of mammalian allergens, in *Proceedings of the Fourth International Paul-Ehrlich-Seminar on Regulatory Control and Standardization of Allergen Extracts* (M. Schaeffer, C. Sisk, and H. D. Brede, eds.), Stuttgart, Gustav Fisher Verlag, 1987, p. 24.
98. Burge, H. A., Simmons, E. G., Muilenberg, M., et al., Intrinsic variability in airborne fungi: implications for allergen standardization, *Experientia*, *51* (suppl.), 143 (1987).
99. Aukrust, L., Selections of source materials for reference preparations of molds, in *Proceedings of the Fourth International Paul-Ehrlich-Seminar on Regulatory Control and Standardization of Allergen Extracts* (M. Schaeffer, C. Sisk, and H. D. Brede, eds.), Stuttgart, Gustav Fisher Verlag, 1987, p. 7.
100. Platts-Mills, T. A. E., and Chapman, M. D., Dust mites: immunology, allergic disease, and environmental control, *J. Allergy Clin. Immunol.*, *80*, 755 (1987).

101. Ackland, J., and Stewart, G. A., Quantitation and thermal stability of the mite allergen DPT 12 in whole mite extracts, *J. Allergy Clin. Immunol.*, *74*, 848 (1984).
102. Spieksma, F. Th. M., Selection of source materials for reference preparations of mites, in *Proceedings of the Fourth International Paul-Ehrlich-Seminar on Regulatory Control and Standardization of Allergen Extracts* (M. Schaeffer, C. Sisk, and H. D. Brede, eds.), Stuttgart, Gustav Fisher Verlag, 1987, p. 14.
103. Coca, A. F., Studies in specific hypersensitiveness. V. The preparation of fluid extracts and solutions for use in the diagnosis and treatment of allergics, *J. Immunol.*, *7*, 163 (1922).
104. Stier, R. F. E., and Hollister, G., Comparative study of pollen antigens as determined by skin reactions, *J. Lab. Clin. Med.*, *12*, 1139 (1927).
105. Marsh, D. G., Different rates of allergen release: an important consideration in the preparation of allergenic extracts, in *Proceedings of the Fourth International Paul-Ehrlich-Seminar on Regulatory Control and Standardization of Allergen Extracts* (M. Schaeffer, C. Sisk, and H. D. Brede, eds.), Stuttgart, Gustav Fisher Verlag, 1987, p. 47.
106. Giessler, W., Maasch, H. J., Winter, G., and Wahl, R., Kinetics of allergen release from house dust mite *Dermatophagoides pteronyssinus*, *J. Allergy Clin. Immunol.*, *77*, 24 (1986).
107. Kauffman, H. F., Van der Heide, S., Hovenga, H., and De Vries, K., Standardization of house dust mite extracts.-Liberation of allergenic and antigenic components in relation to extraction conditions, *Allergy*, *40*, 143 (1985).
108. Bousquet, J., Guérin, B., Furic, R., and Michel, F. B., Standardization of allergenic extracts, in *Provocative Challenge Procedures: Bronchial, Oral, Nasal and Exercise*, Vol. 1 (S. L. Spector, ed.), CRC Press, Boca Raton, Florida, 1983, p. 45.
109. Anderson, M. C., and Baer, H., Extraction procedures for pollen reference preparations, in *Proceedings of the Fourth International Paul-Ehrlich-Seminar on Regulatory Control and Standardization of Allergen Extracts* (M. Schaeffer, C. Sisk, and H. D. Brede, eds.), Stuttgart, Gustav Fisher Verlag, 1987, p. 42.
110. Phillips, P. V., Extraction procedures for reference preparations, in *Proceedings of the Fourth International Paul-Ehrlich-Seminar on Regulatory Control and Standardization of Allergen Extracts* (M. Schaeffer, C. Sisk, and H. D. Brede, eds.), Stuttgart, Gustav Fisher Verlag, 1987, p. 60.
111. Carreira, J., Ratio of major allergens in allergenic extracts. In press.
112. Dreborg, S., Einarsson, R., and Longbottom, J. L., The chemistry and standardization of allergens, in *Handbook of Experimental Immunology*, 4th Ed. (D. M. Weir, L. A. Herzenberg, and C. Blackwell, eds.), Blackwell Scientific Publications, Boston, 1986, p. 165.
113. Norman, P. S., and Marsh, D. G., Human serum albumin and Tween 80 as stabilizers for allergen solutions, *J. Allergy Clin. Immunol.*, *62*, 314 (1980).
114. Nelson, H. S., Effect of preservatives and conditions of storage on the potency of allergy extracts, *J. Allergy Clin. Immunol.*, *67*, 64 (1981).
115. Van Hoeyveld, E. M., and Stevens, E. A., Stabilizing effect of epsilon-aminocaproic acid on allergenic extracts, *J. Allergy Clin. Immunol.*, *76*, 543 (1985).
116. Baer, H., Stability of allergen extracts, in *Regulatory Control and Standardization of*

Allergenic Extracts (H. D. Brede and H. Going, eds.), Gustav Fisher Verlag, Stuttgart, 1980, p. 175.

117. Lowenstein, H., Selection of reference preparation, IUIS reference preparation criteria, in *Proceedings of the Fourth International Paul-Ehrlich-Seminar on Regulatory Control and Standardization of Allergen Extracts* (M. Schaeffer, C. Sisk, and H. D. Brede, eds.), Stuttgart, Gustav Fisher Verlag, 1987, p. 75.
118. Seagroatt, V., and Ford, A., RAST inhibition: a collaborative study on its suitability and reproducibility for the assay of cocksfoot pollen extracts, *Clin. Allergy*, *16*, 213 (1986).
119. Tovey, E. R., and Baldo, B. A., Comparison by electroblotting of IgE-binding components in extracts of house dust mite bodies and spent culture, *J. Allergy Clin. Immunol.*, *79*, 93 (1987).
120. Helm, R. M., Gauerke, M. B., Baer, H., et al., Production and testing of an international reference standard of short ragweed, *J. Allergy Clin. Immunol.*, *73*, 790 (1984).
121. Gjesing, B., Jager, L., Marsh, D. G., and Lowenstein, H., The international collaborative study establishing the first international standard for timothy (*Phleum pratense*) grass pollen allergenic extract, *J. Allergy Clin. Immunol.*, *75*, 258 (1985).
122. Nedergaard, J., Ford, A., Gjesing, B., et al., The collaborative study of the international standard of dog, *Canis domesticus*, hair/dander extract, *J. Allergy Clin. Immunol.*, *82*, 318 (1988).
123. Baer, H., and Anderson, M. C., Preliminary study of the proposed International Reference Bermuda grass pollen, in *Proceedings of the Third International Paul Ehrlich Seminar on Regulatory Control and Standardization of Allergen Extracts* (H. D. Brede and E. Stevens, eds.), Stuttgart, Gustav Fisher Verlag, 1984, p. 241.
124. Helm, R. M., Squillace, D. L., Aukrust, L., Borch, S. M., Baer, H., Bush, R. K., Lowenstein, H., Znamirowski, R., Nitchuk, W., and Yunginger, J. W., Production of an international reference standard *Alternaria* extract. I. Testing of candidate extracts, *Int. Arch. Allergy Appl. Immunol.*, *82*, 178 (1987).
125. Helm, R. M., Squillace, D. L., Yunginger, J. W., and members of the International Collaborative Trial, Production of an international reference standard *Alternaria* extract. II. Results of a collaborative trial, *J. Allergy Clin. Immunol.*, *81*, 651 (1988).
126. Ford, A., National laboratories' reference preparations criteria and availability UK, in *Proceedings of the Fourth International Paul-Ehrlich-Seminar on Regulatory Control and Standardization of Allergenic Extracts* (M. Schaeffer, C. Sisk, and H. D. Brede, eds.), Stuttgart, Gustav Fisher Verlag, 1987, p. 85.
127. Ingemann, I., and Venov, D., Manufacturers' practical consequences of the existence of external standards such as IS, in *Proceedings of the Fourth International Paul-Ehrlich-Seminar on Regulatory Control and Standardization of Allergenic Extracts* (M. Schaeffer, C. Sisk, and H. D. Brede, eds.), Stuttgart, Gustav Fisher Verlag, 1987, p. 118.
128. Maasch, H. H., Geissler, W., and Wahl, R., Quality control for manufacturing standardized allergen extracts. Manufacturers criteria for in-house references, in *Proceedings of the Fourth International Paul-Ehrlich-Seminar on Regulatory Control and Standardization of Allergenic Extracts* (M. Schaeffer, C. Sisk, and H. D. Brede, eds.), Stuttgart, Gustav Fisher Verlag, 1987, p. 118.

129. Einarsson, R., and Dreborg, S., Manufacturers criteria for in-house references, in *Proceedings of the Fourth International Paul-Ehrlich-Seminar on Regulatory Control and Standardization of Allergenic Extracts* (M. Schaeffer, C. Sisk, and H. D. Brede, eds.), Stuttgart, Gustav Fisher Verlag, 1987, p. 122.
130. Overell, B. G., Practicalities of batch control, in *Proceedings of the Third International Paul Ehrlich Seminar on Regulatory Control and Standardization of Allergen Extracts* (H. D. Brede and E. Stevens, eds.), Stuttgart, Gustav Fisher Verlag, 1984, p. 169.
131. Hoffman, D. R., and Golden, D. B. K., Standardized extracts. Stinging and biting insects, *Clin. Rev. Allergy*, *5*, 75 (1987).
132. Ford, A. W., and Platts-Mills, T. A. E., Standardized extracts, dust mite and other arthropods (inhalants), *Clin. Rev. Allergy*, *5*, 49 (1987).
133. Ohman, J. L., Jr., and Sudin, B., Standardized allergenic extracts from mammals, *Clin. Rev. Allergy*, *5*, 37 (1987).
134. Lowenstein, H., and Osterballe, O., Standardized grass pollen extracts, *Clin. Rev. Allergy*, *4*, 405 (1986).
135. King, T. P., and Norman, P. S., Standardized extracts, weeds, *Clin. Rev. Allergy*, *4*, 425 (1986).
136. Belin, L., Standardized extracts, trees, *Clin. Rev. Allergy*, *4*, 389 (1986).
137. Bush, R. K., and Yunginger, J. W., Standardization of fungal allergens, *Clin. Rev. Allergy*, *5*, 3 (1987).
138. Lemanske, R. F., Jr., and Taylor, S. L., Standardized extracts, foods, *Clin. Rev. Allergy*, *5*, 23 (1987).
139. Whal, R., Meineke, D., Oliver, J., Schultze-Werninghaus, G., and Hauck, P. R., Comparison of in-house allergen extracts of Phleum pratense (timothy grass) pollen with the international standard and investigation of IgE specificities of a grass-pollen serum pool from West Germany and of the one recommended by the World Health Organization, *J. Allergy Clin. Immunol.*, *84*, 448 (1989).
140. Yunginger, J. W., Standardization of allergenic extracts, *Ann. Allergy*, *66*, 107 (1991).
141. Norman, P. S., Why standardized extracts? *J. Allergy Clin. Immunol.*, *77*, 405 (1986).
142. Zweig, M. H., Design of protocols to evaluate the efficacy of allergenic extracts and allergy tests, in *Proceedings of the Fourth International Paul-Ehrlich-Seminar on Regulatory Control and Standardization of Allergenic Extracts* (M. Schaeffer, C. Sisk, and H. D. Brede, eds.), Stuttgart, Gustav Fisher Verlag, 1987, p. 239.
143. Van Metre, T. E. Jr., Design of protocols to evaluate the safety and efficacy of allergenic extracts, in *Proceedings of the Fourth International Paul-Ehrlich-Seminar on Regulatory Control and Standardization of Allergenic Extracts* (M. Schaeffer, C. Sisk, and H. D. Brede, eds.), Stuttgart, Gustav Fisher Verlag, 1987, p. 229.
144. Bousquet, J., Guérin, B., and Michel, F. B., Design of protocols to evaluate the safety and efficacy of allergenic extracts, in *Proceedings of the Fourth International Paul-Ehrlich-Seminar on Regulatory Control and Standardization of Allergenic Extracts* (M. Schaeffer, C. Sisk, and H. D. Brede, eds.), Stuttgart, Gustav Fisher Verlag, 1987, p. 213.

145. Bousquet, J., Guérin, B., and Michel, F. B., Clinical trials with standardized extracts, in *Proceedings of the Third International Paul Ehrlich Seminar on Regulatory Control and Standardization of Allergen Extracts* (H. D. Brede and E. Stevens, eds.), Stuttgart, Gustav Fisher Verlag, 1984, p. 290.
146. Adinoff, A. D., Rosloniec, D. M., McCall, L. L., and Nelson, H. S. Immediate skin test reactivity to Food and Drug Administration–approved standardized extracts, *J. Allergy Clin. Immunol.*, *86*, 766 (1990).
147. Lavins, B. J., Dolen, W. K., Nelson, H. S., and Weber, R. W., Use of standardized and conventional allergen extracts in prick skin testing, *J. Allergy Clin. Immunol.*, *89*, 658 (1992).
148. Hunt, K. J., Valentine, M. D., Sobotka, A. K., Benton, A. W., Amoud, F. J., and Lichtenstein, L. M., A controlled trial of immunotherapy in insect hypersensitivity, *N. Engl. J. Med.*, *299*, 157 (1978).
149. Lockey, R. F., Turkeltaub, P. C., Olive, E. S., et al., The hymenoptera venom study III: Safety of venom immunotherapy, *J. Allergy Clin. Immunol.*, *86*, 775 (1990).
150. Bousquet, J., Müller, U. R., Dreborg, S., et al., Immunotherapy with Hymenoptera venoms. Position paper of the European Academy of Allergy, *Allergy*, *42*, 401 (1987).
151. Bousquet, J., and Michel, F. B., Safety considerations in assessing the role of immunotherapy in allergic disorders, *Adis*, 1994, in press.
152. Hejjaoui, J., Ferrando, R., Dhivert, H., Michel, F. B., and Bousquet, J., Systemic reactions occurring during immunotherapy with standardized pollen extracts, *J. Allergy Clin. Immunol.*, *89*, 925 (1992).
153. Bousquet, J., Hejjaoui, A., Dhivert, H., Clauzel, A. M., and Michel, F. B., Specific immunotherapy with a standardized *Dermatophagoides pteronyssinus* extract. III. Systemic reactions during the rush protocol in patients suffering from asthma, *J. Allergy Clin. Immunol.*, *83*, 797 (1989).
154. Stewart, G. E., and Lockey, R. F., Systemic reactions from allergen immunotherapy, *J. Allergy Clin. Immunol.*, *90*, 567 (1992).
155. Malling, H.-J., Dreborg, S., and Weeke, B., Diagnosis and immunotherapy of mould allergy. V. Clinical efficacy and side effects of immunotherapy with *Cladosporium herbarum*, *Allergy*, *41*, 507 (1986).
156. Hejjaoui, A., Dhivert, H., Michel, F. B, and Bousquet, J., Specific immunotherapy with a standardized *Dermatophagoides pteronyssinus* extract. IV. Systemic reactions according to the immuno-therapy schedule, *J. Allergy Clin. Immunol.*, *85*, 473 (1990).
157. Horst, M., Hejjaoui, A., Horst, V., Michel, F. B., and Bousquet, J., Double-blind placebo-controlled rush immunotherapy with a standardized Alternaria extract, *J. Allergy Clin. Immunol.*, *85*, 460 (1991).
158. Turkeltaub, P. S., and Baer, H., The importance of patient skin sensitivity in evaluating dose-dependent adverse reactions during immunotherapy, *J. Allergy Clin. Immunol.*, *75*, 163 (1985).
159. Marsh, D. J., Goodfriend, L., King, T. P., Lowenstein, H., and Platts-Mills, T. A. E., Allergen nomenclature, *J. Allergy Clin. Immunol.*, *80*, 639 (1987).

3

Use of the Skin Blister Model and Intradermal Testing to Explore the Pathogenesis and Pharmacological Control of Cutaneous Allergic Inflammation

William A. Massey and Lawrence M. Lichtenstein

The Johns Hopkins University School of Medicine
Baltimore, Maryland

I. INTRODUCTION

We have explored the pathogenesis of allergic inflammation using in vivo provocation models in the nose, lung, and skin of humans [1–3]. In the skin, two techniques, intradermal skin testing and antigen challenge of skin blisters, were adopted and developed. In this review, studies to examine a number of hypotheses will be discussed, and a detailed description of the basic methods employed will be given.

II. METHODS

A. Subject Selection and Determination of the Optimal Challenge Dose

All study protocols were approved by the Johns Hopkins Institutional Review Committee, and all subjects gave written informed consent. Subjects were healthy adults with allergic rhinitis and/or asthma, between 18 and 50 years of age, who were not taking medications or receiving immunotherapy. They were skin-tested with 0.03 ml ragweed or mixed grass (timothy + orchard) extract in saline diluent with 0.03% human serum albumin and 0.4% phenol in concentrations ranging from 0.1 to 1000 protein nitrogen units (PNU)/ml or, more recently, allergen units (AU). In each subject the concentration of antigen extract used as the optimal challenge dose (OCD) was defined as the concentration of antigen that gave a weal diameter ⩾ 15 mm (or 10 mm with pseudopods) at 15 minutes and an induration diameter ⩾ 30 mm at 8 h during the late-phase reaction (LPR).

B. Skin Blister–Chamber Study

In all but the initial studies, skin blisters were created 14 to 20 h before challenge on the anterior forearm using gentle heat and suction (40°C, 300 mm Hg for 45–60 min) until a complete 1 cm diameter blister was formed. Immediately before challenge, the blisters were unroofed (epidermis was removed), and sterile aluminum chambers with entry and exit ports were aseptically attached. The blister bases were washed by the instillation and removal of two 500-μl aliquots of Ringer's lactate solution. Antigen extract (500 μl) at a concentration ten times that of the OCD (or 1000 PNU/ml for nonallergic subjects), or vehicle control solution, was introduced into separate blister sites. The contents of the chamber were removed hourly during the subsequent 12-h period and replaced each time with a fresh aliquot of buffer consisting of Ringer's lactate with 30 U/ml heparin. The heparin was added to inhibit the formation of a fibrin clot over the denuded dermis. Such clots obstruct the movement of cells into the blister fluid. All subjects were challenged with the same stock solutions of antigen extract. After removal from the chamber, samples were immediately centrifuged to pellet cells, and supernatants were harvested and saved for mediator analysis (stored at −70°C until analyzed). Cell pellets were resuspended in Ringer's lactate buffer and were counted manually using a hemocytometer. After cytocentrifugation, differential counting was performed using a modified Wright-Giemsa stain, and basophil counts were performed by alcian blue staining, as previously described [3].

C. Extracts

Standardized concentrated extracts of ragweed and mixed grass timothy + orchard) in saline with 0.03% human serum albumin and 0.4% phenol were purchased in sufficient quantity to complete all parts of any particular study and stored in 0.5 ml aliquots at −80°C. These stock solutions were diluted in challenge buffer immediately before use. Each lot selected was purchased in sufficient quantity to complete all parts of any particular study.

D. Skin Testing

Simultaneously with the introduction of antigen into the skin chamber, each subject was skin-tested with 0.03 ml of ragweed or mixed grass extract at the concentration that had previously been determined to cause a 4+ reaction followed by a cutaneous LPR. The skin test was placed on the upper arm that was being challenged simultaneously with placement of antigen in the chamber. The erythema and induration at skin test sites was determined by direct inspection and palpation of the skin. An outline of the border of the indurated area was drawn on the skin. Transparent tape was then placed over the lesion and the outline copied onto the tape. This tape, in turn, was placed on white paper, labeled, and placed in the permanent experimental records. For each skin test outline, the long axis and short axis were measured and averaged, and this composite diameter was used to calculate the area of the late-phase erythema and induration.

E. Mediator Assays

Assays for histamine, prostaglandin D_2 (PGD_2), and leukotriene C_4 (LTC_4) have been previously described [3]. In brief, cell-free blister fluid for the histamine assay was frozen immediately after collection and stored at −70°C. Histamine concentrations were determined using a radioenzymatic assay (REA) with a sensitivity of 0.05 ng/ml. The assay is based on the conversion of histamine to ^3H-methylhistamine in the presence of histamine-*N*-methyltransferase and (^3H)-*S*-adenosyl-L-methionine [4]. For measurement of PGD_2, 400 μl of blister fluid, precipitated in 1.6 ml of high-performance liquid chromatography (HPLC)-grade ethyl alcohol, was centrifuged at 5000 rpm for 5 min. The prostanoid-containing supernatants, stored at −70°C until assayed, were transferred to separate tubes and placed in a vacuum-centrifuge until dry and then rehydrated with RIA buffer. A competitive radioimmunoassay (RIA) with a sensitivity of 40 pg/ml, described previously, was then used for the PGD_2 measurements [3]. The identity of the prostanoid measured by the RIA as PGD_2 was confirmed previously by negative-ion gas chromatographic mass spectrophotometry [3,5].

III. RESULTS AND DISCUSSION

The use of the skin blister model for exploring allergic inflammation was pioneered by Drs. Zweiman and Atkins [6,7]. They taught our group their techniques, which we subsequently modified and extended.

Examination of antigen-challenged blisters was first used by our group to determine whether a histamine-releasing factor (HRF) was present in the late-phase inflammatory site [8]. Earlier work in the nose suggested that late-phase histamine release originated in newly arrived basophils [1]. Therefore, it was hypothesized that late-phase reactions in the skin might contain an HRF. Studies were performed in which blister fluid was collected 30 min and 8 h after antigen-E–vs.–buffer challenge of blister bases. In six of nine sensitive subjects challenged with antigen-E, late-phase blister fluids contained an activity that induced greater than 20% histamine release from basophils of multiple donors. Fluids from antigen-E–challenged blister bases collected at 30 min did not contain HRF activity, and fluid from buffer-challenged blister sites at 30 min or 8 h did not have HRF activity. Control experiments with antisera to antigen-E demonstrated that the HRF activity in the blister fluids was not due to retained antigen-E. Further characterization of the HRF activity demonstrated that the activity could be diluted, was synergistic with antigenic stimulation of basophils, was noncytotoxic, was temperature- and Ca^{2+}-dependent, cross-desensitized with anti-IgE, was not active on isolated pulmonary mast cells, and was immunoglobulin E (IgE)-dependent. It was concluded that late-phase allergic reactions in the skin are coincident with the appearance of an IgE-dependent HRF. The identity of this skin-derived IgE-dependent HRF is still unknown. Work in the area of HRFs was recently reviewed by Dr. Susan MacDonald [9].

The skin blister model was next used in a series of studies to describe the presence and kinetics of local mediator release following local antigen stimulation. The goal was to evaluate the determinants of the cutaneous late-phase erythema and induration. It was hypothesized that late-phase size might be determined by late-phase histamine release and the release of newly generated inflammatory lipids. In an early study Pienkowski et al. used a heat suction device to form blisters and sampled directly from the formed blister by needle aspiration [10]. It was demonstrated that blister formation itself led to levels of histamine and PGD_2 comparable to those seen with antigen challenge. Elevated levels of histamine and PGD_2 were seen after blister induction at 30 min and 8.5 h but had returned to baseline by 14 h. Consequently, in this early study, the time interval between blister induction and challenge was greater than 14 h. In most, but not all, subsequent studies a delay of $>$ 14 h between blister formation and antigen challenge was included in the protocols. Also, in these studies by Pienkowski et al., the antigen was injected intracutaneously, directly under the blister base. Subsequent sampling at 0.5, 2.5, 5.5, 8.5 and 24 h was done by tracking a needle under the skin into the blister space and aspirating the blister volume (approximately 0.1 ml).

The subjects were divided into three groups. Group A was nonatopic and had no reactivity to intradermal ragweed. Group B was atopic but had no LPR despite having an immediate response to ragweed. Group C was atopic and had early reactions identical to those of group B but also had late erythema and induration of more than 1 cm in diameter. As expected, the nonatopic group did not release detectable histamine or PGD_2 following antigen challenge with 1000 PNU/ml ragweed solution. The subjects with positive immediate response and negative LPR released less histamine and PGD_2 than subjects who went on to have a positive LPR. In both atopic groups histamine release peaked at 30 min, while PGD_2 release peaked at 2.5 h. In addition, the size of the LPR, in group C, correlated with the peak PGD_2 concentration and with the concentration of histamine at 30 min. From these studies it was concluded that the atopic groups released histamine and PGD_2 into the blister fluids in an antigen-specific manner that was not caused by irritants or contaminants in the antigen solution. It was also noted that the kinetics of PGD_2 release in the skin and nose appeared to be different: Nasal challenge with antigen caused almost simultaneous and immediate histamine and PGD_2 release (much as in experiments with lung mast cells in vitro), while in the skin, PGD_2 release peaked several hours following the initial histamine peak. The correlation of the histamine and PGD_2 peaks with the LPR size suggested that the magnitude of mast cell stimulation might determine the magnitude of the LPR.

Further study of antigen-challenged skin sites was undertaken to examine the kinetic relationship of the mediators released to the physiologic changes of erythema and induration. In these studies by Reshef et al., blisters were formed and were unroofed, and metal chambers with entry and exit ports were placed over the denuded dermis [11]. After washing the blister bases with saline, ragweed and grass antigen solutions at concentrations 10 and 100 times the concentration of the OCD were placed in the chambers. The subsequent release of histamine, PGD_2, and LTC_4 was followed hourly, as was the size of the erythema and induration at the blister site. A simultaneous intradermal skin test with comparable antigen solution at a concentration of 10 to 100 times the OCD was also performed. These studies allowed a more detailed kinetic analysis of the antigen-induced mediator release from the denuded dermis. Histamine release was rapid, with peak levels of 20.6 ± 2.3 ng/ml (mean $\pm$ SEM; $n = 27$) reached during the first hour at antigen-challenged sites and an average release of less than 1 ng/ml at control buffer-challenged sites. At the antigen-challenged sites, though histamine levels declined steadily over the next 8 h to approximately 20% of maximum, there was still, overall, significantly more histamine than at the control sites during the later hours. In five patients chambers were kept in place undisturbed from hour 8 to hour 24. When the fluid was removed from the antigen-challenged sites, histamine levels averaged 77 ± 32 ng/ml, whereas control levels averaged 1 ± 2 ng/ml. This persistent histamine release at the antigen-challenged site resembled the second wave of histamine release previously seen in the nasal model, but with more delayed kinetics.

Release of PGD_2 at antigen-challenged sites was significantly greater than at control buffer-challenged sites, with adjusted (postchallenge–prechallenge) peak levels at hour 5 of 40 ± 17 pg/0.1 ml vs. 0.5 ± 7 pg/0.1 ml at control sites. Once again, the kinetics of the antigen-induced histamine and PGD_2 appearance were clearly different. A broad plateau of LTC_4 appearance was seen at both the antigen-challenged and the buffer-challenged sites between hours 1 to 8. At hours 4, 5, and 6 the concentration of LTC_4 at the antigen-challenged sites was greater than at the control sites. These studies demonstrated that antigen challenge of the skin induced significant immediate and delayed histamine appearance, PGD_2 appearance some hours after maximal histamine release, and a broad low level of LTC_4 appearance over many hours. No direct correlation was seen between the levels of histamine or PGD_2 and the size of the LPR. This was in contrast to the earlier study with intact blisters.

The study by Reshef et al. suggested that histamine release might occur many hours after antigen-challenge in the skin. In addition, the study by Warner et al. demonstrated that an HRF for basophils was present at antigen-challenged sites many hours after antigen had disappeared from the blister. Therefore, a 12-h antigen-challenge study was performed to examine blister fluid for mediator content while simultaneously monitoring the fluid and the underlying dermis for the kinetics and differential of cellular influx [3]. In this study by Charlesworth et al., the blisters were formed 14 to 20 h before unroofing, and the subsequent antigen challenge was for 1 h. Biopsy of antigen- and buffer-challenged blister bases at 8 h demonstrated a sixfold increase in the number of eosinophils at the antigen site as compared with the control site ($p < 0.001$), and a 14-fold increase in the number of basophils and basophil-like cells ($p < 0.01$), a twofold increase in neutrophils ($p < 0.01$), and a 1.4-fold increase in mononuclear cells ($p < 0.03$) [3]. Similar changes were seen in the cells collected hourly in the supernatants overlying the blisters. The number of eosinophils found at the antigen site was 35 times greater than at the buffer site ($p < 0.03$), though the eosinophil totals at antigen sites were only an average of 30% of the totals of neutrophils. Similarly, the basophils at antigen sites were 20 times more numerous than at the buffer sites ($p < 0.03$), though basophils made up less than 10% of the total cell counts at the antigen sites. The number of neutrophils that influxed into the antigen sites was two to three times greater than at the buffer sites ($p < 0.01$), while the number of mononuclear cells was only 1.4 times greater at antigen vs. control sites. Thus, both the biopsy specimens and overlying fluid from antigen-challenged blister sites demonstrated a remarkable preferential recruitment of eosinophils and basophils. An example of cell counts from antigen versus buffer challenge of skin chambers from a later study is given in Figure 1 [12].

The mediators histamine and PGD_2 were measured in supernatants collected hourly. Histamine release peaked within the first hour of antigen exposure and fell to near baseline over the next 6 h, as in previous studies. However, histamine levels rose steadily in hours 8–12, and this was coincident with the basophil influx at the antigen site [3]. Release of PGD_2 was maximal in a broad peak from hour 1 to hour 4, and then levels declined slowly to baseline over hours 5–12. As basophils do not release significant PGD_2 during stimulation, whereas cutaneous mast cells do, these data were interpreted as strong evidence that the histamine measured in hours 8–12 was basophil- rather than mast cell–derived.

The number of basophils appearing in the blister site supernatant at antigen sites during the late phase correlated with the rise in late-phase histamine ($r = 0.81, p < 0.05$) [3]. While this surprisingly tight correlation has not held up in subsequent studies, the arrival of significant numbers of basophils during the time of the late phase is a consistent and reproducible finding. The study also demonstrated that histamine was released later than in the nasal antigen-challenge model. As in previous skin studies, the pattern of PGD_2 release followed different

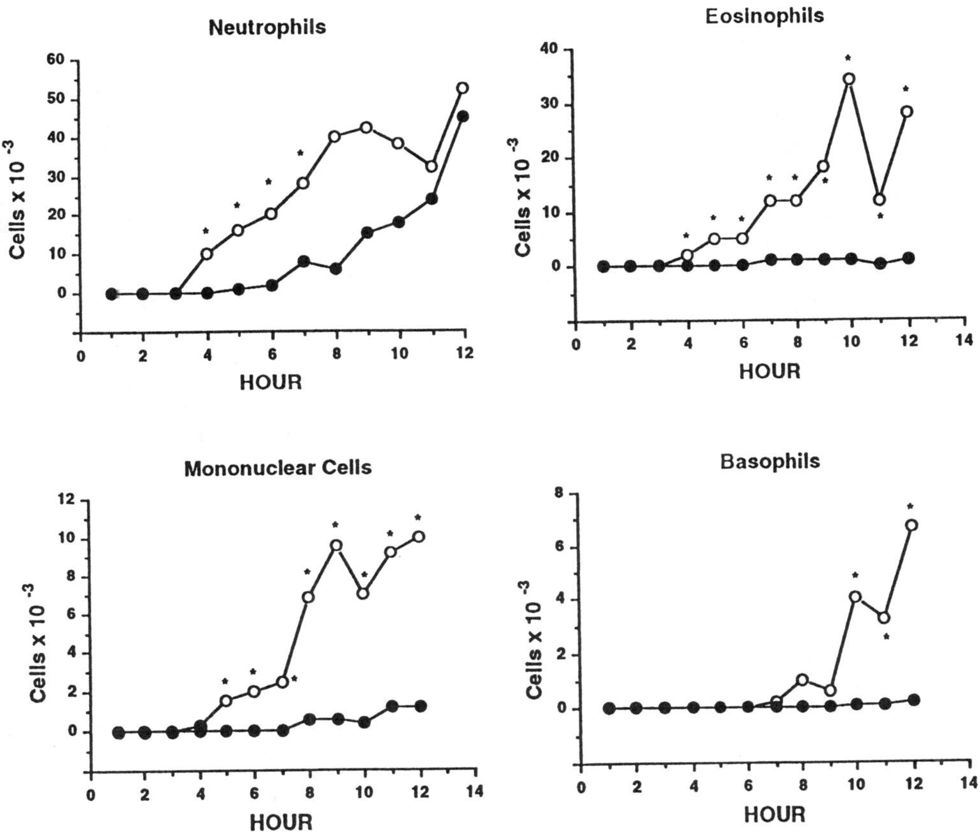

Figure 1 Cells in blister chamber following antigen challenge. Hourly levels of the absolute number of leukocytes in skin-chamber fluids after challenge of atopic subjects with ragweed (○) or control diluent (●). Values presented are the median values from results with eight subjects; $*p < 0.05$ comparing antigen with control values. (From Ref. 12.)

kinetics from those of histamine release, essentially being much more delayed and prolonged. However, the critical finding that PGD_2 levels were falling at the time of late histamine release and basophil influx was similar to the findings in the nasal model. The remarkable preferential arrival of basophils and eosinophils in the site of antigen challenge during the time of the late phase suggested that these cells may participate in the pathogenesis of the reaction. This finding supported the hypothesis that basophil arrival and mediator release may contribute to the late erythema and induration seen many hours after antigen challenge in the skin.

Preliminary work done by Charlesworth et al. suggested that the PGD_2

measured by RIA was indeed authentic as measured by gas chromatography–mass spectrometry (GC-MS) [3]. Therefore, a larger study to examine the levels of PGD_2 with the two different techniques was initiated in order to confirm that the PGD_2 measured by RIA was authentic [5]. Secondary goals of the study were to determine the presence of other potentially relevant prostanoids following antigen challenge. Radioimmunoassay was compared with GC-MS analysis of the prostanoid content of blister fluid in a study with 6 subjects. As GC-MS analysis allowed for simultaneous measurement of a panel of prostanoids, a number of these were also examined, including the biologically active PGD_2 metabolite $9\alpha,11\beta$-PGF_2, $PGE_{2\alpha}$, $PGF_{2\alpha}$, thromboxane B_2, and the prostacyclin metabolite 6κ-$PGF_{1\alpha}$. The RIA and GC-MS analysis of supernatants collected hourly from antigen- and buffer-challenged blister sites demonstrated almost identical quantities of PGD_2 and similar kinetics of appearance. By both techniques peak levels were seen at hour 3 after challenge and decreased steadily to near baseline by hour 8. By GC-MS analysis, levels of the PGD_2 metabolite $9\alpha,11\beta$-PGF_2 were elevated in three of the six subjects and demonstrated kinetics similar to those of PGD_2. Levels of the prostacyclin metabolite 6κ-$PGF_{1\alpha}$ were also significantly elevated, and total 6κ-$PGF_{1\alpha}$ correlated with total histamine release. The parent compound of 6κ-$PGF_{1\alpha}$, prostacyclin (PGI_2), has a number of proinflammatory effects on the vascular endothelium.

More recently, in pursuit of soluble factors that might be critical to the cellular recruitment, activation, and priming seen in late-phase inflammation, studies were conducted to determine whether specific cytokines hypothesized to have a role in allergic inflammation appeared after antigen challenge. As discussed above, earlier studies suggested that a soluble HRF was present in blister fluid from antigen-challenged sites during the time of the LPR. Using the blister model, Bochner et al. examined a group of antigen-challenged atopic subjects for interleukin-1α (IL-1α), IL-1β, and tumor necrosis factor-α (TNFα) [12]. These cytokines were chosen because they are strong activators of the vascular endothelium for increased adhesiveness for circulating leukocytes, a critical event in cellular recruitment. Interleukin-1 bioactivity was found in blister fluids 10–12 h after antigen challenge but not at control sites ($p < 0.05$) (Fig. 2). Interleukin-1β, measured by RIA, was found to peak at hour 1 and again in hours 8–12 ($p < 0.04$). As a control, nonatopic subjects were challenged with high doses of the ragweed antigen solution, and no IL-1 bioactivity or immunoactivity was detected. In addition, the bioactivity found during the LPR in atopic subjects was more than 90% neutralized by antisera to IL-1β. No TNF bioactivity was found. Interleukin-1β is a known inducer of the adhesion molecule E-selectin in cultured human endothelial cells [13]. Previous in vitro studies demonstrated that cultured human vascular endothelial cells acquired increased adhesiveness for neutrophils, eosinophils, and basophils after IL-1β pretreatment [13]. This study extended these previous observations and supported a role for IL-1β in cutaneous late-phase

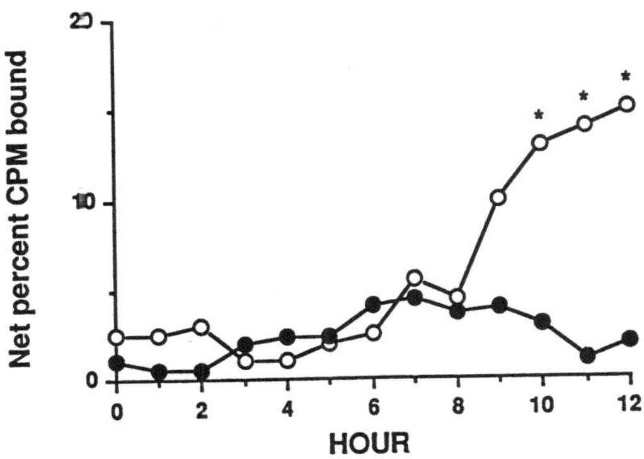

Figure 2 Interleukin-1 (IL-1) bioactivity following antigen challenge. Hourly levels of IL-1 bioactivity in skin-chamber fluids after challenge of atopic subjects with ragweed (○) or control diluent (●). Interleukin-1 bioactivity was determined with the endothelial cell–neutrophil adherence assay, as previously described [27]. Values presented are the median values from results with eight subjects, and ranges for ragweed versus diluent at hours 1, 11, and 12 were 0–13 vs. 1–13, 2–23 vs. 0–18, and 4–24 vs. 0–22 net percent counts per minute (CPM) bound, respectively; $*p < 0.05$ compared with values for ragweed challenge sites at T = 0; comparing antigen with control values for IL-1 bioactivity at hours 10–12, $p < 0.06$; values for ragweed-challenge solution alone, 2 net percent CPM bound; for Ringer's lactate with heparin, 0 net percent CPM; for 1 μg/ml of lipopolysaccharide, 19 net percent CPM. (From Ref. 12.)

reactions. Indeed, biopsy studies have demonstrated upregulation of E-selectin in the microvasculature of cutaneous LPR [14].

A subsequent study was undertaken to determine whether IL-3 and granulocyte-macrophage colony-stimulating factor (GM-CSF), cytokines that promote eosinophil survival and activate and/or prime eosinophils and basophils for proinflammatory activities, were present at antigen-challenged sites during the time of preferential eosinophil and basophil accumulation. The activity of IL-3 and GM-CSF was assayed by bioactivity and ELISA. In addition, experiments were later performed to determine whether IL-5 was present as assayed by ELISA. With an indicator cell line that proliferated to both IL-3 and GM-CSF used as the bioassay, blister fluid from atopic subjects collected over a period of 12 h following antigen and buffer challenge were examined. Activity of IL-3 and GM-CSF began to rise at 4 h, reached a peak at 7 h that was significantly elevated above buffer-control site supernatants ($p < 0.02$), and declined thereafter [15]. Similar antigen challenge of nonatopics revealed no bioactivity (n = 5, p = NS), indicating that the cytokine appearance in the atopic subjects was a specific effect of the allergen solution. Use of neutralizing antisera on hour-4 to -12 pools of late-phase fluids established that the majority of the activity was of GM-CSF. Assay by ELISA of pooled fluids from hour-5 to -10 supernatants confirmed significantly elevated levels of GM-CSF at antigen-challenged as compared with buffer-challenged sites ($p < 0.03$), but IL-3 was not detected (Fig. 3). The concentration of GM-CSF found by both bioassay and immunoassay from fluids overlying antigen-challenged sites during the time of the LPR was several times greater than the 2 to 4 pg/ml required for half-maximal enhancement of eosinophil survival in vitro. In three experiments, fluids from antigen-challenged sites during hours 4–12 were pooled and found to contain no detectable IL-5 by ELISA, with a limit of detection of 10–100 pg/ml (unpublished observation). In contrast to our studies, in which GM-CSF predominates, numerous biopsy studies performed by other groups investigating cutaneous, nasal, and pulmonary antigen-induced late-phase reactions have demonstrated mRNA for IL-3, GM-CSF, and IL-5 [16–20]. The reason for the discrepancy in cytokine mRNA and soluble protein measurements in the skin is unknown. The skin blister model is also an appropriate tool for investigat-

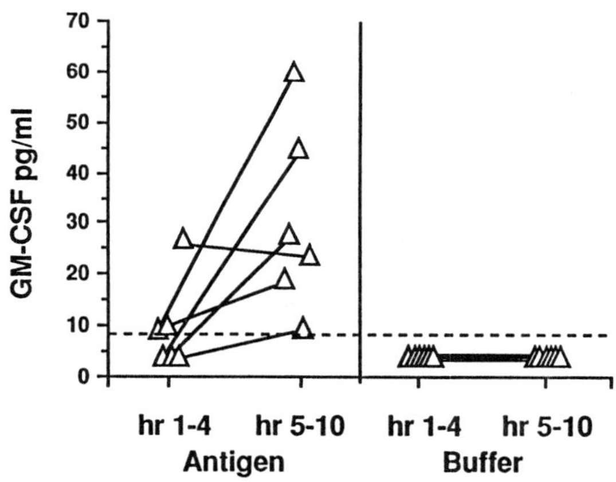

Figure 3 Cytokine levels in concentrated blister fluids measured by ELISA. Antigen-challenged and vehicle control–challenged skin blister site fluid containing no heparin was collected hourly for 10 h. The fluid from hours 1–4 and 4–10 was combined into pools for each subject, (n = 6) concentrated 2.5×, dialyzed, and tested in the granulocyte-macrophage colony-stimulating factor (GM-CSF) ELISA. The concentration of GM-CSF in the 2.5× fluid is indicated on the vertical axis. Granulocyte-macrophage colony-stimulating factor was statistically significantly elevated at the hour 5–10 antigen-challenged site (median 26 pg/ml and range 9–60 pg/ml GM-CSF) compared with the vehicle-challenged site (median < 7.8 pg/ml, and all samples were < 7.8 pg/ml GM-CSF; antigen vs. control $p < 0.03$, n = 6). In a similar assay of interleukin-3 (IL-3) immunoreactivity, the fluids from the six subjects were found to contain no detectable IL-3 (limit of detection 16 pg/ml) at either antigen or control blister sites. (From Ref. 15.)

ing the kinetics of soluble-chemokine production. A recent paper by Gallin's group found elevated levels of IL-8 following plasma-zymosan–induced inflammation at a blister site [21]. In all these studies the critical role of any particular cytokine in the pathogenesis of the LPR is not proved, since in general, specific antagonists are not available for use in humans. However, the demonstration of particular cytokines at these sites of late antigen-induced inflammation is supportive of hypotheses that include these cytokines in key mechanistic roles.

The pharmacological agents used to treat allergic diseases have been examined in cutaneous models of the late-phase reaction. These studies have provided valuable insights into possible mechanisms by which medications, such as prednisone and antihistamines, exert antiallergic effects. Using the skin blister model, our group examined the effects of systemic steroids on early- and late-phase reactions in the skin.

The effect of systemic prednisone therapy on the early- and late-phase skin test size, release of the mediators histamine, PGD_2, and LTC_4, and the influx of leukocytes following antigen challenge was examined [22]. This information was collected from nine subjects enrolled in a double-blind, placebo-controlled, crossover study in which the patients received either 30 mg of prednisone or placebo p.o. twice a day for 3 days. Systemic steroids significantly inhibited the size of the intradermal antigen-induced late-phase skin test area, by as much as 50%, with little effect on the early skin test response ($p < 0.02$, hour 8) (Fig. 4). The effects of steroid pretreatment on histamine release at antigen- vs. buffer-challenged blister sites was also examined by assay of chamber fluid. The immediate histamine release in response to antigen was not affected by the steroid pretreatment. However, the concentration of histamine at antigen sites at hours 10–12 was significantly reduced by prednisone pretreatment from a median of 3.73 to 0.22 ng/ml ($p < 0.02$). Similar results were previously obtained in the nasal model [23]. This study demonstrated that the inhibition of the cutaneous LPR size by prednisone was coincident with a decrease in late-phase mediator release.

The influence of systemic prednisone pretreatment on the antigen-induced arrival of granulocytes during the later hours following challenge was selective for cell type. The influx of eosinophils in hours 6–12 at antigen-challenged sites was essentially abolished by the prednisone pretreatment ($p < 0.02$). The influx of basophils in hours 9–12 into the antigen-challenged site supernatants was also significantly inhibited ($p < 0.02$). The influx of neutrophils, under identical conditions, was not inhibited by the prednisone pretreatment (Fig. 5). It was concluded that the effect of prednisone in selectively inhibiting eosinophil and basophil movement into sites of antigen-induced inflammation might contribute to the clinical suppression of the cutaneous LPR.

The effects of both new nonsedating and older antihistamines on cutaneous allergic reactions were also examined and compared in this model system. In a

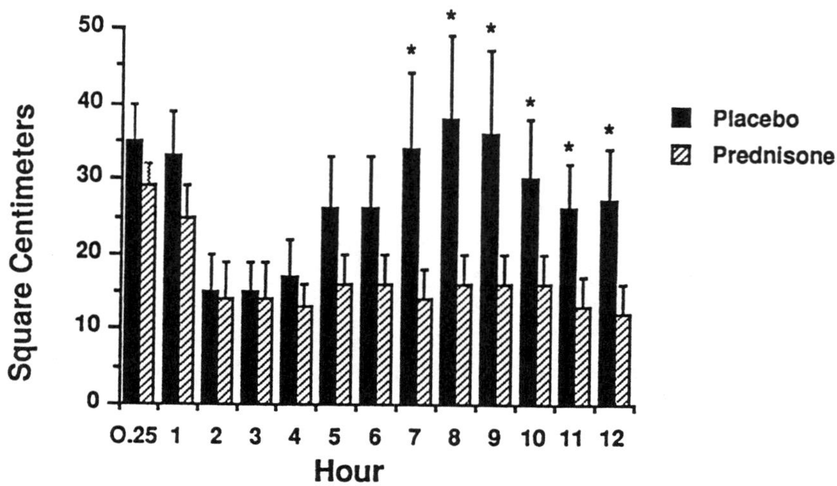

Figure 4 Effect of prednisone on skin test size. Skin test erythema in response to cutaneous ragweed antigen challenge with their optimal challenge dose, in nine allergic subjects receiving placebo or prednisone. The mean ± SEM is shown for all times; $*p < 0.04$. (From Ref. 22.)

series of four separate studies, the new nonsedating antihistamines terfenadine and cetirizine, as well as the older antihistamines promethazine and chlorpheniramine, were given to groups of 10 subjects in a randomized, double-blind, placebo-controlled, crossover fashion [24,25].

As expected, oral terfenadine 60 mg b.i.d. inhibited the initial antigen-induced flare at 15 min by 60%. Over the next 12 h the inhibition of erythema and induration slowly decreased, so that by hour 12 the inhibition was approximately 30%. The area of the antigen-induced erythema and induration over 12 h was significantly different, by analysis of variance, for terfenadine vs. placebo. There was a significant difference between drug and placebo treatment as analyzed by a two-tailed paired *t*-test at every hour from hour 1 to hour 9 ($p < 0.01$, hour 9) [24]. Thus, the inhibition by terfenadine of the cutaneous response to antigen extended well into the period of the LPR. The release of histamine and PGD_2 into blister fluids at antigen-challenged sites was unaffected by terfenadine pretreatment. No significant effect of terfenadine on granulocyte influx was found.

In previous studies we examined the effects of other antihistamines on cutaneous inflammation, using skin testing and antigen challenge of blister bases [25]. Like terfenadine, cetirizine, at usual clinical doses, significantly inhibited the initial antigen-induced flare area by approximately 60% (Fig. 6). The subsequent inhibition of erythema and induration over the next 12 h slowly decreased but was

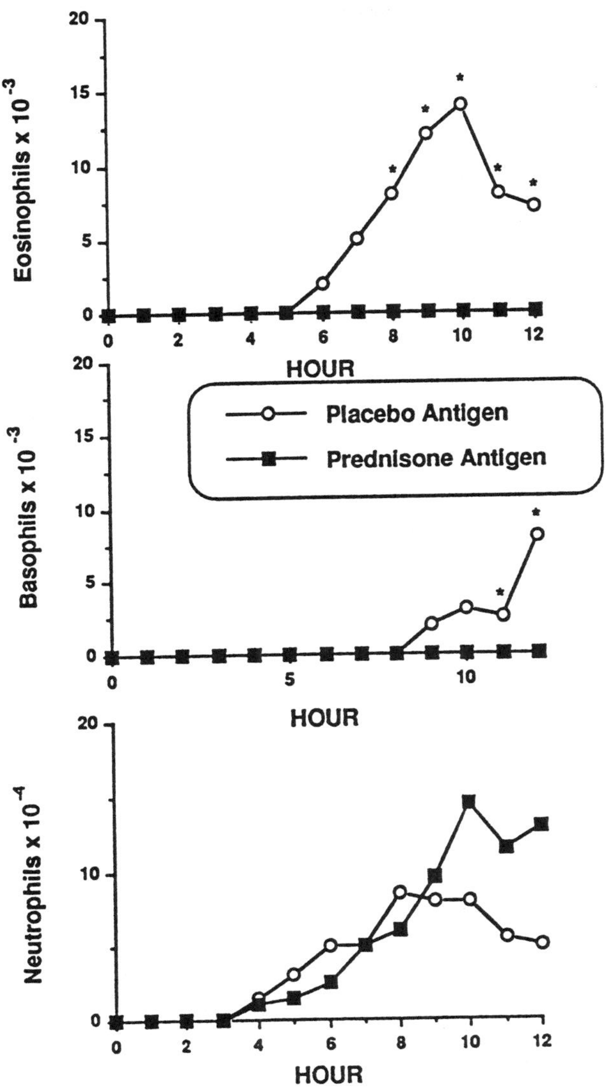

Figure 5 Effect of prednisone on cell migration. The effect of prednisone pretreatment on the median hourly cellular migration into skin chambers in response to antigen challenge with 10 times the optimal challenge dose of antigen in the chambers. No cells were found until 4–6 h. Thereafter, eosinophils and basophils increased specifically in response to the antigen; neutrophils entered under all conditions. The influx of eosinophils and basophils, but not that of neutrophils, was ablated by prednisone pretreatment. Because of very low numbers, only the placebo–antigen curve is visible for eosinophils and basophils. The cell counts at buffer-treated chamber sites is not shown; $*p < 0.05$, n = 9. (From Ref. 22.)

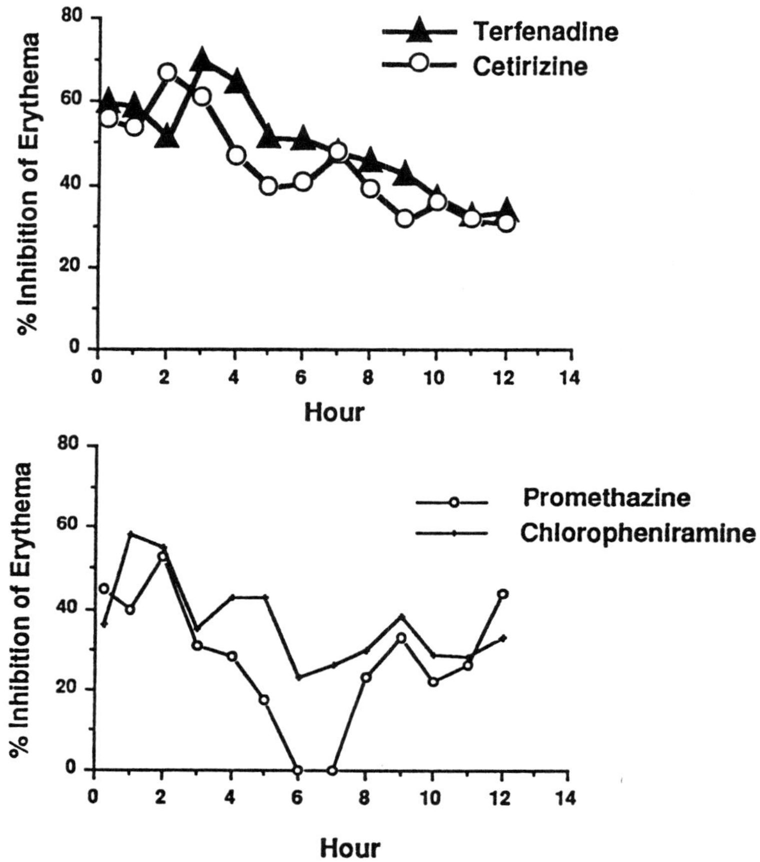

Figure 6 Comparison of the effects of four antihistamines on the skin test response. The skin test reaction area, measured in square millimeters, was used to calculate the percent inhibition using the formula (1 − [area placebo − area antihistamine]/area placebo) × 100. In the top frame the percent inhibition by terfenadine (closed triangles) is compared with that of cetirizine (open circles). Both of these newer antihistamines inhibited approximately 60% of the initial antigen-induced flare area. The subsequent inhibition of erythema and induration over the next 12 h slowly decreased but in each case was still approximately 30% 12 h later. The overall inhibition by promethazine and chlorpheniramine was generally less than that seen with terfenadine and cetirizine and is shown in the second panel. However, a similar pattern of inhibition over many hours can be seen. (From Refs. 24 and 25.)

still approximately 30% 12 h later [25]. The overall inhibition by promethazine and chlorpheniramine of the initial flare was generally less than that seen with terfenadine, but the inhibition was significantly greater than that with placebo over the first 4 h. In the subsequent hours a nonsignificant pattern of inhibition was seen. The mechanism for this inhibition of late-phase erythema and induration is unclear.

Cetirizine, but not the other antihistamines, significantly decreased the late leukocyte migration into antigen-challenged chambers: eosinophils by 68% ($p < 0.04$), basophils by 64% ($p < 0.04$), and neutrophils by 72% ($p < 0.04$) [25]. In addition, none of the antihistamines significantly affected histamine release at antigen-challenged skin test sites. This was surprising, because studies from our nasal antigen challenge model have demonstrated that terfenadine inhibits antigen-induced histamine release from the nasal mucosa [26].

From the antihistamine studies it was concluded that terfenadine may have organ-specific activity on mast cell mediator release. Cetirizine appears to inhibit granulocyte influx to allergen-challenged blister sites. Future studies of newly developed mediator antagonists and novel anti-inflammatory agents, using various models of the late-phase reaction, should help to better define the events underlying chronic allergic inflammation in humans.

In summary, combining antigen challenge of skin blister sites with more traditional intradermal antigen testing and biopsy is a useful method for investigating allergic inflammation. The model allows for simultaneous observation of mediators, cells, and physiologic end points. Mechanisms by which traditional and new antiallergy medication interfere with mediator release, cellular trafficking, and the physiologic end points of erythema and induration can also be examined with this model.

ACKNOWLEDGMENTS

The research discussed in this chapter was supported in part by grants from Marion Merrell Dow, Glaxo, and Pfizer pharmaceutical companies and by NIH grants AI 08270, AI 07290, AR 31891, AI 21036, and AM 31891.

REFERENCES

1. Naclerio, R. M., Proud, D., Togias, A. G., Adkinson, N. F., Jr., Meyers, D. A., Kagey-Sobotka, A., et al., Inflammatory mediators in late antigen-induced rhinitis, *N. Engl. J. Med.*, *313*, 65–70 (1985).
2. Liu, M. C., Hubbard, W. C., Proud, D., Stealey, B., Galli, S., Kagey-Sobotka, A., et al., Immediate and late inflammatory responses to ragweed antigen challenge of the peripheral airways in asthmatics: cellular, mediator, and permeability changes. *Am. Rev. Respir. Dis.*, *144*, 51–58 (1991).

3. Charlesworth, E. N., Hood, A. F., Soter, N. A., Kagey-Sobotka, A., Norman, P. S., and Lichtenstein, L. M., Cutaneous late-phase response to allergen. Mediator release and inflammatory cell infiltration, *J. Clin. Invest.*, *83*, 1519–1526 (1989).
4. Brown, M. J., Ind, P. W., Causon, R., and Lee, T. H., A novel double-isotope technique for the enzymatic assay of plasma histamine: application to estimation of mast cell activation assessed by antigen challenge in asthmatics, *J. Allergy Clin. Immunol.*, *69*, 20–24 (1982).
5. Massey, W. A., Hubbard, W. C., Liu, M. C., Kagey-Sobotka, A., and Lichtenstein, L. M., Profile of prostanoid release following antigen challenge in vivo in the skin of man, *Br. J. Dermatol.*, *125*, 529–534 (1991).
6. Dunsky, E. H., and Zweiman, B., The direct demonstration of histamine release in the skin using a skin chamber technique, *J. Allergy Clin. Immunol.*, *62*, 127–130 (1978).
7. Bedard, P.-M., Atkins, P. C., and Zweiman, B., Antigen-induced local mediator release and cellular inflammatory responses in atopic subjects, *J. Allergy Clin. Immunol.*, *71*, 394–398 (1983).
8. Warner, J. A., Pienkowski, M. M., Plaut, M., Norman, P. S., and Lichtenstein, L. M., Identification of a histamine releasing factor(s) in the late phase of cutaneous IgE-mediated reactions, *J. Immunol.*, *136*, 2583–2587 (1986).
9. MacDonald, S. M., Histamine releasing factors and IgE heterogeneity, in *Allergy Principles and Practice*, (4th ed.) Mosby-Year Book, Inc., St. Louis, 1993.
10. Pienkowski, M. M., Adkinson, N. F. Jr., Plaut, M., Norman, P. S., and Lichtenstein, L. M., Prostaglandin D2 and histamine during the immediate and the late-phase components of allergic cutaneous responses, *J. Allergy Clin. Immunol.*, *82*, 95–100 (1988).
11. Reshef, A., Kagey-Sobotka, A., Adkinson, N. F., Lichtenstein, L. M., and Norman, P. S., The pattern and kinetics in human skin of erythema and mediators during the acute and late-phase response (LPR), *J. Allergy Clin. Immunol.*, *84*, 678–687 (1989).
12. Bochner, B. S., Charlesworth, E. N., Lichtenstein, L. M., Derse, C. P., Gillis, S., Dinarello, C. A., et al., Interleukin-1 is released at sites of human cutaneous allergic reactions, *J. Allergy Clin. Immunol.*, *86*, 830–389 (1990).
13. Bochner, B. S., Luscinskas, F. W., Gimbrone, M. A., Newman, W., Sterbinsky, S. A., Derse-Anthony, C., et al., Adhesion of human basophils, eosinophils, and neutrophils to IL-1–activated human vascular endothelial cells: contribution of endothelial cell adhesion molecules, *J. Exp. Med.*, *173*, 1553–1558 (1991).
14. Leung, D. Y. M., Pober, J. S., and Cotran, R. S., Expression of endothelial-leukocyte adhesion molecule-1 in elicited late phase allergic reactions, *J. Clin. Invest.*, *87*, 1805–1809 (1991).
15. Massey, W., Friedman, B., Kato, M., Cooper, P., Kagey-Sobotka, A., Lichtenstein, L. M., et al., Appearance of granulocyte-macrophage colony-stimulating factor activity at allergen-challenged cutaneous late phase reaction sites, *J. Immunol.*, *150*, 1084–1092 (1993).
16. Kay, A. B., Ying, S., Varney, S. R., Gaga, M., Durham, S. R., Moqbel, R., et al., Messenger RNA expression of the cytokine gene cluster, interleukin-3 (IL-3), IL-4, IL-5, and granulocyte/macrophage colony-stimulating factor, in allergen-induced late-phase cutaneous reactions in atopic subjects, *J. Exp. Med.*, *173*, 775–778 (1991).

17. Broide, D. H., and Firestein, G. S., Endobronchial allergen challenge in asthma: Demonstration of cellular source of granulocyte macrophage colony-stimulating factor by in situ hybridization, *J. Clin. Invest.*, *88*, 1048–1053 (1991).
18. Robinson, D. S., Qutayba, H., Ying, S., Tsicopoulos, A., Barkans, J., Bentley, A. M., et al., Predominant TH2-like bronchoalveolar T lymphocyte population in atopic asthma, *N. Engl. J. Med.*, *326*, 298–304 (1992).
19. Durham, S. R., Ying, S., Varney, V. A., Jacobson, M. R., Sudderick, R. M., Mackay, I. S., et al., Cytokine messenger RNA expression for IL-3, IL-4, IL-5, and granulocyte/macrophage colony-stimulating factor in the nasal mucosa after local allergen provocation: Relationship to tissue eosinophilia, *J. Immunol.*, *148*, 2390–2394 (1992).
20. Broide, D. H., Paine, M. M., and Firestein, G. S., Eosinophils express interleukin 5 and granulocyte-macrophage colony-stimulating factor mRNA at sites of allergic inflammation in asthmatics, *J. Clin. Invest.*, *90*, 1414–1424 (1992).
21. Kuhns, D. B., DeCarlo, E., Hawk, D. M., and Gallin, J. I., Dynamics of the cellular and humoral components of the inflammatory response elicited in skin blisters in humans, *J. Clin. Invest.*, *192*, 1734–1740 (1992).
22. Charlesworth, E. N., Kagey-Sobotka, A., Schleimer, R. P., Norman, P. S., and Lichtenstein, L. M., Prednisone inhibits the appearance of inflammatory mediators and the influx of eosinophils and basophils associated with the cutaneous late-phase response to allergen, *J. Immunol.*, *146*, 671–676 (1991).
23. Pipkorn, U., Proud, D., Lichtenstein, L. M., Schleimer, R. P., Peters, S. P., Adkinson, N. F., Kagey-Sobotka, A., Adams, G. K., III, Norman, P. S., and Naclerio, R. M., Effect of short-term systemic glucocorticoid treatment on human nasal mediator release after antigen challenge, *J. Clin. Invest.*, *80*, 957–961 (1987).
24. Massey, W. A., Charlesworth, E. N., Freidhoff, L., Cooper, P., Kagey-Sobotka, A., and Lichtenstein, L. M., Cutaneous IgE-mediated inflammatory lesion size is inhibited by an H1 antagonist (terfenadine) while mediator release is unaffected in vivo and in vitro, *Clin. Exp. Allergy*, *23*, 399–405 (1993).
25. Charlesworth, E. N., Massey, W. A., Kagey-Sobotka, A., Norman, P. S., and Lichtenstein, L. M., Effect of H1 receptor blockade on the early and late response to cutaneous allergen challenge, *J. Pharmacol. Exp. Ther.*, *262*, 964–970 (1992).
26. Naclerio, R. M., Kagey-Sobotka, A., Lichtenstein, L. M., Freidhoff, L., and Proud, D., Terfenadine, an H1 antihistamine, inhibits histamine release in vivo in the human, *Am. Rev. Respir. Dis.*, *142*, 167–171 (1990).
27. Bochner, B. S., Landy, S. D., Plaut, M., Dinarello, C. A., and Schleimer, R. P., Interleukin 1 production by human lung tissue. I. Identification and characterization, *J. Immunol.*, *139*, 2297–2302 (1987).

4

Experimental Provoked Viral Respiratory Infections in Human Adult Volunteers

Philip Fireman

University of Pittsburgh School of Medicine and Children's Hospital of Pittsburgh Pittsburgh, Pennsylvania

I. INTRODUCTION

Upper respiratory infections (URIs) are the most common illnesses affecting humans, not only children and young adults, but also older patients [1]. The ideal way to define the pathogenesis, pathophysiology, and immunopathology of URIs is to study humans who are experiencing naturally occurring respiratory infections. However, this is difficult to do. It is not always possible to identify precisely the onset of a URI in a particular human subject or to study specific individuals before their natural exposure to a specific infectious agent that naturally causes illness [2]. In the absence of the ability to do this in a predictable fashion, investigators have resorted to studies of human volunteers who are willing to be infected by provocative respiratory challenge with respiratory viruses [3]. These respiratory infections experimentally produced in a standardized, controlled environment also provide the opportunity to control for those variables that exist in everyday living conditions, as well as to design studies to explore the unusual circumstances that may contribute to the expression of the URI [4]. Such well-controlled studies are not possible with naturally acquired infections. It is tempting to draw conclusions from such experimental respiratory infections; however, it is still necessary to validate these changes in the patient with appropriate observations of the naturally acquired disease, to verify their clinical relevance and significance. It is also mandatory that the safety of the infectious agents employed be documented, so that the potential risks to the volunteer are delineated and kept to that minimum of discomfort for which the volunteers provide their informed consent.

Over the past 40 years several laboratories have studied experimentally produced URIs with rhinovirus and influenza viruses, coxsackievirus, coronavirus, and respiratory syncytial virus [5–9]. Investigators have used these studies to explore not only the symptoms and clinical expression of the URI but also the pathophysiology and the effects on host defenses, such as phagocytosis, neutrophil function, ciliary function, T cell function, and cell-mediated immunity [10–13]. Other investigators have used this experimental model to study the efficacy of new or improved viral vaccines as well as other antiviral medications [14–16]. This model has also been useful in studying the efficacy of various symptomatic medications [17–19].

This chapter will describe how our laboratory has performed experimental rhinovirus 39 and influenza A virus challenges in human volunteers. We will also review some of our previously published studies of the effects of both rhinovirus and influenza A virus on a variety of patients' symptoms as well as the changes observed in nasal, pulmonary, and eustachian tube functions [20,21]. We will also describe the changes that occur in nasal secretions and their protein constituents as well as immune parameters during these experimentally provoked URIs [22,23].

II. METHODS OF STUDY

A. Study Population

Healthy adult subjects (aged 18–50 years) were recruited from the adult employees and students of the University of Pittsburgh and the surrounding community. These volunteers were in good general health, and results of ear, nose, and throat (ENT) and general physical examination were normal. A subset of subjects with a history of allergic rhinitis have also been studied. Blood and urine specimens were collected for laboratory tests to confirm that the potential volunteers were in good health. Blood samples were obtained for complete blood counts and assayed for a panel of hepatic enzymes and the presence of human immunodeficiency virus (HIV) and hepatitis virus antibodies. Blood samples were also examined for preexisting antibody to the virus to be studied. Urine samples were submitted for routine urinalysis. Potential subjects were excluded if there was a prior history of nasal or otologic surgery; a history of cardiovascular or lower respiratory tract illness or other serious diseases; a symptomatic upper respiratory infection within the previous 30 days; concurrent nasal or otologic signs and symptoms; abnormal clinical profiles on urinalysis, complete blood count, or assay of blood enzymes; or seropositivity for HIV or hepatitis viruses.

Potential subjects with a history of allergic rhinitis were tested by skin prick with common inhalant allergens including ragweed pollen, grass pollen, tree pollens, dust mite, cat, and dog, and if results were positive, sera were also studied by radioimmunoassay for specific immunoglobulin E (IgE) antibodies. Subjects were enrolled after providing written informed consent. All studies were approved by the institutional review board at the Children's Hospital of Pittsburgh or the University of Pittsburgh School of Medicine.

B. Experimental Plan

The experimental virus challenge study should be conducted before or after the usual late-fall and winter rhinovirus or influenza virus season. During the period of study, the subjects were asked to refrain from taking any over-the-counter or prescription medication, with the exception of birth control pills. Additionally, alcohol consumption was not permitted. Acetaminophen was supplied as a rescue medication for those subjects requiring relief from incurred symptoms of illness such as fever or discomfort, and doses used were recorded by study personnel.

Typically, 1 or 2 days before viral inoculation, susceptible subjects with low preexisting specific viral antibodies reported to the study laboratories during the morning or afternoon hours. At that time a blood sample was taken for desired baseline studies. Preinfection (baseline) symptom scores were recorded, and a battery of baseline physiological tests were administered. A preinfection nasal lavage was performed for viral culture and other assays. The subjects then reported to a nearby hotel or the National Institutes of Health (NIH)-funded General Clinical Research Center of Children's Hospital for a cloister period of 6–9 days. Viral inoculation was usually performed within 24 h after cloistering but may be given 24–48 h before cloistering if the study design does not require measurements before the usual onset of URI symptoms. Symptom scores and measurements of physiological function may also be collected immediately before viral inoculation.

Following intranasal viral inoculation and on each study day, tissues and plastic bags of known weight were supplied to each experimentally infected subject. They were instructed to sneeze into these weighed tissues and return them to the weighed plastic bags, which were collected the following day. A nasal lavage for viral culture and other studies were performed during the morning hours, and symptoms were scored at least once daily. Three times a day, in the evening, morning, and afternoon, oral temperature was recorded. A number of physiological functions were assessed. These might include pulmonary function by spirometry, nasal patency by active posterior rhinomanometry, eustachian tube function by sonotubometry, and middle ear pressure by tympanometry. Additionally, during the afternoon hours, patients underwent ENT physical examinations, and nasal clearance (cilia) function was evaluated by a modification of the saccharin dye test.

Blood samples might be taken for testing at various times during the cloister period, as well as 21 days after viral challenge for convalescent antiviral antibody assay to assess infection.

C. Viral Challenge

Viral challenge was performed with the subject sitting erect with neck hyperextended. Then, 0.25 ml of inoculum/nostril was administered intranasally by pipette as coarse drops. The subject was instructed to perform a lateral head sway to ensure more complete distribution to the nasal mucosa, and to refrain from sneezing or nose blowing for 30 min. The virus to be used should be safety-tested. A safety-tested clinical isolate of rhinovirus 39 (RV39) passaged twice in WI-38 human embryonic lung fibroblasts was provided by Dr. Jack Gwaltney, and a total dose of 100 $TCID_{50}$ was administered. The methodology of RV39 challenge was developed by Dr. Gwaltney as previously described [24].

The influenza A virus used in our studies was a safety-tested clinical isolate of H_1N_1 virus (wild type lot E-262) supplied by the National Institute of Allergy and Infectious Diseases. For each subject, the total intranasal influenza virus dose was estimated to be 10^7 $TCID_{50}$.

D. Assessment of Infection

Nasal lavages were performed for viral culture daily during the cloister period. With the subject sitting erect and neck hyperextended, 5 ml of sterile saline was instilled into each nostril while the subject closed the oral–nasal port. After a period of approximately 30 s, the subject expelled the wash fluid into a cup. Recovered fluids varied in quantity but averaged approximately 6 ml (total) and were immediately transferred to collection tubes, which were placed on ice. Aliquots were submitted to the virology laboratories for culture. Other aliquots were stored frozen at −70°C for other analyses. Methods used for RV39 and influenza virus culture have previously been described [24,25]. Preinoculation and convalescent serum samples were tested for neutralizing antibodies to RV39 or hemagglutination-inhibition antibody assay for influenza virus, as previously described [25,26]. Infection was defined as documented viral shedding with positive viral cultures of nasal lavage on at least one postchallenge day of the cloister period or a fourfold increase in serum antibody titer between prechallenge and convalescent samples.

E. Subjective Assessments of Illness

On each study day, subjects were interviewed regarding the presence and extent of symptoms. Either specific symptoms, including sneezing, nasal discharge, nasal congestion, malaise, headache, chillness, sore throat, and cough, were rated by the subject on a scale of four points (0–3) corresponding to none, mild, moderate, and severe. For analysis, three combined scores were calculated for each subject on each study day: nasal symptom score (sum of scores for sneezing, nasal discharge, and nasal congestion), throat symptom score (sum of scores for sore throat and cough), and systemic symptom score (sum of scores for headache, chilliness, and malaise). Subjects were invited to list additional symptoms not specified on the scoring sheet. The presence of these additional symptoms was recorded by the study technician, but they were not scored. On each study day, the subjects were asked if they believed that they had sufficient illness to qualify was having a cold or flu. These responses were recorded on the diary sheets. A subject was considered to be ill if he or she had reported a cold or flu on at least 2 days.

F. Objective Assessments of Illness

To provide a daily measure of secretion production, subjects were supplied with preweighed tissues at 6:00 p.m. on each study day. The subjects were instructed to expel all nasal secretions into these tissues and seal the expended tissues in plastic bags. These were collected at 6:00 p.m. on the following day and weighed. Secretion weights for each 24-h period were determined by subtraction.

Physiological tests included assessments of middle ear pressure, nasal patency, pulmonary function, eustachian tube function, and nasal clearance function, as previously described. Middle ear pressures were measured with a commercially available automatic digital tympanometer (Teledyne model TA-8A). Instrument output consisted of external canal volume, tympanic membrane compliance, and middle ear pressure. Nasal patency was measured by active posterior rhinomanometry with as custom-built computer-assisted rhinomanometer, previously described [27]. For testing, subjects breathed normally into a mask sealed against the face and serially aligned to a flow sensor. Upstream mask pressure was referenced via a differential transducer to that in the oral cavity. Voltages from the sensors were digitized and routed to the memory of an IBM pcAT computer for editing and analysis. Software programs computed the work performed in moving a liter of air on inspiration. This variable (work/liter) is a direct and linear measure of nasal congestion, and its value was recorded at each test session.

Pulmonary function was measured by a commercial spirometer (Multi Spiro PC, Medical Equipment Design, Inc.) interfaced to an IBM pcAT computer. Forced expiratory maneuvers were performed three times at each testing and the maximum forced expiratory volume in 1 second referenced to a panel of normal values (%FEV_1) was recorded as the test value.

Eustachian tube function was evaluated by sonotubometry with a custom-built instrument development in our laboratories. Briefly, a white noise of known sound pressure was supplied to the nose by a high-volume speaker via a coupling at the nostril [27]. Insert microphones were placed in the external auditory canals and shielded from ambient noises by padded earphones. The subject was asked to swallow, a maneuver triggering activity of the tubal dilatory musculature, and the changes in sound pressure in the ear canals were monitored. Transient (50–500 ms) increases in canal sound pressures of at least 5 dB were recorded as tubal dilations. At each session, the test was performed a total of four times. A tubal dilation on any of the four swallowing attempts was considered to be a positive result.

Nasal clearance function was assessed by the dyed saccharin technique, which has previously been described [20]. For this test, 5 μl of a test solution was placed bilaterally on the mucosa in the anterior part of the nasal cavity just behind the internal ostium. The test solution consisted of 8 mg/ml indigo carmine, 3 mg/ml saccharin, and 45 mg/ml sorbitol (pH adjusted to 7.4). The subjects swallowed as required and were asked to report the first occurrence of a sweet taste; then the pharyngeal cavity was examined for the appearance of the blue dye. Repeat inspections of the pharynx were made at 1-min intervals to a total of 30 min or until the dye was observed unilaterally. The time between administration of the dye and the subject's reporting a sweet taste was recorded as the nasal mucociliary clearance times.

Before each test session, the recording instruments were calibrated. Nasal clearance and pulmonary function were assessed on each of the baseline test days and once daily for the cloister period. Rhinomanometry, tympanometry, and eustachian tube function tests were performed once daily before challenge and three times per day, in morning, afternoon, and evening test sessions, during cloister period. This test battery and sequence has been used in our previous studies of experimental infection without incident or demonstrable effect on measured responses [20–23].

All persons were examined daily by a physician using pneumatic otoscopy. The appearance and mobility of the tympanic membrane and any evidence of abnormalities were recorded. Photographic documentation of the appearance of the tympanic membrane was made on days 4 and 8.

G. Statistical Methods

For analysis, secretion weight, work per liter, clearance time, $\%FEV_1$, the combined symptom score (sum of eight interview symptom scores), and the nasal symptom score (sum of interview scores for rhinorrhea, congestion, and sneezing) were considered to be continuous variables. Middle ear pressures were categorized as abnormal if they were greater than $+30$ or less than -80 mm H_2O. Eustachian tube function test results were classified as normal if dilation occurred on any of four deglutition attempts within a 3-min period. The average values for the continuous variables recorded at baseline testings were compared using Student's *t*-test (two-tailed, evaluated at $p<0.5$). For dichotomous variables, the chi-squared statistic (with Yates correction for continuity) was used for these comparisons.

III. NASAL AND OTOLOGIC CONSEQUENCES OF EXPERIMENTAL VIRUS INFECTION IN ADULT VOLUNTEERS

To understand mechanisms by which viral URI provokes nasal and ear disease, we initiated an experimental program involving intranasal viral challenge of susceptible adult volunteers. Those studies showed that rhinovirus infection causes significant increases in nasal symptoms and signs [20]. Peak symptoms and signs occurred on day 2 and 3 after challenge in both allergic and nonallergic subjects (Fig. 1). Abnormal middle ear (ME) pressures were recorded in the majority of subjects, with a peak in the frequency of negative ME pressures on day 6. Three subjects entered the study with ME pressures of less than 0.100 mm H_2O. Those pressures became significantly more negative in two of the three subjects, and both developed asymptomatic otitis media (OM) by study day 7. These results document a causal relationship between rhinovirus infection and OM in adults and suggest that preexisting eustachian tube (ET) obstruction may be necessary for the expression of that complication. More recently, a total of 96 susceptible subjects were infected with rhinovirus and followed by daily otoscopy for 6 days. Two of these subjects (2%) developed asymptomatic OM during follow-up.

More recently, we challenged a group of 33 subjects with influenza A virus (H_1N_1) and followed the course of illness over a 9-day period [21]. Twenty-six of the subjects were infected with the virus. For those subjects, symptom onset occurred within 2 days of infectious exposure, with a peak symptom load on days 3 and 4 and a resolution by day 8 (Fig. 2). Symptoms were not confined to the nose but extended to the throat, chest, and ME. Systemic symptoms including malaise, fatigue, chills, sweating, headache, body ache, and fever were also reported as an early event of diminishing intensity with increasing time after exposure. The changes in objective measures of nasal pathology, including the nasal work expended in breathing and the weight of expelled nasal secretions, tracked well the temporal course of nasal symptoms (Fig. 3). Other objective tests documented the development of a decreased nasal mucociliary clearance rate, ET dysfunction (Fig. 4), ME underpressures, and the frank expression of asymptomatic OM in five subjects beginning 4 days after viral challenge. One subject with bilateral OM developed symptoms of dizziness and vertigo suggestive of transient inner ear involvement. All signs and symptoms of illness had resolved by 21 days after exposure.

In that study, the rate of documented virus infection was 38% (5 of 13) for subjects with prechallenge specific serum antibody titers of $\geqslant 16$, and 100% (21 of 21) for subjects with lesser antibody titers. Uninfected subjects did not exhibit significant nasal symptoms or signs, though they reported a transient increase in throat and systemic symptoms limited to the second day after challenge. Attendant pathophysiologies documented in the low-titer, infected group, including reduced

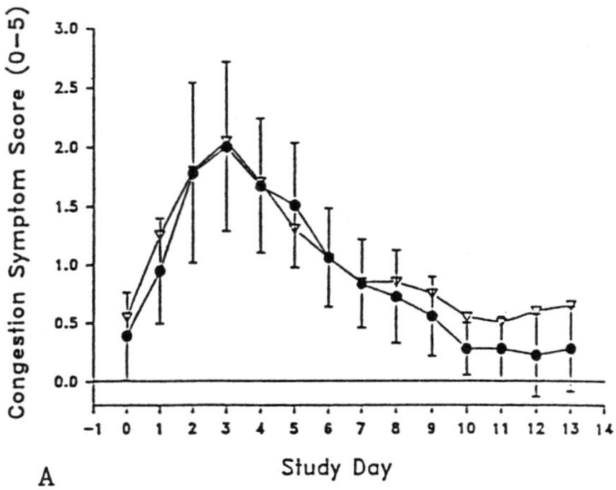

Congestion Symptom Score (0–5)
3.0
2.5
2.0
1.5
1.0
0.5
0.0
−1 0 1 2 3 4 5 6 7 8 9 10 11 12 13 14
Study Day

A

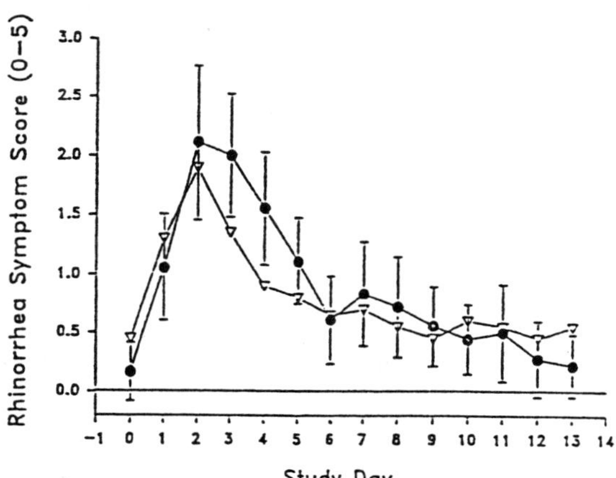

Rhinorrhea Symptom Score (0–5)
3.0
2.5
2.0
1.5
1.0
0.5
0.0
−1 0 1 2 3 4 5 6 7 8 9 10 11 12 13 14
Study Day

B

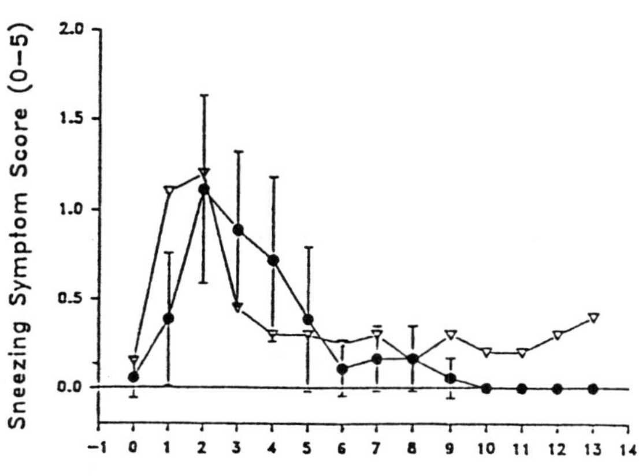

Sneezing Symptom Score (0–5)
2.0
1.5
1.0
0.5
0.0
−1 0 1 2 3 4 5 6 7 8 9 10 11 12 13 14
Study Day

C

mucociliary clearance rates, ET dysfunction, and the development of abnormal ME pressures, were not expressed in the uninfected subjects. Moreover, the symptom load and the frequency and extent of nasal and otologic pathophysiologies were significantly less in infected subjects with high antibody titers than in infected subjects with lower antibody titers. These results suggest that high serum antibody titers protect from infection, minimize the local expression of disease, and limit extension of pathology to anatomically contiguous structures.

Peripheral blood obtained periodically during the course of infection was analyzed for selected immunological components and functions. Early changes observed included increased natural killer cell lytic activity (day 1) and decreased numbers of white blood cells and total and T lymphocytes (day 3), which lasted through day 23. Numbers of activated T lymphocytes increased on days 6 and 7, and a depressed proliferative response to phytohemagglutinin and influenza antigen was observed on days 3 through 7. These results document that experimental influenza infection caused a marked suppression of certain aspects of the immune response.

In a more recent unpublished study, 28 susceptible volunteers were experimentally infected with influenza A virus and followed as described above. The pattern of illness noted for the first study was reproduced. Five of the subjects developed OM on days 4 and 5, with one case characterized by earache and pain. In that subject, tympanometry documented the progressive development of negative ME pressures, to less than −200 mm H_2O, followed by a positive pressure of 30 mm H_2O on the morning of OM diagnosis. At that time, a myringotomy and tympanocentesis was performed to relieve the pain. The effusion was sterile by culture for the presence of bacteria and virus. These results confirm the causal relationship between influenza infection and OM, but fail to document in situ virus infection of the ME mucosa.

IV. SUMMARY

Experimental provocative viral infection has been employed for many years to help define the pathogenesis and mechanisms of URIs. Since it is often not possible to define the onset of viral disease in naturally infected patients, this provocative-challenge model can be employed in clinical investigation to better understand these very common illnesses and develop treatments for their complications. Our laboratory has used this experimental model to document the

---

Figure 1 Means of the diary symptom scores as a function of study day of the allergic rhinitis (AR) (open triangles) and non-AR (filled circles) groups for **(A)** nasal congestion, **(B)** rhinorrhea, and **(C)** sneezing. Vertical bars indicate the 95% confidence interval about the non-AR group's means. (From Ref. 20.)

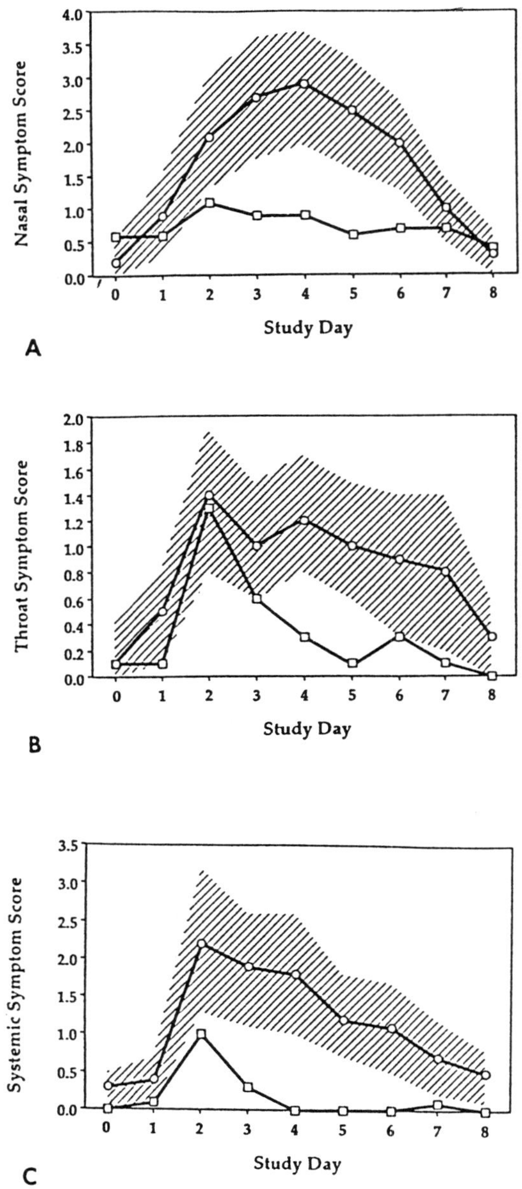

Figure 2 Average daily values of combined **(A)** nasal, **(B)** throat, and **(C)** systemic symptom scores as function of study day for low-titer infected (circles) and uninfected (squares) groups. Cross-hatching indicates 95% confidence interval about low-titer infected group means. (From Ref. 21.)

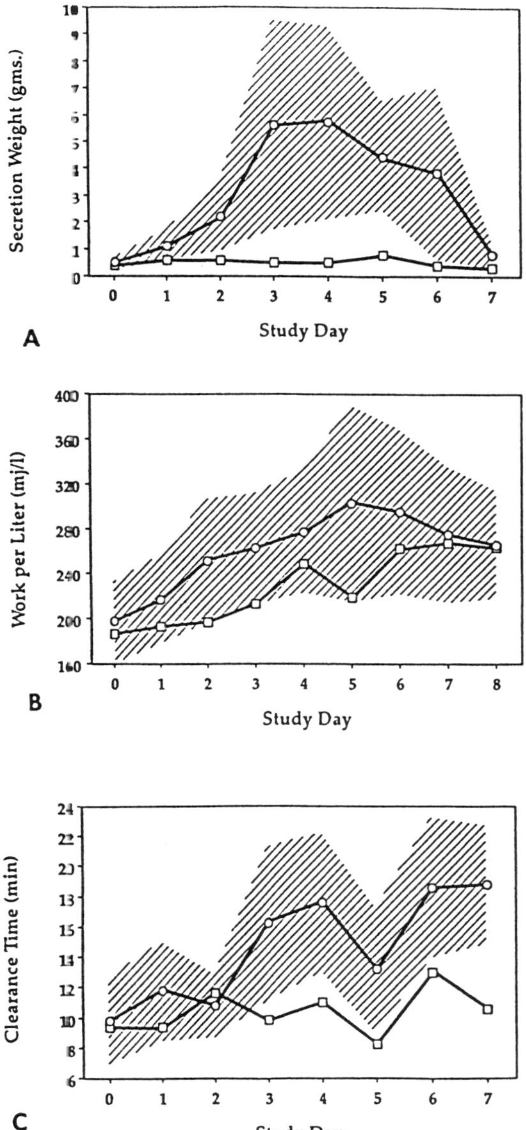

Figure 3 Average daily values of objective measures of **(A)** nasal secretion, **(B)** nasal congestion, and **(C)** nasal clearance times for subjects in low-titer infected (circles) and uninfected (squares) groups. Cross-hatching indicates 95% confidence interval about low-titer infected group means. (From Ref. 21.)

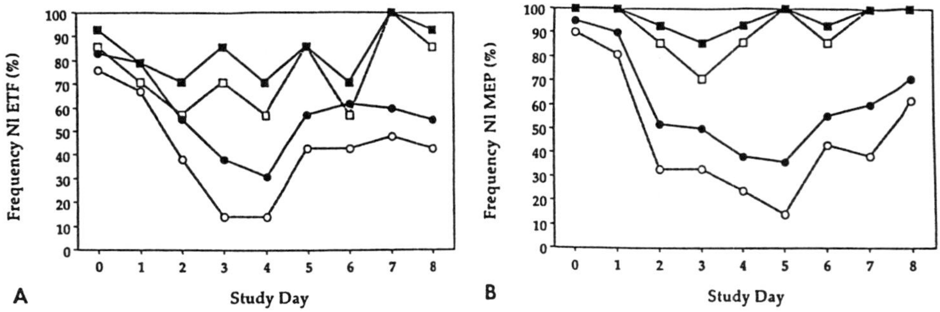

Figure 4 Average daily frequencies of persons (open symbols) and ears (solid symbols) with **(A)** good or normal (N1) eustachian tube function (ETF) and **(B)** normal middle ear pressure (MEP) for subjects in low-titer infected (circles) and uninfected (squares) groups. (From Ref. 21.)

relationship between viral URI and the expression of otitis media. It is our expectation that the information developed will help provide new and better means to treat otitis media, a most common pediatric illness.

ACKNOWLEDGMENTS

The author acknowledges the collaboration and contributions of Drs. David Skoner and William Doyle in their joint clinical investigations. The author also appreciates the help of Carol Wagner in the preparation of this manuscript.

The author's work was supported in part by NIH grants RO1 AI19262 and MO1RR00084.

REFERENCES

1. Andrews, C. H., The natural history of the common cold, *Lancet*, *1*, 71–73 (1949).
2. Tyrrell, D. A. J., A view from the common cold unit, *Antiviral Res.*, *18*, 105–125 (1992).
3. Bynoe, M. L., Hobson, D., Horner, J., et al., Inoculation of human volunteers with a strain of virus isolation from a common cold, *Lancet*, *1*, 1194–1196 (1961).
4. Dowling, H. F., Jackson, G. G., Spiesman, I. G., et al., Transmission of the common cold to volunteers under controlled conditions III. The effect of chilling of the subjects, *Am. J. Hyg.*, *66*, 59–65 (1958).
5. Hendley, J. O., Wenzel, R. P., and Gwaltney, J. M., Transmission of rhinovirus colds by self-inoculation, *N. Engl. J. Med.*, *288*, 1361–1365 (1973).
6. Beare, A. S., Live virus for immunization against influenza, *Prog. Med. Virol.*, *20*, 49–83 (1975).

7. Buchland, F. E., Bynoe, M. L., and Tyrrell, D. A. J., Experiments on the spread of colds II. Studies in volunteers with coxsackie virus A21, *J. Hyg. (Camb.)*, *63*, 327–343 (1965).
8. Bende, M., Barrow, G. I., Heptonstall, J., et al., Changes in human nasal mucosa during experimental coronavirus common colds, *Acta Otolaryngol.*, *107*, 262–269 (1989).
9. Higgins, P. G., Barrow, G. I., Tyrrell, D. A. J., Efficacy of intranasal interferon alpha-2a in respiratory syncytial virus infections in volunteers, *Antiviral Res.*, *14*, 3–10 (1990).
10. Cate, T. R., Couch, R. B., and Johnson, K. M., Studies with rhinovirus in volunteers: production of illness, effect of naturally acquired antibody and demonstration of protective effect not associated with antibody, *J. Clin. Invest.*, *43*, 56–67 (1964).
11. Dolin, R., Richman, D. D., Murphy, B. R., and Fanci, A. S., Cell mediated immune responses in humans after induced infections with influenza A virus, *J. Infect. Dis.*, *135*, 714–719 (1977).
12. Wilson, R., Alton, E., Rutman, E., et al., Upper respiratory tract viral infection and mucociliary clearance, *Eur. J. Respir. Dis.*, *70*, 272–279 (1987).
13. Larson, H. E. and Beades, R., Impairment of human polymorphonuclear function by influenza virus. *Lancet*, *7*, 285–287 (1976).
14. Scientific Committee on Common Cold Vaccines, Prevention of colds by vaccination against rhinoviruses, *Br. Med. J.*, *1*, 1344–1349 (1965).
15. Merrigan, T. C., Hall, T. S., Reed, S., et al., Inhibition of respiratory virus infection by locally applied interferon, *Lancet*, *1*, 563–567 (1973).
16. Dick, E. C., Hossani, S. V., Mink, K. A., et al., Interruption of transmission of rhinovirus cold among human volunteers using viricidal paper handkerchiefs, *J. Infect. Dis.*, *135*, 352–356 (1986).
17. Gaffey, M. J., Hayden, F. G., Boyd, J. C., et al., Ipratropium bromide treatment of experimental rhinovirus infection, *Antimicrob. Agents Chemother.*, *32*, 1644–1647 (1988).
18. Farr, B. M., Gwaltney, J. M., Hendley, J. O., et al., A randomized controlled trial of glucocorticoid prophylaxis against experimental rhinovirus infection, *J. Infect. Dis.*, *162*, 1173–1174 (1990).
19. Doyle, W. J., McBride, T. P., Hayden, D. G., et al., Treatment effects of an atropine/pseudoephedrine combination in rhinovirus colds, *Ann. Otol. Rhinol. Laryngol.*, *102*, 521–527 (1993).
20. Doyle, W. J., Skoner, D. P., Fireman, P., et al., Rhinovirus 39 infection in allergic and non-allergic subjects, *J. Allergy Clin. Immunol.*, *89*, 968–978 (1992).
21. Doyle, W. J., Skoner, D. P., Hayden, D. G., et al., Nasal and otologic effects of experimental influenza A virus infection, *Ann. Otol. Rhinol. Laryngol.*, *103*, 59–69 (1994).
22. Igarashi, Y., Skoner, D. P., Doyle, W. J., et al., Sources of nasal secretion during phases of experimental rhinovirus upper respiratory tract infection, *J. Allergy Clin. Immunol.*, *92*, 772–731 (1993).
23. Skoner, D. P., Whiteside, T. L., Wilson, J. W., et al., Effect of rhinovirus 39 infection on cellular immune parameters in allergic and non-allergic subjects, *J. Allergy Clin. Immunol.*, *92*, 732–743 (1993).

24. Gwaltney, J. M., and Jordan, W., Rhinovirus and respiratory illness in university students, *Am. Rev. Respir. Dis.*, *93*, 362–371 (1966).
25. Tobita, K., Sugiura, A., Enomoto, C., et al., Plaque allergy and primary isolation of influenza A viruses in established line of canine kidney cells (MDCK) in presence of trypsin, *Med. Microbiol. Immunol. (Berlin)*, *162*, 9–14 (1975).
26. Dowdle, W. R., Kendal, A. P., Noble, G. R., Influenza viruses. In *Diagnostic procedures for viral, rickettsial, and chlamydial infections* (Lennette E. H., Schmidt N. J., eds.) 5th ed. Washington, DC: American Public Health Association, 585–609 (1979).
27. Fireman, P., Nasal provocation testing and eustachian tube function, *J. Allergy Clin. Immunol.*, *81*, 953–960 (1988).

5

The Effects of Respiratory Infections on Airway Function

Nizar N. Jarjour, Robert F. Lemanske, Jr., Elliot C. Dick, and William W. Busse

University of Wisconsin School of Medicine
Madison, Wisconsin

William J. Calhoun

University of Pittsburgh
Pittsburgh, Pennsylvania

I. EPIDEMIOLOGY OF VIRUS-INDUCED ASTHMA AND AIRWAY HYPERRESPONSIVENESS

A. Viral-Induced Asthma Exacerbations

Clinicians have noted for many years that acute respiratory tract infections are frequently associated with exacerbations of asthma. Several prospective studies have confirmed this concept and documented that infections with respiratory viruses are responsible for asthma flares. For example, McIntosh and co-workers [1] followed 32 children who were hospitalized at National Jewish Hospital in Denver. Each child was carefully observed for flares of asthma and respiratory infections, which were confirmed by culture and/or a rise in serum antibody titers. Over the 2-year study period, the 32 children had 102 confirmed viral respiratory infections and 139 episodes of wheezing. In 58 of these episodes, wheezing was found in relationship to a viral respiratory infection. Respiratory syncytial virus (RSV) was the most prevalent organism identified in this age group (1–5 years) and the most likely to trigger wheezing. Although other respiratory viruses were found, they were not as prevalent. Furthermore, bacterial infections did not trigger wheezing.

Confirmation of McIntosh and colleagues' findings came from studies at the University of Wisconsin [2]. The 16 children evaluated in this investigation were older, were followed as outpatients, and had a history of wheezing with respiratory infections. Sixty-one episodes of asthma were experienced by these children over the winter months. Of these, 42 episodes were found in conjunction with asymptomatic respiratory infection, and 24 were confirmed as being viral in origin. In this study of older children, rhinovirus was the virus most frequently identified as causing an attack of wheezing, and wheezing was more likely when the patients were symptomatic with their illness. Some patients had episodes of asymptomatic viral infections (virus cultured at a routine follow-up visit) but had no flare of asthma. As in the Denver study, bacterial infections were not a trigger of asthma.

The importance of viral respiratory infection to wheezing is further highlighted by results of an 11-year study in a pediatric outpatient practice [3]. In this extensive project, 6165 lower respiratory illnesses were evaluated, and 1851 (30%) were found to manifest wheezing. Half of the wheezing episodes were found in children less than 2 years old, but wheezing was also noted in a substantial number of older children. In 21% of all children experiencing wheezing, a nonbacterial pathogen was isolated. Of these, RSV, parainfluenza virus, and adenovirus predominated. This frequency of pathogen recovery probably reflects technical difficulties associated with virus isolation, as well as the possibility that other factors may contribute to these episodes of wheezing.

Although adults wheeze with respiratory infections, the frequency of this association in an older age group is not as great as among children [4,5]. Although an explanation for such findings is not clear from available studies, it is possible that asthma exacerbations are more difficult to delineate in adults than in children; this may relate to the fact that the pattern of wheezing is more chronic than episodic in adults.

From these studies, a number of important conclusions can be reached that help us to understand the infectious nature of asthma flares and to provide guidelines for future investigation. First, viral, not bacterial, respiratory infections trigger wheezing in the asthmatic patient. Second, the likelihood of wheezing with a cold is greater if the illness has concomitant constitutional symptoms. Third, viral respiratory infections provoke asthma more frequently in children than adults. Finally, the respiratory virus that triggers asthma is age-related. For example, in small children RSV is most important; for older children, parainfluenza virus and rhinovirus assume greater prevalence. Whether these differences are related to epidemiologic, immunologic, or virologic age-related factors is at present unknown.

B. Influence of Viral Infection on Pulmonary Function in Normal Subjects

Over the years, a number of investigators have examined the effect of uncomplicated respiratory infections on airway function in normal persons [6–11]. By using sensitive pulmonary function testing, i.e., airway resistance, dynamic compliance, and other measures of small-airway function, subtle changes in respiratory physiology have been detected. The changes in lung function are clinically silent, but nonetheless are a consistent finding from study to study. What is also interesting is the persistence of these lung function changes for weeks following the resolution of clinical symptoms of the respiratory illness. The mechanisms causing change in small-airway function are not known; moreover, the effect of certain viral illnesses on lung function is especially intriguing, as the respiratory virus's replication may be confined primarily to the upper airway (e.g., rhinovirus).

Hall and colleagues [12] prospectively studied 10 healthy adults who were infected with RSV while working on an infants' ward. All had symptoms of a severe respiratory infection. More important to our discussion, these patients had an increase in baseline respiratory resistance, heightened airway responsiveness to cholinergic challenges during the acute infection, and persistence of this pattern for up to 8 weeks after infection. None had had a history of asthma or allergic disease. Thus, in addition to subtle obstructive changes in airway function, some severe viral respiratory infections can cause bronchial hyperresponsiveness.

Empey et al. [13] found similar enhancement of airway responsiveness during an acute cold. Sixteen college students were evaluated for signs of increased airway responsiveness during a clinical viral upper respiratory infection (URI). Compared with normal subjects, those with colds showed airway hyperresponsiveness to inhaled histamine. To define the possible site of abnormality, the patients were treated with atropine before a bronchial challenge with histamine. Because atropine blocked the hyperresponsiveness to histamine, the investigators speculated that a vagus-mediated reflex was involved in this enhanced airway reaction. It was further suggested that the cause of this cholinergic-mediated hyperresponsiveness may arise from airway inflammation that sensitizes rapidly adapting sensory fibers of the afferent vagus nerve.

A number of important guidelines for future studies followed from these studies. First, viral respiratory infections can cause mild obstructive changes that are principally detected by tests for "small"-airway function. Second, enhanced airway reactivity may also follow some respiratory infections. Most studies that demonstrate increases in airway responsiveness use measurements of airway resistance that are more sensitive than the forced expired volume in 1 second (FEV_1). Therefore, when changes in bronchial reactivity occur, they can be detected in measures of larger-airway function. Finally, the effects of a URI on lung function and reactivity may persist for weeks (6–8 weeks) after the viral illness. Consequently, if evaluation of optimal function and reactivity, or "baseline" testing in asthmatics, is needed, an appropriate interval is necessary between the viral illness and subsequent testing.

C. Long-Term Effects of Viral Respiratory Infections on Airway Function

In some children there is a continuum of viral bronchiolitis with RSV infection and later episodes of wheezing. Zweiman et al. [14] closely followed 25 children for the development of asthma (or recurrent episodes of wheezing) after a hospitalization for acute bronchiolitis. Five years after the initial episode of bronchiolitis, nearly 50% of the children had recurrent episodes of wheezing. The children who appeared at risk had a higher prevalence of either personal or familial atopic disease. A similar relationship was reported by Rooney and Williams [15] as well as Gurwitz et al. [16]. These studies raised the probability that changes in airway reactivity that follow a respiratory infection can persist for an extended period or even herald the onset of asthma. These observations have not been confirmed in other studies. Nonetheless, numerous observations indicate the potential importance of respiratory infections in the pathogenesis of airway reactivity and underscore the need to study this relationship in detail. Guidelines for such studies are reviewed and discussed in the following sections.

II. EXPERIMENTAL STUDIES OF VIRUS-INDUCED AIRWAY HYPERRESPONSIVENESS

A. Animal Studies

1. Background

To study the effects of virus infection on airway physiology, a number of mammalian species have been studied, including the guinea pig [17–21], ferret [22], dog [23], mouse [24–28], and rat [29–35]. Using these models, a number of factors have been observed that may contribute to virus-induced alterations in airway responsiveness. First, airway tone could be enhanced as a result of effects on sympathetic [24], parasympathetic [21], or noncholinergic/nonadrenergic (NANC) [19,22] pathways. The parasympathetic pathway could be up-regulated through inhibitory effects of the virus on M_2 receptor feedback inhibition of acetylcholine release from postganglionic neurons [21]. The NANC system could contribute through the down-regulation of neutral endopeptidase activity, which would leave neurokinin (substance P) procontractile activity of bronchial smooth muscle unopposed [19,21]. Second, tissue inflammation may also play a role. Virus-induced airway hyperresponsiveness can be passively transferred in vitro using bronchoalveolar lavage cells from infected guinea pigs [20]; although it is unproved, these effects may be related to the production of cytokines that influence airway tone or response [36]. Finally, respiratory infections may enhance neurogenic inflammation, which may secondarily affect airway responses by alterations in airway geometry [34,35].

In our laboratories, in collaboration with Dr. William Castleman of the School of Veterinary Medicine, we have used a rat neonatal and weanling model of pulmonary viral infection to induce a number of pathophysiological alterations relevant to human asthma [29–31,37,38]. Parainfluenza type I (Sendai) virus infection in neonatal rats results in neonatal bronchiolitis and pneumonia that progress to the development of alveolar dysplasia and bronchial hypoplasia [31,37]; these changes are associated with persistent increases in total lung resistance [29,31]. Infected animals also develop bronchiolar mast cell hyperplasia that is associated temporally with airway hyperresponsiveness to methacholine [30]. We have also infected rats with virus as weanlings and have noted similar changes in mast cell hyperplasia, airway resistance, and airway hyperresponsiveness, but no persistent changes in alveolar or bronchiolar architecture [32]. Most of these virus-induced changes can be significantly reversed following short-term corticosteroid therapy [33]. Since these models share many of the features present in both acute and chronic asthma (viral induction, airway inflammation, airway hyperresponsiveness, hypoxemia, and steroid attenuation or abrogation), they are relevant tools for continued study of biological, physiological, and immunological mechanisms by which these changes occur and can be modified in order to better understand their human counterpart.

2. Rat Animal Model

Virus Inoculation. Rats of various strains and ages can be inoculated by aerosols of parainfluenza type 1 (Sendai) virus using an exposure apparatus (Tri-R Instruments, Rockville Center, New York), as described elsewhere [31]. Rats are exposed to the virus (strain P3193 produced in embryonated chicken eggs) or control solution (sterile chorioallantoic fluid) for 15 min. At all times, infected and control rats are housed separately under identical conditions.

Instrumentation and Physiological Measurements. Cannulae are placed in the trachea, jugular vein, and carotid artery of each rat after anesthesia is induced with urethane (1–1.2 g/kg intraperitoneally). Rats are placed supine in a constant-pressure rodent plethysmograph, paralyzed with succinylcholine chloride (4–6 mg/kg intravenously), and ventilated mechanically at 80 breaths/min with the tidal volume adjusted to maintain a normal arterial P_{CO_2} (37 ± 3 [SD] torr). Lungs are inflated to 30 cm H_2O pressure each minute to prevent atelectasis, and accumulated secretions are removed from the airways by suctioning as necessary. Resistance is computed by the isovolume method at 50% tidal volume (Model 6 Pulmonary Mechanics Analyzer, Buxco Electronics, Sharon, Connecticut), using inflation pressure measured at the tracheal cannula and flow and volume obtained for the plethysmograph transducer signal. Dynamic respiratory system compliance (Cdyn) is determined from inflation pressure and tidal volume at points of zero flow. Respiratory system resistance (Rrs) is obtained from the computed resistance by subtracting the resistance of the tracheal cannula and its connector.

Resistance and Cdyn measurements are obtained from an average of 16 breaths, starting at 1 min after inflating the lungs to 30 cm H_2O.

Lung volumes can be measured by the Boyle's law method: the airway opening is occluded at end expiration (functional residual capacity [FRC]), and the simultaneous changes in thoracic volume (plethysmograph signal) and airway opening pressure are recorded for several inspiratory efforts. The FRC is then computed from the relationship of the pressure and volume changes, taking into account the barometric pressure (P_B), the water vapor pressure (P_{H2O}), and the volume of the tracheal tube and connecting tubes (V_{EQ}):

$$FRC = [(\Delta V/\Delta P)(P_B - P_{H2O} - \Delta P)] - V_{EQ}$$

After the occluded breaths, the lungs are inflated from FRC to 30 cm H_2O pressure (total lung capacity [TLC]) and then deflated to -30 cm H_2O (residual lung volume [RV]). Using FRC as the reference point, TLC and RV are computed from the changes in volume occurring with the inflation/deflation maneuver.

Airway responses to methacholine can be obtained following intravenous administration of this agent by recording the subsequent change in resistance using the techniques described above. Methacholine is injected as 1 ml/kg of increasing concentrations of the agent, followed by a flush of 0.3 ml of saline, both being completed in about 5 s. The amount required to produce an increase in resistance of $\geqslant 0.2$ cm H_2O ml^{-1} s is considered a significant end point change, similar to the dose of aerosolized methacholine required to change FEV_1 by 20% in human studies. Additional doses of methacholine can then be given to obtain a maximal change in resistance value. Aerosolized delivery of methacholine can also be performed [39].

Summary. The rat model, as well as others, has provided new and important insight into mechanisms by which viral infections may alter airway biology and physiology. As more sophisticated molecular and immunological probes are developed for the study of immunoinflammatory responses, the changes that viruses can induce in the airway that modulate these responses and their physiological counterparts will no doubt reveal more specific targets for future therapeutic intervention.

B. Human Studies

1. Background

Recent investigations have questioned the ease with which respiratory infections trigger airway reactivity both in normal subjects and in asthma patients. From such studies, it is apparent that not all persons are susceptible to "wheezing" with respiratory infections, and that not all strains of one particular virus are capable of provoking airway hyperresponsiveness. For example, half of a normal adult volunteer population experimentally infected with rhinovirus by Halperin et al. [40] had positive cultures from the lower respiratory tract at bronchoscopy. However, neither spirometry nor bronchoprovocation testing with histamine showed changes during the respiratory illness. Further, when these investigators [41] inoculated asthmatic volunteers with the same rhinovirus strain, only four of the 21 infected asthma patients had a 10% or greater drop in FEV_1 and a concomitant increase in airway sensitivity to inhaled histamine. Although the investigators interpreted their findings as showing that experimental rhinovirus infections aggravate airway reactivity in a minority of adult asthma patients, and that exacerbations of wheezing with other viral pathogens are more likely to play an important role in this relationship, this observed frequency of wheezing with viral URIs is not unusual for adults with asthma [4,5]. Why only some patients are susceptible to virus-induced pathophysiological alterations is not clear from this or other investigations. However, a number of factors appear to influence the ultimate clinical response, including the patient's age, the degree of underlying airway hyperreactivity, the particular respiratory virus, and the degree to which individual patients develop significant clinical symptoms during the respiratory illness. The clinical profile exhibited by patients during a cold may be dictated by a number of mechanisms: airway injury by the infectious pathogen [13,42], diminished β-adrenergic function [43–47], production of virus-specific immunoglobulin E (IgE)-antibodies [48–50], enhanced leukocyte histamine release [51,52], and an increased propensity for the development of late-phase pulmonary reactions that are known to be associated with airway inflammation and hyperresponsiveness [53,54].

2. The Effects of Rhinovirus 16 Infection on Airway Reactivity and Late-Phase Reactions

The following protocol and methods of study were developed to examine the effects of a rhinovirus respiratory infection on airway responsiveness, as well as the pattern of pulmonary response that develops following aerosolized antigen challenge.

Patient Selection. In an initial study [53], the selected patients had a positive immediate skin test reaction by the prick method to an extract of ragweed antigen (1/20, w/v), released leukocyte histamine following an in vitro incubation with ragweed antigen E, and lacked neutralizing antibody in their sera to rhinovirus 16 (RV16). None of the patients smoked, had active clinical asthma, or used any medication at the time of study. All patients gave informed consent before study enrollment, and the study was conducted during periods when they were free of allergic rhinitis symptoms.

For a number of reasons, we first chose to evaluate the effects of a rhinovirus illness in subjects with allergic rhinitis rather than asthma patients. First, although patients with allergic rhinitis do not have clinical asthma, their airway responsiveness is often enhanced in comparison with normal subjects [53]. Second, in patients with allergic rhinitis, it would be unlikely to find abnormal airway smooth muscle with characteristics similar to those noted in asthma (e.g., hypertrophy, hyperresponsiveness, or inflammation) to complicate the effects that a respiratory illness may have on pulmonary function. Third, none of the patients required bronchodilator medication, which could interfere with the interpretation of changes in airway function. Finally, we were concerned that an acute airway infection could provoke an attack of wheezing in patients with underlying asthma.

Study Design. The patients were studied on three separate occasions, separated by 28-day intervals, as indicated by the schematic protocol in Fig. 1: baseline, acute URI, and recovery. At each study period, the patients were evaluated on three consecutive days. Evaluations consisted of, first, spirometry (FEV_1, FVC, $FEF_{25-75\%}$), which was performed before initiating bronchoprovocation studies; second, airway reactivity, which was measured by bronchoprovocation on separate days with aerosols of histamine (preantigen), ragweed antigen, and histamine again (postantigen); and third, leukocyte histamine release, which was measured on each of the three study occasions before any bronchoprovocation (the results of which will not be discussed).

Airway responsiveness to histamine and ragweed antigen was determined in the patients by standard bronchial provocation techniques with increasing concentrations of either histamine or ragweed antigen aerosol delivered through a DeVilbiss nebulizer (DeVilbiss Co., Somerset, Pennsylvania) attached to a French–Rosenthal dosimeter [55]. Bronchial provocation was performed by having the patient inhale from functional residual capacity to vital capacity with a 10-s breath hold [56]. Histamine concentrations (0.03, 0.06, 0.12, 0.25, 0.5, 1.0, 2.0, 5.0, 10.0, and 25.0 mg/ml) were prepared from a stock solution and diluted in buffered saline (pH 7.4). Similarly, extracts of ragweed antigen in increasing concentrations (0.5, 1.0, 5.0, 10.0, 50.0, 100.0, 500.0, and 1,000.0 protein nitrogen units [PNU]/ml) were prepared from a stock solution (20,000 PNU/ml) and diluted in buffered saline (pH 7.4). In a later series of experiments [57], and in a similar fashion, methacholine was inhaled at increasing concentrations (0.04, 0.08, 0.16, 0.32, 0.63, 1.25, 2.5, 5.0, 10.0, and 25.0 mg/ml).

If an initial aerosol of buffered saline did not significantly change the baseline FEV_1, increasing concentrations of histamine or methacholine were given at 5-min intervals until the FEV_1 fell at least 20% from the baseline measurement and was sustained at this level for 5 min. Spirometry was performed, and the best of three efforts for the FEV_1 was selected to construct a dose-response plot for histamine or methacholine aerosol. From this plot, the dose of histamine or methacholine required to produce a 20% decrease in FEV_1 was calculated and defined as the provocative dose 20% (PD_{20}).

The principles for antigen bronchoprovocation challenge with ragweed extract

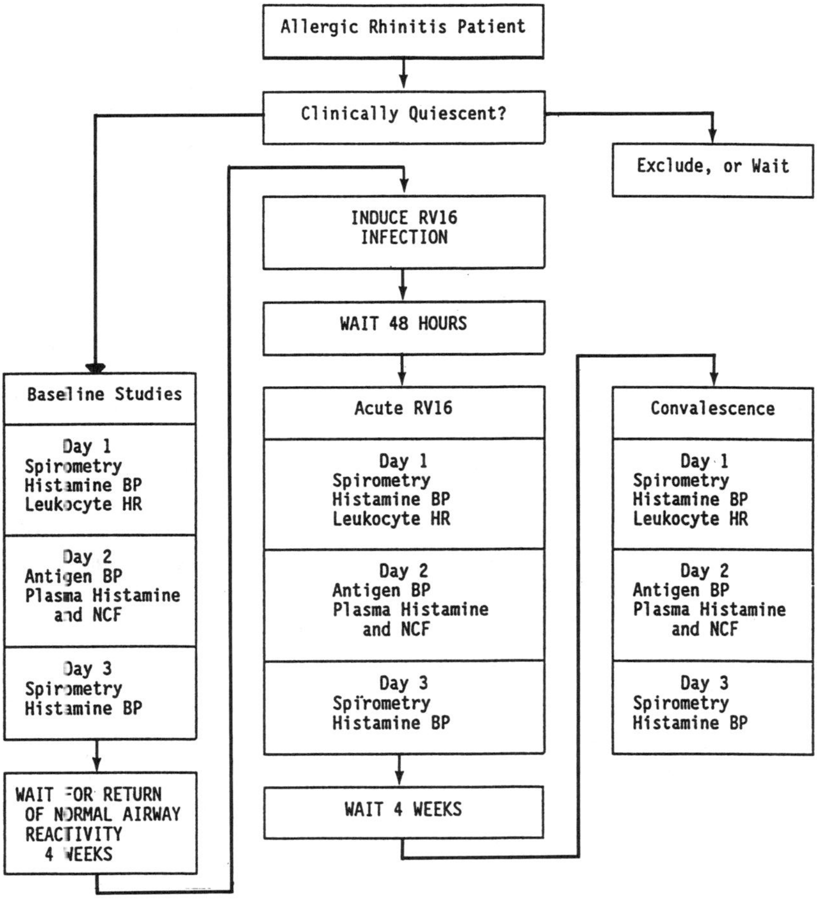

Figure 1 Schematic experimental design for rhinovirus 16 (RV16) inoculation. BP = bronchoprovocation; HR = histamine release; NCF = neutrophil chemotactic factor.

were similar to those described for histamine and methacholine, except that increases in concentration were separated by 10-min intervals. Antigen concentration was increased until the FEV_1 fell at least 20% and was maintained at this level for 10 min. Following antigen challenge, pulmonary function tests were repeated at 0.5, 1, 2, 3, 4, 5, 6, 7, and 8 h to determine whether a late asthmatic response (LAR) occurred (> 15% decrease in FEV_1 from baseline values).

Rhinovirus 16 Inoculation and Confirmation of a Viral Infection. The technique for rhinovirus inoculation followed previously described methods [56,58]. Briefly, no patients had neutralizing antibody in their sera (< 1:1) against a 20–25 tissue culture infective dose 50% ($TCID_{50}$) of RV16 challenge. Rhinoviral colds were induced in the donors by instilling, on 2 successive days, 0.25 ml of RV16 suspension into each nostril by pipette (320–3200 $TCID_{50}$) and then spraying approximately the same amount into each nostril with an atomizer (De Vilbiss, No. 286; De Vilbiss Company, Somerset, Pennsylvania) powered by a De Vilbiss 561 series compressor. The coarse spray coated the nasal cavity well (as visualized by a headlamp).

Colds were evaluated with a questionnaire that was completed by the participant hourly during waking hours [59]. Symptoms evaluated included cough, nasal discharge, sneezing, stuffy nose, headache, malaises, chills, and fever. Symptoms were graded 0 = absent, 1 = mild, 2 = moderate, and 3 = severe. Total symptom scores of ≥12 defined a severe cold, 7–11 a moderate cold, and <7 a mild cold.

Virus being shed by the inoculated subjects was assayed by titration of a nasal wash into diploid (WI-38) cell cultures. Nasal washes were taken by instilling 5 ml of HBSS with 0.5% gelatin into each nostril, holding for 5 s, and then expelling into a sterile petri dish. Nasal washes were inoculated into WI-38, primary rhesus monkey, and HEp-2 cell cultures, and postexperimental washings into WI-38 cells only [58,59]. Etiology was established by at least one identified isolate and/or by a fourfold or greater increase in neutralizing antibody in the convalescent serum specimens [58]. Antibody titers were expressed as initial serum dilutions in which 1:1 = undiluted serum, 1:2 = one part serum and one part diluent, etc.

The Results of Rhinovirus 16 Inoculation. Nine of the ten patients inoculated with RV16 had this virus identified in nasal washes (Table 1). Moreover, eight of the nine patients from whom convalescent sera were available had at least a fourfold rise in RV16-specific antibody. Another patient was shedding a wild rhinovirus at the time of inoculation and continued to shed this virus throughout the experiment. Because he was infected with rhinovirus, his data were included in the study evaluation.

The Effect of Rhinovirus Infection on Pulmonary Function and Airway Responsiveness. Spirometry values (FEV_1, vital capacity, $FEF_{25-75\%}$) were similar at each of the three study periods, preinfection, acute infection, and postinfection, and were ≥95% of the predicted representative values for each patient. Therefore, in no patient was the acute infection associated with a significant change in pulmonary function. This stable level of pulmonary function becomes important in evaluating airway responsiveness in the challenge studies, as changes in baseline levels of airway obstruction may alter the response to inhaled constricting agents independently of altered reactivity.

During the acute rhinovirus infection, airway reactivity to histamine was significantly enhanced from baseline values. The mean value for the histamine PD_{20} has a large standard error, which indicates the wide range of PD_{20} determinations to aerosol histamine, 8.8–300 cumulative breath units, in the allergic rhinitis

Table 1 The Clinical Response to Rhinovirus 16 Inoculation

Patient	Highest symptom score	Highest virus titer ($TCID_{50}$/ml)	Highest mucus index[a]	Convalescent titers
1	6	100,000	2	≥1:45
2	9	3,200	1	1:8
3	5	3,200	0.5	1:32
4	14	320,000	1.5	≥1:45
5	13.5	1,000,000	2	1:23
6	6	320,000	1	1:16
7	6	≥3,200,000	3	ND
8[b]	12	3,200	1	1:23
9	16	10,000	1	1:64
10[c]	5	320	0.25	<1:1

[a]Indicates the amount of nasal mucus in the nasal wash: 0 = none; 1 = ⅓ mucus; 2 = ⅔ mucus; 3 = all mucus.
[b]No data for leukocyte histamine release.
[c]This patient was shedding a wild rhinovirus (not RV16) at the time of inoculation. None of the subsequent isolates were inhibited by RV16 antisera, nor did the patient seroconvert. It appears that the wild rhinovirus prevented inhibition by RV16, but the evidence is not unequivocal; the nasal wash suspensions were not incubated in antisera to this wild rhinovirus and then tested for breakthrough RV16.
$TCID_{50}$ = tissue culture infective dose 50%; ND = Not done.
Source: From Ref. 53.

patients studied (Fig. 2). However, only one of the patients failed to have a fall in the histamine PD_{20} value during the acute rhinovirus respiratory infection. Airway reactivity to ragweed antigen was also significantly enhanced over preinfection values during the acute viral respiratory illness. The relative change in acute airway responsiveness to histamine and ragweed antigen was similar during infection when compared with baseline values. This suggested to us that the acute changes in airway reactivity to inhaled antigen represented changes in nonspecific bronchial responsiveness rather than intrinsic alteration in mast cell secretion. However, to test this possibility, a direct measurement of pulmonary mast cell secretion during antigen provocations would be necessary.

When airway reactivity to histamine was determined 24 h after ragweed antigen challenge, a significant ($p < 0.036$) enhancement in airway reactivity from pre–antigen challenge responses was noted both at baseline and during the acute rhinovirus infection (Fig. 2). During the acute rhinovirus infection, airway reactivity to histamine, after ragweed antigen inhalation challenge, was also significantly enhanced when compared with its baseline counterpart. The relative enhancement of airway reactivity to histamine after antigen challenge during the

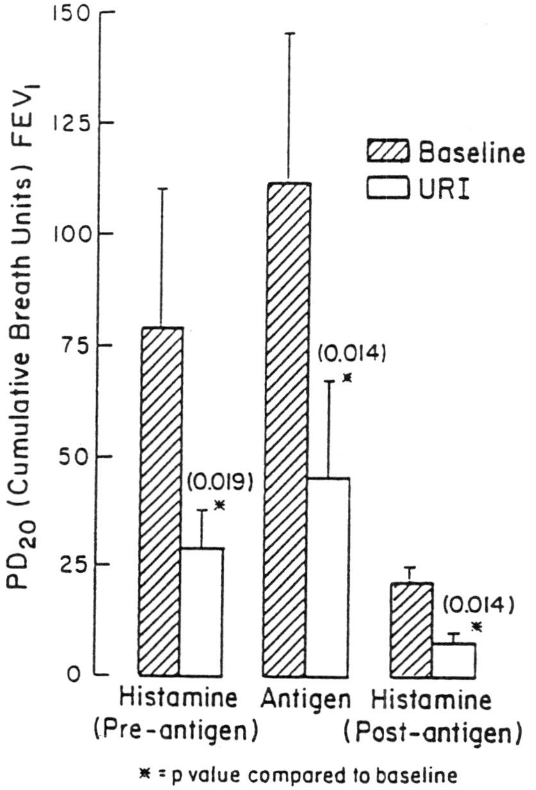

Figure 2 The effect of an acute rhinovirus respiratory infection on airway reactivity to histamine and ragweed antigen (n = 10, mean ± SEM). One inhalation unit = 1 breath of a solution with 1 mg of histamine/ml or 1 breath of antigen extract with 1000 PNU/ml. (From Ref. 53.)

respiratory infection was similar to the changes in histamine reactivity measured before viral infection.

Seven of the patients were available for evaluation of airway reactivity 4 weeks after virus infection (recovery). In these seven patients (Fig. 3), changes in the pattern of airway reactivity to histamine (preantigen) and ragweed antigen (baseline vs. URI) were similar to those described for all 10 patients (Fig. 2). However, 4 weeks after the acute rhinovirus infection, airway reactivity to histamine (preantigen) showed a return toward baseline value but was still significantly different from preinfection determinants. The PD_{20} value for antigen at recovery was less than baseline, but differences were not significant. In contrast, airway

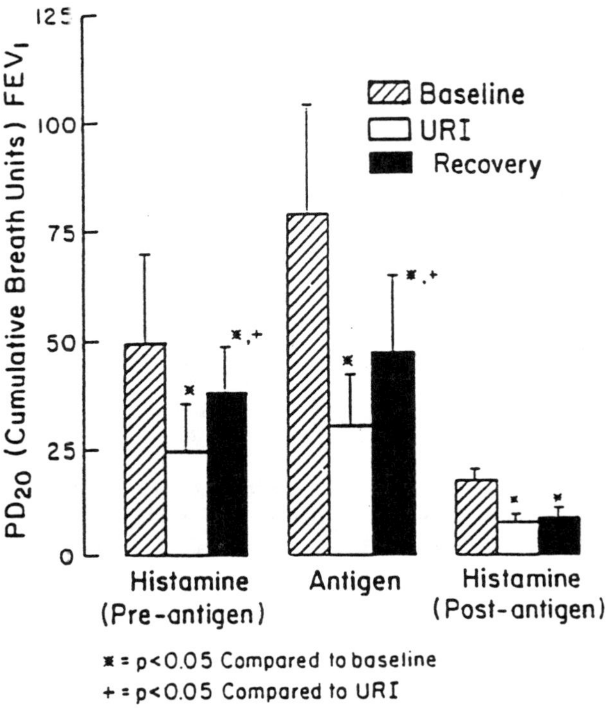

Figure 3 A comparison of the airway response to histamine and ragweed antigen at baseline, during an acute rhinovirus respiratory illness, and 4 weeks later at recovery (n = 7, mean ± SEM). (From Ref. 53.)

reactivity to histamine after antigen challenge remained unchanged from values during the acute URI.

These observations indicate a number of important effects of the preceding viral infection on airway reactivity. First, enhanced nonspecific airway reactivity persisted in the allergic rhinitis patients for at least 4 weeks after infection. Second, the enhanced airway reactivity following antigen challenge did not change 4 weeks after infection. Moreover, these data raised the possibility that events associated with the nonacute reaction to antigen challenge, in particular the late-phase reaction (LPR), were also susceptible to change during the viral infection.

The Effect of Rhinovirus Infection on the Development of Late-Phase Reactions. Following bronchoprovocation with ragweed antigen, all patients were evaluated for the development of LPRs, which we defined as a 15% drop in FEV_1 within 8 h of antigen challenge. At baseline (preinfection) evaluation, only one

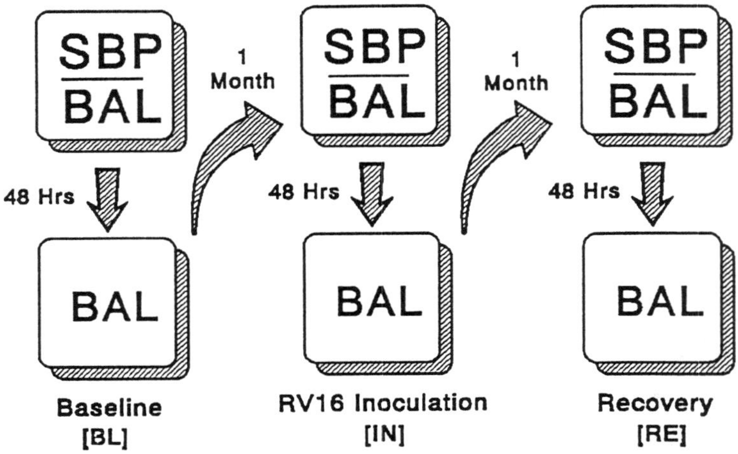

Figure 4 Experimental Design. Each subject underwent paired bronchoalveolar lavage (BAL) studies in each of three phases: baseline (before rhinovirus 16 [RV16] inoculation), RV16 (during acute RV16 infection), and recovery. Each phase was separated in time by 1 month. Segmental bronchoprovocation (SBP) with saline and antigen was performed. Forty-eight hours later, BAL fluids were obtained from each of the previously challenged segments. For details, see text. (Adapted from Ref. 64 with permission.)

of the 10 subjects had an LPR. When the same evaluation was performed during acute RV infection, eight of 10 subjects had LPRs ($p = 0.0085$, McNemar's test). If the relationship between the development of an LPR was compared with indices of airway reactivity, no correlations were found between the LPR and PD_{20} values for histamine or antigen, or between changes in those values from baseline measurements. This indicated that the development of an LPR was independent of enhanced airway reactivity found during the cold. Furthermore, there was no significant difference between the immediate fall in FEV_1 to inhaled antigen at baseline and during the URI. Moreover, there was no correlation between the fall in FEV_1 to antigen at baseline or during the URI and the development of LPRs. Thus, our data indicate that the development of a LPR was also independent of the intensity of the immediate response to antigen.

The Effect of Antigen Provocation on Airway Responsiveness Independent of Rhinovirus 16 Infections. Because antigen provocation caused enhanced airway responsiveness to aerosol histamine, we were interested in the duration of this effect independent of rhinovirus infection. In a subsequent series of experiments, seven of the allergic rhinitis subjects from this study were reevaluated. We found that the enhanced airway responsiveness to histamine that follows antigen provocation lasts less than 2 weeks in these allergic rhinitis patients (Table 2). Since the effects of rhinovirus on airway responsiveness were evaluated 4 weeks after an antigen challenge, the initial antigen challenge at baseline should not have caused enhanced bronchial responsiveness during the acute rhinovirus infection.

3. The Effect of Rhinovirus 16 Infection on Airway Response to Local Antigen Challenge

The previous studies strongly suggested that the airway inflammatory response to antigen was enhanced during the rhinovirus illness. To evaluate this possibility, a more direct assessment of the airway, and its response to antigen, was necessary. Several groups have used bronchoscopy and various bronchoscopic techniques to assess lower airway and pulmonary inflammation in asthma. Recently, we and others have incorporated the techniques of segmental bronchoprovocation (SBP) with antigen to evaluate more precisely mechanisms of airway inflammation in allergic and asthmatic subjects [57,60,61]. We found that antigen SBP in allergic rhinitis subjects is associated with a marked increase in levels of mast cell mediators (histamine and tryptase) 5–10 min after the challenges and cellular inflammation with predominance of eosinophil at 48 h after the challenge [57]. Since viral infections are associated with increased nonspecific airway responsiveness and enhanced LPRs, we postulated that antigen-induced airway inflammation would also be more pronounced following a viral respiratory tract infection. To test this hypotheses, we performed the investigation described below [64].

Patient Selection. Eight subjects with allergic rhinitis (AR) and five normal volunteers (NV) were selected. All had a history of rhinitis and positive prick skin test to one or more common aeroallergens including ragweed (Greer Laboratories, Lenoir, North Carolina) and no serum neutralizing antibody to RV16. Normal

Table 2 The Effect of Ragweed Antigen Challenge on Histamine PD_{20} Values and Their Recovery[a]

	PD_{20} Histamine values	
Baseline	24-Hours post-antigen	2-Weeks post-antigen
76.3 ± 33.3	27.1 ± 10.6*	72.1 ± 27.2

[a]Values are mean ± SEM; n = 7.
$^*p = 0.22$, compared with baseline and 2 weeks after antigen challenge, by Wilcoxon paired analysis.

volunteers had negative skin tests to the same allergens. All subjects were generally healthy, nonsmoking adults who gave informed consent to participation in the following study.

Study Design. Subjects were initially screened with a histamine challenge to determine histamine PD_{20} and an aerosol ragweed antigen challenge to determine antigen PD_{20} [56]. These assessments were completed 1 month before the first bronchoscopy.

Each subject enrolled in this study was evaluated by paired bronchoscopy, antigen SBP, and bronchoalveolar lavage (BAL) on three separate occasions: (1) baseline (before inoculation), (2) during RV16 infection, and (3) during the recovery period (Fig. 4). The three study phases were separated by a minimum of 1-month intervals. In each phase a bronchoscopy was performed, during which SBP was done in two pulmonary segments. The first segment received saline (control), and a second segment (contralateral lung) received ragweed antigen. Bronchoalveolar lavage was done from each segment 5 min after SBP. Forty-eight hours later, a repeat bronchoscopy was performed and BAL done in each of the two previously challenged segments.

Rhinovirus 16 Inoculation. The technique used in RV16 inoculation was described earlier. Viral inoculations were completed 48 h before bronchoscopy. Colds were evaluated by questionnaire as detailed above. Nasal wash, BAL fluid, BAL cells, and BAL fluid supernatant were inoculated onto WI-38 cell line to evaluate viral shedding.

Bronchoscopy Segmental Bronchoprovocation, and Bronchoalveolar Lavage. Bronchoscopy and BAL were done as previously described [62,63]. All procedures were started between 6 and 8 a.m. Spirometry was first obtained, premedication was given (atropine 0.6 mg intramuscularly, midazolam 1.2 mg intramuscularly), and nasopharyngeal anesthesia was achieved with topical cocaine 4% and lidocaine 1%. The fiberoptic bronchoscope was introduced into the airway and wedged into a bronchopulmonary segment. Typically, a segment in the right middle lobe or lingula was selected for study. The SBP with saline was done by instilling 10 ml of 0.9% NaCl followed by a 5-ml air flush. After a 5-min dwell time, BAL was performed by instilling two 60-ml aliquots of sterile saline (37°C). The fluid was immediately withdrawn and the return material pooled. A second segment in the contralateral lung was then identified, and the scope was wedged. Segmental bronchoprovocation instillation of ragweed antigen was done. In these studies, the amount of antigen used was equal to 20% of the calculated cumulative antigen PD_{20}. After a 5-ml air flush and 5-min dwell time, BAL was done as in the saline segment. The two BAL samples were taken to the laboratory for immediate processing. Forty-eight hours later a repeat bronchoscopy was performed, the same two segments were identified, and BAL was done in each of them as described above.

Bronchoalveolar Lavage Processing. The BAL fluid from each segment was analyzed separately. Cells were recovered by centrifugation, washed, and counted in a hemocytometer [57]. The supernatant was frozen (−70°C) until analyzed later for total protein, histamine [62], and tryptase [60,62].

Changes in Pulmonary Function Following Rhinovirus 16 Inoculation. All eight subjects with allergic rhinitis and all five normal volunteers inoculated with RV16 became infected and clinically symptomatic; however, only in one normal volunteer was RV16 detected in the lower airway (a very low titer in this patient).

No significant changes in pulmonary function were noted after RV16 infection in either the allergic rhinitis group or the normal volunteer group. The FEV_1 measured immediately before bronchoscopy was similar on both study days in all three phases.

Changes in Airway Response to Antigen Following Rhinovirus 16 Inoculation. Segmental bronchoprovocation and BAL were performed in all subjects without difficulty. Volume return was similar on both days and in all three phases. Thus, correction for volume was not necessary when expressing mediator or cellular data.

Mediator Response: Histamine and Tryptase. In the saline-challenged segment, histamine content was greater in allergic rhinitis subjects than in normal volunteers immediately following the challenge. Rhinovirus 16 infection did not influence levels of BAL histamine in the saline-challenged segment. In contrast, following antigen SBP, histamine levels were significantly increased in the immediate BAL samples in allergic rhinitis subjects, but not in normal volunteers. There was a further increase in histamine levels following RV-16 infection (inoculation and recovery phases) (Fig. 5). Histamine level in BAL fluid obtained 48 h after SBP (late) were still higher in allergic rhinitis subjects than in normal volunteers.

To determine the possibility that repetitive airway antigen challenge could alter the allergic response, the following study was performed. Four allergic rhinitis subjects had repeat bronchoscopy with antigen SBP alone, without RV16 infection; this did not potentiate the histamine rise seen immediately following antigen SBP.

Bronchoalveolar lavage fluid tryptase levels were higher in allergic rhinitis subjects than in normal volunteers following saline challenge. Immediately following antigen SBP, BAL fluid tryptase levels increased significantly in comparison with saline (Table 3). The rise in tryptase was significantly enhanced following RV-16 infection, but only in allergic rhinitis subjects. Repeated bronchoscopy and antigen SBP in the four allergic rhinitis subjects did not affect tryptase response when there was no intervening respiratory viral illness.

Cellular Response: Total Cells and Eosinophils. Total leukocyte recovery in the immediate BAL fluid was similar in all three phases in both groups of subjects. Rhinovirus 16 infection did not influence the number of cells recovered imme-

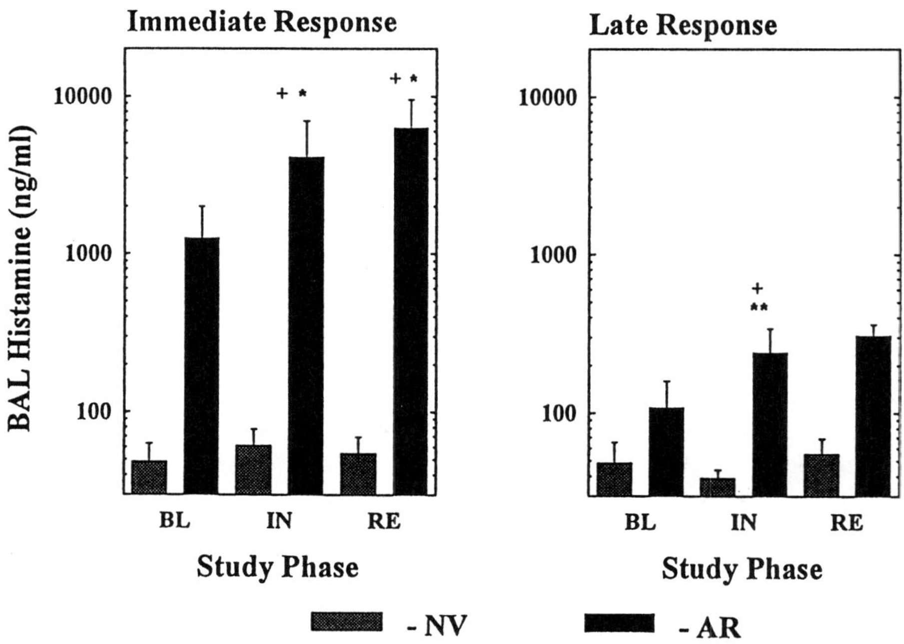

Figure 5 Histamine concentrations in bronchoalveolar lavage (BAL) following antigen challenge. The immediate response (5 min) to antigen challenge is shown in the left panel, and the late (48 h) response is depicted on the right. Solid bars represent allergic rhinitis subjects (AR), and crosshatched bars normal volunteers (NV). Error bars depict the SEM. Statistical significance subjects is indicated:

$*p < 0.05$, $**p < 0.01$, $***p < 0.001$ for AR vs. NV, paired *t*-test or Wilcoxon test
$\dagger p \leqslant 0.05$ vs. baseline phase, post-hoc test

Note the logarithmic scale of the ordinate. Significant enhancement of antigen-driven histamine release is seen in relationship to rhinovirus 16 (RV16) infection in both immediate and late fluids from AR subjects (ANOVA for effect of RV16 infection on histamine concentration in antigen challenged segments: $p < 0.005$, immediate; $p < 0.0001$, late). No effect of virus was observed in NV subjects.

diately following antigen or saline challenge in either group (Fig. 6). However, in the late lavage sample there was a marked increase in recovered cell numbers after antigen challenge in allergic rhinitis subjects; this response was potentiated by the rhinovirus infection. No enhancement in cell recovery to antigen followed rhinovirus infection in normal volunteers (Fig. 3).

The four allergic rhinitis subjects challenged on two separate occasions showed an increase of total cells in the late lavage samples that was similar on both

Table 3 Bronchoalveolar Lavage (BAL) Tryptase Immediately Following Antigen Challenge[a]

Group	Challenge	Baseline	Inoculation	Recovery	p^b
NV	S	0.36 ± 0.06	0.30 ± 0.03	0.33 ± 0.03	>0.9
	A	0.28 ± 0.03	0.28 ± 0.02	0.28 ± 0.03	0.9
AR	S	0.38 ± 0.05	0.43 ± 0.11	0.41 ± 0.06	>0.9
	A	[c]1.26 ± 0.5 [d]	[c]1.74 ± 0.58[d]	[c] 3.24 ± 1.40 [d]	<0.01

[a]Tryptase expressed as ng/ml, mean ± SEM, from BAL fluids obtained 5 min following antigen challenge.
[b]ANOVA for effect of rhinovirus 16 inoculation in indicated subset. Other statistical comparisons: ANOVA for effect of allergy in saline-challenged segments, $p < 0.02$; ANOVA for effect of allergy in antigen-challenged segments, $p < 0.0001$.
[c]$p < 0.05$ AR vs. NV, antigen-challenged segments, Mann-Whitney U-test.
[d]$p < 0.05$, antigen vs. saline, AR subjects, Mann-Whitney U-test.
NV = normal volunteers; AR = allergic rhinitis subjects; S = saline; A = antigen.
(Adapted from Ref. 64 with permission.)

occasions (first challenge, 27.8 ± 6.3 million total cells, vs. second challenge, 52.6 ± 16.4 million, p = NS).

The numbers of eosinophils recovered in BAL fluid immediately after saline challenge were very small, and similar in normal volunteers and allergic rhinitis subjects. Bronchoalveolar lavage fluid obtained 48 h following antigen challenge showed a remarkable increase in eosinophils, but only in allergic rhinitis subjects; this was a significant potentiation of the eosinophil response to antigen with the RV16 infection (Fig. 7).

Repetitive SBP with antigen, without RV16 infection, did not potentiate the eosinophil response to antigen (first challenge, 39 ± 17 million total cells, vs. second challenge, 27 ± 13 million, p = NS).

Summary. A number of significant conclusions can be drawn from these studies. An experimental RV16 infection potentiates mediator release immediately following segmental airway antigen challenge. In addition, cellular inflammation noted 48 h later is also enhanced. These virus-promoted effects were still present 1 month after viral inoculation. This study provides direct evidence that allergic subjects have an enhanced inflammatory airway response to antigen during viral infection. These changes in the airway may explain, at least in part, the increased likelihood of the development of LPRs following antigen challenge seen during viral infection with RV16 [53].

4. Conclusion

Investigations both in animals and humans have provided insight into various immunoinflammatory networks that may affect airway physiological responses during viral infections. These intriguing observations should provide the impetus

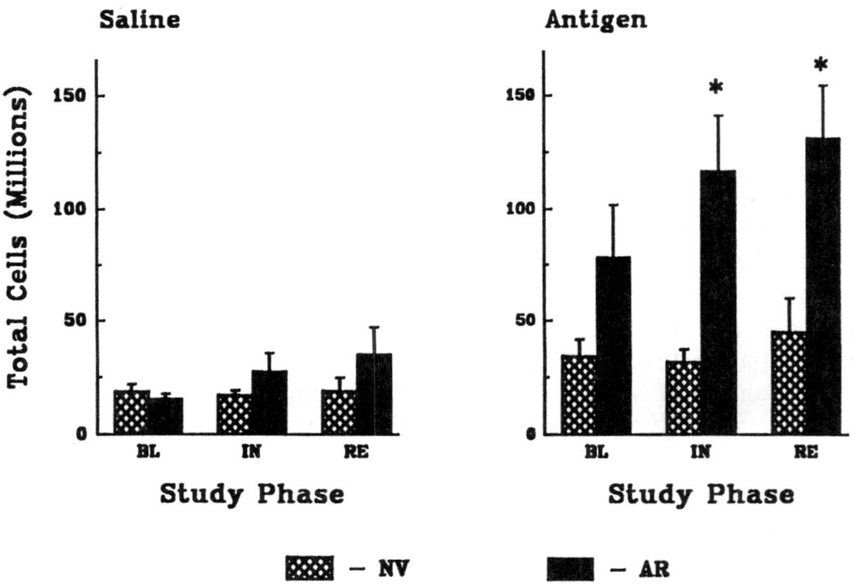

Figure 6 Total cells recovered by bronchoalveolar lavage following antigen and saline challenge. Conventions and format are similar to those described in Fig. 2, except that the 48-h data are shown after saline or antigen challenge. The left panel shows cell recruitment following saline, and the right following antigen challenge. The influence on potentiated cell recovery during and after rhinovirus 16 infection was seen predominantly in late fluids from allergic rhinitis (AR) subjects. Cell recovery was nearly always greater from AR subjects than normal volunteers (NV). A significant effect of RV16 infection was noted only in late samples, and only in AR subjects (ANOVA for effect of RV16 in antigen challenged samples: $p < 0.0001$). BL = baseline; IN = inoculation; RE = recovery.
(Adapted from Ref. 64 with permission.)

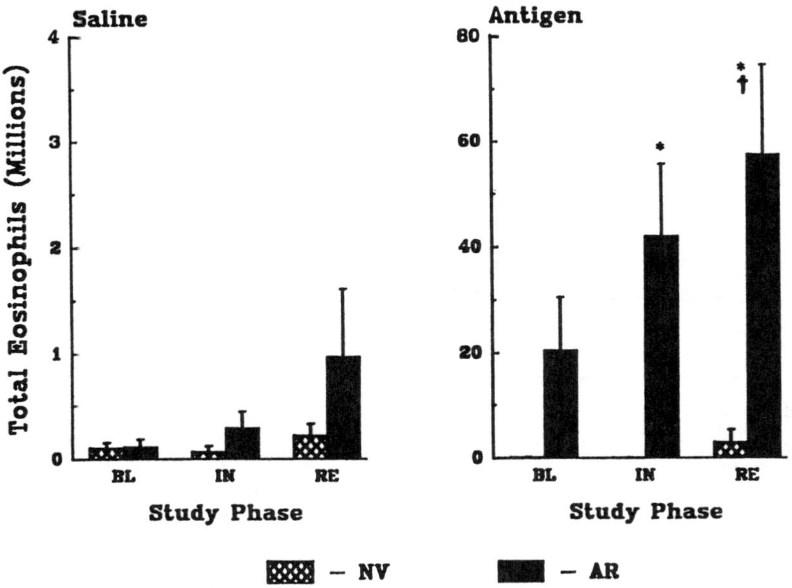

Figure 7 Eosinophil response to rhinovirus 16 (RV16) infection and antigen challenge. Conventions and format are as described in Fig. 3. Note that the scale of the ordinate differs markedly (20-fold) in the two panels. The numbers of recovered eosinophils in normal volunteers (NV) in the right panel during baseline (BL) and inoculation (IN) phases were small, and are not visible at the scale of this axis. Striking increases in eosinophil recovery were seen in late-response fluids from allergic rhinitis (AR) subjects and were potentiated by RV16. The effect of RV16 on eosinophil recruitment was significant only for AR and only in late samples (ANOVA for effect of RV16: $p < 0.0001$). RE = recovery. (Adapted from Ref. 64 with permission.)

for the design of future experiments, which need to address the fact that not all viral infections produce the same end-point clinical responses.

The use of direct evaluation techniques such as bronchoscopy, BAL, and bronchial biopsy and the advent of molecular biological techniques capable of detecting gene products of the virus and inflammatory proteins should allow us to amplify our present knowledge and resolve these perplexing issues.

REFERENCES

1. McIntosh, K., Ellis, E. F., Hoffman, L. S., Lybass, T. G., Eller, J. J., and Fulginiti, V. A., The association of viral and bacterial respiratory infections with exacerbations of wheezing in young asthmatic children, *J. Pediatr.*, *83*, 578–590 (1973).
2. Minor, T. E., Dick, E. C., DeMeo, A. N., Ouellette, J. J., Cohen, M., and Reed,

C. E., Viruses as precipitants of asthmatic attacks in children, *JAMA*, *227*, 292–298 (1974).

3. Henderson, F. W., Clyde, W. A., Jr., Collier, A. M., Denny, F. W., Senior, R. J., Sheaffer, C. I., Conley, W. G., III, and Christian, R. M., The etiology and epidemiologic spectrum of bronchiolitis in pediatric practice, *J. Pediatr.*, *95*, 183–190 (1972).
4. Minor, T. E., Dick, E. C., Baker, J. W., Ouellette, J. J., Cohen, M., and Reed, C. E., Rhinovirus and influenza type A infections as precipitants of asthma, *Am. Rev. Respir. Dis.*, *113*, 149–153 (1976).
5. Hudgel, D. W., Langston, C., Jr., Selner, J. C., and McIntosh, K., Viral and bacterial infections in adults with chronic asthma, *Am. Rev. Respir. Dis.*, *120*, 393–397 (1979).
6. Picken, J. J., Niewoehner, D. E., and Chester, E. H., Prolonged effects of viral infections of the upper respiratory tract upon small airways, *Am. J. Med.*, *52*, 738–746 (1972).
7. Cate, T. R., Roberts, J. S., Russ, M. A., and Pierce, J. A., Effects of common cold on pulmonary function, *Am. Rev. Respir. Dis.*, *108*, 858–865 (1973).
8. Fridy, W. W., Ingram, R. H., Hierholzer, J. C., and Coleman, M. T., Airways function during mild viral respiratory illnesses, *80*, 150–155 (1974).
9. Hall, W. J., Douglas, R. G., Jr., Hyde, R. W., Roth, F. K., Cross, A. S., and Speers, D. M., Pulmonary mechanisms after uncomplicated influenza A infection, *Am. Rev. Respir. Dis.*, *113*, 141–147 (1976).
10. Blair, H. T., Greenberg, S. B., Stevens, P. M., Bilunos, P. A., and Couch, R. B., Effects of rhinovirus infection on pulmonary function of healthy volunteers, *Am. Rev. Respir. Dis.*, *114*, 95–102 (1976).
11. Hall, W. J., and Hall, C. B., Clinical significance of pulmonary function tests. Alteration in pulmonary function following respiratory viral infection, *Chest*, *76*, 458–465 (1976).
12. Hall, W. J., Hall, C. B., and Speers, D. M., Respiratory syncytial virus infection in adults, *Ann. Intern. Med.*, *88*, 203–205 (1978).
13. Empey, D. W., Laitinen, L. A., Jacobs, L., Gold, W. M., and Nadel, J. A., Mechanisms of bronchial hyperreactivity in normal subjects after upper respiratory tract infection, *Am. Rev. Respir. Dis.*, *113*, 131–139 (1976).
14. Zweiman, B., Schoenwetter, W. F., Pappano, J. E., Tempest, B., and Hildreth, E. A., Patterns of allergic respiratory disease in children with a past history of bronchiolitis, *J. Allergy*, *48*, 283–289 (1971).
15. Rooney, J. C., and Williams, H. E., The relationship between proven viral bronchiolitis and subsequent wheezing, *J. Pediatr.*, *79*, 744–747 (1971).
16. Gurwitz, D., Mindorff, C., and Levison, H., Increased incidence of bronchial reactivity in children with a history of bronchiolitis, *J. Pediatr.*, *98*, 551–555 (1981).
17. Saban, R., Dick, E. C., Fishleder, R. I., and Buckner, C. K., Enhancement by parainfluenza 3 infection of contractile responses to substance P and capsaicin in airway smooth muscle from the guinea pig, *Am. Rev. Respir. Dis.*, *136*, 586–591 (1987).
18. Buckner, C. K., Songsiridej, V., Dick, E. C., and Busse, W. W., In vivo and in vitro studies on the use of the guinea pig as a model for virus-provoked airway hyperreactivity, *Am. Rev. Respir. Dis.*, *132*, 305–310 (1985).

19. Dusser, D. J., Jacoby, D. B., Djokic, T. D., Rubinstein, I., Borson, D. B., and Nadel J. A., Virus induces airway hyperresponsiveness to tachykinins: role of neutral endopeptidase, *J. Appl. Physiol.*, *67*, 1504–1511 (1989).
20. Folkerts, G., Verheyen, A., Janssen, M., and Nijkamp, F. P., Virus-induced airway hyperresponsiveness in the guinea pig can be transferred by bronchoalveolar cells, *J. Allergy Clin. Immunol.*, *90*, 364–372 (1992).
21. Fryer, A. D., and Jacoby, D. B., Parainfluenza virus infection damages inhibitory M2 muscarinic receptors on pulmonary parasympathetic nerves in the guinea pig, *Br. J. Pharmacol.*, *102*, 267–271 (1991).
22. Jacoby, D. B., Tamaoki, J., Borson, D. B., and Nadel, J. A., Influenza infection causes airway hyperresponsiveness by decreasing enkephalinase, *J. Appl. Physiol.*, *64*, 2653–2658 (1988).
23. Lemen, R. J., Quan, S. F., Witten, M. L., Sobonya, R. E., Ray, C. G., and Grad, R., Canine parainfluenza type 2 bronchiolitis increases histamine responsiveness in beagle puppies, *Am. Rev. Respir. Dis.*, *141*, 199–207 (1990).
24. Scarpace, P. J., and Bender, B. S., Viral pneumonia attenuates adenylte cyclase but not beta-adrenergic receptors in murine lung, *Am. Rev. Respir. Dis.*, *140*, 1602–1606 (1989).
25. Allan, W., Carding, S. R., Eichelberger, M., and Doherty, P. C., Analyzing the distribution of cells expressing mRNA for T-cell receptor gamma and delta chains in a virus-induced inflammatory process, *Cell Immunol.*, *143*, 55–65 (1992).
26. Scherle, P. A., Palladino, G., and Gerhard, W., Mice can recover from pulmonary influenza virus infection in the absence of class I–restricted cytotoxic T cells, *J. Immunol.*, *148*, 212–217 (1992).
27. Kimsey, P. B., Pecquet, Goad, M. E., Zhi-bo, Z., Brackee, G., and Fox, J. G., Methyl prednisolone acetate modulation of infection and subsequent pulmonary pathology in hamsters exposed to parainfluenza-1 virus (Sendai), *Am. Rev. Respir. Dis.*, *140*, 1704–1711 (1989).
28. Hennet, T., Ziltener, H. J., Frei, K., and Peterhans, E., A kinetic study of immune mediators in the lungs of mice infected with influenza-A virus, *J. Immunol.*, *149*, 932–939 (1992).
29. Sorkness, R., Lemanske, R. F., Jr., and Castleman, W. L., Persistent airway hyperresponsiveness after neonatal viral bronchiolitis in rats, *J. Appl. Physiol.*, *70*, 375–383 (1991).
30. Castleman, W. L., Sorkness, R. L., Lemanske, R. F., Jr., and McAllister, P. K., Viral bronchiolitis during early life induces increased numbers of bronchiolar mast cells and airway hyperresponsiveness, *Am. J. Pathol.*, *137*, 821–831 (1990).
31. Castleman, W. L., Sorkness, R. L., Lemanske, R. F., Jr., Grasee, G., and Suyemoto, M. M., Neonatal viral bronchiolitis and pneumonia induce bronchiolar hypoplasia and alveolar dysplasia in rats, *Lab. Invest.*, *59*, 387–396 (1988).
32. Sorkness, R., Clough, J., Castleman, W., and Lemanske, R. F., Jr., Persistent abnormalities in lung physiology and airway parasympathetic conduction after parainfluenza type 1 infection in adult rats (abstract), *Am. Rev. Respir. Dis.*, *145*, A462 (1992).
33. Sheth, K. K., Sorkness, R. L., Clough, J. J., McAllister, P. K., Castleman, W. L., and

Lemanske, R. F., Jr., Reversal of persistent post-bronchiolitis airway abnormalities with dexamethasone in rats, *J. Appl. Physiol.*, 1993 (in press).

34. Piedimonte, G., Nadel, J. A., Umeno, E., and Mcdonald, D. M., Sendai virus infection potentiates neurogenic inflammation in the rat trachea, *J. Appl. Physiol.*, *68*, 754–760 (1990).
35. Mcdonald, D. M., Respiratory tract infections increase susceptibility to neurogenic inflammation in the rat trachea, *Am. Rev. Respir. Dis.*, *137*, 1432–1440 (1988).
36. Oosterhout, A. J. M., and Nijkamp, F. P., Minireview: lymphocytes and bronchial hyperresponsiveness, *Life Sci.*, *46*, 1255–1264 (1990).
37. Castleman, W. L., Brundage-Anguish, L. J., Kreitzer, L., and Neuenschwander, S. B., Pathogenesis of bronchiolitis and pneumonia induced in neonatal and weanling rats by parainfluenza (Sendai) virus, *Am. J. Pathol.*, *129*, 277–286 (1987).
38. Sorden, S. D., and Castleman, W. L., Brown Norway rats are high responders to bronchiolitis, pneumonia, and bronchiolar mastocytosis induced by parainfluenza virus, *Exp. Lung Res.*, *17*, 1025–1045 (1991).
39. Sorkness, R., Clough, J., Ritter, M., and Lemanske, R. F., Anesthetic effects on pulmonary allergic responses in rats—changes in sensitivity to serotonin, *J. Appl. Physiol.*, *72*, 2157–2161 (1992).
40. Halperin, S. A., Eggleston, P. A., Handley, J. O., Suratt, P. M., Gröschel, D. H. M., and Swaltney, J. M., Jr., Pathogenesis of lower respiratory tract symptoms in experimental rhinovirus infection, *Am. Rev. Respir. Dis.*, *128*, 806–810 (1983).
41. Halperin, S. A., Eggleston, A. A., Beasley, P., Suratt, P., Hendley, J. O., Gröschel, D. H. M., and Gwaltney, J. M., Jr., Exacerbations of asthma in adults during experimental rhinovirus infection, *Am. Rev. Respir. Dis.*, *132*, 976–980 (1985).
42. Saban, R., Dick, E. C., Fishleder, R. I., and Buckner, C. K., Enhancement by parainfluenza 3 infection of contractile responses to substance P and capsaicin in airway smooth muscle from guinea pig, *Am. Rev. Respir. Dis.*, *136*, 586–591 (1987).
43. Buckner, C. K., Clayton, D. E., Ain-Shoka, A. A., Busse, W. W., Dick, E. C., and Shult, P., Parainfluenza 3 infection blocks the ability of a beta-adrenergic receptor agonist to inhibit antigen-induced contraction of guinea pig isolated airway smooth muscle, *J. Clin. Invest.*, *76*, 376–384 (1981).
44. Szentivanyi, A., The beta-adrenergic theory of the atopic abnormality in asthma, *J. Allergy*, *42*, 203–223 (1968).
45. Busse, W. W., Decreased granulocyte response to isoproterenol in asthma during upper respiratory infections, *Am. Rev. Respir. Dis.*, *115*, 783–791 (1977).
46. Busse, W. W., Cooper, W., Warshauer, D. M., Dick, E. C., Wallow, I. H. L., and Albrecht, R., Impairment of isoproterenol, H2 histamine, and prostaglandin E_1 response of human granulocytes after incubation in vitro with live influenza vaccines, *Am. Rev. Respir. Dis.*, *119*, 561–569 (1979).
47. Busse, W. W., Anderson, C. L., Dick, E. C., and Warshauer, D., Reduced granulocyte response to isoproterenol, histamine, and prostaglandin E_1 after in vitro incubation with rhinovirus 16, *Am. Rev. Respir. Dis.*, *122*, 641–646 (1980).
48. Welliver, R. C., Wong, D. T., Sun, M., Middleton, E., Jr., Vaughan, R. S., and Ogra, P. L., The development of respiratory syncytial virus–specific IgE and the release of histamine in nasopharyngeal secretions after infection, *N. Engl. J. Med.*, *305*, 841–846 (1981).
49. Welliver, R. C., Wong, D. T., Middleton, E., Jr., Sun, M., McCarthy, N., and Ogra,

P. L., Role of parainfluenza virus–specific IgE in pathogenesis of croup and wheezing subsequent to infection, *J. Pediatr.*, *101*, 889–896 (1982).

50. Welliver, R. L., Sun, M., Rinaldo, D., and Ogra, P. L., Predictive value of respiratory syncytial virus–specific IgE responses for recurrent wheezing following bronchiolitis, *J. Pediatr.*, *109*, 776–880 (1986).
51. Busse, W. W., Swenson, C. A., Borden, E. C., Treuhaft, M. W., and Dick, E. C., Effect of influenza A virus on leukocyte histamine release, *J. Allergy Clin. Immunol.*, *71*, 382–388 (1983).
52. Ida, S., Hooks, J. J., Siraganian, R. P., and Notkins, A. L., Enhancement of IgE-mediated histamine release from human basophils by viruses: role of interferon, *J. Exp. Med.*, *145*, 892–896 (1977).
53. Lemanske, R. F., Jr., Dick, E. C., Swenson, C. A., et al., Rhinovirus upper infection increases airway hyperreactivity and late asthmatic reactions, *J. Clin. Invest.*, *83*, 1–10 (1989).
54. Lemanske, R. F., Jr., and Kaliner, M., Late phase allergic reactions, in *Allergy: Principles and Practice*, 4th Ed. (E. Middleton, Jr., C. E. Reed, E. F. Ellis, N. F. Adkinson, Jr., J. Yunginger, and W. W. Busse, eds.), Mosby-Year Book, St. Louis, 1993, pp. 320–361.
55. Rosenthal, R. R., Differences in response between hay fever and asthmatic patients, in *Provocative Challenge Procedures: Bronchial, Oral, Nasal and Exercise* (S. Spector, ed.), Vol. I, CRC Press, Boca Raton, Florida, 1983, pp. 113–119.
56. Chai, H., Farr, R., and Froehlich, L. A., Standardization of bronchial inhalation challenge procedures, *J. Allergy Clin. Immunol.*, *56*, 323–327 (1975).
57. Calhoun, W. J., Jarjour, N. N., Gleich, G. L., Stevens, C. A., and Busse, W. W., Increased airway inflammation with segmental versus aerosol antigen challenge, *Am. Rev. Respir. Dis.*, *147*, 1465–1472 (1993).
58. D'Alessio, D. J., Peterson, J. A., and Dick, E. C., Transmission of experimental rhinovirus colds in volunteer married couples, *J. Infect. Dis.*, *133*, 28–36 (1976).
59. D'Alessio, D. J., Meschievitz, C. K., Schultz, S. B., and Dick, E. C., A model for obtaining predictable natural transmission of rhinoviruses in human volunteers, *J. Infect. Dis.*, *150*, 195–201 (1984).
60. Wenzel, S. E., Fowler, A. A., III, and Schwartz, L. B., Activation of pulmonary mast cells by bronchoalveolar allergen challenge, *Am. Rev. Respir. Dis.*, *137*, 1002–1008 (1988).
61. Liu, M. C., Hubbar, W. C., Proud, D., Stealey, B. A., Gali, S. J., Kagey-Sobotka, A., Bleecker, E. R., and Lichtenstein, L. M., Immediate and late inflammatory responses to ragweed antigen challenge of peripheral airways in allergic asthmatics, *Am. Rev. Respir. Dis.*, *144*, 51–58 (1991).
62. Jarjour, N. N., Calhoun, W. J., Schwartz, L. B., and Busse, W. W., Elevated bronchoalveolar lavage fluid histamine levels in allergic asthmatics are associated with increased airway obstruction, *Am. Rev. Respir. Dis.*, *144*, 83–87 (1991).
63. The BAL Study Group, Bronchoalveolar lavage constituents in healthy individuals, idiopathic pulmonary fibrosis and selected comparison groups, *Am. Rev. Respir. Dis.*, *141*, S169–S202 (1990).
64. Calhoun, W. J., Dick, E. C., Schwartz, L. B., and Busse, W. W., A common cold virus, rhinovirus-16, potentiates airway inflammation following segmental bronchoprovocation in allergic subjects, *J. Clin. Invest.*, (in press).

6

Air Pollutants as a Provocative Challenge in Humans

Henry Gong, Jr.

Rancho Los Amigos Medical Center, Downey, California and University of Southern California, Los Angeles, California

I. INTRODUCTION

The study of the effects of respirable pollutants in humans has been stimulated by scientific and public health implications of prior pollution catastrophes (e.g., London in late 1952) and lower but persistent contemporary levels of ambient pollutants. Current ambient concentrations of pollutants have been implicated as causes or facilitators of acute and chronic morbidity, abnormal lung structure and function, and mortality [1]. This potential for human injury is an important rationale for establishing air quality standards, but the process must be based on a credible scientific foundation. The development of this data base relies on a multidisciplinary and complementary approach utilizing animal inhalation toxicology, epidemiology, and controlled human exposures.

The direct approach of exposing human volunteers, under controlled laboratory conditions, to a small amount of inhaled pollutant for relatively brief periods has gained great acceptance and significance as a useful and efficient research tool. The capability of an exposure system or facility to control and alter pollutant concentrations, particle size, temperature, humidity, and physical activity greatly facilitates a systematic evaluation of the individual roles and interactions of these factors in producing a measured response. As a result, controlled exposures to air pollutants are conceptually similar in operation and purpose to standard nonspecific bronchial challenges, i.e., they represent provocative challenges to derive information about human airway responses.

This chapter will present an overview of the methodology and experimental design of controlled human exposure studies with air pollutants. This chapter can realistically provide only a framework and insights into methodology, capabilities, and limitations, since a standardized format for conducting controlled exposures in humans does not exist. Specifically, this chapter will explore major issues involved in planning and conducting controlled-exposure studies, such as subject selection, pollutant types, delivery systems, environmental conditions, frequency and duration of exposures, physical activities, outcome variables, statistical analysis, and safety aspects. These aspects will be reviewed from the perspective of a clinician-investigator who uses a chamber exposure facility primarily for applied research in this area. A comprehensive review of the pulmonary responses of humans to air pollutants is beyond the scope of this chapter and is addressed elsewhere [2–6]. Nevertheless, results from selected studies will be used to illustrate findings from exposures or tests and to support the rationale for experimental designs with common outdoor pollutants, e.g., ozone, sulfur dioxide, sulfuric acid, and carbon monoxide.

II. GOALS OF CONTROLLED EXPOSURES

Human health effects from inhaled pollutants do not always coincide with preconceived notions or general predictions of their specific nature, intensity, or likelihood of occurrence. Effects must be systematically evaluated to obtain specific and relevant experimental evidence. For the most part, exposure studies are largely empirical and descriptive. Controlled human exposures are largely performed to provide relevant scientific and health information about short-term effects for use in the development or review of regulatory and policy decisions. Laboratory-based studies can effectively establish the presence (or absence) of acute reversible responses and characterize exposure–or dose–response relationships [7,8]. This technique also can be employed in the investigation of occupation-related health effects. In addition to empirical dose–response research, controlled exposures can be designed to investigate the mechanisms of pollutant-induced injury in humans, by incorporating other bronchoprovocation tests, drug interventions, or bronchoalveolar lavage.

III. METHODOLOGY

A. Subjects

1. General

Volunteers for exposure studies can originate from a variety of different population samples or groups at risk (Table 1), depending on the experimental question. Selection of the appropriate type(s) of subjects is an important consideration in any

Table 1 Types of Population Sample Evaluated in Controlled Human Exposure Studies

Healthy volunteers
• Children and adolescents
• Young and elderly adults
• Different sexes and races
• Well-trained atheletes
Otherwise healthy volunteers
• Atopy
• Current or past history of smoking or passive smoking
• Acute viral upper respiratory infections
Patients with
• Asthma
• Chronic obstructive pulmonary disease
• Interstitial lung disease
• Coronary artery disease
• Occupational exposure

study, i.e., whether they are from an overall population (e.g., "adults aged 18–40 years"), a well-defined subgroup of that population (e.g., "asthmatics who use bronchodilators daily"), or a smaller subset that has been further selected on the basis of one or more rigid criteria (e.g., "asthmatics with known ozone responsiveness"). A sample from a general population may be somewhat representative, but their individual characteristics may be variable and less defined because of flexible inclusionary criteria. On the other hand, subjects from a specific subgroup (e.g., asthmatics, athletes) may be more homogeneous and better characterized, but their responses are frequently not applicable to the population as a whole. The representative nature of selected subjects with respect to the larger subgroup or population is always somewhat questionable, although the more information one has about subject characteristics, the better one can generalize to the larger group and make comparisons with data from other studies. Selection is also complicated by the practical difficulty of studying a large number of subjects in a given protocol (typically 10–20 subjects) and wide interindividual variability of response to the same pollutant exposure, suggesting that the responses of the most and least sensitive volunteers are part of a spectrum of biological responses in a putatively normally distributed population. Thus, many studies either evaluate large numbers of a general population to define this variability or focus on a small, well-characterized subgroup that is possibly sensitive to the pollutant in question. Volunteers have generally been recruited from schools or colleges, the community, clinics, or participants from previous studies, via printed or verbal advertisements that generally indicate a participation fee.

Some medications have important interactions with pollutants and must be either temporarily withdrawn or used in a well-standardized manner during a study protocol. For example, indomethacin [9,10], and possibly large doses of vitamins E and C [11] can attenuate pulmonary responses to ozone. Oral theophylline [12], inhaled albuterol [13] and metaproterenol [14,15], cromolyn with or without ipratropium bromide [16–19], and nedocromil [20] can prevent or mitigate responses to sulfur dioxide in asthmatics or subjects with hyperreactive airways. A 3-week course of inhaled beclomethasone dipropionate in asthmatics did not attenuate the bronchoconstrictor effect of 0.75 part per million (ppm) sulfur dioxide via an isocapnic hyperventilation challenge [21]. Anticholinergic agents (atropine and perhaps ipratropium bromide) may prevent the ozone-induced increase in specific airway resistance (SRaw) and partially block the expected decrement in forced expired volume in 1 second (FEV_1) but have no effect on forced vital capacity (FVC), symptoms, or breathing pattern [22]. Vitamin C also appears to block methacholine hyperresponsiveness induced by nitrogen dioxide in normal subjects [23]. However, inhaled albuterol does not prevent ozone-related lung function changes [24]. Thus, proscription of certain medications for appropriate intervals before each exposure is required to detect the direct effects of pollutants. The guidelines for withholding concurrent medications are generally similar to those for standard bronchial inhalation challenges [25].

2. Healthy Subjects

Healthy adults have been most frequently studied in controlled exposures. Their results are used for comparative purposes. The criteria for subjects have been operationally defined in individual protocols. In general, most healthy subjects have been male nonsmokers, aged 18–40 years, with few or no allergies, no history of active cardiopulmonary or other medical disorders, and normal lung function who can safely participate in the required procedures. The bronchial reactivity of healthy subjects has not been systematically tested in many studied. The investigator should address the question whether clinically normal subjects with nonspecific airway hyperreactivity (but without clinical asthma) should be included or excluded.

Different subgroups within the healthy population have been of great interest because they may be more (or less) responsive to air pollutants than a reference group (usually healthy young adults). The search for sensitive groups is stimulated by scientific, public health, and legislative issues (Clear Air Act). Healthy children [26], adolescents [27–29], and elderly adults [30–33] have been experimentally exposed to ozone, sulfur dioxide, and sulfuric acid to determine possible differences in response between cohorts. Some groups (elderly adults, older than 50 years) have generally been less responsive to ozone [31] than young adults and similarly responsive to nitrogen dioxide [30] and sulfur dioxide [32]. In a study of 290 white male healthy nonsmokers, the only personal characteristic that predicted individual acute physiological response to ozone exposure was age; i.e., decreasing response in FEV_1 was associated with increasing age [34].

It has been speculated that groups of healthy persons with small lung volume or body surface area and/or low exercise-ventilation capabilities have significantly increased sensitivity to pollutant exposure as compared with that of healthy adult men. Specifically, children, women, and certain racial and ethnic groups have been evaluated. Children have smaller lungs and ventilation capability than adults, and this may contribute to their apparent greater sensitivity to ozone. However, responses are similar to those of men when compared on a relative-dose basis with normalization of lung size, exercise capability, or body surface area [8]. Although many studies have included female subjects, few have been specifically designed to test for gender differences in response. Whether female subjects are more responsive than aged-matched male subjects remains unclear [35–37]. Gender-related differences in lung function responses are partially reduced with normalization procedures [37]. Few interracial comparisons have been reported. North American and European whites have largely participated in most English-language reports of controlled pollutant exposures. Volunteers from other racial and ethnic groups have participated, but their numbers are too sparse to make generalizations, and their racial backgrounds are typically not reported. The only large-scale evaluation indicated that the pulmonary response of 372 healthy white and black North American men and women, aged 18–35 years, was not significantly different over a range of ozone concentrations (0, 0.12, 0.18, 0.24, 0.30, or 0.40 ppm) across individual gender and race groups [38].

Highly trained or fit athletes are considered a susceptible group because of their frequent exposures and sustained high ventilation during outdoor exercise. Studies using athletes as subjects should characterize their exercise habits, body fat content, exercise ventilation, and maximum oxygen consumption (VO_{2max}), as well as medical histories. Simulations of competitive conditions have demonstrated significant symptoms, lung dysfunction, or bronchial hyperreactivity in athletes exposed to ozone [35,37,39–43]. On the other hand, 30-min exposures to 0.18 and 0.30 ppm nitrogen dioxide via mouthpiece did not impair lung function in healthy athletes [44].

3. Healthy Subjects with Coexisting Conditions

Atopic persons constitute a large proportion of the general population and may respond differently from nonatopic subjects to air pollutant exposure. Nonasthmatic atopic adolescents develop significant exercise-induced bronchospasm following brief exposure to sulfur dioxide (1 ppm) [45]. Nonasthmatic subjects with allergic rhinitis have similar responses in spirometry and nonspecific bronchial reactivity following ozone exposure in comparison with nonatopic adults [46,47].

Although smokers have been considered another susceptible group, they have tended to be less (not more) sensitive than nonsmokers or to have a delayed response to ozone exposure [48–50]. This finding may relate to an increased mucus layer in the airways that acts as an antioxidant barrier and/or to habituation of airway irritant receptors secondary to chronic inhalation of tobacco smoke, which also contains irritants such as oxidants. Symptomatic and spirometric sensitivity to ozone exposure is regained in healthy ex-smokers after 6 months of smoking cessation [50]. On the other hand, nitrogen dioxide exposure can reduce the FEV_1 in some elderly smokers more than in elderly persons who have never smoked [51]. Although the significance of the apparent protective effect of smoking and regained sensitivity with abstinence is not known, smokers and ex-smokers need to be identified and characterized to account for possible variability in pollutant sensitivity. Thus, some protocols monitor exhaled carbon monoxide (CO), venous carboxyhemoglobin (COHb), or salivary cotinine or thiocyanate levels to both characterize and monitor subjects' smoking status.

Healthy persons with viral upper respiratory infections (URIs) may experience airway epithelial damage sufficient to cause temporary nonspecific airway hyperreactivity to inhaled histamine [52] or nitrates [53]. These persons are generally excluded from exposure studies, since the results may reflect the effects of the URI rather than those of the air pollutant in question. On the other hand, a few laboratories have nasally inoculated human volunteers with rhinovirus or influenza A virus, preceded or followed by pollutant exposures (ozone or nitrogen dioxide, respectively) to evaluate the role of oxidant gases in increasing the susceptibility to viral URI [54,55]. The results have been equivocal.

4. Patients with Preexisting Conditions

Patients with asthma constitute an important risk group for evaluation, owing to their large numbers in the population, airway sensitivity to multiple inhalants, and rising incidences of morbidity and mortality, to which air pollutants are considered to contribute. However, this group is also complicated to characterize. Asthma is a very heterogeneous and complex disorder with respect to pathogenesis, functional and physiological severity, temporal patterns, and medication requirements. The definition of asthma remains controversial, although virtually all asthmatics demonstrate nonspecific bronchial hyperreactivity [56]. The baseline status of asthmatic subjects must be documented with screening medical history, including symptomatology and medication use, lung function and airway reactivity, and an index of atopic status, e.g., dermal reactivity to allergens or serum immunoglobulin E (IgE). Unfortunately, medication use and proscription of medications have been neither well defined in most clinical studies nor standardized between laboratories.

Asthmatic subjects in typical controlled exposures constitute a selected subgroup of primarily young adults with stable mild disease who can safely withhold medications before exposures and exercise according to study protocols. Subjects with stable mild to moderate asthma are generally recruited, to avoid serious complications and to reduce the number of intersubject variables such as differences in medication use, baseline lung function, and airway reactivity. The intensity of intermittent exercise during laboratory exposures must be carefully controlled to limit exercise-induced bronchospasm, which may mask the response to pollutants. On the other hand, pollutants such as sulfur dioxide may potentiate the bronchoconstrictive effect of exercise [45]. Ideally, subjects with allergic asthma should undergo allergy skin testing to identify reactive antigens so that exposures can be performed out of season for the allergen(s).

Asthmatic subjects have demonstrated different responses according to the type or concentration of the pollutant. Low-level ozone exposures produce similar lung function changes in both asthmatic and nonasthmatic subjects, despite the preexisting airway hyperreactivity in the asthmatic subjects. However, asthmatics respond significantly more than healthy controls at ozone levels greater than 0.40 ppm [57]. Nitrogen dioxide is a very weak bronchospastic pollutant in healthy and asthmatic volunteers who are exposed to concentrations as high 4 ppm [58], although airway reactivity may increase at lower concentrations [59–61]. Sulfuric acid at 100 [62], 450, and 1000 $\mu g/m^3$ [63] produces significant reduction in lung function in asthmatic subjects. However, other laboratories have not been able to replicate these findings [64–66]. On the other hand, sulfur dioxide rapidly produces symptomatic bronchoconstriction at low concentrations [67], regardless of the clinical severity of the asthma [68]. The magnitude of the response is influenced by mode of breathing, exercise, and thermal stress [69–76].

Patients with chronic obstructive pulmonary disease (COPD) have been evaluated less frequently in controlled exposures. The criteria for COPD have been relatively broad, in part because of its heterogeneous nature. These patients are generally older and have a significant smoking history, low physical fitness, and concomitant medical disorders, e.g., combined COPD and coronary artery disease Patients with established COPD are also likely to have variable baseline lung function and be less able to consistently withhold their prescribed medications for specified intervals before exposures. Thus, as in the selection of asthmatic subjects, clinically stable COPD patients with mild to moderate cardiopulmonary involvement are typically evaluated by investigators, and patients with more severe COPD are excluded for safety considerations.

Patients with chronic cardiopulmonary conditions have been less responsive to inhaled oxidants and sulfur dioxide than healthy nonsmokers. Patients with COPD have similar or lesser response than nonsmokers when exposed to ozone concentrations as high as 0.30 ppm for 1–2 h [77]. Similar findings have been made in this patient population with nitrogen dioxide concentrations as high as 2 ppm [51,78] and sulfur dioxide concentrations as high as 0.8 ppm [79]. Similarly, preliminary results [80] in patients with chronic interstitial lung disease suggest minimal responsiveness to 0.30 ppm ozone. The apparent subresponsiveness to inhaled pollutants may stem from protection by increased airway mucus and/or low exercise ventilation during exposures due to limiting symptoms, impaired cardiopulmonary function, and poor physical fitness. Patients with coronary artery disease (CAD) also appear less responsive to ozone [81]. On the other hand, CAD patients can clearly respond during acute low-level CO exposure with clinically significant cardiac effects, i.e., onset of angina pectoris or changes in electrocardiographic patterns [82–84].

B. Generation and Monitoring of Clean Air and Pollutants

The generation and monitoring of environmental agents largely depend on the goal of the study and the specific pollutant. Generation techniques must be well documented, because interlaboratory differences may occasionally contribute to different experimental conclusions. The basic equipment for exposure studies includes sources of purified air and pollutant, a method of adding and titrating experimental pollutants (gases, aerosols, or both) to the purified air, monitors of pollutant concentrations, and a delivery system. Temperature, humidity, and other physical conditions (lighting, noise level) must also be considered in the study design.

1. Clean Air

The purification or filtration of air for laboratory exposures should result in clean air, i.e, with minimally acceptable amounts of contaminants. Clean air is an appropriate control condition to determine nonpollutant effects and potentially biasing or confounding effects originating from laboratory conditions or expectations of the subjects (e.g., "placebo effect" vs. "smog effect"). The requirements for air purification are highest in a large-volume chamber facility, such as that employed by this investigator (Fig. 1), which will be discussed as a model system. In brief, outside or room air is pumped through a series of a chemical and paper filters to achieve high purity [7,85]. A metal catalytic agent (Hopcalite) is used at high and ambient temperatures to convert CO and low-molecular-weight hydrocarbons to carbon dioxide and to capture oxides of nitrogen (NOx), respectively. The ambient-temperature Hopcalite can be regenerated (purged of NOx) by taking it off line and heating it. Activated carbon adsorbs most organic contaminants and catalytically decomposes ozone to molecular oxygen. Aluminum oxide pellets impregnated with potassium permanganate (Purafil or Unisorb) also effectively remove oxidants (including oxides of nitrogen) and hydrocarbons. High-efficiency paper particulate (HEPA) filters capture 99.9% of particles. Although other prefilters or some redundancies of filters in the purification system can be used, the combination of filters described can produce highly purified air that contains several $\mu g/m^3$ of particles and undetectable or barely detectable levels of common pollutant gases, according to conventional air-monitoring instruments. Less elaborate exposure systems typically use only chemical adsorbents and HEPA filters. Carbon monoxide, however, is not efficiently removed by these systems and

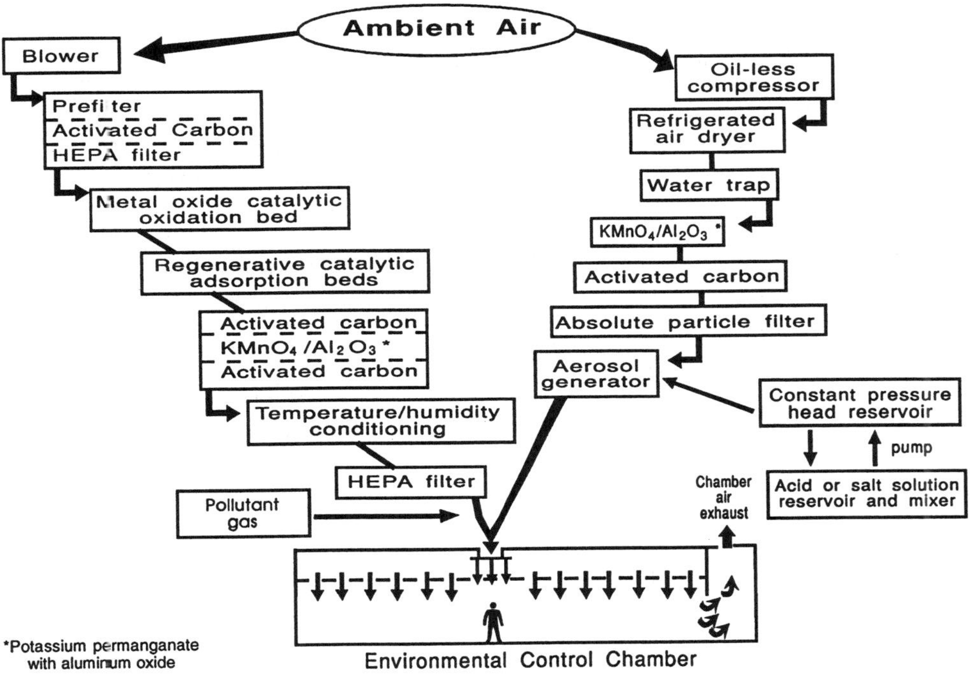

Figure 1 Schematic representation of the exposure facility used by the author for controlled human exposures to gaseous and aerosol air pollutants. The basic components include air purification, pollutant generation, air conditioning, and the exposure chamber. The arrows indicate the direction of airflow. See text for details.

requires a high-temperature catalyst and high-capacity air conditioning. The purified air is subsequently conditioned for temperature and humidity by a dedicated air conditioner, followed by delivery in insulated conduits to the subject.

2. Pollutants

The pollutant(s) to be evaluated will be determined by the specific experimental question. The choice may involve a single gas, particulate aerosol, or a mixture (either simultaneously or sequentially) of gas–gas, gas–soluble particulate, or, rarely, soluble and insoluble particulates. Ozone is generated by either ultraviolet lamps or high-voltage discharge. Either air or 100% oxygen can be used as a source gas, although some prefer the latter because trace amounts of nitrogen oxides may be produced with ozonation of air. Sulfur dioxide, nitrogen dioxide, and CO can be easily generated for exposures from commercially available high-standard source cylinders and appropriate flow meters.

The generation of particulate aerosols for human exposures demands greater preparation and control measures than for gases, as well as some ingenuity and empirical decisions. Water-soluble particulate species such as sulfuric acid or ammonium sulfate may be generated by nebulizing their freshly prepared aqueous solutions. The size (mass median aerodynamic diameter [MMAD]) and range of size distribution (geometric standard deviation [GSD]) are important particle characteristics to control and measure during aerosol exposures. The specific MMAD or GSD for generated particles is largely determined by the nebulizer used. The size of the particles will determine their respirable capabilities and, thus, potential airway effects. Some particulates (e.g., sulfuric acid) may be hygroscopic and increase in size during transit to the airways. Strategies that modify particle size include increasing the air pressure powering the nebulizer (within its technical limits) and/or diluting the solute in solution so that the generated solute particles are small. Circumstances requiring a high ambient particle concentration require increasing the number of nebulizers and/or their flow rates (output) to achieve a nominal steady-state concentration. Manual or automated adjustments in aerosol generation must be driven and confirmed by ongoing particle measurements (discussed subsequently). Rarely, the generation of a mixture of a soluble particulate (e.g., sulfuric acid) and an insoluble particulate (e.g., carbon) is required [86]. This can be aerosolized from an aqueous colloidal dispersion of pure carbon black using Collison nebulizers [86] or spinning-disk aerosol generators. Dry powders can be directly aerosolized by Wright dust-feed generators or fluidized-bed generators. The insoluble particles should be decharged to reverse possible ionic charging imparted during generation.

The generated pollutant is typically injected into the purified air stream and mixed before delivery to the subject (Fig. 1). It is important that all conduits in the system (including a mask or head dome) and, if applicable, chamber walls be as inert as possible to the traversing pollutant to avoid unwanted reactions and contaminants (which may be undetected). Teflon, Plexiglas, and stainless steel are considered reasonable materials for even the most reactive pollutants.

3. Monitoring

Monitoring of the ambient pollutant during exposure is critical for achieving and maintaining a nominal target concentration, for deliberately changing the concentration, and for safety reasons. Ozone is commonly monitored by ultraviolet photometry, CO and hydrocarbons by nondispersive infrared analyzers, and sulfur dioxide by flame or ultraviolet photometry. Oxides of nitrogen are typically measured by chemiluminescent analyzers using the reaction of nitric oxide (NO) with ozone. These gas-monitoring techniques provide rapid response and continuous read-out, and can be automated. However, aerosols are commonly measured by collection of samples on sized fiber filters of Teflon, nylon, glass, or quartz in cascade impactors. Acid samples must be protected from subsequent ammonia neutralization, e.g., ammonia emanating from technicians. The filters subsequently undergo high-precision gravimetric and chemical quantitative analysis, which usually requires hours or days to complete. Strong acidity (H^+) and major particulate ions (SO_4^{2-}, NH_4^+, and NO_3^-) can be determined by the pH method and ion chromatography, respectively. The identity and concentration of the filtered particles can also be measured by high-performance liquid chromatography (HPLC). Particle size can also be characterized by electrostatic precipitators and electron micrographs (e.g., for insoluble particles). Fortunately, optical particle counters (e.g., nephelometers, particle laser spectrometers), electrical-mobility analyzers, or continuous monitors (e.g., for sulfate or ammonia) can provide real-time response and can be used in conjunction with the more common but slower, labor-intensive techniques.

The frequency and duration of sampling must be sufficient to avoid undesired and possibly unknown changes in the nominal concentration. This is rarely an issue with continuous, real-time automated monitors. However, the discrete filter sampling of aerosols depends on the ambient concentration and requires some judgment. Longer sampling times (e.g., hours) may be required when the ambient particle concentration is low, e.g., 100 $\mu g/m^3$ sulfuric acid. On the other hand, filter sampling may be short (e.g., minutes) when the ambient concentration is very high.

Sampling of the environmental air should be representative of the air breathed by the subject, i.e., close to his or her "breathing zone," which is approximately that volume of air within a 1-foot radius of the nose and mouth. Exposure chambers have a set air-turnover rate (10 or more times/h) that may either promote or reduce stagnant air pockets within a chamber, depending on the physical characteristics of the inlet and chamber itself. Different locations within a large chamber should be tested to determine that nominal pollutant levels are well distributed, which implies that the ventilation is also even throughout the chamber.

4. Quality Assurance

Procedures must be incorporated in a specific study and facility in general to assure reliable and accurate measurements. This aspect is beyond the scope of this chapter and will only be briefly discussed. Procedures for quality assurance and control and data validation must be documented and routinely follow guidelines and approved reference methods such as those used by air-quality regulatory agencies, e.g., the U.S. Environmental Protection Agency (EPA). Frequent checks and calibrations of equipment, set routine for measurements, use of positive and negative controls (e.g., with acidic filters), staged data review for consistency, outliers, and errors, and external assessments of quality assurance are some examples. Quality assurance, of course, also applies to subject monitoring and testing.

5. Experimental Modifications

Table 2 summarizes current federal air-quality standards for six outdoor pollutants and the concentration ranges for ozone episodes in the South Coast Air Basin of California. The short-term concentration thresholds indicate not only the considered limits for public health but also bracketing ranges for realistic levels of specific pollutants used in controlled human exposures. It should be noted that second-stage ozone alerts are now rare and that third-stage ozone episodes have not occurred in over 10 years. Sulfuric acid is being considered by the EPA as another criterion pollutant [87].

Laboratory simulations of outdoor pollutant exposure have typically used a single steady-state concentration rather than a triangular concentration profile, i.e., progressive increase, peak, and subsequent decline over hours. The triangular exposure profile may closely simulate a natural exposure and, therefore, be more useful in determining a suitable averaging time for a longer-term air-quality standard. For example, spirometric changes were different between a steady-state 8-h exposure to 0.12 ppm ozone and a triangular exposure pattern, in which the ozone level progressively increased from 0 to 0.24 ppm over the first 4 h and progressively decreased back to 0 by 8 h [88]. Significantly greater peak decreases

Table 2 Air Quality Standards for Criterion Air Pollutants, Including Ozone Episodes in Southern California

Pollutant	Federal primary standard	Averaging time
Ozone (O_3)	0.12 ppm	1 h[b]
	235 μg/m³	
	Alert levels[a]	
	1st-stage: 0.20–0.34 ppm	
	2nd-stage: 0.35–0.49 ppm	
	3rd-stage: >0.50 ppm	
Nitrogen dioxide (NO_2)	0.05 ppm	1 y
	100 μg/m³	
Sulfur dioxide (SO_2)	0.14 ppm	24 h[b]
	365 μg/m³	
Particulates (PM_{10})	150 μg/m³	24 h[b]
	50 μ/m³	1 y
Carbon monoxide (CO)	35 ppm	1 h[b]
	40 mg/m³	
	9 ppm	8 h[b]
	10 mg/m³	
Lead	1.5 μg/m³	24 h

[a]Applicable since 1977 to South Coast Air Quality Management District in California.
[b]May not be exceeded more than once a year.

in FVC and FEV_1 occurred during the last 4 h of the variable exposure as compared with the steady-state condition, even though the time-weighted average exposure was the same in both conditions.

A single pollutant is tested in most controlled human exposures, although its concentration may be varied during separate exposures to evaluate dose-response relationships [38,68]. However, natural exposures are frequently to more than a single pollutant. Concurrent pollutants may interact with each other, producing a complex pollutant mix or different health effects than with either pollutant alone. Laboratory studies with more than one pollutant usually involve only two different pollutants, in addition to clean air, since such protocols are more complex, costly, and time-consuming to conduct. Exposures to each pollutant alone are necessary to identify possible synergistic or additive effects.

Some studies have examined the effects of sequential or concurrent pollutants that are relevant to natural human exposures. For example, prior exposure to ozone (0.12 ppm) can potentiate subsequent lung function responses to sulfur dioxide (0.10 ppm) in adolescent asthmatics, whereas neither gas alone elicits significant responses [89]. Prior exposure to nitrogen dioxide may [90] or may not [91] potentiate airway responsiveness to sulfur dioxide. On the other hand, prior exposure to nitric acid (HNO_3) does not potentiate (and may attenuate) ozone-induced decrements in lung function in ozone-sensitive subjects [92]. Combinations of pollutants such as ozone and peroxyacetyl nitrate (PAN) may result in greater pulmonary decrements than either gas alone, perhaps because of a greater oxidant burden [93]. However, synergism in functional response between ozone and NO_2 [94], sulfuric acid [95,96], sulfur dioxide [97], or CO [98] has not been demonstrated.

Complex atmospheres that simulate community ambient air are very difficult to reproduce and measure in the laboratory. One unique solution to this problem is the use of a mobile exposure chamber [99] that can expose subjects to outside ambient air (with its contaminant mixture), clean air without pollutants, and clean air containing artificially generated concentrations of a pollutant (e.g., ozone) that are comparable to those measured in the ambient environment. As a result, measured health responses in ambient air can be directly compared with those present in more controlled conditions. For example, field studies using a mobile laboratory–chamber have demonstrated that ambient ozone is the agent predominantly responsible for respiratory effects from photochemical air pollution in the Los Angeles area [100].

C. Types of Exposure System

Gaseous or aerosol pollutants can be effectively delivered to the subject by several modalities: by mouthpiece, face mask, or head dome, or within a large-volume or whole-body chamber facility. Each modality offers advantages and disadvantages for the investigator (Table 3). No one modality is perfect for all studies, depending on scientific and nonscientific considerations, such as comfort, duration of exposure, cost, and number of subjects. Individual exposure systems (mouthpiece, face mask, or head dome) will usually suffice for small-scale experiments involving one subject at a time for a short exposure duration. These compact delivery systems have notable advantages over a chamber, with lower costs, simpler equipment, small quantities of purified air and pollutant, and capabilities of rapidly and easily changing temperature, humidity, or pollutant within the delivered air while allowing a continuously comfortable thermal environment for the rest of the body. The small volume of these systems also makes them suitable for studying unstable pollutants or reactive mixtures. Ventilation and breathing patterns can be measured with a pneumotachograph.

Mouthpiece breathing, with blockage of nasal airflow by a nose clip, has significant disadvantages, such as discomfort during prolonged exposure, excessive drying of the mouth with increased salivation, loss of nasal scrubbing of inhaled air, and alteration of the normal upper airway geometry, as well as restricted movement and position. A major disadvantage of the mouthpiece from the regulatory standpoint is that this exposure system is not realistic, except at high exercise levels, and can directly alter breathing patterns and, thus, physiological responses. The pulmonary effects of sulfur dioxide are reduced when subjects are exposed via the nasal or oronasal route vs. the oral route alone [69,101]. The scrubbing of water-soluble sulfur dioxide is reduced or bypassed in the upper airways by mouthpiece breathing (and nose clips). On the other hand, the route of inhaled ozone (0.40 ppm) during moderate and heavy continuous exercise does not appreciably modify acute physiological and symptomatic responses [102,103], indicating similar respiratory removal of ozone by oral, nasal, and oronasal routes under laboratory conditions [104]. Sulfuric acid aerosol is naturally neutralized by endogenous oral ammonia [105,106]. This aspect must be considered to estimate accurately the effect of acid aerosols on airway function [107]. Nasal and oral breathing, as well as humidity, strongly affect acid neutralization and the extent to which acids affect airway function [108]. Oral ammonia is typically reduced or neutralized by lemonade or citrus drinks taken by subjects before and during exposure to acid aerosols [64,66,106,107].

Unidirectional flow or flow-through face masks offer more comfort and unencumbered breathing than mouthpiece systems and can be constructed to separate nasal and oral ventilation. Nonetheless, face masks must be tightly sealed and may alter oral geometry, resulting in an altered oronasal breathing pattern.

Many of the disadvantages of the mouthpiece and face mask systems are avoided or minimized by the head dome or hood [109]. A lightweight, rigid transparent polycarbonate plastic hood for head-only exposure can be constructed with overhead suspension and counter-weighted to rest lightly on the subject's shoulders. A neck seal is attached to the bottom flange of the dome. Inlet air enters

Table 3 Comparison of Types of Exposure System Used in Controlled Human Exposures to Air Pollutants

Characteristic	Mouthpiece (with nose clip)	Head-only exposure (face mask; head dome)	Whole-body exposure (chamber)
Breathing mode	Restricted to oral breathing	Unencumbered	Unencumbered
Alters upper airway configuration	++	−	−
Mobility of subject	+	+	+++
Exercise capability	+	+/++	+++
Comfort	−	+/−	+++
Rebreathing of exhaled air	+	+/++	+
Long duration of exposure possible	+	++	+++
Capability of maintaining steady-state atmosphere	++	+/++	−/++*
Capability for rapid changes in condition (e.g., conc., temp.)	++	++	+
Capability to measure ventilation	+++	++	++
Capability to simulate normal situations	+	++	+++
Capability to study multiple subjects	−	−	+++
Potential effect on outcome variables	+++	++	+
Space requirements	+	+/++	+++
Maintenance needs	+	+	+++
Costs	+	++	+++

− = none or negligible; + = minimal; ++ = moderate; +++ = high

*Depends on engineering capabilities of the chamber, air conditioning, pollutant generation, and ventilation system.

through a diffuser opposite the subject's nose and mouth. Inlet and exhaled air flow upward to exhaust through a pneumotachograph. As a result, this system provides unencumbered breathing, comfort, reasonable mobility and position changes, and capability for accurate measurements of ventilation and for exercise on a bicycle ergometer. Rebreathing of exhaled air is largely dependent on the inlet airflow characteristics as well as the exhaust flow [109]. The head dome remains limited by its restriction of mobility, duration of use, and size (more than one size may be necessary for different subjects). Nonetheless, this modality has promise and has been effectively used in exposures with ozone [109], sulfuric acid [110], and sulfur dioxide (J. Q. Koenig, unpublished data).

More elaborate studies (e.g., long duration of exposures) or those requiring relatively large numbers of subjects are better performed within a room-sized chamber large enough to accommodate two or more subjects simultaneously for extended periods [7,85]. The number of each facilities is limited, owing to their construction and maintenance costs and space requirements. Stainless steel and Plexiglas are typical nonreactive materials used in their construction. The major advantages of the chamber are unencumbered breathing, comfort, mobility, general acceptance by subjects, use of either bicycle ergometer or treadmill, and ability to expose multiple subjects simultaneously for as long as 6–7 h. Above all, the chamber environment can readily simulate many ambient conditions. Some practical disadvantages are related to the large volume of the chamber, which can produce difficulties in rapidly altering chamber conditions (e.g., to achieve cold temperatures, dry air) and the number of air changes per hour. Intense cooling (e.g., to −20°C) or drying (e.g., to 10–20% humidity) may be very difficult or technically impossible, depending on the compressor and air conditioning unit of the chamber. Relatively low air exchange rates in large-volume chambers may not adequately simulate higher outdoor wind speeds. This technical aspect has not been adequately evaluated but may be a factor in interpreting results from sulfuric acid exposures in chambers where endogenous ammonia may transiently persist in the breathing zone and neutralize acid aerosols before inspiration by the subject. If so, the head dome may be superior to the chamber in this regard, but data are not available.

D. Other Environmental Conditions

The typical thermal characteristics of the ambient air in controlled human exposures are similar to those of room air (21°C, 40–50% relative humidity), in order to determine the specific effects of the pollutant alone in a neutral environment. Occasionally, more thermal stress is indicated to simulate natural pollutant episodes, which are frequently associated with specific meteorological conditions. Oxidant episodes typically occur during summer inversions with high temperatures and very low relative humidity. Sulfur dioxide episodes are associated with cool or cold fall or winter conditions, inversions, and high relative humidity. Extreme thermal stress may potentially affect ventilation and airway function, resulting in changes greater than that imposed by the pollutant. Healthy subjects can develop a modest but statistically significant reduction in FVC under hot or dry clean-air conditions [111,112]. The combination of ozone and heat stress impairs exercise performance more severely than ozone at more comfortable temperatures [41,112]. Asthmatics breathing cold (−15°C), dry air with 0.50 ppm sulfur dioxide develop significantly more bronchoconstriction than with either sulfur dioxide (in warm, humid air) or cold air alone [70,72,73,75]. High ambient humidity also significantly affects (increases) the size and size distribution of hygroscopic particles (e.g., sulfuric acid) during delivery to the subject. For example, sulfuric acid particles in a humid atmosphere may be inhaled and impact preferentially in the nose or mouth and/or larynx and have greater likelihood of neutralization by endogenous upper airway ammonia than at lower humidity, resulting in less entry to the lower respiratory tract and minimal perturbation of lung function [108]. Thus, thermal conditions require consideration and appropriate controls during a laboratory study.

E. Duration and Frequency of Exposures

Possible exposure regimens (all including a clean-air control exposure) are continuous single, acute exposures, intermittent exposures on the same day or different days, and repeated continuous, multiday exposures. Separate exposures to pollutant and clean air alone are generally administered in randomized order at least 1 week apart to minimize residual pollutant effects. Their identity must be blinded as much as possible to minimize bias. This may be difficult for some pollutants that have a perceptible odor, e.g., ozone and sulfur dioxide.

The duration and frequency of laboratory exposures depend again on the experimental question and pollutant under consideration. For example, natural daily exposures to pollutants range between seconds and hours and may be repeated daily. Most asthmatics are highly sensitive to less than 1 ppm sulfur dioxide. Only 3–10 min of exposure are necessary to elicit symptomatic bronchoconstriction [67], which is not appreciably increased by 30 min of exposure [76,113]. Responsiveness to sulfur dioxide spontaneously returns to its initial level within 5–6 h [113–115]. Healthy subjects who are responsive to ozone inhalation generally require at least 30 min of exposure during moderate to heavy exercise to elicit a change in lung function [116–119]. As a result, most ozone protocols use an acute-exposure regimen of short duration (generally 2 h). Longer-duration (6–7 h) exposures to ozone at low concentrations (0.08–0.12 ppm) with continuous moderate exercise can progressively decrease lung function and increase symptoms and nonspecific airway reactivity [117–119].

Consecutive daily exposures to air pollutants are feasible in the laboratory setting. However, the experimental design must take into account the possible development of an attenuated response or desensitization ("adaptation") with some pollutants. This attenuation can block subsequent exposure responses, depending on the pollutant and the number and temporal sequence of exposures. For example, less than 60 min between repeated exposures to sulfur dioxide in asthmatics will significantly blunt subsequent exposure effects [113–115]. A single laboratory exposure to ozone (0.40 ppm) in healthy subjects can impair lung function for the following 24–48 h [120]. Attenuation does not occur with single exposures separated by at least 1 week or with repeated exposures to nitrogen dioxide, to our knowledge. If ozone exposures are repeated on a consecutive daily basis for several hours, changes in lung function (as well as symptoms and methacholine sensitivity) will peak by exposure day 2, followed by progressive attenuation. Minimal, if any, responsiveness to ozone occurs by the fourth or fifth exposure day [121], and its persistence varies for 1–2 weeks even without further daily ozone exposures [122]. Whether attenuation occurs naturally is uncertain, although some evidence suggests a diminution of physiological response to acute ozone exposure in chronic residents of a photochemically polluted area and across seasons [123–125]. The time course of response to a particular pollutant, its peak response and temporal recovery, and whether attenuation of pollutant-induced response occurs must be considered to minimize confounding acute or chronic ambient pollutant effects on laboratory-based studies. Thus, recent and chronic ambient pollution exposures must be documented in subjects who participate in laboratory exposures.

F. Activity During Exposure

People usually engage in some type of intermittent physical activity during outdoor conditions and exposures. This activity is commonly simulated during controlled human exposures with some form of exercise, which is a natural method of altering the dose or exposure rate by virtue of increased ventilation and deposition of inhaled pollutants. Exercise enhances pulmonary responses during acute exposures to sulfur dioxide in asthmatics [69,71,74,101] and ozone in healthy subjects [126]. Figure 2 illustrates the effects of intermittent exercise and ozone concentration on FEV_1 during 2-h exposures. Forced vital capacity and maximal midexpiratory flow ($FEF_{25-75\%}$) parallel decrements in FEV_1. Larger physiological decrements occur at higher levels of exercise and at higher ozone concentrations. These changes support the concept of a mean effective dose, which is the product of ozone concentration × ventilation × duration. Thus, low concentrations of ozone can produce effective doses similar to those with higher ozone levels as long as accompanying ventilation and duration are sufficiently increased.

On the other hand, continuous moderate exercise during ozone exposure

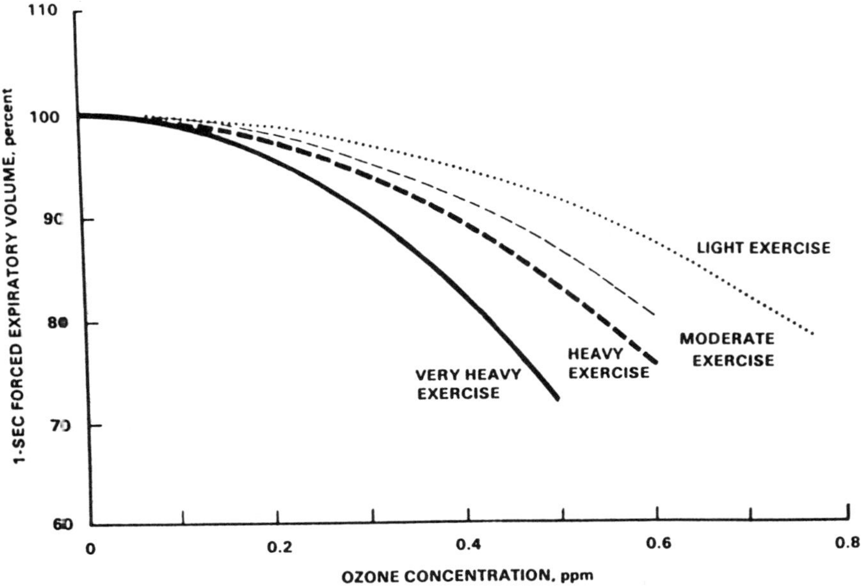

Figure 2 Group mean decrements in forced expired volume in one second (FEV_1) during 2-h ozone exposures with different levels of intermittent exercise: light (minute ventilation ≤23 L/min); moderate (24–43 L/min); heavy (44–63 L/min); and very heavy (≥64 L/min). The intensity of exercise modifies the concentration–response curves. (From Ref. 126.)

(equivalent in duration to the sum of intermittent exercise periods at comparable ozone concentrations and minute ventilation) may elicit greater cumulative changes in lung function than predicted [27,100,127]. This response also appears in 6- to 7-h exposures with nearly continuous moderate exercise [117–119] and may reflect an exponential, rather than linear, nature of dose effects and temporal interactions.

A standardized or best exercise protocol does not exist. Controlled studies using an exercise component have been notably different in the duration, frequency, timing, and intensity of exercise, exercise modality, and achieved or target ventilation (when measured), as well as the exposure duration, concentration of study pollutant, and timing of lung function measurements [128]. These differences may be amplified by the wide interindividual variability in physical fitness and patterns of oronasal breathing during exercise. A number of exercise protocols can be used, but each must have sufficient rationale in terms of the experimental question and related measurements [128]. Although exercise during most controlled exposures is not an outcome variable, attention must be paid to the accurate and timely measurements of ventilation (including at rest), oxygen uptake, lung function, or other variables in relation to exercise periods. Otherwise, the results may be misleading and possibly underestimate the true effect of a pollutant.

Given the above information, some generalities about exercise activities can be stated. Treadmill walking or running and cycle ergometry are the most commonly used exercise modalities in controlled exposures. Activity levels may range from easy walking (e.g., in patients with COPD) to heavy–severe exercise (usually only in fit athletes), which increase ventilation by as little as 10 L/min and as much as over 100 L/min. Some guidelines (Table 4) are available for estimating the ventilation associated with a given intensity of work load, e.g., light, moderate, heavy, very heavy, and severe [126]. The values for oxygen consumption and minute ventilation are approximate estimates for average physically fit men exercising on a bicycle ergometer at 50–60 rpm. Interindividual variability and other factors can greatly modify the estimated values, so that the only precise method for obtaining these data is actual individual measurements. This is especially true when exercise is conducted on a treadmill, in which adequate relative standards for these variables cannot be estimated [128].

Isocapnic hyperventilation in resting subjects can be used in controlled pollutant exposures when altered ventilatory pattern (due to mouthpiece) is not a critical issue and when exercise is contraindicated or not required to increase minute ventilation. Pollutant-induced airway responses with this technique are useful for identifying large numbers of sensitive subjects and in studies emphasizing mechanism of action [69,75], or drug intervention [21].

G. Techniques for Assessing End Points

The measured responses in exposure experiments conceptually represent relevant markers of events in biological systems or samples [129]. These biological markers can reflect effect, exposure, or susceptibility. Markers of effect may be measurable physiological or biochemical responses or other types of response such as health impairment or disease and have been evaluated most frequently in controlled human exposures. The lungs are the initial target organ of inhaled pollutants, so it is not surprising that traditional end points are respiratory symptoms and spirometry. Markers of exposure indicate an exogenous xenobiotic substance or its interaction with target tissues or cells. Markers of susceptibility indicate inherent or acquired excessive or limited capacity to respond to an environmental agent. Markers of exposure and susceptibility will be increasingly evaluated in controlled human exposures as new cellular and molecular biological knowledge and techniques develop [129].

A wide spectrum of techniques (and, thus, end points) can be applied to clinical research studies to document gross or subtle physiological responses, site-specific effects, and mechanisms of action of the pollutant in the lower and upper

Table 4 Ventilation and Oxygen Consumption Levels Associated with Different Types of Exercise

Descriptor of work	Minute ventilation (L/min)	Oxygen consumption (L/min)	Work performed		Representative activities
			watts	kg-m/min	
Light	12–23	0.65–0.96	25–50	150–300	Level walking at 2–3 mph; washing clothes; scrubbing floors
Moderate	23–46	1.25–1.83	75–125	450–750	Dancing; stacking firewood; easy cycling; climbing stairs; playing tennis; digging with spade
Heavy	42–67	2.12–2.47	150–175	900–1050	Cycling at 13 mph; walking on snow; digging trenches; climbing stairs with load
Very heavy	62–100	2.83–3.55	200–250	1200–1500	Cross-country skiing; chopping wood; playing handball; level running at 10 mph; competitive cycling
Severe	>107	>4.27	>300	>1800	Competitive distance running; cross-country skiing

kg-m/min = work performed each minute to move a mass of 1 kg through a vertical distance of 1 m against the force of gravity.
Source: Adapted from Ref. 126.

respiratory tracts (Table 5). The methods vary somewhat in their levels of complexity or sophistication, subject acceptability and safety, invasiveness, advantages and limitations, and costs. Many techniques can be repeated during the same session (before, during, and/or following exposure), except for bronchoprovocation tests, radionuclide imaging procedures involving long-lasting isotopes, and bronchoscopy. However, each can be applied at least once during separate visits, depending on safety, duration of residual testing effects, and subject acceptance. Although most tests in Table 5 are considered relatively safe and repeatable, not all tests can provide accurate or reproducible results, nor are they necessary in all protocols. The investigator must consider the use of specific techniques in relation to the experimental question, available resources, and expertise. Only an overview of these techniques, as applicable to controlled pollutant exposures, will be reviewed here, since a large volume of literature is available for each technique.

1. Symptom Questionnaires

Reported symptoms require careful recording and interpretation. Symptom reports can be obtained repeatedly with some reliability and sensitivity and without significant risk, expense, or resources. However, the well-known disadvantages of symptom data are their qualitative or semiquantitative nature, lack of confirmation, difficult reproducibility and statistical testing, potential for bias, and lack of standardization among subjects and laboratories. Indeed, different methods of symptom reporting are found in the exposure literature, making the interstudy comparison of results impossible [130]. This dimension of response is only as good as the reporting method, which may be simple verbal descriptions, incidence rates, or ordinal scoring systems based on the number of symptoms reported and their severity. The incidence-rate approach may be considerably improved by using a multiple-symptom, ordinal scoring of symptom severity with descriptors such as no symptoms (score of 0) and minimal (5), mild (10), moderate (20), severe (30), and incapacitating symptoms (40) [130]. It is unclear whether summing scores from all symptoms or a group of symptoms is more meaningful or has greater sensitivity in detecting responses than analyzing each symptom separately. Analysis of changes in scores (e.g., difference between preexposure and postexposure scores) may offset criticism related to the typically skewed distribution of scores. Overall, the systematic recording of symptoms remains a useful means of documenting subjective responses, corroborating physiological data, and perhaps understanding biological mechanisms of response.

Symptoms associated with pollutant exposure are considered clinically significant, especially when accompanied by objective functional changes. Questionnaires inquiring about symptoms may identify sensitive and nonsensitive subjects who may then be selected for an exposure protocol or other procedures [131,132]. Symptoms typically reported during exposure to irritant gases (e.g., ozone) are cough, chest tightness, inability to inspire fully, wheeze, shortness of breath, throat irritation, and nasal congestion. Upper airway complaints such as taste or odor predominate in normal subjects exposed to sulfur dioxide, whereas lower respiratory symptoms are most bothersome in asthmatics [133]. Nonrespiratory symptoms such as headache, fatigue, nausea, and eye irritation are also reported from subjects exposed to ozone and volatile organic compounds (VOCs). Symptoms may have modest to good correlation with physiological responses. For example, dose-response studies of healthy volunteers exposed to ozone [100] and asthmatic subjects exposed to sulfur dioxide [101] showed parallel patterns of symptomatic and lung-function changes.

2. Neuropsychological Tests

Psychophysical procedures relate the subject's perceptions of respiratory sensations to semiquantitative estimations of the magnitude of effort during exercise and to the work of breathing [134]. Procedures such as magnitude scaling (e.g., estimation of an inspired volume) and magnitude production (e.g., replication of a predetermined inspired volume) have been used in a limited number of exposure studies. Ozone exposure during exercise was associated with an increased overall perception of effort, which primarily originated from respiratory sensations [135]. Normal subjects' sensitivity to a change in inspired lung volume was greater following ozone exposure than following air exposure [135].

Neuropsychological testing is useful in circumstances in which subjects express upper or lower respiratory tract discomfort but lack objective findings. Frequent recordings of symptoms and severity with a visual analogue scale are readily applicable to VOC exposures [132]. Ozone exposures did not significantly alter visual and auditory attention tasks (vigilance performance) or associated electroencephalographic indices [136,137].

3. Respiratory Function Tests

Spirometry. The forced expiratory maneuver continues to be the most commonly used objective modality to assess acute toxicological responses to inhaled pollutants. The main components of the expiratory curve that represent the flow characteristics of the airways are the FVC, FEV_1, maximal midexpiratory flow (MMEF or $FEF_{25-75\%}$), and flow after 50% or 75% of the volume has been forcibly exhaled ($FEF_{50\%}$ or $FEF_{75\%}$) [129,138]. The simplicity and low coefficient of variation of FVC and FEV_1 in relation to expected changes in the measurement enable the detection of small changes in the same subjects studied repeatedly on the same day or during separate days. Maximal effort with each maneuver and associated effects of total lung capacity or residual volume on forced expiratory results are important considerations. A restrictive pattern has been observed with ozone exposures in which a reduced inspiratory volume (and total lung capacity) decreases FVC and FEV_1 but does not alter the FEV_1/FVC ratio [139]. The forced inspiratory volume (FIV) has been underused, but the FIV in the first 0.5 s of inspiration ($FIV_{0.5}$) is consistently decreased with ozone exposure [117,118], and

Table 5 Some Techniques Used to Measure Responses in Controlled Human Exposures to Pollutants

Technique	Advantages	Disadvantages	Examples of end points
Questionnaire	Safe; subject acceptability; inexpensive	Subjective; difficult to standardize and reproduce	Symptoms: present or absent; severity score
Neuropsychological tests	Safe; generally inexpensive	Largely subjective; difficult to standardize	Visual analogue scaling of effort, breathing, discomfort; vigilance performance; EEG
Respiratory function tests			
Spirometry	Safe; subject acceptability; well established; standardized	Poor specificity and sensitivity for small airways	FVC, FEV_1, MMEF, etc.
Airway mechanics (nasal or lower airways)	Safe; subject acceptability; easy to perform	Large inter-subject variablity; uncertain sensitivity and specificity for small airways	Raw, SRaw, SGaw, R_T
Aerosol probe technique	Simple; sensitive to changes in small-airway and alveolar dimensions	Developmental; lack of standardization; special equipment; high intersubject variability	Dispersion of exhaled aerosol bolus as compared with that on inspiration
Bronchoprovocation tests			
Nonspecific (methacholine, cold air, water aerosol, etc.)	Low risk; standardized; reproducible; results of different methods closely correlate; some stimuli natural or quantifiable	Variable equipment needs; set end point not always present; some lack dose-response capability	Provocative concentration (PC) or dose (PD); dose-response slope
Specific (antigen)	Agent-specific; diagnostic; standardized	Antigen skin test response needed; moderate to high risk in responders; time-consuming	Provocative concentration (PC) or dose (PD)
Tests of epithelial barrier integrity			
Oximetry	Safe, noninvasive; sensitive	Accuracy uncertain in some circumstances or with some models	Arterial oxyhemoglobin saturation (% SaO_2)

Mucociliary clearance	Low risk; nasal or tracheobronchial, regional or whole-organ capabilities; may be more sensitive than pulmonary function tests	Subject cooperation; time-consuming; radiation; limited repeatability; results dependent of deposition pattern and procedure; high intersubject variability; special equipment	Percent particle retention over time in site of interest
Permeability	Low risk; may be more sensitive than pulmonary function tests	Subject cooperation; radiation; results dependent on deposition pattern and procedure; high intersubject variability; special equipment	Percent decrease in activity per minute in lung on gamma camera imaging
Exercise testing for performance	Natural activity; limitation is directly measured; low risk	Related equipment; time-consuming	Ventilation; VO_{2max}; anaerobic threshold; changes in heart rate (ECG), lung function, breathing pattern; duration and work load achieved (performance)
Procedures to collect cellular-biochemical constituents			
Bronchoalveolar Lavage	Low-moderate risk, even in asthmatics; large quantitiy retrieved	Invasive; cooperation needed; special equipment; expensive; not standardized; collection not specific to proximal airways or alveoli	Cells: number, differential, functional assays Fluid: arachidonic acid metabolites; cytokines; histamine; enzymes; protein; complement; antioxidants, etc.
Nasal Lavage	Safe; simple; minimally invasive; no anesthetic needed; more repeatable than BAL; inexpensive	Cooperation needed; small yield; variable baseline; timing is critical	Cells: number, differential Fluid: arachidonic acid metabolites; cytokines; enzymes; histamine; protein, etc.
Blood Collection	Inexpensive; safe; subject acceptability	May not reflect respiratory response	COHb; $PGF_{2\alpha}$; lymphocyte subsets, etc.

FVC = forced vital capacity; FEV_1 = forced expired volume 1 second; MMEF = maximal midexpiratory flow; Raw = airway resistance; SRaw = specific airway resistance; SGaw = specific airway conductance; R_T = total respiratory resistance; VO_{2max} = maximum oxygen consumption; COHb = carboxyhemoglobin; $PGF_{2\alpha}$ = prostaglandin $F_{2\alpha}$.

this may be related to a neurally mediated reduction in maximal inspiratory effort associated with discomfort in taking a deep breath [140].

Partial expiratory flow–volume curves have some advantages over spirometry. Partial expiratory flow–volume curves beginning at 60% of total lung capacity (TLC) can determine maximum expiratory flows in the tidal volume range and avoid potential bronchodilator (in normal subjects) and bronchoconstrictive (in asthmatics) effects of prior deep breaths. Thus, atopic adolescents [45] and asthmatics [141] exposed to sulfur dioxide or sulfuric acid aerosol, respectively, show a true bronchoconstrictive response, according to reductions of partial maximum expiratory flows.

Considerable attention has been paid to the development of respiratory function tests that are sensitive to alterations in the peripheral airways, i.e., the region of terminal and respiratory bronchioles. Structural and functional changes in the small airways can occur with several types of inhaled irritant. The single-breath nitrogen washout test and density-dependence of maximum expiratory flow measure small-airway function [129,138]. Unfortunately, the results from these tests exhibit large inter- and intrasubject variability, and their accuracy and reliability for measuring peripheral physiological events remains uncertain. Further development of tests of peripheral-airway function is required before they can be used reliably in exposure studies.

Airway Resistance. Lung compliance or airway resistance techniques assess mechanical properties during breathing, i.e., the work of breathing [129,138]. The classical measurements of dynamic and static–quasistatic lung compliance have not been used frequently in exposures, owing to their need for placement of an esophageal balloon catheter, subject acceptance, and time-consuming nature. Rather, exposure studies have relied on plethysmographic measurements of airflow resistance or conductance in the nasal or lower respiratory tracts. Measurements of airway resistance are rapid, noninvasive, simple to perform, and fairly reproducible, avoid forced ventilatory maneuvers, and allow simultaneous measurement and correction for thoracic gas volume. However, a body plethysmograph is required for measuring lower-airway resistance. This technique suffers from large variability in values for airway resistance (Raw) and specific airway resistance (SRaw) and the lack of regional specificity, e.g., for the larynx and peripheral airways. Nonetheless, the combination of plethysmography and spirometry has been useful in detecting subtle changes and understanding the pathophysiology of responses when divergent findings are observed. For example, ozone alters spirometry in normal subjects with exposures to 0.18 ppm and higher, but SRaw increases only with high concentrations [22,47,139], suggesting that low levels of ozone initially restrict full inspiration and that higher concentrations produce airway narrowing.

Respiratory system impedance (forced oscillation technique) is a rapid, simple-to-perform technique that measures integrated compliance and resistance of the entire lung and potentially of specific respiratory regions [129,138]. A high-frequency oscillation signal is applied to the airway during normal tidal breathing. The resulting pressure, volume, or flow perturbations in the air column are measured and used to calculate values of components of mechanical impedance (resistance, compliance, and inertance) of the respiratory system. By manipulating the oscillating signal and analyzing the response, one can theoretically obtain data to develop models about central and peripheral airway properties. However, general acceptance and widespread use of this technique will require further technical development. Total respiratory resistance (R_T) is highly dependent on the frequency of the oscillation and is not corrected for lung volume, which affects airway resistance. Studies with sulfur dioxide exposure in asthmatics have shown increased respiratory resistance, suggesting increased resistance in small airways [45,114,142].

Inhaled gases or aerosols may also affect nasal resistance, which can be measured by rhinomanometry. For example, sulfur dioxide is a highly water-soluble gas that is solubilized in the nasal passages. This gas increases nasal resistance in adolescent asthmatics [142]. On the other hand, sulfuric acid aerosol has no effect on nasal resistance [142].

Aerosol Probe Technique. The aerosol bolus technique involves a subject's inhaling a tidal volume of clean air into which a volumetrically small aerosol bolus is injected [129]. The bolus divides as it proceeds through successive bifurcations in the lung and is reassembled during exhalation. Asymmetries in ventilation and variations in regional time constants of the lung influence the reassembly or dispersion of the bolus. Results from this research technique may be influenced by factors such as the bolus volume, particle size, lung volume, and penetration depth, and procedures differ between laboratories. However, the technique can detect proximal airway obstruction and is considered a possible probe of small-airway function [143,144]. The volumetric dispersion of exhaled aerosol boluses increases with the depth of penetration into the lung, using nonhygroscopic triphenyl phosphate aerosol (MMAD 0.47 μm; GSD 1.5) and sophisticated bolus delivery and measurement systems, following 1-h exposure to 0.4 ppm ozone in healthy subjects as compared with that in clean air [144]. These ozone-related changes were accompanied by significant spirometric decreases but no change in Raw and SRaw. However, this technique requires further development and correlation with small-airway structure and function.

4. Bronchoprovocation Tests

Airway hyperreactivity is an exaggerated bronchoconstrictive response to a variety of chemical, physical, and pharmacological stimuli and is a hallmark of clinical asthma and occupationally induced asthma [56]. Nonspecific airway hyperreactivity can be experimentally tested with inhalation of pharmacological agents (e.g., methacholine, histamine, carbachol) or hypertonic or hypotonic aerosols, isocapnic hyperventilation with cold or dry air, and exercise [25]. Challenges are frequently performed during screening procedures to establish baseline reactivity and after exposure to assess the effect of pollutants on the subjects' airway responsiveness. Postexposure challenges should be performed when lung function returns to baseline levels to avoid the confounding effect of altered airway geometry. The response to pharmacological challenges is typically expressed as the provocative concentration or dose necessary to produce a 20% decline in FEV_1 (PC_{20} or PD_{20}). Although this bronchoconstrictor response is easily observed with low concentrations in asthmatics, the response is frequently absent even at maximal concentrations (e.g., 25 mg/ml) in nonasthmatic subjects. The calculation of the dose–response slope [145] provides an index of airway sensitivity in all subjects and eliminates the need to censor data from subjects without a detectable PC_{20} or PD_{20}. Alternatively, some investigators use the provocative concentration or dose that results in a 50% or 100% increase in SRaw as a measure of postexposure nonspecific reactivity [47,114].

Inhalation challenge testing with nonspecific stimuli has been incorporated in many exposure studies as a potentially sensitive probe for assessing pollutant-induced airway reactivity and possibly predicting pollutant responders. Asthmatic and nonasthmatic subjects acutely exposed to nitrogen dioxide [59,61,146], ozone [41,46,117,147], and sulfuric acid [141] have demonstrated increased airway reactivity to cold air–hyperventilation, methacholine or histamine, or carbachol aerosols. Nonspecific hyperreactivity has also been reported to predict individual responsiveness to inhaled gases or aerosols [92,114], although this finding is not universal for ozone [47,117].

Specific airway hyperreactivity is experimentally tested with specific agents such as common antigens, isocyanates, and plicatic acid (from Western red cedar). Their application in human pollutant exposures has been minimal because of their difficult, time-consuming, and risky nature. However, bronchial responsiveness to inhaled allergen in allergic asthmatics can be potentiated with 1-h exposure to 0.12 ppm ozone at rest [148].

5. Tests of Epithelial Integrity

Several methods are available for evaluating the functional integrity of the epithelial barrier in the airways and alveoli. The single-breath technique for measuring diffusing capacity for carbon monoxide (Dco) is a well-established, sensitive clinical index of alveolar–capillary gas-exchange efficiency. The equipment can be automated to improve standardization. However, it has limited applicability in pollutant exposures and, when performed, has not shown significant changes even with high levels of pollutants in COPD patients [51].

Oximetry. An important clinical marker of a pollutant effect would be acute hypoxemia, especially in volunteers with chronic lung disease. Oxygenation status can be readily measured by noninvasive ear or finger oximetry, which avoids invasive arterial punctures for blood gases. Exposure to 4 and 5 ppm nitrogen dioxide produced statistically significant reductions in arterialized oxygen partial pressure (PO_2) in chronic bronchitics [149]. However, subsequent studies could not confirm evidence of ozone- or nitrogen dioxide–induced desaturation in COPD patients and normal subjects [77,78,150]. Monitoring with oximetry should be encouraged as both a safety measure and a marker of effect in subjects with preexisting cardiopulmonary disease.

Mucociliary Clearance. Mucociliary clearance is an important respiratory defense mechanism and a possible sensitive marker of effect. In vivo clearance studies generally measure the rate of transport or removal of tracer particles from the lungs or nose as a whole or from specific regions of the lungs [129]. Tracers are generally introduced into the nasal passage, trachea, or bronchi by an airstream (via nebulization) or instillation (via bronchoscopy or direct placement). Movement of radioactive tracers can be externally monitored with a gamma camera or scintillation detectors. Although this technique can be anatomically specific, many technical variables need to be considered, including the types, configuration, and spatial resolution of detector systems, initial deposition of the tracer aerosol, and type of radioactive isotype [129]. The technical complexities of clearance studies and high intersubject variability have precluded frequent use of this modality in human exposure studies.

Inhaled pollutants can produce small but statistically significant effects on human mucociliary transport. For example, short-term (2-h) exposures to 0.4 ppm ozone can acutely increase mucociliary transport of particle-labeled mucus and enhance mucus clearance from peripheral to central lung regions as compared with clean air rates [151]. Similarly, sulfuric acid exposure acutely increases tracheal and peripheral lung clearance rates in healthy subjects without producing symptoms or effects on spirometry or nonspecific reactivity [110]. Other investigators have reported both transient increases and transient decreases in tracheobronchial clearance that are dependent on concentration, particle size, exposure time, and perhaps subject characteristics [152–154].

Permeability. The protective epithelial integrity of the airways and alveoli relies on tight intercellular junctions. Inhaled pollutants may alter or injure the epithelial barrier, resulting in abnormally increased penetration of inhaled materials into the interstitium and blood. This phenomenon can be evaluated by in vivo tests for tracheobronchial and alveolar permeability, typically with inhalation of radioactively tagged (^{99m}Tc) diethylenetriamine penta-acetic acid (DTPA) aerosol and its subsequent thoracic scanning to obtain clearance half-times [129]. Many of the same technical issues in clearance studies pertain to permeability experiments, such as particle size, breathing pattern, deposition sites, integrity of the molecular tracer, timing of inhalation during the protocol, etc. [129].

Inhaled oxidants appear to modify lung permeability in humans. Ozone exposure (0.4 ppm $\times$ 2 h) sufficient to produce lung function decrements significantly increases ^{99m}Tc-DTPA lung clearance in healthy adults as compared with that in clean air [155]. The faster clearance suggests ozone-induced injury and heightened permeability of the respiratory epithelium, which may be a mechanism for ozone potentiation of subsequent antigen [148] or sulfur dioxide [89] challenges. On the other hand, exposure of healthy subjects to nitrogen dioxide (2.3 ppm × 5 h) produced a delayed decrease in clearance 6 h after exposure relative to clean-air exposure, but no differences at 1 and 18 h following oxidant exposure [156]. The mechanism is unknown, although the subjects did not experience respiratory symptoms or dysfunction. The effects of other pollutants on lung permeability in humans are currently unknown.

6. Exercise Performance

A modification of physical activity by pollutant exposure must be considered clinically significant, especially when accompanied by statistically significant changes in lung function. This issue can be approached in the laboratory with determination of exercise capacity or performance [42,43]. The exercise protocols and end points vary. Some very fit subjects have been unable to complete simulated competitive endurance protocols during exposure to ozone concentrations ranging between 0.18 and 0.35 ppm [39,40]. Other studies have involved athletes who either perform a maximum oxygen consumption (VO_{2max}) test following pollutant exposure or cycle continuously at a high percentage of their VO_{2max} during exposure to low ozone concentrations. Exposure to 0.75 ppm ozone decreases VO_{2max} [157]. Continuously exercising cyclists have reduced VO_{2max}, work time, and workload during exposure to 0.20 ppm ozone but not to 0.12 ppm [41].

7. Bronchoalveolar Lavage

Inhaled agents can produce airway and parenchymal inflammation by direct injury (e.g., ozone), immunological stimulation (e.g., isocyanates, beryllium), or infection [129]. Only lung inflammation due to irritant pollutants will be addressed here, to provide a perspective of how inflammatory markers can be evaluated in human controlled exposure studies. The method of bronchoalveolar lavage (BAL) through a flexible fiberoptic bronchoscope is a widely used and accepted clinical and research tool for sampling pulmonary cells and fluid. The method is technically facile and safe (even in asthmatic subjects) in experienced hands and can obtain large volumes of aspirated BAL fluid for subsequent analysis. The techniques have not been fully standardized, and interlaboratory differences include the amount of saline instilled and aspirated, site(s) of infusion, temperature of the saline, dilution factors, and preparation of BAL cell differentials [158]. An important limitation is the relative lack of specificity in anatomical sampling of cellular and biochemical constituents, e.g., central airways vs. alveoli. The origin of the recovered BAL fluid may be better controlled with a balloon catheter that isolates and lavages a portion of a proximal airway [159] or sequential fractionated aliquots [160,161]. These techniques decrease the mixing of BAL components from proximal and distal regions of the lavaged lung.

Ozone exposures of healthy subjects have consistently demonstrated evidence of an acute pulmonary inflammatory response. Significant increases in BAL polymorphonuclear neutrophils (PMNs), protein, albumin, immunoglobulin G, neutrophil elastase activity, prostaglandin E_2, fibronectin, urokinase plasminogen activator, or lactate dehydrogenase occur after exposures to 0.08–0.60 ppm ozone for periods of 2 or 6.6 h [162–164]. Alveolar macrophages show reduced phagocytic capability for yeast [164]. The temporal pattern of ozone-induced neutrophil influx in humans should be considered in timing BAL sampling [161,165]. Whereas symptoms and FEV_1 decrements occurred and resolved within the first few hours after exposure to 0.3 ppm ozone, the BAL neutrophilia in both proximal and distal aliquots increased more slowly, peaked at about 6 h, and persisted for 24 h after exposure [161].

Other pollutants have different effects on BAL results. For example, healthy volunteers exposed to 8 ppm sulfur dioxide for 20 min showed a time-dependent inflammatory response, i.e., BAL lymphocytes and mast cells increased at 4 and 24 h after exposure and returned to preexposure levels at 72 h [166]. The BAL albumin and FEV_1 were not changed as compared with preexposure values. Ambient levels of nitrogen dioxide elicit a weak inflammatory response or none [167,168], although concentrations as high as 5.5 ppm may significantly increase BAL lymphocytes and mast cells during the initial 24 h following exposure [169,170]. Inflammation-related proteins and mediators were unchanged in these BAL studies, although alterations in alpha-1-protease inhibitor activity [171,172] and macrophage inactivation of influenza virus [173] have been reported. On the other hand, repeated daily exposures to 4 ppm nitrogen dioxide produced a different cellular response, with reduced lymphocyte subsets in BAL fluid and reduced lymphocyte count in peripheral blood but no change in BAL mast cell or lymphocyte numbers [174]. Exposure to sulfuric acid aerosol (1000 $\mu g/m^3$) for 2 h did not elicit an inflammatory cell response or alter components of antimicrobial defense in the BAL performed 18 h after exposure [175].

8. Nasal Lavage

The nose is the primary portal of entry of inspired air and pollutants, and its failure to protect the lower respiratory tract could lead to greater penetration of inhaled pollutants into the lower respiratory tract. Nasal lavage (NAL) offers numerous advantages for measuring the acute nasal response to inhaled pollutants. Nasal lavage is simple to perform, relatively noninvasive and nontraumatic, and does not induce an inflammatory response, as may occur with BAL [129,176]. Multiple samples from the same subject can be obtained during the same exposure visit with safety and subject acceptance. The subject sits upright with head titled back, and sterile phosphate-buffered saline solution (5 ml) is instilled via a syringe into each nostril. The saline solution is held in the nasal passages (with palatal pressure) for 10 s and then forcibly expelled and collected. Approximately 7 ml is routinely recovered. Cellular and biochemical constituents can be analyzed as for BAL fluid.

Nasal lavage is increasingly being used, but the results may be variable. Of 200 volunteers, 50% had less than 10^4 PMNs per milliliter of nasal lavage, and 10% had over 10^5 PMNs/ml, at baseline [177]. The variability in NAL cell numbers may be reduced by taking preexperiment and postexperiment samples on the same day and instructing subjects to avoid intercurrent or concurrent respiratory irritants (e.g., tobacco smoke, chemicals, viruses). Acute exposure to 0.4 and 0.5 ppm ozone significantly increased NAL PMNs [177,178]. Although the PMN counts were increased from NAL and BAL performed 18 h after ozone exposure, their correlation was weak ($r = 0.41, p = 0.24$), and the NAL PMN count did not predict the total number of BAL PMNs [178]. Albumin in NAL was increased after ozone exposure, but other biochemical substances found in BAL were not [178]. A 4-h exposure to 0.5 ppm ozone in subjects with allergic rhinitis revealed increased NAL PMNs, eosinophils, mononuclear cells, epithelial cells, and albumin [179]. Environmental tobacco smoke (ETS) did not increase mediator release in NAL in either sensitive or nonsensitive subjects, despite significant increases in symptoms and posterior nasal resistance in the ETS-sensitive group [131]. A mixture of VOCs (25 mg/m^3 total hydrocarbon), which might be found in new homes and office buildings, significantly increased NAL PMNs both immediately and 18 h after a 4-h exposure, indicating a local inflammatory response [180].

9. Blood Collection

Blood markers of pollutant-related exposure or effect may reflect direct or indirect reactions with pulmonary or extrapulmonary constituents. They are being intensely investigated, since blood collection (via venipuncture) is reasonable and simple for both controlled-exposure and epidemiological studies. Blood levels of COHb are an excellent index of exposure and predictor of effect. Carbon monoxide exposures of patients with coronary artery disease have used COHb as an exposure marker and angina pectoris or electrocardiographic changes as end points [82–84]. Plasma prostaglandin $F_{2\alpha}$ was significantly increased in ozone-sensitive subjects (>24% decrement in FEV_1) during and after 80-min exposure to 0.35 ppm ozone but not in less sensitive subjects who had a reduction of less than 11% in FEV_1 on exposure to ozone [181]. On the other hand, some systemic responses may be delayed. Serum glutathione peroxidase activity significantly decreased, by 14%, at 18 h but not at 8 h following a 5-h exposure to 2.3 ppm nitrogen dioxide [156].

IV. DATA ANALYSIS

Appropriate statistical tests must be applied to determine whether response differences between control (usually clean air) and exposure conditions are meaningful. Testing for a pollutant-related effect and, in some studies, estimating the effect per unit of exposure are fundamental goals of most controlled human exposures. Analytical strategies should be incorporated during the formulation of the experimental design of a new study. Important issues of paired vs. unpaired comparison designs, power calculations of a detectable effect (e.g., for FEV_1), statistical inferences, and dose-response curves are beyond the scope of this review but are considered elsewhere [182]. Greater power of and confidence in the results may be obtained by strategies involving large numbers of subjects, sensitive subjects, optimal stabilization of baseline values (e.g., in asthmatics and COPD subjects), very sensitive tests, high pollutant concentrations, and/or dose–response experiments. However, these possibilities are tempered by the limited number of subjects who can be reasonably studied, available resources, financial and ethical considerations, and other factors.

Careful consideration of the statistical, biological, and clinical significance of the results is essential, since the information may be used in regulatory processes. Some responses may represent an appropriate physiological reaction to a stress or a minor annoyance [183]. Emphasis on these changes for regulatory and clinical purposes may be excessive or premature. On the other hand, failure to detect statistically significant changes does not necessarily rule out a clinical or public health problem (false negative or type II error). Negative or equivocal results may stem from multiple factors: e.g., the subjects may not be sensitive, the sample may be too small (thus enhancing interindividual differences in response), the test procedures may be inadequate to detect a meaningful change, or the pollutant exposure may be insufficient for effect. Negative results from worst-case experimental conditions may not be definitive, since more sensitive or appropriate tests or group of subjects may be found at a future time. For example, ambient levels of sulfur dioxide were not considered a major public health problem until the 1980s. However, asthmatics were subsequently determined to be highly sensitive to low concentrations of the pollutant.

Some investigators have attempted to combine results from multiple exposure studies and develop models of exposure–response for a pollutant for risk assessment [184–186]. This has been difficult because of inconsistent and incomplete reporting of raw data and statistical results. Nonetheless, techniques such as meta-analysis may provide meaningful interpretation of aggregate data.

V. SAFETY ASPECTS

Controlled pollutant exposures of human volunteers must consider the safety and welfare of the subjects as the highest priority. Guidelines should not be inflexible or applicable to all research protocols. Rather, they should allow clinical research to be conducted in a manner that affords research subjects a high degree of protection from unnecessary morbid events. Safety and ethical issues regarding the protocol design, its implementation, and the informed consent process must be carefully considered, despite the excellent track record of controlled exposures. These issues have been reviewed elsewhere [187] and involve the following: identifying risks involved in the research; providing adequate safeguards in the protocol design and during withholding of medications; anticipating risk; minimizing the chances for human error; providing resuscitation equipment; and planning for medical support for problems ranging from minor side effects to a life-threatening emergency. This process should facilitate approval of protocols by the governing institutional review board.

Controlled-exposure studies involve exposures, exercise, and possibly uncomfortable or invasive procedures, e.g., venipuncture, bronchoprovocation challenges, bronchoscopy, or lung scanning with radioactive substances. The safety aspects related to these procedures are familiar to clinician–investigators experienced in their use. The safety aspects of exposures, e.g., using a chamber facility, must be routinely multiple and perhaps even redundant. Early studies used relatively high, unrealistic concentrations of pollutants to determine human responses. However, current research has emphasized the short-term health effects of low to very low pollutant concentrations that simulate ambient conditions. Agents with known or suspected capabilities for irreversible or malignant responses are obviously excluded from studies of human volunteers for ethical reasons. Pollutant generation and monitoring should have strict quality-control measures, ample ventilation and pressure alarms, backup monitors, an engineer, and a quality assurance program. All subjects should be screened for medical contraindications and have diligent monitoring for possible acute and delayed side effects, as well as access to appropriate medical care.

VI. CONCLUSION

Controlled human exposure to pollutants is an important and powerful research tool for direct assessment of the acute effects of inhaled pollutants, dose-response relationships, mechanisms of action of pollutants, and comparison of normal subjects' responses with those of more susceptible groups. These aims can be pursued with a wide variety of conditions and subject groups through the use of traditional and new end points. Data from such studies may be directly relevant to basic sciences, clinical medicine, public health, and the promulgation of air quality standards. Nonetheless, exposure studies frequently generate new questions or unexpected results and have certain inherent limitations that must be acknowledged. Studies with negative or equivocal results still provide important contributions to the data base and help establish threshold information. Finally, credible experimental data must possess the scientific rigor of peer review, relevance to real-world situations, and replication by independent investigators [7]. As a result, these data will strongly complement and strengthen results from animal toxicology and epidemiological studies and contribute to the overall understanding of the health effects of air pollutants.

REFERENCES

1. Bates, D. V., Health indices of the adverse effects of air pollution: the question of coherence, *Environ. Res.*, *59*, 336–349 (1992).
2. Lippmann, M., *Environmental Toxicants. Human Exposure and Their Health Effects*, Van Nostrand Rheinhold, New York, 1992.
3. Samet, J. M., Marbury, M. C., and Spengler, J. D., Health effects and sources of indoor air pollution, *Am. Rev. Respir. Dis.*, *136*, 1486–1508 (1987) (Part I); *137*, 221–242 (1988) (Part II).
4. Gong, H., Jr., Health effects of air pollution. A review of clinical studies, *Clin. Chest Med.*, *13*, 201–214 (1992).
5. Lippmann, M., Health effects of ozone. A critical review, *J. Air Pollut. Cont. Assoc.*, *39*, 672–695 (1989).
6. Samet, J. M., and Utell, M. J., The risk of nitrogen dioxide: What we have learned from epidemiological and clinical studies? *Toxicol. Indust. Health*, *6*, 247–262 (1990).
7. Hackney, J. D., Linn, W. S., and Avol, E. L., Assessing health effects of air pollution, *Environ. Sci. Technol.*, *18*, 115A–122A (1984).
8. Folinsbee, L. J., Human clinical inhalation exposures. Experimental design, methodology, and physiological responses, in *Toxicology of the Lung* (D. E. Gardner, J. D. Grapo, and E. J. Massaro, eds.), Raven Press, New York, 1988, pp. 175–199.
9. Schelegle, E. S., Adams, W. C., and Siefkin, A. D., Indomethacin pretreatment reduces ozone-induced pulmonary function decrements in human subjects, *Am. Rev. Respir. Dis.*, *136*, 1350–1354 (1987).
10. Ying, R. L., Gross, K. B., Terzo, T. S., and Eschenbacher, W. L., Indomethacin does not inhibit the ozone-induced increase in bronchial responsiveness in human subjects, *Am. Rev. Respir. Dis.*, *142*, 817–821 (1990).
11. Chatham, M. D., Eppler, J. H., Sauder, L. R., Greene, D., and Kulle, T. J., Effects of vitamin C, E, and aspirin in normal subjects exposed to ozone (abstract), *Am. Rev. Respir. Dis.*, *135*, A57 (1987).
12. Koenig, J. O., Dumler, K., Rebolledo, V., Williams, P. V., and Pierson, W. E., Theophylline mitigates the bronchoconstrictor effects of sulfur dioxide in subjects with asthma, *J. Allergy Clin. Immunol.*, *89*, 789–794 (1992).
13. Koenig, J. O., Marshall, S. G., Horike, M., Shapiro, G. G., Furukawa, C. T., Bierman, C. W., and Pierson, W. E., The effects of albuterol on sulfur dioxide–induced bronchoconstriction in allergic adolescents, *J. Allergy Clin. Immunol.*, *79*, 54–58 (1987).
14. Linn, W. S., Avol, E. L., Shamoo, D. A., Spier, C. E., Smith, M. N., and Hackney, J. D., Effect of metaproterenol sulfate on mild asthmatics' response to sulfur dioxide exposure and exercise, *Arch. Environ. Health*, *43*, 399–406 (1988).
15. Linn, W. S., Shamoo, D. A., Peng, R.-C., Clark, K. W., Avol, E. L., and Hackney, J. D., Responses to sulfur dioxide and exercise by medication-dependent asthmatics: effect of varying medication levels, *Arch. Environ. Health*, *45*, 24–30 (1990).

16. Sheppard, D., Nadel, J. A., and Boushey, H. A., Inhibition of sulfur dioxide–induced bronchoconstriction by disodium cromoglycate in asthmatic subjects, *Am. Rev. Respir. Dis.*, *124*, 257–259 (1981).
17. Koenig, J. O., Marshall, S. G., van Belle, G., McManus, M. S., Bierman, C. W., Shapiro, G. G., Furukawa, C. T., and Pierson, W. E., Therapeutic range cromolyn dose-response inhibition and complete obliteration of SO_2-induced bronchoconstriction in atopic adolescents, *J. Allergy Clin. Immunol.*, *81*, 897–901 (1988).
18. Myers, D. J., Bigby, B. G., and Boushey, H. A., The inhibition of sulfur dioxide–induced bronchoconstriction in asthmatic subjects by cromolyn is dose-dependent, *Am. Rev. Respir. Dis.*, *133*, 1150–1153 (1986).
19. Myers, D. J., Bigby, B. G., Calvayrac, P., Sheppard, D., and Boushey, H. A., Interaction of cromolyn and a muscarinic antagonist in inhibiting bronchial reactivity to sulfur dioxide and to eucapnic hyperpnea alone, *Am. Rev. Respir. Dis.*, *133*, 1154–1158 (1986).
20. Dixon, C. M. S., Fuller, R. W., and Barnes, P. J., Effect of nedocromil sodium on sulphur dioxide induced bronchoconstriction, *Thorax*, *42*, 462–465 (1987).
21. Wiebicke, W., Jorres, R., and Magnussen, H., Comparison of the effects of inhaled corticosteroids on the airway response to histamine, methacholine, hyperventilation, and sulfur dioxide in subjects with asthma, *J. Allergy Clin. Immunol.*, *86*, 915–923 (1990).
22. Beckett, W. S., McDonnell, W. F., Horstman, D. H., and House, D. E., Role of the parasympathetic nervous system in acute lung response to ozone, *J. Appl. Physiol.*, *59*, 1879–1885 (1985).
23. Mohsenin, V., Effect of vitamin C on NO_2-induced airway hyperresponsiveness in normal subjects. A randomized double-blind experiment, *Am. Rev. Respir. Dis.*, *136*, 1408–1411 (1987).
24. Gong, H., Jr., Bedi, J. F., and Horvath, S. M., Inhaled albuterol does not protect against ozone toxicity in nonasthmatic athletes, *Arch. Environ. Health*, *43*, 46–53 (1988).
25. Spector, S. L., Bronchial provocation tests, in *Bronchial Asthma. Mechanisms and Therapeutics*, 3rd Ed., (E. B. Weiss and M. Stein, eds.), Little, Brown, and Company, Boston, 1993, pp. 501–516.
26. McDonnell, W. F., III, Chapman, R. S., Leigh, M. W., Strope, G. L., and Collier, A. M., Respiratory responses of vigorously exercising children to 0.12 ppm ozone exposure, *Am. Rev. Respir. Dis.*, *132*, 875–879 (1985).
27. Avol, E. L., Linn, W. S., Shamoo, D. A., Valencia, L. M., Anzar, U. T., Venet, T. G., and Hackney, J. D., Respiratory effects of photochemical oxidant air pollution in exercising adolescents, *Am. Rev. Respir. Dis.*, *132*, 619–622 (1985).
28. Koenig, J. Q., Pierson, W. E., Horike, M., and Frank, R., Effects of inhaled sulfur dioxide (SO_2) on pulmonary function in healthy adolescents: exposure to SO_2 alone or SO_2 + sodium chloride droplet aerosol during rest and exercise, *Arch. Environ. Health*, , *37*, 5–9 (1982).
29. Koenig, J. Q., Covert, D. S., and Marshall, S. G., The effects of ozone and nitrogen dioxide on pulmonary function in healthy and in asthmatic adolescents, *Am. Rev. Respir. Dis.*, *136*, 1152–1157 (1987).

30. Drechsler-Parks, D. M., Bedi, J. F., and Horvath, S. M., Pulmonary function responses of older men and women to NO_2, *Environ. Res.*, *44*, 206–212 (1987).
31. Drechsler-Parks, D. M., Bedi, J. F., and Horvath, S. M., Pulmonary function responses of older men and women to ozone, *Exp. Gerontol.*, *22*, 91–101 (1987).
32. Rondinelli, R. C. A., Koenig, J. Q., and Marshall, S. G., The effects of sulfur dioxide on pulmonary function in healthy nonsmoking male subjects aged 55 years and older, *Am. Ind. Hyg. Assoc. J.*, *48*, 299–303 (1987).
33. Reisenauer, C. S., Koenig, J. Q., McManus, M. S., Smith, M. S., Kusic, G., and Pierson, W. E., Pulmonary response to ozone exposures in healthy individuals aged 55 years or greater, *J. Air. Pollut. Cont. Assoc.*, *38*, 51–55 (1988).
34. McDonnell, W. F., Muller, K. E., Bromberg, P. A., and Shy, C. M., Predictors of individual differences in acute response to ozone exposure, *Am. Rev. Respir. Dis.*, *147*, 818–825 (1992).
35. Lauritzen, S. K., and Adams, W. C., Ozone inhalation consequent to continuous exercise in females: comparison with males, *J. Appl. Physiol.*, *59*, 1601–1606 (1985).
36. Adams, W. C., Brookes, K. A., and Schelegle, E. S., Effects of NO_2 alone and in combination with O_3 on young men and women, *J. Appl. Physiol.*, *62*, 1698–1704 (1987).
37. Messino, T. D., and Adams, W. C., Ozone inhalation effects in females varying widely in lung size: comparison with males, *J. Appl. Physiol.*, *69*, 96–103 (1990).
38. Seal, E., Jr., McDonnell, W. F., House, D. E., Salaam, S. A., Dewitt, P. J., Butler, S. O., Green, J., and Raggio, L., The pulmonary response of white and black adults to six concentrations of ozone, *Am. Rev. Respir. Dis.*, *147*, 804–810 (1993).
39. Adams, W. C., and Schelegle, E. S., Ozone and high ventilation effects on pulmonary function and endurance performance, *J. Appl. Physiol.*, *55*, 805–812 (1983).
40. Schelegle, E. S., and Adams, W. C., Reduced exercise time in competitive simulations consequent to low level ozone exposure, *Med. Sci. Sports Exerc.*, *18*, 408–414 (1986).
41. Gong, H., Jr., Bradley, P. W., Simmons, M. S., and Tashkin, D. P., Impaired exercise performance and pulmonary function in elite cyclists during low-level ozone exposure in a hot environment, *Am. Rev. Respir. Dis.*, *134*, 726–733 (1986).
42. Gong, H., Jr., Effects of ozone on exercise performance, *J. Sports Med. Physical Fitness*, *27*, 21–29 (1987).
43. Adams, W. C., Effects of ozone exposure at ambient air pollution episode levels on exercise performance, *Sports Med.*, *4*, 395–424 (1987).
44. Kim, S. U., Koenig, J. Q., Pierson, W. E., and Hanley, Q. S., Acute pulmonary effects of nitrogen dioxide exposure during exercise in competitive athletes, *Chest*, *99*, 815–819 (1991).
45. Koenig, J. Q., Pierson, W. E., Horike, M., and Frank, R., Bronchoconstrictor responses to sulfur dioxide or sulfur dioxide plus sodium chloride droplets in allergic, nonasthmatic adolescents, *J. Allergy Clin. Immunol.*, *69*, 339–344 (1982).
46. Holtzman, M. J., Cunningham, J. H., Sheller, J. R., Irsigler, G. B., Nadel, J. A., and

Boushey, H. A., Effect of ozone on bronchial reactivity in atopic and nonatopic subjects, *Am. Rev. Respir. Dis.*, *120*, 1059–1067 (1979).

47. McDonnell, W. F., Horstman, D. H., Abdul-Salaam, S., Raggio, L .J., and Green, J. A., The respiratory responses of subjects with allergic rhinitis to ozone exposure and their relationship to nonspecific airway reactivity, *Toxicol. Ind. Health*, *3*, 507–517 (1987).
48. Kerr, H. D., Kulle, T. J., McIlhany, M. L., and Swidersky, P., Effects of ozone on pulmonary function in normal subjects, *Am. Rev. Respir. Dis.*, *111*, 763–773 (1975).
49. Shephard, R. J., Urch, B., Silverman, F., and Corey, P. N. J., Interaction of ozone and cigarette smoke exposure, *Environ. Res.*, *31*, 125–137 (1983).
50. Emmons, K., and Foster, W. M., Smoking cessation and acute airway response to ozone, *Arch. Environ. Health*, *46*, 288–295 (1991).
51. Morrow, P. E., Utell, M. J., Bauer, M. A., Smeglin, A. M., Frampton, M. W., Cox, C., Speers, D. M., and Gibb, F. R., Pulmonary performance of elderly normal subjects and subjects with chronic obstructive pulmonary disease exposed to 0.3 ppm nitrogen dioxide, *Am. Rev. Respir. Dis.*, *145*, 291–300 (1992).
52. Empey, D. W., Laitinen, L. A., Jacobs, L., Gold, W. M., and Nadel, J. A., Mechanisms of bronchial hyperreactivity in normal subjects after upper respiratory tract infection, *Am. Rev. Respir. Dis.*, *113*, 131–139 (1976).
53. Utell, M. J., Aquilina, A. T., Hall, W. J., Speers, D. M., Douglas, R. G., Jr., Gibb, F. R., Morrow, P. E., and Hyde, R. W., Development of airway reactivity to nitrates in subjects with influenza, *Am. Rev. Respir. Dis.*, *121*, 233–241 (1980).
54. Henderson, F. W., Dubovi, E. J., Harder, S., Seal, E., Jr., and Graham, D., Experimental rhinovirus infection in human volunteers exposed to ozone, *Am. Rev. Respir. Dis.*, *137*, 1124–1128 (1988).
55. Goings, S. A. J., Kulle, T. J., Bascom, R., Sauder, L. R., Green, D. J., Hebel, J. R., and Clements, M. L., Effect of nitrogen dioxide exposure on susceptibility to influenza A virus infection in healthy adults, *Am. Rev. Respir. Dis.*, *139*, 1075–1081 (1989).
56. Boushey, H. A., Holtzman, M. J., Sheller, J. R., and Nadel, J. A., Bronchial hyperreactivity, *Am. Rev. Respir. Dis.*, *121*, 389–413 (1990).
57. Kreit, J. W., Gross, K. B., Moore, T. B., Lorenzen, T. J., D'Arcy, J., and Eschenbacher, W. L., Ozone-induced changes in lung function and bronchial responsiveness in asthmatics, *J. Appl. Physiol.*, *66*, 217–222 (1989).
58. Linn, W. S., Shamoo, D. A., Avol, E. L., Whynot, J. D., Anderson, K. R., Venet, T. G., and Hackney, J. D., Dose-response study of asthmatic volunteers exposed to nitrogen dioxide during intermittent exercise, *Arch. Environ. Health*, *41*, 292–296 (1986).
59. Bauer, M. A., Utell, M. J., Morrow, P. E., Speers, D. M., and Gibb, F. R., Inhalation of 0.30 ppm nitrogen dioxide potentiates exercise-induced bronchospasm in asthmatics, *Am. Rev. Respir. Dis.*, *134*, 1203–1208 (1986).
60. Bylin, G., Hedenstierna, G., Lindvall, T., and Sundin, B., Ambient nitrogen dioxide concentrations increase bronchial responsiveness in subjects with mild asthma, *Eur. Respir. J.*, *1*, 606–612 (1988).

61. Mohsenin, V., Airway responses to 2.0 ppm nitrogen dioxide in normal subjects, *Arch. Environ. Health*, *43*, 242–246 (1988).
62. Koenig, J. Q., Pierson, W. E., and Horike, M., The effects of inhaled sulfuric acid on pulmonary function in adolescent asthmatics, *Am. Rev. Respir. Dis.*, *128*, 221–225 (1983).
63. Utell, M. J., Morrow, P. E., Speers, D. M., Draling, J., and Hyde, R. W., Airway responses to sulfate and sulfuric acid aerosols in asthmatics. An exposure-response relationship, *Am. Rev. Respir. Dis.*, *128*, 444–450 (1983).
64. Linn, W. S., Avol, E. L., Anderson, K. R., et al., Effect of droplet size on respiratory responses to inhaled sulfuric acid in normal and asthmatic volunteers, *Am. Rev. Respir. Dis.*, *140*, 161–166 (1989).
65. Aris, R., Christian, D., Sheppard, D., and Balmes, J. R., Lack of bronchoconstrictor response to sulfuric acid aerosols and fogs, *Am. Rev. Respir. Dis.*, *143*, 744–750 (1991).
66. Avol, E. L., Linn, W. S., Shamoo, D. A., Anderson, K. R., Peng, R. C., and Hackney, J. D., Respiratory responses of young asthmatic volunteers in controlled exposures to sulfuric acid aerosol, *Am. Rev. Respir. Dis.*, *142*, 343–348 (1990).
67. Balmes, J. R., Fine, J. M., and Sheppard, D., Symptomatic bronchoconstriction after short-term inhalation of sulfur dioxide, *Am. Rev. Respir. Dis.*, *136*, 1117–1121 (1987).
68. Linn, W. S., Avol, E. L., Peng, R.-C., Shamoo, D. A., and Hackney, J. D., Replicated dose-response study of sulfur dioxide effects in normal, atopic, and asthmatic volunteers, *Am. Rev. Respir. Dis.*, *136*, 1127–1134 (1987).
69. Bethel, R. A., Erle, D. J., Epstein, J., Sheppard, D., Nadel, J. A., and Boushey, H. A., Effect of exercise rate and route of inhalation on sulfur-dioxide-induced bronchoconstriction in asthmatic subjects, *Am. Rev. Respir. Dis.*, *128*, 592–596 (1983).
70. Bethel, R. A., Sheppard, D., Epstein, J., Tam, E., Nadel, J. A., and Boushey, H. A., Interaction of sulfur dioxide and dry cold air in causing bronchoconstriction in asthmatic subjects, *J. Appl. Physiol.*, *57*, 419–423 (1984).
71. Bethel, R. A., Sheppard, D., Geffroy, B. N., Tam, E., Nadel, J. A., and Boushey, H. A., Effect of 0.25 ppm sulfur dioxide on airway resistance in freely breathing, heavily exercising, asthmatic subjects, *Am. Rev. Respir. Dis.*, *131*, 659–661 (1985).
72. Linn, W. S., Shamoo, D. A., Venet, T. G., Bailey, R. M., Wighman, L. H., and Hackney, J. D., Comparative effects of sulfur dioxide exposures at 5° C and 22° C in exercising asthmatics, *Am. Rev. Respir. Dis.*, *129*, 234–239 (1984).
73. Linn, W. S., Shamoo, D. A., Anderson, K. R., Whynot, J. D., Avol, E. L., and Hackney, J. D., Effects of heat and humidity on the response of exercising asthmatics to sulfur dioxide exposure, *Am. Rev. Respir. Dis.*, *131*, 221–225 (1985).
74. Sheppard, D., Saisho, A., Nadel, J. A., and Boushey, H. A., Exercise increases sulfur dioxide–induced bronchoconstriction in asthmatic subjects, *Am. Rev. Respir. Dis.*, *123*, 486–491 (1981).
75. Sheppard, D., Eschenbacher, W. L., Boushey, H. A., and Bethel, R. A., Magnitude of the interaction between the bronchomotor effects of sulfur dioxide and those of dry (cold) air, *Am. Rev. Respir. Dis.*, *130*, 52–55 (1984).

76. Kehrl, H. R., Roger, L. J., Hazucha, M. J., and Horstman, D. H., Differing response of asthmatics to sulfur dioxide exposure with continuous and intermittent exercise, *Am. Rev. Respir. Dis.*, *135*, 350–355 (1987).
77. Kehrl, H. R., Hazucha, M. J., Solic, J. J., and Bromberg, P. A., Responses of subjects with chronic obstructive pulmonary disease after exposures to 0.3 ppm ozone, *Am. Rev. Respir. Dis.*, *131*, 719–724 (1985).
78. Linn, W. S., Shamoo, D. A., Spier, C. E., Valencia, L. M., Anzar, U. T., Venet, T. G., Avol, E. L., and Hackney, J. D., Controlled exposure of volunteers with chronic obstructive pulmonary disease to nitrogen dioxide, *Arch. Environ. Health*, *40*, 313–317 (1985).
79. Linn, W. S., Fischer, D. A., Shamoo, D. A., Spier, C. E., Valencia, L. M., Anzar, U. T., and Hackney, J. D., Controlled exposures of volunteers with chronic obstructive pulmonary disease in sulfur dioxide, *Environ. Res.*, *37*, 445–451 (1985).
80. Paulo, M. T., Gong, H., Jr., Clements, P., and Clark, J. J. J., Respiratory response of patients with interstitial lung disease to inhaled ozone (abstract), *Am. Rev. Respir. Dis.*, *143*, A91 (1991).
81. Superko, H. R., Adams, W. C., and Daly, P. W., Effects of ozone inhalation during exercise in selected patients with heart disease, *Am. J. Med.*, *77*, 463–470 (1984).
82. Anderson, E. W., Andelman, R. J., Strauch, J. M., Fortuin, N. J., and Knelson, J. H., Effect of low-level carbon monoxide exposure on onset and duration of angina pectoris, *Ann. Intern. Med.*, *79*, 46–50 (1973).
83. Sheps, D. S., Herbst, M. C., Hinderliter, A. L., Adams, K. F., Ekelund, L. G., O'Neil, J. J., Goldstein, G. M., Bromberg, P. A., Dalton, J. L., Ballenger, M. N., Davis, S. M., and Koch, G. G., Production of arrhythmias by elevated carboxyhemoglobin in patients with coronary artery disease, *Ann. Intern. Med.*, *113*, 343–351 (1990).
84. Allred, E. N., Bleecker, E. R., Chaitman, B. R., Dahms, T. E., Gottlieb, S. O., Hackney, J. D., Pagano, M., Selvester, R. H., Walden, S. M., and Warren, J., Short-term effects of carbon monoxide exposure on the exercise performance of subjects with coronary artery disease, *N. Engl. J. Med.*, *321*, 1426–1432 (1989).
85. Utell, M. J., Morrow, P. E., Hyde, R. W., and Schreck, R. M., Exposure chamber for studies of pollutant gases and aerosols in human subjects: design considerations, *J. Aerosol Sci.*, *15*, 219–221 (1984).
86. Anderson, K. R., Avol, E. L., Edwards, S. A., Shamoo, D. A., Peng, R.-C., Linn, W. S., and Hackney, J. D., Controlled exposures of volunteers to respirable carbon and sulfuric acid aerosols, *J. Air Waste Manage. Assoc.*, *42*, 770–776 (1992).
87. Lipfert, F. W., Morris, S. C., and Wyzga, R. E., Acid aerosols: the next criteria air pollutant? *Environ. Sci. Technol.*, *23*, 1316–1322 (1989).
88. Hazucha, M. J., Folinsbee, L. J., and Seal, E., Jr., Effects of steady-state and variable ozone profiles on pulmonary function, *Am. Rev. Respir. Dis.*, *146*, 1487–1493 (1992).
89. Koenig, J. Q., Covert, D. S., Hanley, Q. S., Van Belle, G. M., and Pierson, W. E., Prior exposure to ozone potentiates subsequent response to sulfur dioxide in adolescent asthmatic subjects, *Am. Rev. Respir. Dis.*, *141*, 377–380 (1990).
90. Jorres, R., and Magnussen, H., Airways response of asthmatics after 30 min

exposure, at resting ventilation, to 0.25 ppm NO_2 or 0.5 ppm SO_2, *Eur. Respir. J.*, *3*, 132–137 (1990).

91. Rubinstein, I., Bigby, B. G., Reiss, T. F., and Boushey, H. A., Jr., Short-term exposure to 0.3 ppm nitrogen dioxide does not potentiate airway responsiveness to sulfur dioxide in asthmatic subjects, *Am. Rev. Respir. Dis.*, *141*, 381–385 (1990).
92. Aris, R., Christian, D., Sheppard, D., and Balmes, J. R., The effects of sequential exposure to acidic fog and ozone on pulmonary function in exercising subjects, *Am. Rev. Respir. Dis.*, *143*, 85–91 (1991).
93. Drechsler-Parks, D. M., Bedi, J. F., and Horvath, S. M., Interaction of peroxyacetyl nitrate and ozone on pulmonary functions, *Am. Rev. Respir. Dis.*, *130*, 1033–1037 (1984).
94. Koenig, J. Q., Covert, D. S., Smith, M. S., Van Belle, G., and Pierson, W. E., The pulmonary effects of ozone and nitrogen dioxide alone and combined in healthy and asthmatic adolescent subjects, *Toxicol. Ind. Health*, *4*, 521–532 (1988).
95. Kulle, T. J., Kerr, H. D., Farrell, B. P., Sauder, L. R., and Bermel, M. S., Pulmonary function and bronchial reactivity in human subjects with exposure to ozone and respirable sulfuric acid aerosol, *Am. Rev. Respir. Dis.*, *126*, 996–1000 (1982).
96. Horvath, S. M., Folinsbee, L. J., and Bedi, J. F., Combined effect of ozone and sulfuric acid on pulmonary function in man, *Am. Ind. Hyg. Assoc. J.*, *48*, 94–98 (1987).
97. Bedi, J. F., Folinsbee, L. J., Horvath, S. M., and Ebenstein, R. S., Human exposure to sulfur dioxide and ozone: absence of a synergistic effect, *Arch. Environ. Health*, *34*, 233–239 (1979).
98. DeLucia, A. J., Whitaker, J. H., and Bryant, L. R., Effects of combined exposure to ozone and carbon monoxide (CO) in humans, in *The Biomedical Effects of Ozone and Related Photochemical Oxidants. Advances in Modern Environmental Toxicology, Volume V* (S. D. Lee, M. G. Mustafa, and M. A. Mehlman, eds.), Princeton Scientific Publishers, Princeton, New Jersey, 1983, pp. 145–159.
99. Avol, E. L., Wightman, L. H., Linn, W. S., and Hackney, J. D., A movable laboratory for controlled clinical studies of air pollution exposure, *J. Air Pollut. Cont. Assoc.*, *29*, 743–745 (1979).
100. Avol, E. L., Linn, W. S., Venet, T. G., Shamoo, D. A., and Hackney, J. D., Comparative respiratory effects of ozone and ambient oxidant pollution exposure during heavy exercise, *J. Air Pollut. Cont. Assoc.*, *34*, 804–809 (1984).
101. Linn, W. S., Venet, T. G., Shamoo, D. A., Valencia, L. M., Anzar, U. T., Spier, C. E., and Hackney, J. D., Respiratory effects of sulfur dioxide in heavily exercising asthmatics, *Am. Rev. Respir. Dis.*, *127*, 278–283 (1983).
102. Hynes, B., Silverman, F., Cole, P., and Corey, P., Effects of ozone exposure: a comparison between oral and nasal breathing, *Arch. Environ. Health*, *43*, 357–360 (1988).
103. Adams, W. C., Schelegle, E. S., and Shaffrath, J. D., Oral and oronasal breathing during continuous exercise produce similar responses to ozone inhalation, *Arch. Environ. Health*, *44*, 311–316 (1989).
104. Gerrity, T. R., Weaver, R. A., Berntsen, J., House, D. E., and O'Neil, J. J.,

Extrathoracic and intrathoracic removal of O_3 in tidal-breathing humans, *J. Appl. Physiol.*, *65*, 393–400 (1988).
105. Larson, T. V., Covert, D. S., Frank, R., and Charlson, R. J. Ammonia in the human airways: neutralization of inspired acid sulfate aerosols, *Science*, *197*, 161–163 (1977).
106. Norwood, D. M., Wainman, T., Lioy, P. J., and Waldman, J. M., Breath ammonia depletion and its relevance to acidic aerosol exposure studies, *Arch. Environ. Health*, *47*, 309–313 (1992).
107. Utell, M. J., Mariglio, J. A., Morrow, P. E., Gibb, F. R., and Speers, D. M., Effects of inhaled acid aerosols on respiratory function: The role of endogenous ammonia, *J. Aerosol Med.*, *2*, 141–147 (1989).
108. Larson, T. V., The influence of chemical and physical forms of ambient air acids on airway doses, *Environ. Health Perspect.*, *79*, 7–13 (1989).
109. Bowes S. M., III, Frank, R., and Swift, D. L., The head dome: a simplified method for human exposures to inhaled air pollutants, *Am. Ind. Hyg. Assoc. J.*, *51*, 257–260 (1990).
110. Laube, B. L., Bowes, S. M., III, Links, J. M., Thomas, K. K., and Frank, R., Acute exposure to acid fog. Effects on mucociliary clearance, *Am. Rev. Respir. Dis.*, *147*, 1105–1111 (1993).
111. Drinkwater, B. L., Raven, P. B., Horvath, S. M., Gliner, J. A., Ruhling, R. O., Bolduan, N. W., and Taguchi, S., Air pollution, exercise, and heat stress, *Arch. Environ. Health*, *28*, 177–181 (1974).
112. Gibbons, S. I., and Adams, W. C., Combined effects of ozone and ambient heat on exercising females, *J. Appl. Physiol.*, *57*, 450–456 (1984).
113. Hackney, J. D., Linn, W. S., Bailey, R. M., Speir, C. M., and Valencia, L. M., Time course of exercise-induced bronchoconstriction in asthmatics exposed to sulfur dioxide, *Environ. Res.*, *34*, 321–327 (1984).
114. Roger, L. J., Kehrl, H. R., Hazucha, M., and Horstman, D. H., Bronchoconstriction in asthmatics exposed to sulfur dioxide during repeated exercise, *J. Appl. Physiol.*, *59*, 784–791 (1985).
115. Sheppard, D., Epstein, J., Bethel, R. A., Nadel, J., and Boushey, H. A., Tolerance to sulfur dioxide–induced bronchoconstriction in subjects with asthma, *Environ. Res.*, *30*, 412–419 (1983).
116. Adams, W. C., Savin, W. M., and Christo, A., Detection of ozone toxicity via the effective dose concept, *J. Appl. Physiol.*, *51*, 415–422 (1981).
117. Folinsbee, L. J., McDonnell, W. F., and Horstman, D. H., Pulmonary function and symptom responses after 6.6-hour exposure to 0.12 ppm ozone with moderate exercise, *J. Air Pollut. Cont. Assoc.*, *38*, 28–35 (1988).
118. Horstman, D. H., Folinsbee, J., Ives, P. J., Abdul-Salaam, S., and McDonnell, W. F., Ozone concentration and pulmonary response relationships for 6.6-hour exposures with five hours of moderate exercise to 0.08, 0.10, and 0.12 ppm, *Am. Rev. Respir. Dis.*, *142*, 1158–1163.
119. McDonnell, W. F., Kehrl, H. R., Abdul-Salaam, S., Folinsbee, L. J., Devlin, R. B., O'Neil, J. J., and Horstman, D. H., Respiratory response of humans exposed to low levels of ozone for 6.6 hours, *Arch. Environ. Health*, *46*, 145–150 (1991).

120. Folinsbee, L. J., and Horvath, S. M., Persistence of the acute effects of ozone exposure, *Aviat. Space Environ. Med.*, *57*, 1136–1143 (1986).
121. Folinsbee, L. J., Bedi, J. F., and Horvath, S. M., Respiratory responses in humans repeatedly exposed to low concentrations of ozone, *Am. Rev. Respir. Dis.*, *121*, 431–439 (1980).
122. Horvath, S. M., Gliner, J. A., and Folinsbee, L. J., Adaptation to ozone: duration of effect, *Am. Rev. Respir. Dis.*, *123*, 496–499 (1981).
123. Hackney, J. D., Linn, W. S., Karuza, S. K., Buckley, R. D., Law, D. C., Gates, D. V., Hazucha, M., Pengelley, L. D., and Silverman, F., Effects of ozone exposure in Canadians and Southern Californians, *Arch. Environ. Health*, *32*, 110–116 (1977).
124. Linn, W. S., Avol, E. L., Shamoo, D. A., Peng, R. C., Valencia, L. M., Little, D. E., and Hackney, J. D., Repeated laboratory ozone exposures of volunteer Los Angeles residents: an apparent seasonal variation in response, *Toxicol. Ind. Health*, *4*, 505–420 (1988).
125. Hackney, J. D., Linn, W. S., Shamoo, D. A., and Avol, E. L., Responses of selected reactive and nonreactive volunteers to ozone exposure in high and low pollution seasons, *Atmospheric Ozone Research and Its Policy Implications* (T. Schneider, S. D. Lee, G. J. R. Walters, and L. D. Grant, eds.), Elsevier Science Publishers, Amsterdam, 1989, pp. 311–318.
126. U.S. Environmental Protection Agency, *Air Quality Criteria for Ozone and Other Photochemical Oxidants*. EPA/600/8-84/020eF (Vol. V). Environmental Criteria and Assessment Office, Research Triangle Park, North Carolina, 1986.
127. Folinsbee, L. J., Bedi, J. F., and Horvath, S. M., Pulmonary function changes after 1 h continuous heavy exercise in 0.21 ppm ozone, *J. Appl. Physiol.*, *57*, 984–988 (1984).
128. Horvath, S. M., Design and measurement considerations for exercise protocols in human air pollution inhalation studies, in *Inhalation Toxicology of Air Pollution: Clinical Research Considerations* (R. Frank, J. J. O'Neill, M. J. Utell, J. D. Hackney, J. Van Ryzin, and P. E. Brubaker, eds.), American Society for Testing and Materials, Philadelphia, 1985, pp. 25–35.
129. National Research Council (U.S.), Subcommittee on Pulmonary Toxicology, *Biologic Markers in Pulmonary Toxicology*. National Academy Press, Washington, D.C., 1989.
130. Hackney, J. D., and Linn, W. S., Collection and analysis of symptom data in clinical air pollution studies, in *Inhalation Toxicology of Air Pollution: Clinical Research Considerations* (R. Frank, J. J. O'Neill, M. J. Utell, J. D. Hackney, J. Van Ryzin, and P. E. Brubaker, eds.), American Society for Testing and Materials, Philadelphia, 1985, pp. 73–82.
131. Bascom, R., Kulle, T., Kagey-Sobotka, A., and Proud, D., Upper respiratory tract environmental tobacco smoke sensitivity, *Am. Rev. Respir. Dis.*, *143*, 1304–1311 (1991).
132. Harving, H., Dahl, R., and Molhave, L., Lung function and bronchial reactivity in asthmatics during exposure to volatile organic compounds, *Am. Rev. Respir. Dis.*, *142*, 751–754 (1991).
133. Witek, T. J., Schachter, E. N., Beck, G. J., Cain, W. S., Colice, G., and Leaderer,

B. P., Respiratory symptoms associated with sulfur dioxide exposure, *Int. Arch. Occup. Environ. Health*, *55*, 179–183 (1985).

134. Mihevic, P. M., Sensory cues for perceived exertion: a review, *Med. Sci. Sports Exerc.*, *13*, 150–163 (1981).
135. Mihevic, P. M., Gliner, J. A., and Horvath, S. M., Perception of effort and respiratory sensitivity during exposure to ozone, *Ergonomics*, *24*, 365–374 (1987).
136. Gliner, J. A., Matsen-Twisdale, J. A., and Horvath, S. M., Auditory and visual sustained attention during ozone exposure, *Aviat. Space Environ. Med.*, *50*, 906–910 (1979).
137. Gliner, J. A., Horvath, S. M., Sorich, R. A., and Hanley, J., Psychomotor performance during ozone exposure: spectral and discriminant function analysis of EEG, *Aviat. Space Environ. Med.*, *51*, 344–351 (1980).
138. Bates, D. V., *Respiratory Function in Disease*, 3rd Ed., W. B. Saunders, Philadelphia, 1989.
139. McDonnell, W. F., Horstman, D. H., Hazucha, M. J., Seal, E., Jr., Haak, E. D., Salaam, S. A., and House, D. E., Pulmonary effects of ozone exposure during exercise: dose-response characteristics, *J. Appl. Physiol.*, *54*, 1345–1352 (1983).
140. Hazucha, M. J., Bates, D. V., and Bromberg, P. A., Mechanism of action of ozone on the human lung, *J. Appl. Physiol.*, *67*, 1535–1541 (1989).
141. Utell, M. J., Morrow, P. E., and Hyde, R. W., Airway reactivity to sulfate and sulfuric acid aerosols in normal and asthmatic subjects, *J. Air Pollut. Cont. Assoc.*, *34*, 931–935 (1984).
142. Koenig, J. Q., Morgan, M. S., Horicke, N., and Pierson, W. E., The effects of sulfur oxides on nasal and lung function in adolescents with extrinsic asthma, *J. Allergy Clin. Immunol.*, *76*, 813–818 (1985).
143. McCawley, M., and Lippmann, M., Development of an aerosol dispersion test to detect early changes in lung function, *Am. Ind. Hyg. Assoc. J.*, *49*, 357–366 (1988).
144. Keefe, M. J., Bennett, W. D., Dewitt, P., Seal, E., Strong, A. A., and Gerrity, T. R., The effect of ozone exposure on the dispersion of inhaled aerosol boluses on healthy human subjects, *Am. Rev. Respir. Dis.*, *144*, 23–30 (1991).
145. O'Connor, G., Sparrow, D., Taylor, D., Segal, M., and Weiss, S., Analysis of dose-response curves to methacholine. An approach suitable for population studies, *Am. Rev. Respir. Dis.*, *136*, 1412–1417 (1987).
146. Frampton, M. W., Morrow, P. E., Gibb, F. R., Speers, D. M., and Utell, M. J. Effects of nitrogen dioxide exposure on pulmonary function and airway reactivity in normal humans, *Am. Rev. Respir. Dis.*, *143*, 522–527 (1991).
147. Golden, J. A., Nadel, J. A., and Boushey, H. A., Bronchial hyperirritability in healthy subjects after exposure to ozone, *Am. Rev. Respir. Dis.*, *118*, 287–294 (1978).
148. Molfino, N. A., Wright, S. C., Katz, I., Tarlo, S., Silverman, F., McClean, P. A., Szalao, J. P., Raizenne, M., Slutsky, A. S., and Zamel, N., Effect of low concentrations of ozone on inhaled allergen responses in asthmatic subjects, *Lancet*, *338*, 199–203 (1991).
149. Von Nieding, G., and Wagner, H. M., Effects of NO_2 on chronic bronchitis, *Environ. Health Perspect.*, *29*, 137–142 (1979).

150. Linn, W. S., Jones, M. P., Bachmayer, E. A., Clark, K. W., Karuza, S. K., and Hackney, J. D., Effect of low-level exposure to ozone on arterial oxygenation in humans, *Am. Rev. Respir. Dis.*, *119*, 731–740 (1979).
151. Foster, W. M., Costa, D. L., and Langenback, E. G., Ozone exposure alters tracheobronchial mucociliary function in humans, *J. Appl. Physiol.*, *63*, 996–1002 (1987).
152. Leikauf, G. D., Spektor, D. M., Albert, R. E., and Lippmann, M., Dose-dependent effects of submicrometer sulfuric acid aerosol on particle clearance from ciliated human lung airways, *Am. Ind. Hyg. Assoc. J.*, *45*, 285–292 (1984).
153. Spektor, D. M., Leikauf, G. D., Albert, R. E., and Lippmann, M., Effects of submicrometer sulfuric acid aerosols on mucociliary transport and respiratory mechanics in asymptomatic asthmatics, *Environ. Res.*, *37*, 174–191 (1985).
154. Spektor, D. M., Yen, B. M., and Lippmann, M., Effect of concentration and cumulative exposure of inhaled sulfuric acid on tracheobronchial particle clearance in healthy humans, *Environ. Health Perspect.*, *79*, 167–172 (1989).
155. Kehrl, H. R., Vincent, L. M., Kowalsky, R. J., Horstman, D. H., O'Neil, J. J., McCartney, W. H., and Bromberg, P. A., Ozone exposure increases respiratory epithelial permeability in humans, *Am. Rev. Respir. Dis.*, *135*, 1124–1128 (1987).
156. Rasmussen, T. R., Kjaergaard, S. K. J., Tarp, U., and Pedersen, O. F., Delayed effects of NO_2 exposure on alveolar permeability and glutathione peroxidase in healthy humans, *Am. Rev. Respir. Dis.*, *146*, 654–659 (1992).
157. Folinsbee, L. J., Silverman, F., and Shephard, R. J., Decrease of maximum work performance following ozone exposure, *J. Appl. Physiol.*, *42*, 531–536 (1977).
158. The BAL Cooperative Group Steering Committee, Bronchoalveolar lavage constituents in healthy individuals, idiopathic pulmonary fibrosis, and selected comparison groups, *Am. Rev. Respir. Dis.*, *141* (suppl), S169–S202 (1990).
159. Eschenbacher, W. L., and Gravelyn, T. R., A technique for isolated airway segment lavage, *Chest*, *92*, 105–109 (1987).
160. Rennard, S. I., Ghafouri, M., Thompson, A. B., Linder, J., Baughan, W., Jones, K., Ertl, R. F., Christensen, K., Prince, A., Stahl, M. G., and Robbins, R., Fractional processing of sequential bronchoalveolar lavage to separate bronchial and alveolar samples, *Am. Rev. Respir. Dis.*, *141*, 208–217 (1990).
161. Schelegle, E. S., Siefkin, A. D., and McDonald, R. J., Time course of ozone-induced neutrophilia in normal humans, *Am. Rev. Respir. Dis.*, *143*, 1353–1358 (1991).
162. Seltzer, J., Bigby, B. G., Stulbarg, M., Holtzman, M. J., Nadel, J. A., Ueki, I. F., Leikauf, G. D., Goetzl, E. J., and Boushey, H. A., O_3-induced change in bronchial reactivity to methacholine and airway inflammation in humans, *J. Appl. Physiol.*, *60*, 1321–1326 (1986).
163. Koren, H. S., Devlin, R. B., Graham, D. E., Mann, R., McGee, M. P., Horstman, D. H., Kozumbo, W. J., Becker, S., House, D. E., McDonnell, W. F., and Bromberg, P. A., Ozone-induced inflammation in the lower airways of human subjects, *Am. Rev. Respir. Dis.*, *139*, 407–415 (1989).
164. Devlin, R. B., McDonnell, W. F., Mann, R., Becker, S., House, D. E., Schreinemachers, D., and Koren, H. S., Exposure of humans to ambient levels of ozone for

6.6 hours causes cellular and biochemical changes in the lung, *Am. J. Respir. Cell Mol. Biol.*, *4*, 72–81 (1991).

165. Koren, H. S., Devlin, R. B., Becker, S., Perez, R., and McDonnell, W. F., Time-dependent changes of markers associated with inflammation in the lungs of humans exposed to ambient levels of ozone, *Toxicol. Pathol.*, *19*, 406–411 (1991).

166. Sandstrom, T., Stjernberg, N., Andersson, M.-C., Kolmodin-Hedman, B., Lundgren, R., Rosenhall, L., and Angstrom, T., Cell response in bronchoalveolar lavage fluid after exposure to sulfur dioxide. A time-response study, *Am. Rev. Respir. Dis.*, *140*, 1828–1831 (1989).

167. Frampton, M. W., Finkelstein, J. N., Roberts, N. J., Jr., Smeglin, A. M., Morrow, P. E., and Utell, M. J., Effects of nitrogen dioxide exposure on bronchoalveolar lavage proteins in humans, *Am. J. Respir. Cell. Mol. Biol.*, *1*, 499–505 (1989).

168. Rubinstein, I., Reiss, T. F., Bigby, B. G., Stites, D. P., and Boushey, H. A., Jr., Effects of 0.6 ppm nitrogen dioxide on circulating and bronchoalveolar lavage lymphocyte phenotypes in healthy subjects, *Environ. Res.*, *55*, 18–30 (1991).

169. Sandstrom, T., Andersson, M. C., Kolmodin-Hedman, B., Stjernberg, N., and Angstrom, T., Bronchoalveolar mastocytosis and lymphocytosis after nitrogen dioxide exposure in man: a time-kinetic study, *Eur. Respir. J.*, *3*, 138–143 (1990).

170. Sandstrom, T., Stjernberg, N., Andersson, M.-C., Bjermer, L., Eklund, A., Kolmodin-Hedman, B., Lindstrom, K., Rosenhall, L., and Angstrom, T., Inflammatory cell response in bronchoalveolar lavage fluid after nitrogen dioxide exposure of healthy subjects. A dose-response study, *Eur. Respir. J.*, *3*, 332–339 (1990).

171. Mohsenin, V., and Gee, B. L., Acute effect of nitrogen dioxide exposure on the functional activity of alpha-1-protease inhibitor in bronchoalveolar lavage fluid of normal subjects, *Am. Rev. Respir. Dis.*, *136*, 646–650 (1987).

172. Johnson, D. A., Frampton, M. W., Winters, R. S., Morrow, P. E., and Utell, M. J., Inhalation of nitrogen dioxide fails to reduce the activity of human lung alpha-1-proteinase inhibitor, *Am. Rev. Respir. Dis.*, *142*, 758–762 (1990).

173. Frampton, M. W., Smeglin, A. M., Roberts, N. J., Jr., Finkelstein, J. N., Morrow, P. E., and Utell, M. J., Nitrogen dioxide exposure in vivo and human alveolar macrophage inactivation of influenza virus in vitro, *Environ. Res.*, *48*, 179–192 (1989).

174. Sandstrom, T., Helleday, R., Bjermer, L., and Stjernberg, N., Effects of repeated exposure to 4 ppm nitrogen dioxide on bronchoalveolar lymphocyte subsets and macrophages in healthy men, *Eur. Respir. J.*, *5*, 1092–1096 (1992).

175. Frampton, M. W., Voter, K. Z., Morrow, P. E., Roberts, N. J., Jr., Culp, D. J., Cox, C., and Utell, M. J., Sulfuric acid aerosol exposure in humans assessed by bronchoalveolar lavage, *Am. Rev. Respir. Dis.*, *146*, 626–632 (1992).

176. Koren, H. S., Hatch, G. E., and Graham, D. E., Nasal lavage as a tool in assessing acute inflammation in response to inhaled pollutants, *Toxicology*, *60*, 15–25 (1990).

177. Graham, D., Henderson, F. and House, D., Neutrophil influx measured in nasal lavages of humans exposed to ozone, *Arch. Environ. Health*, *43*, 228–233 (1988).

178. Graham, D. E., and Koren, H. S., Biomarkers of inflammation in ozone-exposed humans. Comparison of the nasal and bronchoalveolar lavage, *Am. Rev. Respir. Dis.*, *142*, 152–156 (1990).

179. Bascom, R., Naclerio, R. M., Fitzgerald, T. K., Kagey-Sobotka, A., and Proud, D., Effect of ozone inhalation on the response to nasal challenge with antigen of allergic subjects, *Am. Rev. Respir. Dis.*, *142*, 594–601 (1990).
180. Koren, H. S., Graham, D. E., and Devlin, R. B., Exposure of humans to a volatile organic mixture. III. Inflammatory response, *Arch. Environ. Health*, *47*, 39–44 (1992).
181. Schelegle, E. S., Adams, W. C., Giri, S. N., and Siefkin, A. D., Acute ozone exposure increases plasma prostaglandin $F_{2\alpha}$ in ozone-sensitive human subjects, *Am. Rev. Respir. Dis.*, *140*, 211–216 (1989).
182. Von Ryzin, J., Statistical considerations in designing, analyzing, and reporting of clinical pulmonary studies, in *Inhalation Toxicology of Air Pollution: Clinical Research Considerations* (R. Frank, J. J. O'Neill, M. J. Utell, J. D. Hackney, J. Van Ryzin, P. E. Brubaker, eds.), American Society for Testing and Materials, Philadelphia, 1985, pp. 109–116.
183. American Thoracic Society, Guidelines as to what constitutes an adverse respiratory health effect, with special reference to epidemiologic studies of air pollution, *Am. Rev. Respir. Dis.*, *131*, 666–668 (1985).
184. Hazucha, M. J., Relationship between ozone exposure and pulmonary function changes, *J. Appl. Physiol.*, *62*, 1671–1680 (1987).
185. Ostro, B. D., Lipsett, M. J., and Jewell, N. O., Predicting respiratory morbidity from pulmonary function tests: a reanalysis of ozone chamber studies, *J. Air Pollut. Cont. Assoc.*, *39*, 1313–1318 (1989).
186. Larsen, R. I., McDonnell, W. F., Horstman, D. H., and Folinsbee, L. J., An air quality data analysis system for interrelating effects, standards, and needed source reductions: Part II. A lognormal model relating human lung function decrease to O_3 exposure, *J. Air Waste Manage. Assoc.*, *41*, 455–459 (1991).
187. Hamilos, D. L., Oppenheimer, J. J., Nelson, H. S., Wenzel, S., Driscoll, S., Lockey, R. F., Golden, D. B. K., Fan, L., Sanks, R. J., Bock, S. A., Yunginger, J. W., Stevenson, D., Sulivan, T., and Corbridge, T., Suggested approaches for research protocols involving the potential for life-threatening reactions, *J. Allergy Clin. Immunol.*, *91*, 1101–1109 (1993).

7

Deposition and Fate of Inhaled Pharmacological Aerosols

Joseph D. Brain and James D. Blanchard

Harvard School of Public Health
Boston, Massachusetts

I. INTRODUCTION

Inhaled aerosols provide important information about the respiratory tract. The major theme of this book is the use of aerosols for provocation testing. There is considerable interest in the distribution of airway responsiveness in human populations, especially as it relates to the diagnosis of asthma. Frequently, skin tests have little relation to airway reactivity; provocation tests with agents such as methacholine or antigens are more reliable. We expect that pharmacological aerosols will be increasingly used as probes of lung function, for studies in experimental pharmacology and pathology, and especially for therapeutic purposes All these applications depend on the ability of the investigator to deliver known amounts of aerosol into people or animals. It is essential to quantify aerosol deposition and retention accurately; only then can results among different investigators and laboratories be compared. All these factors conspire to make considerations of dose, how much and where, an important endeavor.

The availability of pharmacological aerosols in respiratory therapy illustrates some of the key issues. Pharmaceutical companies manufacture and promote aerosols that are intended to relieve bronchospasm, congestion, edema, allergy, and inflammation, as well as reduce the viscosity of mucus, treat sinus infection, activate macrophages, inhibit proteases, and so on. Other aerosolized agents can elicit bronchoconstriction.

A major concern with most inhaled aerosols is whether they deposit at the desired location in the respiratory tract. Deposition site is highly dependent on the particle size of the aerosol and the breathing pattern used. These are not always adequately controlled. Particles may be too large or individuals may inhale too quickly to allow particles to pass the oropharynx and larynx into the lungs. Thus, in many cases it is problematic to estimate or calculate the dose of a drug given to a patient by aerosol.

Aerosols for challenge tests and drug therapy may be produced by nebulizers, pressurized metered-dose inhalers (MDIs), or dry-powder inhalers. Challenge tests for occupational agents sometimes simply involve the person's handling the suspected material [1]. Although a variety of aerosol generators are made, in many cases there are insufficient data regarding the size distribution of the particles produced and the efficiency of generation. Furthermore, nebulizers of the same design and model may not perform alike [2,3]. Accurate characterization of many freshly generated therapeutic aerosols is complex because the size of the particles may change rapidly as a result of evaporation, hygroscopic growth, or agglomeration. A large fraction of the fresh aerosol may be too large to penetrate into the lungs. Unfortunately, data on particle size distribution often are collected by methods that fail to account for these dynamic changes.

Dose estimation is further complicated by other factors. Many devices require intelligent use by the patient, and they are frequently misused [4,5]. Often, little is known about the distribution and metabolism of the drugs given. Comprehensive studies describing the accumulation of drugs in blood or urine, or the site of action within the respiratory tract, are seldom available. Also lacking is adequate knowledge of the anatomical distribution of receptor sites throughout the respiratory tract. Thus, even when a drug is delivered to the lungs, one often does not know if it has reached the desired region. For example, fibrotic areas or regions served by obstructed airways would receive little or no drug.

Much of this book deals with the careful assessment of the responses to provocative challenge. Changes in pulmonary function are a common response to a challenge. Responses can also be measured at the level of a cell (degranulation of mast cells), an enzyme (increased phosphodiesterase), or a receptor (the leukotriene D_4 receptor on the plasma membrane). Descriptions of responses are of little value, however, without accurate measurements of the dose, preferably at the site of action. Aerosol exposures present a special problem, since the actual dose retained is often difficult to determine. Many investigators fail even to try. They report the dose administered to a person as the concentration in the nebulizer fluid, the amount of aerosol generated, or the amount in the exposure chamber. Since exposure dose does not equal retained dose, it is important to describe adequately the variables that determine exposure–dose relationships.

In this review we summarize particle deposition and clearance mechanisms and how they both influence retention. We consider strategies that can be used to deliver aerosols, discuss approaches that can be used to describe the amount and distribution of dose, and review some factors that are known to influence the amount and distribution of retained particles. Although gases accompanying inhaled drugs and gas–particle interactions are sometimes important, the effects and uptake of inhaled gases are not covered.

II. PARTICLE TRANSPORT AND DEPOSITION MECHANISMS

Deposition is the process that determines the fraction of the inspired particles that is caught in the respiratory tract and thus fails to exit with expired air. Deposited dose equals the amount of material inhaled multiplied by the fraction of material that deposits. All particles that touch a surface are assumed to deposit at the site of initial contact. Distinct physical mechanisms operate on inspired particles to move them across streamlines of air and toward the surface of the respiratory tract; these are gravitational sedimentation, inertia, Brownian diffusion, and electrostatic forces. Which mechanisms contribute to the deposition of a specific particle depends on the particle's aerodynamic and physicochemical characteristics, the subject's breathing pattern, the geometry of the respiratory tract, and the flow and mixing pattern of the aerosol. For most aerosols the first three mechanisms are most important. Detailed treatments on particle deposition are available [6–14], as are comprehensive treatises on the physics of aerosol behavior [15–21].

A. Aerodynamic Equivalent Diameter

The transport and deposition of a particle larger than 1 μm in the respiratory system are largely determined by aerodynamic characteristics: particle size, density, and shape plus gas velocity [22]. A sphere of 3-μm diameter with a density of 4 g/cm^3 behaves aerodynamically the same as a 6-μm sphere with a density of 1 g/cm^3. Such particles may be compared by their aerodynamic equivalent diameter (d_{ae}). The aerodynamic equivalent diameter is the diameter of the unit-density (1 g/cm^3) sphere that has the same gravitational settling velocity in air as the particle in question. Aerodynamic diameter is proportional to $d_p\rho^{1/2}$, where d_p is the geometric particle diameter and ρ is the particle density. In the above example, both particles have a d_{ae} of 6 μm. The d_{ae} is used to describe the size of particles larger than 0.4 μm, the particle size that deposits least in the respiratory tract [23]. For particles of unknown density or shape, d_{ae} must be determined experimentally.

B. Deposition Mechanisms

1. Gravitational Settling

Gravity accelerates falling bodies downward, and a particle reaches its terminal settling velocity when the gravitational force equals the opposing viscous resistive forces of the air. Particles small enough to enter the lungs reach their terminal settling velocity in less than 0.1 ms. Particles deposit when they have enough time to settle onto airway walls or alveolar surfaces. Thus the probability that a particle deposits by gravitational settling increases with increasing $d_{ae}2t$, where t is the residence time in the respiratory tract [22]. Breath holding enhances deposition by sedimentation. Sedimentation is important for particles larger than about 0.1 μm that enter the peripheral airways and alveoli, where air flow rates are slow, residence times are long, and distances to lung surfaces are short [10].

2. Inertial Impaction

Inertia is the tendency of a moving particle to resist changes in speed and direction. It is related to momentum, the product of the particle's mass and velocity. High air velocities and abrupt changes in airflow direction occur in the nose and oropharynx and at central airway bifurcations. Inertia causes a particle entering bends at these sites to continue in its original direction instead of following the curvature of the airflow. If the particle has sufficient mass and velocity it crosses airflow streamlines and impacts on the airway wall. The probability that a particle deposits by inertial impaction increases with increasing product of $d_{ae}{}^2Q$, where Q is the respired flow rate [22,24]. Impaction probability also increases with increasing angle of airstream deflection. Inertial impaction is an important deposition mechanism for particles with a d_{ee} larger than 2 μm [22] and may occur during both inspiration and expiration in the extrathoracic airways (oropharynx, nasopharynx, and larynx) and central airways. In obstructed airways, the enhanced linear velocities at narrowed sites may cause smaller particles to deposit by impaction as well.

3. Diffusion

Aerosol particles also undergo Brownian diffusion, a random motion in three dimensions caused by their collisions with gas molecules; this motion can lead to contact and deposition on respiratory surfaces. Diffusion is significant for particles with diameters less than 1 μm, so that their size is similar to the mean free path of gas molecules. Unlike inertial or gravitational displacement, diffusion is independent of air flow rate and particle density; however, it is affected by particle shape and size [25]. For diffusing particles that measure 0.4 μm and smaller, size can be expressed in terms of the thermodynamic equivalent diameter (d_{te}), the diameter of a sphere that has the same average diffusional velocity in air as the actual particle [23]. The probability that a particle deposits by diffusion increases with decreasing particle size and decreasing values of $(t/d_{te})^{1/2}$ [22]; thus, deposition is dependent on the square root of residence time. Diffusion, like sedimentation, is usually most important in the peripheral airways and alveoli [10] but can also occur in the nose and mouth [26].

As particle size decreases, inertia and sedimentation become less important, but diffusion increases in importance. For example, a particle with a d_{ae} of 2 μm moves by diffusion (Brownian displacement) only about 9 μm in 1 s; it settles by gravity about 125 μm in the same period. However, as particle size drops to 0.2 μm, the diffusional displacement increases to 37 μm, whereas gravitational displacement decreases to only 2.1 μm. Table 1 shows a comparison of settling and diffusion displacements for a range of particle sizes. Generally, gravity and inertia dominate the transport and deposition of particles larger than 1.0 μm in diameter, and diffusion dominates the transport and deposition of particles smaller than 0 1 μm. For particles between 0.1 and 1.0 μm, sedimentation and diffusion are both important [23,25].

4. Electrostatic Attraction

Electrical forces may cause charged particles to deposit in the respiratory tract. The surfaces of the respiratory tract are uncharged but electrically conducting. When an electrically charged particle approaches the lung surface, the particle induces on that surface an image charge of the opposite polarity that attracts the

Table 1 Root Mean Square Brownian Displacement in 1 s Compared with Distance Fallen in Air in 1 s for Unit-Density Particles of Different Diameters[a]

	Diameter (μm)	Brownian displacement in 1 s (μm)	Distance fallen in 1 s (μm)
Settling greater in 1 s	50	0.978	71,700
	20	1.55	11,500
	10	2.20	2,910
	5	3.14	740
	2	5.10	124
	1	7.50	33.7
Diffusion greater in 1 s	0.5	11.4	9.71
	0.2	21.6	2.23
	0.1	38.1	0.871
	0.05	71.4	0.382
	0.02	172	0.141
	0.01	339	0.0689
	0.00037[b]	9060	0.00249

[a]Values are for inspired air at 37°C and 100% humidity; air viscosity = 1.906×10^{-5} Pa s; air density = 1.112 kg/m^3; Cunningham slip correction calculated according to Jennings [10].

[b]Diameter of typical "air molecule" [8].

Source: From Weiss, E. B., Stein, M., eds., *Bronchial Asthma: Mechanisms and Therapeutics*, 3d Ed., Little, Brown, and Company, Boston, 1993.

particle. This attraction may cause the particle to deposit, and thus the deposition of charged particles relative to that of neutral particles is increased. Experimental [27] and theoretical [28] studies show that electrostatic attraction may be an important deposition mechanism in the lung periphery for particles (especially fibers) that are charged above a certain threshold and have a diameter of 0.1–1.0 μm [29]. Melandri et al. [27] established that the probability of electrostatic deposition is proportional to $(q^2/d)^{1/3}$, where q is the electrical charge on the particle. For charged 1-μm particles, deposition is increased over that of uncharged particles once there are about 40 charges on the particle; for 0.3-μm particles only 10 charges are needed.

5. Interception and Other Forces

Deposition can also occur in the lungs when particles have dimensions that are significant relative to those of the air spaces. As particles move into smaller and smaller air spaces, some may reach a point where the distance to a surface from the center of a particle is less than the particle size. The resulting contact is called interception. Interception is particularly important for the deposition of fibers [30,31]. Other forces acting to affect deposition, such as acoustic forces, magnetic forces, or thermal forces, are normally not significant in the respiratory tract.

III. CHARACTERIZING AND DELIVERING AEROSOLS

Important considerations for challenge testing with aerosols include techniques of aerosol generation; characterization of the aerosol mass, size distribution, and dynamic properties; delivery of the aerosol; and delineation of the factors that influence the amount of material deposited in the lungs, including breathing pattern and subject characteristics [32–34]. Different subjects breathing the same aerosol frequently retain quite different amounts, and variations in breathing pattern are often responsible. Thus, an important challenge for physicians is to train patients to use proper aerosol inhalation technique.

A. Aerosol Generation and Delivery

The common devices to generate liquid and solid pharmacological aerosols are jet and ultrasonic nebulizers, MDIs, and dry-powder inhalers. Nebulizers are commonly used for bronchoprovocation testing, since these devices allow the clinician to prepare challenge solutions over a wide concentration range that are then aerosolized for testing. Metered-dose inhalers and dry-powder inhalers are more commonly used for therapeutic purposes, since they are convenient and allow good control of the dosing regimen. Nebulizers can aerosolize a wide variety of water-soluble materials; MDIs and dry powder inhalers can aerosolize only those compounds compatible with the special formulation requirements of these devices. One must keep in mind that all devices within the same class have different output characteristics in terms of mass, size distribution, and constancy [34]. Devices of the same model may have unit-to-unit variability; it is also possible that the same unit has dose-to-dose variability [2,34]. Close attention to the manufacturer's operating instructions or an established laboratory protocol will minimize variability. Several texts describe both theoretical and practical aspects of aerosol generation and measurement [15,19–21,35–43]. Surveys of typical medical devices are also published [34,35,40,44–50]. Since MDIs and dry-powder inhalers are not usually used for bronchoprovocation testing, in this review we will limit our discussion of these devices.

Methods to nebulize substances for challenge testing are continuous flow and intermittent generation with a dosimeter or a squeeze bulb. The continuous-flow method [51,52] involves nebulizing the aerosol continuously while the subject breathes for a preset length of time. One modification places one-way valves between the nebulizer and the subject. The intermittent-generation methods deliver a bolus of aerosol during inspiration only. The automated dosimeter [53] has a solenoid valve between the compressed air source and the nebulizer. The valve is triggered open by the change in mouth pressure or flow direction at the onset of inspiration. The valve remains open for a preset length of time, usually 0.6 s. To favor deposition in the proximal lung, the opening of the valve can be delayed. Another intermittent method, sometimes called the "Yan method" [32,54], uses a hand-held nebulizer with a squeeze bulb to force air manually through the nebulizer at the beginning of a breath.

To test for airway responsiveness to occupational dusts, vapors, or gases, one can expose a person in a chamber [1,32] or with a closed-circuit delivery system [55]. One crude way to generate a cloud of dust is to have the person transfer powder (with or without lactose powder as a diluent) from one pan to another in a chamber [1]. If this approach is used, the dust concentration must remain below the short-term exposure limit (TLV-STEL) established by the American Conference of Governmental Industrial Hygienists [32,56]. An improved dust-generation method, which allows greater control and quantification of dose, is to aspirate the powder off a rotating brush that is partially immersed in the powder [57,58]. The suspended dust is carried within tubing to the mouthpiece and a nearby aerosol photometer that continuously monitors inhaled particle concentration. For exposures to paint sprays or fumes from heated materials the subject can handle prepared quantities of the material in a chamber [55].

B. Particle Size and Mass Distributions

To estimate total and regional lung doses, it is necessary to characterize the aerosol in terms of the particle size distribution and the mass concentration. Particle size is a prime factor governing the fraction of inhaled particles that penetrates past the oropharynx and enters the lungs, and the particle fraction that deposits in each lung region. The mass concentration is proportional to the actual amount of particles that deposits in each region. Size distributions can be described in terms of particle number, surface area, or mass; most dose estimates use mass. Particle mass distributions are often characterized by two values: the mass median aerodynamic diameter ($d_{ae,mm}$ or MMAD) and the geometric standard deviation (σ_g or GSD) [23]. The $d_{ae,mm}$ denotes the particle size at which half of the total aerosol mass is contained in larger particles and half in smaller particles. Since the $d_{ae,mm}$ is expressed as an aerodynamic diameter, it describes how the overall aerosol behaves in the respired air and can be used to estimate where and by what processes particles deposit in the respiratory tract. Another frequently encountered particle size parameter is the mass median diameter (d_{mm} or MMD), which is the same as the $d_{ae,mm}$ except that the particle size is expressed in terms of the particle's actual density.

The σ_g denotes the spread of particle sizes. Most aerosols have particle sizes that are distributed lognormally; that is, on a plot of frequency distribution vs. log particle diameter, the distribution looks Gaussian. An aerosol with all identically sized particles has a σ_g of 1.0. An aerosol with a $\sigma_g \leq 1.22$ is considered monodisperse [59]: to a first approximation all the particles behave aerodynamically alike. An aerosol with a $\sigma_g > 1.22$ is polydisperse: there are appreciable differences in aerodynamic behavior among the particles. Most therapeutic aerosols are polydisperse. An aerosol with a $d_{ae,mm}$ of 2 μm and a σ_g of 2 has ± 1 geometric standard deviation or 68% of its mass contained between particles of 1 and 4 μm. An important implication of a lognormal distribution is that most of the aerosol mass is contained in the large particles, since mass is proportional to the cube of diameter. Where these large particles deposit in the respiratory tract governs where much of the dose deposits.

1. Factors Affecting the Particle Size and Mass Distribution of the Aerosol Produced by Nebulizers

Jet Nebulizer Characteristics and Air Flow Rate. The operation of jet nebulizers is well described [60,61]. A typical jet nebulizer uses compressed air exiting a nozzle at high velocity to draw liquid from a second, closely adjacent orifice into the airstream. The liquid enters the accelerating airstream as a thin stream that quickly elongates to the point where it breaks into droplets. The droplets then impact onto a nearby surface and shatter into smaller droplets. Fewer than 0.5% of the resultant droplets are small enough to leave the nebulizer; the larger droplets drip back into the liquid to start the process again.

The size distribution of aerosol droplets from a jet nebulizer depends on the diameter of the liquid inlet orifice, the air velocity at the nozzle, and the ratio of the mass flow rate of air to liquid [60]. The droplets at the nebulizer outlet become smaller with increasing air velocity and increasing ratio of the mass flow rate of air to liquid. Increasing the nebulizer flow rate also increases the aerosol output rate [61]. The formation of droplets depends on the proper alignment and placement of the jet nozzle, liquid inlet, and impaction surface; many nebulizers have baffles to remove larger particles by impaction. Thus, the internal orientation and geometry of the jet nebulizer is critical to maintaining a reproducible output and size distribution. The output and size distribution are also affected by droplets' impacting and settling onto the tubing downstream of the nebulizer [62]. Some nebulizers have vents that allow air to enter the nebulizer via the Bernoulli effect that is created either during inspiration (e.g., the Medic-Aide Sidestream or the Pari IS-2) or by the nebulizer jet. The additional air can boost the mass of the aerosol output, but if the flow rate of the additional air exceeds the aerosol output, as is often the case, the aerosol concentration actually decreases [61,63,64]. The additional airflow can also keep larger particles suspended and thus shift the size distribution to larger sizes [63]. Other factors that in some situations affect the droplet size are the gas density and the liquid surface tension and viscosity; however, with jet nebulizers used with dilute aqueous solutions in normal clinical settings these three factors are unimportant [60]. The solution concentration itself has no effect on the size distribution of the droplets except to the extent that it changes the physical characteristics of the solution [61,63].

Evaporation. The nebulizing action cause continual reflux of a large volume (and surface area) of water, which promotes extensive water evaporation and saturates the air emerging from the jet nebulizer. Consequently, the total water output of the nebulizer is the sum of the output of droplets and water vapor. Depending on the nebulizer, the water vapor output comprises 20–85% of the total water loss, so that the droplet output may be as little as 15% or as much as 80% of the total water output [66–68]. The evaporating water cools and concentrates the solution, causing isotonic solutions and the resultant droplets to become increasingly hypertonic over time [61,63,66,67,69–71]. The rate of evaporation-induced solute concentration depends on the air flow rate and the ratio of the volume of water vapor to the total volume of both droplets and water vapor leaving the nebulizer per unit volume of air [60]. Evaporative losses from the solution can be decreased by using air from a compressor, which supplies air at ambient humidity, rather than from a compressed gas cylinder, which supplies air that is totally dry. Using cold solutions also decreases evaporative losses without changing the aerosol output [67], but the droplets are also affected by the cold, which is discussed next.

An important consequence of the evaporative cooling of the solution is that the freshly generated droplets are cold, which indirectly causes their size to decrease and their solute concentration to increase, sometimes dramatically [70]. As the cold droplets warm to ambient temperature, they evaporate water until the droplet vapor pressure equals the vapor pressure of the surrounding air [72]. The greater the temperature gradient between the droplets and the surrounding air, the greater the evaporative loss and droplet shrinkage and the more concentrated the droplets.

Evaporation is enhanced when dry compressed gas is used, because the dry air promotes more evaporative loss from the solution and in turn a lower solution temperature and a larger temperature gradient. Further droplet shrinkage and solute concentration occurs if any supplemental air inhaled with the aerosol—e.g., through a T-piece—is not saturated [73]. Thus, solutions in jet nebulizers that are initially isotonic can produce droplets that are hypertonic by the time they reach the mouth [70]. For aerosols produced from an isotonic saline solution, Ferron and Gebhart [74] report that for selected jet nebulizers [63], the effect of droplet evaporation on inhaled droplet size can vary from modest to dramatic. In cases where the relative humidity at nebulizer outlet is greater than 99%, the consequent shrinkage in droplet diameter from the point of formation is between 2% and 14%. Yet if the relative humidity at the nebulizer outlet is 95% (which was the case for one nebulizer they analyzed), the shrinkage in droplet diameter is as much as 55%.

The time needed to evaporate to a stable droplet size depends primarily on the initial droplet diameter, being less than 0.5 s for a 1-μm droplet but as long as 10 s for a 10-μm droplet [72]. Since a droplet may be airborne for only a few seconds before it is inhaled, larger droplets undergo less change in solute concentration.

In summary, the size and solute concentration of droplets are affected by any difference in vapor pressure between the droplet and the surrounding air and the time available for equilibration. Thus gradients of relative humidity and temperature do affect the droplets and can cause the solute concentration in the droplets to be different from that of the nebulized fluid [63,70]. The change in the droplet solute concentration can be minimized by keeping the nebulizer fluid at room temperature and using airflows that are as close as possible to the temperature and humidity of the aerosol [70]. Furthermore, droplet shrinkage and increased tonicity will be reversed, partly or wholly, when droplets enter the nearly saturated air of the lungs and grow hygroscopically (discussed later).

Droplet Size Distributions from Jet Nebulizers. Size distribution data for jet nebulizers come from a number of studies [e.g., 61–63,69,73,75]. Sterk and coworkers [63] analyzed the aerosols generated by 11 jet nebulizers from physiologically isotonic saline and found that the initial droplets had $d_{ae,mm}$'s from 1.6 to 4.9 μm and σ_g's from 1.8 to 2.3. For the Wright nebulizer, which is commonly used for provocation testing, the $d_{ae,mm}$ and σ_g were 1.6 μm and 1.84 at a driving pressure of 249 kPa (36 psi). For the DeVilbiss model 645, a discontinued model but with the same jet design as the popular model 646, the $d_{ae,mm}$ and σ_g were 1.9 μm and 1.88 with a closed vent and at a driving pressure of 135 kPa (20 psi).

Ultrasonic Nebulizers. Ultrasonic nebulizers use mechanical energy from a rapidly vibrating piezoelectric crystal to produce an aerosol [60]. At the solution surface, the vibrations create an liquid fountain that forms smaller capillary waves at the surface that break into aerosol droplets. The droplet size distribution from an ultrasonic nebulizer is directly related to the liquid surface tension and inversely related to the liquid density and the oscillation frequency. In comparison with jet nebulizers, ultrasonic nebulizers have these general features: (1) they produce aerosols with larger droplets and have a higher output rate; (2) they may heat instead of cool the solution; and (3) the evaporative losses are lower, and with some models negligible, since they aerosolize two to 10 times more water per unit volume of air, with much of the water used to produce larger droplets, but there is still sufficient water vapor to saturate both the air above the solution and any supplemental air [60,63,67,69,70,75–77]. Furthermore, although the freshly generated aerosol is warm and must cool as it moves through the tubing, the water vapor tends to condense on the cooler walls of the tubing instead of the droplets, preventing the droplets from becoming hypotonic [76]. Thus, droplets from ultrasonic nebulizers tend to maintain their initial size after production, shrinking 10% or less after production [63,70,74]. One occasional drawback of ultrasonic nebulizers is that the intense ultrasonic energy can cause some substances to degrade [78]. Ultrasonic nebulizers are recommended for bronchoprovocation testing with nonisotonic aerosols [32].

Several studies report the aerosol outputs from ultrasonic nebulizers [e.g., 63,69,76,77]. Sterk and co-workers [63] found the aerosols generated from physiologically isotonic saline by nine ultrasonic nebulizers to have $d_{ae,mm}$'s from 3 to 7 μm and σ_g's from 1.8 to 2.2.

2. Droplet Size Distributions at the Mouthpiece Versus in the Lungs

There are two particle size distributions of interest in calculating inhaled drug dose: the distribution at the mouthpiece and the distribution in the lungs. The size distribution at the mouthpiece determines the fraction of particles that is small enough to be inhaled past the oropharynx and enter the lungs. Fewer than half the particles larger than 8 μm get past the larynx during tidal breathing [10]. As mentioned above, for nebulized aerosols the size distribution at the mouthpiece depends on the extent of droplet evaporation and losses between the nebulizer and the mouth.

The particle size distribution within the lungs determines the fraction of particles that deposit in the airways versus the parenchyma. For insoluble hydrophobic particles, the size distribution at the mouth is also the size distribution in the lungs so long as agglomeration is minimal. For hydrophilic particles, however, estimating the size distribution in the lungs is more complex because of hygroscopic growth. The relative humidity in the lungs beyond the first 10 generations is about 99.5% [79], which causes dry NaCl particles with d_{ae} from 0.1 to 10 μm to increase in diameter by factors of 2.5 to 4.4, respectively [80]. For nebulized droplets, which enter the lungs already wet, the extent of hygroscopic growth in the lungs is less than 2 (discussed below).

C. Measuring Aerosol Output from Devices

1. Inhaled Aerosol Mass

The dose from nebulizers is often calculated on the basis of the initial dose of drug in the nebulizer (the nebulizer charge) and the change in nebulizer weight from the beginning to the end of the delivery period [51]. Although weighing the nebulizer before and after challenge may be adequate for routine clinical protocols [32], this approach is flawed for exact research, since it ignores both the extensive weight loss due to evaporation of the nebulized solution and the droplet losses by sedimentation and impaction within the nebulizer, tubing, and valves upstream of the patient [62,67,70,73]. The actual value of interest is the inhaled aerosol mass per unit time or air volume [60,81]. A common way to measure the inhaled aerosol mass is to collect the aerosolized drug output on an absolute filter [67,75]. Additional refinements are to collect the aerosol at the mouthpiece under actual or simulated breathing conditions [62] or to add an artificial oropharynx and measure the mass of drug that penetrates [82]. The collected mass on the filter can be weighed. However, if the drug is labile or combined with other ingredients, it is more meaningful to assay for bioactivity, the drug itself, or the presence of a chemical, fluorescent, or radioactive tracer [61,62,67–69]. Nebulized proteins can be collected on a Buchner funnel combined with a cold collection flask [83].

2. Delivery Efficiency

On the basis of the inhaled aerosol mass from a nebulizer, one can calculate the device's delivery efficiency. The delivery efficiency is the fraction of drug initially within the nebulizer that is delivered to the mouthpiece over the challenge period [62]. Delivery efficiency helps one determine how much drug to aerosolize and can help to select among different nebulizers, especially when expensive drugs are aerosolized. Different models of nebulizer have marked differences in delivery efficiency: for one ultrasonic and two jet nebulizers the efficiencies ranged from 5% to 22%, with much of the losses occurring within the tubing and internal nebulizer surfaces [62]. Nebulizer efficiency can be improved by minimizing the internal surface area and adding surfactant to the nebulized solution, which makes it easier for drops that have deposited on the internal nebulizer surface to drip back to the nebulizer fluid and be reaerosolized [84].

3. Particle Size Distribution

The particle size distributions from devices are based on measurements of either the freshly generated spray droplets or the particles remaining after liquid evaporation [41]. Techniques to analyze droplet sizes directly within the nebulized spray are available [39,85–87] and include high-speed photography [88] and Fraunhofer diffraction [89]. An advantage of these methods is that they directly analyze the spray and are free from sampling biases. However, as mentioned previously, the size distribution of a droplet is heavily dependent on the relative humidity of the surrounding air. Thus, the applicability of any measurement of a wet droplet depends on having the suspending air at a controlled, relevant humidity. Recently, an experimental system has been developed to generate stable atmospheres with relative humidities of 99% and higher that are suitable to determine particle sizes at the nebulizer outlet and in the lung [90]. However, to the extent that the maintenance and measurement of high-humidity atmospheres is complex, it may be preferable to make these measurements at a well-controlled lower humidity after allowing sufficient time for the droplets to reach their equilibrium size [72].

A robust way to circumvent the relative humidity problem is to base the size distribution on the diameter of the dry particles after evaporation [61,63,69]. Drying offers the following important advantages: (1) the size distribution is stable, so that expensive, fast-responding devices are not needed and artifacts, such as evaporation of liquid droplets as they pass through a cascade impactor, are less likely [41]; (2) one can calculate the initial droplet size distribution on the basis of the composition of the nebulized solution [61,63,69]; (3) for hygroscopic particles, one can calculate the equilibrium droplet size in the lungs on the basis of the molar composition of the solution and the physicochemical properties of the solute [80]; and (4) for hydrophobic particles, the dry particle size distribution is the size distribution in the lungs.

A common way to measure the size distribution of particles is to mix the wet droplets with a dry airflow in a chamber and, after drying to extract the particles from the chamber, size them with an inertial, centrifugal, electrical, or optical analytical method [61,63,69,91]. Incorporating an artificial oropharynx upstream of the sizing device is an option [82]. Inertial and centrifugal methods are popular and well described [19,92]; these methods include cascade impactors [93–95], centrifugal aerosol spectrometers [96], inertial spectrometers [97], and liquid impingers [98,99]. Impactors are a recommended reference method to characterize the aerosol from MDIs [100]. Impingers maintain the collected droplets in solution, which is advantageous for chemical analysis and when it is desired to keep the drug hydrated, but in comparison with cascade impactors, impingers have less size resolution and can have a lower collection efficiency for submicrometer particles [101].

A differential mobility analyzer is appropriate for sizing dry particles, 0.01–1 μm, on the basis of their movement in an electrical field [102]. Optical methods for size analysis have been reviewed [85,103,104] and include single-particle counters that size particles on the basis of the amount of light they scatter [105,106]; phase Doppler analyzers, which can also be used for sprays [107]; time-of-flight analyzers [108]; and electrical single-particle aerodynamic relaxation time (E-SPART) analyzers [109]. Another method is to collect the particles on slides and then analyze them with light or electron microscopy combined with an image analysis system [110]. Most optical methods provide particle size distributions based on particle cross-sectional area, which reveals little about the particles' aerodynamic properties. However, the time-of-flight and E-SPART analyzers measure aerodynamic equivalent diameter.

A caveat with any device that extracts an aerosol sample from the nebulized cloud is that one must use isokinetic sampling when appropriate and try to minimize losses of large particles to the walls of the sampling inlet [111].

IV. FACTORS INFLUENCING PARTICLE DEPOSITION

The physical mechanisms responsible for deposition have already been discussed. The effectiveness of these mechanisms depends on various factors, some of which can be controlled by the clinician or scientist, such as particle size and breathing pattern. Others such as airway geometry and disease are uncontrollable. Many aspects of particle deposition in the respiratory tract have captured the energy and imagination of investigators; these studies are reviewed in many papers and books [6–14, 22,112]. Other excellent sources of information on deposition are published works from the International Symposia on Inhaled Particles [113–119]. Deposition from a more clinical perspective was featured at recent symposia on respiratory drug delivery [120–122], congresses of the International Society for Aerosols in Medicine [123–125], and a symposium on pharmaceutical aerosols [125a], and in reviews [6,8,126]. Some major influences on the fraction of the inspired particles that deposits within the respiratory tract and the anatomical distribution of retained particles are now discussed.

A. Anatomy of the Respiratory Tract

The configuration of the lungs and airways is important because the efficiency of deposition depends in part on the diameters of the airways, their angles of branching, and the average distances of particles to lung surfaces in the acini. Along with the volumetric flow rate, airway anatomy specifies the local linear velocity of the airstream and thus determines whether the flow is laminar or turbulent. For example, at the laryngeal aperture an air jet is formed that creates turbulent and unstable airflows that enhance particle impaction in the trachea [127,128]. There are interspecies and intraspecies differences in lung morphometry [49,129–131]; even within the same individual, the dimensions of the respiratory tract change with lung volume, age, and pathological processes. Among normal subjects breathing in the same manner, total deposition fraction has a coefficient of variation as large as 27%. This is largely due to intersubject differences in airway geometry [132–135]. Gender differences in laryngeal and airway geometries may cause women to have greater upper airway deposition by impaction as compared with men [136,137]. For any person, decreasing lung volume not only increases the deposition fraction but also causes the major site of particle deposition within the airways to shift from the lung periphery to more central airways [6]. At low lung volumes, airways have smaller cross-sectional areas, higher linear velocities, and thus enhanced deposition by impaction in central airways for a given flow rate. As a person ages, anatomical changes of the respiratory tract also affect deposition fraction [138]. Children under 8 years old who are breathing at rest have higher total, head, and tracheobronchial deposition fractions and lower alveolar deposition fraction than adults [139–142]. The higher airway deposition may help explain why some children have a greater response than adults to a given dose of a provocation agent [143].

B. Choice of Pathway

Most people breath nasally at rest. As ventilation rate rises above 35–40 L/min, the high-resistance nasal pathway starts to be combined with the low-resistance oral pathway [144–146]. With continuing increases in ventilation rate, the oral path takes on a greater percentage of the total ventilation, but this percentage varies considerably among subjects, ranging from only 10% to as much as 80% [144,147,148].

A highly significant change in the effective anatomy of the respiratory tract occurs when air is inhaled through the mouth instead of the nose or when the nose is bypassed because of a tracheostomy or an endotracheal tube. The nose has a major role as an upstream filter that prevents inhaled particles from penetrating into the lungs. The smallest total cross-sectional area of the respiratory tract also occurs in the nose. High velocities, sharp curves, nasal hairs, and secondary flows all combine to collect inhaled particles in the nose. Excellent reviews of particle inhalability and deposition in the nose are available [e.g., 11,13,112,149–152]. The inhalability, deposition, and clearance of particles in the head during nasal breathing have been studied by several investigators [e.g., 10,152–160]. Collectively, these reports indicate that the anterior portion of the nose collects particles larger than 1 μm by impaction, with the probability of impaction increasing with increasing $d_{ae}{}^2Q$, though there is some evidence that impaction probability is better described by $d_{ae}{}^2p^{2/3}$, where p is the pressure drop across the nose [13,156]. Most studies show that particles larger than 10 μm are completely trapped in the nose. The actual fraction of inhaled material trapped in the nose varies considerably among individuals and is more variable than the deposition fraction in the lungs [159]. These intersubject differences may be due to variations in nasal distensibility and geometry, including the number and shape of nasal hairs.

Besides being an upstream filter, the nose also humidifies the inspired air; it is a more effective humidifier than the mouth because the inhaled air passes by the large surface area of the highly vascular nasal turbinates. Because of this humidification, hygroscopic particles (d_{ae}>1 μm) grow more rapidly when inhaled through the nose than when inhaled through the mouth and thus have enhanced deposition fraction [80].

The nose is an efficient filter for large particles, but the mouth, because of its simpler geometry, is not. The shift from a higher filtering efficiency during nasal breathing to lower filtering efficiency during oronasal breathing may potentiate asthma attacks during exercise. During exercise, large volumes of air are inhaled by the mouth, so that more and more antigenic particles, such as pollens, penetrate to and deposit in the lungs. This increased exposure of airways increases the risk of allergic responses. With exercise the amount of particles depositing in the lungs may increase more than predicted by the increased ventilation. Although airway cooling and drying are central features of exercise-induced asthma [161], if allergens are present in the inspired air, increased deposition of allergens because of mouth breathing may also be involved.

When a subject breathes orally through a tube, few particles smaller than 10 μm deposit in the mouth itself, but a substantial fraction of inhaled particles can impact at the larynx. Rudolf et al. [162] found that the probability of particles' depositing at the larynx is related to the modified impaction parameter $d_{ae}^2Q^{2/3}V^{-1/4}$, where V is the tidal volume. The tidal volume term accounts for how vocal cord geometry, which changes during breathing, influences deposition fraction. Such sensitivity to the vocal cords could explain why there are large intersubject differences in particle deposition in the oropharynx [137,152,163]. When a subject breathes oronasally without a tube, the oral deposition fraction of particles is higher but also sensitive to oral configuration, which changes with ventilation level [164]. Reviews of particle deposition in the oropharynx are available [13,152]. When a subject breathes through an endotracheal tube, so that the larynx is bypassed, both the airway and the pulmonary deposition fractions of particles are increased relative to nasal breathing [165].

C. Particle Size and Size Distribution

As mentioned earlier, a major factor governing the effectiveness of deposition mechanisms is the size of the inspired particles. The importance of particle size is seen in Table 2, which lists the total and regional deposition fraction as a function of particle size in three healthy subjects. Regional deposition fraction is the fraction of the total inhaled mass that deposits in a defined region. For deposition studies, the typical respiratory tract regions are the oropharynx, nose, larynx, central airways, peripheral airways, and acini. Depending on particle size, total deposition fraction is similarly sensitive [10]. As is discussed later, proper selection of particle size is one way to target particles to a desired lung region.

In Table 2, one can compare the particle size corresponding to the highest deposition fraction for each lung compartment. It can be seen how during oral breathing the larynx and airways act as sequential upstream filters for the acini. The larynx, which collects particles by impaction, consistently removes more particles than the airways. The laryngeal deposition fraction maximum is at a d_{ae}

Table 2 Total and Regional Deposition Fraction of Stable Unit-Density Spheres in the Human Respiratory Tract During Oral Breathing from Functional Residual Capacity at Two Flow Rates (Q) and Tidal Volumes (V)

Particle diameter (μm)	Deposition fraction (%) Q = 0.25 L/s, V = 0.5 L				Q = 0.75 L/s, V = 1.5 L			
	Total	Larynx	Airways[a]	Acini[a]	Total	Larynx	Airways	Acini
0.005	67				87			
0.01	62				84			
0.05	33	0	0	33	45	0	0	45
0.1	21	0	0	21	25	0	0	25
0.2	13	0	0	13	14	0	0	14
0.4	11	0	0	11	11	0	0	11
0.7	12	0	0	12	12	0	0	12
1	15	0	0	15	15	0	0	15
2	28	2	1	25	39	1	1	37
3	44	8	4	32	63	8	5	50
4	56	16	7	33	77	21	11	45
5	65	24	11	30	86	40	17	29
6	72	34	15	23	90	52	20	18
7	78	43	18	17	93	61	22	10
8	82	52	20	10	95	69	21	5
9	84	59	19	6	96	77	17	2
10	86	65	17	4	97	82	14	1
12	87	74	12	1	98	89	9	0
15	89	81	8	0				

[a]The airway and acinar region designations are based on fast and slow clearing compartments, respectively.
Source: Modified from Ref. 10.

greater than 15 μm, since impaction efficiency increases with increasing d_{ae}. For the airways, which collect particles by impaction and sedimentation, the deposition maximum is at a d_{ae} of 7–8 μm. Larger particles are removed upstream in the larynx, while smaller particles have lower impaction and sedimentation efficiencies. For the acini, which collect particles by sedimentation and diffusion, there are actually two maxima. One maximum occurs at a d_{ae} of 3–4 μm. Again, larger particles are removed upstream in the larynx and airways, while smaller particles have lower sedimentation efficiencies. The other maximum occurs at d_{ae} less than 0.005 μm, since diffusional displacement increases with decreasing particle size. A deposition fraction minimum exists at a d_{ae} of 0.4 μm, the particle size with the lowest combined settling and diffusional displacements (see Table 1).

Our ability to estimate deposition fraction on the basis of particle size is confounded by the fact that most therapeutic aerosols are polydisperse. One can calculate total and regional deposition fraction on the basis of the aerosol's $d_{ae,mm}$ regardless of the geometric standard deviation, but theoretical studies show that for many $d_{ae}s_{,mm}$'s this approach significantly overestimates or underestimates total and regional deposition fractions [166–169]. Diu and Yu [166] found that increasing polydispersity increases the deposition fraction for aerosols with $d_{ae,mm}$'s between 0.04 and 2 μm and decreases the deposition fraction for aerosols with $d_{ae,mm}$'s outside this range. Thus, the overall effect of increasing polydispersity is to decrease the dependency of deposition fraction on particle size. Another way to calculate total and regional deposition for polydisperse aerosols is to use an approach that combines the aerosol's $d_{ae,mm}$ and σ_g with semiempirical deposition equations [169].

D. Hygroscopicity and Evaporation

Many types of particle undergo size changes as they move through the delivery system and the respiratory tract. Water droplets shrink through evaporation, while hygroscopic droplets, such as NaCl particles, may undergo dramatic hygroscopic growth, especially as the relative humidity nears 100% [80,170,171]. Since the relative humidity in the lungs beyond the upper airways is 99.5% [79], hygroscopicity can substantially affect particle size and deposition fraction. Many inhaled drugs are hygroscopic [172,173]; for example dry 1-μm particles of atropine sulfate and histamine grow in the lungs by factors of 2.2 and 3.5, respectively [172].

The effect of hygroscopicity on deposition fraction has been studied both experimentally [e.g., 174–177] and theoretically [80,142,168,171,172,178–180], and has been reviewed [181–183]. These studies show that with increasing particle hygroscopicity and relative humidity, the function between deposition fraction and particle size shifts to smaller particle sizes. Whereas the deposition minimum for nonhygroscopic particles is about 0.4 μm (see Table 2), the minimum for initially dry NaCl particles is about 0.1 μm. Consequently, hygroscopic NaCl particles, which are dry and larger than 0.1 μm when inhaled, deposit more than nonhygroscopic particles of the same size. Table 3 illustrates this effect by comparing the deposition fraction of hygroscopic NaCl particles and stable nonhygroscopic particles. The greatest hygroscopicity-related increases in deposition occur for particles with dry diameters of about 1 μm, the total deposition fraction for the NaCl particles being almost three times that of stable particles. Hygroscopicity also affects regional deposition fraction; it can more than double the airway and acinar deposition fraction of drug particles with initial dry sizes of about 0.5–2 μm [172].

The rate of hygroscopic-particle growth depends on particle size. Dry particles less than 1 μm reach full size in about 2 s, but particles 3 μm and larger take more

Table 3 Total and Regional Deposition Fraction of Stable, Nonhygroscopic Unit-Density Spheres and NaCl Particles in the Human Respiratory Tract During Oral and Nasal Breathing from Functional Residual Capacity (Tidal Volume = 1 L, Flow Rate = 0.25 L/s)

Initial particle diameter (μm)	Type	Deposition fraction (%) Oral breathing				Nasal breathing			
		Total	Larynx	Airways[a]	Acini[a]	Total	Larynx	Airways	Acini
0.1	Stable	43	0	8	35	43	0	8	35
	NaCl	22[b]	0	4	18	22	0	4	18
0.4	Stable	17	0	3	15	19	2	2	14
	NaCl	37	0	4	34	40	3	4	33
1.0	Stable	25	0	3	22	28	4	3	21
	NaCl	76	0	11	65	79	15	10	54
2.0	Stable	52	0	6	46	62	23	5	35
	NaCl	84	0	24	61	89	31	17	40
5.0	Stable	84	11	23	50	91	53	12	26
	NaCl	90	11	50	28	94	55	26	12
10.0	Stable	91	30	47	15	96	77	19	5
	NaCl	93	30	60	3	96	77	19	0

[a]The airway and acinar region designations are based on fast and slow clearing compartments, respectively.
[b]Deposition fraction after complete hygroscopic growth in air at 99.5% relative humidity.
Source: Modified from Ref. 83.

than 10 s [80]. The time lag for the growth of large particles offers an attractive means to enhance deposition in the airways and pulmonary region while minimizing deposition in the oropharynx. Fifty percent of 5-μm (initially dry) NaCl particles deposit in the airways during tidal oral breathing, whereas only 23% of nonhygroscopic 5-μm particles deposit there, even though both particles have the same oropharyngeal deposition fraction [80].

When an aqueous solution is nebulized, the hygroscopic growth of the droplets can be predicted on the basis of the solution osmolality. Inhaled hygroscopic droplets reach equilibrium size when the water vapor pressure at the droplet surface equals the water vapor pressure of the air in the lungs. The water vapor pressure in the lungs is, in turn, controlled by the osmolality of the liquid layer on the lung surface, which is approximately isosmotic with serum [184]. Thus, inhaled droplets absorb or desorb water until the droplet solution is isosmotic with the surface liquid: solid hygroscopic particles or hyperosmotic droplets gain water and grow, hyposmotic droplets lose water and shrink (pure water droplets completely evaporate), and isosmotic droplets maintain their size. The measurement and adjustment of the osmolality of the nebulized solution constitute a valuable, yet underutilized, strategy to target and optimize drug delivery [173,185].

However, marked hyposmotic or hyperosmotic concentrations may also cause bronchoconstriction in asthmatics [186].

E. Breathing Pattern

1. Flow Rate and Lung Volume

When a subject changes breathing pattern, deposition fraction may change profoundly. Minute volume determines the total number of particles entering the lungs. Flow rate affects the probability of particle impaction and the extent of turbulent flow, which enhances particle deposition in the upper airways. The combination of flow rate, tidal volume, breath-holding time, and lung volume affects particle residence time in each lung region and hence the probability of deposition by gravitational and diffusional forces [22]. Tidal volume and flow rate also influence the motion of the larynx and affect particle deposition there [162]. Changing lung volume also alters the dimensions of the airways and parenchyma. High levels of ventilation and breath holding represent extremes of breathing patterns; they give rise to markedly different deposition patterns.

Many of these breathing-pattern interactions are represented in Table 2, which shows total and regional deposition fraction data for two breathing patterns differing in flow rate and tidal volume by a factor of 3. The larger tidal volume increases the proportion of the breath that goes to the acini, and the higher flow rate causes the particles to spend less time in the airways and more time in the acini. Both of these factors enhance deposition by sedimentation and diffusion for particles less than 5 μm in diameter in the acini. The higher flow rate also enhances deposition by impaction for particles 4 μm and larger at the larynx. However the large change in breathing pattern has little effect on the deposition fraction in the airways. This insensitivity is related to the upstream filtering action of the larynx that was mentioned earlier.

Generally, when airflow velocities increase, as during physical exertion or labored respiration consequent to an asthma attack, inertial deposition increases. During slow, relaxed breathing, particle sedimentation and diffusion are the primary deposition processes, and particle collection in the acini increases because of the proximity of lung surfaces there.

2. Breathing Patterns During Provocation Testing

The various bronchoprovocation protocols use different breathing patterns to deliver the challenge aerosol. For the tidal-breathing method [32,51,52], the aerosol is delivered continuously during quiet tidal breathing. For the dosimeter method [32,53], the aerosol is delivered as a bolus at the onset of an inspiratory capacity breath of 5 s duration. For the "Yan method" [32,54], the aerosol is delivered at the onset of an inspiratory capacity breath of 1–2 s duration, followed by 3-s breath hold at total lung capacity. To estimate the flow rates during these maneuvers, the physiological breathing parameters for modeling particle deposition in the respiratory tract can be used [187]. The mean tidal volume and inspiratory time are 750 ml and 2.5 s, respectively, for a typical adult man and 464 ml and 4.25 s for a woman. During the tidal-breathing test the mean inhaled flow rates would be 300 ml/s for the man and 217 ml/s for the woman. The mean inspiratory capacity is 3.68 L for an adult man and 2.29 L for a woman. During performance of the dosimeter test with a 5-s inhalation, the mean flow rates would be 736 and 458 ml/s, respectively. During performance of the Yan method with a 2-s inhalation, the mean inhaled flow rates would be 1840 and 1145 ml/s, respectively.

Do the great disparities in inspiratory flow rate and volume among the three provocation protocols create appreciable differences in regional deposition? To address this question, we calculated the regional deposition of polydisperse isotonic droplets by using the semiempirical deposition equations of Rudolf et al. [162,169] and the size distribution data for droplets from four nebulizers: a Wright nebulizer, a DeVilbiss 645 nebulizer (with the same jet design as the model 646), a hypothetical jet nebulizer with a $d_{ae,mm}$ of 4μm and a σ_g of 2, and a DeVilbiss Pulmosonic ultrasonic nebulizer with a $d_{ae,mm}$ of 6.7 μm and a σ_g of 1.55 [63]. The droplet size distribution from the hypothetical jet nebulizer represents an upper limit for most models of jet nebulizer [63]. The comparisons are best used to illustrate the relative deposition probabilities of droplets in each lung region. Two caveats concerning the comparisons are (1) that they are based on data from healthy persons with unconstricted airways and (2) that the semiempirical equations are based on the data obtained when the aerosol was inhaled over the entire breath, as is done with the tidal breathing method, whereas the dosimeter and Yan methods use aerosol boluses inhaled at the onset of inspiration. We assume that the relative regional distribution of particle deposition for droplets in a bolus approximates that for particles inhaled over an entire breath. In addition, we neglect both the effect of the breath hold for the Yan method, since the equations do not account for this, and the effect of hygroscopic growth, which entails only a slight error, since the droplets are assumed to be from isotonic saline [74].

Table 4 shows that for the tidal breathing and dosimeter methods the Wright and DeVilbiss 645 nebulizers produce about the same levels of particle deposition in the larynx and airways, but that the dosimeter method, because of its greater inhaled volume, enhances deposition in the acini. The droplets from the DeVilbiss 645, being slightly larger than those from the Wright nebulizer, have slightly greater deposition in some lung compartments. The Yan method, with its extremely high flow rates, has a two- to three-fold increase in laryngeal deposition and a two- to fourfold increase in airway deposition. The increases are less pronounced in the typical woman because of lower flow rates. The breath hold in the Yan method, which is neglected in these calculations, would mainly increase acinar deposition, since the bolus would be deep within the acini during the breath

Table 4 Predicted Total and Regional Deposition of Droplets from Selected Nebulizers in a Standard Man and Woman with Three Bronchoprovocation Protocols[a]

		Man				Woman			
Nebul	Test	Total	Larynx	Airways	Acini	Total	Larynx	Airways	Acini
Wright	Tidal	35	3	2	30	28	3	2	23
	Dosi	58	4	3	50	56	3	2	50
	Yan	47	9	8	30	44	7	5	32
D 645	Tidal	40	5	3	32	32	4	2	25
	Dosi	61	5	3	53	61	5	3	53
	Yan	53	12	11	30	50	10	6	33
Jet	Tidal	63	22	9	32	54	20	8	27
	Dosi	83	27	13	43	81	23	10	47
	Yan	79	39	20	21	75	35	15	26
Pulmo	Tidal	80	40	15	25	72	36	14	22
	Dosi	95	48	22	25	93	42	18	33
	Yan	95	64	23	7	92	59	21	13

[a]Deposition values are based on the semiempirical formulas of Rudolf et al. [162, 169] using standard lung volume and breathing values from the ICRP Task Group [187]. The respective $yd_{ae,mm}$ and σ_g of the nebulizers (Nebul) are: Wright: 1.6 μm, 1.84; DeVilbiss 645 (D 645): 1.9 μm, 1.88; Hypothetical jet nebulizer (Jet): 4 μm, 2; DeVilbiss Pulmosonic ultrasonic (Pulmo): 6.7, 1.55 [63]. See text for further details.

Dosi = dosimeter.

hold. In comparison with the Wright and DeVilbiss 645 nebulizers, the hypothetical jet nebulizer and the Pulmosonic ultrasonic nebulizer produce greater airway deposition and show more disparity between the deposition values for the tidal breathing and the dosimeter methods. The airway deposition with the tidal breathing and dosimeter methods is seven to nine times greater with the Pulmosonic than with the Wright nebulizer. There is enhanced airway deposition with the Pulmosonic, since this device's $d_{ae,mm}$ of 6.7 μm is close to the size that maximally deposits in the airways (see Table 2). The deposition trends found here generally agree with data from studies that compared difference provocation protocols [34,188].

3. Breathing Patterns for Drug Delivery

The optimal breathing pattern when delivering drugs depends on the type of device used. For jet nebulizers, experimental data show that the inspiratory flow rate should be slow (<0.55 L/s), as higher flow rates enhance drug deposition in the oropharynx [189]. The flow rate should be about 0.2 L/s for optimum deposition of particles ($d_{ae,mm}$ = 1.1 μm) in obstructed patients [190], though deposition is less dependent on ventilation in restricted patients [3]. To enhance the dose of drug delivered to the pulmonary region, tidal breaths should be moderate (1–2 L) [185,191]. If nebulization is continuous, breath holding wastes drug that is aerosolized during the breath hold, and this causes the total dose delivered to be less than if the drug were inhaled continuously over the same length of time [185]. Overall, jet nebulizers deposit about 10% of the nebulized drug in the lungs, with most of the drug being lost in the nebulizer apparatus and tubing [126,190,192–195].

For MDIs containing bronchodilators, it is recommended that the inspiratory flow rate be less than 0.5 L/s, that the inspired volume be large but below total lung capacity, and that there be a 10-s breath hold at end-inspiration [196]. With this maneuver, 10–20% of the aerosolized drug deposits in the lungs; a large amount of the drug impacts in the oropharynx because of the high velocity of the aerosol as it leaves the MDI [196–198]. In contrast to MDIs and nebulizers, dry-powder inhalers require rapid inspirations. Peak inspiratory flow rates of 0.5 L/s and greater help to disperse the drug powder into smaller particles that enter the lungs and improve the effectiveness of the drug delivered; however, breath holding or inspirations from residual volume have no added benefit [199,200]. The deposition fraction of drug in the lungs with dry-powder inhalers ranges from 15% to 20% [201–203].

F. Disease

The distribution of diseased portions of the lungs, which influences the distribution and deposition pattern of inspired particles, is often heterogeneous. Bronchoconstriction and obstruction of airways due to mucus or inflammation diverts more airflow to unobstructed airways. With advancing disease, the remaining healthy airways and acini are increasingly exposed to inspired particles. In these healthy regions, higher flow rates enhance particle impaction in the airways, and longer residence times in the lung periphery promote deposition by sedimentation and diffusion [204–206]. Often there is enhanced deposition at the obstructed sites despite the reduced airflow through these regions; however, the regions downstream of these obstructions have less deposition [205–211]. Such heterogeneous deposition patterns are found in asthmatic subjects [212–214], patients with cystic fibrosis [215], and smokers [216,217]. In restrictive disease such as diffuse interstitial fibrosis, there is an irregular peripheral deposition pattern [208]. Sweeney et al. [218–220] studied the progressive influence of emphysema, chronic bronchitis, and fibrosis on the distribution of deposition of submicrometric particles throughout rodent lungs. One common result in all three diseases is that the presence of detectable pulmonary disease always results in less uniform patterns of particle deposition throughout the lungs. In obstructed patients, total deposition fraction is greater than in healthy persons and increases with the severity of disease, as indicated by pulmonary function or clinical diagnosis [217,221–224].

V. DEPOSITION OF CHALLENGE AEROSOLS AND AIRWAYS RESPONSIVENESS DURING PROVOCATION TESTING

In contrast to the enhanced deposition fraction seen in patients with airway obstruction, when the airways are constricted during provocation testing with methacholine, total deposition fraction at the onset of testing is about the same in both responsive and nonresponsive subjects [193,213,225,226]. Furthermore, deposition fraction remains about the same in responders and nonresponders over the course of the testing [225,227]. Although total deposition is fairly constant during provocation testing, there is a distinct change in the regional deposition pattern. With increasing doses of the challenge agent there is a marked increase in deposition in the central airways and less deposition in peripheral lung regions in both responders and nonresponders [213,228–230]. On the basis of the similar characteristics of particle deposition in responders and nonresponders, several investigators conclude that a subject's initial responsiveness to an inhaled methacholine challenge is more dependent on intrinsic properties of the airways than on the amount or pattern of deposition of methacholine in the lungs [193,213, 225,229].

While there is agreement that the total deposition fraction of a methacholine challenge aerosol is not related to responsiveness in asthmatic subjects, there are data supporting a relation between total deposition fraction and responsiveness in normal subjects [226]. The challenge agent and the type of pharmacological response evoked may also be important [193]. With inhaled histamine the deposition fraction is related to responsiveness only in normal subjects [231]; but with inhaled atropine the deposition fraction is related to responsiveness in both normal and asthmatic subjects [193].

In addition, the measurement of responsiveness within a person can be altered by changing the pattern of deposition of the challenge aerosol. A person's responsiveness is enhanced when the challenge aerosol is inhaled so that the droplets deposit either in a more heterogeneous pattern [232] or preferentially in the central airways rather than the lung periphery [213,233–235]. Thus, it is important to control the method of inhalation when comparing test results among and within individuals [34,188].

VI. REGIONAL AND LOCAL PATTERNS OF DEPOSITION

A. Targeting Drugs to Specific Regions of the Respiratory Tract

Some of the factors that are known to influence particle deposition can be exploited to target drugs to diseased lung regions with greater control of dose while simultaneously decreasing systemic side effects. For example, when delivering aerosolized drugs it is often desirable to minimize oral deposition to avoid side effects such as gagging, cough, bronchospasm, and, in the case of aerosolized steroids, hoarseness, oropharyngeal candidiasis, [236], and in children suppressed bone growth. A powerful approach to targeting drugs is to combine a preselected breathing pattern with a particular particle size. Stahlhofen et al. [237], on the basis of their studies in healthy subjects, recommend that to target the acini, one take slow, deep breaths (1 L, 8/min) of an aerosol with a $d_{ae,mm}$ of 2 μm. This pattern enhances particle settling and deposits about 50% of the inhaled mass in the lung periphery, which most of the remaining mass being exhaled. To target the nose, oropharynx, or larynx, they suggest using rapid breaths ($Q > 0.75$ L/s) and a $d_{ae,mm}$ of 9 μm or larger. This strategy deposits more than 80% of the inhaled mass in these upper airway regions as a result of enhanced particle impaction. However, the data from Stahlhofen et al. show that we are less able to target the tracheobronchial region by selecting breathing pattern and particle size because there is always appreciable deposition in other lung regions. Particles with $d_{ae,mm}$ of 6 to 8 μm are useful, since about 20% of the mass deposits in the airways. Nonetheless, when these particles are inhaled with rapid, shallow breathing, there is also enhanced oropharyngeal and laryngeal deposition; whereas when inhaled with slow, deep breathing, there is enhanced acinar deposition.

Several investigators have tailored particle size, breathing pattern, or both in attempts to enhance drug or particle deposition in the airways or lung periphery [189–191,212,232,234,235,238–246]. Many studies appeared successful; those that failed many have done so because the range of particle sizes, breathing patterns, or lung penetrations were insufficient to favor deposition in one region over another.

One proven way to target the airways is to inhale 2- to 3-μm particles and use forced exhalations or coughing to enhance deposition near flow-limiting segments [233,247–250]. Furthermore, in diseased patients with narrowed or obstructed airways, enhanced deposition of particles at sites of obstruction helps to target these areas [205], while particles may need to be smaller than 1 μm to pass successfully through obstructed sites to reach downstream lung regions.

There are other strategies to target particles [47,251]. Breath holding increases both airway and alveolar deposition fraction of particles. Increased aerosol monodispersity allows better prediction and control of deposition sites [166–168], or certain $d_{ae,mm}$'s such as 2 μm, that have deposition patterns independent of polydispersity could be used [166,169]. Hygroscopic particles that are initially small enough to escape deposition in the mouth or nose, but that grow in the airways and enhance the deposition fractions in the airways and acini, may be useful [185]. Conversely, hygroscopic growth can be decreased when particles are mixed with hydrophobic materials [181,252–254]. To minimize deposition fraction in conducting airways, the aerosolized drug can be delivered at the beginning of inspiration or as an aerosol bolus that is followed by clean air [188,222,234, 251,255,256]. Boluses introduced at the end of the breath favor deposition in the airways. Aerosol boluses offer the advantages of reducing the total dose of drug delivered to the lungs as well as decreasing the likelihood of side effects and cost. Bolus delivery may also help those patients who are unable to do the respiratory gymnastics required for targeted delivery. Finally, there is the possibility, mostly theoretical at this time, that one could enhance deposition mechanisms locally and thus influence local collection efficiency and regional deposition fraction. Magnetic and acoustic forces such as shock waves are possibilities.

B. Factors Affecting Regional Dose

When using challenge or therapeutic aerosols, one needs to calculate delivered drug dose and the regional distribution of dose. One can calculate delivered drug dose on the basis of inhaled mass per unit time and the fraction that deposits in each region, using data such as those shown in Table 2. Yet this compartmental approach neglects the substantial disparity in the surface area of the airways and parenchyma. For example, Sweeney et al. [257] analyzed the deposition of drug from an MDI on the basis of anatomical compartments and surface area. About half of the drug deposited in the lungs; of this, 82% deposited in the parenchyma and only 18% in the intrapulmonary airways. However, when surface area was accounted for, the dose per unit of surface area was about 280 times greater in the airways than in the parenchyma. Often the deposition of particles is enhanced in certain airway generations, in which case the disparity between airway and parenchymal surface dose is even greater [258].

C. Local Distribution of Deposited Dose

1. Effect of the Larynx

The anatomical distribution of particles deposited on the respiratory tract surface is influenced by the airway geometry, deposition mechanism, and disease. The distribution of deposition has been measured most precisely in studies of aerosol transport in hollow casts of the upper airways or in bifurcating tubes; some studies also included an artificial larynx. As air passes through the larynx, a laryngeal jet forms that causes particles to impact on the tracheal wall about 2 cm downstream of the larynx [127,259]. Many particles deposit at the larynx itself, since the abrupt change in local airflow also favors impaction [10,127]. The combined upstream filtering action of the larynx and laryngeal jet causes less deposition in the first three airway generations then there would be if the larynx were absent [128].

2. Effect of Deposition Mechanism

Localized areas of high deposition can occur at airway bifurcations along the cardinal ridge, because of impaction or secondary flows [260–262]. In the deeper lung, sedimentation causes particles to deposit only on the bottom half of lung surfaces, while diffusion deposits particles on all surfaces. In humans and dogs, theoretical studies suggest there is a uniform pattern of deposition at alveolar ducts [263], but in rodents experimental studies show there is nonuniform deposition at duct bifurcations [264] and among ducts and alveoli [265].

3. Effect of Bifurcations on Exhaled Airflow Pattern

Particle deposition during exhalation can also create "hot spots." Model studies show that when airflows converge at a bifurcation, two pairs of helical vortices form in the parent branch immediately downstream of the bifurcation [266]. These radial currents cause particles to impact on the walls that are perpendicular to the plane of convergence and thus create two focal, triangular areas of high deposition located opposite to each other in the parent branch [267]. In addition, studies in hollow airway casts show that there may be enhanced particle deposition on the parent airway wall directly opposite the opening for the daughter airways [268]. The magnitude of these expiratory deposition patterns in vivo is probably less than those for inspiration because particles are filtered out of the airways during the previous inspiration; however, they may be important for rapid, shallow breathing [267].

4. Effect of Obstructive Disease

Deposition "hot spots" also develop downstream of airway obstructions or constrictions [204,269,270]. At sites of mild to severe obstruction, high linear velocities and flow turbulence enhance particle deposition by impact and turbulent diffusion, which combine to create "hot spots" immediately downstream [204, 205,207,209,269]. Sites of obstruction may also be dynamic: the passing air flow can create waves in the mucous layer that increase particle losses due to turbulent diffusion [271]; similarly, flow limitation and dynamic compression of airways during exhalation enhance particle deposition fraction in patients with bronchitis or emphysema [272]. There is decreased particle deposition in the lung regions downstream of obstructions, as a result of the filtering of the constricted sites plus the lower airflow entering these regions [205].

VII. CLEARANCE AND RETENTION OF PARTICLES

The lungs' response to particles depends not only on the amount of particles deposited but also on the amount retained over time. Retention is the amount of material present in the lungs at any time and equals deposited mass minus cleared mass. During continuous aerosol exposure, the lungs reach a steady state of retention when the rate of deposition equals the rate of clearance. It is both the amount of particles retained over time within a specific lung region and the physicochemical properties of the retained particles that determine the magnitude of the lungs' response.

As discussed before, such factors as particle size, hygroscopicity, and breathing pattern affect the site of deposition within the respiratory tract. In turn, where particles deposit in the lungs determines which mechanisms are used to clear them, how fast they are cleared, and the amount retained over time. The implications of particle characteristics for integrated retention are described by Brain and Valberg [273] on the basis of the model developed by the Task Group on Lung Dynamics [274]. They show that the total amount and the distribution of retained dose among the nose and pharynx, trachea and bronchi, and pulmonary and lymphatic compartments are dramatically altered by particle size and solubility.

Particles that deposit on the ciliated airways are cleared primarily by the mucociliary escalator. Those particles that penetrate to and deposit in the peripheral, nonciliated areas of the lungs can be cleared by many mechanisms, including phagocytosis by alveolar macrophages, particle dissolution, or movement of free particles or particle-containing cells directly into the interstitium or the lymphatics. Excellent reviews discuss these clearance processes in detail [12,14,112, 275–285].

A. Mucociliary Transport

1. Physiology

The ciliated epithelial cells of the airways and nasal passages are covered by a two-layered mucous blanket: a top high-viscosity gel layer and a bottom low-viscosity serous layer. The gel-mucous blanket along with any less soluble particles that deposit on it are moved toward the pharynx by the cilia. Also present in this moving mucous carpet are cells and particles that have been transported from the nonciliated alveoli to the ciliated airways. Mucus, cells, and debris coming from the nasal cavities and the lungs meet at the pharynx, mix with salivary secretions, are swallowed, and enter the gastrointestinal tract. In humans the ciliated epithelium extends form the trachea down to the terminal bronchioles. The particles are removed with half-times of minutes to hours; the rate depends on the speed of the mucous blanket. The speed is faster in the trachea than in the small airways [286] and is affected by factors influencing either the cilia or the amount and quality of mucus. In the airways there is little time for solubilization of slowly dissolving materials. In contrast, particles deposited in the nonciliated compartments have much longer residence times; there, small differences in solubility can result in significantly different clearance rates.

Ciliary action may be affected by the number of strokes per minute, the amplitude of each stroke, the time course and form of each stroke, the length of the cilia, the ratio of ciliated to nonciliated area, and the susceptibility of the cilia to intrinsic and extrinsic agents that modify their rate and quality of motion. The characteristics of the mucous layer are critically important. The thickness of the mucous layer and its rheological properties may vary widely. In asthmatic subjects, tracheobronchial clearance can be retarded in comparison with normal subjects, possibly because of a combination of ciliary dysfunction and altered mucous rheological properties [287]. In the peripheral bronchioles, for example, the gel layer is less evident. Another factor influencing mucociliary clearance in asthmatics is the presence or absence of flow-limiting segments during tidal breathing [288]. Flow-limiting segments may mechanically disturb the local mucociliary layer, thus slowing clearance [248]. Asthmatics without flow-limiting segments may have normal or even faster-than-normal mucociliary clearance rates [288]. Many of the factors that influence mucociliary clearance, and their clinical implications, have been reviewed [289–291].

2. Measuring Mucociliary Transport

Mucociliary transport has been studied by a variety of techniques, such as monitoring the movement of inert or radiolabeled particles deposited on the tracheal mucus via either a bronchoscope or an inhaled bolus. One can estimate tracheal mucous velocity from the distance the particles move over time as observed either with movies filmed through the bronchoscope or with a gamma camera [292,293]. Bronchoscopic techniques yield higher numbers for tracheal mucous velocity (15–21 mm/min) than do the noninvasive bolus techniques (4.4 mm/min). These values are characteristic only for the trachea and large central airways. Transport in the terminal bronchioles is about 0.1–0.6 mm/min [294].

Many investigators have estimated mucociliary transport from whole-lung clearance curves. These curves are generated by first having a subject inhale a radiolabeled aerosol and then monitoring the amount of radioactivity in the lungs over time (hours to days). Albert and Arnett [295] first used this method and noted that the clearance curve can be divided into two phases, a fast and a slow phase. The fast phase is complete within 24–48 h and has generally been attributed to tracheobronchial clearance; the slow phase has been attributed to alveolar clearance [24,294,296]. This approach has been used to study clearance in normal and abnormal subjects [297–301].

There is now evidence that clearance from the airways may be incomplete in the first 24 h; this may be even more pronounced in patients with lung disease. Gore and Patrick [302] noted that particles instilled into the trachea can be sequestered in epithelial cells. Geiser et al. [303] found latex particles trapped in the periciliary sol fluid below the gel-mucous blanket. The particles may have been displaced there by surface tension forces created by surfactant [304,305]. Stahlhofen et al. [306] noted both fast and slow phases of clearance even in humans given a bolus of particles delivered only 45 ml beyond the larynx. Wolff et al. [307] delivered radiolabeled particles with a bronchoscope to airway generations 6 through 10 in dogs and found that about 20% of the particles were cleared slowly.

Another approach to measuring mucociliary clearance is to examine the deposition and clearance of particles in central vs. peripheral lung regions [308], which is referred to as the aerosol penetrance or the airways penetration index [216,309]. The appropriate interpretation of such clearance curves has been noted [309,310].

More studies are needed to elucidate the best methodology to model mucociliary clearance and to understand its role and importance in patients with pulmonary disease. Clearly it is also essential to understand the initial deposition pattern of inhaled particles to determine the importance of mucociliary clearance for the disappearance of the particles from the lungs.

B. Nonciliated Regions

Particles that deposit in the nonciliated portion of the lungs are cleared mechanically, by dissolution, or by the combined action of these processes. During mechanical clearance most particles move toward the ciliated region within alveolar macrophages. It is possible that particles also move as a result of a surface tension gradient due to surfactant that extends from the alveoli to the airways [311]. Other particles may enter the interstitial tissues, particularly when deposited levels are high [279]. Macrophages are credited with keeping the alveolar surfaces clean and sterile. These cells rest on the continuous epithelial layer of the lung. It is their phagocytic and lytic potentials that provide most of the bactericidal properties of the lungs. Rapid endocytosis prevents particle penetration through the alveolar epithelia and facilitates alveolar-bronchiolar transport. Particle clearance by alveolar macrophages was the focus of a recent international symposium [312]. In addition, the biology of lung macrophages has been reviewed [313–320], and the various kinds of lung macrophage have been described [321]. These include alveolar, airway, connective tissue, pleural, and intravascular macrophages.

Particles enter the lung connective tissue by translocation through type I epithelial cells [322], though there are some data indicating that alveolar macrophages carry particles into the interstitium as well [323]. Once in the interstitium, most particles are phagocytosed by interstitial macrophages, though some particles may temporarily remain free. Interstitial particles are cleared eventually through either dissolution [324] or transportation to regional lymph nodes through lymphatic pathways. In tissues, particles are cleared with half-times ranging from a few days to thousands of days, depending on their solubility. In contrast, particles remaining on alveolar surfaces in humans are cleared with biological half-times estimated to be days to weeks.

VIII. MEASURING PARTICLE RETENTION

Once particles are introduced into the respiratory tract, the challenge of quantifying the amount and distribution of dose must be faced. Not only are the technological solutions frequently complex, but also the nature of the problem to be solved is often obscure. How should the dose to the respiratory tract be calculated? Should it be averaged over the whole lung, or should the local airway or alveolar epithelial dose be estimated?

At the outset it is essential to remember that the initial deposition pattern is continuously modified by clearance processes. Loss and redistribution of deposited particles is the rule, not the exception, unless the aerosol-exposure period is brief and the interval between exposure and analysis is short.

A. Noninvasive vs. Invasive Methods

An extensive menu of measurement techniques is available. The approaches vary in expense, resolution, and the extent to which the subject must be disturbed. There are advantages to using nondestructive, noninvasive methods of detection. These methods allow repeated measurements on the same person or animal and thus permit replicative and serial measurements. For human experimentation such detection methods are essential. However, measurements of retention in whole animals may provide inadequate details about the distribution of dose to structures of interest. The greatest precision is achieved by killing and dissecting animals. The lungs can be made rigid by freezing or drying and then sliced or dissected. It is then possible to divide the respiratory tract physically into individual pieces or specific lung compartments and analyze the particle content of each piece. Depending on one's patience and the sensitivity of the detection method, the distribution of particle retention can be described with increasing detail. These approaches permit an identification of the anatomical location of retained particles. Articles and a review from our laboratory describe these methods [220,265,325].

Actual detection of particles in the lungs can rely on any distinctive property of the particles. Particles may be radioactive, fluorescent, radioopaque, magnetic, or pharmacologically active. They may have a characteristic visual appearance that can be identified with light or electron microscopy. Their elemental or molecular nature may be identified by a repertoire of techniques including colorimetry, atomic absorption, neutron activation, nuclear magnetic resonance, and electron energy loss spectrometry, among mothers. The type of question suggests which properties of the particle can be exploited for ease and specificity of detection.

Various approaches one can use are reviewed in greater detail by Brain and Valberg [7] and in the accompanying references. The first approach is to estimate the dose on the basis of measurements of inspired particle size and concentration. The minimum characterization of any aerosol exposure should include its concentration, size, and composition. Although it is essential to describe the aerosol inhaled, it is important to realize that many factors such as species, age, level of activity, and disease influence the fraction and distribution of the inspired particles deposited in each subject.

B. Modeling

If ventilation is measured well, one can estimate deposition fraction on the basis of theoretical predictions and models. Current deposition models include those of Egan and Nixon [326]; Koblinger and Hofmann [327,328]; and Taulbee, Yu, and Diu [329,330]. The deposition of hygroscopic particles has also been modeled [80,168,172,179,180]. The general concepts of several deposition models, including some just mentioned, are explained in a review by Heyder and Rudolf [331].

The International Commission on Radiological Protection (ICRP) Task Group is developing a new deposition model [187] that incorporates the deposition formalism of Egan and co-workers [326,332] and new anatomical, deposition, and clearance data. A major advance of this model is that it is broadly applicable: deposition and clearance estimates can be made for most people on the basis of their age, race, and breathing level and the presence or absence of lung disease [333–335]. The considerations that enter dosimetric modeling of inhaled particles were the focus of recent meetings [37,336–339].

Prediction of total and regional deposited dose in healthy persons has become easier with recently developed semiempirical deposition formulas that are based on data such as those shown in Table 2 [13,162,169]. These formulas are designed for subjects breathing well-characterized aerosols in a known manner and are customized for each subject on the basis of his or her functional residual capacity. Other equations have been developed to predict the total and regional deposition fraction of particles in persons of different ages [340] and in adults breathing oronasally and at different activity levels [341]. There also exists a simplified estimation method to predict the deposition of hygroscopic particles [178].

C. Photometry and Filter Collection

Another approach to quantifying inhaled dose is to measure the difference in the particle concentration of inspired and expired air using light-scattering methods [342]. By adding a measurement of ventilation, one can determine the deposition fraction in the respiratory tract [223,224,301]. Although this technique is both sensitive and accurate, it is suitable only for well-characterized, monodisperse, nonhygroscopic aerosols that act as surrogates for challenge, environmental or therapeutic aerosols [225]. By modifying this method, information can be obtained regarding airway size and convective transport in the respiratory tract [132,222,343,344]. Alternatively, total deposition fraction can be measured by using a filter to collect the inhaled particles and then repeating the measurement using a different filter to collet the exhaled particles [3,81,190,226,231]. The filters are then assayed for the drug or an appropriate label. An advantage of the filter method is that one can use actual aerosols that are polydisperse and hygroscopic. However, neither the photometric nor the filter method provides information regarding the regional sites of deposition.

D. Bronchoalveolar Lavage

Bronchoalveolar lavage can provide information about retention of drugs that are not rapidly absorbed across the lung epithelium. Smaldone et al. [3] found that deposition of pentamidine was correlated with the drug concentration lavaged from the middle lobe airways 24 h after exposure.

E. Radioactivity

Radioactivity has been used frequently for studies of particle deposition because of its potential for noninvasive measurement and its sensitivity and resolution. Hundreds of radioisotopes are produced, and labeled drugs can be synthesized with a wide spectrum of energies, types of radiation (alpha, beta, gamma, positrons), and half-lives. Gamma emitters penetrate through tissue and are therefore suitable for making measurements externally. Alpha or beta emitters are better suited for producing autoradiographs; their short path-lengths, which make them unsuitable for external detection, produce high resolution images on film that is in contact with particle-laden tissue.

Descriptions of the technologies involves are widely available. Several books summarize the applications of radioactivity to imaging [345,346]. Restricting the field of view of the detector to a region of interest is frequently useful. This can be achieved with a collimator constructed of lead, which blocks most radiation coming to the detector except that from a selected region of the body. A variety of shielded counters that employ large sodium iodide crystals and appropriate lead shielding have been constructed [347,348].

1. Gamma Cameras

Gamma cameras employ a stationary radioactivity detector that simultaneously collects information from a large area. As first described by Anger [349], this device uses a single large scintillation crystal, which is masked with a honeycomb parallel-hold lead collimator with as many as 15,000 holes. Each part of the crystal looks at a small area of the patient or animal, and scintillations are produced in different parts of the crystal. An array of phototubes senses the light pulses produced in the crystal by incoming gamma rays, and the relative pulse sizes from different photomultiplier tubes give the position of the scintillation. From this the two-dimensional position of the labeled particle in the respiratory tract can be estimated and displayed on a cathode-ray tube screen or stored in a computer. Images are often divided into central and peripheral lung regions; a penetration index that represents the relative deposition in these two areas can then be calculated [216,309]. Methodological considerations for the use of gamma cameras to measure lung dose were recently discussed [3,350,351]. Itoh et al. [352] have shown that total deposition measurements made by gamma camera agree well with deposition measurements made by photometry and filter collection.

2. Tomography

Tomography is used to map and follow the distribution of retained particles in three dimensions. In the two-dimensional view of the lung provided by a gamma camera, the central lung region, which is taken to represent the central airways, in actuality also contains overlapping small airways and acini. Thus, one cannot discriminate particle deposition among these regions, and deposition fraction in central airways may be overestimated [353]. Alternatively, tomography can resolve particles within central airways and peripheral lung regions. There are two types of tomography appropriate for measuring regional particle retention: single-photon emission computed tomography (SPECT) and positron emission tomography (PET).

Single-Photon Emission Computed Tomography. With SPECT [353–355], the subject inhales gamma-emitting radionuclide particles and then the gamma camera makes one scan. The camera is then rotated a few degrees and another scan is made; the process is repeated until the lung has been scanned from as many as 64 angles. Since each deposited radiolabelled particle released multiple photons, which the camera detects from different positions, there are several emission lines, with the particle at their intersection. After the scans, a computer program reconstructs the series of two-dimensional scans into a three-dimensional image, and particle retention in desired lung slices can be compared. One drawback of SPECT is that it requires levels of radioactivity about ten times higher than two-dimensional gamma camera imaging [309]. It may also take up to 15 min to complete all the scans, which is enough time for particles within the central airways to redistribute via mucociliary clearance [354].

Positron Emission Tomography. To use PET [356] for particle retention studies, the subject would inhale particles labeled with a positron-emitting radionuclide, such as ^{11}C or ^{68}Ga. A positron travels 2–5 mm before it combines with an electron; the ensuing annihilation process produces two photons that travel at nearly 180° relative to each other. A series of paired scintillation detectors surrounding the subject record the site of interaction of these photons; then the line along which decay events originated can be reconstructed [357]. Since a particle creates multiple photon pairs, which other detector paris detect, there are several emission lines, with the particle at their intersection. After the scan is complete, these multiple emission lines are analyzed by tomographic computer analysis to generate the three-dimensional particle-deposition pattern [357]. Since PET determines the origin of photo emission on the basis of coincident detection by detector pairs, as opposed to the collimation required by SPECT, PET ignores less of the emitted radiation and is more efficient than SPECT [356]. Other advantages are that PET is relatively fast and that many of the positron-emitting isotopes have short half-lives, so it is easier to make repeated studies in the same subject. By using drugs labeled with positron-emitting radionuclides, PET can locate the distribution of receptor sites within the respiratory tract [358].

F. Magnetopneumography

Some aerosol particles are magnetizable, and sensitive magnetopneumography can measure their concentration and distribution in the lungs [359]. This technique applies a magnetic field to the whole thorax or to localized areas and detects the resultant alignment of ferromagnetic domains in retained lung particles. Accumulations of magnetic particles have been measured in foundry workers, arc welders, coal miners, and asbestos miners [360–362]. The greatest advantage of this technique is that the duration of measurement is not limited by radioactive decay. Measurements can be made as long as sufficient dust remains in the lungs. Thus one can noninvasively describe clearance kinetics over years [363]. Two magnetic dusts suitable for studying retention of dust in the lung are Fe_3O_4 (magnetite) and γ-Fe_2O_3 (a magnetic form of hematite). Both are inert, are relatively insoluble at physiological pH, and can be aerosolized. The magnitude of the remnant field quantifies the amount of dust remaining in the lungs.

IX. CONCLUSIONS

Even if specific deposition patterns of drug particles can be selected, we are left with the key question: Does it make a difference? If deposition is mainly in large airways, does the distribution of response differ importantly from that seen when the same drug or allergen is placed in small airways or alveoli? The answer may well depend on the mechanisms and pathways involved.

For example, if one changes the particle deposition pattern and the resultant distribution of responses is relatively uniform, this would suggest that there may be a uniform reflex response such as bronchoconstriction. It could also suggest that there is drug absorption and transport via the bronchial circulation. It should be remembered that the anatomical distribution of response depends not exclusively on the distribution of particle deposition, but also on the distribution of mast cells and other inflammatory cells in the airways and the distribution of receptors throughout the airway epithelia. The regional distributions of many receptor classes are still too ill defined to evaluate the effectiveness of targeting strategies. Furthermore, the properties of the mucus and the bronchial epithelium are important, since many drugs or antigens must breach these barriers to come into contact with more reactive cells, nerves, or smooth muscle. It remains to be shown conclusively whether widely varying retention patterns importantly influence the extent and distribution of the airway responsiveness.

Measuring the distribution of pharmacological particles within the respiratory tract is one segment of the more general problem of correlating concentrations of a drug at its site of action with a measured response. Much of the variability in drug responses among different pharmaceutical preparations, different individuals, and various animal species may result from differences in concentration of the drug at the site of action rather than to variations in responsiveness of specific active tissues. Different drug preparations may be deposited at different sites and absorbed at different rates from airway and alveolar surfaces. The chemical stability of the drug at various sites within the respiratory tract is important, as are enzymes throughout the respiratory tract that may be involved in drug metabolism. Looking for the drug's metabolites in blood, urine, and feces may provide important clues to its fate. Such studies of drug disposition and metabolism within the respiratory tract will continue to be central to the use of therapeutic drugs; they will be an essential step to determine the proper form of the drug and the appropriate dosages. Such considerations will also be crucial to the search for mechanisms that underlie drug effects, interactions between drugs, and adverse drug reactions. Investment in a thorough description of the location of deposited particles in the respiratory tract will be rewarded, since improved understanding of the effects of aerosols stems from the recognition of factors important to their uptake and fate.

REFERENCES

1. Pepys, J., and Hutchcroft, B. J., Bronchial provocation tests in etiological diagnosis and analysis of asthma, *Am. Rev. Respir. Dis.*, *112*, 829–859 (1975).
2. Lux, C., Ahrens, R., and Hoefer, J., Evaluation of jet nebulizers available in the U.S. for antibiotic delivery to patients with cystic fibrosis (abstr.), *J. Aerosol Med.*, *6* (suppl.), 71 (1993).
3. Smaldone, G. C., Fuhrer, J., Steigbigel, R. T., and McPeck, M., Factors determining pulmonary deposition of aerosolized pentamidine in patients with human immunodeficiency virus infection, *Am. Rev. Respir. Dis.*, *143*, 727–737 (1991).
4. Crompton, G. K., Problems patients have using pressurised aerosol inhalers, *Eur. J. Respir. Dis.*, *63* (suppl. 119), 101–104 (1982).
5. Saunders, K. B., Misuse of inhaled bronchodilator agents, *Br. Med. J.*, *1*, 1037–1038 (1965).
6. Agnew, J. E., Physical properties and mechanisms of deposition of aerosols, in *Aerosols and the Lung: Clinical and Experimental Aspects* (S. W. Clarke and D. Pavia, eds.), Butterworths, London, 1984, pp. 49–70.
7. Brain, J. D., and Valberg, P. A., Deposition of aerosol in the respiratory tract, *Am. Rev. Respir. Dis.*, *120*, 1325–1373 (1979).
8. Gerrity, T. R., Pathophysiological and disease constraints on aerosol delivery, in

Respiratory Drug Delivery (P. R. Byron, ed.), CRC Press, Boca Raton, Florida, 1990, pp. 1–38.

9. Heyder, J., Gebhart, J., and Stahlhofen, W., Inhalation of aerosols: particle deposition and retention, in *Generation of Aerosols and Facilities for Exposure Experiments* (K. Willeke, ed.), Ann Arbor Science, Ann Arbor, Michigan, 1980, pp. 65–103.
10. Heyder, J., Gebhart, J., Rudolf, G., Schiller, C. F., and Stahlhofen, W., Deposition of particles in the human respiratory tract in the size range 0.005–15 μm, *J. Aerosol Sci.*, *17*, 811–825 (1986).
11. Lippmann, M., Regional deposition of particles in the human respiratory tract, in *Handbook of Physiology, Section 9: Reactions to Environmental Agents* (D. H. K. Lee, H. L. Falk, and S. D. Murphy, eds.), American Physiological Society, Bethesda, Maryland, 1977, pp. 213–232.
12. Raabe, O. G., Deposition and clearance of inhaled aerosols, in *Mechanisms in Respiratory Toxicology*, Vol. 1 (H. Witschi and P. Nettesheim, eds.), CRC Press, Boca Raton, Florida, 1982, pp. 27–75.
13. Stahlhofen, W., Rudolf, G., and James, A. C., Intercomparison of experimental regional deposition data, *J. Aerosol Med.*, *2*, 285–308 (1989).
14. Stuart, B. O., Deposition and clearance of inhaled particles, *Environ. Health Perspect.*, *55*, 369–390 (1984).
15. Davies, C. N., ed., *Aerosol Science*, Academic Press, New York, 1966.
16. Friedlander, S. K., *Smoke, Dust, and Haze: Fundamentals of Aerosol Behavior*, Wiley, New York, 1977.
17. Fuchs, N. A., *The Mechanics of Aerosols*, Dover, New York, 1989.
18. Hesketh, H. E., *Fine Particles in Gaseous Media*, 2d Ed., CRC Press, Boca Raton, Florida, 1986.
19. Hinds, W. C., *Aerosol Technology—Properties, Behavior, and Measurement of Airborne Particles*, Wiley-Interscience, New York, 1982.
20. Reist, P. C., *Introduction to Aerosol Science*, MacMillan, New York, 1984.
21. Willeke, K., and Baron, P. A., eds., *Aerosol Measurement: Principles, Techniques, and Applications*, Van Nostrand Reinhold, New York, 1993.
22. Heyder, J., Particle transport onto human airway surfaces, *Eur. J. Respir. Dis.*, *63* (suppl. 119), 29–50 (1982).
23. Heyder, J., Definitions and standards related to aerosols in medicine: aerosols, *J. Aerosol Med.*, *4*, 217–221 (1991).
24. Lippmann, M., and Albert, R. E., The effect of particle size on the regional deposition of inhaled aerosols in the human respiratory tract, *Am. Ind. Hyg. Assoc. J.*, *30*, 257–275 (1969).
25. Heyder, J., and Scheuch, G., Diffusional transport of nonspherical aerosol particles, *Aerosol Sci. Technol.*, *2*, 41–44 (1983).
26. Gradon, L., and Yu, C. P., Diffusional particle deposition in the human nose and mouth, *Aerosol Sci. Technol.*, *11*, 213–220 (1989).
27. Melandri, C. V., Tarroni, G., Prodi, V., DeZaiacomo, T., Formignani, M., and Lombardi, C. C., Deposition of charged particles in the human airways, *J. Aerosol. Sci.*, *14*, 657–669 (1983).

28. Yu, C. P., Theories of electrostatic lung deposition, *Ann. Occup. Hyg.*, *29*, 219–227 (1985).
29. Vincent, J. H., On the practical significance of electrostatic lung deposition of isometric and fibrous aerosols, *J. Aerosol Sci.*, *16*, 511–519 (1985).
30. Harris, R. L., and Fraser, D. A., A model for deposition of fibers in the human respiratory tract, *Am. Ind. Hyg. Assoc. J.*, *37*, 73–89 (1976).
31. Timbrell, V., The inhalation of fibrous dusts, *Ann. N.Y. Acad. Sci.*, *132*, 255–273 (1965).
32. Eiser, N. M., Kerrebijn, K. F., and Quanjer, P. H., Guidelines for standardization of bronchial challenges with (nonspecific) bronchoconstricting agents, *Bull. Eur. Physiopathol. Resp.*, *19*, 495–514 (1983).
33. Sterk, P. J., Fabbri, L. M., Quanjer, P. H., Cockcroft, D. W., O'Byrne, P. M., Anderson, S. D., Juniper, E. F., and Malo, J. L., Airway responsiveness: standardized challenge testing with pharmacological, physical and sensitizing stimuli in adults, *Eur. Respir. J.*, *6* (suppl. 16), 53–83 (1993).
34. Ryan, G., Dolovich, M. B., Obminski, G., Cockcroft, D. W., Juniper, E., Hargreave, F. E., and Newhouse, M. T., Standardization of inhalation provocation tests: influence of nebulizer output, particle size and method of inhalation, *J. Allergy Clin. Immunol.*, *67*, 156–161 (1981).
35. Byron, P. R., Aerosol formulation, generation, and delivery using nonmetered systems, in *Respiratory Drug Delivery* (P. R. Byron, ed.), CRC Press, Boca Raton, Florida, 1990, pp. 143–165.
36. Byron, P. R., Aerosol formulation, generation, and delivery using metered systems, in *Respiratory Drug Delivery* (P. R. Byron, ed.), CRC Press, Boca Raton, Florida, 1990, pp. 167–205.
37. Crapo, J. D., Smolke, E. D., Miller, F. J., Graham, J. A., and Hayes, A. W., eds., *Extrapolation of Dosimetric Relationships to Inhaled Particles and Gases*, Academic Press, San Diego, 1989.
38. Dennis, R., ed., *Handbook on Aerosols*. National Technical Information Services, U.S. Department of Commerce, Washington, D.C., 1976.
39. Lefebvre, A. H., *Atomization and Sprays*, Hemisphere, New York, 1989.
40. Mercer, T. T., *Aerosol Technology in Hazard Evaluation*, Academic Press, New York, 1973.
41. Swift, D. L., Aerosol measurement in the health care field, in *Aerosol Measurement: Principles, Techniques, and Applications* (K. Willeke and P. A. Baron, eds.), Van Nostrand Reinhold, New York, 1993,pp. 816–832.
42. Vincent, J. H., *Aerosol Sampling: Science and Practice*, John Wiley & Sons, New York, 1989.
43. Willeke, K., ed., *Generation of Aerosols and Facilities for Exposure Experiments*, Ann Arbor Science, Ann Arbor, Michigan, 1980.
44. Clarke, S. W., and Pavia, D., eds., *Aerosols and the Lung*, Butterworths, London, 1984.
45. Dolovich, M., Physical properties underlying aerosol therapy, *J. Aerosol Med.*, *2*, 171–186 (1989).

46. Ganderton, D., and Jones, T., eds., *Drug Delivery to the Respiratory Tract*, VCH, New York, 1987.
47. Gonda, I., Aerosols for delivery of therapeutic and diagnostic agents to the respiratory tract, *Crit. Rev. Therapeutic Drug Carrier Systems*, *6*, 273–313 (1990).
48. Morén, F., Newhouse, M. T., Dolovich, M. B., and Newman, S. P., eds., *Aerosols in Medicine: Principles, Diagnosis, and Therapy*, 2d Ed., Elsevier Science Publishers, Amsterdam, 1993.
49. Phalen, R. F., ed., *Inhalation Studies: Foundations and Techniques*, CRC Press, Boca Raton, Florida, 1984.
50. Wilson, A. F., Aerosol delivery systems, in *Bronchial Asthma: Mechanisms and Therapeutics* (E. B. Weiss and M. Stein, eds.), Little, Brown, Boston, 1993, pp. 749–755.
51. Cockcroft, D. W., Killian, D. N., Mellon, J. J. A., and Hargreave, F. E., Bronchial reactivity to inhaled histamine: a method and clinical survey, *Clin. Allergy*, *7*, 235–243 (1977).
52. Juniper, E. F., Frith, P. A., Dinnett, C., Cockcroft, D. W., and Hargreave, F. E., Reproducibility and comparison of responses to inhaled histamine and methacholine, *Thorax*, *33*, 703–710 (1978).
53. Bruce, C. A., Rosenthal, R. R., Lichtenstein, L. M., and Norman, P. S., Diagnostic tests in ragweed allergic asthma: a comparison of direct skin tests, leukocyte histamine release and quantitative bronchial challenge, *J. Allergy Clin. Immunol.*, *53*, 230–239 (1974).
54. Yan, K., Salome, C. M., and Woolcock, A. J., Rapid method for measurement of bronchial responsiveness, *Thorax*, *38*, 760–765 (1983).
55. Vandenplas, O., Malo, J. L., Cartier, A., Perrealt, G., and Cloutier, I., Closed-circuit methodology for inhalation challenge tests with isocyanates, *Am. Rev. Respir. Dis.*, *145*, 582–587 (1992).
56. American Conference of Governmental Industrial Hygienists, *Threshold Limit Values for Chemical Substances and Biologic Exposure Indices*, American Conference of Governmental Industrial Hygienists, Cincinnati, 1992.
57. Cloutier, Y., Lagier, F., Lemieux, R., Blais, M. C., St.-Arnaud, C., Cartier, A., and Malo, J. L., New methodology for specific inhalation challenges with occupational agents in powder form, *Eur. Respir. J.*, *2*, 769–777 (1989).
58. Cloutier, Y., and Malo, J.-L., Update on an exposure system for particles in the diagnosis of occupational asthma, *Eur. Respir. J.*, *5*, 887–890 (1992).
59. Fuchs, N. A., and Sutugin, A. G., Generation and use of monodisperse aerosols, in *Aerosol Science* (C. N. Davies, ed.), Academic Press, New York, 1966, pp. 1–30.
60. Mercer, T. T., Production of therapeutic aerosols. Principles and techniques, *Chest*, *80* (suppl.), 813–818 (1981).
61. Mercer, T. T., Tillery, M. I., and Chow, H. Y., Operating characteristics of some compressed-air nebulizers, *Am. Ind. Hyg. Assoc. J.*, *29*, 66–78 (1968).
62. Smaldone, G. C., Perry, R. J., and Deutsch, D. G., Characteristics of nebulizers used in the treatment of AIDS-related Pneumocystis carinii pneumonia, *J. Aerosol Med.*, *1*, 113–126 (1988).

63. Sterk, P. J., Plomb, A., Van de Vate, J. F., and Quanjer, P. H., Physical properties of aerosols produced by several jet- and ultrasonic nebulizers, *Bull. Eur. Physiopathol. Respir.*, *20*, 65–72 (1984).
64. Collis, G. C., Cole, C. H., and LeSouef, P. N., Dilution of nebulized aerosols by air entrainment in children, *Lancet*, *336*, 341–343 (1990).
65. Mercer, T. T., Goddard, R. F., and Flores, R. L., Effect of auxiliary air flow on the output characteristics of compressed-air nebulizers, *Ann. Allergy*, *27*, 211–217 (1969).
66. Cockcroft, D. W., Hurst, T. S., and Gore, D. P., Importance of evaporative water losses during standardized nebulized inhalation challenge tests, *Chest*, *96*, 505–508 (1989).
67. Dennis, J. H., Stenton, S. C., Beach, J. R., Avery, A. J., Walters, E. H., and Hendrick, D. J., Jet and ultrasonic nebulizer output: use of a new method for direct measurement of aerosol output, *Thorax*, *45*, 728–732 (1990).
68. O'Callaghan, C., Clarke, A. C., and Milner, A. D., Inaccurate calculation of drug output from nebulizers, *Eur. J. Pediatr.*, *148*, 473–474 (1989).
69. Ferron, G. A., Weber, J., and Kerrebijn, K. F., Properties of aerosols produced with three nebulizers, *Am. Rev. Respir. Dis.*, *114*, 899–908 (1976).
70. Phipps, P. R., and Gonda, I., Droplets produced by medical nebulizers: some factors affecting their size and solute concentration, *Chest*, *97*, 1327–1332 (1990).
71. Schöni, M. H., and Kraemer, R., Osmolality changes in nebulizer solutions, *Eur. Respir. J.*, *2*, 887–892 (1989).
72. Ferron, G. A., and Soderholm, S. C., Estimation of times for evaporation of pure water droplets and for stabilization of salt solution particles, *J. Aerosol. Sci.*, *21*, 415–429 (1990).
73. Porstendörfer, J., Gebhart, J., and Röbig, G., Effect of evaporation on the size distribution of nebulized aerosols, *J. Aerosol Sci.*, *8*, 371–380 (1977).
74. Ferron, G. A., and Gebhart, J., Estimation of the lung depositions of aerosol particles produced with medical nebulizers, *J. Aerosol Sci.*, *19*, 1083–1086 (1988).
75. Mercer, T. T., Goddard, R. F., and Flores, R. L., Output characteristics of several commercial nebulizers, *Ann. Allergy*, *23*, 314–326 (1965).
76. Mercer, T. T., Goddard, R. F., and Flores, R. L., Output characteristics of three ultrasonic nebulizers, *Ann. Allergy*, *29*, 66–78 (1968).
77. Newman, S. P., Pellow, P. G. D., and Clarke, S. W., In vitro comparison of DeVilbiss jet and ultrasonic nebulizers, *Chest*, *92*, 991–994 (1987).
78. Waldman, D. L., Weber, D. A., Oberdörster, G., Drago, S. R., Utell, M. J., Hyde, R. W., and Morrow, P. E., Chemical breakdown of technetium-99m DPTA during nebulization, *J. Nucl. Med.*, *28*, 378–382 (1987).
79. Ferron, G. A., Haider, B., and Kreyling, W. G., Inhalation of salt aerosol particles. I. Estimation of the temperature and relative humidity of the air in the human upper airways, *J. Aerosol Sci.*, *19*, 343–363 (1988).
80. Ferron, G. A., Kreyling, W. G., and Haider, B., Inhalation of salt aerosol particles. II. Growth and deposition in the human respiratory tract, *J. Aerosol Sci.*, *19*, 611–631 (1988).
81. Smaldone, G. C., Drug delivery via aerosol systems: concept of "aerosol inhaled," *J. Aerosol Med.*, *4*, 229–235 (1991).

82. Kim, C. S., Eldridge, M. A., and Sackner, M. A., Oropharyngeal deposition and delivery aspects of metered-dose inhaler aerosols, *Am. Rev. Respir. Dis.*, *135*, 157–164 (1987).
83. Cipolla, D., and Gonda, I., Method for recovery of nebulized proteins (abstr.), *J. Aerosol Med.*, *6* (suppl.), 15 (1993).
84. Smye, S. W., Shaw, A., Norwood, H. M., and Littlewood, J. M., Some factors influencing the efficiency of a jet nebuliser system, *Clin. Phys. Physiol. Meas.*, *11*, 167–175 (1990).
85. Rader, D. J., and O'Hern, T. J., Optical direct-reading techniques: In situ sensing, in *Aerosol Measurement: Principles, Techniques, and Applications* (D. J. Rader and T. J O'Hern, eds.), Van Nostrand Reinhold, New York, 1993,pp. 345–380.
86. Tishkoff, J. M., Ingebo, R. D., and Kennedy, J. B., eds., *Liquid Particle Size Measurement Techniques*, ASTM STP 848, American Society for Testing and Materials, Philadelphia, 1984.
87. Hirleman, E. D., Bachalo, W. D., and Felton, P. G., eds., *Liquid Particle Size Measurement Techniques*, ASTM STP 1083, American Society for Testing and Materials, Philadelphia, 1990.
88. Lavergne, G., Biscos, Y., Bismes, F., and Hebrard, P., Optical particle sizing: Digital video image processing application, in *Optical Particle Sizing* (G. Lavergne, Y. Biscos, and F. Bismes, eds.), Plenum Press, New York, pp. 471–482.
89. Felton, P. G., A review of the Fraunhofer diffraction particle sizing technique, *Liquid Particle Sizing Measurement Techniques*, ASTM STP 1083 (E. D. Hirleman, W. D. Bachalo, and P. G. Felton, eds.), American Society for Testing and Materials, Philadelphia, 1990, pp. 47–59.
90. Martonen, T. B., Development of surrogate lung systems with controlled thermodynamic environments to study hygroscopic particles: air pollutants and pharmacologic drugs, *Part. Sci. Technol.*, *8*, 1–20 (1990).
91. Gebhart, J., Roth, C., and Bernhard, F., Output characterization of medical nebulizers by means of the residual technique (abstr.), *J. Aerosol Med.*, *6* (suppl.), 73 (1993).
92. Marple, V. A., Rubow, K. L., and Olson, B. A., Inertial, gravitational, centrifugal, and thermal collection techniques, in *Aerosol Measurement: Principles, Techniques, and Applications* (K. Willeke and P. A. Baron, eds.), Van Nostrand Reinhold, New York, 1993, pp. 206–232.
93. Hickey, A. J., Factors influencing aerosol deposition in inertial impactors and their effect on particle size characterization, *Pharmacol. Technol.*, *14*, 118–130 (1990).
94. Lodge, J. P., Jr., and Chan, T. L., eds., *Cascade Impactor: Sampling and Data Analysis*, American Industrial Hygiene Association, Akron, Ohio, 1986.
95. Vaughan, N. P., The Andersen impactor: calibration, wall losses and numerical simulation, *J. Aerosol Sci.*, *20*, 67–90 (1989).
96. Stöber, W., Design performance and applications of spiral duct aerosol centrifuges, in *Fine Particles, Aerosol Generation, Measurement Sampling and Analysis* (B. Y. H. Lin, ed.), Academic Press, New York, 1976, pp. 351–398.
97. Prodi, V., Melandri, C., Tarroni, G., de Zaiacomo, T., and Formignani, M., An inertial spectrometer for aerosol particles, *J. Aerosol Sci.*, *10*, 411–419 (1979).

98. Hallworth, G. W., and Westmoreland, D. G., The twin impinger: a simple device for assessing the delivery of drugs from metered dose pressurized aerosol inhalers, *J. Pharm. Pharmacol.*, *39*, 966–972 (1987).
99. May, K. R., Multistage liquid impinger, *Bacteriol. Rev.*, *30*, 559–570 (1966).
100. Dolovich, M., and Smaldone, G. C., Standards for in vitro/in vivo measurements of MDI characteristics (abstr.), *J. Aerosol Med.*, *69* (suppl.), 103 (1993).
101. Miller, N. C., Marple, V. A., Schultz, R. K., and Poon, W. S., Assessment of the twin impinger for size measurement of metered-dose inhaler sprays, *Pharm. Res.*, *9*, 1123–1127 (1992).
102. Knutson, E. O., and Whitby, K. T., Aerosol classification by electric mobility: apparatus, theory, and applications, *J. Aerosol Sci.*, *6*, 443–451 (1975).
103. Baron, P. A., Mazumder, M. K., and Cheng, Y. S., Direct-reading techniques using optical particle detection, in *Aerosol Measurement: Principles, Techniques, and Applications* (K. Willeke and P. A. Baron, eds.), Van Nostrand Reinhold, New York, 1993, pp. 381–409.
104. Gebhart, J., Optical direct-reading techniques: light intensity systems, in *Aerosol Measurement: Principles, Techniques, and Applications* (K. Willeke and P. A. Baron, eds.), Van Nostrand Reinhold, New York, 1993, pp. 313–344.
105. Knollenberg, R. G., Techniques for probing cloud microstructure, in *Clouds: Their Formation, Optical Properties, and Effects* (P. V. Hobbs and A. Deepak, eds.), Academic Press, New York, 1981, pp. 15–89.
106. Holve, D. J., and Annen, K. D., Optical particle counting, sizing, and velocimetry using intensity deconvolution, *Opt. Eng.*, *23*, 591–603 (1984).
107. Bachalo, W. D., and Houser, M. J., Phase Doppler spray analyzer for simultaneous measurements of drop size and velocity distributions, *Opt. Eng.*, *23*, 583–590 (1984).
108. Chen, B., Cheng, Y. S., and Yeh, H. C., Performance of a TSI aerodynamic particle sizer, *Aerosol Sci. Technol.*, *4*, 89–97 (1985).
109. Renninger, R. G., Mazumder, M. K., and Testerman, M. K., Particle sizing by electrical single particle aerodynamic relaxation time analyzer, *Rev. Sci. Instrum.*, *52*, 242–246 (1981).
110. Fletcher, R. A., and Small, J. A., Analysis of individual collected particles, in *Aerosol Measurement: Principles, Techniques, and Applications* (K. Willeke and P. A. Baron, eds.), Van Nostrand Reinhold, New York, 1993, pp. 260–295.
111. Brockman, J. E., Sampling and transport of aerosols, in *Aerosol Measurement: Principles, Techniques, and Applications* (K. Willeke and P. A. Baron, eds.), Van Nostrand Reinhold, New York, 1993, pp. 77–111.
112. Vincent, J. H., The fate of inhaled aerosols: a review of observed trends and some generalizations, *Ann. Occup. Hyg.*, *34*, 623–637 (1990).
113. Davies, C. N., ed., *Inhaled Particles and Vapours*, Pergamon Press, New York, 1961.
114. Davies, C. N., ed., *Inhaled Particles and Vapours II*, Pergamon Press, New York, 1967.
115. Dodgson, J., McCallum, R. I., Bailey, M. R., and Fisher, D. R., eds., *Inhaled Particles VI*, *Ann. Occup. Hyg.*, *32* (suppl 1) (1988).

116. Dodgson, J., ed., *Inhaled Particles VII*, Pergamon Press, Oxford, in press.
117. Walton, W. H., ed., *Inhaled Particles III*, Unwin Bros., Surrey, England, 1971.
118. Walton, W. H., ed., *Inhaled Particles IV*, Pergamon Press, Oxford, 1977.
119. Walton, W. H., ed., *Inhaled Particles V*, *Ann. Occup. Hyg.*, 26 (1982).
120. Byron, P. R., ed., *Respiratory Drug Delivery*, CRC Press, Boca Raton, Florida, 1990.
121. Byron, P. R., ed., *Proceedings of Respiratory Drug Delivery II*, University of Kentucky College of Pharmacy, Lexington, Kentucky, 1991.
122. Byron, P. R., ed., *Proceedings of Respiratory Drug Delivery III*, *J. Biopharm. Sci.*, *3* (1–2), (1992).
123. Smaldone, G. C., ed., *Proceedings of the 7th Congress on Aerosols in Medicine*, *J. Aerosol Med.*, *2*, 81–245 (1989).
124. Smaldone, G. C., ed., Definitions and standards related to aerosols in medicine, *J. Aerosol Med.*, *4*, 217–273 (1991).
125. Smaldone, G. C., ed., *Proceedings of the 9th Congress on Aerosols in Medicine*, *J. Aerosol Med.*, *6* (suppl.) (1993).
125a. Dahneke, B., Oberdörster, G., and Wolff, R., eds., *Symposium on Pharmaceutical Aerosols*, *Aerosol Sci. Technol.*, *18*, 221–304 (1993).
126. Newman, S. P., Therapeutic aerosol deposition in man, in *Aerosols in Medicine: Principles, Diagnosis, and Therapy*, 2d Ed. (F. Morén, M. T. Newhouse, M. B. Dolovich, and S. P. Newman, eds.), Elsevier Science Publishers, Amsterdam, 1993, pp. 375–399.
127. Chan, T. L., Shreck, R. M., and Lippmann, M., Effect of the laryngeal jet on particle deposition in the human trachea and upper bronchial airways, *J. Aerosol Sci.*, *11*, 447–459 (1980).
128. Lippmann, M., and Altshuler, B., Regional deposition of aerosols, in *Air Pollution and the Lung* (E. F. Aharonson, A. Ben-David, and M. A. Klingberg, eds.), Halsted Press–Wiley, New York, 1976, pp. 25–48.
129. Nikiforov, A. T., and Schlesinger, R. B., Morphometric variability of the human upper bronchial tree, *Respir. Physiol.*, *59*, 289–299 (1985).
130. Schlesinger, R. B, and McFadden, L., Comparative morphometry of the upper bronchial tree in six mammalian species, *Anat. Rec.*, *199*, 99–108 (1981).
131. Soong, T. T., Nicolaides, P., Yu, C. P., Soong, S. C., A statistical description of the human tracheobronchial tree geometry, *Respir. Physiol.*, *37*, 161–172 (1979).
132. Blanchard, J. D., Heyder, J., O'Donnell, C. R., and Brain, J. D., Aerosol-derived lung morphometry: comparisons with a lung model and lung function indexes, *J. Appl. Physiol.*, *71*, 1216–1224 (1991).
133. Heyder, J., Gebhart, J., Stahlhofen, W., and Stuck, B., Biological variability of particle deposition in the human respiratory tract during controlled and spontaneous mouth-breathing, *Ann. Occup. Hyg.*, *26* (Inhaled Particles V), 137–147 (1982).
134. Heyder, J., Gebhart, J., and Scheuch, G., Influence of human lung morphology on particle deposition, *J. Aerosol Med.*, *1*, 81–88 (1988).
135. Yu, C. P., and Diu, C. K., A probabilistic model for intersubject deposition variability of inhaled particles, *Aerosol Sci. Technol.*, *1*, 355–362 (1982).
136. Pritchard, J. N., Jefferies, S. J., and Black, A. Sex differences in the regional

deposition of inhaled particles in the 2.5–75. μm size range, *J. Aerosol Sci.*, *17*, 385–389 (1986).
137. Svartengren, M., Anderson, M., Bylin, G., Philipson, K., and Camner, P., Mouth and throat deposition of 3.6 μm radiolabelled particles in asthmatics, *J. Aerosol Med.*, *4*, 313–321 (1991).
138. Phalen, R. F., Oldham, M. J., and Schum, G. M., Growth and aging of the bronchial tree: implications for particle deposition calculations, *Radiat. Prot. Dosim.*, *38*, 15–21 (1991).
139. Becquemin, M. H., Yu, C. P., Roy, M., and Bouchikhi, A., Total deposition of inhaled particles related to age: comparison with age-dependent model calculations, *Radiat. Prot. Dosim.*, *38*, 23–28 (1991).
140. Hofmann, W., Martonen, T. B., and Graham, R. C., Predicted deposition of nonhygroscopic aerosols in the human lung as a function of subject age, *J. Aerosol Med.*, *2*, 49–68 (1989).
141. Xu, G. B., and Yu, C. P., Effects of age on deposition of inhaled aerosols in the human lung, *Aerosol Sci. Technol.*, *5*, 349–357 (1986).
142. Yu, C. P., and Xu, G. B., Deposition of hygroscopic aerosol particles in growing human lungs, in *Deposition and Clearance of Aerosols in the Human Respiratory Tract* (W. Hofmann, ed.), Facultas, Vienna, 1987, pp. 111–117.
143. LeSouëf, P. N., Validity of methods used to test airway responsiveness in children, *Lancet*, *339*, 1282–1284 (1992).
144. Chadha, T. S., Birch, S., and Sackner, M. A., Oronasal distribution of ventilation during exercise in normal subjects and patients with asthma and rhinitis, *Chest*, *92*, 1037–1041 (1987).
145. Niinimaa, V., Cole, P., Mintz, S., and Shephard, R. J., The switching point from nasal to oronasal breathing, *Respir. Physiol.*, *42*, 62–71 (1980).
146. Saibene, F., Mognoni, P., Lafortune, C. L., and Mostardi, R., Oronasal breathing during exercise, *Pflügers Arch*, *378*, 65–69 (1978).
147. Niinimaa, V., Cole, P., Mintz, S., and Shephard, R. J., Oronasal distribution of respiratory airflow, *Respir. Physiol.*, *43*, 69–75 (1981).
148. Wheatley, J. R., Amis, T. C., and Engel, L. A., Oronasal partitioning of ventilation during exercise, *J. Appl. Physiol.*, *71*, 546–551 (1991).
149. Hounam, R. F., and Morgan, A., Particle deposition, in *Respiratory Defense Mechanisms. Vol. 5. Lung Biology in Health and Disease* (J. D. Brain, D. F. Proctor, and L. M. Reid, eds.), Marcel Dekker, New York, 1977, pp. 125–156.
150. Martonen, T. B., and Zhang, Z., Comments on recent data for particle deposition in human nasal passages, *J. Aerosol Sci.*, *23*, 667–674 (1992).
151. Sato, Y., A review of aerosol therapy in otorhinolaryngology, *J. Aerosol Med.*, *1*, 133–145 (1988).
152. Yu, C. P., Diu, C. K., and Soong, T. T., Statistical analysis of aerosol deposition in nose and mouth, *Am. Ind. Hyg. Assoc. J.*, *42*, 726–733 (1981).
153. Becquemin, M. H., Swift, D.L., Bouchikhi, A., Roy, M., and Teillac, A., Particle deposition and resistance in the noses of adults and children, *Eur. Respir. J.*, *4*, 694–702 (1991).

154. Breysse, P. N., and Swift, D. L., Inhalability of large particles into the human nasal passage: in vivo studies in still air, *Aerosol Sci. Technol.*, *13*, 459–464 (1990).
155. Heyder, J., and Rudolf, G., Deposition of aerosol particles in the human nose, in *Inhaled Particles IV* (W. H. Walton, ed.), Pergamon Press, Oxford, 1977, pp. 107–125.
156. Hounam, R. F., Black, A., and Walsh, M., The deposition of aerosol particles in the nasopharyngeal region of the human respiratory tract, *J. Aerosol Sci.*, *2*, 47–61 (1971).
157. Lippmann, M., Deposition and clearance of inhaled particles in the human nose, *Ann. Otol. Rhinol. Laryngol.*, *79*, 519–528 (1970).
158. Pattle, R. E., The retention of gases and particles in the human nose, in *Inhaled Particles and Vapours II* (C. N. Davies, ed.), Pergamon Press, Oxford, 1961, pp. 302–309.
159. Rasmussen, T. R., Swift, D. L., Hilberg, O., and Pedersen, O. F., Influence of nasal passage geometry on aerosol particle deposition in the nose, *J. Aerosol Med.*, *3*, 15–25 (1990).
160. Schiller, C. F., Gebhart, J., Heyder, J., Rudolf, G., and Stahlhofen, W., Deposition of monodisperse insoluble aerosol particles in the 0.005 to 0.2 μm size range within the human respiratory tract, *Ann. Occup. Hyg.*, *32* (suppl 1, Inhaled Particles VI), 41–49 (1988).
161. Godfrey, S., Controversies in the pathogenesis of EIA, *Eur. J. Respir. Dis.*, *68*, 81–88 (1986).
162. Rudolf, G., Gebhart, J., Heyder, J., Schiller, C. F., and Stahlhofen, W., An empirical formula describing aerosol deposition in man for any particle size, *J. Aerosol Sci.*, *17*, 350–355 (1986).
163. Anderson, M., Svartengren, M., Bylin, G., Philipson, K., and Camner, P., Deposition in asthmatics of particles inhaled in air or in helium-oxygen, *Am. Rev. Respir. Dis.*, *147*, 524–528 (1993).
164. Bowes, S. M., III, and Swift, D. L., Deposition of inhaled particles in the oral airway during oronasal breathing, *Aerosol Sci. Technol.*, *11*, 157–167 (1989).
165. Knight, V., Yu, C. P., Gilbert, B. E., and Divine, G., Ribavirin aerosol dosage according to age and other variables, *J. Infect. Dis.*, *158*, 443–448 (1988).
166. Diu, C. K., and Yu, C. P., Respiratory tract deposition of polydisperse aerosols in humans, *Am. Ind. Hyg. Assoc. J.*, *44*, 62–65 (1983).
167. Gonda, I., Study of the effects of polydispersity of aerosols on regional deposition in the respiratory tract, *J. Pharm. Pharmacol.*, *33* (suppl.), 52P (1981).
168. Persons, D. D., Hess, G. D., Muller, W. J., and Scherer, P. W., Airway deposition of hygroscopic heterodispersed aerosols: results of computer calculation, *J. Appl. Physiol.*, *63*, 1195–1204 (1987).
169. Rudolf, G., Gebhart, J., Heyder, J., Scheuch, G., and Stahlhofen, W., Mass deposition from inspired polydisperse aerosols, *Ann. Occup. Hyg.*, *32* (suppl. 1, Inhaled Particles VI), 919–938 (1988).
170. Cinkotai, F. F., The behavior of sodium chloride particles in moist air, *J. Aerosol Sci.*, *2*, 325–329 (1971).

171. Ferron, G. A., The size of soluble aerosol particles as a function of the humidity of the air: application to the human respiratory tract, *J. Aerosol Sci.*, *8*, 251–267 (1977).
172. Ferron, G. A., Oberdörster, G., and Henneberg, R., Estimation of the deposition of aerosolized drugs in the human respiratory tract due to hygroscopic growth, *J. Aerosol Med.*, *2*, 271–284 (1989).
173. Groom, C. V., and Gonda, I., Equilibrium diameters of inhalation aerosol droplets, *J. Pharm. Pharmacol.*, *32* (suppl.), 1P (1980).
174. Blanchard, J. D., and Willeke, K., Total deposition of ultrafine sodium chloride particles in human lungs, *J. Appl. Physiol.*, *57*, 1850–1856 (1984).
175. Gebhart, J., Anselm, A., Ferron, G., Heyder, J., and Stahlhofen, W., Experimental data on the total deposition of hygroscopic particles in the human respiratory tract, in *Aerosols: Science, Industry, Health and Environment* (S. Masuda and K. Takahashi, eds.), Pergamon Press, Oxford, 1990, pp. 1299–1302.
176. Hicks, J. F., Pritchard, J. N., Black, A., and Megaw, W. J., Experimental evaluation of aerosol growth in the human respiratory tract, in *Aerosols: Formation and Reactivity* (W. Schikarski, H. J. Fissan, and S. K. Friedlander, eds.), Pergamon Press, Oxford, 1986, pp. 244–247.
177. Tu, K. W., and Knutson, E. O., Total deposition of ultrafine hydrophobic and hygroscopic aerosols in the human respiratory system, *Aerosol Sci. Technol.*, *3*, 453–465 (1984).
178. Ferron, G. A., Dua, S. K., Karg, E., Kreyling, W. G., Tuch, T., and Heyder, J., Estimation of the deposition of polydisperse hygroscopic aerosol particles in the respiratory tract, *J. Aerosol Sci.*, *22* (suppl. 1), s863–s866 (1991).
179. Martonen, T. B., Analytical model of hygroscopic particle behavior in human airways, *Bull. Math. Biol.*, *44*, 425–442 (1982).
180. Xu, G. B., and Yu, C. P., Theoretical lung deposition of hygroscopic NaCl aerosols, *Aerosol Sci. Technol.*, *4*, 455–461 (1985).
181. Hickey, A. J., and Martonem, T. B., Behavior of hygroscopic pharmaceutical aerosols and the influence of hydrophobic additives, *Pharm. Res.*, *10*, 1–7 (1993).
181a. Hiller, F. C., Health implications of hygroscopic particle growth in the human respiratory tract, *J. Aerosol Med.*, *4*, 1–23 (1991).
182. Morrow, P. E., Factors determining hygroscopic aerosol deposition in airways, *Physiol. Rev.*, *66*, 330–376 (1986).
183. Pritchard, J. N., Particle growth in the airways and the influence of airflow, in *A New Concept in Inhalation Therapy* (S. P. Newman, F. Morén, and G. K. Crompton, eds.), Medicom, Brussels, 1987, pp. 3–24.
184. Boucher, R. C., Stutts, M. J., Bromberg, P. A., and Gatzy, J. T., Regional difference in airway liquid composition, *J. Appl. Physiol.*, *50*, 613–620 (1981).
185. Persons, D. D., Hess, G. D., and Scherer, P. W., Maximization of pulmonary hygroscopic aerosol deposition, *J. Appl. Physiol.*, *63*, 1205–1209 (1987).
186. Schoeffel, R. E., Anderson, S. D., and Altounyan, R. E. C., Bronchial hyperreactivity in response to inhalation of ultrasonically nebulized solutions of distilled water and saline, *Br. Med. J.*, *283*, 1285–1287 (1981).
187. International Commission on Radiological Protection Respiratory Tract Task Group,

Human Respiratory Tract Model for Radiological Protection, International Commission on Radiological Protection, in press.

188. Ryan, G., Dolovich, M. B., Roberts, R. S., Frith, P. A., Juniper, E. F., Hargreave, F. E., and Newhouse, M. T., Standardization of inhalation provocation tests: two techniques of aerosol generation and inhalation compared, *Am. Rev. Respir. Dis.*, *123*, 195–199 (1981).
189. Laube, B. L., Swift, D. L., and Adams, G. K., III, Single-breath deposition of jet-nebulized saline aerosol, *Aerosol. Sci. Technol.*, *3*, 97–102 (1984).
190. Ilowite, J. S., Gorvoy, J. D., and Smaldone, G. C., Quantitative deposition of aerosolized gentamicin in cystic fibrosis, *Am. Rev. Respir. Dis.*, *136*, 1445–1449 (1987).
191. Pavia, D., Thomson, M. L., Clarke, S. W., and Shannon, H. S., Effect of lung function and mode of inhalation on penetration of aerosol into the human lung, *Thorax*, *32*, 194–197 (1977).
192. Thomas, S. H. L., O'Doherty, M. J., Page, C. J., Nunan, T. O., and Bateman, N. T., Which apparatus for inhaled pentamidine? A comparison of pulmonary deposition via eight nebulisers, *Eur. Respir. J.*, *4*, 616–622 (1991).
193. Gillett, M. K., Briggs, B. A., and Snashall, P. D., The influence of aerosol retention and pattern of deposition on bronchial to atropine and methacholine in humans, *Am. Rev. Respir. Dis.*, *140*, 1727–1733 (1989).
194. Nieminen, M. M., Holli, H., Lahdensuo, A., Muittari, A., and Karvonen, J., Aerosol deposition in automatic dosimeter nebulization, *Eur. J. Respir. Dis.*, *71*, 145–152 (1987).
195. Lewis, R. A., and Fleming, J. S., Fractional deposition from a jet nebulizer: how it differs from a metered dose inhaler, *Br. J. Dis. Chest*, *79*, 361–367 (1985).
196. Newman, S. P., Pavia, D., Garland, N., and Clarke, S. W., Effects of various inhalation modes on the deposition of radioactive pressurised aerosols, *Eur. J. Respir. Dis.*, *63* (suppl. 119), 57–68 (1982).
197. Dolovich, M., Ruffin, R. E., Roberts, R., and Newhouse, M. T., Optimal delivery of aerosols from metered dose inhalers, *Chest*, *80* (suppl.), 911–915 (1981).
198. Spiro, S. G., Singh, C. A., Tolfree, S. E. J., Partridge, M. R., and Short, M. D., Direct labeling of ipratropium bromide aerosol and its deposition pattern in normal subjects and patients with chronic bronchitis, *Thorax*, *39*, 432–435 (1984).
199. Hansen, O. R., and Pedersen, O. R., Optimal inhalation technique with terbutaline Turbuhaler, *Eur. Respir. J.*, *2*, 637–639 (1989).
200. Pedersen, S., and Steffensen, G., Fenoterol powder inhaler technique in children: influence of inspiratory flow rate and breath-holding, *Eur. J. Respir. Dis.*, *68*, 207–214 (1986).
201. Newman, S. P., Morén, F., Trofast, E., Talaee, N., and Clarke, S. W., Deposition and clinical efficacy of terbutaline sulphate from Turbuhaler, a new multi-dose powder inhaler, *Eur. J. Respir. Dis.*, *2*, 247–252 (1989).
202. Newman, S. P., Morén, F., Trofast, E., Talaee, N., and Clarke, S. W., Terbutaline sulphate Turbuhaler: effect of inhaled flow rate on drug deposition and efficacy, *Int. J. Pharmacol.*, *74*, 209–213 (1991).
203. Vidgren, M., Karkkainen, A., Karjalainen, P., Nuutinen, J., and Paronen, P., In-

vitro and in-vivo deposition of drug particles inhaled from pressurised aerosol and dry powder inhalers, *Drug Dev. Ind. Pharm.*, *14*, 2649–2665 (1988).

204. Kim, C. S., Brown, L. K., Lewars, G. G., and Sackner, M. A., Deposition of aerosol particles and flow resistance in mathematical and experimental airway models, *J. Appl. Physiol.*, *55*, 154–163 (1983).

205. Kim, C. S., Eldridge, M. A., Garcia, L., and Wanner, A., Aerosol deposition in the lungs with asymmetric airways obstruction: in vivo observation, *J. Appl. Physiol.*, *67*, 2579–2585 (1989).

206. Trajan, M., Logus, J. W., Enns, E. G., and Man, S. P. F., Relationship between regional ventilation and aerosol deposition in tidal breathing, *Am. Rev. Respir. Dis.*, *130*, 64–70 (1984).

207. Isawa, T., Wasserman, K., and Taplin, G. V., Lung scintigraphy and pulmonary function studies in obstructive airway disease, *Am. Rev. Respir. Dis.*, *102*, 161–172 (1970).

208. Itoh, H., Ishii, Y., Maeda, H., Todo, G., Torizuka, K., and Smaldone, G. C., Clinical observations of aerosol deposition in patients with airways obstruction, *Chest*, *80* (suppl.), 837–840 (1981).

209. Lourenço, R. V., Loddenkemper, R., and Cargon, R. W., Patterns of distribution and clearance of aerosols in patients with bronchiectasis, *Am. Rev. Respir. Dis.*, *106*, 857–866 (1972).

210. Ramanna, L., Tashkin, D. P., Taplin, G. V., Elam, D., Detels, R., Coulson, A., and Rokaw, S. N., Radioaerosol lung imaging in chronic obstructive pulmonary disease, *Chest*, *68*, 634–640 (1975).

211. Taplin, G. V., Taskin, D. P., Chopra, S. K., Anselmi, O. E., Elam, D., Calvarese, B., Coulson, A., Detels, R., and Rokaw, S. N., Early detection of chronic obstructive pulmonary disease using radionuclide lung-imaging procedure, *Chest*, *71*, 567–575 (1977).

212. Agnew, J. E., Bateman, R. J. M., Pavia, D., and Clarke, S. W., Radionuclide demonstration of ventilatory abnormalities in mild asthma, *Clin. Sci.*, *66*, 525–531 (1984).

213. Chung, K. F., Jeyasingh, K., and Snashall, P. D., Influence of airway calibre on the intrapulmonary dose and distribution of inhaled aerosol in normal and asthmatic subjects, *Eur. Respir. J.*, *1*, 890–895 (1988).

214. Laube, B. L., Swift, D. L., Wagner, H. N., Jr., Norman, P. S., and Adams, G. K. III, The effect of bronchial obstruction on central airway deposition of a saline aerosol in patients with asthma, *Am. Rev. Respir. Dis.*, *133*, 740–743 (1986).

215. Laube, B. L., Links, J. M., LaFrance, N. D., Wagner, H. N., Jr., and Rosenstein, B. J., Homogeneity of bronchopulmonary distribution of ^{99m}Tc aerosol in normal subjects and cystic fibrosis patients, *Chest*, *95*, 822–830 (1989).

216. Dolovich, M. B., Sanchis, J., Rossman, C., and Newhouse, M. T., Aerosol penetrance: a sensitive index of peripheral airways obstruction, *J. Appl. Physiol.*, *40*, 468–471 (1976).

217. Lippmann, M., Albert, R. E., and Peterson, H. T., Jr., The regional deposition of inhaled particles in man, in *Inhaled Particles III* (W. H. Walton, ed.), Unwin Bros., Surrey, England, 1971, pp. 105–122.

218. Sweeney, T. D., Brain, J. D., Tryka, A. F., and Godleski, J. J., Retention of inhaled particles in hamsters with pulmonary fibrosis, *Am. Rev. Respir. Dis.*, *128*, 138–143 (1983).
219. Sweeney, T. D., Brain, J. D., Skornik, W. A., and Godleski, J. J., Chronic bronchitis produced by SO_2 alters the deposition pattern of inhaled aerosol in rats (abstr.), *Am. Rev. Respir. Dis.*, *131*, A195 (1985).
220. Sweeney, T. D., Brain, J. D., Leavitt, S. A., and Godleski, J. J., Emphysema alters the deposition pattern of inhaled particles in hamsters, *Am. J. Pathol.*, *128*, 19–28 (1987).
221. Albert, R. E., Lippmann, M., Peterson, H., Berger, J., Sanborn, K., and Bohning, D., Bronchial deposition and clearance of aerosols, *Arch. Intern. Med.*, *131*, 115–127 (1973).
222. Anderson, P. J., Blanchard, J. D., Brain, J. D., Feldman, H. A., McNamara, J. J., and Heyder, J., Effect of cystic fibrosis on inhaled aerosol boluses, *Am. Rev. Respir. Dis.*, *140*, 1317–1324 (1989).
223. Kim, C. S., Lewars, G. A., and Sackner, M. A., Measurement of total lung aerosol deposition as an index of lung abnormality, *J. Appl. Physiol.*, *64*, 1527–1537 (1988).
224. Love, R. G., and Muir, D. C. F., Aerosol deposition and airway obstruction, *Am. Rev. Respir. Dis.*, *114*, 891–897 (1976).
225. Anderson, P. J., Garshick, E., Blanchard, J. D., Feldman, H. A., and Brain, J. D., Intersubject variability in particle deposition does not explain variability in responsiveness to methacholine, *Am. Rev. Respir. Dis.*, *144*, 649–654 (1991).
226. Donna, E., Danta, I., Kim, C. S., and Wanner, A., Relationship between deposition of an responsiveness to inhaled methacholine in normal and asymptomatic subjects, *J. Allergy Clin. Immunol.*, *83*, 456–461 (1989).
227. Svartengren, M., Linnman, L., Philipson, K., and Camner, P., Regional deposition in human lung of 2.5 μm particles, *Exp. Lung Res.*, *12*, 265–279 (1987).
228. Clague, H., Ahmad, D., Chamberlain, M. J., Morgan, W. K. C., and Vinitski, S., Histamine bronchial challenge: effect of regional challenge and aerosol deposition, *Thorax*, *38*, 668–675 (1983).
229. O'Riordan, T. G., Walser, L., and Smaldone, G. C., Changing patterns of aerosol deposition during methacholine bronchoprovocation, *Chest*, *103*, 1385–1389 (1993).
230. Richards, R., Haas, A., Simpson, S., Britten, A., Renwick, A., and Holgate, S., Effect of methacholine induced bronchoconstriction on the pulmonary distribution and plasma pharmacokinetics of inhaled sodium cromoglycate in subjects with normal and hyperreactive airways, *Thorax*, *43*, 611–616 (1988).
231. Wanner, A., Brodnan, J. M., Perez, J., Henke, K. G., and Kim, C. S., Variability of airway responsiveness to histamine aerosol in normal subjects, *Am. Rev. Respir. Dis.*, *131*, 3–7 (1985).
232. Laube, B. L., Norman, P. S., and Adams, G. K. III, The effect of aerosol distribution on airway responsiveness to inhaled methacholine in patients with asthma, *J. Allergy Clin. Immunol.*, *89*, 510–518 (1992).
233. Guillemi, S., Jones, A. L., and Paré, P. D., Effect of breathing pattern during inhalation challenge on the shape and position of the dose-response curve, *Lung*, *167*, 95–106 (1987).

234. Ruffin, R. E., Dolovich, M. B., Wolff, R. K., and Newhouse, M. T., The effects of preferential deposition of histamine in the human airway, *Am. Rev. Respir. Dis.*, *117*, 485–492 (1978).
235. Strohl, K. P., O'Cain, C. F., Ingram, R. H., Jr., Yanta, M. A., Kaplan, W. D., and McFadden, E. R., Jr., Inhalation pattern and predominant site of bronchoconstriction in healthy subjects, *J. Appl. Physiol.*, *50*, 575–579 (1981).
236. Newhouse, M., Aerosol therapy of obstructive and parenchymal pulmonary disease: principles and clinical aspects, *J. Aerosol Med.*, *2*, 187–200 (1989).
237. Stahlhofen, W., Gebhart, J., Heyder, J., and Scheuch, G., Deposition pattern of droplets from medical nebulizers in the human respiratory tract, *Bull. Eur. Physiopathol. Respir.*, *19*, 459–463 (1983).
238. Clay, M. M., Pavia, D., and Clarke, S. W., Effect of aerosol particle size on bronchodilation with nebulized turbutaline in asthmatic patients, *Thorax*, *41*, 364–368 (1986).
239. Clay, M. M., and Clarke, S. W., Effect of nebulized aerosol size on lung deposition in patients with mild asthma, *Thorax*, *42*, 190–194 (1987).
240. Dolovich, M., Ryan, G., and Newhouse, M. T., Aerosol penetration into the lung: influence of airway responses, *Chest*, *80* (suppl.), 834–836 (1981).
241. Gayrard, P., Badier, M., Vervloet, D., and Orehek, J., Different bronchoconstrictor effects of carbachol boluses inhaled near residual volume or total lung capacity, *Respiration*, *51*, 81–85 (1987).
242. Johnson, M. A., Bloom, R., Newman, S., and Clarke, S. W., The optimum aerosol size and dose of salbutamol in the treatment of asthma (abstr.), *Thorax*, *42*, 730 (1987).
243. Mitchell, D. M., Solomon, M. A., Tolfree, S. E. J., Short, M., and Spiro, S. G., Effect of particle size on bronchodilator aerosols on lung distribution and pulmonary function in patients with chronic asthma, *Thorax*, *42*, 457–461 (1987).
244. Kaw, J. L., and Waseem, M., Some advances in dust-related pulmonary toxicology during the last decade, *J. Sci. Ind. Res.*, *51*, 791–801 (1992).
245. Newhouse, M. T., and Ruffin, R. E., Deposition and fate of aerosolized drugs, *Chest*, *73*, 936–943 (1978).
246. Simonds, A. K., Newhouse, S. P., Johnson, M. A., Talaee, N., Lee, C. A., and Clarke, S. W., Alveolar targeting of aerosol pentamidine, *Am. Rev. Respir. Dis.*, *141*, 827–829 (1990).
247. Bennett, W. D., and Ilowite, J. S., Dual pathway clearance of Tc99m-DPTA from the bronchial mucosa, *Am. Rev. Respir. Dis.*, *139*, 1132–1138 (1989).
248. Foster, W. M., Langenback, E. G., Smaldone, G. C., Bergofsky, E. H., and Bohning, D. E., Flow limitation on expiration induces central particle deposition and disrupts effective flow of airway mucus, *Ann. Occup. Hyg.*, *32* (suppl. 1, Inhaled Particles VI), 101–111 (1988).
249. Smaldone, G. C., and Messina, M. S., Enhancement of particle deposition by flow-limiting segments in humans, *J. Appl. Physiol.*, *59*, 509–514 (1985).
250. Swift, D. L., A new method for aerosol delivery to the bronchial airways, *Deposition and Clearance of Aerosols in the Human Respiratory Tract* (W. Hofmann, ed.), Facultas, Vienna, 1987, pp. 207–211.

251. Bennett, W. D., Targeting respiratory drug delivery with aerosol boluses, *J. Aerosol Med.*, *4*, 69–78 (1991).
252. Otani, Y., and Wang, C. S., Growth and deposition of saline droplets covered with a monolayer of surfactant, *Aerosol Sci. Technol.*, *3*, 155–166 (1984).
253. Wojciak, J. F., Notter, R. H., and Oberdörster, G., Size stability of phosphatidylcholine-phosphatidylglycerol aerosols and a dynamic film compression state from their interfacial tension, *J. Colloid Interface Sci.*, *106*, 547–557 (1985).
254. Hickey, A. J., Gonda, I., Irwin, W. J., and Fildes, F. J. T., The effect of hydrophobic coating upon the behavior of a hygroscopic aerosol powder in an environment of controlled temperature and humidity, *J. Pharm. Sci.*, *79*, 1009–1014 (1990).
255. Nieminen, M. M., Holli, H., Lahdensuo, A., Muittari, A., and Karvonen, J., Aerosol deposition in automatic dosimeter nebulization, *Eur. J. Respir. Dis.*, *71*, 145–152 (1987).
256. Ruffin, R. E., Dolovich, M. B., Oldenburg, F. A., Jr., and Newhouse, M. T., The preferential deposition of inhaled isoproterenol and propranolol in asthmatic patients, *Chest 80*(suppl.), 904s–906s (1981).
257. Sweeney, T. D., Blanchard, J. D., Zeltner, T. B., Carter, J. E., and Brain, J. D., Delivery of aerosolized drugs to the lungs with a metered-dose inhaler: quantitative analysis of regional deposition, *J. Aerosol Sci.*, *21*, 350–354 (1990).
258. Gerrity, T. R., Lee, P. S., Hass, F. J., Marinelli, A., Werner, P., and Lourenço, R. V., Calculated deposition of inhaled particles in the airway generations of normal subjects, *J. Appl. Physiol.*, *47*, 867–873 (1979).
259. Martonen, T. B., Measurement of particle dose distribution in a model of a human larynx and tracheobronchial tree, *J. Aerosol. Sci.*, *14*, 11–22 (1983).
260. Gurman, J. L., Lippmann, M., and Schlesinger, R. B., Particle deposition in replicate casts of the human upper respiratory tree under constant and cyclic inspiratory flow. I. Experimental, *Aerosol Sci. Technol.*, *3*, 245–252 (1984).
261. Kim, C. S., and Garcia, L., Particle deposition in cyclic bifurcating tube flow, *Aerosol Sci. Technol.*, *14*, 302–315 (1991).
262. Schlesinger, R. B., Bohning, D. E., Chan, T. L., and Lippmann, M., Particle deposition in a hollow cast of the human tracheobronchial tree, *J. Aerosol Sci.*, *8*, 429–445 (1977).
263. Yu, C. P., and Cai, F. S., Calculated particle deposition at the alveolar duct, *J. Aerosol Med.*, *2*, 69–75 (1989).
264. Brody, A. R., and Roe, M. W., Deposition pattern of inorganic particles at the alveolar level in the lungs of mice and rats, *Am. Rev. Respir. Dis.*, *128*, 724–729 (1983).
265. Zeltner, T. B., Sweeney, T. D., Skornik, W. A., Feldman, H. A, and Brain, J. D., Retention and clearance of 0.9-mm particles inhaled by hamsters during rest and exercise, *J. Appl. Physiol.*, *70*, 1137–1145 (1991).
266. Schroter, R. C., and Sudlow, M. F., Flow patterns in models of the human bronchial airways, *Respir. Physiol.*, *7*, 341–355 (1969).
267. Kim, C. S., and Garcia, L., Particle deposition in cyclic converging tube flow, *Aerosol Sci. Technol.*, *14*, 322–330 (1991).
268. Schlesinger, R. B., Concato, J., and Lippmann, M., Particle deposition during

exhalation: a study in replicate casts of the human upper tracheobronchial tree, in *Aerosols in the Mining and Industrial Work Environments* (V. A. Marple and B. Y. H. Liu, eds.), Ann Arbor Science, Ann Arbor, Michigan, 1983, pp. 165–176.

269. Christensen, W. D., and Swift, D. L., Aerosol deposition and flow limitation in a compliant tube, *J. Appl. Physiol.*, *60*, 630–637 (1986).
270. Kim, C. S., Lewars, G. A., Eldridge, M. A., and Sackner, M. A., Deposition of aerosol particles in a straight tube with an abrupt obstruction, *J. Aerosol Sci.*, *15*, 167–176 (1984).
271. Kim, C. S., Abraham, W. M., Chapman, G. A., and Sackner, M. A., Influence of two-phase gas-liquid interaction on aerosol deposition in airways, *Am. Rev. Respir. Dis.*, *131*, 618–623 (1985).
272. Smaldone, G. C., and Messina, M. S., Flow limitation, cough, and patterns of aerosol deposition in humans, *J. Appl. Physiol.*, *59*, 515–520 (1985).
273. Brain, J. D., and Valberg, P. A., Models of lung retention based on the ICRP Task Group, *Arch. Environ. Health*, *28*, 1–11 (1974).
274. Task Group on Lung Dynamics, Deposition and retention models for internal dosimetry of the human respiratory tract, *Health Phys.*, *12*, 173–207 (1966).
275. Byron, P. R., and Phillips, E. M., Absorption, clearance, and dissolution in the lung, in *Respiratory Drug Delivery* (P. R. Byron, ed.), CRC Press, Boca Raton, Florida, 1990, pp. 107–141.
276. Cuddihy, R. G., and Yeh, H. C., Respiratory tract clearance of particles and substances dissociated from particles, in *Inhalation Toxicology* (U. Mohr, ed.), Springer-Verlag, New York, 1988, pp. 167–193.
277. Jones, J. G., Clearance of inhaled particles from the alveoli, in *Aerosols and the Lung: Clinical and Experimental Aspects* (S. W. Clarke and D. Pavia, eds.), Butterworths, London, 1984, pp. 170–196.
278. King, M., Mucus, mucociliary clearance, and coughing, in *Respiratory Function in Disease*, 3d Ed. (D. V. Bates, ed.), W.B. Saunders, Philadelphia, 1989, pp. 69–78.
279. Lehnert, B. E., Lung defense mechanisms against deposited dusts, *Prob. Respir. Care*, *3*, 130–162 (1990).
280. Lippmann, M., and Schlesinger, R. B., Interspecies comparison of particle deposition and mucociliary clearance in the tracheobronchial airways, *J. Toxicol. Environ. Health*, *13*, 441–469 (1984).
281. Lippmann, M., Yeates, D. B, and Albert, R. E., Deposition, retention, and clearance of inhaled particles, *Br. J. Ind. Med.*, *37*, 337–362 (1980).
282. Oberdörster, G., Lung clearance of inhaled insoluble and soluble particles, *J. Aerosol Med.*, *1*, 289–330 (1988).
283. Pavia, D., Lung mucociliary clearance, in *Aerosols and the Lung: Clinical and Experimental Aspects* (S. W. Clarke and D. Pavia, eds.), Butterworths, London, 1984, pp. 127–155.
284. Schlesinger, R. B., Clearance from the respiratory tract, *Fund. Appl. Toxicol.*, *5*, 435–450 (1985).
285. Sleigh, M. A., Blake, J. R., and Liron, N., The propulsion of mucus by cilia, *Am. Rev. Respir. Dis.*, *137*, 726–741 (1988).
286. Serafini, S. M., Wanner, A., and Michaelson, E. D., Mucociliary transport in central

and intermediate size airways: effect of aminophyllin, *Bull. Eur. Physiopathol. Respir.*, *12*, 415–422 (1976).

287. Mezey, R. J., Cohn, M. A., Fernandez, R. J., Januszkiewicz, A. J., and Wanner, A., Mucociliary transport in allergic patients with antigen-induced bronchospasm, *Am. Rev. Respir. Dis.*, *118*, 677–684 (1978).
288. O'Riordan, T. G., Zwang, J., and Smaldone, G. C., Mucociliary clearance in adult asthma, *Am. Rev. Respir. Dis.*, *146*, 598–603 (1992).
289. Camner, P., and Mossberg, B., Mucociliary disorders: a review, *J. Aerosol Med.*, *1*, 21–28 (1988).
290. Satir, P., and Sleigh, M. A., The physiology of cilia and mucociliary interactions, *Annu. Rev. Physiol.*, *52*, 137–155 (1991).
291. Wanner, A., Clinical aspects of mucociliary transport, *Am. Rev. Respir. Dis.*, *116*, 73–125 (1977).
292. Sackner, M. A., Rosen, M. J., and Wanner, A., Estimation of tracheal mucous velocity by bronchofiberscopy, *J. Appl. Physiol.*, *34*, 495–499 (1973).
293. Yeates, D. B., Aspin, N., Levison, H., Jones, M. T., and Bryan, A. C., Mucociliary transport rates in man, *J. Appl. Physiol.*, *39*, 487–495 (1975).
294. Morrow, P. E., Gibb, F. R., and Gazioglu, K.M., A study of particulate clearance from the human lungs, *Am. Rev. Respir. Dis.*, *96*, 1209–1221 (1967).
295. Albert, R. E., and Arnett, L. C., Clearance of radioactive dust from the lung, *Arch. Environ. Health*, *12*, 99–106 (1955).
296. Booker, D. V., Chamberlain, A. C, Rudo, J., Muir, D. C., and Thompson, M. L., Elimination of 5 micron particles from the human lung, *Nature*, *215*, 30–33 (1967).
297. Camner, P., and Philipson, M. S., Human alveolar deposition of 4 micron teflon particles, *Arch. Environ. Health*, *33*, 181–185 (1978).
298. Lourenço, R. V., Klimek, M. F., and Borowski, C. J., Deposition and clearance of 2 micron particles in the tracheo-bronchial tree of normal subjects—smokers and nonsmokers, *J. Clin. Invest.*, *50*, 1411–1420 (1971).
299. Poe, N. D., Cohen, M. B., and Yanda, R. L., Application of delayed lung imaging following radioaerosol inhalation, *Radiology*, *122*, 739–746 (1977).
300. Sanchis, J, Dolovich, M., Chalmers, R., and Newhouse, M., Quantitation of regional aerosol clearance in the normal human lung, *J. Appl. Physiol.*, *33*, 757–762 (1972).
301. Stahlhofen, W., Gebhart, J., and Heyder, J., Experimental determination of the regional deposition of aerosol particles in the human respiratory tract, *Am. Ind. Hyg. Assoc. J.*, *41*, 385–399 (1980).
302. Gore, D. J., and Patrick, G., A quantitative study of the penetration of insoluble particles into the tissues of the conducting airways, *Ann. Occup. Hyg.*, *26*, 149–161 (1982).
303. Geiser, M., Im Hof, V., Gehr, P., and Cruz-Orive, L. M., Histological and stereological analysis of particle deposition in the conducting airways of hamster lungs, *J. Aerosol Med.*, *3*, 131–145 (1990).
304. Gehr, P., Im Hof, V., Geiser, M., and Schürch, S., The fate of particles deposited in the intrapulmonary conducting airways, *J. Aerosol Med.*, *4*, 349–361 (1991).
305. Schürch, S., Gehr, P., Im Hof, V., Geiser, M., and Green, F., Surfactant displaces

particles toward the epithelium in airways and alveoli, *Respir. Physiol.*, *80*, 17–32 (1990).

306. Stahlhofen, W., Gebhart, J., Rudolf, G., and Scheuch, G., Measurement of lung clearance with pulses of radioactively labelled aerosols, *J. Aerosol Sci.*, *17*, 333–336 (1986).
307. Wolff, R. K., Tillquist, H., Muggenburg, B. A., Harkema, J. R., and Mauderly, J. L., Deposition and clearance of radiolabeled particles from small ciliated airways in beagle dogs, *J. Aerosol Med.*, *2*, 261–270 (1989).
308. Smaldone, G. C., Perry, R. J., Bennett, W. D., Messina, M. S., Zwang, J., and Ilowite, J., Interpretation of "24 hour lung retention" in studies of mucociliary clearance, *J. Aerosol Med.*, *1*, 11–20 (1988).
309. Agnew, J. E., Characterizing lung aerosol penetration, *J. Aerosol Med.*, *4*, 237–249 (1991).
310. Foster, W. M., Is 24 hour lung retention an index of alveolar deposition? (editorial), *J. Aerosol Med.*, *91*, 1–9 (1988).
311. Rensch, H., Von Seefeld, H., Gebhart, K. F., Renzow, D., and Sell, P. J., Stop and go particle transport in the peripheral airways? A model study, *Respiration*, *44*, 346–350 (1983).
312. Morgan, A., ed., Particle clearance by alveolar macrophages, *Environ. Health Perspect.*, 97 (1992).
313. Bowden, D. H., Macrophages, dust, and pulmonary disease, *Exp. Lung Res.*, *12*, 89–107 (1987).
314. Brain, J. D., Macrophages in the respiratory tact, in *Handbook of Physiology, Section 3: The Respiratory System*, Vol. 1 (A. P. Fishman and A. B. Fisher, eds.), American Physiological Society, Bethesda, Maryland, 1985, pp. 447–471.
315. Du Bois, R. M., The alveolar macrophage, *Thorax*, *40*, 321–327 (1986).
316. Fels, A. O. S., and Cohn, Z. A., The alveolar macrophage, *J. Appl. Physiol.*, *60*, 353–369 (1986).
317. Herscowitz, H. B., In defense of the lung: paradoxical role of the pulmonary alveolar macrophage, *Ann. Allergy*, *5*, 634–650 (1985).
318. Reynolds, H. Y., Immunologic system of the respiratory tract, *Physiol. Rev.*, *71*, 1117–1133 (1991).
319. Sibelle, Y., and Reynolds, H. Y., Macrophages and polymorphonuclear neutrophils in lung defense and injury, *Am. Rev. Respir. Dis.*, *141*, 471–501 (1990).
320. Valberg, P. A., and Blanchard, J. D., Pulmonary macrophage physiology: origin, motility, and endocytosis, in *Comprehensive Treatise on Pulmonary Toxicology: Comparative Biology of the Normal Lung*, Vol. 1 (R. A. Parent, ed.), CRC Press Boca Raton, Florida, 1991, pp. 681–724.
321. Brain, J. D., Lung macrophages—How many kinds are there? What do they do? *Am. Rev. Respir. Dis.*, *137*, 507–509 (1988).
322. Adamson, I. Y. R., and Bowden, D. H., Dose response of the pulmonary macrophagic system to various particulates and its relationship to transepithelial passage of free particles, *Exp. Lung Res.*, *2*, 165–175 (1981).
323. Harmsen, A. G., Muggenberg, B. A., Snipes, M. B., and Bice, D. E., The role of

macrophages in particle translocation from lungs to lymph nodes, *Science*, *230*, 1277–1280 (1985).
324. Kreyling, W. G., André, S., Collier, C. G., Ferron, G. A., Métivier, H., and Schumann, G., Interspecies comparison of lung clearance after inhalation of monodisperse, solid cobalt oxide aerosol particles, *J. Aerosol Sci.*, *22*, 509–535 (1991).
325. Sweeney, T. D., and Brain, J. D., Pulmonary deposition: Determinants and measurement techniques, *Toxicol. Pathol.*, *19*, 384–392 (1991).
326. Egan, M. J., and Nixon, W., A model of aerosol deposition in the lung for use in halation dose assessments, *Radiat. Prot. Dosim.*, *11*, 5–17 (1985).
327. Hofmann, W., and Koblinger, L., Monte Carlo modeling of the aerosol deposition in human lungs. Part II: Deposition fractions and their sensitivity to parameter variations, *J. Aerosol Sci.*, *21*, 675–688 (1990).
328. Koblinger, L., and Hofmann, W., Monte Carlo modeling of aerosol deposition in the human lungs. Part I: Simulation of particle transport in a stochastic lung structure, *J. Aerosol Sci.*, *21*, 661–674 (1990).
329. Taulbee, D. B., and Yu, C. P., A theory of aerosol deposition in the human respiratory tract, *J. Appl. Physiol.*, *38*, 77–85 (1975).
330. Yu, C. P., and Diu, C. K., A probabilistic model for intersubject deposition variability of inhaled particles, *Aerosol Sci. Technol.*, *1*, 355–362 (1982).
331. Heyder, J., and Rudolf, G., Mathematical models of particle deposition in the human respiratory tract, *J. Aerosol Sci.*, *15*, 697–707 (1984).
332. Egan, M. J., Nixon, W., Robinson, N. I., James, A. C., and Phalen, R. F., Inhaled aerosol transport and deposition calculations for the ICRP Task Group, *J. Aerosol Sci.*, *20*, 1305–1308 (1989).
333. Bair, W. J., Overview of the ICRP respiratory tract model, *Radiat. Prot. Dosim.*, *38*, 147–152 (1991).
334. James, A. C., Stahlhofen, W., Rudolf, G., Egan, M. J., Nixon, W., Gehr, P., and Briant, J. K., The respiratory tract deposition model proposed by the ICRP Task Group, *Radiat. Prot. Dosim.*, *38*, 159–166 (1991).
335. Bailey, M. R., Birchall, A., Cuddihy, R. G., James, A. C., and Roy, M., Respiratory tract clearance model for dosimetry and bioassay of inhaled radionuclides, *Radiat. Prot. Dosim.*, *38*, 153–158 (1991).
336. Dahl, A. R., Schlesinger, R. B., Heck, H. D., Medinsky, M. A., and Lucier, G. W., Comparative dosimetry of inhaled materials: differences among animal species and extrapolation to man. Symposium overview, *Fundam. Appl. Toxicol.*, *16*, 1–13 (1991).
337. Guilmette, R. A., and Boecker, B., eds., Respiratory tract dosimetry, *Radiat. Prot. Dosim.*, *38* (1991).
338. Mchaffey, J. A., ed., Modeling for scaling to man: biology, dosimetry and response. 26th Hanford Life Sciences Symposium, *Health Phys.*, *57* (suppl. 1) (1989).
339. Oberdörster, G., Lung dosimetry and extrapolation of results of animal inhalation studies to man, *J. Aerosol Med.*, *4*, 335–347 (1991).
340. Yu, C. P., Zhang, L., Becquemin, M. H., Roy, M., and Bouchikhi, A., Algebraic

modeling of total and regional deposition of inhaled particles in the human lung of various ages, *J. Aerosol Sci.*, *23*, 73–79 (1992).

341. Miller, F. J., Martonen, T. B., Ménachie, M. G., Graham, R. C., Spektor, D. M., and Lippmann, M., Influence of breathing mode and activity level on the regional deposition of inhaled particles and implications for regulatory standards, *Ann. Occup. Hyg.*, *32* (suppl. 1, Inhaled Particles VI), 3–10 (1988).
342. Gebhart, J., Heigwer, G., Heyder, J., Roth, C., and Stahlhofen, W., The use of light scattering photometry in aerosol medicine, *J. Aerosol Med.*, *1*, 89–112 (1988).
343. Heyder, J., Blanchard, J. D., Feldman, H. A., and Brain, J. D., Convective mixing in human respiratory tract: estimates with aerosol boli, *J. Appl. Physiol.*, *64*, 1273–1278 (1988).
344. Heyder, J., Assessment of airway geometry with inert aerosols, *J. Aerosol Med.*, *2*, 89–97 (1989).
345. Early, P. J., and Sodee, D. B., *Principles and Practice of Nuclear Medicine*, C. V. Mosby, St. Louis, 1985,
346. Sorenson, J. A., and Phelps, M. E., eds., *Physics in Nuclear Medicine*, 2d Ed., Grune and Stratton, Orlando, Florida, 1987.
347. Cuddihy, R. G., and Boecker, B. B., Controlled administration of respiratory tract burdens of inhaled radioactive aerosols in beagle dogs, *Toxicol. Appl. Pharmacol.*, *25*, 597–605 (1973).
348. Morsy, S. M., Werner, F., Stahlhofen, W., and Pholit, W., A detector of adjustable response for the study of lung clearance, *Health Phys.*, *32*, 243–251 (1977).
349. Park, R. P., Smith, P. H. S., and Taylor, D. M., *Basic Science of Nuclear Medicine*, Churchill Livingstone, New York, 1978.
350. Cross, C. E., Hornof, W. J., Koblik, P. D., and Fisher, P. E., Aerosol deposition: practical considerations of methodology for the direct measurement of aerosol delivery to the lung bronchiolar–alveolar surfaces, *J. Aerosol Med.*, *5*, 39–45 (1992).
351. Thomas, S. H. L., O'Doherty, M. J., Page, C. J., and Nunan, T. O., Variability in the measurement of nebulized aerosol deposition in man, *Clin. Sci.*, *81*, 767–775 (1991).
352. Itoh, H., Smaldone, G. C., Swift, D. L., and Wagner, H. N., Jr., Quantitative measurement of total lung deposition: comparison of three different techniques, *J. Aerosol Sci.*, *16*, 367–371 (1985).
353. Phipps, P. R., Gonda, I., Bailey, D. L., Borham, P., Bautovich, G., and Anderson, S. D., Comparison of planar and tomographic gamma scintigraphy to measure the penetration of inhaled aerosols, *Am. Rev. Respir. Dis.*, *139*, 1516–1523 (1989).
354. Chan, H.-K., Use of single photon emission computed tomography in aerosol studies, *J. Aerosol Med.*, *6*, 23–36 (1993).
355. Logus, J. W., Trajan, M., Hooper, H. R., Lentle, B. C., and Mann, S. F. P., Single photon emission tomography of lungs imaged with Tc-labeled aerosol, *J. Can. Assoc. Radiol.*, *35*, 133–138 (1984).
356. Schuster, D. P., Positron emission tomography: theory and its applications to the study of lung disease, *Am. Rev. Respir. Dis.*, *139*, 818–840 (1989).
357. Koeppe, R. A, and Hutchins, G. D., Instrumentation for positron emission tomogra-

phy: tomographs and data processing and display systems, *Semin. Nucl. Med.*, *22*, 162–181 (1992).

358. Vanwaarde, A., Meeder, J. G., Blanksma, P. K., Brodde, O. E., Visser, G. M., Elsinga, P. H., Paans, A. M. J., Vaalburg, W., and Lie, K. I., Uptake of radioligands by rat heart and lung in vivo—CGP-12177 does and CGP-26505 does not reflect binding to beta-adrenoreceptor, *Eur. J. Pharmacol.*, *222*, 107–112 (1992).
359. Valberg, P. A., and Brain, J. D., Lung particle retention and lung macrophage function evaluated using magnetic aerosols, *J. Aerosol Med.*, *1*, 331–349 (1988).
360. Cohen, D., Crowther, T. S., Gibbs, G. W., and Becklake, M. R., Magnetic lung measurements in relation to occupational exposure in asbestos miners and millers of Quebec, *Environ. Res.*, *26*, 535–550 (1981).
361. Freedman, A. P., Robinson, S. E., and Johnston, R. J., Noninvasive magnetopneumographic estimation of lung dust loads and distribution in bituminous coal workers, *J. Occup. Med.*, *26*, 613–618 (1980).
362. Kalliomäki, K., Kalliomäki, P.-L., Kelhä, V., and Vaaranen, V., Instrumentation for measuring the magnetic lung contamination of steel workers, *Ann. Occup. Hyg.*, *23*, 175–184 (1980).
363. Cohen, D., Arai, S., and Brain, J. D., Smoking impairs longterm dust clearance from the lungs, *Science*, *204*, 514–517 (1979).

8

Methodologies of Aerosol Delivery

Richard R. Rosenthal

Consultant
Fairfax, Virginia

I. INTRODUCTION

The challenge procedures detailed in this chapter may serve as a useful adjunct to routine pulmonary function testing for the diagnosis of asthma or for objective measurement of the airway hyperreactivity that is the hallmark of that illness. Now that methacholine has been approved by the U.S. Food and Drug Administration (FDA), inhalation challenge, a type of bronchoprovocation, is in widespread use for both clinical and research purposes. Inhalation challenge with methacholine (or histamine) may be safely conducted in an outpatient setting using the procedures described here. Provocation testing, both for diagnostic purposes and in clinical trials of pharmaceutical agents, is now routine in many settings.

Inhalation challenge with methacholine is a sensitive and specific means by which to assess the presence and extent of airway hyperreactivity in patients with asthma [1–5] as well as others who may have airway hyperreactivity. Numerous authors have demonstrated that methacholine or histamine challenge can be used both to identify patients with asthma and to quantify the severity of hyperresponsiveness as an index of disease severity [6–9]. Inhalation challenge with an autacoid such as histamine [10] or methacholine, together with a history of dyspnea, is probably the simplest and most objective method for determining the presence of asthma in different populations. Well-standardized histamine or methacholine inhalation tests should be available in all major pulmonary function laboratories, and the tests, ideally, should be reproducible and comparable between investigators [9]. Pratter et al. [11] demonstrated that among a group of patients who were referred as diagnostic dilemmas, methacholine challenge was more effective than a history of wheezing, a prior clinical diagnosis of asthma, physical examination, or pulmonary function testing in predicting the presence or absence of symptomatic asthma. Dales et al. [12] have shown that physicians could not accurately predict the presence of increased airway responsiveness in patients with symptoms suggestive of airway asthma, and that a methacholine challenge was required to properly guide subsequent patient management. Others have similarly confirmed the utility of inhalation challenge with methacholine for diagnostic purposes [13–15] and have shown it to be sufficiently well tolerated to be a practical office procedure if carefully done in properly chosen patients [16]. Challenge with methacholine has been established as a safe and effective means of identifying the presence of asthma and monitoring the state of disease for follow-up [17,18]. It is useful in children with normal resting spirometric values who present with problems suggesting lower-airway hyperreactivity [19] and children with cough who are likely to benefit from specific bronchodilator therapy [20]. Conversely, measurement of bronchial responsiveness is both feasible and clinically valuable in elderly subjects [21]. Patients with conditions other than asthma, such as chronic obstructive bronchitis [22], bronchopulmonary dysplasia [23], and sarcoidosis [24], may also have hyperreactive airways that will respond to bronchodilator therapy, and this can be evaluated with the methacholine challenge. Ahrens et al. [25] have suggested that methacholine responsiveness may be a useful measure of the protection afforded by bronchodilators, in addition to traditional methods such as longitudinal measures of forced expired volume in 1 second (FEV_1), especially insofar as there may be discordance between the two. In summary, methacholine challenge is a means by which one can identify patients with hyperreactive airways, regardless of cause, and measure the extent of such hyperreactivity when appropriate.

II. METHODOLOGIES OF AEROSOL DELIVERY

Two methods are commonly used to administer methacholine for inhalation challenge, the tidal-breathing method and the intermittent method.

The tidal-breathing method [26] involves the nebulization of aerosol, usually from a Wright nebulizer, during tidal breathing of escalating concentrations of agonist for 2-min intervals. Pulmonary function is measured after each such dose. The concentrations of methacholine (or histamine) are plotted against the FEV_1, and the concentration of agonist that causes a 20% drop in FEV_1, known as the provocative concentration or PC_{20}, is interpolated from the dose–response curve.

The intermittent method requires that discrete inhalations (breaths) of aerosol be given in a sequence of five inhalations, each five-breath sequence of escalating concentration of agonist being followed by a pulmonary function determination.

METHACHOLINE CHALLENGE

Name:____________________________ Date:__________

Study:____________Age:____Sex:____Height:____Weight:____Temperature:____Humidity:____Barometric Pressure:____

Conditions	Time	# of Breaths	FEV1	FEV1 % Pred.	FVC	MMEF	PEFR	FEV1 % Control	Cumul. Units *	Comments
Baseline		N/A						N/A	N/A	BP: P:
Control		5						100%	0	
Meth. Conc. 0.025 mg/ml		5							0.125	
0.075 mg/ml		5							0.50	
0.25 mg/ml		5							1.75	
0.75 mg/ml		5							5.50	
2.5mg/ml		5							18.0	
7.5 mg/ml		5							55.5	
25.0mg/ml		5							180.5	
Bronchodilator										

Target : 20% reduction of Control FEV1______ * 1 Breath Unit =1 inhalation of 1 mg/ml of Methacholine

PD20 FEV1:______

Impression:

____

Physician's Name

Figure 1 The methacholine challenge flow sheet may be used to list the doses of methacholine used and to document the response at each dose. The cumulative units are the product of the breaths and the concentration if the output of the nebulizer in weight of methacholine is not known. After five breaths of saline (control) the forced expired volume in 1 second (FEV_1) is determined, and the target of a 20% reduction from that value is determined. The procedure is stopped when that target is reached or exceeded by the administration of any combination of full and partial doses.

Figure 1 illustrates a suggested flow sheet and dosage schedule. Modified (shortened) protocols have been used in epidemiological studies and have been validated against the longer standard protocol. Shorter protocols starting at higher doses might be useful in populations with a low probability of hyperresponsiveness [27] but entail the danger that an excessively high starting dose may cause profound changes after the first dose, putting patients unnecessarily at risk and precluding the construction of proper dose–response curves. With the intermittent method, the actual dose delivered can be determined (see below). In this method, the provocative dose that causes a 20% drop in the FEV_1 ($PD_{20}FEV_1$ or simply PD_{20}) is interpolated from the dose–response curve. The intermittent method has been recommended by the standardization committee of the National Institute of Allergy and Infectious Disease [28] and is embodied in the FDA-approved methodology for the Provocholine (Roche) brand of methacholine.

A hand-held nebulizer fitted with a T piece is sometimes used to administer discrete inhalations of aerosol but requires that the patient coordinate the inspiratory effort with occlusion of the T piece by one finger. While this technique is simple, there is no means of ensuring regularity in dose administration, and the consistency of dosing with regard to volume inhaled is poor. To better implement the intermittent administration of aerosol, a nebulization dosimeter may be used. The dosimeter (Fig. 2) is a breath-actuated air-metering device that when attached to a standard jet nebulizer (DeVilbiss #646) may be used to administer reproducible volumes of aerosol. The Digidoser (Pulmonary Data Services Inc., Louisville, Colorado) is a dosimeter configured into a personal computer–based spirometer and uses the pneumotachygraph as a breath sensor (Fig. 3). The DeVilbiss #646 nebulizer is configured so that the air from the dosimeter enters the bowl of the nebulizer under pressure and is throttled through a jet, the airstream from which is at an angle to a hollow "straw" that sits in the liquid in the bowl. The low pressure

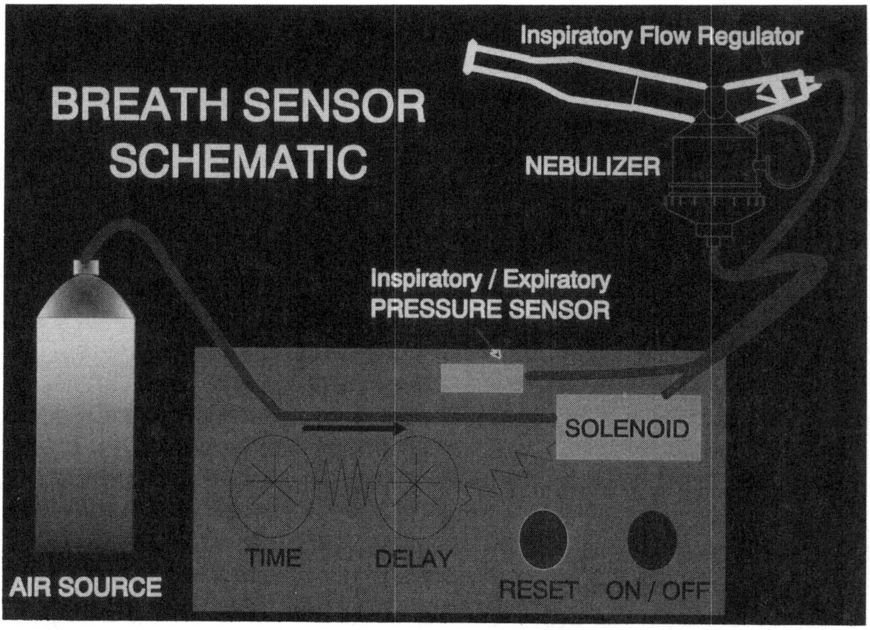

Figure 2 The dosimeter is a breath-actuated air-metering device that can deliver a reproducible amount of aerosol on demand. (Courtesy of Pulmonary Data Services Inc., Louisville, Colorado).

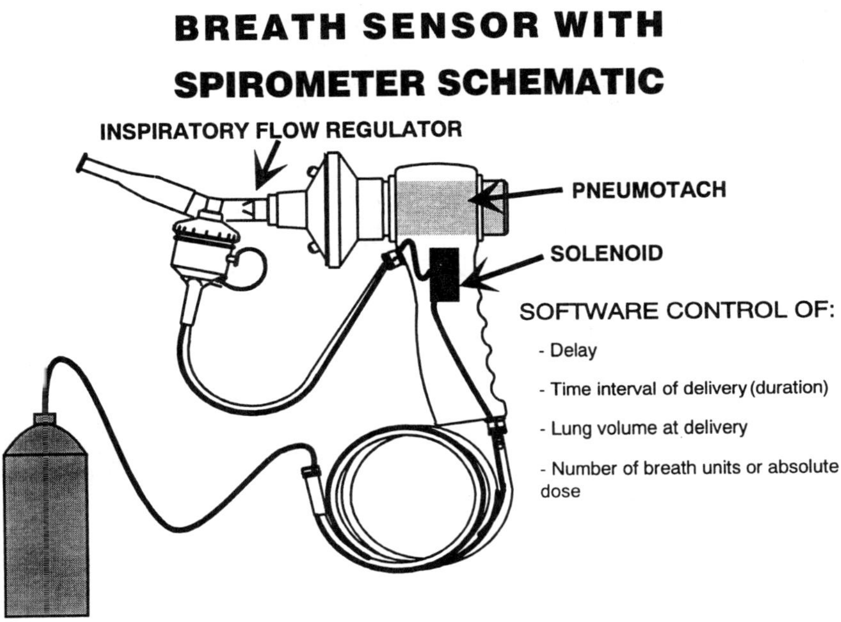

Figure 3 The Digidoser is a dosimeter configured into a personal computer–based spirometer that enables both control and documentation of all the determinants of reproducibility of aerosol generation. (Courtesy of Pulmonary Data Services Inc., Louisville, Colorado).

created by the high-velocity jet stream sucks the liquid up through the straw and entrains it into the jet stream, which is then impacted against the bulbous end of the "baffle". Upon contact with the baffle, the liquid-laden jet stream is virtually exploded into small aerosol droplets, forming the aerosol mist that is inhaled (Fig. 4).

A number of sources of variability both between and within nebulizers have been identified. They include patency of the jet, position of the straw and baffle relative to the jet [29], the amount of solution in the nebulizer bowl, the driving gas flow and pressure from the dosimeter, the duration of aerosol generation, the duration of inhalation, and the inspiratory flow rate.

Table 1 lists the factors affecting reproducibility of aerosol administration. These sources of variability can be addressed as follows. The breath-actuated dosimeter provides aerosol administration for a variable but consistent, operator-selected time interval, which can be initiated at the onset of inspiration or at any settable interval thereafter. If the patient inspires from residual volume or reliably

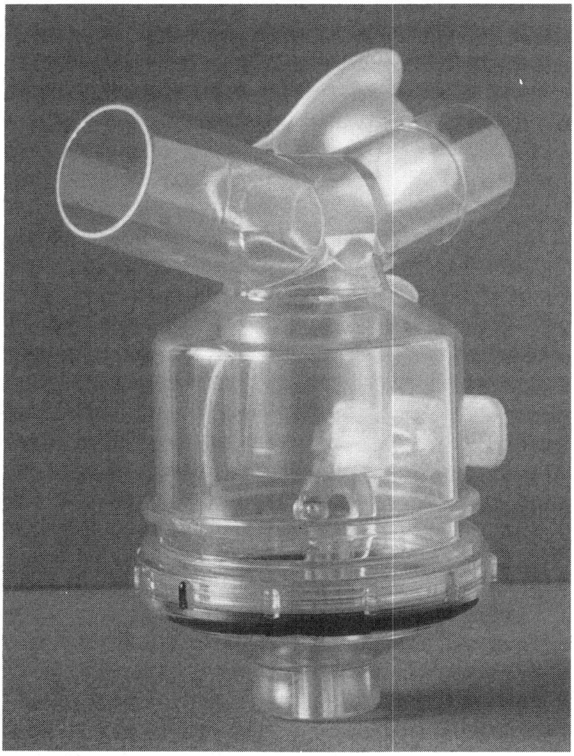

Figure 4 The DeVilbiss #646 nebulizer is a jet nebulizer that can be fitted to the dosimeter.

Table 1 Factors Affecting Reproducibility of Aerosol Administration

Interval of aerosol administration
Inspiratory flow rate
Lung volume during aerosol administration
Aerosol residence time
Configuration of nebulizer

at functional residual capacity, the lung volume at which aerosol is administered is similarly consistent. If the position of the straw and baffle is fixed, either by gluing them in place or by using a registration mark (Fig. 5) on the outside of the top section of the nebulizer as a means of lining up the straw and baffle in the same orientation, the variability of nebulizer output is significantly improved. A newly developed valve, when added to the nebulizer, regulates the inspiratory flow rate through the nebulizer, adding even considerably more consistency to nebulizer output [30]. The nebulizer jet must be kept clean, and a stylus is provided for this by the manufacturer. The nebulizer bowl must be filled with 2 ml of each concentration before nebulizer discharge and must be kept in a horizontal position during discharge. Finally, rather than a compressor, which can produce uneven

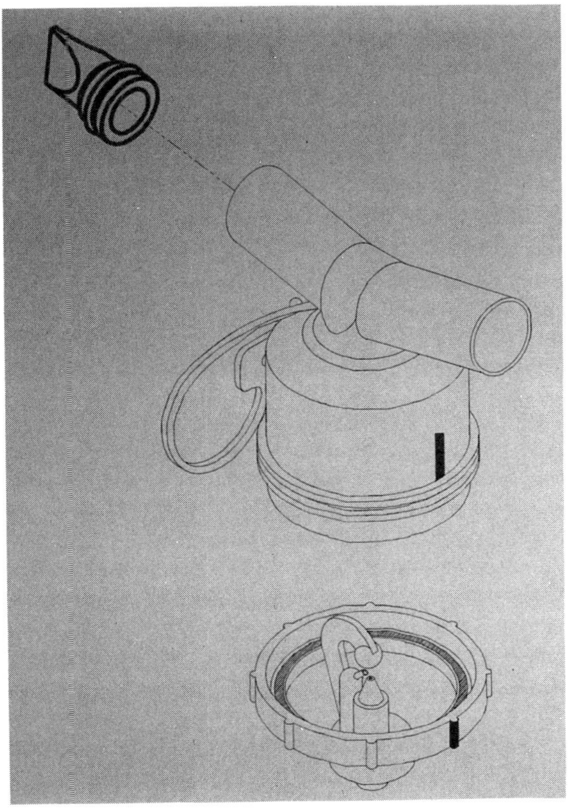

Figure 5 Registration marks on the bowl and body of the DeVilbiss #646 nebulizer can be used to fix the position of the straw and baffle, which, in the presence of a flow-regulating valve, will ensure consistent output of the nebulizer when configured with a dosimeter.

pressures over the time course of nebulizer discharge, it is desirable to use a cylinder of gas fitted with a regulator designed to maintain a constant pressure regardless of flow. When these elements are controlled, nebulizers may be calibrated by weighing before and after discharge under the conditions defined by the above parameters, such as inspiratory flow rate of 0.5 L/s, discharge time of 0.6 s, and pressure to the nebulizer of 30 psi. When the volume of output of the nebulizer is known, the dose of agonist (in milligrams) can be computed from the concentration in the nebulizer. Before the invention of the inspiratory flow regulator, dosage units were so-called breath units, defined as the amount of methacholine or histamine contained in one breath (volume of aerosol unknown) of a solution containing 1 mg/ml of methacholine or histamine. This unitage is still in common use, and several studies have shown very good reproducibility [31,32].

The intermittent method is carried out as follows. First, a baseline pulmonary function test is performed. Although there is no significant correlation between the baseline FEV_1 and the degree of hyperreactivity [33], the FEV_1 must generally be 70% of the predicted value or better. Then, five inhalations of buffered saline (preserved with 0.04% phenol) are given as "saline control." Any subject with a decrease of more than 15% from baseline should be excluded from challenge that day. A 20% decrease in FEV_1 is then computed from the saline control value and designated as the target. The challenge is terminated when the subject's FEV_1 matches or is lower than that value. Patients are given five successive inhalations of the concentrations of methacholine shown, with replicate pulmonary function measurements performed within 5 min of each dose sequence, until the target is reached or exceeded. Partial doses (fewer than five inhalations) may be given if, in the opinion of the investigator, the next dose would overshoot the target significantly. If wheezing, chest tightness, or other symptoms persist for more than 1–15 min after the last dose or are excessive at the conclusion of the study, the patient may be given an inhaled bronchodilator to reverse the induced bronchospasm. Doses are quantified as accumulated breath units, defined above, or, if a calibrated nebulizer (requiring a flow-regulator valve) is used, as milligrams of methacholine or histamine. From the data on the flow sheet, a dose–response curve is constructed that relates the FEV_1 in terms of percent of the saline control value to the dose of methacholine administered. From this dose–response curve the provocative dose necessary for a 20% decrease in FEV_1 is interpolated (Fig. 6) and used as a measure of methacholine sensitivity. Other parameters such as midexpiratory flow rate (FEF_{25-75}%) may be useful as well [34]. The results of challenge with the tidal-breathing method and the intermittent method are generally comparable [35,36], although there is considerable variability between and within subjects when the tidal-breathing method is used, since the respiratory frequency, the inspiratory flow rate, and the inspiratory time are all unregulated and subject to variability [37]. Although the reproducability of the intermittent method has been

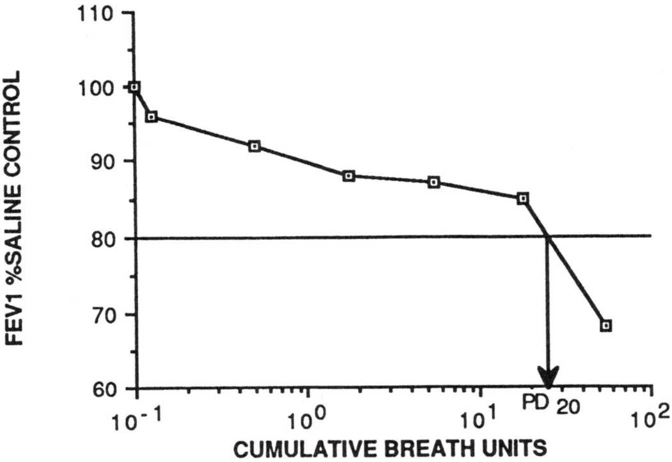

Figure 6 The methacholine dose–response curve is generated from the sequential measurements of the forced expired volume in 1 second (FEV_1) after each dose of methacholine. The PD_{20} is the interpolated dose of methacholine that caused a 20% decrease in the FEV_1 as a percent of the saline control value.

shown to be better than that of the tidal-breathing method [38], regulation of the tidal volume and ventilatory rate has been found to improve reproducibility of the PC_{20}. Regulation of flow to the Wright nebulizer is also an important issue, since output is not linear to the input flow; accordingly, calibration of the Wright nebulizer may be in order [39]. If a dosimeter is configured to implement aerosol delivery for the tidal-breathing method, losses outside the respiratory tract are minimized, since there is no aerosol discharge during the expiratory phase; this increases the efficacy of the challenge and enhances reproducibility [40]. In any case, if ad libitum tidal breathing is used, the volume history (inspiratory volumes) is not regulated and there is no opportunity to reproduce all of the parameters of the challenge.

Regardless of the method chosen, a detailed description of the equipment and procedures used and the inclusion criteria for the patients should be provided in all publications, including the dosing schedule, which pulmonary function tests were done, and how the data were analyzed [41].

III. INTERPRETATION OF DATA

Histamine [42] and methacholine are the excitatory autacoids most useful for distinguishing normal from asthmatic subjects, and the FEV_1 is the best test [28,43] for making this distinction. It is recommended that the entire dose–

response curve be reported, with the percent change in FEV_1 from the saline control value plotted against the dose delivered in cumulative units, the former on a linear ordinate and the latter on a logarithmic abscissa [28,44,45]. Connolly et al. have suggested that the bronchoconstrictor effect of histamine depends on both the cumulative dose and the number of component doses, and that the PD_{20} is more accurately expressed on a cumulative scale [45]. When the tidal-breathing method is used, the PC_{20} must be interpolated from the concentrations delivered, and when the intermittent method is used, the PD_{20} is interpolated from the doses given as either milligrams or breath units. Most asthmatics will have a PC_{20} of 8 mg/ml or less or a PD_{20} on the order of 65 cumulative breath units. Fetters and Matthews [46] have suggested that the diagnosis of asthma can be excluded if the methacholine test is negative, but that the sensitivity could be enhanced if the cutoff for asthma were 20 cumulative breath units. The linear dose–response relationship between the dose of methacholine and the FEV_1 response provides a comprehensive summary of the methacholine bronchoprovocation and is useful in epidemiological surveys [47].

Alternative methods of expression of the dose–response curve include area under the curve (AUC) [48,49], which may be of use if there is a plateau phenomenon wherein additional doses cause little or no subsequent decrease in airway function. The PD_{20} has been shown, however, to correlate with the overall slope and the AUC [22]. Yet another dose–response parameter is the slope of the curve, and Orehek has opined that differences between asthmatics and normal subjects were related to differences in the slope of the curve. He suggested that the provocative dose be regarded as a measure of sensitivity and the slope a measure of reactivity [50]. Chung pointed out that the slope of the dose–response curve is related to the starting airway caliber, the slope being steeper the more dilated the patient's airways are. Accordingly, increases in the provocative dose after treatment with a bronchodilator/antagonist such as atropine reflect both bronchodilation and specific antagonist activity [51], an observation similarly born out in our laboratory [52].

IV. RELEVANCE OF METHACHOLINE CHALLENGE

Methacholine and histamine challenges are thought of as measures of nonspecific (nonimmunological) airway hyperreactivity. Challenge with either agent gives comparable results in asthmatics, and steroids do not influence the procedure [53]. Of critical importance is the observation that methacholine and histamine sensitivity as measured by bronchoprovocation dose–response curves is related to the degree of asthma [3,17,54,55]. Moreover, relatively greater airway hyperreactivity is more likely to be associated with the early onset of illness [56,57].

Methacholine and histamine sensitivity is also related to antigen sensitivity [18,58]. A relationship between the degree of histamine sensitivity and cat dander sensitivity has been documented in cat-sensitive children [59], and a similar relationship has been noted in occupational asthma due to exposure to grain dust [60].

Finally, methacholine and histamine challenges have been compared with other nonspecific challenges including cold air [13], which seems to act through an exclusive mechanism [61], and exercise [62] as well as ultrasonically nebulized distilled water [63,64]. While all are specific for asthma, bronchoprovocation with methacholine and histamine seems to have the highest sensitivity. Although comparable in terms of sensitivity and specificity, histamine challenge may be less desirable than methacholine challenge because of the potential side effects of flushing, headache, and tachycardia, which are not noted with methacholine. Moreover, methacholine is FDA-approved for bronchoprovocation by inhalation challenge and is packaged, labeled, and marketed as such.

REFERENCES

1. Rosenthal, R. R., The emerging role of bronchoprovocation, *J. Allergy Clin. Immunol.*, *64* (suppl.), 564 (1979).
2. Fish, J. E., Rosenthal, R. R., Batra, G., Menkes, H., Summer, W., Permutt, S., and Norman, P., Airway responses to methacholine in allergic and nonallergic subjects, *Am. Rev. Respir. Dis.*, *113*, 579 (1976).
3. Hargeave, F. E., Ryan, G., Thomson, N. C., O'Byrne, P. M., Latimer, K., Juniper, E. F., and Dolovich, J., Bronchial responsiveness to histamine or methacholine in asthma: measurement and clinical significance, *J. Allergy Clin. Immunol.*, *68*, 347 (1981).
4. Townley, R. G., Ryo, U. Y., Kolotkin, B. M., and Kang, B., Bronchial sensitivity to methacholine in current and former asthmatic and allergic rhinitis patients and control subjects, *J. Allergy Clin. Immunol.*, *56*, 429 (1975).
5. Hopp, R. J., Bewtra, A. K., Nair, N. M., and Townley, R. G., Specificity and sensitivity of methacholine inhalation challenge in normal and asthmatic children, *J. Allergy Clin. Immunol.*, *74*, 154 (1984).
6. Rosenthal, R. R., Norman, P. S., and Summer, W. R., Bronchoprovocation: effect on priming and desensitization phenomenon in the lung, *J. Allergy Clin. Immunol.*, *56*, 338–346 (1975).
7. Orehek, J., Gayrard, P., Smith, A. P., Grimaud, C., and Charpin, J., Airway response to carbachol in normal and asthmatic subjects: distinction between bronchial sensitivity and reactivity, *Am. Rev. Respir. Dis.*, *115*, 937–943 (1977).
8. Hargeave, F. E., Ramsdale, E. H., Sterk, P. J., and Juniper, E. F., Advances in the use of inhalation provocation tests in clinical evaluation, *Chest*, *87* (suppl. 1), 32S–35S (1985).
9. Cockcroft, D. W., Bronchial inhalation tests. I. Measurement of nonallergic bronchial responsiveness, *Ann. Allergy*, *55*, 527–534 (1985).
10. Woolcock, A. J., Dowse, G. K., Temple, K., Stanley, H., Alpers, M. P., and Turner, K. J., The prevalence of asthma in the South-Fore people of Papua New Guinea. A

method for field studies of bronchial reactivity, *Eur. J. Respir. Dis.*, *64*, 571–581 (1983).
11. Pratter, M. R., Hingston, D. M., and Irwin, R. S., Diagnosis of bronchial asthma by clinical evaluation. An unreliable method, *Chest*, *84*, 42 (1983).
12. Dales, R. E., Nunes, F., Partyka, D., and Ernst, P., Clinical prediction of airways hyperresponsiveness, *Chest*, *93*, 984–986 (1988).
13. Rosenthal, R. R., Inhalation challenge, *NER Allergy Proc*, *9*, 113–122 (1988).
14. Hargreave, F. E., Sterk, P., Adelroth, E. C., Ramsdale, E. H., and O'Byrne, P. M., Airway responsiveness to histamine or methacholine: advances in measurement and interpretation, *Respiration*, *50* (suppl. 2) 72–76 (1986).
15. Alberts, W. M., and Goldman, A. L., Clinical use of methacholine bronchial challenge testing, *South Med. J.*, *80*, 827–830 (1987).
16. Easton, J. G., The value of inhalation challenge testing as an office procedure, *Ann. Allergy*, *51*, 252–258 (1975).
17. Fourie, P. R., and Joubert, J. R., Determination of airway hyperreactivity in asthmatic children: a comparison among exercise, nebulized water, and histamine challenge, *Paediatr. Pulmonol.*, *4*, 245 (1988).
18. Adinoff, A. D., Schlosberg, R. T., and Strunk, R. C., Methacholine inhalation challenge in young children: results of testing and follow-up, *Ann. Allergy*, *61*, 282–286 (1988).
19. Shapiro, G. G., Furukawa, C. T., Pierson, W. E., and Bierman, C. W., Methacholine bronchial challenge in children, *J. Allergy Clin. Immunol.*, *69*, 365–369 (1982).
20. de Benedictis, F. M., Canny, G. J., and Levinson, H., Methacholine inhalation challenge in the evaluation of chronic cough in children, *J. Asthma*, *23*, 303–308 (1986).
21. Pratter, M. R., and Irwin, R. S., Usefulness and safety of pharmacologic bronchoprovocation challenge in evaluating patients with normal spirometric tests who are suspected of having asthma, *Chest*, *93*, 898–900 (1988).
22. Kopferschmitt-Kubler, M. C., Bigot, H., and Pauli, G., Allergen bronchial challenge tests: variability and reproducibility of the early response, *J. Allergy Clin. Immunol.*, *80*, 730–740 (1987).
23. Malo, J. L., Cartier, A., L'Archevêque, J., Ghezzo, H., and Martin, R. R., Bronchoconstriction due to isocapnic cold air inhalation minimally influences bronchial hyperresponsiveness to methacholine in asthmatic subjects, *Bull. Eur. Physiopathol. Respir.*, *22*, 473–477 (1986).
24. Bechtel, J. J., Starr, T. III, Dantzuen, D. R., and Bower, J. S., Airway hyperreactivity in patients with sarcoidosis, *Am. Rev. Respir. Dis.*, *124*, 759–761 (1981).
25. Ahrens, R. C., Bonham, A. C., Maxwell, G. A., and Weinberger, M. M., A method for comparing the peak intensity and duration of action of aerosolized bronchodilators using bronchoprovocation with methacholine, *Am. Rev. Respir. Dis.*, *129*, 903–906 (1984).
26. Cockroft, D. W., Killian, D. N., Mellon, J. J. A., and Hargreave, F. E., Bronchial reactivity to inhaled histamine. A method and clinical survey, *Clin. Allergy*, *7*, 235 (1977).
27. Hendrick, D. J., Fabbri, L. M., Hughes, J. M., Banks, D. E., Barkman, H. W., Jr.,

Connolly, M. J., Jones, R. N., and Weill, H., Modification of the methacholine inhalation test and its epidemiologic use in polyurethane workers, *Am. Rev. Respir. Dis.*, *133*, 600–604 (1986).
28. Chai, H., Farr, R. S., Froehlich, L. A., Mathison, D. A., McLean, J. A., Rosenthal, R. R., Sheffer, A. L., Spector, S. L., and Townley, R. G., Standardization of bronchial inhalation challenge procedures, *J. Allergy Clin. Immunol.*, *56*, 323 (1975).
29. Hollie, M. C., Malone, R. A., Skufca, R. M., and Nelson, H. S., Extreme variability in aerosol output of the DeVilbiss 646 jet nebulizer, *Chest*, *100*, 1339–1344 (1991).
30. Rosenthal, R. R., Gelman, M., Balsamo, J., Lehman, A., and Sheridan, M., Enhancing reproducibility of aerosol administration, *J. Allergy Clin. Immunol.*, *91*, 375 (1993).
31. Gerritsen, J., Hoëter, G. H., Akkerboom, H. J., and Knol, K., Recovery of FEV_1 after histamine challenge in asthmatic children, *Clin. Allergy*, *17*, 119–126 (1987).
32. Weiss, M., Wheeler, B., Eggleston, P., and Adkinson, N. F., Jr., A protocol for performing reproducible methacholine inhalation tests in children with moderate to severe asthma, *Am. Rev. Respir. Dis.*, *139*, 67–72 (1989).
33. Asher, M. I., Bertrand, J. M., Beaudry, P. H., and Coates, A. L., Histamine inhalation challenge in children: a comparison of two methods, *Ann. Allergy*, *50*, 389–392 (1983).
34. Murray, A. B., and Furguson, A. C., A comparison of spirometric measurements in allergen bronchial challenge testing, *Clin. Allergy*, *11*, 87–93 (1981).
35. Ryan, G., Dolovich, M. B., Roberts, R. S., Frith, P. A., Juniper, E. F., Hargreave, F. E., and Newhouse, M. T., Standardization of inhalation provocation tests: two techniques of aerosol generation and inhalation compared.
36. Frolund, L., Svendsen, U. G., Nielsen, N. H., Weeke, B., and Madsen, F., Bronchial allergen challenge: comparison between two different methods of provocation, *Clin. Allergy*, *17*, 439–448 (1987).
37. Madsen, F., Frolund, L., Nielsen, N. H., Svendsen, U. G., and Weeke, B., Bronchial challenge: ventilation during 'tidal volume breathing' inhalation is not constant. *Bull. Eur. Physiopathol. Respir.*, *22*, 517–522 (1986).
38. Madsen, F., Nielsen, N. H., Frolund, L., Svendsen, U. G., and Weeke, B., Bronchial challenge: a small reservoir for the Wright jet nebulizer, *Bull. Eur. Physiopathol. Respir.*, *23*, 67–71 (1987).
39. Nieminen, M. M., Lahdensuo, A., Kellamaeki, L., Karvonen, J., and Muittari, A., Methacholine bronchial challenge using a dosimeter with controlled tidal breathing, *Thorax*, *43*, 896–900 (1988).
40. Weeke, B., Madsen, F., and Frolund, L., Reproducibility of challenge tests at different times, *Chest*, *91* (suppl.), 83S–89S (1987).
41. Popa, V., and Singleton, J., Provocation dose and discriminant analysis in histamine bronchoprovocation. Are the current predictive data satisfactory? *Chest*, *94*, 466–475 (1988).
42. Kanner, R. E., Schenker, M. B., Munoz, A., and Speizer, F. E., Spirometry in children. Methodology for obtaining optimal results for clinical and epidemiologic studies, *Am. Rev. Respir. Dis.*, *127*, 720–724 (1983).
43. Woolcock, A. J., Yan, K., and Salome, C., Methods for assessing bronchial reactivity, *Eur. J. Respir. Dis. Suppl.*, *128*, 181–195 (1983).

44. Cropp, G. J., Bernstein, I. L., Boushey, H. A., Jr., Hyde, R. W., Rosenthal, R. R., Spector, S. L., and Townley, R. G., Guidelines for bronchial inhalation challenges with pharmacologic and antigenic agents, *ATS News*, 1980, pp. 11–19.
45. Connolly, M. J., Avery, A. J., Walters, E. H., and Hendrick, D. J., The use of sequential doses of inhaled histamine in the measurement of bronchial responsiveness: cumulative effect and distortion produced by shortening the test protocol, *J. Allergy Clin. Immunol.*, *82*, 863–868 (1988).
46. Fetters, L. J., and Matthews, J. I., Methacholine challenge test, *Arch. Intern. Med.*, *144*, 938–940 (1984).
47. Enarson, D. A., Schulzer, M., Vedal, S., and Chan-Yeung, M., Summarizing methacholine bronchoprovocation data in epidemiologic surveys, *Bull. Eur. Physiopathol. Respir.*, *23*, 387–389 (1987).
48. Hopp, R. J., Bewtra, A. K., Nair, N. M., Watt, G. D., and Townley, R. G., Methacholine inhalation challenge studies in a selected pediatric population, *Am. Rev. Respir. Dis.*, *134*, 994–998 (1986).
49. Townley, R. G., Bewtra, A., Wilson, A. F., Hopp, R. J., Elston, R. C., Nair, N., and Watt, G. D., Segregation analysis of bronchial response to methacholine inhalation challenge in families with and without asthma, *J. Allergy Clin. Immunol.*, *77*, 101–107 (1986).
50. Cerveri, I., Bruschi, C., Zoia, M. C., Zanon, P., Maccarini, L., Grassi, M., and Rampulla, C., Distribution of bronchial nonspecific reactivity in the general population, *Chest*, *93*, 26–30 (1988).
51. Madsen, F., Frolund, L., Nielsen, N. H., Svendsen, U. G., and Weeke, B., Fixed ventilation during tidal volume breathing bronchial challenge may improve repeatability, *Allergy*, *42*, 535–540 (1987).
52. Rosenthal, R. R., Summer, W. R., Menkes, H., Norman, P. S., and Permutt, S., The effect of atropine on acute antigen mediated airway constriction in subjects with allergic asthma, *Am. Rev. Respir. Dis.*, *115*, 371–379 (1977).
53. Spector, S. L., and Farr, R. S., A comparison of methacholine and histamine inhalations in asthmatics, *J. Allergy Clin. Immunol.*, *56*, 308–316 (1975).
54. Spector, S. L., and Kinsman, R. A., More implications of reactivity characteristics to methacholine and histamine in asthmatic patients, *J. Allergy Clin. Immunol.*, *64*, 587–589 (1979).
55. Amaro-Galvez, R., McLaughlin, F. J., Levison, H., Rashed, N., Galdes-Sebaldt, M., and Zimmerman, B., Grading severity and treatment requirements to control symptoms in asthmatic children and their relationship with airway hyperreactivity to methacholine, *Ann. Allergy*, *59*, 298–302 (1987).
56. Spector, S. L., Staudenmayer, H., Kinsman, R. A., Fukuhara, J., and Westmoreland, C., Methacholine and histamine inhalation challenges in asthma: relationships to age of onset, length of illness, and pulmonary functions, *Allergy*, *34*, 167–173 (1979).
57. Weiss, S. T., Tager, I. B., Múnoz A., and Speizer, F. E., The relationship of respiratory infections in early childhood to the occurrence of increased levels of bronchial responsiveness and atopy, *Am. Rev. Respir. Dis.*, *131*, 573–578 (1985).
58. Cockroft, D. W., Ruffin, R. E., Frith, P. A., Cartier, A., Juniper, E. F., Dolovich, J., and Hargreave, F. E., Determinants of allergen-induced asthma: dose of allergen,

circulating IgE antibody concentration, and bronchial responsiveness to inhaled histamine, *Am. Rev. Respir. Dis.*, *120*, 1053–1058 (1979).

59. Neijens, H. J., Degenhart, H. J., Raatgeep, H. C., and Herrebijn, K. F., Study on the significance of bronchial hyperreactivity in the bronchus obstruction after inhalation of cat dander allergen, *J. Allergy Clin. Immunol.*, *64*, 507–515 (1979).
60. Enarson, D. A., Chan-Yeung, M., Kus, J., Vedal, S., and Lam, S., Predictors of bronchial hyperexcitability in grainhandlers, *Chest*, *87*, 452–455 (1985).
61. Malo, J. L., Cartier, A., L'Archevêque, J., Ghezzo, H., and Martin, R. R., Bronchoconstriction due to isocapnic cold air inhalation minimally influences bronchial hyperresponsiveness to methacholine in asthmatic subjects, *Bull. Eur. Physiopathol. Respir.*, *22*, 473–477 (1986).
62. Mellis, C. M., Kattan, M., Keens, T. G., Levison, H., Comparative study of histamine and exercise challenges in asthmatic children, *Am. Rev. Respir. Dis.*, *117*, 911–915 (1978).
63. Galdes-Sebalt, M., McLaughlin, F. J., and Levison, H., Comparison of cold air, ultrasonic mist, and methacholine inhalations as tests of bronchial reactivity in normal and asthmatic children, *J. Pediatr.*, *107*, 526–530 (1985).
64. Hopp, R. J., Christy, J., Bewtra, A. K., Nair, N. M., and Townley, R. G., Incorporation and analysis of ultrasonically nebulized distilled water challenges in an epidemiology study of asthma and bronchial reactivity, *Ann. Allergy*, *60*, 129–133 (1988).

9

Bronchial Challenge Testing: In Vivo–In Vitro Correlations

Carol A. Hirshman

The Johns Hopkins University
Baltimore, Maryland

I. INTRODUCTION

Animal models have been useful and will continue to be useful in testing hypotheses about mechanisms of airway hyperresponsiveness that are untestable in humans. In animal models, invasive studies are feasible, airway tissue is easily obtained, and environmental and genetic factors can be reasonably well controlled. Studies in animal models provide important insights into the pathogenesis and treatment of airway hyperresponsiveness. The species chosen for use in a particular study depends on the question to be answered.

In the search for a defect in the airway smooth muscle underlying the airway hyperresponsiveness of asthma, mechanical and biochemical properties of airway smooth muscle have been compared in sensitized and unsensitized animals of several species. Although differences in contractile responses to drugs have been found [1–5], these studies are difficult to interpret because the animals lacked nonspecific airway hyperresponsiveness and the observed differences probably reflected changes associated with atopy, rather than airway hyperresponsiveness. Another approach is to acutely induce airway hyperresponsiveness in experimental animals using air pollutants such as ozone, infectious agents such as viruses and bacteria, inflammatory mediators, or irritants and to compare pharmacological and biochemical properties in the challenged and unchallenged animals. In a recent review of this topic, airway smooth muscle showed increased sensitivity to contractile agonists after some, but not all, types of acute challenge [6]. Moreover, the relevance of studies of acute transient airway hyperresponsiveness to the chronic hyperresponsiveness of human asthma is questionable.

This chapter focuses on the use of the basenji–greyhound (BG) dog model of persistent airway hyperresponsiveness to identify an abnormal biochemical pathway in the airway smooth muscle that may play an important role in the genesis or expression of airway hyperresponsiveness in human asthma.

II. CHARACTERISTICS OF THE BASENJI–GREYHOUND DOG MODEL OF AIRWAY HYPERRESPONSIVENESS

We originally selected, from a colony of basenji dogs crossed with greyhounds, offspring that were unusually sensitive to *Ascaris suum* antigen aerosols [7]. Further breeding has resulted in a line of BG dogs with persistent airway hyperresponsiveness and atopy [8]. We have also bred a small colony of allergic dogs that lack nonspecific airway hyperresponsiveness (purebred basenjis), which we use as a control population.

Basenji–greyhound dogs demonstrate nonspecific airway hyperresponsiveness to methacholine (Fig. 1), histamine (Fig. 1), calcium chelators, and hypotonic aerosols [9–11], as compared with basenjis, greyhounds, or mongrels. As in patients with asthma, propranolol increases airway responsiveness to bronchoconstrictors in BG dogs [12], whereas it is without effect in mongrels, and large-volume ventilation results in bronchoconstriction in BG dogs but results in bronchodilitation in mongrel dogs [13]. Atopy in the BG dog is manifested by a chronic relapsing dermatitis [14] and multiple positive skin tests to allergens common in their native environment [15]. The allergic component can be passively transferred to nonallergic dogs [8,15].

The mechanisms underlying the airway hyperresponsiveness in this model are not yet known. Airway hyperresponsiveness in the BG dog is not related to a decrease in baseline airway caliber [9], to a grossly defective lung epithelial barrier [9,16], or to parasympathetic nervous system predominance [10,17]. Although mononuclear leukocytes from BG dogs show reduced cyclic adenosine monophosphate (cAMP) responses to β-adrenergic agonist [9,11], similar responses are seen in leukocytes from the allergic control dogs [15,18]. Similarly, mast cells from the bronchoalveolar lavage fluid of both BG and allergic control dogs show increased spontaneous histamine release and histamine releasability to the calcium ionophore A23184 [19], indicating that atopy rather than nonspecific airway hyperresponsiveness modified these responses.

These characteristics make the BG dog model of airway hyperresponsiveness a unique means of elucidating a smooth muscle defect underlying airway hyperresponsiveness separate from atopy, drug therapy, and acute disease.

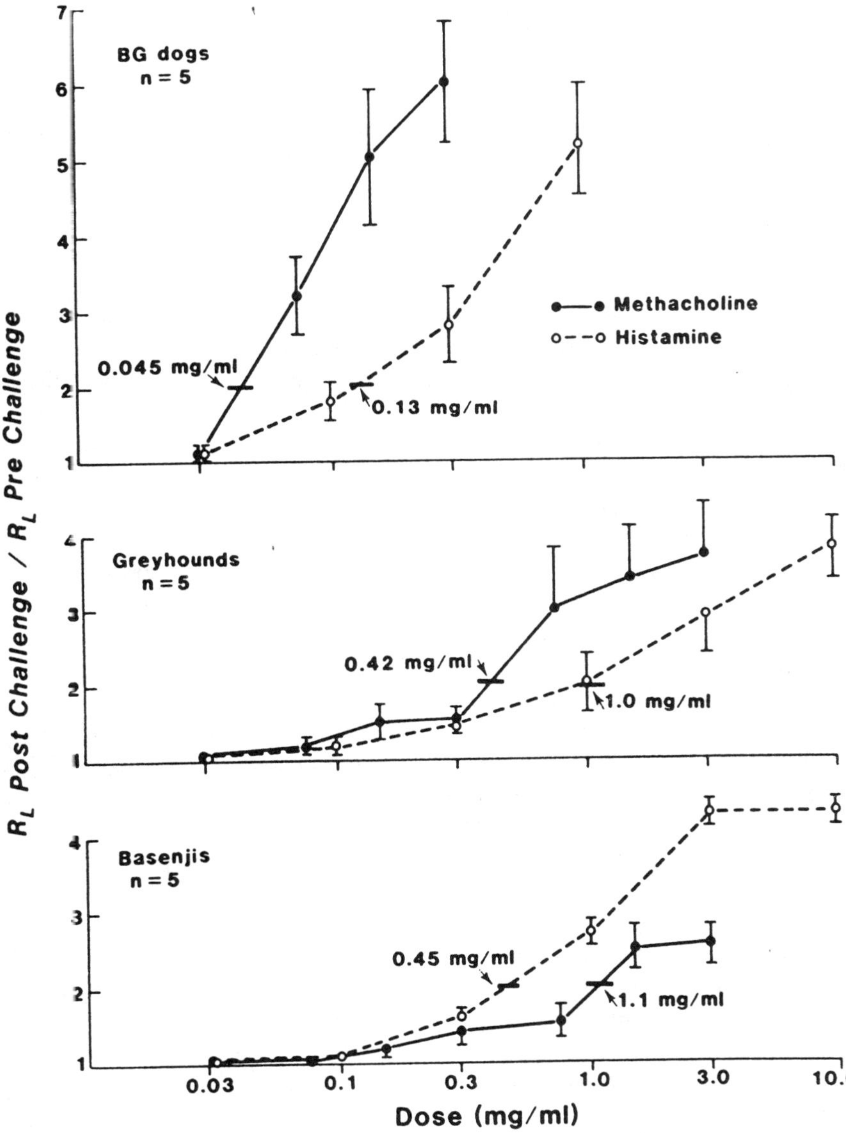

Figure 1 Increase in pulmonary resistance (R_L) to increasing doses of methacholine and histamine. The dose of agonist that increases R_L to twice that of the prechallenge value in basenji–greyhound (BG), basenji, and greyhound dogs is indicated on the graph. (From Ref. 10.)

III. CONTRACTILE RESPONSES

Airway smooth muscle is responsive to a variety of agents. This responsiveness depends on the presence of membrane receptors that are activated by specific agonists and blocked by specific antagonists. The major pharmacological agents used to elicit experimental bronchoconstriction are histamine and cholinergic agonists.

Histamine acting at H_1 receptors can trigger bronchoconstriction in the dog, as in the human, by stimulation of vagal pathways [20–22] as well as by a direct action on bronchial smooth muscle [23,24]. In addition, histamine acting at H_2 receptors has been shown to increase cAMP levels and relax airway smooth muscle [25]. The component of the constrictor response to histamine that is vagally mediated can be prevented by vagal block, vagotomy, or anticholinergic drug pretreatment. In some studies in the dog these interventions have virtually abolished the pulmonary response to histamine [20,26], suggesting that the major effect of histamine in these studies was vagally mediated. Other investigators, however, found that vagal block or vagotomy had no consistent effect on the pulmonary response to histamine in the dog [23,24], or that massive doses of atropine (1 mg/kg intravenously) produced only a slight shift to the right (dose ratio, 3.6) of the dose–response curve for histamine-induced increases in pulmonary resistance [27]. These discrepancies perhaps are explained best on the basis of individual variation, since in dogs, large differences have been demonstrated in both the extent and the character of histamine–vagal interactions [28,29].

Constrictor responses to histamine may be partially antagonized by histamine-stimulated release of catecholamines from the adrenal medulla [30] or intrapulmonary nerve endings [31]. Evidence for an inhibitory effect of H_2 receptors on histamine aerosol challenge in the dog has been obtained only indirectly by the potentiation of histamine-induced airway constriction by H_2 receptor antagonists [21,32].

Cholinergic agonists (methacholine, carbachol, and acetylcholine), on the other hand, are believed to have little or no reflex effect but are thought to act directly on cholinergic receptors on smooth muscle. Binding studies show both M_2 and M_3 muscarinic receptor subtypes in tracheal smooth muscle, with M_2 receptors predominating [33]. Contraction is thought to be mediated by M_3 receptors [34], while inhibition of relaxation is thought to be mediated by M_2 receptors [33].

Despite pharmacological dissimilarities between histamine and cholinergic agonists, and their predilections for different sites of action in the airway, pulmonary responses to cholinergic agonists and histamine are closely correlated, in both experimental animals [10,24] and humans [35]. This indicates that airway hyperresponsiveness is not restricted to responses initiated by a specific receptor.

In a large group of mongrel dogs, Snapper and co-workers [36] showed a wide range in pulmonary responses to histamine, which were unrelated to age, sex, weight, and baseline pulmonary function. Moreover, responses to histamine in individual animals were reproducible over 20 months and, in this population of 102 dogs, were distributed in a unimodal fashion, with animals that were unusually responsive falling at one extreme of the distribution, rather than in a bimodal fashion, with a normal and an abnormal population.

Most dog models of asthma fail to demonstrate the airway hyperresponsiveness characteristic of human asthma [37], most likely because the animals are often selected for use on the basis of allergic sensitivity to *Ascaris* antigen rather than airway hyperresponsiveness. By selecting dogs at the responsive end of the distribution that were in addition atopic, we thought we would come closer to identifying a mechanism underlying the airway hyperresponsiveness of asthma. We have shown marked airway hyperresponsiveness to aerosols of methacholine and histamine in an inbred population of BG dogs, as compared with purebred greyhounds, which were not atopic, and purebred basenjis, which were atopic [10,15] (Table 1, Fig. 1).

At 2 years of age, dogs of each breed were sacrificed, and responses to methacholine and histamine in vitro were compared with the in vivo responses obtained within the prior 6 weeks. We found that trachealis muscle from the BG dogs and from the allergic control dogs (basenjis) was significantly less sensitive (not more sensitive) to methacholine than trachealis muscle from the nonallergic control dogs (greyhounds) (Fig. 2) and that trachealis muscle from all three breeds showed similar sensitivity to histamine [38,39]. Broadstone and colleagues [40] had similar findings in horses. In vitro, the airway smooth muscle from horses with in vivo cholinergic airway hyperresponsiveness showed decreased, not increased, sensitivity to acetylcholine. Similarly, Weinmann and associates [41] found that tracheal tissue from mice with in vivo cholinergic airway hyperresponsiveness [42] did not show increased in vitro cholinergic sensitivity. It is interesting to note that several studies that examined the relationship of in vivo airway hyperreactivity and pharmacological responsiveness of human asthmatic airway tissue in vitro also failed to find a positive correlation between in vivo and in vitro contractile responses [43–47]. In fact, Whicker and co-workers [47] and Goldie and associ-

Table 1 Characteristics of Dog Populations

Breed	Hyperresponsive to histamine and methacholine	Atopic
BG	Yes	Yes
Greyhounds	No	No
Basenjis	No	Yes

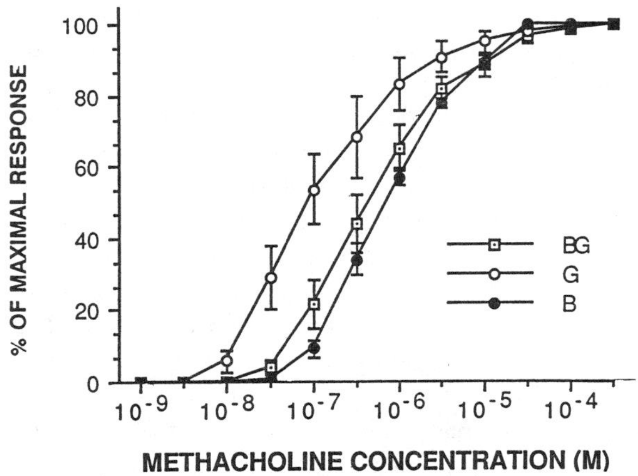

Figure 2 Cumulative dose–response curves for methacholine-induced contraction in thoracic trachealis muscle from five basenji–greyhounds (BG) dogs, greyhounds, and basenjis. Methacholine was less potent in trachealis preparations from the BG dogs and basenjis than in those from the greyhounds ($p < .05$). (From C. A. Hirshman and H. Downes: Experimental asthma in animals, in *Bronchial Asthma: Mechanisms and Therapeutics*, 3rd Ed. [E. W. Weiss, M. S. Segal, and M. Stein, eds.], Little, Brown, & Co., Boston, 1993.)

ates [45] showed decreased in vitro sensitivity to cholinergic agonists in bronchial preparations obtained from asthmatic subjects. These studies, however, unlike the studies in animal models, have been difficult to interpret because of the confounding factors of prior drug therapy and end-stage disease.

IV. RELAXANT RESPONSES

Two types of adrenergic receptor have been described in canine airway smooth muscle: α and β_2 receptors. Stimulation of α receptors constricts airway smooth muscle, whereas stimulation of β_2 receptors relaxes it. Studies support the existence of α receptors in the airway muscle of the dog [48], although the response generated by stimulation of these receptors is small (10–20% of the maximal response elicited by acetylcholine). Thus, α receptor stimulation probably produces only mild bronchoconstriction.

Although stimulation of adrenergic nerve fibers causes relaxation of airway smooth muscle, adrenergic innervation of the lung is sparse; and norepinephrine, the predominant neurotransmitter released, is much less potent than epinephrine as a β_2-adrenergic agonist [49]. Therefore, it seems likely that the major sympathetic control of bronchomotor tone is mediated by circulating epinephrine. This view is supported by similar effects of adrenalectomy and β-adrenergic blockade on the pulmonary response to airway challenge [50,51].

Mongrel dogs do not develop airway constriction after administration of propranolol [52,53], nor does propranolol potentiate the pulmonary responses to administered agonists [53] in mongrel dogs. In contrast, the BG dog does develop baseline airway constriction [12] as well as enhanced pulmonary responses to aerosols of antigen, citric acid, and methacholine after β-adrenergic blockade with propranolol [12,54].

The intracellular events involved in the relaxation of airway smooth muscle are not completely understood, but increased accumulation of cAMP is thought to play a pivotal role. β-Adrenergic agonists increase cAMP levels in airway muscle via activation of the catecholamine-sensitive adenylyl cyclase complex. Since Szentivanyi [55] proposed in 1968 that asthma might be due to an inherited or acquired deficit in β-adrenergic function, much research has focused on the β-adrenergic receptor and the β-adrenergic cascade. However, over 20 years later the question is still unsettled, because research has largely focused on the leukocyte, and a great deal of evidence indicating that the leukocyte is a poor model of human asthma has accumulated. Although several studies have demonstrated that leukocytes from asthmatic patients and allergic dogs with chronic airway hyperresponsiveness show reduced cAMP response to β agonists, similar responses are seen in leukocytes from normal subjects following treatment with β agonists, in leukocytes from atopic subjects who do not have asthma, and in leukocytes from atopic dogs [15] that do not have airway hyperreactivity. In addition, leukocytes from some asthmatic patients show this β deficit only after allergen exposure [56]. Moreover, β-adrenergic receptors on lung tissue and on leukocytes show markedly different susceptibilities to desensitization by β agonists [57].

However, compelling evidence in favor of decreased β-adrenergic sensitivity in asthma comes from studies of bronchial muscle tissue obtained from animal models of asthma [1,2,38–40,58,59] and from studies of tissues of asthmatic subjects (obtained either at surgery or at autopsy) that showed a deficit in β-adrenergic function. These results have largely been buried in studies showing a poor correlation between in vivo and in vitro responses to contractile agonists [43–46] in asthma and have led to the present bias that an intrinsic defect does not reside in the smooth muscle of the airway. However, close examination of these data reveals significant differences in relaxation between tissue from asthmatic and nonasthmatic subjects. Cerrina and associates [44] related airway responsiveness to aerosolized histamine in vivo to the effects produced by isoproterenol in histamine-preconstricted airways in vitro. Four of the 19 subjects were asthmatic. Airways from asthmatic subjects showed in vitro insensitivity to isoproterenol, with an inverse relationship to in vivo responses, suggesting that β-adrenergic function decreased as the level of in vivo airway hyperresponsiveness increased.

Goldie and co-workers [45], using human bronchial preparations obtained at autopsy from 32 nonasthmatic and seven asthmatic subjects and preconstricted with carbachol, found that asthmatic tissue was three to 20 times less sensitive to isoproterenol than control tissue, whereas sensitivity to theophylline was comparable.

Similarly, trachealis muscle obtained from the BG dog model showed decreased sensitivity to isoproterenol as compared with trachealis from control dogs when the muscle was precontracted with methacholine [38,39] (Fig. 3). This decreased sensitivity to isoproterenol could not be related to prior drug therapy, since no animal had ever received therapy with β-adrenergic agonists or steroids. Moreover, this β-adrenergic deficit in the airway smooth muscle was not seen in a control population of allergic dogs lacking airway hyperresponsiveness, suggesting that the decreased sensitivity to β-adrenergic agonists was related in some way to airway hyperresponsiveness to cholinergic agonists.

Dr. C. G. Emala in our laboratory [60] has recently characterized the biochemical pathway from the β-adrenergic receptor through the G protein to activation of adenylyl cyclase in trachealis muscle membranes of the BG dog. He found

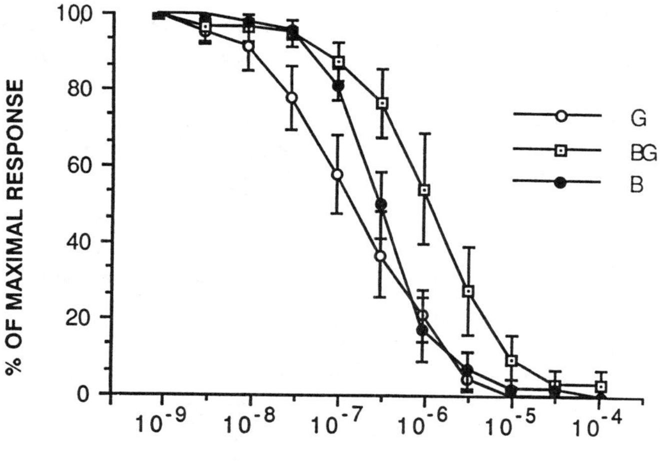

Figure 3 Cumulative dose–response curves for isoproterenol-induced relaxation in thoracic trachealis muscle from five basenji–greyhound (BG) dogs, greyhounds, and basenjis. Preparations were precontracted with methacholine (EC_{50}). Isoproterenol was less potent in trachealis preparations from the BG dogs than in those from the basenjis and greyhounds ($p < .05$). (From C. A. Hirshman and H. Downes: Experimental asthma in animals, in *Bronchial Asthma: Mechanisms and Therapeutics*, 3rd Ed. [E. W. Weiss, M. S. Segal, and M. Stein, eds.], Little, Brown & Co., Boston, 1993.)

biochemical evidence for impaired generation of cAMP in response to β-adrenergic agonists in muscle membranes from the BG dog. Agents that bypassed the β-adrenergic receptor, such as forskolin, prostaglandin E, and aluminum fluoride activated adenylyl cyclase to a similar extent in BG and control muscle membranes, and the quantities of $G_s\alpha$ were similar. However, β-adrenergic receptor numbers were increased, not decreased, in the muscle membranes of BG dogs as compared with control dogs, with no difference in agonist binding, suggesting that the impaired generation of cAMP was due to a defect in coupling between the β-adrenergic receptor and the $G_s\alpha$.

The increased numbers of β-adrenergic receptors seen in our study are in contrast to at least five reports of reduced numbers of β-adrenergic receptors seen in animal models of allergic inflammation [61–63], suggesting that the mechanism underlying the β-adrenergic agonist impairment in the BG dog is not simply an inflammatory process. Our studies, however, agree well with three studies of human asthmatic airways that showed increased numbers of β-adrenergic receptors in the same airway tissues, which were hyporesponsive to β-adrenergic agonists in organ bath studies. Tissues from nonasthmatic subjects [64–66] were used as controls.

These data are not consistent with β-adrenergic receptor desensitization by prior adrenergic drug therapy, where decreased, not increased, numbers of β-adrenergic receptors would be expected. Consistent with this view, the dogs in our study had never received β agonist drugs. Two asthmatic subjects in the study by Goldie et al. [45] whose airway tissue showed decreased sensitivity to β-adrenergic drugs were not receiving β-adrenergic drugs, and β-adrenergic drugs had been withdrawn two weeks before surgery in the study by Cerrina et al. [44]; yet airway tissue from the subjects with asthma again showed decreased sensitivity to β-adrenergic agonists.

In vivo evidence for impaired β-adrenergic–mediated bronchodilation in mild asthma in humans has been conflicting [67,68]. However, during acute exacerbations in severe asthma, bronchodilation in response to parenteral or inhaled β-adrenergic agonists is significantly impaired [69]. Three important questions remain to be addressed: Where is the site of the defect in the airway smooth muscle in human asthmatics? If it is not a genetic defect, how is it induced? Does the defect contribute to morbidity and mortality in human asthmatics?

V. MODULATION OF CONTRACTILE RESPONSES BY β-ADRENERGIC AGONISTS AND CORTICOSTEROIDS

A second way that impaired β-adrenergic responsiveness may contribute to morbidity and mortality is by failing to decrease sensitivity of the muscle to constrictor stimuli. This is an area that is still poorly understood. Several studies have looked at changes in bronchial responsiveness in subjects with mild asthma after a single dose of a β-adrenergic agonist and found decreases in bronchial responsiveness as measured by shifts to the right of the dose–response curves to histamine and methacholine [70]. However, two recent studies [71] have observed tolerance to this effect after chronic use, and a recent study be Bel et al. [72] showed that β-adrenergic agonists failed to protect against excessive airway narrowing in asthmatics, but did protect in patients with chronic obstructive pulmonary disease. These studies, although interesting, are difficult to interpret because the study subjects are usually mild asthmatics in whom asthma therapy has been discontinued for the duration of the study, and the control group, if present, is not studied at the same degree of airway constriction.

We have addressed this issue recently by comparing the ability of the β-adrenergic agonist albuterol to attenuate airway responses to methacholine and histamine in BG and mongrel dogs. We found that when the airway was constricted with methacholine, β-adrenergic agonists were significantly less effective in protecting against the development of airway constriction (Fig. 4) [73] in BG than in control dogs. This was also observed in Lindeman et al. [74] in the small airways of the lung periphery in these same animals.

Trachealis and bronchial smooth muscle from these animals showed similar impaired responses. Pretreatment with the β-adrenergic agonist failed to modify methacholine sensitivity in the muscle from the BG dog, whereas it significantly decreased sensitivity in muscle from the mongrel control dogs [75]. Pretreatment with agonists that bypassed the β-adrenergic receptor significantly decreased methacholine sensitivity in airway muscle of the BG dog. This functional impairment correlated well with the decreased generation of cAMP in response to β-adrenergic agonists in membranes from the same muscle. These studies provide further evidence that impaired responses to β-adrenergic agonists modify contractile responses to cholinergic agonists differently, both in vivo and in vitro in BG dogs.

Although long-term treatment with corticosteroids is associated with reduced responses to constrictor stimuli such as histamine and methacholine, the magnitude of the reduction in airway responsiveness in studies in human asthmatics has been variable [76]. Similar results were found in the BG dog. Administration of methylprednisolone (2 mg/kg/d) for 6 weeks had little effect on methacholine responsiveness in BG dogs [77–79]. However, corticosteroids restored the protective effect of β-adrenergic agonists on airway responses to contractile agonists in the same BG dogs [78] (Fig. 5). The mechanisms involved are not known. Corticosteroids may prevent development of the decreased sensitivity to β agonists or may enhance β-adrenergic–mediated smooth muscle function by increasing the numbers of receptors or improving coupling between the receptor and the G protein.

Although numerous studies have looked at the effects of corticosteroids on airway responsiveness, few studies have addressed the issue of steroid withdrawal

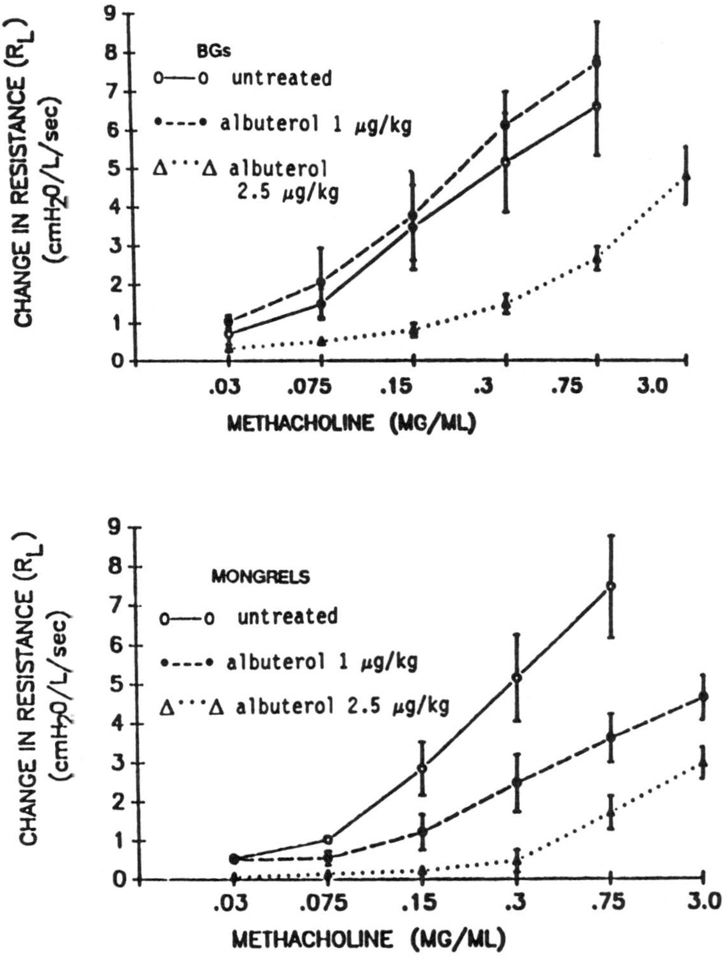

Figure 4 Change in pulmonary resistance (R_L) with increasing concentrations of methacholine in basenji–greyhound (BG) dogs (above) and mongrel dogs (below) untreated and pretreated with albuterol 1 and 2.5 μg/kg. Each point represents mean ± SEM of five dogs. (Modified from Ref. 73.)

and airway responsiveness. In a recent study in the BG dog in which 4 weeks of treatment with methylprednisolone had no beneficial effect on cholinergic responsiveness, corticosteroid withdrawal was associated with an increase in cholinergic responsiveness, which persisted for up to 2 weeks in this model [79]. This enhancement did not reflect a seasonal increase in airway responsiveness, since responses in untreated control animals were not altered during the same period.

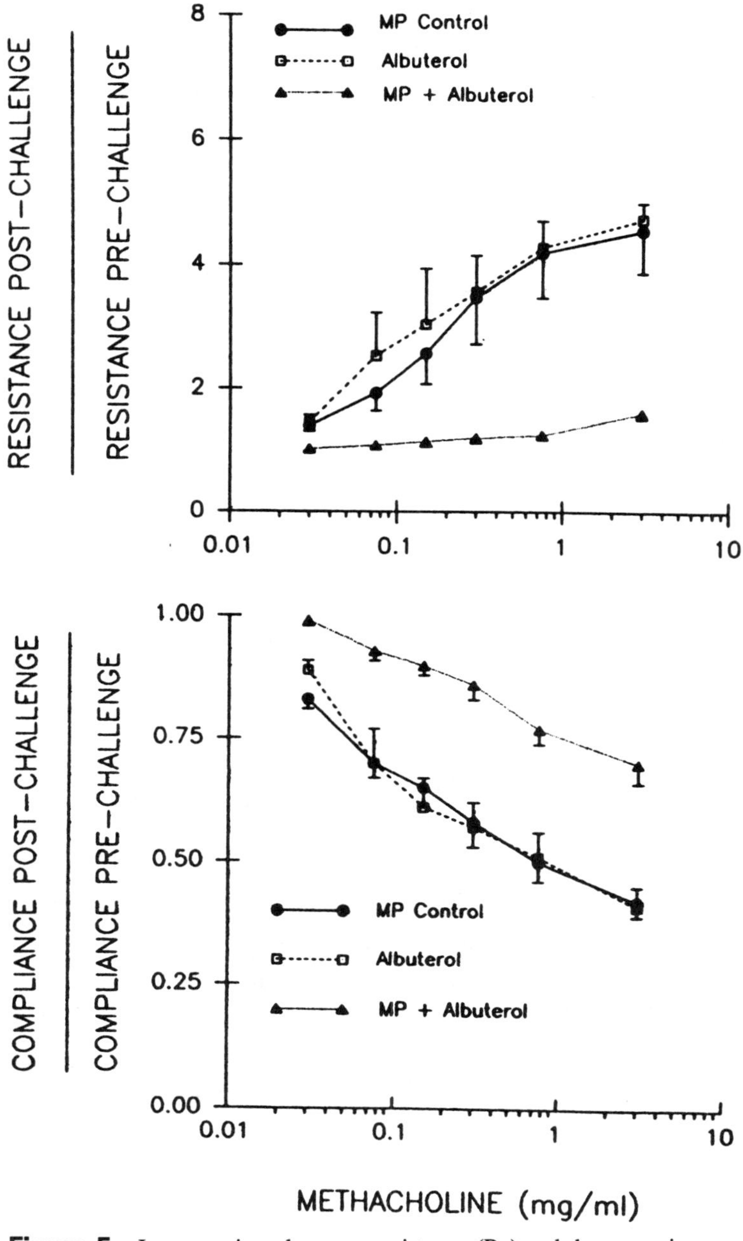

Figure 5 Increases in pulmonary resistance (R_L) and decreases in compliance (C_{dyn}) with increasing concentrations of methacholine in basenji–greyhound (BG) dogs during week 3 of chronic methylprednisolone (MP) treatment, during week 3 of chronic MP treatment and pretreatment with albuterol (1 μg/kg), and after pretreatment with albuterol (1 μg/kg) before chronic MP treatment. Each point represents mean ± SEM of five dogs. (From Ref. 78.)

This may be in some way related to the phenomenon of asthma relapse, in which some steroid-dependent asthmatics develop life-threatening asthma after abrupt steroid withdrawal [80].

VI. SUMMARY

Studies demonstrate that the airways of BG dogs show an impaired response to β-adrenergic agonists. This is manifested both in vivo and in vitro by decreased sensitivity to relaxing agonists and failure of β agonists to protect against the development of constriction. The impairment in the airway smooth muscle of this model has some striking similarities to findings of studies of airways of patients with asthma showing decreased generation of cAMP but increased numbers of β receptors, suggesting impaired β receptor–G protein coupling. It is possible that a genetic defect exists in the β receptor gene. A more likely possibility is that this defect is induced as a result of the disease process. The activation of immune mechanisms and chemoattractants or the release of proteoglycans, and of cytokines from inflammatory cells, may play a role in inducing this defect.

REFERENCES

1. Souhrada, J. F., Changes of airway smooth muscle in experimental asthma. *Respir. Physiol.*, *32*, 79–90 (1978).
2. Rubinfeld, A. R., Rinard, G. A., and Mayer, S. E., Responsiveness of isolated tracheal smooth muscle in a canine model of asthma, *Lung*, *160*, 99–107 (1982).
3. Antonissen, L. A., Mitchell, R. W., Kroeger, R. W., Kepron, E. A., Tse, K. S., and Stephens, N. L., Mechanical alterations of airway smooth muscle in a canine asthmatic model, *J. Appl. Physiol.*, *46*, 681–687 (1979).
4. Kaukel, E., Beier, W., Fedderson, C., Schrum, C., and Koppermann, G., Mechanical and biochemical alterations in guinea pig tracheae caused by sensitization, *Respiration*, *45*, 255–261 (1984).
5. Morcillo, E., Perpina, J., and Esplugues, J., Hyperresponsiveness to autocoids and autonomic drugs in lung parenchymal strips from sensitized animals, *Am. Rev. Respir. Dis.*, *129*, 948–951 (1984).
6. Black, J. L., and Armour, C. L., Induction of hyperresponsiveness in human airways in vivo and in vitro, *Pulm. Pharmacol.*, *2*, 169–178 (1989).
7. Hirshman, C. A., Asthma. *Comp. Pathol. Bull.*, *7*, 3–4 (1985).
8. Hirshman, C. A., Downes, H., and Veith, L., Airway responses in offspring of dogs with and without airway hyperreactivity, *J. Appl. Physiol.*, *56*, 1272–1277 (1984).
9. Hirshman, C. A., Malley, A., and Downes, H., The basenji–greyhound dog model of asthma: reactivity to *Ascaris suum*, citric acid and methacholine, *J. Appl. Physiol.*, *49*, 953–957 (1980).
10. Hirshman, C. A., and Downes, H., Airway responses to methacholine and histamine in basenji–greyhound and other purebred dogs, *Respir. Physiol.*, *63*, 339–346 (1986).
11. Osborne, M. L., Evans, T. W., Sommerhoff, C. P., Chung, K. F., Hirshman, C. A.,

Boushey, H. A., and Nadel, J. A., Hyptonic and isotonic aerosols increase bronchial reactivity in basenji–greyhound dogs, *Am. Rev. Respir. Dis.*, *135*, 345–349 (1987).

12. Hirshman, C. A., Downes, H., Leon, D. A., and Peters, J. E., The basenji–greyhound dog model of asthma: pulmonary responses after β-adrenergic blockade, *J. Appl. Physiol.*, *51*, 1423–1427 (1981).
13. Davidson, A. B., Hirshman, C. A., Downes, H., and Drazen, J. M., Large volume ventilation results in bronchoconstriction in basenji–greyhound crossbred dogs, *J. Appl. Physiol.*, *62*, 2308–2313 (1987).
14. Butler, J. M., Peters, J. E., Hirshman, C. A., White, C. R., Margolin, L. B., and Hanifin, J. M., Pruritic dermatitis in asthmatic basenji–greyhound dogs: a model for human atopic dermatitis, *J. Am. Acad. Dermatol.*, *8*, 33–38 (1983).
15. Hirshman, C. A., Leu, D. B., Austin, D. R., Chan, S. C., Veith, L., and Hanifin, J. M., Elevated mononuclear leukocyte phosphodiesterase in allergic dogs with and without airway hyperresponsiveness, *J. Allergy Clin. Immunol.*, *79*, 46–53 (1987).
16. Taylor, S. M., Downes, H., Hirshman, C. A., Peters, J. E., and Leon, D., Pulmonary uptake of mannitol as an index of lung epithelial permeability, *J. Appl. Physiol.*, *55*, 614–618 (1983).
17. Hirshman, C. A., and Downes, H., The basenji–greyhound dog model of asthma: influence of atropine on antigen-induced bronchoconstriction, *J. Appl. Physiol.*, *50*, 761–765 (1981).
18. Chan, S. C., Hanifin, J. M., Holden, C. A., Thompson, W. J., and Hirshman, C. A., Elevated leukocyte phosphodiesterase as a basis for depressed cyclic adenosine monophosphate responses in the basenji–greyhound dog model of asthma, *J. Allergy Clin. Immunol.*, *76*, 148–158 (1985).
19. Hirshman, C. A., Austin, D. R., and Kettelkamp, N. S., Enhanced bronchoalveolar lavage cell histamine releasability in allergic dogs with and without airway hyperresponsiveness, *J. Allergy Clin. Immunol.*, *81*, 829–835 (1988).
20. Dain, D., and Gold, W. M., Mechanical properties of the lungs and experimental asthma in conscious allergic dogs, *J. Appl. Physiol.*, *38*, 96–100 (1975).
21. Yamatake, Y., Sasagawa, S., and Yanaura, S., Involvement of histamine H_1- and H_2-receptors in induced asthma in dogs, *Jpn. J. Pharmacol.*, *27*, 791–797 (1977).
22. Dixon, M., Jackson, D. M., and Richards, I. M., The effects of histamine, acetylcholine and 5-hydroxytryptamine on lung mechanics and irritant receptors in the dog, *J. Physiol. (Lond.)*, *287*, 393–403 (1979).
23. Loring, S. H., Drazen, J. M., and Ingram, R. H., Canine pulmonary response to aerosol histamine: direct versus vagal effects, *J. Appl. Physiol.*, *42*, 946–952 (1977).
24. Snapper, J. R., Drazen, J. M., Loring, S. H., Braasch, P. S., and Ingram, R. H., Vagal effects on histamine, carbachol, and prostaglandin $F_{2\alpha}$ responsiveness in the dog, *J. Appl. Physiol.*, *47*, 13–16 (1979).
25. Florio, C., Flezar, M., Martin, J. G., and Heisler, S., Identification of adenylate cyclase–coupled histamine H_2 receptors in guinea pig tracheal smooth muscle cells in culture and the effect of dexamethasone, *Am. J. Respir. Cell. Mol. Biol.*, *7*, 582–589 (1992).
26. Gold, W. M., Kessler, G.-F., and Yu, D. Y. C., Role of vagus nerves in experimental asthma in allergic dogs, *J. Appl. Physiol.*, *33*, 719–725 (1972).

27. Krell, R. D., Charkrin, L. W., and Wardell, J. R., The effect of cholinergic agents on a canine model of allergic asthma, *J. Allergy Clin. Immunol.*, *58*, 19–30 (1976).
28. Loring, S. H., Drazen, J. M., Snapper, J. R., and Ingram, R. H., Vagal and aerosol histamine interactions on airway responses in dogs, *J. Appl. Physiol.*, *45*, 40–44 (1978).
29. Vanta, M. A., Loring, S. H., Ingram, R. H., and Drazen, J. M., Direct and reflex bronchoconstriction induced by histamine aerosol inhalation in dogs, *J. Appl. Physiol.*, *50*, 869–873 (1981).
30. Staszewska-Barczak, J., and Vane, J. R., The release of catecholamine from the adrenal medulla by histamine, *Br. J. Pharmacol.*, *25*, 728–742 (1965).
31. Maengwyn-Davies, G. D., The dual mode of action of histamine in the cat isolated tracheal chain, *J. Pharm. Pharmacol.*, *20*, 572–573 (1968).
32. Snapper, J. R., Braasch, P. S., Ingram, R. H., Loring, S. H., and Drazen, J. M., In vivo effect of cimetidine on canine pulmonary responsiveness to aerosol histamine, *J. Allergy Clin. Immunol.*, *66*, 70–74 (1980).
33. Fernandes, L. B., Fryer, A. D., and Hirshman, C. A., M_2 muscarinic receptors inhibit isoproterenol-induced relaxation of canine airway smooth muscle, *J. Pharmacol. Exp. Ther.*, *262*, 119–126 (1992).
34. Roffel, A. D., Elzing, C. R. S., Van Amsterdam, G. M., deZeeuw, R. A., and Zaagsma, J., Muscarinic M_2 receptors in bovine tracheal smooth muscle: discrepancies between binding and function, *Eur. J. Pharmacol.*, *153*, 73–82 (1988).
35. Spector, S. L., and Farr, R. S., A comparison of methacholine and histamine inhalations in asthmatics, *J. Allergy Clin. Immunol.*, *56*, 308–316 (1975).
36. Snapper, J. R., Drazen, J. M., Loring, S. H., Schneider, W., and Ingram, R. H., Distribution of pulmonary responsiveness to aerosol histamine in dogs, *J. Appl. Physiol.*, *44*, 738–742 (1978).
37. Krell, R. D., and Chakrin, L. W., Canine airway responses to acetylcholine, prostaglandin $F_{2\alpha}$, histamine, and serotonin after chronic antigen exposure, *J. Allergy Clin. Immunol.*, *58*, 664–675 (1976).
38. Downes, H., Austin, D. R., Parks, C. M., and Hirshman, C. A., Comparison of drug responses in vivo and in vitro in airways of dogs with and without airway hyperresponsiveness, *J. Pharmacol. Exp. Ther.*, *237*, 214–219 (1986).
39. Downes, H., Austin, D. R., Parks, C. M., and Hirshman, C. A., Comparison of in vitro drug responses in airways of atopic dogs with and without in vivo hyperresponsiveness, *Pulm. Pharmacol.*, *2*, 209–216 (1989).
40. Broadstone, R. V., LeBlanc, P. H., Derkson, F. J., and Robinson, N. E., In vitro responses to acetylcholine and electrical stimulation of airways from horses with recurrent obstructive pulmonary disease, *Physiologist*, *32*, 180 (1989).
41. Weinmann, C. G., Black, C. M., Levitt, R. C., and Hirshman, C. A., In vitro tracheal responses from mice chosen for in vivo lung cholinergic sensitivity, *J. Appl. Physiol.*, *69*, 274–280 (1990).
42. Levitt, R. C., and Mitzner, W., Expression of airway hyperreactivity to acetylcholine as a simple autosomal recessive trait in mice, *FASEB J.*, *2*, 2605–2608 (1988).
43. Bai, T. R., Abnormalities in airway smooth muscle in fatal asthma, *Am. Rev. Respir. Dis.*, *141*, 552–557 (1990).

44. Cerrina, J., Ladurie, M. L. R., Labat, C., Raffestin, B., Bayol, A., and Brink, C., Comparison of human bronchial muscle responses to histamine in vivo with histamine and isoproterenol agonists in vitro, *Am. Rev. Respir. Dis.*, *134*, 57–61 (1986).
45. Goldie, R. G., Spina, D., Henry, P. J., Lulich, K. M., and Patterson, J. W., In vitro responsiveness of human asthmatic bronchus to carbachol, histamine, β-adrenoceptor agonists and aminophylline, *Br. J. Clin. Pharmacol.*, *22*, 669–676 (1986).
46. Thomson, N. C., Airway disease and bronchodilators: in vivo versus in vitro human airway responsiveness to different pharmacologic stimuli, *Am. Rev. Respir. Dis.*, *136*, S58–S73 (1987).
47. Whicker, S. D., Armour, C. L., and Black, J. L., Responsiveness of bronchial smooth muscle from asthmatic patients to relaxant and contractile agonists, *Pulm. Pharmacol.*, *2*, 25–31 (1989).
48. Leff, A. R., and Munoz, N. M., Evidence for two subtypes of alpha-adrenergic receptors in canine airway smooth muscle, *J. Pharmacol. Exp. Ther.*, *217*, 530–535 (1981).
49. Chahl, L. A., and O'Donnell, S. R., The interaction of cocaine and propranolol with catecholamines on guinea pig trachea, *Eur. J. Pharmacol.*, *2*, 77–82 (1967).
50. Colebatch, H. J. H., and Mitchell, C. A., Constriction of isolated living liquid-filled dog and cat lungs with histamine, *J. Appl. Physiol.*, *30*, 691–702 (1971).
51. Diamond, L., Potentiation of bronchomotor responses by beta-adrenergic agonists, *J. Pharmacol. Exp. Ther.*, *181*, 434–445 (1972).
52. Nisam, M. R., Zbinden, A., Chesrown, S., Barnett, D., and Gold, W. M., Distribution and pharmacological release of histamine in canine lung in vivo, *J. Appl. Physiol.*, *44*, 455–463 (1978).
53. Snapper, J. R., Braasch, P. S., Ingram, R. H., Loring, S. H., and Drazen, J. M., Effects of beta-adrenergic blockade on muscarinic and prostaglandin responsiveness in the dog, *J. Allergy Clin. Immunol.*, *67*, 199–205 (1981).
54. Tobias, J. D., Sauder, R. A., and Hirshman, C. A., Pulmonary reactivity to methacholine during β-adrenergic blockade: propranolol vs. esmolol, *Anesthesiology*, *73*, 132–136 (1990).
55. Szentivanyi, A., The beta-adrenergic theory of the atopic abnormality in bronchial asthma, *J. Allergy*, *42*, 203–232 (1968).
56. Meurs, H., Köeter, G. H., de Vries, K., and Kaufman, H. F., The beta-adrenergic system and allergic bronchial asthma: changes in lymphocyte beta-adrenergic number and adenylate cyclase activity after an allergen asthmatic attack, *J. Allergy Clin. Immunol.*, *70*, 272–280 (1982).
57. Hasegawa, M., and Townley, R. G., Difference between lung and spleen susceptibility of beta-adrenergic receptors to desensitization by terbutaline, *J. Allergy Clin. Immunol.*, *71*, 230–238 (1983).
58. Mirbahar, K. B., and Eyre, P., Autacoid and autonomic reactivity of bovine and ovine bronchus: modifications by antigenic sensitization, *Arch. Int. Pharmacodyn.*, *258*, 60–70 (1982).
59. Robinson, E. H., Broadstone, R. V., LeBlanc, P. H., and Derkson, F. J., Isoproterenol and electrically stimulated relaxation of airways from horses with recurrent obstructive pulmonary disease, *Physiologist*, *32*, 179 (1989).

60. Emala, C., Park, G., Levine, M. A., and Hirshman, C. A., Altered β-adrenergic G protein coupling in tracheal muscle of the BG dog (abstr.), *Am. Rev. Respir. Dis.*, *145*, A567 (1992).
61. Bai, T. R., Beta$_2$-adrenergic receptors in asthma: a current perspective, *Lung*, *170*, 125–141 (1992).
62. Motojima, S., Yukawa, T., Fulcade, T., and Mukino, S., Changes in airway responsiveness and β and α_1 adrenergic receptors in the lungs of guinea pigs with experimental asthma, *Allergy*, *44*, 66–69 (1989).
63. Szentivanyi, A., Heim, O., and Schultz, P., Changes in adrenoceptor densities in membranes of lung tissue and lymphocytes from patients with atopic disease, *Ann. NY Acad. Sci.*, *332*, 295–298 (1979).
64. Bai, T. R., Mak, J. C. W., and Barnes, P. J., A comparison of β-adrenergic receptors and in vitro relaxant responses to isoproterenol in asthmatic airway smooth muscle, *Am. J. Respir. Cell. Mol. Biol.*, *6*, 647–651 (1992).
65. Spina, D., Rigby, P. J., Paterson, J. W., and Goldie, R. G., Autoradiographic localization of beta-adrenoceptors in asthmatic human lung, *Am. Rev. Respir. Dis.*, *140*, 1410–1415 (1989).
66. Sharma, P. K., and Jeffry, P. K., Airway β-adrenoceptor number in cystic fibrosis and asthma, *Clin. Sci.*, *78*, 409–417 (1990).
67. Barnes, P. J., and Pride, N. B., Dose-response curves to inhaled β-adrenoceptor agonists in normal and asthmatic subjects, *Br. J. Clin. Pharmacol.*, *15*, 677–682 (1983).
68. Cheung, D., Timmers, M. C., Zwinderman, A. H., Bel, E. H., Dijkman, J. H., and Sterk, P. J., Long term effects of a long acting β_2-adrenoceptor agonist, salmeterol, on airway hyperresponsiveness in patients with mild asthma, *N. Engl. J. Med.*, *327*, 1198–1203 (1992).
69. Rebuck, A. S., and Read, J., Assessment and management of severe asthma, *Am. J. Med.*, *51*, 788–798 (1971).
70. Tattersfield, A. E., Effect of beta agonists and anticholinergic drugs on bronchial reactivity, *Am. Rev. Respir. Dis.*, *136*, S64–S68 (1987).
71. O'Connor, B. J., Aikman, S. L., and Barnes, P. J., Tolerance to the nonbronchodilator effects of inhaled β_2 agonists in asthma, *N. Engl. J. Med.*, *327*, 1204–1208 (1992).
72. Bel, E. H., Zwinderman, A. H., Timmers, M. C., Dijkman, J. H., and Sterk, P. J., The protective effect of a beta$_2$ agonist against excessive airway narrowing in response to bronchoconstrictor stimuli in asthma and chronic obstructive lung disease, *Thorax*, *46*, 9–14 (1991).
73. Tobias, J. D., Sauder, R. A., and Hirshman, C. A., Reduced sensitivity to β-adrenergic agonists in basenji–greyhound dogs, *J. Appl. Physiol.*, *69*, 1212–1219 (1990).
74. Lindeman, K. S., Hirshman, C. A., and Freed, A. N., Functional antagonism of airway constriction in the canine lung periphery, *J. Appl. Physiol.*, *68*, 1114–1120 (1990).
75. Black, C., Curry, C., and Hirshman, C. A., Mechanism of decreased sensitivity to β agonists in trachealis of basenji–greyhounds (abstr.), *FASEB J.*, *5*, A1237 (1991).
76. Tattersfield, A. E., and Barnes, P. J., Beta$_2$ agonists and corticosteroids, new developments and controversies, *Am. Rev. Respir. Dis.*, *146*, 1637–1641 (1992).
77. Darowski, M. J., Hannon, V. M., and Hirshman, C. A., Corticosteroids decrease

airway hyperresponsiveness in the basenji–greyhound dog model of asthma, *J. Appl. Physiol.*, *66*, 1120–1126 (1989).

78. Sauder, R. A., Tobias, J. D., and Hirshman, C. A., Methylprednisolone restores sensitivity to beta-adrenergic agonists in basenji–greyhound dogs, *J. Appl. Physiol.*, *72*, 694–698 (1992).
79. Lindeman, K. S., and Hirshman, C. A., Glucocorticoids reduced mediator release in canine peripheral airways (abstr.), *Am. Rev. Respir. Dis.*, *145*, A380 (1992).
80. Toogood, J. H., Complications of topical steroid therapy for asthma, *Am. Rev. Respir. Dis.*, *141*, S89–S96 (1990).

10

The Use of Nonisotonic Aerosols for Evaluating Bronchial Hyperresponsiveness

Sandra D. Anderson, Christine M. Smith, Leanne T. Rodwell, and Jacqueline I. du Toit

Royal Prince Alfred Hospital, Sydney, Australia

Josef Riedler and Colin F. Robertson

Royal Children's Hospital, Melbourne, Australia

I. INTRODUCTION

It is 25 years since it was first proposed that nonisotonic aerosols (NIAs) be used for identifying bronchial hyperresponsiveness (BHR) [1,2]. It was not until 1980, when a technique was described for bronchial challenge with distilled water, that interest was taken in using nonisotonic aerosols for the laboratory diagnosis and assessment of severity of asthma [3]. In 1981, Schoeffel and colleagues [4] reported that in patients with asthma an attack could be provoked by aerosols of hypertonic saline as well as water. They demonstrated that the sensitivity to these aerosols was increased as the osmolarity of the aerosol increased or decreased from normal (308 mOsm/L) (Fig. 1). It was appreciated at that time that the airway surface liquid volume covering the first 10 generations of airways was less than 1 ml (Fig. 2) and that deposition of aerosols onto this small fluid layer could cause a rapid and profound change in osmolarity [5]. Thus, bronchial provocation tests using NIAs became known as "osmotic" challenges.

II. THE CHALLENGE

Since that time we have characterized and standardized methods used to challenge with nonisotonic aerosols [6–12]. The use of (1) a single concentration of saline or water, (2) forced expired volume in 1 second (FEV_1) to record airway response, (3) 15 ml as the dose, (4) time of exposure as a means to assess the dose for each

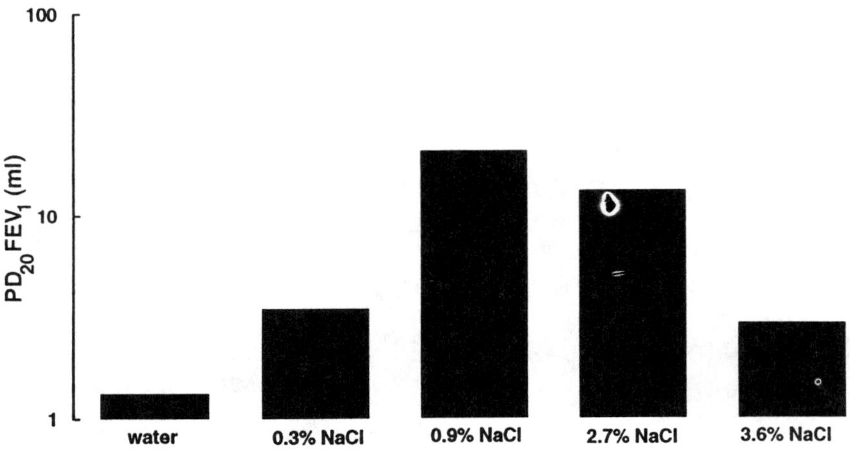

Figure 1 The geometric mean of the provocative dose of ultrasonically nebulized water and hypotonic, isotonic, and hypertonic solutions required to induce a 20% reduction in forced expired volume in 1 second from the prechallenge value (PD_{20} FEV_1) in 10 asthmatic patients. Only three of the subjects achieved a 20% fall with 0.9% saline, and the highest dose delivered was taken to express the PD_{20} for the other seven subjects. The data are redrawn from the observations made by Schoeffel et al. [4].

interval of exposure, and (5) gravimetric measurement as an estimate of total dose, has enabled the challenge to be used routinely in the lung function laboratory. The sensitivity of the challenge has been improved by taking as abnormal a fall in FEV_1 greater than 15% [7,13], a value based on measurements in healthy subjects (see below).

Bronchial provocation tests with nonisotonic aerosols are practical to use in the identification and assessment of the bronchial responsiveness associated with moderate to severe asthma. Challenges with NIAs require little patient cooperation, and the equipment required is portable, relatively cheap, and readily available. Bronchial challenge by inhaling aerosols of hyperosmolar saline and distilled water has obvious appeal from an ethical standpoint and provides an attractive and cheap alternative to pharmacological agents, allergens, or sensitizing agents. They can also be used in children [13–15]. There may be an advantage in using these challenges in that they provoke airway narrowing indirectly by causing the endogenous release of mediators to which the subject is sensitive. Although challenge with NIAs is less sensitive for detecting BHR than challenge with methacholine and histamine, it has a high positive predictive value for identifying BHR associated with moderate to severe asthma [13,15]. There have been no reports of false-positive tests with NIAs in healthy subjects. This is in contrast to histamine and methacholine challenges, which have low specificity but

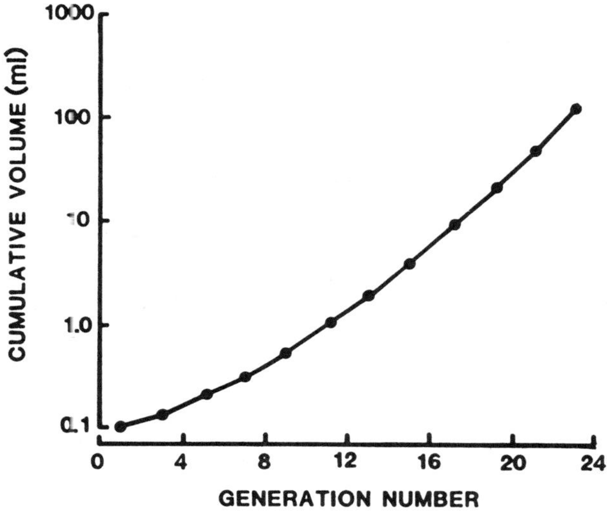

Figure 2 Cumulative volume in milliliters of airway surface liquid in relation to airway generation. The airway surface liquid depth is assumed to be 10 μm. This is likely to be an exaggeration, as the actual depth is probably 5–6 μm and is always less than the length of the cilia. The total volume in the first 10 generations (where the aerosol is likely to deposit) is calculated as being 0.75 ml. Thus, only a small volume of hyperosmolar/hypo-osmolar aerosol needs to deposit to increase or decrease the osmolarity of the airway surface liquid. (From Ref. 9)

a high negative predictive value. In population studies it has been reported that approximately 30% of persons with hyperresponsiveness to methacholine and histamine have no symptoms of asthma [16–18].

III. MECHANISM FOR AIRWAY NARROWING BY OSMOTIC STIMULI

That challenge with NIAs may be more specific for detecting the BHR associated with asthma is probably related to the way in which these aerosols cause airway narrowing. The bronchial smooth muscle does not contract directly in response to a change in osmolarity [19], as it is likely to do with the inhalation of methacholine or histamine. Rather, a change in osmolarity of the airway surface liquid causes the production and release of substances from cells in the airway epithelium and mucosa [20–22]. These substances act either directly on smooth muscle, causing it to contract, or indirectly by activation of other cells and initiation of other events, such as edema, the end result of which is airway narrowing [8]. It may be that challenges with NIAs also stimulate the sensory nerve endings [23] and initiate local responses via axon reflexes [24]. The tachykinins have been implicated in airway inflammation, and the recent development of antagonists may provide important insights into the mechanism whereby changes in airway osmolarity can cause the airways of asthmatics to narrow.

One of the cells that appears to be important is the mast cell. The mast cell releases histamine in vitro in response to an increase in osmolarity, and the release is enhanced in the presence of anti-IgE [25–28]. By a technique of isolating and lavaging airway segments in vivo [29], mediator release in the airways in response to a change in osmolarity has now been studied in patients with asthma. Studies using this technique have demonstrated that, in conjunction with histamine, other substances such as prostaglandin D_2 are released [20,22]. Thus, both preformed and newly formed mediators are released from mucosal mast cells in response to NIA challenges. Other studies have demonstrated increases in neutrophil chemotactic activity in serum of asthmatics following challenge with both water [30,31] and hyperosmolar saline [32], suggesting that cell activation is also a consequence of osmotic challenge. Although in this and other respects challenge with NIAs is similar to allergen challenge, there is an important difference in that any increase in bronchial responsiveness following challenge with NIAs is only small and very transient [33–37].

IV. DRUG EFFECTS AND REFRACTORINESS TO CHALLENGE WITH NONISOTONIC AEROSOLS

Some important features of osmotic challenges make them different from challenge with histamine and methacholine. First, the response to these challenges is inhibited by the acute administration of cromolyn sodium [6], nedocromil sodium [38,39], and furosemide [40,41]. The protective effect of these drugs may be due not only to their action on mast cells [42–44] but also to their putative effect on sensory nerves [45,46]. Second, there is a refractory period within an hour or two after challenge in about 50% of subjects [6,47–49]. The mechanism for refractoriness is unknown. There has been a suggestion that prostaglandins are involved, because pretreatment with indomethacin for 3 days prevented some subjects from becoming refractory [50,51]. However, we have found this to be the case in only a minority of patients [49].

The potential to harvest cells and mediators from the sputum induced by challenge with hyperosmolar aerosols [52,53] makes this technique attractive for studying patients with asthma. Not only can the airway responsiveness to these aerosols be measured, but it is also possible to collect sputum induced by the same challenge. It is hoped that in this way the numbers of inflammatory cells and their type, state of activation, and mediators can be quantified. Although this technique is currently used only for research, success will undoubtedly bring this application to routine laboratory use. The sputum can be induced by the osmotic movement of water into the airways in response to the deposition of hyperosmolar saline. The sputum can be more easily induced at higher osmolarities that may also induce cough. The data currently available on bronchial responsiveness to hyperosmolar saline provide indirect evidence for the presence in the airway of cells that are associated with airway inflammation, the hallmark of asthma [54,55]. In this respect, challenges with NIAs give additional information as compared with challenges that measure sensitivity of smooth muscle alone.

Challenge with NIAs may be useful for evaluating the contribution of epithelial cells and cells present in the submucosa to the development and modulation of BHR. By comparing airway responses to methacholine and histamine with airway responses to NIAs, before and after acute or long-term therapy, it may become possible to distinguish the effect of a drug in modifying smooth muscle responses from the effect it may have on cell-mediated events. The long-term effects of corticosteroids given as aerosols on the airway response to hyperosmolar saline support this concept [56,57]. Further, these studies suggest that there may be important differences between formulations of aerosol steroids. For example, treatment with beclomethasone dipropionate for up to 6 months reduces the sensitivity to 4.5% saline but does not prevent the airways from narrowing at higher doses of the same concentration [56]. By contrast, treatment with budesonide has, in the majority of subjects, resulted in a plateau or a complete block in the airway response to 4.5% saline after 3 months [57].

V. A CHANGE IN AIRWAY OSMOLARITY—A COMMON STIMULUS

Perhaps one of the greatest advantages of using NIAs to assess the presence of BHR associated with asthma is that events that can change the osmolarity of the respiratory tract are frequently encountered in everyday life. For example, inhaling aerosol particles of water or salt from showers, mist, or sea spray could easily and rapidly change the osmolarity of the airway surface liquid. When the intrathoracic airways are used to humidify the airways during exercise there is potential for the osmolarity to change quickly over minutes. Aspiration of sea water or fresh water while snorkeling or scuba diving is not uncommon [58]. Infections of the respiratory tract can also change osmolarity of the secretions by the presence of osmotically active substances within bacteria, or the cells recruited in their defence, or the mucus produced by the glands. Therapeutic substances are now commonly delivered by aerosol from nebulizers to patients with lung disease. The volume delivered is small, but if the aerosol is nonisotonic, it can provoke an attack of asthma in sensitive people [59–62]. Local anesthetics are also commonly given by aerosol before bronchoscopy. Again, there is the potential to alter the tonicity of the respiratory tract, and bronchoconstriction has been reported [63,64]. As bronchoalveolar lavage is a popular technique for collecting cells, care must be taken to prevent unwanted bronchoconstriction [65]. Substances such as water [66] or acetylcysteine that are administered by transtracheal catheters to induce cough in postoperative patients also have the potential to cause bronchoconstriction.

VI. DELIVERY AND DEPOSITION OF THE AEROSOL

A. Equipment

Ultrasonic nebulizers are used to generate NIAs because they produce dense aerosols with concentrations of between 66 and 100 μL or mg/L. Compared with jet nebulizers, ultrasonic nebulizers deliver between two and four times more aerosol over the same period. The droplet size generated by the nebulizer is important and may differ according to the purpose for which it was designed, i.e. either for delivery of drugs or the humidification of air. The droplet size distribution may also vary, but within a frequency of 0.5–4 MHz it remains fairly constant [67]. Ultrasonic nebulization of a given liquid should produce droplet sizes that vary inversely with two-thirds the power of the acoustic frequency. This has been shown to be true for frequencies of about 10 kHz to 3 MHz [68]. Thus the ultrasonic nebulizers used for inhalation therapy will generate smaller droplets at higher operating frequencies. The manufacturers' specifications will usually include the droplet size and distribution. However, this can vary with the viscosity and vapor pressure of the nebulizer fluid, the flow rates generated, and the nature of the apparatus connecting the patient to the ultrasonic nebulizer.

Most ultrasonic nebulizers have a variable output that determines the density of the aerosol produced. There is an enormous reduction in this output from the reservoir to the mouthpiece or face mask when tubing is used. In order to standardize testing between laboratories, nebulizer outputs should be measured at the end of the tubing rather than at the reservoir, and this value should be reported. The output of the nebulizer may also vary with the volume of fluid in the reservoir, and this should be kept constant for each patient [69]. For these challenges the nebulizer should be able to deliver at least 1.5 ml/min to the valve or mouthpiece. We have found that coughing frequency increases with the density of the aerosol, and for this reason we are satisfied using a nebulizer with an output of between 1.2 and 2.6 ml/min delivered to the mouthpiece.

The aerosol may be delivered via a two-way valve or by face mask. As excessive condensation occurs in small valves, it is mandatory to use large valves with low resistance to flow if the output of the nebulizer is to keep closer to specification. We have preferred to use a large valve (Hans Rudolph No. 2700, Kansas City, Missouri) rather than a face mask because the inspiratory valve closes during expiration. Thus the aerosol is not dissipated but included in the next inspiration. Using this technique and by weighing the reservoir and tubing, but not the valve, before and after challenge, we have been able to measure the output delivered to the valve. Because of the accumulation of saliva during challenge, the valve is not weighed. The precise amount of aerosol inhaled is not known for each subject. However, from some carefully performed studies we have found that 47% of the amount delivered to the valve reaches the mouth. It is 15–35% of this volume that deposits in the lower airways and changes the osmolarity of the airway surface liquid.

The bore of the tubing attached to the reservoir is important and will reduce or increase the amount of aerosol delivered to the mouthpiece. In our system the aerosol from the nebulizer passes via a tubing 60–70 cm long with a smooth interior surface and internal bore size of 22 mm. Other workers use bore sizes larger than this. It is likely that there will be major differences in the distribution of aerosol particles delivered from wide-bored tubing and face masks as compared with valves. We have measured the mass median aerodynamic diameter of the particles coming out of the Hans Rudolph No. 2700 valve mouthpiece and found them to be remarkably monodispersed—3.6 μm with a geometric mean less than 1.1. Presumably our equipment has filtered out the other particles, as the distribution specified by the manufacturer is 2–12 μm. If a wider tube and face mask are used there may be a larger distribution of particles, and this could be advantageous under some conditions.

It is strongly recommended that once the characteristics of the system have been worked out, no changes be made in tubing bore or length. We have also found that the output of nebulizers declines over time, and we recommend that it be checked frequently and the crystal replaced if necessary. We recommend that the output of the nebulizer be measured, by weighing, for each patient.

The dose of aerosol delivered by the nebulizer we use is a function of time, although the actual density of the aerosol within each breath will vary according to the tidal volume. We have found a close correlation between the time for which the aerosol is inhaled and the dose of aerosol delivered. This is illustrated for one nebulizer in Fig. 3. In order to obtain the total dose, we always measure change in weight of the canister and tubing before and after challenge. The total dose is then divided by the time of exposure, so that the dose for each interval of exposure can be estimated. From this a dose–response curve can be drawn relating cumulative dose delivered (ml) to a change in lung function (Fig. 4).

From the data published on deposition of aerosol particles of varying mass median diameter, it is predicted that approximately 15–35% of the 3.6-μm particles will deposit in the tracheobronchial tree (Fig. 5) [70,71]. The distribution of aerosol within the airways may also vary according to the tonicity of the aerosol and the relative humidity of the airways. There is some experimental evidence [72] to support the theoretical predictions [73] that water particles could

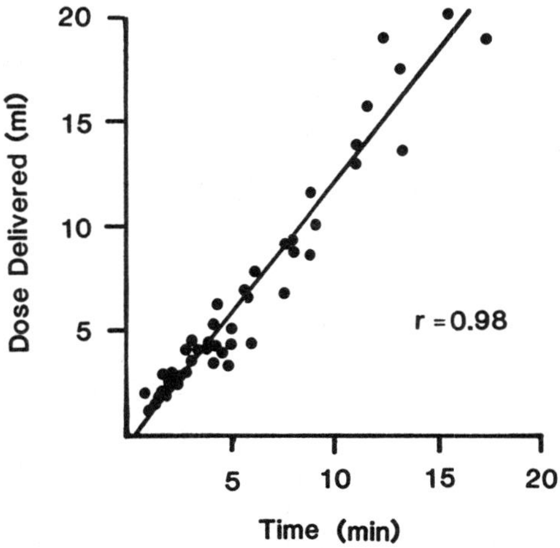

Figure 3 The dose delivered from one MistO_2gen ultrasonic nebulizer 143A (Timeter, Oregon Pike, Pennsylvania) in relation to time. The dose delivered was measured gravimetrically and was the amount delivered to the inspiratory port of the Hans Rudolph No. 2700 valve.

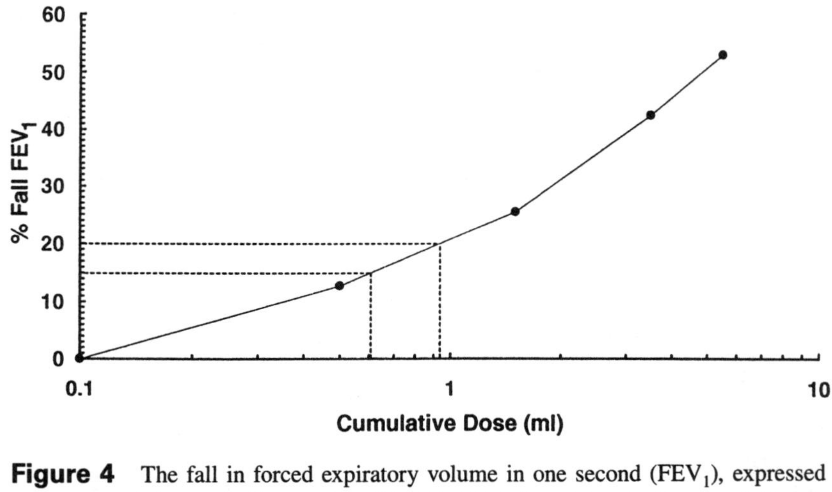

Figure 4 The fall in forced expiratory volume in one second (FEV_1), expressed as a percentage of the prechallenge value (% Fall FEV_1), in relation to the cumulative dose of 4.5% saline. The broken lines represent the values for the provocative dose of 4.5% saline required to induce a 15% (PD_{15}) and 20% (PD_{20}) fall in FEV_1.

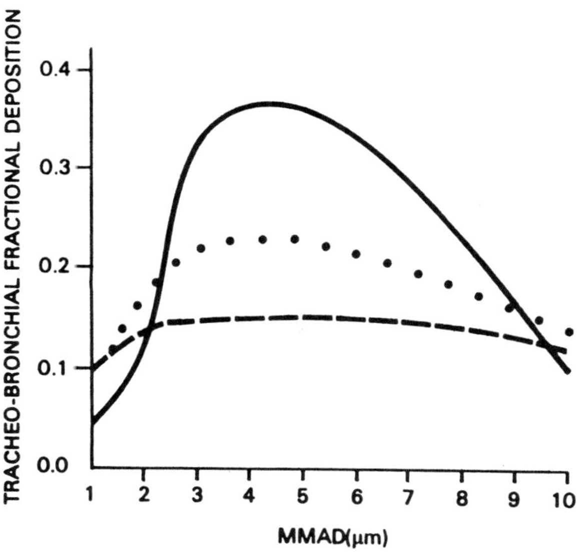

Figure 5 Estimation of fractional deposition of an inhaled dose vs. the mass median aerodynamic diameter (MMAD) in the tracheobronchial region of the human respiratory tract for a monodispersed (solid line, geometric standard deviation [σ_g] = 1), mildly polydispersed (dotted line, σ_g = 2), and polydispersed (broken line, σ_g = 3.5) aerosol. (From Ref. 70.)

shrink and hypertonic particles grow as they traverse the humid airways. Thus, there may be regional differences in the deposition of hypotonic and hypertonic aerosols.

For the nebulizer and settings that we use (MistO$_2$gen 143A, Timeter, Oregon Pike, Pennsylvania; 1.5–2.6 ml/min), it is predicted that approximately 0.08–0.43 ml/min will deposit in the lower airways. Even at the much lower rate of deposition, an osmolarity of 640 mOsm, required for the optimal release of histamine from mast cells by NaCl [26], would be achieved in less than 5 min. It is not known how quickly water will move from the epithelial cells to the airway lumen to compensate for the change in osmolarity. We do know that it is the rate of change in osmolarity rather than the dose of NaCl that is the major determinant of the airway response. This is illustrated in Fig. 6 for one subject who inhaled three different concentrations of saline. The actual dose of NaCl in millimoles did not result in the same airway response under these conditions, and the airway response was more rapidly induced by the highest concentration. This may be explained by the difference in rate of change of osmolarity and possibly the rate of return of water to the airway surface liquid from the airway submucosa. However,

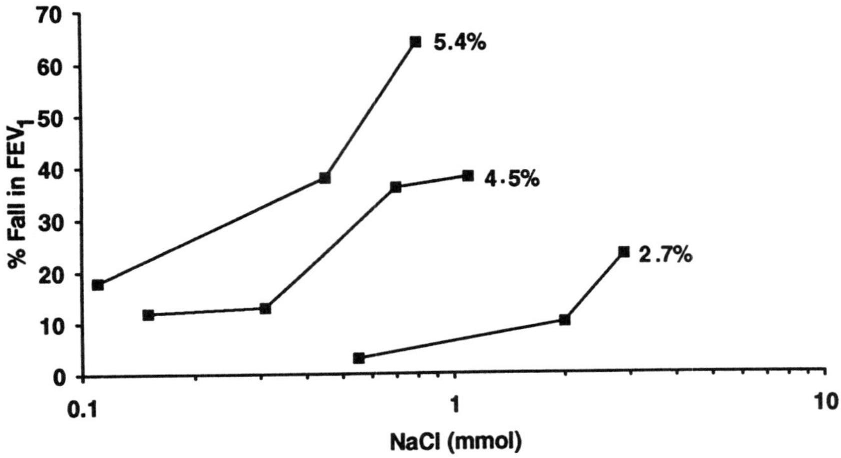

Figure 6 Relationship between the % fall in FEV_1 and the number of millimoles of NaCl delivered during challenge with 2.7%, 4.5%, and 5.4% saline in a patient with asthma.

studies of prolonged and intermittent challenge with the same concentration of saline suggest that the dose is cumulative over the short time of challenge [9,10,32]. There is evidence from in vitro studies to show that the apical membrane of human nasal epithelial cells is more permeable to water than is the basement membrane [74]. If this is also the case in vivo, a lag may occur between water loss to the lumen and water replacement in the epithelial cell. In this situation, a change in the osmolarity or volume of the epithelial cells themselves may become the crucial event that initiates the response to these aerosols.

B. Technique

In the development of these challenge tests for routine use in the laboratory, a number of different techniques have been used. Some of the earlier studies reported using single-dose exposures for periods of between 5 and 10 min [3,75, 76]. Because many asthmatic patients are very sensitive to the effects of these aerosols, we do not recommend such prolonged exposure times. For our initial exposure we use 30 s and double the time for each exposure if the change in FEV_1 does not exceed 10%. Thus, 30 s, 1 min, 2 min, 4 min, and 8 min are the standard exposure times for routine testing in our laboratory. If changes in FEV_1 are more than 10%, we repeat the exposure for the same time or less. A similar technique was also used by Groot [77], who modified the original protocol described by Schoeffel et al. [4] and increased sensitivity by doubling ventilation volumes (3, 5, 10, 20, 40, 80, 160 L). This technique is slow, as a 5-min interval occurs between exposures. By contrast, Simone et al. [78] and Robuschi et al. [38] used an exposure time of 120 s and measured specific airway resistance (SRaw), making their challenge relatively short.

We have found that the maximum response occurs within 1–2 min after exposure to hyperosmolar saline, and for this reason we have an interval of at least 90 s between exposures. Allegra and Bianco [3] had an interval of 3 min between exposures for challenge with distilled water.

There are other techniques that are less commonly used. These include increasing the output of the nebulizer while keeping the time of exposure constant [34,79] and increasing the dose geometrically by increasing the length of challenge and the output of the nebulizer. We have also increased the osmolarity of the solution from 0.9% to 1.8%, 2.7%, 3.6%, 4.5%, and 5.4% NaCl [80] or by doubling the concentration (0.9%, 1.8%, 3.6%, 7.2%, 14.4% NaCl) [81]. The patient inhales each concentration for a period of 3 min, and between each exposure and the next a period of 3 min elapses, which is sufficient time to change solutions (Fig. 6) [82]. In routine laboratory investigation this technique is less practical, as it requires changing the fluid in the canister every few minutes. However, it may have some advantages in research or in the evaluation of drugs. We have also investigated the responses to repeated 60-s aerosol exposures

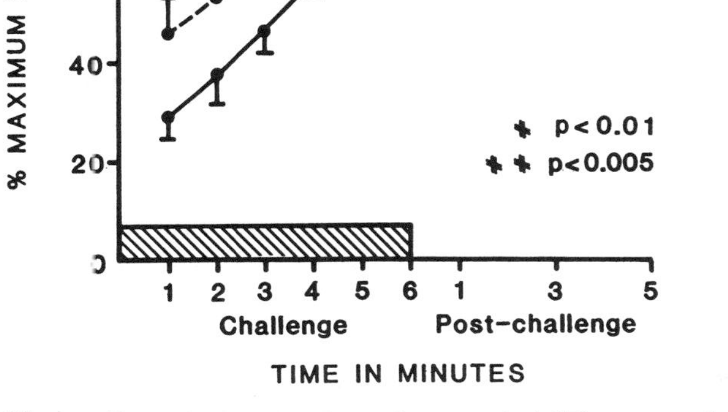

Figure 7 This diagram shows the mean (±1 SE) response (expressed as a percentage of the maximum response) to hyperosmolar saline (dashed line) and isocapnic hyperventilation (solid line) during the last 6 min of challenge and the first 5 min following challenge. (Data obtained from Ref. 9.)

followed immediately by measurement of lung function [9]. Using this technique has made it possible to obtain a plateau in response to the inhalation of hyperosmolar saline in most patients after six to ten 1-min exposures. This plateau represented approximately 86% of the final airway response measured within 3 min of the final exposure (Fig. 7). The dose–response curve generated by this technique exhibits a well-defined slope because of the large number of points obtained, and it is characterized by a plateau in the majority of subjects. We have found both these techniques useful for assessing drug action and for research. However, they are not yet used in the laboratory for routine assessment, as we prefer to challenge with water or saline in a single concentration (2.7%, 3.6%, or 4.5%) and progressively increase the time of exposure.

VII. MEASUREMENT OF LUNG FUNCTION

Changes in lung function in response to inhaling NIAs have been recorded in a number of ways. Specific airways resistance has been used by Bianco et al. [83,84] and Sheppard et al. [79,83,84]. An increase in SRaw of 100% or 6 cm H_2O/L/s is considered a positive response.

Forced expiratory volume in 1 second and the flow rates through the middle half of the vital capacity are also used [34,69]. As the changes in these flow rates are well correlated with FEV_1, we now report only changes in FEV_1. Although we have previously considered a reduction of 20% or more in FEV_1 abnormal, we now take a fall of 15% or more, and as the numbers of healthy subjects studied increases, this may be lowered to as little as 12%. The mean percent fall in FEV_1 in healthy subjects was 3.3% (SD<4.7%) after inhalation of 15–56 ml of water (n = 37) and 4.6% (SD 3.1%) after inhalation of 15–56 ml of 4.5% saline (n = 75). Others, studying normal children, have found similar results and also believe a 20% decrease in FEV_1 is unnecessarily stringent to define abnormality [13].

VIII. RESPONSES IN PATIENTS WITH OTHER RESPIRATORY DISEASES

We have measured responses to 4.5% saline in a selected group of 17 asymptomatic smokers who had abnormal responsiveness to histamine but no symptoms of asthma. Of these, 11 had a PD_{20} to saline that was less than 18 ml (mean PD_{20} ± 1 SD was 5.2 ± 6.2 ml). Of these 11, five had a PD_{20} to histamine less than 2 μmol. Because smoking is associated with inflammatory changes in the airway mucosa [85], measurements of abnormal responsiveness to NIAs in smokers are in keeping with the concept that responsiveness to NIAs is related to airway inflammation. We have found no bronchial responsiveness to 4.5% saline in patients with interstitial lung disease (mean % fall in FEV_1 ± 1 SD, 6.8% ± 4%; n = 8) [86]. The only patients with cystic fibrosis who have recorded a 20% fall in

FEV_1 to 4.5% saline have been those who have been clinically recognized and treated for asthma.

IX. FACTORS AFFECTING THE RESPONSE

There is no strong relationship between the prechallenge level of lung function and the sensitivity to NIAs [6,10]. In patients with normal lung function a 20% fall in FEV_1 can be provoked by less than 2 ml of aerosol delivered to the valve, while in others with abnormal lung function as much as 10 ml may be required to provoke the response.

Because the medications used in the treatment of asthma—e.g., bronchodilators, sodium cromoglycate, and nedocromil sodium—can inhibit the response to these aerosols [3,6,38,56,78,87], it is preferable to challenge 6–8 h after aerosol medication was last taken. The observation by Mattoli et al. [51] that indomethacin could prevent the refractory period to water encouraged investigators to document carefully current medications of all types. The effect of a number of drugs on the responses to aerosols of distilled water has been reviewed [7].

It has been reported that the response to water aerosol is enhanced following allergen challenge [88]. The responsiveness to water was apparently increased during the late response to the allergen, because it was not recorded after the immediate response but rather after 5 h, remaining high for at least 3 h (Fig. 8). This study has important implications for use of these aerosols for diagnosis of

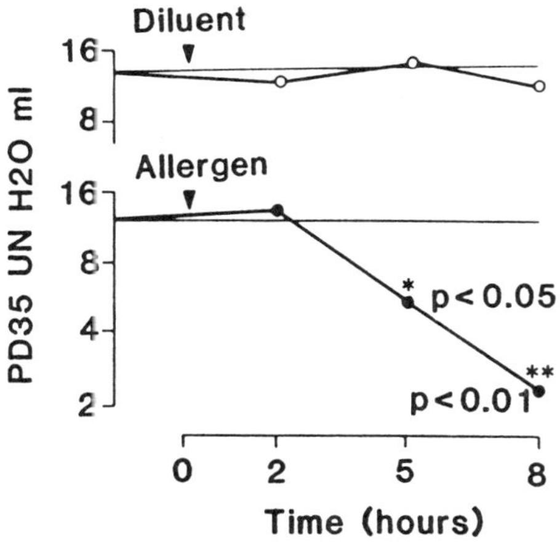

Figure 8 The provocative dose of ultrasonically nebulized water required to induce a 35% reduction in specific conductance following diluent, and after challenge with inhaled grass or cat allergen. At 5 and 8 h after allergen challenge, there is a marked increase in sensitivity to inhaled water. (From Ref. 88.)

occupational asthma. Measuring the airway response to water or a hyperosmolar aerosol before and after exposure to a sensitizing agent may be a practical and ethically appealing way to identify occupationally related changes in BHR.

The tonicity of the aerosol may affect the airway response, and we have found discordant responses in a proportion of patients who have been challenged with both water and saline [10,35]. This is discussed in detail below but must be considered when interpreting results and considering the factors affecting response.

From the small numbers of subjects studied, it does not appear that the temperature of the aerosol has a significant effect on the airway response to NIAs [69]. Because tidal breathing is used, the aerosol is probably close to body temperature by the time it reaches the pharynx. The temperature of the aerosol increases as the nebulizer reservoir heats up with time, so that the longer the challenge is, the closer the inspired aerosol will be to body temperature. We have investigated temperature only over the range of 22–37°C, and it may be that cooling the aerosol would increase the response.

Coughing as a result of inhaling NIAs has been a problem for some patients and in itself could affect the volume of the aerosol inhaled and deposited. The frequency of cough is greater with water than with hyperosmolar aerosols. It has been reported that cough will increase with a reduction in chloride ion concentration [89], but increasing chloride ion concentration can also cause cough. The cough problem is transitory, and most patients stop coughing after several minutes. For this reason, we have been unable to include an assessment of cough along with challenge with NIAs. The mechanism of the cough and constriction are probably different, as iso-osmolar solutions deficient in a permeant anion can cause cough without causing constriction [79,89,90].

One of the major factors affecting the deposition of, and therefore response to, these aerosols is the dynamic change in lung function with increasing doses. Regional deposition of the aerosol may well change in patients whose lung function is reduced from 90% to 65% of predicted value during the challenge.

X. CHOICE OF AEROSOL

The early studies using NIAs to challenge patients with asthma employed aerosols of water, and there is a considerable data base on hypotonic aerosol challenge, which has been reviewed [7,77]. There are now many different groups of investigators who have studied the effects of hyperosmolar aerosols [6,15,47,55, 91–94]. Although sodium chloride has been most commonly used, potassium chloride is more potent for provoking responses at the same, or even lower, osmolarity [95]. The reason that potassium ions are more potent than sodium ions is unknown, but effects of potassium on membrane depolarization may be important [95]. The permeability coefficient of a substance is also important.

Eggleston et al. [26] have shown that the release of histamine from human lung mast cells is greater the lower the permeability coefficient of the substance. Although ion concentration and its permeability can modify the response to these aerosols [90], it is the osmolarity that is of major importance. We found no significant difference between response to 3.6% saline and to 20% dextrose in a group of asthmatics [69], and this has been confirmed by others [90]. We have chosen to use sodium chloride solutions or water for practical and ethical reasons.

We originally studied a large number of clinically recognized asthmatic patients using either water or 4.5% NaCl aerosol and found 80–90% to have a 20% fall in FEV_1 with less than 33 ml (Fig. 9). Our initial study [4] suggested that there was no difference in potency between water and 3.6% saline (Fig. 1). However, as the number of subjects receiving both hypo-osmolar and hyperosmolar challenge has increased, we now find a proportion of subjects who are not equally sensitive to aerosols of water and 4.5% saline (Fig. 10). Other investigators have reported similar discrepancies between water and 10% KCl [96].

There are a number of differences between challenges with water and hyperosmolar saline that lead us to suggest that these challenges should be considered separately. For example, water increases sensitivity to methacholine and histamine [33,34]. In another study we confirmed this finding, but we did not find an increase in responsiveness after 4.5% saline [35]. This suggested to us that different mediators may be released in response to these challenges [35]. Some recent studies, however, have reported small increases in sensitivity to methacholine after hyperosmolar challenge [36,37]. It would seem that a systematic

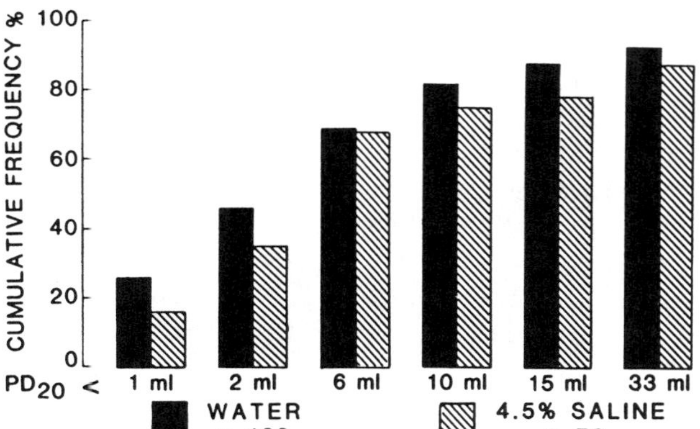

Figure 9 The cumulative frequency distribution of the responses to ultrasonically nebulized aerosols of water and 4.5% saline in two separate groups of patients with clinically recognized asthma.

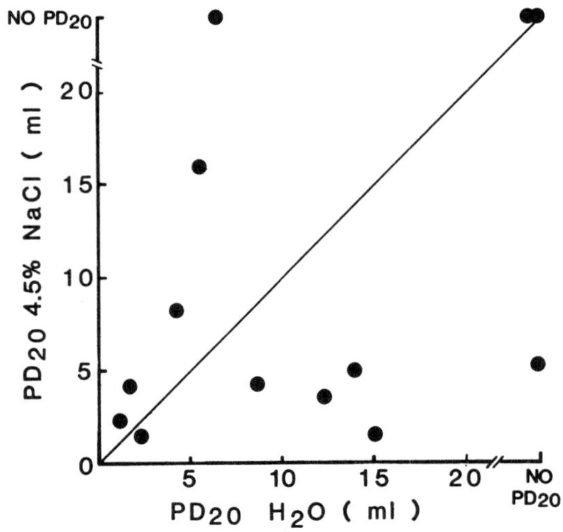

Figure 10 The provocative dose of ultrasonically nebulized 4.5% saline required to induce a 20% reduction in FEV_1 from prechallenge value (PD_{20}) in relation to the PD_{20} for water aerosol in a group of 18 asthmatic subjects.

study of patients with disparate responses to salt and water is warranted to determine the nature of the differences.

The presence of ions, changes in membrane permeability, the site of deposition of the aerosol particle, and the type of mediators released could all account for the differences between responses to water and hyperosmolar saline. This does not change the concept that inflammation needs to be present for BHR to these aerosols to be recorded. Despite these differences, there are a number of similarities between the responses to hypo- and hyperosmolar aerosols, particularly in relation to the effects of drugs [3,6,7,81,87]. The presence of a refractory period in some subjects [6,47–49], and the documentation of an increase in neutrophil chemotactic activity [30–32], suggest that common pathways are involved whereby these NIAs provoke airway narrowing.

We have found a normal distribution of log PD_{20} to 4.5% NaCl challenge within the asthmatic population attending our laboratory for research studies (Fig. 11). Unfortunately, in our early studies we used 1 min for the initial exposure, so that we have less discrimination within the group of very sensitive subjects. Although there are differences in the sensitivity to saline and water in the same individual, for the population the distribution of sensitivity is very similar (Fig. 9). Originally we continued a challenge until a PD_{20} was recorded or 30 ml of aerosol had been delivered to the valve. Using a 20% fall in FEV_1 as the abnormal response,

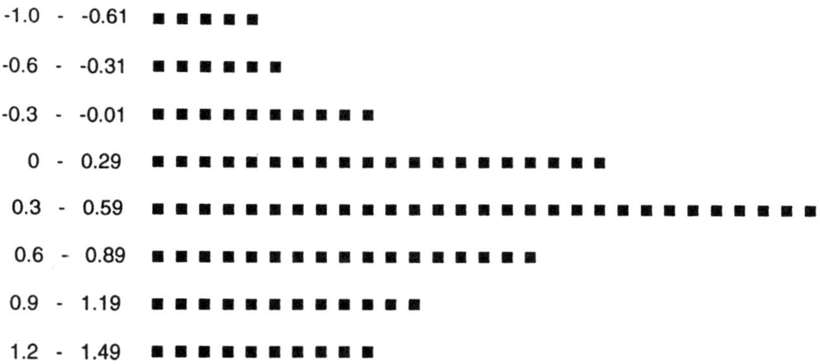

Figure 11 Distribution of the log values for PD_{20} recorded in 109 asthmatic subjects who volunteered for research studies investigating the bronchoconstricting effects of 4.5% saline.

between 80% and 85% of the clinically recognized patients responded to 15 ml of water, 3.6% saline, or 4.5% saline. Over the time of our challenge (30 s and 1, 2, 4, and 8 min), between 15 and 30 ml of aerosol is delivered. We terminate the test after this volume because increasing the dose has not greatly increased the number of positive tests (Fig. 9). The amount of 4.5% saline aerosol required to induce a 20% fall in FEV_1 in a group of 109 asthmatic subjects is illustrated in Fig. 12.

XI. COMPARISON WITH OTHER CHALLENGES

A number of studies have investigated the relationship between responses to NIAs and other challenge tests, particularly exercise, isocapnic hyperventilation, and the inhalation of methacholine and histamine. Again there appear to be some differences and some similarities between hypo-osmolar and hyperosmolar challenges. For example, several investigators have not found a significant relationship between water and methacholine [35,97], whereas a significant relationship is found between saline and methacholine [10].

We have compared the airway responses to methacholine and 4.5% saline (n = 26) and to histamine and 4.5% saline (n = 28) (Fig. 13). These data demonstrate that a PD_{20} to saline of less than 15 ml is associated with a PD_{20} to histamine of less than 2 μmol (PC_{20} of 4 mg/ml). For the majority of patients the PD_{20} for methacholine was also less than 2 μmol. In those patients with a PD_{20} to 4.5% saline less than 15 ml we have always observed responsiveness to methacholine or histamine. By contrast, responsiveness to methacholine and histamine is not necessarily accompanied by responsiveness to NIAs. In another group of patients, when water and methacholine were compared the results were less

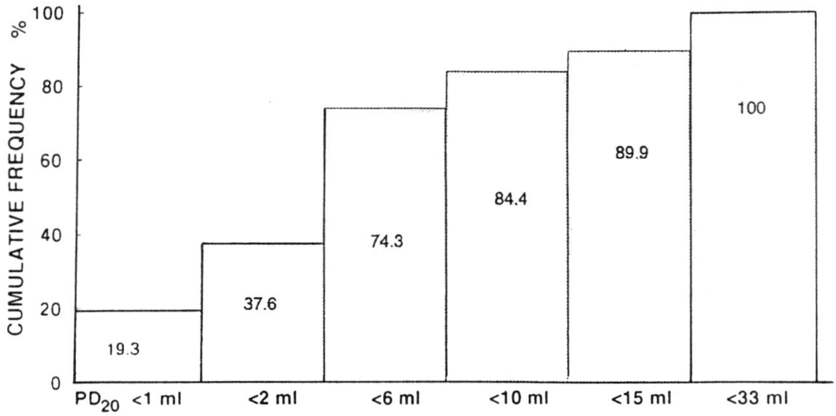

Figure 12 The cumulative frequency (%) of 109 asthmatic subjects with a PD_{20} < than 1, 2, 6, 10, 15, and 33 ml. The majority of these subjects responded after less than 10 min of exposure to the aerosol.

concordant, but again responsiveness to water indicated a PD_{20} to methacholine also below 2 μmol.

The proposal that evaporative water loss from hyperpnea induces an increase in ion concentration in the periciliary fluid and a subsequent increase in osmolarity [5,98] has encouraged us and other investigators to compare responses to exercise and isocapnic hyperventilation with inhalation of hyperosmolar saline [9,10,47, 99–103]. Not surprisingly, the sensitivity to water loss by evaporation is similar to the dehydrating effects of inhaling hyperosmolar aerosols (Fig. 14). Remarkable similarities have been found in both position and shape of the dose–response curves when the osmotic load has been expressed as water loss [99]. The concordance in position and shape of these curves may simply relate to the volume of water lost by evaporation from below the pharynx (about 25% of the total) [104,105]. This volume loss would cause changes in periciliary fluid osmolarity similar to those caused by the deposition of small volumes of hyperosmolar aerosol in the same regions of the lower respiratory tract. Other workers have found a relationship between water and exercise [97,106]. This finding may not be surprising, as there are predicted to be regional differences in water transport in the airways in that condensation and evaporation both occur [104,105,107].

XII. SUMMARY AND RECOMMENDATIONS FOR CHALLENGE WITH NIA

For the routine investigation of patients in the laboratory we make the following suggestions.

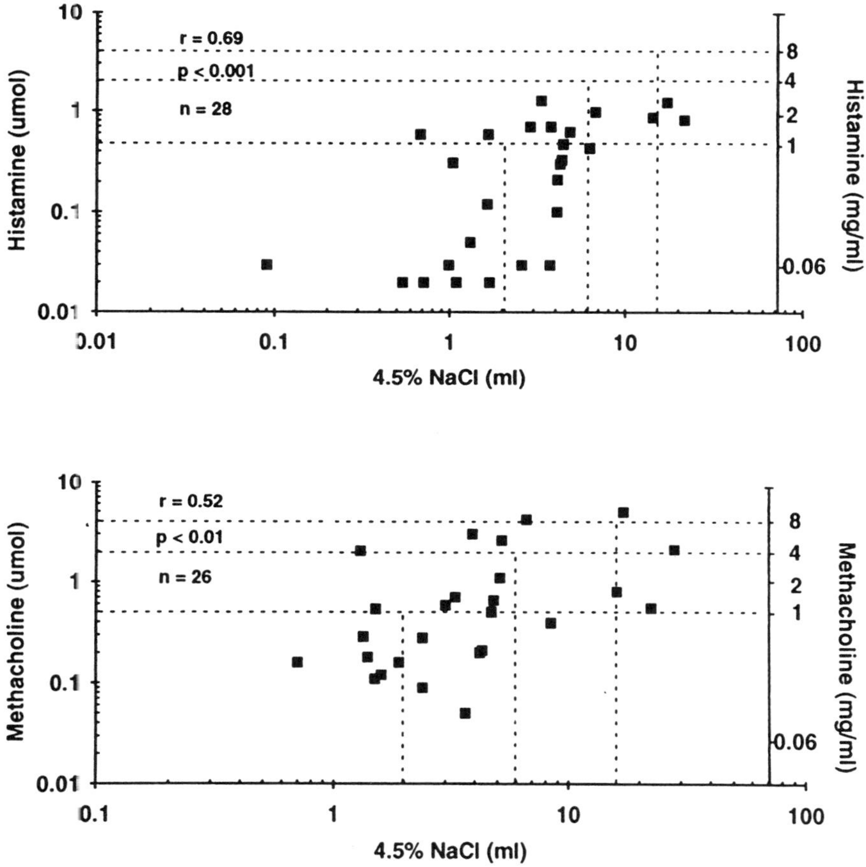

Figure 13 The relationship between the airway sensitivity (PD_{20}) to histamine and 4.5% saline and methacholine and 4.5% saline in two separate groups of asthmatic subjects.

A. Safety

As with any other bronchial provocation tests, challenge using NIAs leads to airway narrowing that can be of sudden onset and cause a marked reduction in arterial oxygen tension. We recommend that the precautions set out in detail by Sterk et al. [12] be taken. In brief, we do not recommend a challenge with NIAs in persons with severe airflow limitation or those with an FEV_1 less than 1.2 L. Any person with a medical condition that may be affected adversely by a fall in arterial oxygen should also be excluded from testing. The usual equipment required to reverse an acute attack of asthma (bronchodilators, oxygen), cardiopulmonary resuscitation equipment, and drugs such as antihistamines, epinephrine, and

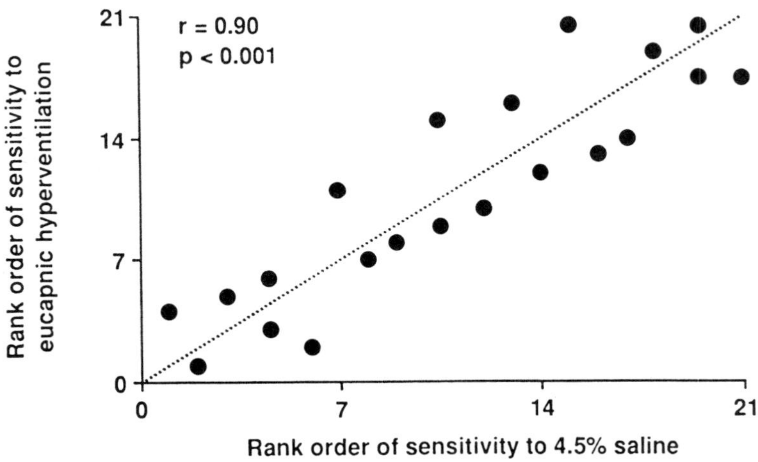

Figure 14 Sensitivity to isocapnic hyperventilation with dry air and to 4.5% saline in 21 asthmatic subjects. (From Ref. 11.)

intravenous corticosteroids should all be at hand. Trained personnel only should administer these challenges, and immediate access to medical help should be available. Patients should never be left unattended, and their airway narrowing should be reversed to within 90% of baseline before they leave the laboratory. The initial exposure time should be only 30 s, and for a person known to be hyperresponsive, a challenge with 2.7% NaCl rather than 4.5% aerosol may be all that is required to demonstrate sensitivity to hyperosmolarity.

B. Equipment

A suitable ultrasonic nebulizer is needed, with a canister that has a volume fill of 100–200 ml and can be easily detached and weighed. The output of the nebulizer should be sufficient to deliver at least 1.5 ml/min to the mouthpiece after passing through the tubing and generate a particle size of 3–6 μm. Other equipment required is a large two-way valve, a spirometer, and a scale for weighing.

C. Solution

A single concentration, i.e., water or 4.5% saline (close to sea water), is recommended, as 85% of clinically recognized asthmatics respond and the test is relatively faster if these concentrations are used. We use sterile distilled pyrogen-free water and add pharmacopeia (USB or BP)-grade sodium chloride to this. This solution is kept in the refrigerator for 1 week only before being discarded.

D. Protocol

The time of inhalation of the aerosol is progressively increased, from 30 s initially to 1, 2, 4, and 8 min, until there has been a fall in FEV_1 of 20% or more or until 15 g of solution has been delivered to the inspiratory port. The FEV_1 is measured 60 s after each inhalation period, and the challenge is continued within 3 min.

E. Expression of the Response

A dose–response curve is constructed by plotting the change in FEV_1, expressed as a percentage of the baseline value or the predicted value, against the cumulative dose of aerosol delivered, expressed in ml (Fig. 4).

A value for PD_{15} or PD_{20} can be obtained by linear interpolation (Fig. 4). A PD_{20} of less than 2.0 ml is consistent with severe hyperresponsiveness, one of 2.1–6.0 ml with moderate hyperresponsiveness, and one greater than 6.0 ml with mild hyperresponsiveness (Fig. 15). Within the asthmatic population the PD_{20} is log-normally distributed (Fig. 11). To assess changes in sensitivity to an intervention, the values for PD_{20} are compared after log transformation. The repeatability of the test is good (Fig. 16), with the fold difference for PD_{20}, between test days being 1.64 and the 95% confidence intervals 0.94–2.88. Because baseline lung function can change over time or in response to therapy, a reactivity or slope of the dose-response curve can be measured [56]. This is taken as the change in lung function (either % fall or actual fall % predicted) divided by the cumulative dose of aerosol

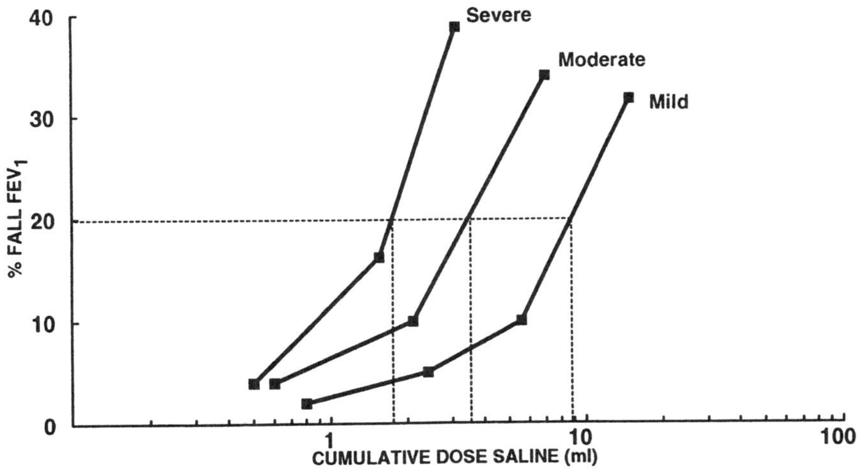

Figure 15 The fall in FEV_1, expressed as a percentage of prechallenge value, in relation to the cumulative dose of 4.5% saline aerosol in three asthmatic subjects.

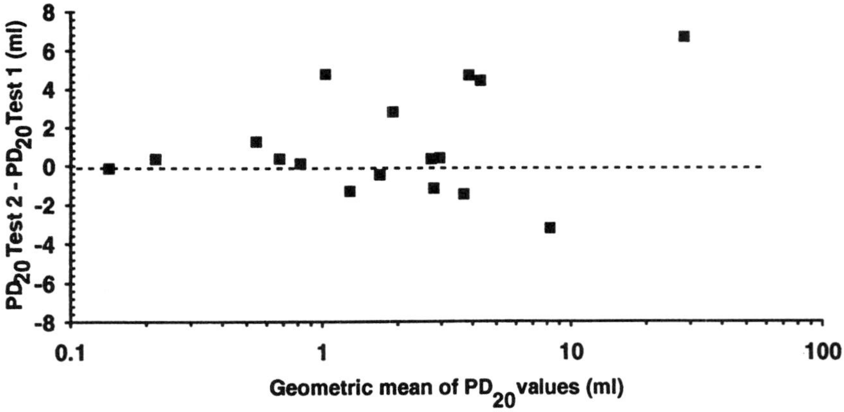

Figure 16 The repeatability of the 4.5% NaCl challenge test is shown by the small difference between the two PD_{20} values (ml) as a function of the geometric mean of the two values for most subjects. Ten of the 17 subjects differed by less than 2 ml on the two test days, which were 31.1 ± 16 days (mean ± 1 SD) apart.

that caused that change in lung function. This index can be used even if a 20% fall in FEV_1 is not obtained, as is the case after acute treatment with sodium cromoglycate or nedocromil sodium and chronic treatment with some inhaled corticosteroids.

F. Bronchial Challenge Using Hyperosmolar Saline in Children

The well-standardized protocol for performing bronchial challenges with hyperosmolar saline in adults has been slightly modified for its use in children. We recommended a smaller valve with more appropriate dead space and more convenient size for children to hold. Using a Starling pump attached to a Hans Rudolph 1410 valve, together with a Timeter ultrasonic nebulizer, we measured an adequate nebulizer output to the mouth, ranging from 1.9–2.5 ml/min. With this simulated breathing system the mass median aerodynamic diameter ranged from 2.3–2.9 microns with a geometric standard deviation of 1.2 microns over a range of tidal volumes from 300–500 ml and a respiratory rate of 20 breaths/min [108].

We assessed the reproducibility of the response to inhaled 4.5% NaCl in 17 children with mild to severe asthma who had two or three challenge tests within a 10 day period. The difference for PD_{15} FEV_1 between these measurements was 0.85 doubling dose, which reflects good reproducibility. Sensitivity to the challenge to identify current asthma in these selected children was 94% [109].

Traditionally, for epidemiological surveys of asthma in children, pharmacological agents have been used to assess bronchial responsiveness as an objective measure of asthma. As these agents become less available in some communities there has been an increasing interest in the use of nonpharmacological agents. Hyperosmolar saline challenge has a very high specificity of 92% for clinical asthma in epidemiological studies but has a sensitivity of approximately 50% [110]. The difference in sensitivity between laboratory and field studies is a reflection of the range of severity of asthma in the community. The majority of children with asthma have infrequent episodic asthma and it was this group who accounted for most of the negative responses to challenge. In field studies the acute effects of medication on the response to hyperosmolar saline can be overcome by withholding the medication. However, regular treatment with inhaled steroids may attenuate, and in some cases inhibit, the response in some subjects [110].

Inhalation of hyperosmolar saline stimulates the release of endogenous mediators and identifies current asthma. It is a relatively inexpensive test that is safe, well tolerated and reproducible in children, and can be performed readily in the field.

XIII. CONCLUSION

Bronchial provocation testing using aerosols of nonisotonic solutions is a cheap and rapid technique for identifying bronchial hyperresponsiveness associated with asthma. Challenges with aerosols of water and hyperosmolar saline have obvious appeal from an ethical standpoint and provide useful information to both the patient and physician. The osmolarity of the respiratory tract can be rapidly changed by events commonly encountered in daily life. Thus, identifying bronchial hyperresponsiveness to a change in osmolarity can help the patient to recognize an important stimulus for provoking an attack of asthma and aid physicians in their choice of preventative medication [57].

REFERENCES

1. Cheney, F. W., and Butler, J., The effects of ultrasonically-produced aerosols on airway resistance in man, *Anesthesiology*, *29*, 1099–1106 (1968).
2. De Vries, K., Booij-Noord, H., Goei, J. T., Grobler, N. J., Sluiter, H. J., Tammeling, G. J., and Orie, N. G. M., Hyperreactivity of the bronchial tree to drugs, chemical and physical agents, in *Bronchitis II* (N. G. M. Orie and H. J. Sluiter, eds.), Royal Vangorocum, Assen, the Netherlands, 1964, pp. 167–180.
3. Allegra, L., and Bianco, S., Non-specific bronchoreactivity obtained with an ultrasonic aerosol of distilled water, *Eur. J. Respir. Dis.*, *61*, 41–49 (1980).
4. Schoeffel, R. E., Anderson, S. D., and Altounyan, R. E., Bronchial hyperreactivity in response to inhalation of ultrasonically nebulised solutions of distilled water and saline, *Br. Med. J.*, *283*, 1285–1287 (1981).

5. Anderson, S. D., Schoeffel, R. E., Follet, R., Perry, C. P., Daviskas, E., and Kendall, M., Sensitivity to heat and water loss at rest and during exercise in asthmatic patients, *Eur. J. Respir. Dis.*, *63*, 459–471 (1982).
6. Anderson, S. D., Schoeffel, R. E., and Finney, M., Evaluation of ultrasonically nebulised solutions as a provocation in patients with asthma, *Thorax*, *38*, 284–291 (1983).
7. Anderson, S. D., Bronchial challenge by ultrasonically nebulized aerosols, *Clin. Rev. Allergy*, *3*, 427–439 (1985).
8. Smith, C. M., and Anderson, S. D., Inhalation provocation tests using non-isotonic aerosols, *J. Allergy Clin. Immunol.*, *84*, 781–790 (1989).
9. Smith, C. M., and Anderson, S. D., A comparison between the airway response to isocapnic hyperventilation and hypertonic saline in subjects with asthma, *Eur. Respir. J.*, *2*, 36–43 (1989).
10. Smith, C. M., and Anderson, S. D., Inhalation challenge using hypertonic saline in asthmatic subjects: a comparison with responses to hyperpnoea, methacholine and water, *Eur. Respir. J.*, *3*, 144–151 (1990).
11. Anderson, S. D., Asthma provoked by exercise, hyperventilation, and the inhalation of non-isotonic aerosols, in *Asthma: Basic Mechanisms and Clinical Management*, 2nd Ed. (P. J. Barnes, I. W. Rodger, and N. C. Thompson, eds.), Academic Press, London, 1992, pp. 473–490.
12. Sterk, P. J., Fabbri, L. M., Quanjer, Ph. H., Cockcroft, D. W., O'Byrne, P. M., Anderson, S. D., Juniper, E. F., and Malo, J.-L., Airway responsiveness. Standardized challenge testing with pharmacological, physiological and sensitizing stimuli in man, *Eur. Respir. J.*, *6* (suppl. 16), 53–83 (1993).
13. Galdes-Sebalt, M., McLaughlin, F. J., and Levison, H., Comparison of cold air, ultrasonic mist, and methacholine inhalations as tests of bronchial reactivity in normal and asthmatic children, *J. Pediatr.*, *107*, 526–530 (1985).
14. Hopp, R. J., Christy, J., Bewtra, A. K., Nair, N. K., and Townley, R. G., Incorporation and analysis of ultrasonically nebulized distilled water challenges in an epidemiological study of asthma and bronchial reactivity, *Ann. Allergy*, *60*, 129–133 (1990).
15. Araki, H., and Sly, P., Inhalation of hypertonic saline as a bronchial challenge in children with mild asthma and normal children, *J. Allergy Clin. Immunol.*, *84*, 99–107 (1989).
16. Woolcock, A. J., Peat, J. K., Salome, C. M., Yan, K., Anderson, S. D., Schoeffel, R. E., McCowage, G., and Killalea, T., Prevalence of bronchial hyperresponsiveness and asthma in a rural adult population, *Thorax*, *42*, 361–8 (1987).
17. Casale, T. B., Rhodes, B. J., Donnelly, A. L., and Weiler, J. M., Airway reactivity to methacholine in nonatopic asymptomatic adults, *J. Appl. Physiol.*, *64*, 2558–2561 (1988).
18. Cockcroft, D. W., Murdock, K. Y., Berscheid, B. A., and Gore, B. P., Sensitivity and specificity of histamine PC_{20} determination in a random selection of young college students, *J. Allergy Clin. Immunol.*, *89*, 23–30 (1992).
19. Finney, M. J. B., Anderson, S. D., and Black, J. L., The effect of non-isotonic solutions on human isolated airway smooth muscle, *Respir. Physiol.*, *69*, 277–286 (1987).
20. Eschenbacher, W. L., and Gravelyn, T. R., Mediator release after local osmolar

challenge to the airways, in *Mechanisms in Asthma: Pharmacology, Physiology, and Management*. Alan R Liss, New York, 1988, pp. 355–363.

21. Gravelyn, T. R., Pan, P. M., and Eschenbacher, W. L., Mediator release in an isolated airway segment in subjects with asthma, *Am. Rev. Respir. Dis.*, *137*, 641–646 (1988).
22. Maxwell, D. L., Atkinson, B. A., Barros, M., and Lee, T. H., Histamine release in isolated large airway segments of normal and asthmatic subjects in vivo, *Thorax*, *45*, 309P (1990).
23. Pisarri, T. E., Jonson, A., Coleridge, H. M., and Coleridge, J. C. G., Intravenous injection of hypertonic NaCl solutions stimulates pulmonary C-fibres in dogs, *Am. J. Physiol.*, *260* (Heart Circ Physiol 29), H1522–1530 (1991).
24. Umeno, E., McDonald, O. M., and Nadel, J. A., Hypertonic saline increases vascular permeability in the rat trachea by producing neurogenic inflammation, *J. Clin. Invest.*, *851*, 1905–1908 (1990).
25. Eggleston, P. A., Kagey-Sobotka, A., Schleimer, R. P., et al., Interaction between hyperosmolar and IgE-mediated histamine release from basophils and mast cells, *Am. Rev. Respir. Dis.*, *130*, 86–91 (1984).
26. Eggleston, P. A., Kagey-Sobotka, A., and Lichtenstein, L. M., A comparison of the osmotic activation of basophils and human lung mast cells, *Am. Rev. Respir. Dis.*, *135*, 1043–1048 (1987).
27. Eggleston, P. A., Kagey-Sobotka, A., Proud, D., Adkinson, N. F., and Lichtenstein, L. M., Disassociation of the release of histamine and arachidonic acid metabolites from osmotically activated basophils and human lung mast cells, *Am. Rev. Respir. Dis.*, *141*, 960–964 (1990).
28. Silber, G., Proud, D., Warner, J., Naclerio, R., Kagey-Sobotka, A., Lichtenstein, L., and Eggleston, P., *In vivo* release of inflammatory mediators by hyperosmolar solutions, *Am. Rev. Respir. Dis.*, *137*, 606–612 (1988).
29. Eschenbacher, W. L., and Gravelyn, T. R., A technique for isolated airway segment lavage, *Chest*, *92*, 105–109 (1987).
30. Shaw, R. J., Anderson, S. D., Durham, S. R., Taylor, K. M., Schoeffel, R. E., Green, W., Torzillo, P., and Kay, A. B., Mediators of hypersensitivity and "fog"-induced asthma, *Allergy*, *40*, 48–57 (1985).
31. Moscata, G., Rampulla, C., Dellabianca, A., Zanotti, E., and Candura, S., Effect of salbutamol and inhaled sodium cromoglycate on the airway and neutrophil chemotactic activity in 'fog'-induced bronchospasm, *J. Allergy Clin. Immunol.*, *82*, 382–388 (1988).
32. Belcher, N. G., Murdoch, R. D., Dalton, N., House, F. R., Clark, T. J. H., Rees, J., and Lee, T. H., A comparison of mediator and catecholamine release between exercise- and hypertonic saline–induced asthma, *Am. Rev. Respir. Dis.*, *137*, 1026–1032 (1988).
33. Black, J. L., Schoeffel, R. E., Sundrum, R., Berend, N., and Anderson, S. D., Increased responsiveness to methacholine and histamine after challenge with ultrasonically nebulised water in asthmatic subjects, *Thorax*, *40*, 427–432 (1985).
34. Mattoli, S., Foresi, A., Corbo, G., et al., Increase in bronchial responsiveness to methacholine and late asthmatic response after the inhalation of ultrasonically nebulized distilled water, *Chest*, *90*, 726–732 (1986).

35. Smith, C. M., Anderson, S. D., and Black, J. L., Methacholine responsiveness increases after ultrasonically nebulized water, but not after ultrasonically nebulized hypertonic saline, *J. Allergy Clin. Immunol.*, *79*, 85–92 (1987).
36. O'Hickey, S. P., Arm, J. P., Rees, P. J., and Lee, T. H., Airway responsiveness to methacholine after inhalation of nebulized hypertonic saline in bronchial asthma, *J. Allergy Clin. Immunol.*, *83*, 472–476 (1989).
37. Bussieres, S., Turcotte, H., and Boulet, L.-P., Hyperosmolarity-induced increases in airway responsiveness and late asthmatic responses, *Eur. Respir. J.*, *4*, 290–295 (1991).
38. Robuschi, M., Vaghi, A., Simone, P., et al., Prevention of fog-induced bronchospasm by nedocromil sodium, *Clin. Allergy*, *17*, 69–74 (1987).
39. Rodwell, L. T., Anderson, S. D., du Toit, J. I., and Seale, J. P., Nedocromil sodium inhibits the airway response to hyperosmolar challenge in patients with asthma, *Am. Rev. Respir. Dis.*, *146*, 1149–1155 (1992).
40. Robuschi, M., Vaghi, A., Gambaro, G., Spagnotto, S., and Bianco, S., Inhaled furosemide (F) is effective in preventing ultrasonically nebulized 5.8% NaCl bronchoconstriction, *Eur. Respir. J.*, *1* (suppl. 2), 194S (1988).
41. Rodwell, L. T., Anderson, S. D., du Toit, J. I., and Seale, J. P., Inhaled furosemide reduces airway sensitivity to inhaled 4.5% NaCl aerosol in asthmatic subjects, *Thorax*, *48*, 208–213 (1993).
42. Leung, K. B. P., Flint, K. C., Brostoff, J., Hudspith, B. N., Johnson, N. Mc. I., Lau, H. Y. A., Liu, W. L., and Pearce, F. L., Effects of sodium cromoglycate and nedocromil sodium on histamine secretion from human lung mast cells, *Thorax*, *43*, 756–761 (1988).
43. Romanin, C., Reinsprecht, M., Pecht, I., and Schindler, H., Immunologically activated chloride channels involved in degranulation of rat mucosal mast cells, *EMBO J.*, *10*, 3603–3608 (1991).
44. Reinsprecht, M., Pecht, I., Schindler, H., and Romanin, C., Potent block of Cl^- channels by antiallergic drugs, *Biochem. Biophys. Res. Comm.*, *188*, 957–963 (1992).
45. Jackson, D. M., and Richards, I. M., The effects of sodium cromoglycate on histamine aerosol–induced reflex bronchoconstriction in the anaesthetized dog, *Br. J. Pharmacol.*, *61*, 257–262 (1977).
46. Jackson, D. M., Pollard, C. E., and Roberts, S. M., The effect of nedocromil sodium on the isolated rabbit vagus nerve, *Eur. J. Pharmacol.*, *221*, 175–177 (1992).
47. Belcher, N. G., Rees, P. J., Clark, T. J. H., et al., A comparison of the refractory periods induced by hypertonic airway challenge and exercise in bronchial asthma, *Am. Rev. Respir. Dis.*, *135*, 822–825 (1987).
48. Mattoli, S., Foresi, A., Corbo, G. M., et al., Refractory period to ultrasonic mist of distilled water: relationship to methacholine responsiveness, atopic status, and clinical characteristics, *Ann. Allergy*, *58*, 134–140 (1987).
49. Rodwell, L. T., Anderson, S. D., Spring, J. F., and Seale, J. P., Indomethacin and airway responsiveness to repeated 4.5% NaCl challenges *Aust. NZ J. Med.*, Abstract of the Thoracic Society of Australia and New Zealand Annual Scientific Meeting 1993, *Eur. Respir. J.*, *6*, (Suppl. 17), 200s (1993).

50. Hawksworth, R. J., O'Hickey, S., and Lee, T. H., The effects of indomethacin on hypertonic saline–induced bronchoconstriction and the refractory period, *Eur. Respir. J.*, *5*, 963–966 (1992).
51. Mattoli, S., Foresi, A., Corbo, G. M., et al., The effect of indomethacin on the refractory period occurring after the inhalation of ultrasonically nebulized distilled water, *J. Allergy Clin. Immunol.*, *79*, 678–683 (1987).
52. Gibson, P. G. Girgis-Gabardo, A., Morris, M. M., Mattoli, S., Kay, J. M., Dolovich, J., Denburg, J., and Hargreave, F. E., Cellular characteristics of sputum from patients with asthma and chronic bronchitis, *Thorax*, *44*, 693–699 (1989).
53. Pin, I., Gibson, P. G., Kolendowicz, R., Girgis-Gabardo, A., Denburg, J. A., Hargreave, F. E., and Dolovich, J., Use of induced sputum cell counts to investigate airway inflammation in asthma, *Thorax*, *47*, 25–29 (1992).
54. Gibson, P. G., Saltos, N., Hopkins, Y. J., and Borgas, T., Airway epithelial mast cells are associated with persisting airway hyperresponsiveness to methacholine and hypertonic saline in asthma, Personal communication, 1993.
55. Gibson, P. G., Salton, N., Hopkins, Y. J., Borgas, T., and Saunders, N. A., Repair of airway inflammation in asthma: the role of mast cells in persisting airway hyperresponsiveness (abstr.), *Am. Rev. Respir. Dis.*, *145*, A19 (1992).
56. Rodwell, L. T., Anderson, S. D., and Seale, J. P., Inhaled steroids modify bronchial responses to hyperosmolar saline, *Eur. Respir. J.*, *5*, 953–962 (1992).
57. Anderson, S. D., du Toit, J. I., Rodwell, L. T., and Jenkins, C. R., Acute effect of sodium cromogylcate on airway narrowing induced by 4.5 percent saline aerosol, *Chest*, *105*, 673–680 (1994).
58. Jenkins, C., Anderson, S. D., Wong, R., and Veale, A., Compressed air diving and respiratory disease, *Med. J. Aust.*, *158*, 275–279 (1993).
59. Bernstein, L., and Audensmoore, R. W., Iatrogenic bronchospasm occurring during clinical trials of a new mucolytic agent, acetylcysteine, *Dis. Chest*, *46*, 469–473 (1964).
60. Mann, J. S., Howarth, P. H., and Holgate, S. T., Bronchoconstriction induced by ipratropium bromide in asthma: relation to hypotonicity, *Br. Med. J.*, *289*, 469 (1984).
61. O'Callaghan, C., Milner, A. D., and Swarbrick, A., Paradoxical deterioration in lung function after nebulised salbutamol in wheezy infants, *Lancet*, *20*, 1424–1425 (1986).
62. Chua, H. L., Collis, G. G., and LeSouef, P. N., Bronchial response to nebulized antibiotics in children with cystic fibrosis, *Eur. Respir. J.*, *3*, 1114–1116 (1990).
63. Miller, W. C., and Awe, R., Effect of nebulized lidocaine on reactive airways, *Am. Rev. Respir. Dis.*, *111*, 7399–7441 (1975).
64. Loehning, R. W., Waltemath, C. L., and Bergman, N. A., Lidocaine and increased respiratory resistance produced by ultrasonic aerosols, *Anesthesiology*, *41*, 306–310 (1976).
65. Rankin, J. A., Snyder, R. R. T., Schachter, E. N., and Matthay, R. A., Broncho-alveolar lavage; its safety in subjects with mild asthma, *Chest*, *85*, 723–728 (1984).
66. Waltemath, C. L., and Bergman, N. A., Increased respiratory resistance provoked by endotracheal administration of aerosols, *Am. Rev. Respir. Dis.*, *108*, 520–525 (1973).

67. Boucher, R. M. G., and Kreuter, J., The fundamentals of the ultrasonic atomization of medicated solutions, *Ann. Allergy*, *26*, 591–600 (1968).
68. Mercer, T. T., Production of therapeutic aerosols; principles and techniques, *Chest*, *80*, 813S–818S (1981).
69. Anderson, S. D., and Schoeffel, R. E., The inhalation of ultrasonically nebulized aerosols as a provocation test for asthma, in *Airway Responsiveness: Measurement and Interpretation, Proceedings of a Workshop* (F. E. Hargreave and A. J. Woolcock, eds.), Astra Pharmaceuticals Canada Ltd., Ontario, Canada, 1985, pp. 39–50
70. Gonda, I., Pharmaceutical developments in therapeutic and diagnostic aerosols, *Pharm. Tech. Japan*, *2*, 883–893 (1986).
71. Gerrity, T. R., Lee, P. S., Hass, F. J., Marinelli, A., Werner, P., and Lourenço, R. V., Calculated deposition of inhaled particles in the airway generations of normal subjects, *J. Appl. Physiol. Respirat. Environ. Exercise Physiol.*, *47*, 867–873 (1979).
72. Phipps, P. R., Characteristics and pulmonary deposition of therapeutic and diagnostic aqueous aerosols, Ph.D. Thesis, University of Sydney, 1990.
73. Ferron, G. A., Haider, B., and Kreyling, W. G., Inhalation of salt aerosol particles. 1. Estimation of the temperature and relative humidity of the air in the human upper airways, *J. Aerosol Sci.*, *19*, 343–363 (1988).
74. Boucher, R. C., and Willumsen, N. J., Effects of raised osmolality on human nasal epithelium (HNE) (abstr.), *FASEB J.*, *2*, A706 (2379) (1988).
75. Fabbri, L. M., Hendrick, D. J., and Diem, J. E., Effect of atropine on the bronchial response of asthmatic subjects to the inhalation of ultrasonically nebulized distilled water, *J. Allergy Clin. Immunol.*, *71*, 468–472 (1983).
76. Fabbri, L. M., Mapp, C. E., and Hendrick, D. J., Comparison of ultrasonically nebulized distilled water and hyperventilation with cold air in asthma, *Ann. Allergy*, *53*, 172–177 (1984).
77. Groot, C., Lammers, J. W., Festern, J., van Herwaarden, C., Refractoriness for ultrasonically nebulized distilled water and histamine challenge, *J. Appl. Physiol.*, *70*, 1011–1115 (1991).
78. Simone, P., Robuschi, M., Vaghi, A., et al., Prevention of fog-induced bronchospasm by Duovent and its components (fenoterol, ipratropium bromide) in asthmatics, *Respiration*, *50* (suppl. 2), 192–195 (1986).
79. Sheppard, D., Rizk, N. W., Boushey, H. A., et al., Mechanisms of cough and bronchoconstriction induced by distilled water aerosols, *Am. Rev. Respir. Dis.*, *127*, 691–694 (1983).
80. Finney, M. J. B., Anderson, S. D., and Black, J., Terfenadine modifies airway narrowing induced by the inhalation of nonisotonic aerosols in subjects with asthma, *Am. Rev. Respir. Dis.*, *141*, 1151–1157 (1990).
81. Rodwell, L. T., Anderson, S. D., and Seale, J. P., Inhaled clemastine, an H_1 antihistamine inhibits airway narrowing caused by aerosols of non-isotonic saline, *Eur. Respir. J.*, *4*, 1128–1134 (1991).
82. Smith, C. M., Physical agents in bronchial provocation tests, in *Methods in Asthmology* (L. Allegra, P. Braga, and R. Dal Negro, eds.), Springer-Verlag, New York, 1993, pp. 226–237.
83. Bianco, S., Robuschi, M., Caeserani, R., et al., Effects of prostacyclin on aspecifi-

cally and specifically induced bronchoconstriction in asthmatic patients, *Eur. J. Respir. Dis.*, *61* (suppl. 106), 81–87 (1980).

84. Bianco, S., Robuschi, M., and Damonte, C., Drug effect on bronchial response to PGF_2 alpha and water inhalation: Proceedings of the Symposium on the Nose and Bronchi, *Eur. J. Respir. Dis.*, *64* (suppl. 28), 213–221 (1983).
85. Hogg, J. C., Hulbert, W. C., Armour, C., et al., The effect of mucosal inflammation on airways reactivity, in *Asthma: Physiology, Immunopharmacology and Treatment* (A. B. Kay, K. F. Austen, and L. M Lichtenstein, eds.), Academic Press, London, 1984, pp. 327–338.
86. Anderson, S. D., and Rodwell, L. T., Lung function before and after challenge with an aerosol of 4.5% NaCl in patients with sarcoidosis and healthy subjects, *Aust. N.Z. J. Med.*, *20*, 517S (1990).
87. Boulet, L.-P., Turcotte, H., and Tennina, S., Comparative efficacy of salbutamol, ipratropium and cromoglycate in the prevention of bronchospasm induced by exercise and hyperosmolar challenges, *J. Allergy Clin. Immunol.*, *83*, 882–887 (1989).
88. Mormile, F., Mattoli, S., Rosati, G., et al., Allergen-induced increase in non-allergic bronchial responsiveness to ultrasonic mist, *Prog. Resp. Res.*, *19*, 256–265 (1985).
89. Higenbottam, T., Cough induced by changes of ionic composition of airway surface liquid, *Bull. Eur. Physiopathol. Respir.*, *20*, 553–562 (1984).
90. Eschenbacher, W. L., Boushey, H. A., and Sheppard, D., Alteration in osmolarity of inhaled aerosols cause bronchoconstriction and cough, but absence of a permeant anion causes cough alone, *Am. Rev. Respir. Dis.*, *129*, 211–215 (1984).
91. Kivity, S., Ganem, R., Greif, J., and Topilsky, M., The combined effect of nifedipine and sodium cromoglycate on the airway response to inhaled hypertonic saline in patients with bronchial asthma, *Eur. Respir. J.*, *2*, 513–516 (1989).
92. O'Hickey, S. P., Belcher, N. G., Rees, P. J.,and Lee, T. H., Role of histamine release in hypertonic saline induced bronchoconstriction, *Thorax*, *44*, 650–653 (1989).
93. Finnerty, J. P., Wilmont, C., and Holgate, S. T., Inhibition of hypertonic saline–induced bronchoconstriction by terfenadine and flurbiprofen: evidence for the predominant role of histamine, *Am. Rev. Respir. Dis.*, *140*, 593–597 (1989).
94. Boulet, L.-P., Legris, C., Thibault, L., and Turcotte, H., Comparative bronchial responses to hyperosmolar saline and methacholine in asthma, *Thorax*, *42*, 953–958 (1987).
95. Magyar, P., Dervaderics, M., Toth, A., et al., Inhalation of hypertonic potassium chloride solution: a specific bronchial challenge for asthma, *Ital. J. Chest Dis.*, *37*, 29–34 (1983).
96. Magyar, P., Dervaderics, M., and Toth, A., Bronchial challenge with hypertonic KCL solution in the diagnosis of bronchial asthma, *Schweiz Med. Wschr.*, *114*, 910–913 (1984).
97. Bascom, R., and Bleeker, E. R., Bronchostriction induced by distilled water: sensitivity in asthmatics and relationship to exercise-induced bronchospasm, *Am. Rev. Respir. Dis.*, *134*, 248–253 (1986).
98. Anderson, S. D., Is there a unifying hypothesis for exercise-induced asthma? *J. Allergy Clin. Immunol.*, *73*, 660–665 (1984).

99. Smith, C. M., and Anderson, S. D., Hyperosmolarity as the stimulus to asthma induced by hyperventilation, *J. Allergy Clin. Immunol.*, *77*, 729–736 (1986).
100. Smith, C. M., and Anderson, S. D., An investigation of the hyperosmolar stimulus to exercise-induced asthma (abstr.), *Aust. N.Z. J. Med.*, *17*, A513 (1987).
101. Kivity, S., Greif, J., Reisner, B., Fireman, E., and Topilsky, M., Bronchial inhalation challenge with ultrasonically nebulized saline; comparison to exercise-induced asthma, *Ann. Allergy*, *57*, 355–358 (1986).
102. Belcher, N. G., Lee, T. H., and Rees, P. J., Airway responses to hypertonic saline, exercise and histamine challenges in bronchial asthma, *Eur. Respir. J.*, *2*, 44–48 (1989).
103. Boulet, L.-P., and Turcotte, H., Comparative effects of hyperosmolar saline inhalation and exercise in asthma, *Immunol. Allergy Pract.*, *11*, 93–100 (1989).
104. Foresi, A., Mattoli, S., Corbo, G. M., et al., Comparison of bronchial responses to ultrasonically nebulized distilled water, exercise, and methacholine in asthma, *Chest*, *90*, 822–826 (1986).
105. Daviskas, E., Gonda, I., and Anderson, S. D., Mathematical modelling of heat and water transport in human respiratory tract, *J. Appl. Physiol.*, *69*, 362–372 (1990).
106. Daviskas, E., Gonda, I., and Anderson, S. D., Local airway heat and water vapour losses, *Respir. Physiol.*, *84*, 115–132 (1991).
107. Hanna, L. M., and Scherer, P. W., Regional control of local airway heat and water vapor losses, *J. Appl. Physiol.*, *61*, 624–632 (1986).
108. Riedler, J., and Robertson, C. F., Effect of tidal volume on the output and particle size distribution of hypertonic saline from an ultrasonic nebulizer, *Eur. Respir. J.*, *7*, 998–1002 (1994).
109. Riedler, J., Reade, T., and Robertson, C. F., Repeatibility of the response to 4.5% NaCl challenge in children with mild to severe asthma, *Pediatr. Pulmonol.*, 1994 (in press).
110. Riedler, J., Reade, T., Dalton, M., Holst, Di, and Robertson, C. F., Hypertonic saline challenge in an epidemiological survey of asthma in children, *Am. J. Respir. Crit. Care Med.*, 1994 (in press).

11

Inhalation Challenges with Lipid Mediators (Leukotrienes, Prostaglandins, and PAF-Acether) and Adenosine

Jonathan P. Arm

Brigham and Women's Hospital and Harvard Medical School
Boston, Massachusetts

Tak H. Lee

Guy's Hospital
London, England

I. LEUKOTRIENES, PROSTAGLANDINS, AND PAF-ACETHER

Arachidonic acid (AA) released from membrane phospholipids during cell activation may be oxidatively metabolized by the enzymes of the cyclooxygenase or lipoxygenase pathway [1] (Fig. 1). Arachidonic acid is metabolized by the cyclooxygenase pathway to prostaglandin (PG) G_2 and PGH_2. These cyclic endoperoxides are metabolized by specific synthetases to PGE_2 PGD_2, $PGF_{2\alpha}$, PGI_2 (prostacyclin), and thromboxane (TX) A_2. The 5-lipoxygenase (5-LO) pathway, which has a more limited distribution than the cyclooxygenase cascade, generates 5-hydroperoxyeicosatetraenoic acid (5-HPETE) from AA. 5-HPETE is reduced to 5-hydroxyeicosatetraenoic acid (5-HETE) or is converted enzymatically to leukotriene (LT) A_4. Leukotriene A_4 is processed enzymatically to LTB_4 or to LTC_4. Leukotriene C_4 is cleaved by γ-glutamyl transpeptidase to LTD_4, and by a dipeptidase to LTE_4. Leukotriene C_4, LTD_4, and LTE_4 constitute the activity previously recognized as slow-reacting substance of anaphylaxis (SRS-A).

The phospholipid mediator platelet activating factor (PAF or PAF-acether) was initially described as generated by rabbit basophils [2]. Phospholipase A_2 generates the immediate precursor lyso-PAF from ether phospholipids [3]. Lyso-PAF is then acetylated by acetyltransferase to PAF-acether. PAF-acether is metabolized by acetylhydrolase back to lyso-PAF. PAF-acether is synthesized by many different cells, including platelets, neutrophils, eosinophils, monocytes, and macrophages.

The contribution of lipid mediators to the pathophysiology of bronchial asthma

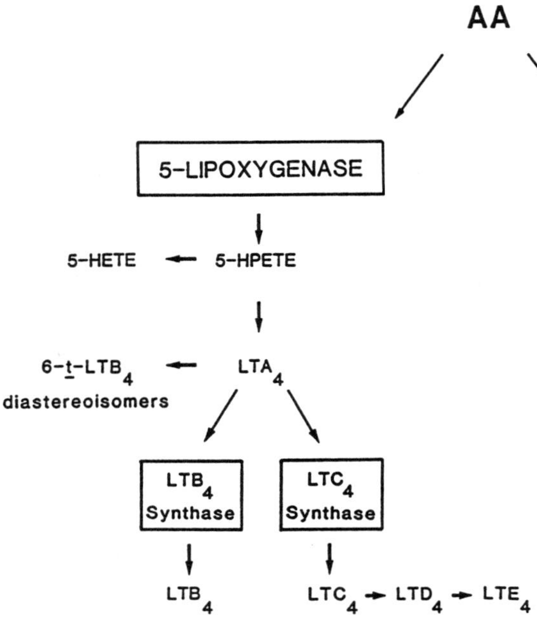

Figure 1 Metabolism of arachidonic acid (AA) by the 5-lipoxygenase and cyclooxygenase pathways. 5-HETE = 5-hydroxyeicosatetraenoic acid; 5-HPETE = 5-hydroperoxyeicosatetraenoic acid; 6-*t*-LTB_4 = 6-*trans*-LTB_4 diastereoisomers; LT = leukotriene; PG = prostaglandin.

is suggested by their potent biological properties, their generation by a diverse variety of inflammatory cells, their identification in the bronchoalveolar lavage fluid of asthmatic subjects both at rest and following experimentally provoked asthma, and studies demonstrating the capacity of 5-LO inhibitors and leukotriene antagonists to attenuate the asthmatic response.

A. Methodology

1. Leukotrienes and Prostaglandins

Inhalation challenges with leukotrienes and prostaglandins are performed using modifications of well-established and standardized techniques developed for inhalation challenges with histamine and methacholine. They fall broadly into two types. In the method described by Cockroft et al. [4], a flow of compressed air is passed continuously through a nebulizer to generate an aerosol that the subject inhales during tidal breathing over 1–2 min, wearing a nose clip. In the method described by Chai et al. [5], the nebulizer is linked to a dosimeter that delivers a pulse of compressed air to the nebulizer, each pulse lasting for between 0.5 and 1.0 s. The dosimeter is triggered by the start of inspiration. In both methods the control saline diluent is inhaled, and this is followed by the inhalation of geometrically increasing concentrations of agonist until the desired decrement in pulmonary function is achieved. The importance of selecting a nebulizer that generates particles of a suitable size, the importance of delivering air to the nebulizer under suitable conditions of flow and pressure, and the effects of different rates and patterns of inhalation have been reviewed extensively elsewhere [6]. Airway response is measured using standard techniques of pulmonary function such as forced expired volume in 1 second (FEV_1), airway resistance (Raw), specific airway conductance (SGaw), or measurements of flow derived from maximal or partial forced expiratory flow volume curves such as $V_{30}P$ and $V_{40}P$. The timing of measurements should be made so that the time of the expected maximal airway response is encompassed. Leukotriene D_4 has a rapid onset of action, within 2–3 min of inhalation, comparable to that of histamine [7]. In contrast, LTC_4 and LTE_4 have a slower onset of action, reaching a peak at 5–15 minutes [8,9]. The response to the sulfidopeptide leukotrienes is sustained, and relaxation starts at 20–30 min following inhalation. Prostaglandin $F_{2\alpha}$ and PGD_2 and its immediate metabolite, $9\alpha,11\beta\text{-PGF}_2$, have a rapid onset of bronchoconstriction, with a maximal effect at between 3 and 10 min [10–12].

In our laboratory, inhalation challenges are performed using a Hudson nebulizer linked to a breath-activated dosimeter [13–15]. Delivery of air to the nebulizer is regulated to a pressure of 138 kPa (20 pounds per square inch), for a duration of 0.6 s from the start of inspiration of each breath. Under these conditions the Hudson nebulizer delivers droplets with a mass median aerodynamic diameter of 1.6 μm, and the output of the nebulizer is 2.6 μl per breath. Changes in airway caliber are determined by measurements of SGaw, residual volume, and $V_{25}P$ in a total body plethysmograph linked to a digital computer [16]. Four to six measurements of SGaw are recorded at each time point, and the mean value for each parameter is calculated. Baseline SGaw is $>0.9\ s^{-1}kPa^{-1}$ before each challenge. Following baseline measurements of SGaw, the subject inhales 10 breaths of phosphate-buffered saline (PBS) as a control. Each inhalation starts at functional residual capacity and terminates at approximately 70% of baseline vital capacity; a 5-s breath hold is maintained at the end of each inhalation. Provided the decrease in SGaw is <10%, the patient is subjected to inhalation challenge. Threefold increasing concentrations of LTE_4 are inhaled, starting at a concentration of 4×10^{-7} mol/L (180 ng/ml) in asthmatic subjects and 1×10^{-5} mol/L (4.4 μg/ml) in normal subjects. Specific airway conductance is measured every 5 min for 15 min. If the desired decrease in SGaw is not achieved within 15 min, the concentration of LTE_4 in the nebulizer is increased threefold and the protocol is repeated. The starting concentrations of LTC_4 and LTD_4 used for inhalation challenge are 4×10^{-8} mol/L (25 and 20 ng/ml, respectively) in asthmatic subjects and 4 × 10^{-7} mol/L (250 and 200 ng/ml, respectively) in normal subjects.

It is essential that the purity and identity of the agonists used for challenge be established. In our own studies, leukotrienes are prepared by total chemical synthesis [17] and frozen under argon at −70°C. Their authenticities are confirmed by nuclear magnetic resonance analysis. The products are analyzed before inhalation challenge by reverse-phase high-performance liquid chromatography (RP-HPLC) using a 10-μm C_{18} ultrasil-ODS column (4.6 × 250 mm) at a flow rate of 1 ml/min with 65% methanol, 34.9% water, and 0.1% acetic acid, pH 5.6, as solvent. Absorbance is monitored with an on-line spectrophotometer linked to an integrator. The purities of the leukotrienes before challenge are confirmed by their elution as single peaks at their unique retention times in this solvent system. The concentrations of the stock solutions are assessed by ultraviolet (UV) scanning at 280 nM, assuming a molar extinction coefficient of 40,000 cm^{-1} M^{-1}, and dilutions of the compounds are prepared in PBS. On different occasions, samples of the solution remaining in the nebulizer after the highest concentration of the leukotriene has been administered are analyzed by RP-HPLC and by measurement of UV absorbance at 280 nM to determine whether the purity or concentration of the product has changed during nebulization.

Because the sulfidopeptide leukotrienes are not readily available in large quantities, Bel and colleagues described a technique for challenges with LTD_4 in which more efficient use is made of the agonist [18]. They reported the results of inhalation challenges with LTD_4 in nonasthmatic subjects using relatively small quantities at low concentrations. Leukotriene D_4 was dissolved in a volatile medium that was nebulized through an efficient jet nebulizer. One-half of a milliliter of the desired concentration was nebulized by compressed nitrogen over 1 min into a 30-L drying chamber. The droplets were reported to have a mass median aerodynamic diameter of 2.5 μm and to evaporate rapidly to dry particles. The aerosol in the drying chamber was inhaled by tidal breathing while oxygen was delivered to the mouthpiece at 4 L/min. With this technique it was possible to administer 385 nmol of LTD_4 as a single dose nebulized from 0.5 ml of a 0.77 mmol/L solution. By comparison, when the dosimeter method described above is used, a minimum volume of 1.5 ml of solution is required to ensure a consistent output from the nebulizer, and 10 breaths of a 0.77 mmol/L solution would generate a dose of 20 nmol at the mouth. Bel and colleagues also compared their technique with a conventional tidal breathing technique for methacholine challenge. Close agreement was found between the two techniques in determining both the dose of methacholine required to elicit a 10% fall in FEV_1 and the dose required to elicit a 40% fall in $V_{40}P$. Between-day reproducibility was reported as ± 1.6 doubling doses.

Starting concentrations for inhalation challenges with $PGF_{2\alpha}$ have varied widely between studies, depending on selection of subjects and method of challenge. Using a tidal-breathing method, Thomson et al. reported a starting concentration of 0.07 μg/ml [19], and Hardy and colleagues used a concentration of 39 μg/ml [11]. Using a dosimeter, Beasley and co-workers reported starting concentrations for PGD_2, $PGF_{2\alpha}$, and $9\alpha,11\beta$-PGF_2 of 2.8×10^{-6} mol/L [12]. In our own studies, we have administered $PGF_{2\alpha}$ from a starting concentration of 0.7 μg/ml.

2. PAF-Acether

Inhalation challenges with PAF-acether are somewhat different from those with other bronchoconstrictor substances in two major respects. Bronchial smooth muscle exhibits a variable and sometimes marked tachyphylaxis to PAF-acether [20,21]. This may lead to an attenuation of the bronchoconstrictor response to sequential increasing doses of PAF-acether. Furthermore, the airway response to PAF-acether is not marked and is best determined with sensitive measurements of changes in airway caliber, such as SGaw or $V_{30}P$. Platelet activating factor is diluted in a suitable buffer, such as phosphate-buffered saline. Human serum albumin may be added to minimize adherence to the nebulizer and to other surfaces [20,22–24]. Starting concentrations have varied between 0.1 μg/ml and 2 mg/ml. In asthmatic subjects, Rubin and colleagues used a starting concentration of 0.1 μg/ml [20], increasing concentrations being given up to 1 mg/ml. However, as noted below, asthmatic subjects do not appear to exhibit a marked degree of airway hyperresponsiveness to PAF, and other investigators have begun inhalation challenges with PAF at higher concentrations [23,25]. Inhalation of PAF-acether may be associated with a sensation of flushing and warmth and a small increase in heart rate. Maximal bronchoconstriction occurs within 2–3 min of inhalation and is relatively short-lived, airway caliber returning to baseline by 15–45 min [20].

B. Experimental Results

1. Leukotrienes

Potency. The sulfidopeptide leukotrienes are potent bronchoconstrictor agents when inhaled. Griffin and colleagues [26] reported that the concentration of LTD_4 required to elicit bronchoconstriction in six asymptomatic asthmatic subjects was on average one-third of that necessary to elicit a response in normal subjects. Adelroth and co-workers [27] demonstrated a significant correlation between airway responses to methacholine, LTC_4, and LTD_4 in 12 asthmatic and six nonasthmatic subjects, as shown by measurements of FEV_1 and $V_{40}P$ indicating that asthmatic subjects were hyperresponsive to LTC_4 and LTD_4 as compared with normal control subjects. They also demonstrated a correlation between airway responsiveness to methacholine and relative responsiveness to LTC_4 and LTD_4. Subjects with the most responsive airways demonstrated the lowest relative responsiveness to LTC_4 and LTD_4 as compared with methacholine. For example, LTC_4 was 38 times more potent than methacholine in eliciting bronchoconstriction in the asthmatic subject with the most responsive airways, and 2500 times more potent than methacholine in the normal subject with the least responsive airways. Thus, experience with LTC_4 and LTD_4 suggests that asthmatic subjects, as compared with normal subjects, are relatively less hyperresponsive to the sulfido-peptide leukotrienes than to histamine and methacholine. It has been suggested that this may reflect a down-regulation of specific leukotriene receptors due to the presence of leukotrienes in the airways [27,28].

The airway responses to LTE_4 were compared with those to histamine and methacholine in 20 asthmatic subjects and 6 normal subjects [15]. There was a correlation between the dose of LTE_4 causing a 35% fall in SGaw (PD_{35} SGaw) and both the histamine PD_{35} SGaw and the methacholine PD_{35} SGaw. In contrast to the results reported for LTC_4 and LTD_4, we found that LTE_4 was on average 73 times more potent than methacholine and 112 times more potent than histamine in asthmatic subjects, and 20 and 58 times more potent than methacholine and histamine, respectively, in nonasthmatic subjects. These studies were extended in a direct comparison of the potency of LTC_4, LTD_4, and LTE_4 with that of histamine and methacholine in normal and asthmatic subjects [29]. The airways of asthmatic subjects were 14, 15, 6, 9, and 219 times more responsive than those of normal subjects to histamine, methacholine, LTC_4, LTD_4 and LTE_4, respectively. The airways of asthmatic subjects therefore possess a relative hyporesponsiveness to LTC_4 and LTD_4 as compared with histamine and methacholine and exhibit a marked and selective hyperresponsiveness to LTE_4 (Fig. 2).

Airway responsiveness to histamine and LTE_4 was also evaluated in subjects with aspirin-induced asthma (AIA), before and after desensitization [30]. In subjects without aspirin sensitivity, LTE_4 was between 51 and 550 times more potent than histamine on a molar basis. By comparison, the airways of four of five subjects with AIA were between 920 and 6600 times more sensitive to LTE_4 as compared with histamine. Subjects were desensitized through a conventional oral desensitization regime and took 600 mg of aspirin daily while airway responsiveness to LTE_4 and histamine was reassessed. Following desensitization, there were no significant changes in airway responsiveness to histamine, but the dose of LTE_4 required to elicit a 35% fall in SGaw increased between 5- and 100-fold (Fig. 3), and the relative potency of LTE_4 compared with histamine decreased a mean of 15-fold. These preliminary findings suggest that a selective airway hyperresponsiveness to LTE_4 may contribute to the mechanisms of AIA, and that the efficacy of desensitization may be due in part to a decrease in the sensitivity of the airways to LTE_4.

Site Selectivity. The site selectivity of airway hyperresponsiveness to the SRS-A leukotrienes has been evaluated by a number of investigators. Bisgaard et al. [31] reported that the airways of eight asthmatic subjects were more responsive to LTD_4

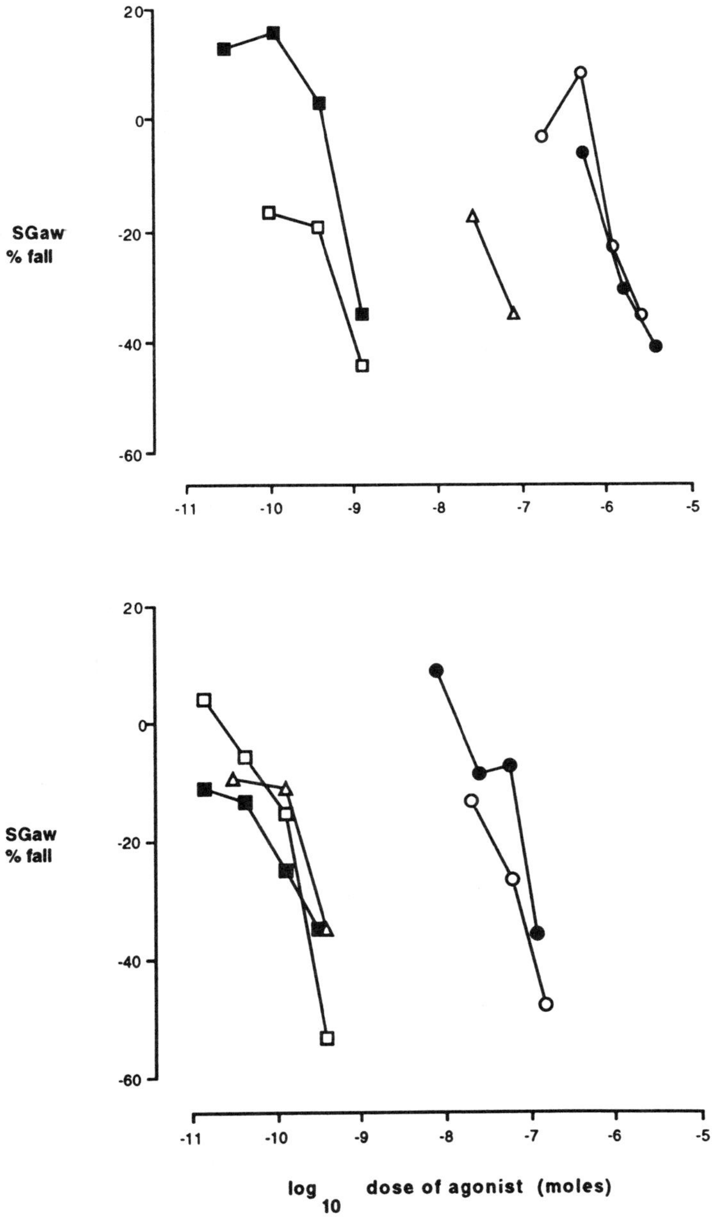

Figure 2 Dose–response curves to histamine (open circles), methacholine (solid circles), leukotriene (LT) C_4 (open squares), LTD_4 (solid squares), and LTE_4 (open triangles) in a normal subject (top panel) and an asthmatic subject (bottom panel). SGaw = specific airway conductance. (From Ref. 83.)

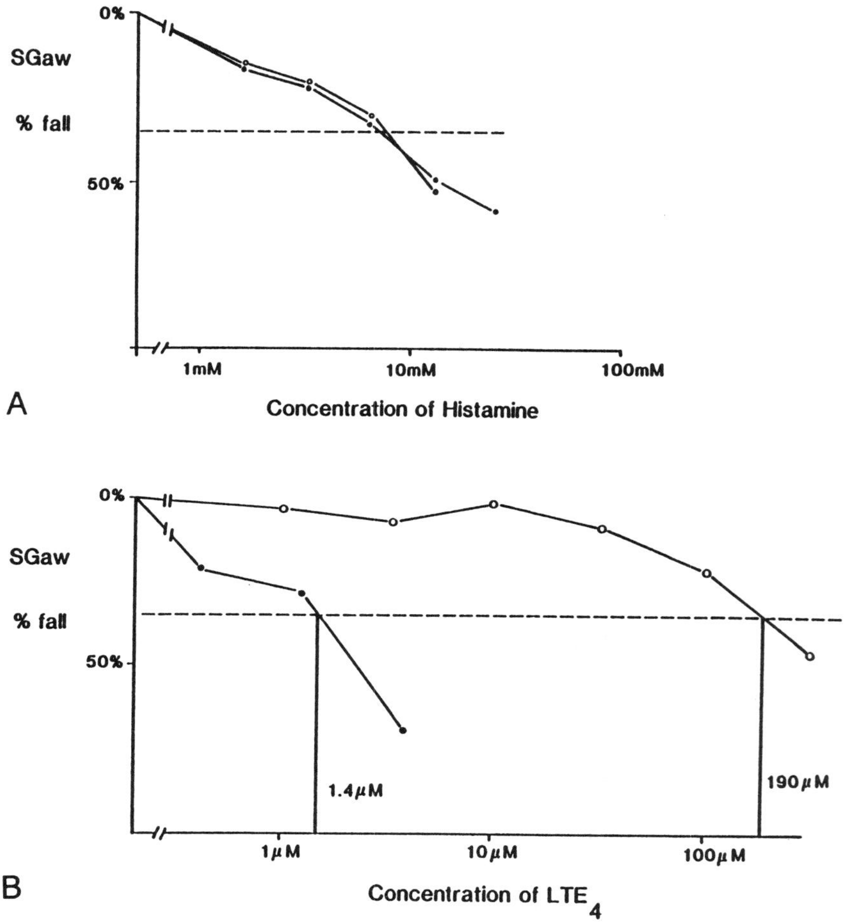

Figure 3 Dose–response curves to histamine (Panel A) and to leukotriene E (LTE_4) (Panel B) in a subject with aspirin-induced asthma before (solid circles) and after (open circles) oral aspirin desensitization.

than those of nine healthy controls. However the differences were 100- to 1000-fold for FEV_1 but only 15-fold for V_{30}. Smith et al. [32] demonstrated that a 30% fall in V_{30} in response to LTD_4 was accompanied by a 60% fall in SGaw in asthmatic subjects and a 30% fall in SGaw in normal control subjects. Davidson et al. [9] reported that a 30% fall in V_{30} in response to histamine was accompanied by a 10% and 13% fall in FEV_1 in asthmatic and normal subjects, respectively. In contrast, when the subjects inhaled LTE_4, a 30% fall in V_{30} was accompanied by a

17% fall in FEV_1 in asthmatic subjects and a 3% fall in FEV_1 in normal control subjects. Thus, the cumulative data suggest that hyperresponsiveness to the leukotrienes may be more marked in the central than in the peripheral airways of asthmatic subjects.

Induction of Hyperresponsiveness. The finding that SRS-A could enhance the contractile response of guinea pig ileum to histamine [33] has prompted a number of investigators to evaluate the capacity of the sulfidopeptide leukotrienes to enhance airways smooth muscle responsiveness both in vitro and in vivo. Pretreatment of guinea pig tracheal spirals with LTE_4, but not LTC_4 or LTD_4, in the presence of 1.3 mmol/L of calcium enhanced the subsequent contractile response to histamine [34]. Twenty-three nanomoles per liter of LTE_4 produced a mean 0.4 log decrease in the concentration of histamine required to elicit 50% maximal contraction. In contrast, LTC_4 and LTD_4 at concentrations that elicited the same contractile response as LTE_4 did not augment the contractile response of guinea pig tracheal spirals to histamine. Further work has demonstrated that LTE_4 augments the airway response to histamine in vitro through the secondary generation of prostanoids that act via the thromboxane (TP) receptor to facilitate cholinergic neurotransmission [35].

In healthy human subjects, inhalation of LTD_4 did not enhance airway responsiveness to histamine [36], to isocapnic hyperventilation, or to exercise challenge [37]. In contrast, LTD_4 increased airway responsiveness to inhaled $PGF_{2\alpha}$ [38] and to methacholine [39]. The effect of LTD_4 on airway responsiveness to methacholine was comparable in extent and duration to that elicited by PAF [22], persisting for up to 2 weeks. Normal airways differ from asthmatic airways not only in their sensitivity to a range of pharmacological and irritant stimuli [40] but also by the presence of maximal airway narrowing [41]. Bel and colleagues have demonstrated that in normal subjects the maximal airway narrowing is greater in response to LTD_4 than to methacholine. Furthermore, the degree of maximal airway narrowing in response to methacholine is augmented by preinhalation of LTD_4 [18], an effect that was prevented by pretreatment with inhaled budesonide [42].

In asthmatic subjects, inhalation of bronchoconstricting doses of LTC_4 did not increase the airway responses to ultrasonically nebulized distilled water [43]. Since LTC_4 and LTD_4 are converted to LTE_4, and because LTE_4 may persist at the site of contraction for the longest period of time [44], the capacity of LTE_4 to enhance airway histamine responsiveness was studied in both asthmatic and normal subjects [14]. Inhalation of LTE_4 to produce a mean fall in SGaw of 41% led to a mean 3.5-fold decrease in the dose of histamine required to elicit a 35% fall in SGaw ($p < 10^{-5}$). There was no significant change in airway histamine responsiveness following inhalation of methacholine that elicited a comparable fall in SGaw. Changes in airway histamine responsiveness were maximal at 4–7 h after inhalation of LTE_4 (Fig. 4) and had returned to baseline values by 1 week. In

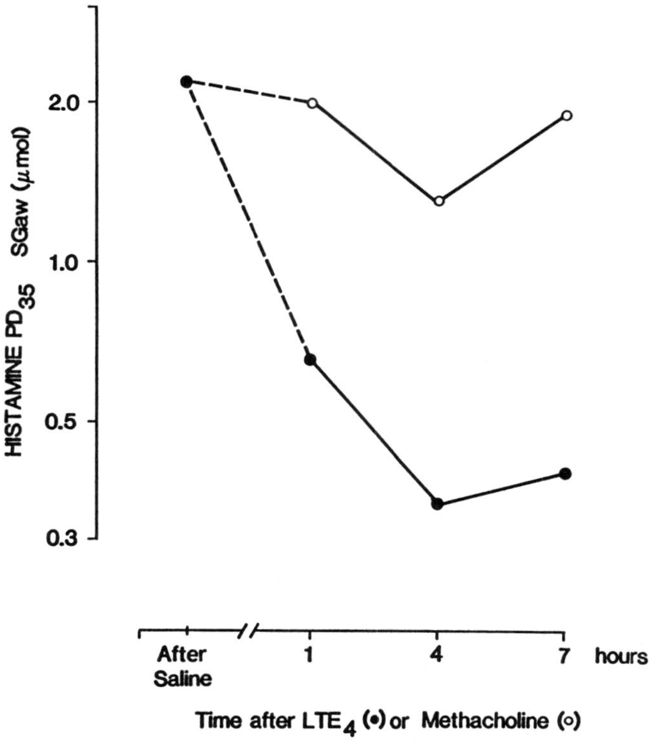

Figure 4 Representative example of the time course of changes in airway hyperresponsiveness to histamine following inhalation of leukotriene E_4 (LTE_4) in one asthmatic subject. Results are expressed as the dose of histamine required to elicit a 35% fall in specific airway conductance (SGaw) after inhalation of saline, and at 1, 4, and 7 h after inhalation of bronchoconstricting doses of methacholine (open circles) and LTE_4 (solid circles).

addition, a 50 times lower dose of LTE_4, which elicited a mean 7% fall in SGaw, decreased the histamine PD_{35} SGaw 1.5-fold ($p < 0.005$). In a further study, inhalation of bronchoconstricting doses of LTC_4 and LTD_4 by asthmatic subjects led to an increase in airway responsiveness to histamine similar to that elicited by LTE_4 [45]. Inhalation of LTC_4, LTD_4, and LTE_4 in normal subjects to produce at least a 35% fall in SGaw did not enhance airway responsiveness to histamine. In addition to their capacity to enhance airway histamine responsiveness in asthmatic subjects, leukotrienes may act synergistically with histamine during the acute bronchoconstrictor response [46].

Leukotriene Antagonists and 5-Lipoxygenase Inhibitors. In the last few years, a number of potent and selective leukotriene antagonists and 5-LO inhibitors have become available and have been evaluated in bronchial asthma. As more potent drugs have been developed, substantial evidence has accumulated suggesting a role for leukotrienes in the pathophysiology of bronchial asthma. Administration of leukotriene antagonists before LTD_4 challenge of asthmatic subjects has been reported to produce up to 120-fold rightward shift in the LTD_4 dose–response curve [47–49]. Several studies have reported bronchodilatation following administration of leukotriene antagonists to asthmatic, but not normal, subjects, an effect that is additive to that elicited by albuterol [50]. These drugs have been shown to antagonize the asthmatic response to exercise [51,52], allergen [53,54], cold, dry air [55], and aspirin [56] (Fig. 5), and to attenuate the increase in airway hyperresponsiveness that accompanies the late asthmatic response to allergen [53]. There are more limited data on the effects of 5-LO inhibitors in experimentally provoked asthma. Administration of these drugs has led to a substantial inhibition of whole-blood LTB_4 generation [57,58] and of the allergen-induced rise in urinary LTE_4 excretion [58]. The heat exchange required to cause a 20% fall in FEV_1 increased by 47% following treatment with 800 mg A-64077 [57]. The same drug administered 3 h before allergen challenge was without significant effect [58]. However, the inhibition of the acute asthmatic response to allergen

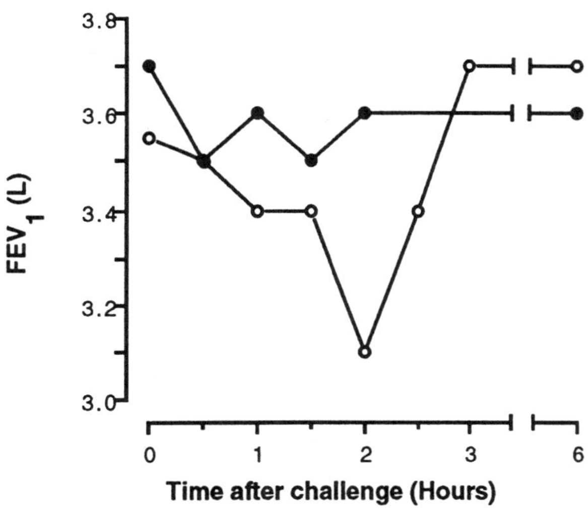

Figure 5 Time course of changes in forced expired volume in 1 second (FEV_1) in response to oral aspirin challenge, following administration of placebo (open circles) and SK&F 104353 (solid circles), in a single subject with aspirin-induced asthma.

correlated with the inhibition of urinary LTE_4 excretion, suggesting that the lack of effect may have been due to underdosing.

LY 171883 is a comparatively weak leukotriene antagonist. Nevertheless, administration of 600 mg twice daily for 6 weeks led to a small but significant improvement in FEV_1, reduction in symptoms, and reduction in bronchodilator use [59]. Preliminary data have also been reported suggesting a beneficial effect of both leukotriene antagonists and a 5-LO inhibitor in chronic asthma [60–62].

2. Prostaglandins

Potency. Initial studies on the bronchoconstrictor effects of prostaglandins were directed to the properties of $PGF_{2\alpha}$. Prostaglandin $F_{2\alpha}$ was shown to contract human airways in vivo, and asthmatics were shown to be more sensitive to $PGF_{2\alpha}$ than were normal control subjects. Smith et al. [63] studied 10 asthmatic subjects and five healthy control subjects and showed that, whereas asthmatics were approximately eight times more responsive to histamine than normal subjects, they were 160 times more responsive to $PGF_{2\alpha}$. Mathé et al. [10] compared airways responses to histamine and $PGF_{2\alpha}$ in 10 asthmatic subjects and 10 normal control subjects. Whereas asthmatics were 10 times more sensitive to histamine that the control subjects, they were 8000 times more sensitive to $PGF_{2\alpha}$. In this study, $PGF_{2\alpha}$ was 2400 times more potent than histamine in asthmatic subjects, and 2.6 times more potent than histamine in normal healthy control subjects. Thomson et al. [19] demonstrated that airway responsiveness to $PGF_{2\alpha}$ correlated with that to methacholine, but that the range of responsiveness to $PGF_{2\alpha}$ was greater than that to methacholine. Challenges with $PGF_{2\alpha}$ were found to be as reproducible as those with methacholine, and a cumulative dose effect was noted. However, the airway response to $PGF_{2\alpha}$ may not be as simple as originally described. Both Fish et al. [64] and Beasley and colleagues [12,65] have reported complex biphasic or triphasic responses to inhaled $PGF_{2\alpha}$ and have suggested that this may be due to the action of $PGF_{2\alpha}$ on separate receptors mediating bronchodilatation and bronchoconstriction. Studies of the effects of cholinergic blockade on airways responses to $PGF_{2\alpha}$ have yielded conflicting results [64–69], but the cumulative data suggest that the contribution of cholinergic pathways to $PGF_{2\alpha}$-induced bronchoconstriction is small. Neither α-adrenergic blockade [67] nor pretreatment with disodium cromoglycate (DSCG) [67,68] inhibited airway responses to $PGF_{2\alpha}$. In conclusion, airway responsiveness to $PGF_{2\alpha}$ correlates with that to methacholine; asthmatic subjects are relatively more hyperresponsive to $PGF_{2\alpha}$ than to histamine or methacholine; and the action of $PGF_{2\alpha}$ is likely to be mediated through a direct effect on smooth muscle, with little contribution from cholinergic pathways or secondary mediator generation.

Prostaglandin D_2 is the major cyclooxygenase product of the mast cell [70,71]. It is released after immunoglobulin E (IgE)-dependent challenge of human lung fragments [72] and is the major cyclooxygenase product generated by human lung mast cells after both immunological and ionophore-induced activation [71,72]. Prostaglandin D_2 contracts pulmonary smooth muscle, stimulates neutrophil chemokinesis [73], causes vasodilatation, and increases postcapillary venular permeability [74]. It acts synergistically with LTB_4 in promoting neutrophil infiltration of human skin [74]. In normal and asthmatic subjects, PGD_2 is a potent contractile agent when inhaled [11,12,65]. Hardy et al. [11] studied seven normal and seven asthmatic subjects. In asthmatic subjects the potency of PGD_2 was approximately 3.5 times and 10 times greater than that of $PGF_{2\alpha}$ and histamine, respectively. In addition, there was a significant correlation between airway responsiveness to PGD_2 and to histamine. Normal subjects were substantially less sensitive to PGD_2. Five hundred micrograms per milliliter of PGD_2 produced a mean 20% fall in SGaw; by comparison, the same dose of $PGF_{2\alpha}$ had no discernible effect in normal subjects.

$9\alpha,11\beta$-PGF_2, the major metabolite of PGD_2, is a potent contractile agonist for human airways both in vitro and in vivo [12]. $9\alpha,11\beta$-PGF_2 was found to be approximately four times more potent than PGD_2 in contracting human bronchial smooth muscle in vitro, but these two agonists were equipotent in eliciting bronchoconstriction in vivo, suggesting that some of the contractile activity of PGD_2 may be mediated through its metabolite, 9α-11β-PGF_2. The same authors also demonstrated a significant correlation between airway responses to $9\alpha,11\beta$-PGF_2 and those to both PGD_2 and histamine. In addition, they found that when subjects were pretreated with 1 mg of ipratropium bromide by inhalation, the airway response to methacholine was attenuated 70- to 200-fold, and the response to PGD_2 and $9\alpha,11\beta$-PGF_2 was inhibited 12- to 23-fold [65]. This suggests that some of the action of these prostaglandins was mediated through cholinergic pathways.

Both in vitro and in vivo studies suggest that the bronchoconstrictor actions of prostaglandins are mediated through the TP receptor [75,76]. A single 80-mg dose of GR 32191, a specific TP receptor antagonist, increased the dose of PGD_2 required to cause a 20% fall in FEV_1 more than tenfold but had no effect on the airway response to methacholine [76]. Because of the short half-life of TXA_2, it is not possible to study its direct bronchoconstrictor properties. Nevertheless, a stable thromboxane mimetic, U 46619, is available. U-44619 was found to be 178 times more potent than methacholine in asthmatic subjects, airways responses to U 46619 correlated with those to methacholine, and no tachyphylaxis was observed [77].

Induction of Hyperresponsiveness. Several studies have investigated the capacity of prostaglandins to enhance airway responsiveness in both normal and asthmatic subjects. Walters et al. [78] demonstrated that inhalation of a subthreshold dose of $PGF_{2\alpha}$ enhanced the airway response to a subsequent histamine challenge in nine nonatopic normal subjects. Heaton et al. [79] extended these observations in a study of similar design. In six normal subjects they found that a subthreshold dose of $PGF_{2\alpha}$ inhaled 10 min before challenge enhanced airway responsiveness to histamine approximately fourfold but had no effect on the airway response to methacholine. Consistent with this study is the report that 50 mg of flurbiprofen, a potent cyclooxygenase inhibitor, given three times daily for 3 days, led to a threefold decrease in the airway response to histamine but had no effect on the airway response to methacholine in the same subjects [80]. A subthreshold dose of the thromboxane mimetic U 46619 led to a transient increase in the airway response to methacholine [77]. The effect was apparent within 1 min of inhalation of U 46619 and had resolved by 1 h. The effect on histamine responsiveness was not assessed. The effects of PGD_2 on airways responses to histamine and methacholine were investigated by Fuller et al. [81]. Six atopic asthmatic subjects inhaled a single breath of either saline, histamine, bradykinin, or PGD_2, in doses that produced no measurable bronchoconstriction, immediately before each dose of histamine or methacholine. Fuller et al. found that PGD_2, but not saline, bradykinin, or histamine enhanced airways responses to subsequent histamine and methacholine challenge approximately twofold. Hardy et al. [82] confirmed the potentiating effect of PGD_2 on airway histamine responsiveness in three asthmatic subjects but indicated that the results may represent a physiological rather than a pharmacological effect of PGD_2. They investigated the effect on the bronchoconstrictor response of equipotent doses of two mediators given sequentially. Histamine or PGD_2 was inhaled by asthmatic subjects to produce a 25% fall in SGaw, followed immediately by equipotent doses of histamine or PGD_2. The airway response to histamine given as the second agonist was the same irrespective of whether PGD_2 or histamine was given as the first agonist. Histamine and PGD_2 were therefore additive and not synergistic in their effects on the airways of asthmatic subjects.

Therapeutic Intervention. There have been numerous studies of the action of cyclooxygenase inhibitors, thromboxane synthetase inhibitors, and thromboxane-receptor antagonists in bronchial asthma. We have recently reviewed these data [83], which suggest that prostanoids make little contribution to resting airway tone in either asthmatic or normal airways in vivo. Cyclooxygenase inhibition or administration of TP-receptor antagonists has had at best a small effect on the acute airway response to allergen and exercise. It is interesting to note that in one study, inhibition of cyclooxygenase led to an exaggerated acute airway response to allergen in atopic nonasthmatic subjects. There is also experimental data from human pulmonary tissue in vitro [84] and from in vivo animal studies [85] suggesting that inhibition of cyclooxygenase may lead to increased generation of leukotrienes and an augmented acute allergic response. In addition to the well-documented idiosyncratic reaction to aspirin and other nonsteroidal anti-inflammatory drugs that may occur in a small proportion of asthmatic persons, these data provide grounds for caution in the prescription of these agents to asthmatic subjects. The data regarding the late asthmatic response to allergen is conflicting, but prostanoids may contribute to the allergen-induced increase in airway hyperresponsiveness. As suggested above, prostanoids may contribute to the resting airway hyperresponsiveness in asthma. Prostanoids also play an important role in the refractory period that may occur after asthma provoked by exercise, hypertonic saline, or distilled water.

3. Platelet Activating Factor

Potency. PAF-acether is a potent platelet-aggregating agent, causes the formation of neutrophil aggregates resulting in a neutropenia, elicits neutrophil chemotaxis and lysozyme release, is also a potent eosinophil chemotactic agent, and is a potent bronchoconstrictor [86,87]. The immediate precursor of PAF, lyso-PAF, is biologically inactive. In the skin, injection of PAF-acether causes a delayed response similar to the late cutaneous response seen after antigen challenge [88]. In animals, inhalation of PAF-acether causes bronchospasm and produces intense and prolonged inflammation in the airways, increased microvascular permeability, and edema [89]. In addition, it induces a platelet-dependent bronchial hyperresponsiveness that persists for several days [90].

Bronchoconstriction in response to PAF is maximal within 2 min of inhalation and is relatively short-lived, persisting for between 15 and 45 min [20]. Tachyphylaxis to PAF-acether makes it difficult to elicit reproducible dose–response curves and to determine reliably the true sensitivity of the airways to PAF-acether. Nevertheless, early studies in humans reported that PAF was 100 times more potent than methacholine in eliciting a 40% fall in $V_{40}P$ [91] and between 5 and 836 times more potent than methacholine in eliciting a 35% fall in SGaw [20]. No correlation was found between airway responsiveness to PAF-acether and that to methacholine [20]. Further studies have confirmed the potency of PAF as a bronchoconstrictor in both asthmatic and normal subjects. However, the airways of asthmatic subjects are not especially hyperresponsive to PAF in comparison with those of normal subjects [20,21]. In the study by Rubin and co-workers [20], increasing doses of PAF were given, up to a concentration of 1 mg/ml. At this dose only three of six asthmatic subjects and five of six normal subjects had achieved a 35% fall in SGaw. Nevertheless, the mean PC_{35} SGaw in the three asthmatic responders was 0.19 mM as compared with 0.88 mM in the five normal responders. In the same study, the normal subjects did not have a significant fall in FEV_1 or $V_{30}P$, while the asthmatic subjects had a mean 10.5% fall in FEV_1 without an accompanying change in $V_{30}P$. Thus, the bronchoconstrictor effect that is observed in response to PAF depends not only on the method of challenge but also on the parameter of airway caliber that is measured. In a separate study, the airways of seven asthmatic children were more sensitive to inhaled PAF than those of seven normal children, when FEV_1 was measured [25]. A direct comparison of individual PD_{20} values was not given, nor was the potency of PAF compared with that of methacholine or histamine.

The mechanism of PAF-induced bronchoconstriction in not completely elucidated. There is evidence in animal studies that it may be platelet-dependent [90].

It may also depend on the secondary generation of other mediators. Leukotriene release was reported following treatment of isolated perfused rat lungs with PAF [92]. Furthermore, inhalation of 2 mg/ml PAF by normal subjects, which elicited a mean 48% fall in SGaw (range 25%–69%), led to a tenfold rise in urinary LTE_4 excretion and a 2.4-fold rise in the urinary excretion of 2,3-dinor TXB_2, the major urinary metabolite of TXA_2 [93]. It is therefore not surprising that PAF-induced bronchospasm has been shown to be inhibited by cysteinyl-leukotriene receptor antagonists [94,95]. Chlorpheniramine has also been reported to attenuate the bronchoconstrictor response to PAF [96], although ketotifen was without effect [23]. Inhalation of atropine led to an increased response to PAF, with a decrease in the PC_{35} SGaw and an increase in the slope of the dose–response curve to PAF [96]. The possible role of thromboxane is suggested by the observation that the thromboxane synthase inhibitor OKY-046 inhibited PAF-induced bronchospasm and hyperresponsiveness in dogs [97], and by the finding of increased thromboxane metabolites in the urine in humans after PAF inhalation [93]. Nevertheless, indomethacin did not inhibit the acute bronchoconstrictor response to PAF [96].

Induction of Airways Hyperresponsiveness. Cuss et al. [91] observed that the inhalation of PAF-acether in six nonasthmatic subjects led to a decrease in the concentration of methacholine required to cause a 40% fall in $V_{40}P$ from a mean of 10.8 mg/ml before to 4.3 mg/ml at 3 days after inhalation of PAF-acether. The increase in nonspecific hyperresponsiveness was maximal between 1 and 3 days and lasted for 1–2 weeks. Inhalation of lyso-PAF together with methacholine to elicit a similar degree of bronchoconstriction was not followed by any change in airway responses to methacholine. Subsequent studies have yielded inconsistent results. Rubin et al. confirmed that PAF increases airway responsiveness to methacholine in a study of six healthy nonasthmatic subjects [20]. Kaye and Smith also reported that inhalation of PAF to elicit a mean 25% fall in SGaw led to an increase in airway responsiveness to methacholine in six of eight normal subjects, which persisted for up to 14 days [22]. However, other studies have not been able to reproduce this effect [98,99]. A consistent finding is the inability of PAF to increase airway hyperresponsiveness in asthmatic subjects [20,21,24]. The observation of increased generation of cysteinyl leukotrienes and thromboxane following inhalation of PAF [93] suggests that these mediators may play a role in PAF-induced airway hyperresponsiveness in humans. Consistent with this suggestion is the finding that a thromboxane synthase inhibitor inhibited PAF-induced bronchoconstriction and airway hyperresponsiveness in the dog [97]. To our knowledge, no studies of leukotriene or prostanoid inhibitors or antagonists have been conducted to assess directly the role of these mediators in PAF-induced hyperresponsiveness.

PAF Antagonists. Extracts of the leaves of *Ginkgo biloba* have been found to contain naturally occurring PAF antagonists. These compounds include the gingkolides BN-52020, BN-52021, and BN-52022. BN-52063, a mixture of all three gingkolides, had no effect on the airway response to isocapnic hyperventilation or on the immediate response to exercise [100]. Nevertheless, the degree of bronchoconstriction at 20 and 30 min after exercise was less following BN-52063 than following placebo, indicating a more rapid recovery from exercise-induced asthma. The effect of BN-52021 (gingkolide B) was studied in asthmatic children [25]. Inhalation of 50 mg/ml of the active drug had no effect on PAF-induced bronchoconstriction. At a concentration of 450 mg/ml there was a significant reduction in PAF-induced bronchoconstriction in both asthmatic and normal children. This dose also led to a rightward shift in the dose–response curve to antigen in all seven subjects tested.

Synthetic analogues of PAF have also been developed as PAF antagonists. Despite demonstrating potency against inhaled PAF, the results of studies in antigen-induced asthma have been disappointing. Administration of 200 mg of WEB 2086 three times daily for 1 week [101], or of a single 500-mg dose of MK-287 1 h before challenge [102], had no significant effect on allergen-induced early or late asthmatic responses or on the allergen-induced increase in airway histamine responsiveness. WEB 2086 administered over a 12-week period had no steroid-sparing effect in the management of asthmatic subjects requiring treatment with inhaled corticosteroids [103].

The ability of PAF to elicit many of the events that are characteristic of asthma, including eosinophil chemotaxis, bronchoconstriction, mucosal edema, and airway hyperresponsiveness, led to the suggestion that this mediator may play an important role in the pathophysiology of the disease. Nevertheless, the recent studies with PAF antagonists cast doubt on this hypothesis. Thus, in spite of the biological properties of PAF, at present its role in the pathophysiology of asthma remains unclear and unproved. Further studies with more potent antagonists, and perhaps with antagonists capable of antagonizing the putative intracellular functions of PAF, are required to elucidate further the role of this potent mediator in asthma.

II. ADENOSINE

Adenosine is a naturally occurring purine nucleoside formed from the cleavage of adenosine 5′-monophosphate (AMP) by 5-nucleotidase [104]. Large amounts of extracellular adenosine are generated when cells use adenosine triphosphate (ATP) for energy, especially under hypoxic conditions [105]. As an extracellular mediator, adenosine regulates cell function via surface receptors that either stimulate or inhibit adenylate cyclase activity via A_2 receptors or A_1 receptors, respectively [106]. In vitro studies suggest that adenosine may modulate the release of mast cell–derived mediators. Pretreatment of rat peritoneal mast cells with adenosine had no effect on spontaneous histamine release but led to an increased release of histamine in response to the calcium ionophore A23187, cross-linking of the high-affinity IgE receptor (FCεRI), concanavalin A, or compound 48/80 [107]. The effect was dose- and time-dependent, being apparent at nanomolar doses, and maximal after a 5-min preincubation with 10 μM adenosine. Studies in human mast cells and basophils also demonstrated that adenosine could enhance histamine release in response to cross-linking of FCεRI, but only when added from 2 min before challenge to 5 min after challenge [108,109]. When it was added 5 min or more before challenge, there was inhibition of mast cell degranulation. These effects were mediated via cell-surface A_2-purinoceptors. Björck and colleagues investigated the responses of isolated airway smooth muscle to adenosine [110]. It was shown that isolated airway smooth muscle from asthmatic subjects was more responsive in vitro to adenosine than smooth muscle from nonasthmatic subjects. This is in contrast to studies that have failed to demonstrate in vitro hyperresponsiveness of asthmatic airway smooth muscle to histamine, cholinergic stimulation, and leukotrienes. Of interest was the observation that the in vitro response to adenosine was mediated by both histamine and leukotrienes and was completely abolished by treatment with a combination of an H_1-receptor antagonist and either the cysteinyl-leukotriene receptor antagonist ICI 198,615 or the 5-lipoxygenase activating protein inhibitor MK-886 [110]. The possible role of adenosine in bronchial asthma is suggested by its bronchoconstrictor properties, and by the findings that plasma levels of adenosine rose significantly after allergen inhalation in parallel with the fall in FEV_1 [111].

A. Methodology

Bronchial challenges with adenosine or with adenosine monophosphate (AMP), which is rapidly transformed to adenosine when inhaled, are performed in a similar manner to those for histamine. Using a tidal-breathing method, previous investigators have reported starting concentrations for adenosine and AMP of 0.11 μmol/ml (0.03 mg/ml) and 0.12 μmol/ml (0.04 mg/ml), respectively [111–115]. Doubling concentrations were inhaled until the desired decrement in pulmonary function was achieved. Maximal bronchoconstriction occurred between 2 and 5 min after inhalation [111]. In our experience with a dosimeter method, as described above, challenges with AMP commence from starting concentrations of 0.3 mg/ml. Adenosine monophosphate is more soluble than adenosine and is therefore the preferred agonist.

B. Experimental Results

1. Mechanism of Action

In vivo studies suggest that the bronchoconstrictor response to adenosine depends on the release of mast cell–derived mediators. In a group of nine subjects with mild atopic asthma, Rafferty et al. demonstrated that AMP-induced bronchoconstriction is almost entirely inhibited by the specific H_1 receptor antagonists terfenadine and astemizole [115]. In response to a single dose of AMP, previously shown to cause a 30% fall in FEV_1, preadministration of the H_1 receptor antagonists resulted in a mean 86% inhibition of bronchoconstriction. Phillips et al. [116] also demonstrated that adenosine-induced bronchoconstriction was attenuated by 80% when subjects with nonatopic asthma were pretreated with 180 mg terfenadine, a dose that completely abolished the bronchoconstrictor response to the PC_{20} of histamine. A higher dose of 600 mg terfenadine did not lead to any further inhibition of the bronchoconstrictor response to adenosine. In a further study, 180 mg terfenadine shifted the mean PC_{20} values of histamine and AMP from 0.4 mg/ml and 9.3 mg/ml to 20.2 mg/ml and 150 mg/ml, respectively; a mean shift in the dose–response curve to histamine of 50-fold and in that to AMP of 16-fold [117].

The contribution of prostanoids to the bronchoconstrictor response to AMP has been evaluated through the administration of cyclooxygenase inhibitors. When the PC_{20} of AMP was inhaled, 180 mg terfenadine led to a 50% inhibition of the airway response, 100 mg flurbiprofen led to a 36% inhibition of the response, and both drugs combined inhibited the response by 60% [118]. No effect of flurbiprofen on the airway response to histamine was noted. Pretreatment with 50 mg indomethacin twice daily for 3 days led to a modest but significant shift in the PC_{20} of AMP to 1.28 mg/ml, as compared with 0.91 mg/ml following placebo [119]. In this study, changes in airway histamine responsiveness were not studied, and it is possible that a cyclooxygenase-dependent component of histamine hyperresponsiveness may have been attenuated [80,120].

Bronchoconstriction induced by adenosine is selectively antagonized by theophylline, which acts as a competitive adenosine-receptor antagonist in doses that do not inhibit cyclic-AMP activity [113]. Adenosine-induced bronchoconstriction was potentiated by dipyridamole, an adenosine-uptake inhibitor [114]. This is compatible with mediation of adenosine-induced bronchoconstriction by stimulation of cell-surface purinoceptors.

The contribution of neural mechanisms to the bronchoconstrictor response to AMP has also been evaluated. Following treatment with 1 mg nebulized ipratropium bromide, there was an increase in FEV_1 of 11–15%, an increase in SGaw of 69–73%, and a 196-fold shift in the dose response curve to methacholine. This was accompanied by a modest shift in the PC_{20} FEV_1 and PC_{35} SGaw to AMP of 1.5-fold ($p < 0.05$) and 1.3-fold ($p > 0.05$), respectively [112]. Subsequent studies have also shown a small shift in the dose–response curve to AMP following inhalation of ipratropium bromide [121,122]. A comparable change in the airway response to histamine was also demonstrated [122], consistent with the action of histamine both directly at H_1 receptors on smooth muscle and indirectly through cholinergic mechanisms. However, the effect of bronchodilatation on the airway response to AMP was not controlled for, and it is possible that the small changes in airway response to AMP seen following anticholinergic agents is due to changes in resting airway caliber. The contribution of peptidergic neural mechanisms to AMP-induced bronchoconstriction was evaluated in a study in which the effect of bradykinin on AMP responsiveness was evaluated [123]. Marked refractoriness is observed following either AMP or bradykinin challenges. If these agents share a common mode of action, refractoriness to bradykinin challenge should be accompanied by a similar reduction in the response to AMP. Following an initial bradykinin challenge, the dose–response curve to a second bradykinin challenge was shifted to the right 15-fold, and that to AMP twofold, with no change in histamine responsiveness. These studies suggest that neural mechanisms are not a major component of AMP-induced bronchoconstriction. It is also unlikely that the response to inhaled adenosine is mediated by a down-regulation of β-adrenoreceptor responsiveness, as the airway response to inhaled isoproterenol is not altered after inhalation of adenosine [112].

These results suggest that the bronchoconstrictor response to AMP is mediated through cell-surface purinoceptors leading to the generation of the preformed mast cell mediator histamine, accompanied by some generation of arachidonic acid–derived mediators. Consistent with this hypothesis is the observation that cromolyn and nedocromil sodium attenuated the airway response to AMP seven- to ninefold and 22- to 27-fold, respectively [124,125], although the mechanism of action of these "mast cell–stabilizing" drugs remains unclear. There may be a small neural contribution to AMP-induced bronchoconstriction.

2. Potency

The potency of adenosine was compared with that of histamine in both atopic and nonatopic asthmatic subjects. Mann et al. [111] reported that the dose of adenosine and histamine causing a 20% fall in FEV_1 in 31 atopic asthmatic subjects ranged from 0.30 to 30.5 μmol/ml and 0.07 to 6.19 μmol/ml, respectively. In the same subjects, airway responsiveness to adenosine correlated with that to histamine with respect to both the dose required to produce a 20% fall in FEV_1 ($r = 0.60$) and the dose required to produce a 40% fall in SGaw ($r = 0.64$, $p < 0.01$). Responses to adenosine, AMP, and adenosine diphosphate were comparable, the geometric mean concentrations of each that caused a 20% fall in FEV_1 being 2.34, 4.27, and 2.19 μmol/ml, respectively. In a separate study of nine nonatopic asthmatic subjects [116], the geometric mean concentrations of AMP and histamine required to produce a 20% fall in FEV_1 were 13 μmol/ml and 1.82 μmol/ml, respectively. In subsequent studies [117,118,122,123,126–128], the relative potency of adenosine compared with histamine has varied between eightfold [122] and 50-fold [128].

3. Refractoriness to Adenosine Monophosphate

Refractoriness to challenge with adenosine and AMP is well recognized. In 10 nonatopic asthmatic subjects, the PC_{20} FEV_1 of AMP was 332 mg/ml [126]. After a first AMP challenge, all subjects showed a diminished response to a second AMP challenge, and in five of the 10 subjects less than a 20% fall in FEV_1 was achieved with the highest concentration of adenosine. In the remaining five subjects, the PC_{20} FEV_1 increased from 110 mg/ml to 583 mg/ml [126]. In eight atopic asthmatic subjects, refractoriness to AMP was also demonstrated, the PC_{20} FEV_1 increasing from 275 mg/ml during an initial AMP challenge to 1154 mg/ml and 1976 mg/ml during a second and third AMP challenge, respectively [127]. The same subjects did not show any refractoriness to sequential histamine challenges. In the same study there was a tendency to an increased response to allergen after two sequential AMP challenges, as compared with that seen after two sequential histamine challenges. These findings suggest that refractoriness to AMP is not due either to changes in airway histamine responsiveness or to mast cell mediator depletion. The increased response to allergen after AMP challenge may be related to an accompanying increase in nonspecific airway hyperresponsiveness following AMP inhalation [129].

Following an initial episode of bronchospasm elicited by exercise or by osmotic challenge to the airways, approximately 50% of subjects will demonstrate a refractory period of 2–4 h during which a second identical challenge will elicit substantially less bronchoconstriction. It has been suggested that refractoriness may be due to mast cell mediator depletion. Adenosine appears to induce bronchoconstriction predominantly via the release of preformed mediators from mast cells. Therefore, if refractory behavior is due to depletion of preformed mast cell mediators, airway responses to adenosine should be diminished during the refractory period. Changes in airway responsiveness to AMP were therefore examined following the inhalation of hypertonic saline in nine asthmatic subjects who demonstrated varying degrees of refractory behavior [130]. The PD_{35} SGaw of AMP at baseline was 2.4 μmol (geometric mean). Following hypertonic saline challenge, the airway responsiveness to AMP was increased, and the geometric mean PD_{35} SGaw of AMP was 1.3 μmol ($p < 0.05$, n = 9). These results suggest that the mechanism of refractoriness to hypertonic saline is unlikely to be due to depletion of histamine from airway mast cells.

III. CONCLUSIONS

The sulfidopeptide leukotrienes, selected prostaglandins, and PAF-acether are potent bronchoconstrictor agonists. The possible role of these lipid mediators in the pathogenesis of bronchial asthma is suggested by their presence in asthmatic airways, by their potent proinflammatory and bronchoconstrictor properties, and by the efficacy of specific receptor antagonists and 5-LO inhibitors in inhibiting asthmatic responses to a range of bronchoconstrictor stimuli. Inhalation challenges with these substances may be performed safely and reproducibly and have proved to be a valuable tool in the investigation of the pathogenetic mechanisms in bronchial asthma.

Adenosine is another putative mediator of bronchial asthma, though its contribution remains unclear. Its predominant mode of action in causing bronchoconstriction appears to be through an effect on purinoceptors leading to the release of histamine from airway mast cells. Inhalation challenges with adenosine have been used to explore mechanisms of refractory behavior in asthma.

REFERENCES

1. Samuelsson, B., Leukotrienes: mediators of hypersensitivity reactions and inflammation, *Science*, *220*, 568–575 (1983).
2. Benveniste, J., Henson, P. M., and Cochrane, C. G., Leukocyte dependent histamine release from rabbit platelets: the role of IgE, basophils and a platelet-activating factor, *J. Exp. Med.*, *136*, 1356–1377 (1972).
3. Snyder, F., Biochemistry of platelet activating factor, in *Perspectives in Asthma III* (G. Holme and J. Morley, eds.), Academic Press, New York, 1986.
4. Cockcroft, D. W., Killian, D. N., Mellon, J. J. A., and Hargreave, F. E., Bronchial reactivity to inhaled histamine: a method and clinical survey. *Clin. Allergy*, *7*, 235–243 (1977).
5. Chai, H., Farr, R. S., Fröehlich, L. A., Matheson, D. A., McLean, J. A., Rosenthal, R. R., Sheffer, A. L., Spector, S. L., and Townley, R. G., Standardization of bronchial inhalation procedures, *J. Allergy Clin. Immunol.*, *56*, 323–327 (1975).
6. Eiser, N. M., Kerrebijn, K. F., and Quanjer, P. H., Guidelines for standardisation of bronchial challenges with (nonspecific) bronchoconstricting agents, *Bull. Eur. Physiopathol. Respir.*, *19*, 495–514 (1983).
7. Weiss, J. W., Drazen, J. M., Coles, N., McFadden, E. R., Jr., Weller, P., Corey, E. J., Lewis, R. A., and Austen, K. F., Airway constriction in normal humans produced by inhalation of leukotriene D. Potency, time course, and effect of aspirin therapy, *JAMA*, *249*, 2814–2817 (1983).
8. Weiss, J. W., Drazen, J. M., McFadden, E. R., Jr., Weller, P., Corey, E. J., Lewis, R. A., and Austen, K. F., Bronchoconstrictor effects of leukotriene C in humans, *Science*, *216*, 196–198 (1982).
9. Davidson, A. B., Lee, T. H., Scanlon, P. D., Solway, J., McFadden, E. R., Jr., Ingram, R. H., Jr., Corey, E. J., Austen, K. F., and Drazen, J. M., Bronchoconstrictor effects of leukotriene E_4 in normal and asthmatic subjects, *Am. Rev. Respir. Dis.*, *135*, 333–337 (1987).
10. Mathé, A. A., Hedqvist, P., Holmgren, A., and Svanborg, N., Bronchial hyperreactivity to prostaglandin $F_{2\alpha}$ and histamine in patients with asthma, *Br. Med. J.*, *1*, 193–196 (1973).
11. Hardy, C. C., Robinson, C., Tattersfield, A. E., and Holgate, S. T., The bronchoconstrictor effect of inhaled prostaglandin D_2 in normal and asthmatic men, *N. Engl. J. Med.*, *311*, 209–213 (1984).
12. Beasley, C. R. W., Robinson, C., Featherstone, R. L., Varley, J. G., Hardy, C. C., Church, M. K., and Holgate, S. T., $9\alpha,11\beta$-prostaglandin F_2: a novel metabolite of prostaglandin D_2 is a potent contractile agonist of human and guinea-pig airways, *J. Clin. Invest.*, *79*, 978–983 (1987).

13. Eiser, N. M., Mills, J., McRae, K. D., Snashall, P. D., and Guz, A., Histamine receptors in normal human bronchi, *Clin. Sci.*, *58*, 537–544 (1980).
14. Arm, J. P., Spur, B. W., and Lee, T. H., The effects of inhaled leukotriene E_4 on the airway responsiveness to histamine in subjects with asthma and normal subjects, *J. Allergy Clin. Immunol.*, *82*, 654–660 (1988).
15. O'Hickey, S. P., Arm, J. P., Rees, P. J., Spur, B. W., and Lee, T. H., The relative responsiveness to inhaled leukotriene E_4, methacholine and histamine in normal and asthmatic subjects, *Eur. Respir. J.*, *1*, 913–917 (1988).
16. Chowiencyzk, P. J., Rees, P. J., Payne, J., and Clark, T. J. H., A new method for computer-assisted determination of airways resistance, *J. Appl. Physiol.*, *50*, 672–678 (1981).
17. Lewis, R. A., Drazen, J. M., Austen, K. F., Clark, D. A., and Corey, E. J., Identification of the C(6)-S-conjugate of leukotriene A with cysteine as a naturally occurring slow reacting substance of anaphylaxis (SRS-A). Importance of the 11-cis-geometry for biological activity, *Biochem. Biophys. Res. Commun.*, *96*, 271–277 (1980).
18. Bel, E. H., van der Veen, H., Kramps, J. A., Dijkman, J. H., and Sterk, P. J., Maximal airway narrowing to inhaled leukotriene D4 in normal subjects. Comparison and interaction with methacholine, *Am. Rev. Respir. Dis.*, *136*, 979–984 (1987).
19. Thomson, N. C., Roberts, R., Bandouvakis, J., Newball, H., and Hargreave, F. E., Comparison of bronchial responses to prostaglandin $F_{2\alpha}$ and methacholine, *J. Allergy Clin. Immunol.*, *68*, 392–398 (1981).
20. Rubin, A-H. E., Smith, L. J., and Patterson, R., The bronchoconstrictor properties of platelet-activating factor in humans, *Am. Rev. Respir. Dis.*, *136*, 1145–1151 (1987).
21. Chung, K. F., and Barnes, P. J., Effects of platelet activating factor on airway calibre, airway responsiveness, and circulating cells in asthmatic subjects, *Thorax*, *44*, 108–115 (1989).
22. Kaye, M. G., and Smith, L. J., Effects of inhaled leukotriene D_4 and platelet-activating factor on airway reactivity in normal subjects, *Am. Rev. Respir. Dis.*, *141*, 993–997 (1990).
23. Chung, K. F., Minette, P., McCusker, M., and Barnes, P. J., Ketotifen inhibits the cutaneous but not the airway responses to platelet-activating factor in man, *J. Allergy Clin. Immunol.*, *81*, 1192–1198 (1988).
24. Hopp, R. J., Bewtra, A. K., Nabe, M., Agrawal, D. K., and Townley, R. G., Effect of PAF-acether inhalation on nonspecific bronchial reactivity and adrenergic response in normal and asthmatic subjects, *Chest*, *98*, 936–941 (1990).
25. Hsieh, K.-H., Effects of PAF antagonist, BN52021, on the PAF-, methacholine-, and allergen-induced bronchoconstriction in asthmatic children, *Chest*, *99*, 877–882 (1991).
26. Griffin, M., Weiss, J. W., Leitch, A. G., McFadden, E. R., Jr., Corey, E. J., Austen, K. F., and Drazen, J. M., Effects of leukotriene D on the airways in asthma, *N. Engl. J. Med.*, *308*, 436–439 (1983).
27. Adelroth, E., Morris, M. M., Hargreave, F. E., and O'Byrne, P. M. Airway responsiveness to leukotrienes C_4 and D_4 and to methacholine in patients with asthma and normal controls, *N. Engl. J. Med.*, *315*, 480–484 (1986).

28. Drazen, J. M., and Austen, K. F., Leukotrienes and airway responses, *Am. Rev. Respir. Dis.*, *136*, 985–998 (1987).
29. Arm, J. P., O'Hickey, S. P., Hawksworth, R. J., Fong, C. Y., Crea, A. E. G., Spur, B. W., and Lee, T. H., Asthmatic airways have a disproportionate hyperresponsiveness to LTE_4, as compared with normal airways, but not to LTC_4, LTD_4, methacholine, and histamine, *Am. Rev. Respir. Dis.*, *142*, 1112–1118 (1990).
30. Arm, J. P., O'Hickey, S. P., Spur, B. W., and Lee, T. H., Airway responsiveness to histamine and leukotriene E_4 in subjects with aspirin-induced asthma, *Am. Rev. Respir. Dis.*, *140*, 148–153 (1989).
31. Bisgaard, H., Groth, S., and Madsen, F., Bronchial hyperreactivity to leucotriene D_4 and histamine in exogenous asthma, *Br. Med. J.*, *290*, 1468–1471 (1985).
32. Smith, L. J., Greenberger, P. A., Patterson, R., Krell, R. D., and Bernstein, P. R., The effect of inhaled leukotriene D_4 in humans, *Am. Rev. Respir. Dis.*, *131*, 368–372 (1985).
33. Brocklehurst, W. E., Slow reacting substance and related compounds, *Prog. Allergy*, *6*, 539–558 (1962).
34. Lee, T. H., Austen, K. F., Corey, E. J., and Drazen, J. M., Leukotriene E_4-induced airway hyperresponsiveness of guinea pig tracheal smooth muscle to histamine and evidence for three separate sulfidopeptide leukotriene receptors, *Proc. Natl. Acad. Sci. USA*, *81*, 4922–4925 (1984).
35. Jacques, C. A., Spur, B. W., Johnson, M., and Lee, T. H., Mechanism of LTE_4-induced histamine hyperresponsiveness in guinea-pig tracheal and human bronchial smooth muscle, *in vitro*, *Br. J. Pharmacol.*, *104*, 859–866 (1991).
36. Barnes, N. C., Watson, A., Piper, P. J., and Costello, J. F., Action of inhaled leukotriene C and D on large and small airways, Effect of pre-inhalation of leukotriene D on histamine dose–response curve (abstr.), *Am. Rev. Respir. Dis.*, *129*, A1 (1984).
37. Bisgaard, H., and Groth, S., Bronchial effects of leukotriene D_4 inhalation in normal human lung, *Clin. Sci.*, *72*, 585–592 (1987).
38. Barnes, N. C., Piper, P. J., and Costello, J. F., Actions of inhaled leukotrienes and their interactions with other allergic mediators, *Prostaglandins*, *28*, 629–630 (1984).
39. Kern, R., Smith, L. J., Patterson, R., Krell, R. D., and Bernstein, P. R., Characterization of the airway response to inhaled leukotriene D_4 in normal subjects, *Am. Rev. Respir. Dis.*, *133*, 1127–1132 (1986).
40. Holgate, S. T., Beasley, C. R. W., and Twentyman, O. P., The pathogenesis and significance of bronchial hyperresponsiveness in airways disease, *Clin. Sci.*, *73*, 561–572 (1987).
41. Woolcock, A. J., Salome, C. M., and Yan, K., The shape of the dose response curve to histamine in asthmatic and normal subjects, *Am. Rev. Respir. Dis.*, *130*, 71–75 (1984).
42. Bel, E. H., van der Veen, H., Dijkman, J. H., and Sterk, P. J., The effect of inhaled budesonide on the maximal degree of airway narrowing to leukotriene D4 and methacholine in normal subjects in vivo, *Am. Rev. Respir. Dis.*, *139*, 427–431 (1989).

43. Bianco, S., Robuschi, M., Vaghi, A., Simone, P., Folco, G., Berti, F., and Pasargiklian, M., Effects of leukotriene C_4 on the bronchial response to an ultrasonic mist of water, in *Progress in Respiratory Research. Volume 19: Asthma and Bronchial Hyperreactivity* (H. Herzog and A. P. Perruchoud, eds.), Karger, Basel, 1985, pp. 82–86.
44. Sautebin, L., Vigano, T., Grassi, E., Crivellani, M. T., Galli, G., Berti, F., Mezzetti, M., and Folco, G., Release of leukotrienes induced by the calcium ionophore A23187 from human lung parenchyma in vitro, *J. Pharmacol. Exp. Ther.*, *234*, 217–221 (1985).
45. O'Hickey, S. P., Hawksworth, R. J., Fong, C. Y., Arm, J. P., Spur, B. W., and Lee, T. H., Leukotrienes C_4, D_4, and E_4 enhance histamine responsiveness in asthmatic airways, *Am. Rev. Respir. Dis.*, *144*, 1053–1057 (1991).
46. Phillips, G. D., and Holgate, S. T., Interaction of inhaled LTC_4 with histamine and PGD_2 on airway calibre in asthma, *J. Appl. Physiol.*, *66*, 304–312 (1989).
47. Kips, J. C., Joos, G. F., De Lepeleire, I., Margolskee, D. J., Buntinx, A., Pauwels, R. A., and Van Der Straeten, M. E., MK-571, a potent antagonist of leukotriene D_4–induced bronchoconstriction in the human, *Am. Rev. Respir. Dis.*, *144*, 617–621 (1991).
48. Smith, L. J., Geller, S., Ebright, L., Glass, M., and Thyrum, P. T., Inhibition of leukotriene D_4–induced bronchoconstriction in normal subjects by the oral LTD_4 receptor antagonist ICI 204,219, *Am. Rev. Respir. Dis.*, *141*, 988–992 (1990).
49. Christie, P. E., Spur, B. W., and Lee, T. H., The effect of inhalation of the leukotriene receptor antagonist SK&F 104353 on LTC_4 and LTE_4-induced bronchoconstriction in asthmatic subjects, *J. Allergy Clin. Immunol.*, *88*, 193–198 (1991).
50. Hui, K. P., and Barnes, N. C., Lung function improvement in asthma with a cysteinyl-leukotriene antagonist, *Lancet*, *1*, 1062–1063 (1991).
51. Manning, P. J., Watson, R. M., Margolskee, D. J., Williams, V. C., Schwartz, J. I., and O'Byrne, P. M. Inhibition of exercise-induced bronchoconstriction by MK-571, a potent leukotriene D_4 antagonist, *N. Engl. J. Med.*, *323*, 1736–1739 (1990).
52. Finnerty, J. P., Wood-Baker, R., Thomson, H., and Holgate, S. T., Role of leukotrienes in exercise-induced asthma; inhibitory effect of ICI 204219, a potent leukotriene D_4 receptor antagonist, *Am. Rev. Respir. Dis.*, *145*, 746–749 (1992).
53. Taylor, I. K., O'Shaughnessy, K. M., Fuller, R. W., and Dollery, C. T., Effect of cysteinyl-leukotriene receptor antagonist ICI 204.219 on allergen-induced bronchoconstriction and airway hyperreactivity in atopic subjects, *Lancet*, *337*, 690–694 (1991).
54. Findlay, S. R., Barden, J. M., Easley, C. B., and Glass, M., Effect of the oral leukotriene antagonist, ICI 204,219, on the antigen-induced bronchoconstriction in subjects with asthma, *J. Allergy Clin. Immunol.*, *89*, 1040–1045 (1992).
55. Israel, E., Juniper, E. F., Callaghan, J. T., Mathur, P. N., Morris, M. M., Dowell, A. R., Enas, G. G., Hargreave, F. E., and Drazen, J. M., Effect of a leukotriene antagonist, LY171883, on cold air–induced bronchoconstriction in asthmatics, *Am. Rev. Respir. Dis.*, *140*, 1348–1353 (1989).
56. Christie, P. E., Smith, C. M., and Lee, T. H., The potent and selective sulfidopep-

tide leukotriene antagonist, SK&F 104353, inhibits aspirin-induced asthma, *Am. Rev. Respir. Dis.*, *144*, 957–958 (1991).

57. Israel, E., Dermarkarian, R., Rosenberg, M., Sperling, R., Taylor, G., Rubin, P., and Drazen, J. M., The effects of a 5-lipoxygenase inhibitor on asthma induced by cold, dry air, *N. Engl. J. Med.*, *323*, 1740–1744 (1990).

58. Hui, K. P., Taylor, I. K., Taylor, G. W., Rubin, P., Kesterson, J., Barnes, N. C., and Barnes, P. J., Effect of a 5-lipoxygenase inhibitor on leukotriene generation and airway responses after allergen challenge in asthmatic patients, *Thorax*, *46*, 184–189 (1991).

59. Cloud, M. L., Enas, G. G., Kemp, J., Platts-Mills, T., Altman, L. C., Townley, R., Tinkelman, D., King, T., Jr., Middleton, E., Sheffer, A. L., McFadden, E. R., Jr., and Farlow, D. S., A specific LTD_4/LTE_4-receptor antagonist improves pulmonary function in patients with mild, chronic asthma, *Am. Rev. Respir. Dis.*, *140*, 1336–1339 (1989).

60. Wahedna, I., Wisniewski, A. F. Z., Wong, C. S., and Tattersfield, A. E., Effect of multiple doses of RG 12525, an oral leukotriene D_4 antagonist, in chronic asthma (abstr.), *Am. Rev. Respir. Dis.*, *145*, A16 (1992).

61. Spector, S. L., Glass, M., and Minkwitz, M. C., ICI Asthma Trial Group. The effect of six weeks of therapy with oral doses of ICI 204,219 in asthmatics (abstr.), *Am. Rev. Respir. Dis.*, *145*, A16 (1992).

62. Israel, E., Rubin, P., Kemp, J. P., Grossman, J., Pierson, W., Siegel, S. C., Tinkelman, D., Murray, J. J., Busse, W., and Segal, A. T., The effect of inhibition of 5-lipoxygenase by zileuton in mild-to-moderate asthma. *Ann. Intern. Med.*, *119*, 1059–1066 (1993).

63. Smith, A. P., Cuthbert, M. F., and Dunlop, L. S., Effects of inhaled prostaglandins E_1, E_2 and $F_{2\alpha}$ on the airway resistance of healthy and asthmatic man, *Clin. Sci.*, *48*, 421–430 (1975).

64. Fish, J. E., Newball, H. H., Norman, P. S., and Peterman, V. I., Novel effects of $PGF_{2\alpha}$ on airway function in asthmatic subjects, *J. Appl. Physiol.*, *54*, 105–112 (1983).

65. Beasley, R., Varley, J., Robinson, C., and Holgate, S. T., Cholinergic-mediated bronchoconstriction induced by prostaglandin D_2 and its initial metabolite 9α,11β-PGF_2 and $PGF_{2\alpha}$ in asthma, *Am. Rev. Respir. Dis.*, *136*, 1140–1144 (1987).

66. Mathé, A. A., and Hedqvist, P., Effects of prostaglandins $F_{2\alpha}$ and E_2 on airway conductance in healthy subjects and asthmatic patients, *Am. Rev. Respir. Dis.*, *111*, 313–320 (1975).

67. Patel, K. R., Atropine, sodium cromoglycate and thymoxamine in $PGF_{2\alpha}$-induced bronchoconstriction in extrinsic asthma, *Br. Med. J.*, *2*, 360–362 (1975).

68. Newball, H. H., and Lenfant, C., The influence of atropine and cromolyn on human bronchial hyperreactivity to aerosolized prostaglandin $F_{2\alpha}$. *Respir. Physiol.*, *30*, 125–136 (1977).

69. Orehek, J., Gayrard, P., Grimaud, C., and Charpin, J., Bronchial response to inhaled prostaglandin $F_{2\alpha}$ in patients with common or aspirin-sensitive asthma, *J. Allergy Clin. Immunol.*, *59*, 414–419 (1977).

70. Lewis, R. A., Soter, N. A., Diamond, P. T., Austen, K. F., Oates, J. A., and Roberts,

L. J., Prostaglandin D_2 generation after activation of rat and human mast cells with anti-IgE, *J. Immunol.*, *129*, 1627–1631 (1982).

71. Holgate, S. T., Burns, G. B., Robinson, C., and Church, M. K., Anaphylactic- and calcium-dependent generation of prostaglandin D_2 (PGD_2), thromboxane B_2 and other cyclooxygenase products of arachidonic acid by dispersed human lung mast cells and relationship to histamine release, *J. Immunol.*, *133*, 2138–2144 (1984).
72. Schulman, E. S., Newball, H. H., Demers, L. M., Fitzpatrick, F. A., and Adkinson, N. F., Anaphylactic release of thromboxane A_2, prostaglandin D_2, and prostacyclin from human lung parenchyma, *Am. Rev. Respir. Dis.*, *124*, 402–406 (1981).
73. Goetzl, E. J., Weller, P. F., and Valone, F. H., Biochemical and functional bases of the regulatory and protective roles of the human eosinophil, in *Advances in Inflammation Research*, Vol. 1 (G. Weissman, B. Samuelson, and R. Paoletti, eds.), Raven Press, New York, 1976, pp. 157–167.
74. Soter, N. A., Lewis, R. A., Corey, E. J., and Austen, K. F., Local effects of synthetic leukotrienes (LTC_4, LTD_4, LTE_4 and LTB_4) in human skin, *J. Invest. Dermatol.*, *80*, 115–119 (1983).
75. Coleman, R. A., and Sheldrick, R. L. G., Prostanoid-induced contraction of human bronchial smooth muscle is mediated by TP-receptors, *Br. J. Pharmacol.*, *96*, 688–692 (1989).
76. Beasley, R. C. W., Featherstone, R. L., Church, M. K., Rafferty, P., Varley, J. G., Harris, A., Robinson, C., and Holgate, S. T., Effect of a thromboxane receptor antagonist on PGD_2- and allergen-induced bronchoconstriction, *J. Appl. Physiol.*, *66*, 1685–1693 (1989).
77. Jones, G. L., Saroea, H. G., Watson, R. M., and O'Byrne, P. M., Effect of an inhaled thromboxane mimetic (U46619) on airway function in human subjects, *Am. Rev. Respir. Dis.*, *145*, 1270–1274 (1992).
78. Walters, E. H., Parrish, R. W., Bevan, C., and Smith, A. P., Induction of bronchial hypersensitivity: evidence for a role for prostaglandins, *Thorax*, *36*, 571–574 (1981).
79. Heaton, R. W., Henderson, A. F., Dunlop, L. S., and Costello, J. F., The influence of pretreatment with prostaglandin $F_{2\alpha}$ on bronchial sensitivity to inhaled histamine and methacholine in normal subjects, *Br. J. Dis. Chest*, *78*, 168–173 (1984).
80. Curzen, N., Rafferty, P., and Holgate, S. T., Effects of a cyclo-oxygenase inhibitor, flurbiprofen, and an H_1 histamine receptor antagonist, terfanadine, alone and in combination on allergen induced immediate bronchoconstriction in man, *Thorax*, *42*, 946–952 (1987).
81. Fuller, R. W., Dixon, C. M. S., Dollery, C. T., and Barnes, P. J., Prostaglandin D_2 potentiates airway responsiveness to histamine and methacholine, *Am. Rev. Respir. Dis.*, *133*, 252–254 (1986).
82. Hardy, C. C., Bradding, P., Robinson, C., and Holgate, S. T., The combined effects of two pairs of mediators, adenosine with methacholine and prostaglandin D_2 with histamine, on airway calibre in asthma, *Clin. Sci.*, *71*, 385–392 (1986).
83. Arm, J. P., and Lee, T. H., Chemical mediators II: leukotrienes and eicosanoids, in *Bronchial Asthma*, 3rd Ed. (E. B. Weiss and M. Stein, eds.), Little, Brown, Boston, 1993, pp. 112–134.

84. Undem, B. J., Pickett, W. C., Lichtenstein, L. M., and Adams, G. K., The effect of indomethacin on the immunologic release of histamine and sulfidopeptide leukotrienes from human bronchus and lung parenchyma, *Am. Rev. Respir. Dis.*, *136*, 1183–1187 (1987).
85. Lee, T. H., Austen, K. F., Leitch, A. G., Israel, E., Robinson, D. R., Lewis, R. A., Corey, E. J., and Drazen, J. M., The effects of a fish-oil enriched diet on pulmonary mechanics during anaphylaxis, *Am. Rev. Respir. Dis.*, *132*, 1204–1209 (1985).
86. Page, C. P., Archer, C. B., and Morley, J., PAF-acether: a mediator of inflammation and asthma, *Trends Pharmacol. Sci.*, *5*, 239–241 (1984).
87. Wardlaw, A. J., Moqbel, R., Cromwell, O., and Kay, A. B., Platelet-activating factor. A potent chemotactic and chemokinetic factor for human eosinophils, *J. Clin. Invest.*, *78*, 1701–1706 (1986).
88. Archer, C. B., Page, C. P., Paul, W., Morley, J., and MacDonald, D. M., Inflammatory characteristics of platelet activating factor (PAF-acether) in human skin, *Br. J. Dermatol.*, *110*, 45–50 (1984).
89. Mojarad, M., Hamasaki, Y., and Said, S. I., Platelet activating factor increases pulmonary microvascular permeability and induces pulmonary oedema, *Bull. Eur. Physiopathol. Respir.*, *19*, 253–256 (1983).
90. Mazzoni, L., Morley, J., Page, C. P., and Sanjar, S., Induction of airway hyperreactivity by platelet activating factor in the guinea pig, *J. Physiol.*, *365*, 107P (1985).
91. Cuss, F. M., Dixon, C. M. S., and Barnes, P. J., Effects of platelet-activating factor on pulmonary function and bronchial responsiveness in man, *Lancet*, *2*, 189–192 (1986).
92. Voelkel, N. F., Worthen, S., Reeves, J. T., Henson, P. M., and Murphy, R. C., Nonimmunological production of leukotrienes induced by platelet-activating factor, *Science*, *218*, 286–288 (1982).
93. Taylor, I. K., Ward, P. S., Taylor, G. W., Dollery, C. T., and Fuller, R. W., Inhaled PAF simulates leukotriene and thromboxane A_2 production in humans, *J. Appl. Physiol.*, *71*, 1396–1402 (1991).
94. Spencer, D. A., Evans, J. M., Green, S. E., Piper, P. J., and Costello, J. F., Participation of the cysteinyl leukotrienes in the acute bronchoconstrictor response to inhaled platelet activating factor in man, *Thorax*, *46*, 441–445 (1991).
95. Kidney, J. C., Ridge, S., Chung, K. F., and Barnes, P. J., Inhibition of PAF-induced bronchoconstriction by the leukotriene D4 receptor antagonist ICI 204,219, *Am. Rev. Respir. Dis.*, *147*, 215–217 (1993).
96. Smith, L. J., Rubin, A.-H. E., and Patterson, R., Mechanism of platelet activating factor–induced bronchoconstriction in humans, *Am. Rev. Respir. Dis.*, *137*, 1015–1019 (1988).
97. Chung, K. F., Aizawa, H., Leikauf, G. D., Ueki, I. F., Evans, T. W., and Nadel, J. A., Airway hyperresponsiveness induced by platelet-activating factor: role of thromboxane generation, *J. Pharmacol. Exp. Ther.*, *236*, 580–584 (1986).
98. Hopp, R. J., Bewtra, A. K., Agrawal, D. K., and Townley, R. G., Effect of platelet-activating factor inhalation on nonspecific bronchial reactivity in man, *Chest*, *96*, 1070–1072 (1989).

99. Lai, C. K. W., Jenkins, J. R., Polosa, R., and Holgate, S. T., Inhaled PAF fails to induce airway hyperresponsiveness to methacholine in normal human subjects, *J. Appl. Physiol.*, *68*, 919–926 (1990).
100. Wilkens, J. H., Wilkens, H., Uffmann, J., Bövers, J., Fabel, H., and Frölich, J. C., Effects of a PAF-antagonist (BN52063) on bronchoconstriction and platelet activation during exercise induced asthma, *Br. J. Clin. Pharmacol.*, *29*, 85–91 (1990).
101. Freitag, A., Watson, R. M., Matsos, G., Eastwood, C., and O'Byrne, P. M., Effect of a platelet activating factor antagonist, Web 2086, on allergen induced asthmatic responses, *Thorax*, *48*, 594–598 (1993).
102. Bel, E. H., De Smet, M., Rossing, T. H., Timmers, M. C., Dijkman, J. H., and Sterk, P. J., The effect of a specific oral PAF-antagonist, MK-287, on antigen-induced early and late asthmatic reactions in man (abstr.), *Am. Rev. Respir. Dis.*, *143*, A811 (1991).
103. Johnston, S., Spence, D., Calverley, P., Winter, J., Dhillon, P., Winning, A., Ramhamadany, E., Higgins, C., Turner, S., and Holgate, S. T., Web 2086, a platelet activating factor (PAF) antagonist, has no steroid sparing effect in asthmatic patients requiring inhaled corticosteroids, *Thorax*, *47*, 871 (1992).
104. Fain, J. N., and Malbon, C. C., Regulation of adenylate cyclase by adenosine, *Mol. Cell. Biochem.*, *25*, 143–169 (1979).
105. Arch, J. R. S., and Newsholme, E. A., The control of the metabolism and the hormonal role of adenosine, in *Essays in Biochemistry*, Vol. 14 (P. N. Campbell and W. N. Aldridge, eds.), Academic Press, New York, 1978, pp. 82–123.
106. Wolff, J., Londos, C., and Cooper, D. M. R., Adenosine receptors and the regulation of adenylate cyclase, *Adv. Cyclic Nucleotide Res.*, *19*, 1635–1643 (1981).
107. Marquardt, D. L., Parker, C. W., and Sullivan, T. J., Potentiation of mast cell mediator release by adenosine, *J. Immunol.*, *120*, 871–878 (1978).
108. Hughes, P. J., Holgate, S. T., and Church, M. K., Adenosine inhibits and potentiates IgE-dependent histamine release from human lung mast cells by an A_2-purinoceptor mediated mechanism, *Biochem. Pharmacol.*, *33*, 3847–3852 (1984).
109. Church, M. K., Holgate, S. T., and Hughes, P. J., Adenosine inhibits and potentiates IgE-dependent histamine release from human basophils by an A_2-receptor mediated mechanism, *Br. J. Pharmacol.*, *80*, 719–726 (1983).
110. Björck, T., Gustafsson, L. E., and Dahlén, S.-E., Isolated bronchi from asthmatics are hyperresponsive to adenosine, which apparently acts indirectly by liberation of leukotrienes and histamine, *Am. Rev. Respir. Dis.*, *145*, 1087–1091 (1992).
111. Mann, J. S., Holgate, S. T., Renwick, A. G., and Cushley, M. J., Airway effects of purine nucleosides and nucleotides and release with bronchial provocation in asthma, *J. Appl. Physiol.*, *61*, 1667–1676 (1986).
112. Mann, J. S., Cushley, M. J., and Holgate, S. T., Adenosine-induced bronchoconstriction in asthma: Role of parasympathetic stimulation and adrenergic inhibition, *Am. Rev. Respir. Dis.*, *132*, 1–6 (1985).
113. Cushley, M. J., Tattersfield, A. E., and Holgate, S. T., Adenosine-induced bronchoconstriction in asthma: antagonism by inhaled theophylline, *Am. Rev. Respir. Dis.*, *129*, 380–384 (1984).
114. Cushley, M. J., Tallant, N., and Holgate, S. T., The effect of dipyridamole on

histamine- and adenosine-induced bronchoconstriction in normal and asthmatic subjects, *Eur. J. Respir. Dis.*, *67*, 185–192 (1985).

115. Rafferty, P., Beasley, R., and Holgate, S. T., The contribution of histamine to immediate bronchoconstriction provoked by inhaled allergen and adenosine 5′-monophosphate in atopic asthma, *Am. Rev. Respir. Dis.*, *136*, 369–373 (1987).
116. Phillips, G. D., Rafferty, P., Beasley, R., and Holgate, S. T., Effect of oral terfenadine on the bronchoconstrictor response to inhaled histamine and adenosine 5′-monophosphate in non-atopic asthma, *Thorax*, *42*, 939–945 (1987).
117. Phillips, G. D., Polosa, R., and Holgate, S. T., The effect of histamine-H_1 receptor antagonism with terfenadine on concentration-related AMP-induced bronchoconstriction in asthma, *Clin. Exp. Allergy*, *19*, 405–409 (1989).
118. Phillips, G. D., and Holgate, S. T., The effect of oral terfenadine alone and in combination with flurbiprofen on the bronchoconstrictor response to inhaled adenosine 5′-monophosphate in nonatopic asthma, *Am. Rev. Respir. Dis.*, *139*, 463–469 (1989).
119. Crimi, N., Palermo, F., Polosa, R., Oliveri, R., Maccarrone, C., Palermo, B., and Mistretta, A., Effect of indomethacin on adenosine-induced bronchoconstriction, *J. Allergy Clin. Immunol.*, *83*, 921–925 (1989).
120. Walters, E. H., Effect of inhibition of prostaglandin synthesis on induced bronchial hyperresponsiveness, *Thorax*, *38*, 195–199 (1983).
121. Crimi, N., Palermo, F., Oliveri, R., Polosa, R., Settinieri, I., and Mistretta, A., Protective effects of inhaled ipratropium bromide on bronchoconstriction induced by adenosine and methacholine in asthma, *Eur. Respir. J.*, *5*, 560–565 (1992).
122. Polosa, R., Phillips, G. D., Rajakulasingam, K., and Holgate, S. T., The effect of inhaled ipratropium bromide alone and in combination with oral terfenadine on bronchoconstriction provoked by adenosine 5′-monophosphate and histamine in asthma, *J. Allergy Clin. Immunol.*, *87*, 939–947 (1991).
123. Polosa, R., Rajakulasingam, K., Church, M. K., and Holgate, S. T., Repeated inhalation of bradykinin attenuates adenosine 5′-monophosphate (AMP) induced bronchoconstriction in asthmatic airways, *Eur. Respir. J.*, *5*, 700–706 (1992).
124. Richards, R., Phillips, G. D., and Holgate, S. T., Nedocromil sodium is more potent than sodium cromoglycate against AMP-induced bronchoconstriction in atopic asthmatic subjects, *Clin. Exp. Allergy*, *19*, 285–291 (1989).
125. Phillips, G. D., Scott, V. L., Richards, R., and Holgate, S. T., Effect of nedocromil sodium and sodium cromoglycate against bronchoconstriction induced by inhaled adenosine 5′-monophosphate, *Eur. Respir. J.*, *2*, 210–217 (1989).
126. Daxun, Z., Rafferty, P., Richards, R., Summerell, S., and Holgate, S. T., Airway refractoriness to adenosine 5′-monophosphate after repeated inhalation, *J. Allergy Clin. Immunol.*, *83*, 152–158 (1989).
127. Phillips, G. D., Bagga, P. K., Djukanovic, R., and Holgate, S. T., The influence of refractoriness to adenosine 5′-monophosphate on allergen-provoked bronchoconstriction in asthma, *Am. Rev. Respir. Dis.*, *140*, 321–326 (1989).
128. Ghosh, S. K., and Rafferty, P., Effect of felodipine on histamine and adenosine induced bronchoconstriction in patients with asthma, *Eur. J. Clin. Pharmacol.*, *41*, 73–74 (1991).

129. Rosati, G., Hargreave, F. E., and Ramsdale, E. H., Inhalation of adenosine 5′-monophosphate increases methacholine airway responsiveness, *J. Appl. Physiol.*, *67*, 792–796 (1989).
130. O'Hickey, S. P., Rees, P. J., and Lee, T. H., Airway responsiveness to adenosine 5′-monophosphate following inhalation of hypertonic saline, *Eur. Respir. J.*, *2*, 923–928 (1989).

12

Airway Challenges with Inhaled Constrictor Mediators

Paul M. O'Byrne

McMaster University
Hamilton, Canada

Noe Zamel

University of Toronto
Toronto, Canada

I. INTRODUCTION

Inhalation challenges with airway constrictor agonists, such as histamine or methacholine, are widely used in both clinical and research laboratories to measure airway responsiveness. This is because airway hyperresponsiveness has been identified as an important feature in patients with current symptomatic asthma and indeed has been included among the defining characteristics of asthma by the American Thoracic Society [1]. Airway responsiveness is the ability of the airways to narrow after exposure to constrictor agonists. Thus, airway hyperresponsiveness is an increased ability to develop this response. Airway hyperresponsiveness consists of an increased sensitivity of the airways to constrictor agonists, so that a smaller concentration of a constrictor agonist is needed to initiate the bronchoconstrictor response [2]; a steeper slope of the dose–response curve; and a greater maximal response to the agonist [3] (Fig. 1).

Airway hyperresponsiveness has been the focus of extensive clinical and research interest over the past 30 years. This is because most clinicians and investigators interested in asthma have come to recognize that airway hyperresponsiveness is an important, perhaps even a cardinal, feature of asthma. In populations of asthmatic patients, the severity of airway hyperresponsiveness correlates with the severity of asthma [4] and with the amount of treatment needed to control symptoms [5]. Research in this area has examined a variety of methods of measuring airway responsiveness, the clinical significance of and the effects of

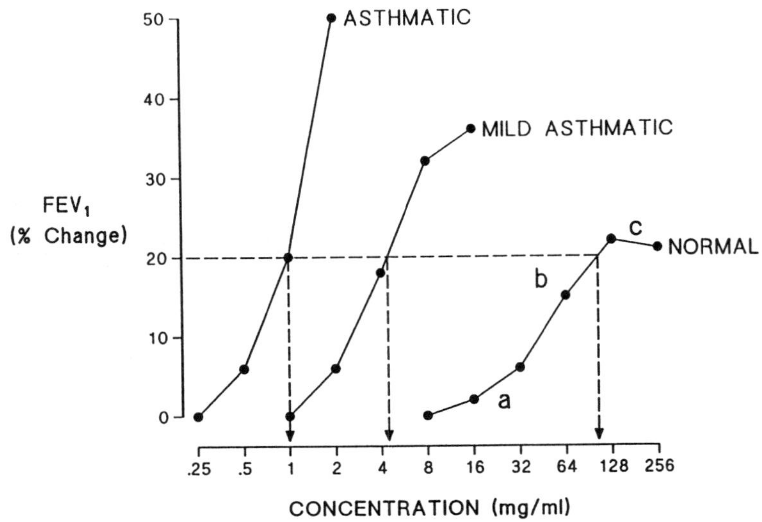

Figure 1 Dose–response curves obtained in a normal subject and asthmatic subjects with increasing severity of airway hyperresponsiveness, by inhaling increasing concentrations of a constrictor agonist. In normal subjects and subjects with mild asthma, **(a)** a threshold response (sensitivity), **(b)** a slope of the dose-response (reactivity), and **(c)** a maximal response (plateau) can be obtained. In most subjects with current asthma, a plateau response cannot be obtained. For clinical purposes, the response is usually measured as the percent change from baseline in forced expired volume in 1 second (FEV_1) and is expressed as the provocation concentration of the agonist causing a 20% fall in FEV_1 (PC_{20}).

antiasthma medications on these measurements, and the pathophysiology and pathogenesis of airway hyperresponsiveness in asthmatic patients. As a result of this research, the methods of its measurement have been standardized and are widely accepted. The two commonly used methods of measuring airway responsiveness in North America have been carefully characterized and compared [6]. These will be fully described in this chapter, together with the methods of measuring the responses and expressing the results. One further method, which is more rapid to perform and may be more useful in large epidemiological studies, will also be briefly described.

Other methods of measuring airway responsiveness to sensitizing stimuli, such as inhaled allergen [7], occupational sensitizing agents, [8], or nonsensitizing naturally occurring stimuli—e.g., exercise [9] and isocapnic hyperventilation [10]—have also been described. Inhalation challenges with sensitizing stimuli, such as allergen, are indicated in very specific circumstances. They are most commonly used in identifying occupational sensitizing agents. Chemical agonists, which are easier to administer and produce short-lived airway constrictor responses, should be used to routinely measure airway responsiveness.

II. HISTORICAL PERSPECTIVE

The initial observation that bronchoconstriction occurs more readily in asthmatic than in nonasthmatic subjects after exposure to a constrictor agonist was made in 1921 by Alexander and Paddock [11], who demonstrated an "asthmatic breathing" in asthmatic subjects, but not in nonasthmatic ones, after subcutaneous administration of the cholinergic agonist pilocarpine. This observation was confirmed by Weiss et al. [12], who reported in 1932 that asthmatic subjects, but not nonasthmatic ones, developed bronchoconstriction, as measured by changes in the vital capacity, after being given intravenous histamine. Later, Curry [13] noted that this increased bronchoconstrictor response to histamine occurred with intramuscular, intravenous, and nebulized histamine, again only in asthmatic patients. Tiffeneau and Beauvallet [14] were the first to describe the use of acetylcholine inhalation tests to determine the degree of airway responsiveness in asthmatics.

It is now known that in asthmatic subjects airway hyperresponsiveness is present to many chemical stimuli, such as histamine [15]; the cholinergic agonists acetylcholine [16], methacholine [17], and carbachol [18]; the peptide leukotrienes [19]; prostaglandin D_2 [20] and prostaglandin $F_{2\alpha}$ [21]; and adenosine [22]; and to physical stimuli such as exercise [23], hyperventilation of cold, dry air [10], and both hypotonic and hypertonic solutions [24].

III. METHODS OF MEASURING AIRWAY RESPONSIVENESS

The two most widely used methods of measuring airway responsiveness employ inhalation of an aerosolized agonist, generated by a nebulizer, to provoke generally mild, short-lived airway constriction. In one method [4], which is a modification of a method originally described by de Vries et al. [25], aerosol is generated by a Wright nebulizer, delivered to either a face mask or a mouthpiece, and inhaled by tidal breathing for 2 min. In the second method [26], aerosol is generated by a DeVilbiss 646 nebulizer attached to a Rosenthal–French dosimeter, delivered to a mouthpiece, and inhaled by five inspiratory-capacity breaths. These two methods have been compared, and with the appropriate standardization of features that influence the response, the two methods give very similar results and are of similar reproducibility [6].

A more recent method of measuring airway responsiveness has been described by Yan et al. [27]. This method uses a hand-operated nebulizer, with the aerosol being generated by squeezing the bulb of the nebulizer. This removes the necessity of a source of compressed air. The potential advantages of this method are that its equipment is portable and that it can be performed more quickly than the other

Table 1 Inhalation Tests with Histamine or Methacholine

Indications:	Evaluation of symptoms suggestive of asthma (in patients with normal airway caliber)
	Evaluation of the presence of occupational asthma (together with other parameters)
	Evaluation of the severity of asthma (together with other parameters)
	Research studies in asthma
Contraindications:	Severe airflow obstruction ($FEV_1 < 40\%$ predicted or < 1.5 L).
Factors that enhance response:	Recent exposure to relevant inhaled allergens
	Recent exposure to relevant occupational agents
	Recent respiratory viral infections
	Exposure to atmospheric pollutants (ozone)
Factors that reduce response:	Avoidance of relevant allergens or occupational agents
	Bronchodilator drugs (β_2-adrenoceptor agonists, theophylline)
	Specific antagonists (antihistamines, anticholinergics)
	Regular treatment with corticosteroids
	Previous inhalation challenge with histamine (within 6 h)

FEV_1 = forced expired volume in 1 second.

methods. These reasons make it an attractive alternative for use in epidemiology studies in which measurements of airway responsiveness are being made.

IV. FACTORS THAT AFFECT INHALATION TESTS

The important technical factors that influence the response to inhalation tests and must be standardized for accurate interpretation of the results are nebulizer output [28], the particle size of the aerosol, the speed and volume of inspiration [28], and the temperature of the solution. Nebulizer output varies among different types of nebulizers and even among different nebulizers of the same type. Therefore, each nebulizer needs to be calibrated before use. This is done by weighing the nebulizer before and after operation with compressed air at a constant pressure but with different flow rates, to obtain the flow rate of compressed air that achieves the desired output. With the Wright nebulizer, an output of 0.13 ml/min is used. The particle size of the aerosol does not appear to be an important variable, once it is in the range 1.5–4.0 μm [28]. The volume and speed of inspiration is not an important variable if the tidal-breathing method is used; however, it may be more important in the method that uses inspiratory-capacity breaths.

Bronchodilator medications must be avoided before the inhalation test, as they will antagonize the response to the constrictor aerosol. It is standard practice to withhold short-acting β_2-adrenoceptor agonists and anticholinergic agents for at least 8 h, short-acting xanthines for at least 24 h, and long-acting xanthines, β_2

agonists, and some antihistamines for at least 48 h; the longer-acting antihistamines may influence the response to inhaled histamine for several weeks. Regular treatment with inhaled corticosteroids [29,30] or nedocromil sodium [31] has been demonstrated to improve airway responsiveness in asthmatic patients. The effects of inhaled corticosteroids are slowly progressive over time and may persist in subjects with mild asthma for more than 3 months after use of the agents is discontinued [32]. For these reasons, use of inhaled or oral corticosteroids, cromolyn, or nedocromil is continued without interruption during the inhalation test. However, it must be understood that the results obtained may be different (almost always improved) from a measurement made when the patient is not taking these medications.

In research studies, where the reproducibility of the inhalation test is an important consideration, other factors need to be considered. For example, inhalation of allergens [33] or atmospheric pollutants such as ozone [34], or recent viral respiratory infections [35], can cause airway hyperresponsiveness. The duration of this effect varies among stimuli and among individual subjects. Therefore, in research studies, inhalation tests are not performed within 6 weeks of exposure to these stimuli. In certain clinical situations, however, it may be important to perform inhalation tests both before and during exposure to an allergen or occupational sensitizing agent, to determine whether this exposure is important in causing symptoms. Other stimuli known to cause bronchoconstriction, such as exercise or cold air, should be avoided before all inhalation tests. If all of the factors that can influence the response to inhaled bronchoconstrictor agonists are standardized, inhalation tests to measure airway responsiveness are very reproducible from day to day [17].

V. CHOICE OF CONSTRICTOR AGONIST

Inhaled histamine and methacholine have been the constrictor agonists most widely used in clinical laboratories to measure airway responsiveness. Many other aerosol agonists have been used, as described above, but mainly in research studies. Airway responsiveness to histamine correlates extremely well with airway responsiveness to methacholine [17]. There are, however, inherent disadvantages to inhaled histamine that make inhaled methacholine a more useful agonist for many research studies. These disadvantages include the development of systemic side effects, such as flushing, headache, and tachycardia, when high concentrations (albeit concentrations not required in most asthmatic subjects) are inhaled. These side effects are generally not seen with even high concentrations of inhaled methacholine. Also, at high concentrations (>32mg/ml) histamine precipitates out of solution. However, as all of these disadvantages exist only with high concentrations, histamine is as useful as methacholine for measuring airway responsiveness in clinical practice, where lower concentrations are used.

A second potential problem with using histamine in research studies is that tachyphylaxis (a decreased response to repeated stimulation) occurs following repeated challenges with inhaled histamine in subjects with mild asthma when challenges are separated by up to 6 h [36]. Tachyphylaxis does not occur to repeated challenges with inhaled acetylcholine in asthmatic subjects [36]. These results suggest that histamine tachyphylaxis in asthmatics is specific to histamine stimulation and not due to bronchoconstriction per se. However, prior histamine inhalation reduces airway responsiveness to other bronchoconstrictor stimuli such as acetylcholine [37] and exercise [38]. Therefore, repeated histamine inhalation tests should be separated by 1 day, and histamine inhalation should not precede other inhalation challenges. Tachyphylaxis does not appear to occur to inhaled methacholine at the concentrations used in asthmatic subjects [39], but it does occur when higher concentrations are inhaled by nonasthmatic subjects [39,40].

Prolonged bronchoconstriction has been reported following methacholine inhalation challenge [41]. This occurs only if very high concentrations of methacholine are used. Also, methacholine is unstable when diluted in phosphate-buffered saline; therefore, normal saline must be used as the diluent. Other cholinergic agonists, such as acetylcholine [16] and carbachol [18], have been used to measure airway responsiveness in human subjects. A major disadvantage of acetylcholine is that it must be prepared freshly before the inhalation challenge and kept cool, to keep the solutions stable. Both histamine and methacholine are stable in solution for up to 3 months at the concentrations commonly used.

VI. MEASUREMENT OF THE RESPONSE

The response of the airways to an inhalation challenge can be measured in a number of different ways. Mostly, the response is measured with noninvasive methods such as the forced expired volume in 1 second (FEV_1), airway resistance, maximum expiratory flow–volume curves, or total respiratory resistance. The FEV_1 is the most commonly used method of measuring response in clinical practice. However, other methods may have advantages in certain situations, depending on the objective of the test, and are used mostly in research studies.

A. Forced Expired Volume in 1 Second

The FEV_1 is the most popular test of pulmonary function, being extensively used for detection of airflow limitation, for evaluating the effects of bronchodilators, and in epidemiological surveys. The main advantages of this test are that it is simple to perform, requires relatively less expensive equipment than other tests, and is very reproducible. The main disadvantages are, first, that the FEV_1 requires a full inspiration, which may alter the measurement, as described above. Also, with measurements of airways resistance, the FEV_1 is relatively insensitive to obstruction of the peripheral airways. Finally, although most of the flow expired in the first second of the forced vital capacity is effort-independent, the initial part of the forced vital capacity is effort-dependent, which may slightly affect the FEV_1.

B. Airway Resistance

The measurement of airway resistance with a whole-body plethysmograph was introduced by DuBois et al. [42]. Airway resistance can be measured during either panting or resting breathing. Since some of the agonists used may cause laryngeal narrowing and panting, in part, overcomes this, it appears that measurement of airway resistance during panting is preferable. Airway resistance measured in the body plethysmograph includes the resistance of the central and peripheral airways. Since central airway resistance is the predominant component of total airway resistance, the measurement of airway resistance is not very sensitive to change in resistance of the smaller airways. In addition, as already described, some bronchoconstrictor agonists cause laryngeal constriction, and measurements of airway resistance may therefore reflect laryngeal more than lower airway changes. The main advantage of measuring airway resistance is that the measurements can be obtained while avoiding a deep inspiration, which is known to alter airway smooth muscle tone in both normal and asthmatic subjects during inhalation challenges. In normal subjects, a deep inspiration causes airway dilation, while in asthmatic subjects the effect ranges from no effect, to airway dilation in some asthmatics, to airway constriction in others. Since airway resistance varies with lung volume, it is important to relate changes in resistance to changes in lung volume. This can be done by calculating either specific airway resistance (SRaw) or specific airway conductance (SGaw). The SRaw is obtained by multiplying airway resistance by the corresponding lung volume (usually close to functional residual capacity) at which the resistance is measured. The SGaw is obtained by taking the reciprocal of the airway resistance, the airway conductance, and dividing it by the corresponding lung volume. Thus, with increasing severity of airways constriction during an inhalation challenge, the SRaw will increase while the SGaw will decrease. The only advantage of one method over the other is that the scale of SRaw tends to be bigger than that of SGaw, so that changes are easier to recognize. Measurements of airway resistance and functional residual capacity require a whole-body plethysmograph, which is expensive and relatively complex to use.

C. Maximum Expiratory Flow–Volume Curves

1. Complete Flow–Volume Curves

Maximum expiratory flow–volume curves were first described by Hyatt et al. [43]. The flow–volume curves can be obtained by using either a variable-volume whole-body plethysmograph or a spirometer. The complete flow–volume curves require a full inspiration and are affected by this maneuver in the same way as the

FEV_1. The data from the flow–volume curves are usually expressed as one or two flows measured at given volumes. When total lung capacity (TLC) is measured, the maximum flows are determined at a fixed percentage of TLC, usually 60% or 40%. If TLC is not measured, the flows are determined at a given percentage of vital capacity (VC), usually 50% or 25%. However, this has the disadvantage that VC falls as airway constriction occurs, and therefore the flows are not measured at the same lung volume during an inhalation challenge. To overcome this problem, considering that TLC does not change significantly during airway constriction, flows can be measured at a fixed distance from the beginning of the complete flow–volume curve, even if TLC is not measured. In this way, flows are measured at the same lung volume during the inhalation challenge. The main advantage of maximum expiratory flow–volume curves is that the flows in the last portion of the vital capacity are determined by the geometry of the peripheral airways. Also, the equipment, if a electronic spirometer and an X-Y plotter are used, is relatively simple.

2. Partial Flow–Volume Curves

Bouhuys et al. (44) demonstrated in 1969 that in the presence of induced airway constriction, flow–volume curves following a partial inspiration had lower flows than after a complete inspiration. This difference between partial and complete curves has been attributed to airway dilation following lung inflation. Thus, partial flow–volume curves, which avoid a deep inspiration, have the same advantages as measurements of airway resistance, with the additional advantage of reflecting the geometry of the peripheral airways. Therefore, measurements of SRaw will reflect more the effect of a constrictor agonist on the more central airways, while partial flow volume curves will reflect more the effect on peripheral airways. Since the airway dilation following lung inflation depends on the degree of inflation, the partial flow–volume curves should be started at a fixed lung volume. A standard method of obtaining partial flow–volume curves has been described, in which the partial maneuver starts from the same lung volume, with TLC as the reference volume [45].

D. Total Respiratory System Resistance

DuBois [46] in 1953 described a method of measuring total respiratory system resistance, $R_{(rs)}$, by sinusoidally oscillating the system at its resonant frequency. The method was further modified so that $R_{(rs)}$ was measured by oscillatory frequencies of 3 and 5 cycle/s. Takishima et al. [47] have developed a fully automated method of aerosol delivery and continuous recording of $R_{(rs)}$. The major advantage of this method is its simplicity, in that the subject just has to breath with resting tidal volume. However, $R_{(rs)}$ measures the resistance of the total respiratory system, including the chest wall, and while it is a sensitive method of measuring the response, it is not specific regarding the different components of the respiratory system.

VII. EXPRESSING THE RESULTS

Most recent studies in which airway responsiveness has been measured have plotted the changes in lung function against the log of the concentration of the agonist administered (Fig. 1). There are several ways of expressing the results from these semi-log dose–response curves. The most usual way is to determine the provocative concentration (PC) or provocative dose (PD) of the agonist that causes a predetermined change in lung function, usually a fixed percentage of baseline. If FEV_1 is the parameter used to assess lung function, a 20% fall from baseline is usually used, and the results are expressed as the PC_{20} FEV_1, i.e., the concentration of the agonist that causes a 20% fall in FEV_1 (Fig. 1). For SGaw, a 35% reduction is usually used, because of the greater variability of the measurement.

Other ways of expressing the results include applying a curve-fitting equation to the dose–response curve and obtaining various parameters from the equation. Woolcock et al. [3] have described parameters related to the position, slope, and plateau of the dose–response curve. They found differences in all parameters between normal and asthmatic subjects. Normal subjects and subjects with mild asthma have a plateau response at higher concentrations of inhaled agonists. By contrast, subjects with more severe asthma do not demonstrate a plateau response, even with very severe degrees of airway constriction. The use of parameters such as these may be very useful in studies of mechanisms of airway responsiveness. However, for most clinical applications of measurements of airway responsiveness, the simpler method of expressing results, such as PC_{20} FEV_1, is the most useful.

VIII. SIGNIFICANCE OF AIRWAY HYPERRESPONSIVENESS

Airway hyperresponsiveness can be demonstrated in almost all patients with current symptomatic asthma [4]. With the method described by Cockcroft et al. [4], asthmatic subjects generally have a histamine or methacholine PC_{20} (using FEV_1) of less than 8 mg/ml. Most nonasthmatics will have a PC_{20} of greater than 16 mg/ml. There is some overlap, however, and defining an exact level of airway responsiveness that would distinguish asthmatic subjects from nonasthmatic subjects is not possible. This is because there appears to be a continuous distribution of nonspecific airway responsiveness in the general population, with asthmatic subjects in one tail of this distribution [48]. In addition, even subjects with normal histamine or methacholine airway responsiveness can develop symptoms of asthma if exposed to specific stimuli to which they are sensitized, such as inhaled allergen or toluene diisocyanate [49].

As has already been described, the severity of airway hyperresponsiveness generally correlates with the severity of asthma. The degree of airway hyperresponsiveness correlates with variations in peak expiratory flow rates [50], which are another important variable in asthma, and with the improvement of FEV_1 after inhalation of a bronchodilator [50]. Last, the degree of airway constriction caused by exercise or hyperventilation of cold, dry air in asthmatic subjects is related to the level of airway hyperresponsiveness [10]. As these stimuli are considered to act through release of endogenous mediators, it is likely that hyperresponsiveness of asthmatic airways to these released constrictor mediators plays a role in causing symptoms in asthmatic patients.

Airway hyperresponsiveness to inhaled agonists such as histamine or methacholine can also be demonstrated in patients with airflow obstruction apparently due to chronic bronchitis [51]. The degree of airflow obstruction, as indicated by the reduction of FEV_1 and the FEV_1/VC ratio, correlates with the increase in airway responsiveness [51]. This suggests that in patients with airflow obstruction, the airway hyperresponsiveness demonstrated is a result of reduced airway caliber. By contrast, many patients with airway hyperresponsiveness and asthma have normal airway caliber at the time the inhalation challenge is being performed. However, this can pose a problem in interpreting the result of an inhalation challenge with a constrictor agonist in a patient with significant airflow obstruction at the time of the study. Recent results from McClean et al. [52] have demonstrated that the only parameter extracted from the methacholine dose–response curve that is not associated with baseline lung function is the dose–response threshold (defined as the concentration that produces a statistically significant change in FEV_1 or $V_{40}P$). Therefore, the threshold concentration may be a more specific measure of airway hyperresponsiveness than the PC_{20}; however, this independence of the dose–response threshold from the baseline lung function needs to be studied in populations of asthmatic subjects.

The likelihood of identifying the presence of airway hyperresponsiveness in patients suspected of having asthma, on the basis of history and physical examination, and in whom airway caliber is normal is only slightly better than chance alone, even for physicians experienced in treating asthma [53]. Therefore, objective measurements of airway responsiveness are particularly useful in such patients with normal airway caliber in whom a diagnosis of asthma is being considered. Another important application of measuring airway responsiveness is the diagnosis of occupational asthma [54]. Last, it has been suggested that measurement of airway responsiveness is useful in determining the optimal treatment requirements of asthmatics, but this requires further study.

IX. CONCLUSIONS

Measurements of airway responsiveness to the inhaled bronchoconstrictor mediators histamine and methacholine can be useful in making a diagnosis of asthma, particularly in patients with symptoms consistent with asthma who have no evidence of airflow obstruction. Histamine or methacholine inhalation tests can be performed quickly, safely, and reproducibly by experienced technicians, once the factors known to influence the tests are appropriately controlled.

REFERENCES

1. American Thoracic Society, Standards for the diagnosis and care of patients with chronic obstructive pulmonary disease (COPD) and asthma, *Am. Rev. Respir. Dis.*, *136*, 225–244 (1987).
2. Hargreave, F. E., Ryan, G., Thomson, N. C., O'Byrne, P.M., Latimer, K., Juniper, E. F., and Dolovich, J., Bronchial responsiveness to histamine or methacholine in asthma: measurement and clinical significance, *J. Allergy Clin. Immunol.*, *68*, 347–355 (1981).
3. Woolcock, A. J., Salome, C. M., and Yan, K., The shape of the dose–response curve to histamine in asthmatic and normal subjects, *Am. Rev. Respir. Dis.*, *130*, 71–75 (1984).
4. Cockcroft, D. W., Killian, D. N., Mellon, J. J. A., and Hargreave, F. E., Bronchial reactivity of inhaled histamine: a method and clinical survey, *Clin. Allergy*, *7*, 235–243 (1977).
5. Juniper, E. F., Frith, P. A., and Hargreave, F. E., Airway responsiveness to histamine and methacholine: relationship to minimum treatment to control symptoms of asthma, *Thorax*, *36*, 575–579 (1981).
6. Ryan, G., Dolovich, M. B., Roberts, R. S., Frith, P. A., Juniper, E. F., Hargreave, F. E., Newhouse, M. T., Standardization of inhalation provocation tests: two techniques of aerosol generation and inhalation compared, *Am. Rev. Respir. Dis.*, *123*, 195–199 (1981).
7. Cockcroft, D. W., Ruffin, R. E., Dolovich, J., and Hargreave, F. E., Allergen-induced increase in non-allergic bronchial reactivity, *Clin. Allergy*, *7*, 503–513 (1977).
8. Chan-Yeung, M., and Lam, S., Occupational asthma: state of the art, *Am. Rev. Respir. Dis.*, *133*, 686–703 (1986).
9. Anderson, S. D., Silverman, M., Godfrey, S., and Konig, P. Exercise-induced asthma: a review, *Br. J. Dis. Chest*, *69*, 1–39 (1975).
10. O'Byrne, P. M., Ryan, G., Morris, M., McCormack, D., Jones, N. L., Morse, J. L. C., and Hargreave, F. E., Asthma induced by cold air and its relation to nonspecific bronchial responsiveness to methacholine, *Am. Rev. Respir. Dis.*, *125*, 281–285 (1982).
11. Alexander, H. L., and Paddock, R., Bronchial asthma: response to pilocarpine and epinephrine, *Arch. Intern. Med.*, *27*, 184–191 (1921).
12. Weiss, S., Robb, G. P., and Ellis, L. B., The systemic effects of histamine in man, *Arch. Intern. Med.*, *49*, 360–396 (1932).
13. Curry, J. J., The action of histamine on the respiratory tract in normal and asthmatic subjects, *J. Clin. Invest.*, *25*, 785–791 (1946).
14. Tiffeneau, R., and Beauvallet, P., Epreuve de bronchoconstriction et de bronchodilatation par aerosols, *Bull. Acad. Med.*, *129*, 165–168 (1945).
15. Juniper E. F., Frith, P. A., and Hargreave, F. E., Long term stability of bronchial responsiveness to histamine, *Thorax*, *37*, 288–291 (1982).

16. Simonssen, B. G., Clinical and physiological studies on chronic bronchitis III. Bronchial reactivity to inhaled acetylcholine, *Acta Allergol.*, *20*, 325–348 (1965).
17. Juniper, E. F., Frith, P. A., Dunnett, C., Cockcroft, D. W., and Hargreave, F. E., Reproducibility and comparison of responses to inhaled histamine and methacholine, *Thorax*, *33*, 705–710 (1978).
18. Sotomayor, H., Badier, M., Vervloet, D., and Orehek, J., Seasonal increase of carbachol airway responsiveness in patients allergic to grass pollen, *Am. Rev. Respir. Dis.*, *130*, 56–58 (1984).
19. Adelroth, E., Morris, M. M., Hargreave, F. E., and O'Byrne, P. M., Airway responsiveness to leukotrienes C4 and D4 and to methacholine in patients with asthma and normal controls, *N. Engl. J. Med.*, *315*, 480–484 (1986).
20. Hardy, C. C., Robinson, C., Tattersfield, A. E., and Holgate, S. T., The bronchoconstrictor effect of inhaled prostaglandin D2 in normal and asthmatic men, *N. Engl. J. Med.*, *311*, 209–213 (1984).
21. Thomson, N. C., Roberts, R., Bandouvakis, J., Newball, H., and Hargreave, F. E., Comparison of bronchial responses to prostaglandin F2α and methacholine, *J. Allergy Clin. Immunol.*, *68*, 392–398 (1981).
22. Holgate, S. T., Mann, J. S., and Cushley, M. J., Adenosine as a bronchoconstrictor mediator in asthma and its antagonism by methylxanthines, *J. Allergy Clin. Immunol.*, *74*, 302–306 (1984).
23. Anderton, R. C., Cuff, M. T., Frith, P. A., Cockcroft, D. W., Morse, J. L. C., Jones, N. L., and Hargreave, F. E., Bronchial responsiveness to inhaled histamine and exercise, *J. Allergy Clin. Immunol.*, *63*, 315–320 (1979).
24. Anderson, S., Schoeffel, R., and Finney, M., Evaluation of ultrasonically nebulized solutions for provocative testing in patients with asthma, *Thorax*, *38*, 284–291 (1983).
25. De Vries, K., Goei, J. T., Booy-Noord, H., and Orie, N. G. M., Changes during 24 hours in the lung function and histamine hyperreactivity of the bronchial tree in asthmatic and chronic bronchitis patients, *Int. Arch. Allergy*, *20*, 93–99 (1962).
26. Chai, H., Farr, R. S., Froehlich, L. A., Mathison, D. A., McLean, J. A., Rosenthal, R. R., Scheffes, A. L., Spector, S. L., Townley, R. G., Standardization of bronchial inhalation challenge procedures, *J. Allergy Clin. Immunol.*, *56*, 323–327 (1975).
27. Yan, K., Salome, C. M., and Woolcock, A. J., Rapid method for measurement of bronchial responsiveness, *Thorax*, *38*, 760–765 (1983).
28. Ryan, G., Dolovich, M. B., Obminski, G., Cockcroft, D. W., Juniper, E. F. Hargreave, F. E., Newhouse, M. T., Standardization of inhalation provocation tests: influence of nebulizer output, particle size, and methods of inhalation, *J. Allergy Clin. Immunol.*, *67*, 156 (1981).
29. Krahn, J., Koeter, van der Mark, T. W., Sluiter, H. J., and de Vries, K., Changes in bronchial hyperreactivity induced by 4 weeks of treatment with anti-asthmatic drugs in patients with asthma: a comparison between budesonide and terbutaline, *J. Allergy Clin. Immunol.*, *76*, 628–636 (1985).
30. Juniper, E. F., Kline, P. A., Vanzieleghem, M. A., Ramsdale, E. H., O'Byrne, P. M., and Hargreave, F. E., Effect of long-term treatment with inhaled corticosteroids on airway hyperresponsiveness and clinical asthma in nonsteroid dependent asthmatics, *Am. Rev. Respir. Dis.*, *142*, 832–836 (1990).

31. Bel, E. H., Timmers, M. C., Hermans, J., Dijkman, J. H., and Sterk, P. J., The long-term effect of nedocromil sodium and beclomethasone diproprionate on bronchial responsiveness to methacholine in nonatopic asthmatic subjects, *Am. Rev. Respir. Dis.*, *141*, 21–28 (1990).
32. Juniper, E. F., Kline, P., Vanzieleghem, M., and Hargreave, F., Reduction of budesonide after a year of increased use: a randomized controlled trial to evaluate whether improvements in airway responsiveness and clinical asthma are maintained, *J. Allergy Clin. Immunol.*, *87*, 483–489 (1991).
33. Cartier, A., Thomson, N. C., Frith, P. A., Roberts, R., and Hargreave, F. E., Allergen-induced increase in bronchial responsiveness to histamine: relationship to the late asthmatic response and change in airway caliber, *J. Allergy Clin. Immunol.*, *70*, 170–177 (1982).
34. Golden, J. A., Nadel, J. A., and Boushey, H. A., Bronchial hyperirritability in healthy subjects after exposure to ozone, *Am. Rev. Respir. Dis.*, *118*, 287–294 (1978).
35. Empey, D. W., Laitinen, L. A., Jacobs, L., Gold, W. M., and Nadel, J. A., Mechanisms of bronchial hyperreactivity in normal subjects after upper respiratory tract infections, *Am. Rev. Respir. Dis.*, *113*, 131–139 (1976).
36. Manning, P. J., Jones, G. L., and O'Byrne, P. M., Tachyphylaxis to inhaled histamine in asthmatic subjects, *J. Appl. Physiol.*, *63*, 1572–1577 (1987).
37. Manning, P. J., and O'Byrne, P. M., Histamine bronchoconstriction reduces airway responsiveness in asthmatic subjects, *Am. Rev. Respir. Dis.*, *137*, 1323–1325 (1988).
38. Hamilec, C. M., Manning, P. J., and O'Byrne, P. M., Exercise refractoriness post histamine bronchoconstriction in asthmatic subjects, *Am. Rev. Respir. Dis.*, *138*, 794–798 (1988).
39. Stevens, W. H., Manning, P. J., and O'Byrne, P. M., Tachyphylaxis to inhaled methacholine in normal but not asthmatic subjects, *J. Appl. Physiol.*, *69*, 875–879 (1990).
40. Beckett, W. S., McDonnell, W. F., and Wong, N. D., Tolerance to methacholine inhalation challenge in nonasthmatic subjects, *Am. Rev. Respir. Dis.*, *137*, 1499–1501 (1988).
41. Thomson, N. C., O'Byrne, P. M., and Hargreave, F. E., Prolonged asthmatic responses to inhaled methacholine, *J. Allergy Clin. Immunol.*, *71*, 357–362 (1983).
42. DuBois, A. B., Botelho, S. Y., and Comroe, J. H., Jr., A new method for measuring airway resistance in man using a body plethysmograph: values in normal subjects and in patients with respiratory disease, *J. Clin. Invest.*, *35*, 327–335 (1956).
43. Hyatt, R. E., Schilder, D. P., and Fry, D. L., Relationship between maximum expiratory flow and degree of lung inflation, *J. Appl. Physiol.*, *13*, 331–336 (1958).
44. Bouhuys, A., Hunt, V. R., Kim, B. M., and Zapletal, A., Maximum expiratory flow rates in induced bronchoconstriction in man, *J. Clin. Invest.*, *48*, 1159–1168 (1969).
45. Zamel, N., Partial flow-volume curves, *Bull. Eur. Physiopathol. Respir.*, *20*, 471–475 (1984).
46. DuBois, A. B., Resistance to breathing measured by driving the chest at 6cps, *Fed. Proc.*, *12*, 35–36 (1953).
47. Takishima, T., Hida, W., Sasaki, H., Suzuki, S., and Sasaki, T., Direct writing recorder of dose–response curves of airways to methacholine—clinical application, *Chest*, *80*, 600–606 (1981).

48. Cockcroft, D. W., Berscheid, B. A., and Murdock, K. Y., Unimodal distribution of bronchial responsiveness to inhaled histamine in a random human population, *Chest*, *83*, 751–754 (1983).
49. Hargreave, F. E., Ramsdale, E. H., and Pugsley, S. O., Occupational asthma without bronchial hyperresponsiveness, *Am. Rev. Respir. Dis.*, *130*, 513–515 (1984).
50. Ryan, G., Latimer, K. M., Dolovich, J., and Hargreave, F. E., Bronchial responsiveness to histamine: relationship to diurnal variation of peak flow rate, improvement after bronchodilator, and airway caliber, *Thorax*, *37*, 423–429 (1982).
51. Ramsdale, E. H., Morris, M. M., Roberts, R. S., and Hargreave, F. E., Bronchial responsiveness to methacholine in chronic bronchitis: relationship to airflow obstruction and cold air responsiveness, *Thorax*, *39*, 912–918 (1984).
52. McClean, P. A., VanderDoelen, J., and Zamel, N., Dose response threshold is independent of baseline lung function, *Am. Rev. Respir. Dis.*, 1994, in press.
53. Adelroth, E., Hargreave, F. E., and Ramsdale, E. H., Do physicians need objective measurements to diagnose asthma? *Am. Rev. Respir. Dis.*, *134*, 704–707 (1986).
54. Vedal, S., Enarson, D. A., Chan, H., Ochnio, J., Tse, K. S., and Chan-Yeung, M., A longitudinal study of the occurrence of bronchial hyperresponsiveness in Western red cedar workers, *Am. Rev. Respir. Dis.*, *137*, 651–655 (1988).

13

Allergen Inhalation Challenges

Sheldon L. Spector

*Allergy Medical Clinic and Allergy Research Foundation
Los Angeles, California*

I. BACKGROUND AND INTRODUCTION

Although allergen inhalation challenges have been performed for a variety of reasons, they probably are more frequently used at present in clinical research, especially to better understand the pathogenesis of immunoglobulin E (IgE)-mediated airway reactions (Table 1). They can serve to clarify the role of a particular allergenic substance in producing asthmatic symptoms. They also play an indisputable role in establishing a cause-and-effect relationship with a newly suspected causative agent in an occupational setting. Like any procedure, allergen challenges have limitations and should be interpreted along with a good history and other diagnostic tests, such as skin tests. The ability of a new pharmacological agent or immunotherapy treatment to block an allergen challenge, especially the late-phase reaction [1,2], has some important implications for treatment. The greatest interest in the late airway reactions is based on the recognition that such reactions are associated with increases in nonspecific airway reactivity and are also associated with IgE-mediated airway inflammation.

II. ALLERGENIC EXTRACTS USED

Most of the available allergenic extracts are still not adequately standardized, and their potency has not been confirmed. There are several ways to quantify allergen extracts. Weight per volume (w/v), which is the weight of an allergen that has been

Table 1 Inhalation Tests with Histamine or Methacholine

Indications	Evaluation of symptoms suggestive of asthma (in patients with normal airway caliber)
	Evaluation of the presence of occupational asthma (together with other parameters)
	Evaluation of the severity of asthma (together with other parameters)
	Research studies in asthma
Contraindications	Severe airflow obstruction (FEV_1 < 40% predicted or < 1.5 L)
Factors that enhance response	Recent exposure to relevant inhaled allergens
	Recent exposure to relevant occupational agents
	Recent respiratory viral infections
	Exposure to atmospheric pollutants (ozone)
Factors that reduce response	Avoidance of relevant allergens or occupational agents
	Bronchodilator drugs (β_2-adrenoceptor agonists, theophylline)
	Specific antagonists (antihistamines, anticholinergics)
	Regular treatment with corticosteroids
	Previous inhalation challenge with histamine (within 6 h)

FEV_1 = forced expired volume in 1 second.

extracted by a given volume of liquid, is a common expression of concentration. Thus, a 1:100 w/v of an extract would contain the quantity of allergen that could be extracted from 1 g of pollen by 100 ml of extracting fluid. Protein nitrogen units (PNU) per milliliter are another common expression of contents. Although one can approximate in many instances that a 1:100 weight per volume extract contains about 10,000 PNU, in reality this is a gross estimation and nothing more. Neither of the above units is an exact indicator of potency. In vivo methods are best used for this purpose. Europeans have favored testing based on a comparison with the histamine wheal. The quantity of the extract producing a wheal that is the same size as the wheal produced by a given concentration of histamine, formerly expressed as a histamine equivalent potency (HEP) unit, now usually is expressed as biological units. In the United States, the Food and Drug Administration (FDA) has suggested a technique that uses intradermal testing with threefold dilutions of an extract, with subsequent measurement of the flare rather than the wheal size [3]. This "intradermal end point" is expressed as the number of threefold dilutions that produce a summed erythema diameter of 50 mm. The mean value for 15 individuals defines the potency of the extract, which is expressed in allergy units (AU) [3]. Other measures of potency, such as radioimmunoassay inhibition [4], leukocyte histamine release [5], or characterizing the content of a known major allergen, such as antigen E in ragweed, have also been used [5]. If reagents for quantifying major allergen content are not available, IgE allergen–binding properties of extracts can be quantified by radioallergosorbent test (RAST) inhibition. The relative potency of mite extracts based on RAST inhibition is predictable and correlates well with the relative potency by skin testing. A more detailed discussion of many of these methods is found in Chapter 1 by Yunginger and Chapter 2 by Bousquet and Michel. New antigens are being appreciated all the time. There is recent interest in latex as a cause of immediate hypersensitivity reactions, including bronchial reactions [6]. Suphioglu and co-workers have reported evidence that starch granules, e.g., ryegrass pollens, that are less than 3 μm in diameter have provoked asthma [7]. Pollen, mite, and mold extracts all have appreciable enzymatic activity, including proteases and sugar-cleaving enzymes, which may be important in the degradation of the extracts with time. Temperature accentuates the degradation effect of time. At room temperature, extracts can lose potency within weeks, and at higher temperatures within days. When extracts are stored at 4°C there is very little, if any, effect in the first 3 months with concentrated extracts, and a small fall-off by the end of 1 year.

A. Additives

Agents such as thimerosal and parabens may be effective in preventing bacterial growth but do not stabilize potency.

B. Buffers

Bicarbonate or phosphate buffers are not good stabilizers; thus, the traditional Coca's solution of sodium bicarbonate buffer with 0.4% phenol not only does not insure extract stability but may actually adversely affect the stability.

C. Stabilizers

Phenol can actually have a deleterious effect on the extract and speed its degradation. Although its effect is minimal at 1:100 w/v, at 1:1000 w/v and in more dilute concentrations it may have a significant effect.

Glycerol is a very effective stabilizer of extract potency at a concentration of 50% [8]. A 10% or even a 25% solution of glycerol is not very effective after a 3-month period. A possible disadvantage of 50% glycerol is its irritating effect in intradermal skin testing. Solutions of 25% glycerol or less have been used for immunotherapy and are fairly well tolerated.

Serum albumin (0.03% HSA) has been used as an effective protein stabilizer [9], although it is less effective than glycerol. Since there is some concern about intradermal testing and immunotherapy with 50% glycerol, it has been suggested that a mixture of HSA 0.3% and glycerol 10% might be a reasonable combination for allergen immunotherapy and intradermal skin testing.

III. SAFETY OF ALLERGEN CHALLENGES

Inhalation challenges with concentrated antigens can cause severe or prolonged asthmatic attacks. A number of precautions are therefore necessary when performing allergen challenges (Table 1). A physician, nurse, or technician familiar with the intricacies of an antigen-challenge procedure should perform them. This should not be done as a routine procedure in an office setting with inexperienced personnel. The necessary equipment for cardiopulmonary resuscitation should be available immediately. This includes oxygen, epinephrine, and aerosol bronchodilators, i.e., any medication necessary to appropriately treat an immediate asthmatic or anaphylactic reaction. Baseline pulmonary function should be adequate, so that the patient does not already have a compromised pulmonary status. Ideally, technicians who administer allergen challenges should not have an allergic background or a personal or family history of asthma. A well-ventilated room helps prevent excessive antigen exposure from the air. Subjects should avoid allergens that might sensitize during an upper respiratory infection some weeks thereafter [10].

IV. STORAGE OF ALLERGENS

Most allergenic mixtures come as concentrated solutions or lyophilized products, although many of the lyophilized solutions have an expiration date of years. These preparations probably can last almost indefinitely. As mentioned, glycerin (glycerol)-containing extracts, which have a concentration of 50%, also protect the antigens from degradation and prolong the original strength. Phenol can be used as an alternative but may have a deleterious effect on antigenicity at higher dilutions. Other stabilizers, such as albumin, may improve extract stability, as can a nonionic detergent, polysorbate 80, and may be used to dilute mixtures that contain protein subject to loss due to adsorption on the surface of the glass or plastic container. This ability is also favored with storage at 4°C or below.

V. INDICATIONS FOR ALLERGEN CHALLENGE

A. A Clarification of the Role of Specific Allergens

Although there are cells that are common to both the lung and the skin, there are enough differences between these two organs, in terms of the orientation of the mast cells, eosinophils, vascular components, and the presence of bronchial tissue in the lungs, to make the lung quite different from another organ such as the skin or the nose. For this reason, many investigators feel that the target organ itself should be challenged to determine the role that the allergen may play in producing symptoms in that organ [11,12]. In fact, many studies show that the allergen inhalation challenge (AIC) provides different information than does a skin test or in vitro test. Various investigators have examined the relationship between IgE, mast cells, and basophils in various parts of the body [11–13]. In one study, mast cells from monkeys' respiratory tracts responded to ragweed antigens, although the same monkeys had no skin-test reactivity to ragweed antigens [14]. Other investigators have found differences in the cutaneous and respiratory response to cromolyn sodium [15]. Not only do mast cells differ in their response as compared with basophils, but mast cells in one part of the body differ as well from mast cells in other parts of the body. May and Williams showed a difference in blood basophil response as compared with tissue mast cell response [16]. They demonstrated that basophils became unresponsive to antigen challenge at a time when clinical sensitivity, skin-test reactivity, and IgE levels remained the same.

Another possible dissociation of response is local production of IgE in a particular organ. Thus, Aas [11] found nasal allergies to pollens in patients who had a positive skin-test response to that pollen and a negative response to bronchial challenge. Huggins and Brostoff [17] actually measured the local production of IgE in nasal secretions. They studied a certain number of patients with negative skin-test and negative serum RAST results to *Dermatophagoides pteronyssinus*. These same patients had specific IgE in their nasal secretions, which corresponded to a strong clinical history and positive response to nasal provocation with house dust mite. A similar local conjunctival sensitization to allergen has been described in the eye [18]. Fish and co-workers [19] have postulated that the site of response in asthmatic vs. rhinitic patients need not be the same. The allergic rhinitic patients have large-airway involvement, while the asthmatics have both peripheral- and central-airway involvement. Another interpretation, however, would be that the pulmonary function test used to measure this response was itself responsible for the differences seen in patients with rhinitis vs. asthma.

A single study favored the conclusion that bronchial challenge offered no more than skin (or other) tests in confirming the diagnosis of allergic asthma [20]. These investigators examined patients with ragweed hay fever and asthmatic patients with comparable skin-test reactivity and leukocyte histamine release. There was no difference in the mean PD_{35} (i.e., the provocative dose necessary to elicit a 35% fall in specific airway conductance [SGaw]) AIC response; i.e., antigen challenge did not differentiate the two groups, nor did skin test reactivity or in vitro testing. The PD_{35} procedure itself partly explains their results, since it is a highly variable test, susceptible to suggestion and other factors [21]. The maximum dose used for AIC has not been well characterized. In some studies, in fact, when a new antigen was being tested in an asthmatic patient, the investigators have not seriously considered the proper control for that antigen, namely an asthmatic with comparable nonspecific reactivity. A decision regarding the maximum dose of antigen used should consider the cause-and-effect relationship between such a dose and a clinical response. For example, Townley and co-workers [22] performed AIC in normal subjects and patients with hay fever and asthma. When they used an antigen concentration of 10,000 PNU and the forced expired volume in 1 second

(FEV_1), 11 of 14 patients with hay fever who had never wheezed before had a positive AIC. The FEV_1 separated hay fever patients from asthmatic subjects; nevertheless, 10,000 PNU caused hay fever patients to wheeze. This implies that too high a dose was used to draw meaningful conclusions regarding the role of antigen in hay fever, a condition not characterized by wheezing. Cavanaugh and colleagues [23] reported similar results and commented that the subjects who responded only to a high concentration of antigen behaved as a separate population, demonstrating a higher incidence of negative skin test reactions in comparison with other subjects tested.

We observed two patients in whom severe asthma lasting for days developed after they received an allergen extract at a concentration of 10^{-2} w/v, which is somewhat analogous to the PNU data mentioned [24]. The observations cited above have prompted the recommendation that bronchial challenges should be done with concentrations of antigen lower than 10^{-2} w/v or 10,000 PNU.

Killian and associates [25] and Cockcroft and co-workers [26] have observed an inverse relationship between the level of nonspecific reactivity as measured by histamine challenge and the intensity of the allergic reaction. When responsiveness to histamine is great, only a mild allergic reaction is required in the airways to trigger asthma. When the responsiveness is low, a more severe allergic reaction is required. Thus, asthma could be expected to be triggered by AIC in sensitized subjects without a history of asthma if the allergic reaction produced is severe enough. This has been shown when allergen inhalation did provoke asthma in subjects with allergic rhinitis and in asymptomatic subjects with positive results in allergic skin tests. One can only question the clinical meaning of such observations and caution investigators against using antigen concentrations that are too great, because of safety considerations. In addition, a late asthmatic response has not been well characterized by the relationship between the allergen dose and nonspecific bronchial reactivity.

B. An Alternative to or Comparison With Skin Tests, In Vitro Tests, or Other Diagnostic Methods

Bronchial challenges have been employed when there is insufficient information or discrepancies between history, skin test results, and/or in vitro results. As stated, certain in vitro tests may yield negative results with the same antigen that causes a positive skin test or inhalation challenge response. In vitro tests are also more costly than skin testing. Skin tests may not measure locally concentrated IgE attached to mast cells in a particular organ [17]. Skin tests may not be possible if severe eczema or other skin disorders are present in an area to be tested.

Although provocation tests have been touted as an absolute standard with which other tests should be compared, provocation testing also has its limitations, as will be discussed later.

Aas [11] compared pollen and house dust reactivity as assessed by skin tests and AIC (Table 2); both the type of antigen and the degree of skin-test reactivity influence a subsequent positive AIC response. Patients with pollen reactivity are more likely to have a positive bronchial challenge result than those with house-dust reactivity. Interestingly, patients with positive skin test results and negative bronchial challenge responses had nasal allergies to the pollen. The implication is that skin tests reveal IgE reactivity but not which organ is susceptible to the IgE effect.

Table 2 also summarizes the results of our study of the relationship between

Table 2 Allergy Skin Tests Compared with Bronchial Inhalation Challenges: Data of Spector et al. and Aas

Skin test results	No. of patients studied	No. (%) with positive response to bronchial challenge[a]
Spector et al. [27]		
Prick (puncture) test (1:10 or 1:20 w/v)		
Wheal greater than 9 mm	32	33 (61)
Wheal greater than 5 mm	68	24 (35)
Wheal greater than 2 mm with erythema of 14 mm	101	25 (25)
Wheal less than or equal to 2 mm	77	2 (3)
Intradermal[b]		
Positive at 10^{-5} w/v	54	33 (61)
Positive at 10^{-4} w/v	102	36 (35)
Positive at 10^{-3} w/v	131	35 (27)
Negative at 10^{-3} w/v	245	9 (4)
Aas [11]		
Pollen skin test		
1+ to 2+	128	85 (66)
3+ to 4+	188	174 (93)
Negative	71	8 (11)
House dust skin test		
1+	159	70 (44)
2+	117	74 (63)
3+	93	81 (87)
4+	33	26 (85)
Negative	132	40 (30)

[a]With 0.001 w/v antigen.

[b]Positive response defined as wheal 6 mm in diameter larger than that produced by diluent alone.

w/v = weight per volume.

skin test reactivity and AIC [27]. In this case, two types of skin test were used: the prick or puncture test and the intradermal skin test [27]. With the latter, if dilute antigens produced a positive reaction (defined by a wheal diameter 6 mm greater than that of the diluent control), the chance for a subsequent positive AIC was relatively great. Only 4% of the subjects tested had a positive AIC despite a negative skin test. This low incidence can partially be explained by our definition of a positive skin test result, which was a wheal 6 mm greater than that produced by its diluent control. If this definition had been less stringent, there would have been more positive skin test results related to a subsequent positive challenge response. Our study [27] was done with subjects who usually gave a history of perennial symptoms, so that the historic relationship to certain antigens was often unclear. If a patient has a positive skin test result that accompanies a strong history of reaction to the antigen, than an AIC may not be necessary, since the history allows for a reasonable prediction of a subsequent response to bronchial inhalation challenge. For example, 25 of 27 patients had a predictably positive AIC response in a previous study [13].

The degree of organ reactivity itself, whether of the nasal passages or the bronchial airways, partly influences the degree of the positive challenge response. Organ hyperreactivity as measured by methacholine or histamine inhalation challenge has already been mentioned as a factor that influences a positive response to AIC with an antigen [28,29]. Hill and associates [30] believed they could predict the results of AIC with whole ryegrass and house dust mite from the levels of skin sensitivity to undiluted extract and the percent fall in PEFR after exercise, the latter representing the degree of nonspecific bronchial reactivity.

C. Clarification of Mediators and Mechanisms

Antigen challenge has been associated with elevated histamine levels [31]. Deal and associates [32] could not demonstrate kinetic release after either antigen or thermal challenge, although there were random elevations in arterial blood histamine after both of these challenges. Allergen inhalation challenge produces a sustained or biphasic release of neutrophil chemotactic factor, but its measurement requires complicated bioassay techniques [32,33]. Ahmed and co-workers [34] described the liberation of slow-reacting substance of anaphylaxis (SRS-A) after ragweed AIC that impaired mucus transport. Marom and colleagues [35] found that the two major components of SRS-A, leukotrienes C_4 (LTC_4) and LTD_4, are potent contributors to mucus secretions observed during allergic reactions in vitro and in vivo. Allergen inhalation challenge is associated with release of LTE_4 and thromboxane A_2 into the urine [36]. Platelet activating factor (PAF) may also be involved, in view of the ability of the PAF antagonist BN52021 to inhibit PAF and (in some subjects) allergen-induced bronchoconstriction [37]. Additionally, circulating platelets are significantly decreased during an allergen-induced, but not a methacholine-induced, early asthmatic reaction [38]. Yet some investigators doubt the role of platelets in allergen-induced bronchial obstruction [39]. Wenzel and co-workers found prostaglandin D_2, thromboxane B_2, LTC_4, and histamine in the bronchoalveolar lavage (BAL) fluid after allergen instillation [40,41].

Schwartz and co-workers described a method to assess mast cell activation in vivo as contrasted with the activation of basophils. They found that an elevated plasma or serum tryptase level has diagnostic value for indicating mast cell–related events such as would occur with anaphylactic reactions [42]. Alveolar macrophage (AM) activation occurs immediately after antigen challenge. The late airway response to an allergen is associated with the appearance of high-density AMs, which potentiates superoxide release and may thereby contribute to increased airway injury [43]. Eosinophils and their products, as well as macrophages, probably play a significant role in this injury during the late phase [44]. The adhesion molecule L-selectin may play a role regarding homing of eosinophils into the lung during the asthmatic reaction after allergen challenge [45].

Dorsch and co-workers [46], analyzing the skin blister fluid from patients with dual skin reactions after intradermal allergen injection, found a complex array of mediators, including histamine, active kallikrein, thromboxane B_2, and PAF. Lavage fluid from an isolated endobronchial challenge showed a close association between immediate hypersensitivity events and the appearance of active kallikrein, kininogen substrate, and the liberation of kinin [47]. Platelet factor 4 also is released, and radioimmunoassay of this substance provides enough precision to differentiate clearly between asthmatic subjects and nonallergic control subjects [48]. The kinetics of its release are similar to those of neutrophil chemotactic factor in the circulation after AIC. Although serum complement fell during bronchospasm induced by antigen and not by methacholine, according to Arroyave and associates [49], a decrease in complement also occurred in some of the controls, making interpretation of these data difficult. Pryjma and colleagues [50] also reported a drop in hemolytic complement level after AIC in 8 of 22 patients. In four of seven patients, cromolyn sodium prevented the complement change. Castro et al. [51] reported that among ten different allergens, house dust extract proved to be the most potent complement activator.

Deal and co-workers [52] have contrasted AIC with hyperventilation after cold air. The former challenge produced a prolonged release of neutrophil chemotactic factor; the latter did not. Weiler-Ravell and Godfrey [53] postulated at least two different pathways for mechanisms to explain the fact that one-half of their 12 asthmatic subjects were rendered almost totally unresponsive to exercise-induced asthma after antigen-induced bronchospasm and one-half were not. On the other hand, Boulet and co-workers [54] induced a late response to exercise only in a subgroup of patients who the previous day had developed a late asthmatic response to allergen challenge and not in those who had experienced only an immediate allergic response.

D. Evaluation of New Allergens in Pulmonary Disease

The literature is replete with studies of new allergens that can produce pulmonary disease. Although most of these are organic substances, many are not.

E. Evaluation of New Treatments and Blocking Agents

Pharmaceutical manufacturers generally test new medications for their ability to block an antigen inhalation challenge, since this is advocated as an ideal model for studying asthma. Although in vitro animal experiments are often done first, the results in humans may differ. For example, Miller and Patterson [55] did not demonstrate bronchial hyperreactivity to physostigmine in rhesus monkeys with reagin-mediated asthma, even though it was seen with physostigmine in asthmatics [56]. Perper and associates [57] were able to inhibit *Ascaris* skin reactivity with the selective β-adrenergic agent albuterol. Yet they and others [58–60] could not demonstrate a block with β-adrenergic agents during allergic skin testing in humans.

Patient selection may be the most important factor in proving clinically meaningful associations in new drug trials. For example, a truly reagin-mediated population is best to demonstrate the effectiveness of a cromolyn-like substance if its action is believed to be inhibitory to mediator release in allergic patients. Asthma is too often equated erroneously with allergies. Furthermore, the technique of the study may influence the conclusions. For example, it was found that ICI 74,917, a phenanthrolene derivative, diminished allergen-induced bronchoconstriction but failed to improve asthma symptoms as compared with placebo [61]. In view of the high concentration of antigens used and the doubtful assumption that response to antigen inhalation challenge alone is a good model for asthma, the usefulness of extrapolating from bronchial-challenge response to a clinically meaningful conclusion is doubtful. A blocking medication should also be administered at a peak, appropriate time in relation to the bronchial inhalation challenge. Thus, timing, among many other factors, is important. Finally, if too high an antigen concentration is used, the specificity or clinical usefulness is questionable.

Reviving concepts of Tiffeneau [62] and Herxheimer [63] that dealt with hyposensitization of patients by the bronchial route, a Russian group suggested another treatment approach. They delivered antigens to the mucous membrane of the bronchi with aerosol inhalers, and they concluded that this direct instillation of antigen to shock the organ was more effective and less reactogenic than intradermal or subcutaneous injections of allergens [64,65].

F. Evaluation of the Therapeutic Effect of Immunotherapy

Allergen challenges have been used to evaluate the benefit of hyposensitization as reflected by a decrease in bronchial reactivity after treatment. As mentioned,

Assem and McAllen [66] gave immunotherapy with certain antigens and found a decrease only in bronchial reactivity in the responding group. This decreased reactivity correlated with clinical improvement. Other parameters had no such correlation. As discussed previously with reference to late reactions, Price and co-workers reported on their continued second year of study of mite immunotherapy in 51 children with perennial asthma and positive bronchial challenge to the antigen [67]. Patients receiving active treatment reduced their use of medication to relieve symptoms more than controls did. If treatment was stopped during the second year, their symptoms deteriorated. Improvement was associated with loss of the late reaction 6 h after bronchial provocation (with antigen), not with a change in the immediate reaction of lungs or skin. Those who improved in the placebo group did not lose their late reaction. Van Beuer and Stevens reported the complete resolution of the late asthmatic response (LAR) in five of 15 children after 1 year of house dust immunotherapy. Ohman compared the efficacy of immunotherapy in cat-induced asthma with that of placebo in a double-blind protocol including nine actively treated subjects. Clinical improvement in ocular and pulmonary symptoms correlated with significant reductions in bronchial sensitivity to cat antigen. There was no significant change in bronchial reactivity to methacholine. In another study, immunotherapy ameliorated both allergen sensitivity to cat dander and histamine bronchial hyperreactivity. Immunotherapy with dog antigen only attenuated the bronchial allergen sensitivity [68].

G. Convincing the Patient of Cause-and-Effect Relationship

Commonly, patients have preconceived ideas about their sensitivity to an allergen in their environment. With bronchial challenge, a relationship between symptoms and exposure can be demonstrated. Thus, an antigen inhalation challenge can help convince the patient of cause-and-effect relationships and the need for eliminating or minimizing exposure, such as exposure to the family pet.

VI. LOCATION OF RESPONSE

Investigators have tried to define the pattern of change in lung mechanics and gas exchange during an AIC. For example, Olive and Hyatt [69] noted that the first effect of the inhaled antigen was to cause a parallel shift in the maximal expiratory flow volume (MEFV) curve with no change in slope. Maximal flow at 60% of control total lung capacity was the most sensitive indicator of response. Actually, there was heterogeneity of response. One-third of the 15 subjects had closure of units with no change in MEFV slope. Another third initially showed the same pattern but at the height of the response showed an MEFV slope change which suggested that other airways increased the resistance. Finally, one-third had an immediate change of slope, with all but one showing an increase in residual volume. These data suggest that the site of airway obstruction may be different among asthmatic subjects. In the patients they studied, Ahmed and co-workers [70] believed that flow isovolume (Viso-V), a sensitive indicator of small-airway response, was a better indicator of airway response to AIC than was SGaw.

Olgiatti and co-workers [71] found a greater decrease in mean arterial oxygen saturation after ragweed challenge than after methacholine challenge for comparable severity of bronchospasm as measured by SGaw. The results suggest greater involvement of peripheral airways after AIC in seven patients studied.

VII. IMMEDIATE VERSUS LATE ASTHMATIC RESPONSE

Late-phase reactions have been described in various organs such as the skin, lung, and nose. After an allergen challenge there is an immediate component within minutes followed by a late-phase reaction. This secondary phase is thought to be an inflammatory response, although it has been investigators have defined it somewhat differently.

In 1987, Dorsch defined late-phase reaction as an inflammatory response lasting 2 h to 2 days [72]. Pelikan defined it as a response 4–12 h after the immediate reaction [73], and Lemanske and Kaliner defined it as beginning 3–4 h after the challenge [74]. Perhaps this lack of a rigid definition is related in part to the various tissues where the reactions have been described, such as the skin, nose, and tracheobronchial tree, and the confusion regarding the mechanism behind these reactions. Although LARs at one time were thought to be Arthus-like reactions mediated by IgG, IgM, and complement (as described with hypersensitivity pneumonitis), most investigators feel that IgE-mediated reactions involving mast cells, other inflammatory cells, and chemotactic factors are primarily responsible. The dosage rather than the concentration of allergen appears to determine the early and late asthmatic response [75]. The time of day of allergen exposure also influences the development of the LAR. In one study [75], an allergen challenge in the morning produced an LAR in four of 10 subjects, whereas the same challenge in the evening caused an LAR in nine of 10 ($p < 0.05$). Premedication with a β agonist can convert early responses to dual allergic responses [76,77].

The prevalence of these late responses also has varied. Since this chapter deals mainly with asthmatic responses, these data will be briefly summarized. A prevalence of greater than 50% has been found by some investigators, such as Warner et al. in studies of house dust in pediatric patients [67,78]. Robertson found LARs in eight of 15 of his ragweed-sensitive patients [79]. Paggiaro and Chan-Yeung found an incidence of dual reactions of 47.3% in 332 patients with Western red cedar asthma [80]. The 43.4% incidence of isolated LARs is unusual but may be more characteristic of low-molecular-weight agents such as plicatic acid and diisocyanates [81,82]. Booij-Noord and co-workers found an incidence of 47% in a study of house dust–sensitive patients [83], and Kim found isolated

LARs in 10 of 22 or 45% of his patients [84]. Pelikan and co-workers found an unusually large number of isolated late responses [73]. In a study of 61 patients with a total of 83 LARs, 35 had isolated LARs and 48 had dual late responses. Bronsky and Ellis, working at the National Jewish Hospital, found an incidence of less than 1% [85]. Our data derived from adult patients at the same institution also showed a low percentage [12,27]. In both of these last studies a large proportion of the patients, because of the severity of their asthma, were taking corticosteroids, which are known to block LARs.

Various factors have contributed to the lack of clarity in the literature regarding the definition and importance of the LAR. For example, which pulmonary function parameter and how much of a decrement should be used to define a positive response? Some investigators have used a fall in FEV_1 of 10%, while others have employed the more stringent 15%. Perhaps another pulmonary function test such as SGaw should be employed if the obstruction involves primarily large airways. Ideally, a placebo should be given to help clarify the characteristic liability of the airways of an asthmatic subject over time.

Bundgaard and Boudet studied reproducibility of LARs in five adult asthmatics after a challenge with *Cladosporium herbarum* [86]. One patient had an early but not a late asthmatic response and another had an early and a late response on one occasion but no late response on the second. One patient with a negative skin test had no early asthmatic response but showed a reproducible LAR after antigen inhalation. This patient also had an LAR after saline but not after histamine. Thus, only one patient had a reproducibly positive allergen challenge as defined by a 20% fall in FEV_1. Ihre et al. could change isolated late reactions following allergen challenges to dual reactions by increasing the allergen dose [87]. There is not necessarily a correlation between the late-onset skin reaction and the late bronchial reaction [88]. The concentration of the allergen will influence the subsequent response. If hay fever patients who have never had an asthmatic response are given a concentrated allergen mixture, both an immediate and late response can be induced. Is this clinically meaningful? Certain antigens such as dust and molds seem to favor the production of an LAR as compared with others [67,85]. The level of circulating IgE and the size of the early response as measured by skin tests or mediator release may also influence results. Although the presence of a late cutaneous response may also be important, there is not a consistently good correlation between cutaneous response and LAR. In fact, Atkins and co-workers tried to correlate the intensity of simultaneously occurring late-onset skin and bronchial reactivity in seven allergic subjects following skin and inhalation challenge with pollen antigen [88]. They found that the LAR correlated with the degree of increase in serum neutrophil chemotactic factor (NCF-A) activity, but the intensity of the late-onset skin responses correlated with the level of specific antigen IgE in the serum. Certain investigators have suggested that if the degree of both methacholine (or histamine) reactivity and immediate skin test reactivity by end-point titration is known, one can accurately predict the bronchial inhalation response to an antigen [89]. Since such predictability does not carry over to the LAR or to occupational allergy due to a new substance, it would appear that AIC is still important for clarifying immediate and late-phase mechanisms and occupational allergy.

There are important implications of the focus on late-phase reactions as an explanation for the chronic clinical features of various allergic diseases such as asthma, allergic rhinitis, urticaria, and even atopic dermatitis. The relationship between bronchial hyperresponsiveness and the late-phase reaction has received considerable attention. Inhalation of allergens either experimentally or through natural exposure can increase nonspecific bronchial responsiveness to histamine and methacholine [90–93]. This increase in reactivity can be demonstrated either shortly after the immediate airway response or during the interval following the LAR [94]. The increased responsiveness may then persist for days or even weeks after the initial exposure. In a study of the time course of hyperreactivity following an antigen challenge, Cockcroft and Murdock [95] confirmed the lack of bronchial responsiveness to inhaled histamine after isolated earlier asthmatic responses, but they found that the 12 subjects with allergen-induced dual responses were significantly more responsive to inhaled histamine 7 and 30, but not 2 h or 5 or 7 days, after AIC. Durham et al. [96] found that in subjects who developed LARs after exposure to occupational agents there was an increase in nonspecific bronchial responsiveness to methacholine 2–3 h after the challenge. Clinically, there is an increased nonspecific bronchial responsiveness during seasonal pollen exposure [92], and reductions in reactivity can occur after prolonged allergen avoidance [97]. In some studies, immunotherapy also seems to be associated with inhibition of late response and clinical improvement [67,98]. Warner and coworkers [78] treated 27 subjects with mite immunotherapy and 24 with placebo in a 12-week double-blind, controlled study. All were asthmatic children with bronchial sensitivity to *D. pteronyssinus*. The treated children not only were clinically better than controls but lost their LARs, even though there was no change in their immediate response. On the other hand, Murray et al. [99] reported that hyposensitization with house dust mites can actually lead to increased airway responsiveness in children.

Neutrophil chemotactic factor activity has been found quite consistently in early and late responses following AIC. It also has been found after exercise challenge [74]. The appearance of NCF-A activity parallels the rise and fall of pulmonary function parameters seen during the development of the dual response [100]. Histamine has been found only sporadically [74]. In fact, Howarth and coworkers [101] studied the response to AIC in two groups of subjects with asthma, one with airways markedly reactive to methacholine and the other with less reactive airways. In the more reactive group there was no significant increase in plasma histamine, whereas in the less reactive group there was a significant increase in plasma histamine 5 min after the allergen challenge. Both groups had a significant increase in serum NCA after the challenge.

Metabolites of arachidonic acid have been noted in association with AIC. Prostaglandin D_2 is released into the human airways during an AIC. It is a major prostaglandin generated by tissue mast cells in vitro and by lung tissue in vivo. Prostaglandin D_2 was found to be released into human airways during acute AIC and when BAL was performed in asthmatic patients after a mite challenge. Release of prostaglandin D_2 occurs as an early event after the instillation of *D. pteronyssinus* in patients sensitive to this allergen [102]. Leukotriene B_4, which is a potent neutrophil chemotactic factor in humans, has been found in plasma specimens obtained during the development of both early and late asthmatic responses following AIC [100,103].

Abraham [104], using a sheep model, found that the lipoxygenase products of arachidonic acid metabolism released during early stages of allergic reactions played an important role in the subsequent development of LARs [104]. The dual responders produced more leukotrienes and were more sensitive to the leukotrienes produced than the acute responders. Other leukotrienes, such as LTC_4 and LTD_4, are good candidates as well, inasmuch as they can induce bronchospasm, enhance vascular permeability, and increase mucus secretion.

Platelet activating factor (PAF) administered by inhalation produces airway obstruction and increases bronchial hyperreactivity. Many of the medications used in the treatment of asthma, such as cromolyn, corticosteroids, ketotifen, and theophylline, also block PAF. Nakamura et al. [105] measured the concentration of the lyso form of PAF in plasma at 0 and 20 min and at 6 and 24 h after AIC among patients with bronchial asthma. Patients with LARs had a significantly increased concentration of lyso-PAF as compared with patients who had a single immediate response 6 h after the antigen challenges. There was no difference in PAF levels at 20 min. These results suggest that PAF may participate in the LAR.

Ito and co-workers [106] performed inhalation challenges with *Dermatophagoides farinae* in 13 mite-sensitive patients. Seven showed dual bronchial reactions, and five showed isolated immediate responses. Six of seven patients with dual reactions had higher IgG_1 antibodies than the five patients with isolated immediate reactions when examined before the challenge, suggesting that there is a close correlation between the presence of high IgG_1 antibodies and the propensity to develop LARs. Gonzalez and co-workers [107] measured the number of helper (OKT_4) and suppressor (OKT_8) T cells in blood and BAL fluid in six patients with early reactions after AIC and in six subjects with dual responses. There was a significant increase in the percentage of OKT_4 cells in the blood of the patients with single early responses. There was a significant decrease in the percentage of OKT_4 cells in the BAL fluid, along with an increase in OKT_8 cells. The percentage of OKT_4 cells was much lower ($p<0.005$) on the antigen-challenge day in those with single early responses than those with late-phase responses. This suggests the possibility that suppressor T cells are mobilized into the lung after allergen-induced single early reactions and that this may be associated with the prevention of a subsequent late-phase response.

Direct instillation of allergen into the bronchi and subsequent BAL can be used as means of studying local mechanisms in cellular inflammation. In one study [108], 11 allergic asthmatics all with a previously demonstrated LAR were compared with six healthy asymptomatic subjects. Allergen instillation caused an immediate pallor followed by reactive hyperemia, edema, and bronchial narrowing. By 48 h neutrophils and eosinophils increased significantly, as did helper T lymphocytes. By 96 h, neutrophil counts returned to normal, whereas eosinophils and helper T cells remained elevated. Other investigators have elaborated on the role of T lymphocytes during an antigen challenge [109] and on the early recruitment of eosinophils [110]. Cookson and co-workers [111] found a strong correlation with the magnitude of the late response and the fall in eosinophil counts. Frick et al. [112] reported an increase in the proportion of peripheral blood eosinophils that are hypodense only in patients with both an immediate and a late asthmatic response. They concluded that the percent of hypodense eosinophils better reflects the severity of asthma than the concentration of total peripheral blood eosinophils. Medications can affect both the immediate and the late response to antigen challenge. Their blocking properties will be detailed subsequently. The pharmaceutical industry has utilized blocking properties to predict possible effectiveness in various allergic diseases, especially asthma.

Corticosteroids taken orally classically block the late response very well but do not block the immediate response in most systems. On the other hand, oral steroids given 3 h before an AIC in sheep blocked both [113], and Martin and co-workers [114] found that prednisone blocked the immediate antigen response to pollens when given at 40 mg orally daily for 7 days before and on the day of the challenge.

In an Italian study, prednisone not only inhibited the LAR and the increased airway responsiveness after toluene diisocyanate exposure but also normalized the number of leukocytes and the concentration of albumin found in the BAL fluid [115]. Unlike oral steroids, steroid aerosols typically have inhibited both the immediate and the late response [116].

Cromolyn is effective in inhibiting both the early phase response and the LAR. In a study by Mattolis et al. [117], two doses of cromolyn were employed to block allergen-induced late responses as well as the increased responsiveness to methacholine. Although the two doses of cromolyn significantly delayed the onset of LAR, cromolyn did not alter the magnitude of LAR. It did prevent the allergen-induced increase in methacholine responsiveness. Both of these effects were greatest at the maximal dose used. Pelikan and co-workers [118] found that cromolyn sodium was highly protective against the immediate asthmatic response to AIC, whereas beclomethasone dipropionate did not significantly block these early responses. Other investigators reported that beclomethasone and theophylline, but not cromolyn, prevented the LAR [119]. Theophylline did not affect the associated increased airway responsiveness to methacholine, while beclomethasone did. In other studies, theophylline blocked the late response and slightly altered the early response [120]. In fact, Pauwels [121] suggests that theophylline has inhibitory activity on airway inflammation induced by allergic and nonallergic stimuli.

Nedocromil given 3 h before AIC in four subjects significantly reduced the bronchoconstrictor response and protected the patients against AIC, as compared with placebo. The highest dose of 2 mg was the most effective [122]. Both nedocromil sodium and cromolyn sodium significantly reduced the early response to antigen and blocked the LAR to antigen in allergic sheep [123]. Classically, β-agonists are thought to affect only early response, but the timing and duration of action of these agents may particularly explain the results. They do block mediators, but have been insufficiently studied (in my opinion) with regard to the late response. Various agents have a differential effect on mediators and pulmonary function, according to Howarth et al. [124]. Ipratropium bromide pretreatment produces bronchodilatation comparable to that achieved with albuterol but has no significant effect on mediator or airway response to challenge. Allergen inhalation challenge was performed in eight atopic subjects during control days and after pretreatment with albuterol 200 μg, cromolyn 20 mg, ipratropium bromide 1 mg, or saline. Pretreatment with albuterol abolished not only the bronchoconstriction but also the increases in levels of plasma histamine and serum NCF that had occurred at baseline and with placebo. Cromolyn attenuated the airway response, but there were still significant falls in the SGaw and FEV_1 and increases in plasma histamine. Cromolyn completely blocked NCF. Ipratropium bromide produced bronchodilatation comparable to that seen with albuterol but had no significant effect on the immediate airway responses to challenge.

Guinot and co-workers [125] assessed the effect of a specific PAF antagonist, BN52063, on the early asthmatic response to inhaled allergen in a double-blind, cross-over study of eight atopic asthmatics. Each received treatment for 3 days with BN52063 or placebo separated by a 1-week wash out. There was a significant antagonism of the early bronchoconstriction and a tendency toward antagonism of the residual bronchial hyperreactivity for 6 h after AIC using acetylcholine as a test for hyperresponsiveness. There were no side effects with the treatment.

The nonsteroidal anti-inflammatory agent indomethacin is reported by some investigators to inhibit the LAR but not the early response [126,127]. It is not considered a useful medication in the treatment of asthma. Although considerable enthusiasm regarding the LAR has been prompted by the assertion that it is a clinical manifestation of airway inflammation, its use as a clinical model has certain limitations. In fact, it may be too big a step to assume that there is a hierarchy of useful medication based only on the ability to block LAR as a measure of this inflammation. Many situations need clarification as they bear on the late response, and many studies must still be done to put the immediate and late responses in the proper perspective, for the following reasons:

1. It is known that the concentration of antigen used is an important determinant of the LAR. Should that concentration be so high as to elicit a response without clinical applicability, it may have little practical meaning. An early allergen response can be converted to a dual response by performing an allergen challenge along with a short-acting β agonist. Interestingly, when a β agonist is employed in such a manner, there is no accompanying increase in nonspecific hyperresponsiveness [76].
2. Hay fever subjects can show methacholine hyperresponsiveness after allergen challenge or allergen exposure. Thus, nonasthmatic allergic subjects showed the same hyperreactivity as asthmatic subjects [128]. Additionally, many nonallergic asthmatics have hyperresponsiveness, so it is unclear what is perpetuating their symptoms and creating their ongoing inflammatory reaction.
3. Rhinovirus infections were induced in 10 patients with allergic rhinitis. Most developed increased late-phase histamine reactivity but not methacholine reactivity after AIC with allergens to which they had shown reactivity. Four weeks later, eight of 10 had developed late-phase reactions, as compared with one of 10 before the viral infection [1].
4. In some studies, allergic or occupational exposure can cause increased airway responsiveness without a measurable late response, only an early response. For example, AIC of 12 subjects resulted in early but not late responsiveness, with the increased methacholine responsiveness occurring 1–6 days later in three of the 12 (25%). Machado studied 21 patients with bronchial inhalation tests to various antigens, including pollens, animals, house dust mites, and molds. He found that an increased methacholine reactivity occurred 6 h after allergen challenge in patients with dual reactions or equivocal reactions and even in three patients with isolated immediate reactions. The increased reactivity was still present 1 week after the challenge [129].
5. Exercise and possibly distilled water have been associated with increased LAR without increased nonspecific responsiveness.
6. Certain medications that inhibit the LAR are not found to be useful in the treatment of asthma. Thus, indomethacin, which has been found to inhibit late responses by many but not all investigators, is not a treatment for asthma [130,131].
7. Certain medications that are extremely useful in treating asthma do not appear to affect the late response (though this may partially be due to the study design). These include β agonists, which are well known to be very effective in the acute management of asthma. Also, cromolyn sodium, although useful in many patients, has not proved to be a panacea for the treatment of asthma in the large majority of patients, despite its consistent inhibition of the late (and early) asthmatic response.

8. In a study by Tak Lee, fish oil was administered to 20 allergic subjects with the hope of ameliorating their asthma by changing arachidonic acid pathways [132]. Although there was no clinical improvement in the asthma, the LARs to inhaled antigens were nevertheless attenuated.

In summary, allergen challenges producing isolated immediate, late, or combination reactions have stimulated much interest. Late-phase reactions may help explain perpetuation of hyperreactivity in certain persons. Pharmacological agents that block early and/or late reactions may be telling us something about mechanisms and the role of these agents in inflammation. However, much more information and further clarification are necessary before we base clinical therapy on the ability of these agents to block the response to AIC.

VIII. RELATIVE CONTRAINDICATIONS AND PRECAUTIONS WITH AN ALLERGEN CHALLENGE PROCEDURE

A person with a fixed moderate to severe impairment of lung function should be tested by bronchial challenge with caution. Those with asthmatic symptoms should not be given a bronchoconstrictor, which would further compromise pulmonary function. In general, if the FEV_1 is 1 L or less, challenge should be discouraged.

The duration of action of histamine by inhalation is minutes; methacholine's effect also is short-lived, although a few subjects have a reaction lasting hours. On the other hand, AIC can provoke prolonged or late reactions and require even more precautions.

During the first inhalation challenge, the initial antigen concentration should be the one that produced a 2+ reaction on intracutaneous injection; this 2+ equals a wheal more than 5 mm in diameter (minus the diameter of the wheal produced by the diluent control). When the prick technique is used, a 5% solution of 1:20 w/v dilution of aqueous solutions of antigen or antigen in 50% glycerol is applied to the skin. A wheal more than 3 mm in diameter is considered equivalent to a positive intradermal test result with a solution having a concentration of antigen of 1:10,000 ± one dilution. Antigen skin tests should include a "negative" diluent control and a "positive" histamine control. When glycerol is used as a diluent, a control must be added. When intradermal tests are used, the injected histamine solution should consist of 0.02 mL of a 0.01% base solution. For prick tests, a 1% solution of histamine base is recommended. Medications should be withheld as discussed in the next section.

IX. PREPARATION OF THE PATIENT FOR A CHALLENGE

Ideally, an investigator should avoid suggesting to the patient that a particular response is expected, since this may influence the results [21,133]. Thus, before a bronchial challenge, a patient should be informed that the inhaled substance may result in an increase, a decrease, or no change in pulmonary function. Subjects are best tested in an asymptomatic state. Smoking and consumption of cola drinks, coffee, and chocolate should be stopped at least 6 h before testing. Air pollution exposure and exercise should be avoided 2 h before bronchial challenge. If possible, medications should be stopped. Granted that this is not always practical or possible for patients requiring chronic medications, Table 3 lists recommendations based on the metabolism and half-lives of the drugs or on clinical experience. An international committee has suggested as a general guideline withholding medications for at least a time equal to 10 half-lives [134]. The metabolism of the medications is often such that a person may remain under the influence of the substance for a longer time than is presumed from the listed recommendations.

Although corticosteroids inhibit the development of late-phase responses to allergen challenge, a dose–response relationship has not been worked out. It is often impossible to withhold corticosteroids, so the question of how long to withhold them is rather academic. In reality, it is uncommon for patients taking

Table 3 Suggested Suspension Times for Commonly Used Medications Before Bronchial Provocation Testing with Allergens

Medication	Withholding time[a]
β Agonists	
Long-Acting	48 h
Short-Acting	8 h
Theophylline	
Long-Acting	72 h
Short-Acting	24 h
α-Adrenergic blocking agents	2–24 h
Anticholinergic agents	2–24 h
Cromolyn sodium	24 h
Nedocromil	24 h
Antihistamines	(48 h)
Terfenadine	3 days
Loratadine	10 days
Cetirizine	5 days
Astemizole	6–8 weeks
Azalastine	2–3 days
Corticosteroids	
Oral	Depending on the clinical situation[b]
Aerosolized	Depending on the clinical situation[b]

[a]Times given are minimums.
[b]Not the day of the test.

oral corticosteroids to be given an allergen challenge. Topical corticosteroids can prevent early reactions if they are administered for at least 1 week before the challenge [135]. They also are known to block late-phase reactions [136].

This effect can be minimized if challenges are done at consistent times in relation to a given medication. This applies in particular to medications such as thyroid preparations or tranquilizers that cannot readily be withdrawn but nevertheless may influence the outcome. Other factors known to affect baseline measurements or subsequent response to bronchoconstrictive substances, such as exposure to natural viruses or vaccines, air pollutants, or recent antigenic challenges, are discussed below.

X. FACTORS AFFECTING RESPONSE

A. Environmental Contacts

Recent contacts with allergens (viruses, vaccines, pollutants) may affect responses to antigen bronchial challenge (as in methacholine and histamine challenges), even if such contacts have not been systematically studied. Herxheimer [137] and Tiffeneau [138] thought that hyposensitization by inhalation could occur. The current technique of bronchial challenge, beginning with dilute antigens and progressing to more concentrated extracts until a positive response is obtained, would theoretically induce hypersensitization [137], with less antigen being required to produce a positive response because of a previous exposure to that antigen. It is similar to the "priming effect" described by Connell [139]. Zwick and co-workers [140] found a higher incidence of allergic disease, subclinical sensitization to aeroallergens, bronchial hyperresponsiveness, and disorders of allergen immunotherapy in competitive swimmers as compared with their control population, and they postulated that this may have been due to exposure to chlorine in swimming pools. Others have commented on the increased bronchial responsiveness to allergen in allergic subjects after exposure to even low ozone concentrations [141] or to parental smoking early in life [142].

Rosenthal and colleagues [143] gave 13 ragweed-sensitive asthmatic patients a ragweed-extract bronchial challenge on four successive days. On a later day during the pollen season, nine patients were rechallenged. None demonstrated an increase in bronchial sensitivity with repeat exposure or during the season. Kelly and co-workers [144] suggested that priming may occur from natural environmental pollen antigens. All four patients studied showed an increase in bronchial reactivity to ragweed antigen on inhalation challenge after the ragweed-pollen season. Similarly, a reduction in bronchial reactivity to inhaled histamine among patients in specially cleaned hospital rooms for 2 months or more was reported; this confinement presumably prevented exposure to the house dust mite antigen to which the patients were sensitive [97]. Unfortunately, a control population was not included.

B. Baseline Values and Airway Caliber

Although not all investigators have noticed a relationship between baseline values and subsequent bronchial challenge response, Hume and Gandevia [145] reported that as the FEV_1 and forced vital capacity (FVC) improve, so does the absolute response until it reaches a maximum. Also, the absolute response was poor if the initial value was low. Goldberg and Cherniack [146] described the greatest changes after therapy as taking place when airway resistance was highest. Initial values may in fact reflect pathogenic mechanisms. At one time mucosal edema may be predominant; at another time bronchospasm may be predominant. Barbato and co-workers [147] postulated that baseline airway caliber has the potential to modify bronchial hyperreactivity during the pollen season. Vedal et al. [148] also postulated that airway caliber and possibly immunological sensitivity to plicatic acid are associated with the occurrence of bronchial hyperresponsiveness in red cedar workers [148].

C. Bronchial Liability Caused by the Pulmonary Function Measurement Itself

Certain pulmonary function maneuvers may affect both normal and asthmatic subjects, but not necessarily in the same manner [149–151]. Reversible hyperinflation may also be induced by a bronchial challenge [152]. Characteristically, two different methods are used to measure airway response: maximal expiratory flow maneuvers and submaximal maneuvers such as airway resistance. A disadvantage of a forced expiratory maneuver as measured by spirometry is the reduction in normal tone that occurs after inspiration to total lung capacity [149,153] or after induced bronchoconstriction in normal [154] and asthmatic [155] subjects. By contrast, a deep inspiration or expiration causes bronchoconstriction in asthmatic patients that is prevented by anticholinergics such as atropine [150,151,156,157].

The ability to abolish changes in bronchomotor tone with a deep inspiration may render the FEV_1 relatively insensitive in those showing this response. Although the FEV_1 maneuver can be criticized because of effort-dependency, it has survived the test of time as a useful, convenient, and minimally variable test of pulmonary function. Unfortunately, the body plethysmograph is expensive to make or purchase and is not widely available. The panting maneuver itself may be affected by laryngeal narrowing induced by a particular drug administered during bronchial provocation. Measurements of airway resistance and maximum flow should be made at the same lung volume [158–160].

D. Body (Circadian) Rhythms

The time of day may influence a bronchial challenge via circadian and body rhythms. Gervais and associates [161] found a 24-h rhythm in bronchial reactivity to house dust in asthmatic patients. At 8:00 a.m. there was the least, and at 11:00 p.m. the greatest, effect in terms of persistence of bronchospasm after challenge. Human susceptibility to antigenic substances may vary also during the menstrual cycle [162].

E. Medications

A review by Pipkorn [163] of the blocking effect of various antiallergic medications on in vivo allergen testing, including some of the newer antihistamines as well as the usual asthma medications, should be consulted. Also, those medications that preferentially block the LAR are summarized earlier in this chapter in the section "Clarification of Mediators and Mechanisms."

1. Anticholinergics

Atropine blockade of AIC became a subject of controversy because of the role of reflex airway constriction in asthma. Yu and associates [164] reported that 1.5–2.5 mg of atropine sulfate given intravenously could block antigen reactions, which indicates dependency on cholinergic pathways. However, atropine did not block antigen-induced bronchoconstriction in other investigations. Thus, Rosenthal and colleagues [165] found no block of AIC with 1.2 or 5.0 mg of atropine (inhaled), although it inhibited bronchoconstriction to aerosolized methacholine and citric acid. Fish and co-workers [166] supported these results by failing to inhibit AIC bronchoconstriction with 5 mg of atropine given before the antigen and 1.2 mg of atropine mixed with antigen to maintain the blockade. Itkin and Anand [167] examined the effect of inhaled and intravenous atropine on AIC. Bronchospasm to at least one antigen developed in each subject. If both 0.8 mg of atropine and antigen were inhaled, the bronchoconstrictor effect of antigen was blocked completely in eight of the 20 subjects and partially in five. In one-third of the 20 subjects the AIC was blocked when 1.5 mg of atropine was given 15 min before the challenge. All demonstrated inhibition of methacholine challenge when 0.8 mg of atropine was mixed with 2.5 mg of methacholine. Rosenthal and colleagues [165] suggested a cholinergic effect with low antigen doses. Interestingly, atropine at low but not high doses inhibited the action of histamine [168].

At least two factors have been shown to be associated with a positive response to bronchial inhalation challenge with a specific antigen: nonspecific airway hyperreactivity and a positive skin test result as an index of specific IgE to an antigen [29,169]. The different results with atropine may be due to subject differences in nonspecific reactivity as measured by methacholine or histamine inhalation. This corresponds to an observation that certain patients show a greater blocking effect to histamine inhalation with aerosolized atropine than do others [170].

2. Antihistamines

Protection against AIC is dependent on the antihistamine dose. Schiller and Lowell [171] did not find pretreatment with 0.06–1.2 mg tripelennamine given intravenously protective against AIC; the same drug in higher doses was successful. Others have reported similar results with larger doses given either by inhalation or intravenously [172].

Popa [173] protected seven of nine asthmatics against allergen-induced bronchoconstriction with 10 mg chlorpheniramine given intravenously. One of the remaining two, unprotected with the lower dose, was protected with 15 mg. Certain antihistamines may be more potent blockers than others. Booij-Noord and co-workers [174,175] found the pure antihistamine mepyramine maleate to be as protective as thiazinamium. Thiazinamium may have other than just antihistaminic properties.

Although the hydroxyzine metabolite cetirizine, which is commercially available in other countries, did not significantly modify the allergen inhalation challenge, it inhibited recruitment of eosinophils as measured in the BAL fluid [176,177]. Terfenadine (180 mg) had a slight inhibitory effect on early and late-phase bronchoconstriction following allergen challenge [178]. However, loratadine failed to attenuate the early and late airway response to inhaled allergen [179].

3. Adrenergic Blocking Agents

Thymoxamine, an α-receptor blocker, inhibited AIC when given intravenously (0.1 mg per kg) in 10 of 11 patients [180]. In two of the same patients, thymoxamine (1.5%) inhalation also effectively inhibited allergen-induced bronchoconstriction.

4. β-Adrenergic Agonists

Epinephrine significantly inhibited the flare of histamine and both the wheal and flare of antigen in six atopic subjects at a dose of 0.3 ml of a 1 mg/ml subcutaneous injection. Histamine and antigen intradermal skin tests were performed 10 min after the epinephrine injection [181]. β-Adrenergic agonists such as inhaled fenoterol (800 μg) are reported to be more effective than cholinergic agonists such as SCH1000 (80 μg) in preventing early allergen-induced bronchospasm [182]. Similar effects were demonstrated with fenoterol by Jorde and associates [183]. Martin and associates [184] reported that terbutaline sulfate (2.5 mg every 6 h for 36 h) significantly blocked AIC. Falliers [185] observed that a combination of ephedrine and theophylline was more effective than either alone in blocking an aerosolized allergenic challenge. The long-acting β agonist salmeterol blocks the early and late response to allergen challenge as well as the hyperreactivity that follows [186]. Even high-dose nebulized albuterol (2.5 mg) can inhibit the early and late asthmatic reaction as well as the increased airway responsiveness provoked by inhaled allergen [187]. β-Agonists have the potential for worsening the allergic symptoms as well. In one study, the early bronchial responsiveness to allergen could be increased following continuous treatment with a β-adrenergic receptor agonist [188]. In another study, the author concluded that antigen deposition may be increased following metered-dose β-agonist treatment [76].

5. Cromolyn Sodium and Cromolyn-Like Agents

Many studies indicate that cromolyn sodium blocks the immediate bronchial challenge response to allergens; however, not all patients demonstrate such an inhibition [189–193]. Cromolyn sodium also blocks late reactions. It is effective as micronized powder with lactose, micropellets without lactose, and aerosol solution [191]. Nedocromil sodium inhibits the early and late response to allergen challenge as well as the allergen-induced increase in bronchial hyperreactivity [194,195].

6. Corticosteroids and Corticosteroid Aerosols

In several studies, oral corticosteroids did not block bronchoconstriction from high concentrations of house dust and wheat flour antigens [192,196]. However, Martin and co-workers [184] did find that 40 mg oral prednisone for 7 days inhibited the immediate reaction to bronchial challenge with pollen antigens. Aerosol beclomethasone dipropionate given 30 min before the allergen challenge inhibited the late but not the immediate allergen-induced reaction, as has been mentioned [193].

7. Theophylline

Theophylline reduced antigen-induced bronchospasm and inhibited the rise of plasma histamine and serum neutrophil chemotactic activity [184]. The protective effect correlates with the serum theophylline level [120,185]. Theophylline slightly but significantly blocks early and late-phase reactions to allergen challenge as well as the increased airway responsiveness to methacholine that follows, according to some investigators [197], but according to others it does not inhibit allergen-induced increase in airway responsiveness to methacholine [198].

8. Other Medications

Although some investigators report no blocking effect or a minimal blocking effect of inhibitors of prostaglandin synthesis after AIC in asthmatic patients [199,200], Hamid et al. [178] reported that flurbiprofen, a cyclooxygenase inhibitor, had a mild blocking effect on the early and late-phase allergen challenge response. A thromboxane synthetase inhibitor has a small but significant blocking effect on the early response to antigen challenge (but not the late response or resultant hyperreactivity) [201]. ICI 204,291, an antileukotriene, was found to inhibit early and late-phase reactions to allergen challenge as well as the hyperreactivity to histamine that followed [202]. Inhaled furosemide effectively prevents the early response to allergen and inhibits the increase in reactivity to methacholine that follows the early response [203]. Inhaled prostaglandin E_2 (PGE_2) inhibits the early and late response to allergen as well as the allergen-induced increase in bronchial reactivity [204]. This is interesting, since PGE_2 is a substance produced in the lung itself. Gallopomil, a potent calcium channel blocker, given as an inhaled dose of 20 mg, or verapamil in another study, had a mild effect on blocking early response to allergen challenge [205,206], yet gallopomil does not seem to block the late-phase reaction or subsequent increased airway reactivity [205]. Dietary supplements with fish oil lipids can attenuate the late allergen response, but this does not appear to alter clinical severity [207].

F. Emotional and Other Factors

The influence of emotional factors, location of the responding cells, and the measurement itself are discussed above.

XI. REPRODUCIBILITY AND VARIABILITY OF THE ANTIGEN CHALLENGE

Various investigators have commented on the reproducibility of an antigen challenge. In one study that evaluated the early response to house dust mite in 28 patients, the authors believed that PD_{20} was significantly reproducible in a range of one doubling dose (twofold variation) in a 2-week interval [208]. In a group of 16 subjects with asthma, Tiffeneau [209] found that there was satisfactory repeatability in the antigen dose responsible for a given modification of spirometry. The correlation between the "threshold doses" of on different days was at $r = 0.85$, $p < 0.01$. Rosenthal and co-workers [143] performed a bronchial inhalation challenge to ragweed pollen in 13 patients during four successive days. He found that the allergen dose required to reduce SGaw by 35% demonstrated a one-decimal logarithmic variation from day to day (a tenfold variation). Frolund and colleagues [210] compared AIC performed by the standard method of tidal-volume breathing with a dosimeter method of inhalation and found good comparability between the two methods, even though the total allergen doses inhaled were different. The reproducibility of the late-phase reaction is not as good as that of the early-phase reaction.

XII. DECIDING ON THE PROPER PULMONARY FUNCTION TESTS

Ideally, the investigator should chose the pulmonary function test or tests that best reflect the site or sites of involvement. Practically, the choice of test may depend on available equipment; however, properly chosen tests with and without the use of bronchodilators by different routes of administration can provide considerable information about the site of airway obstruction and the alteration in lung mechanisms elicited by a challenge test [158,159]. It is also important to determine the history and timing of recent bronchodilator use, the baseline pulmonary function, and the nature of the disease influencing that baseline, as well as the challenge technique and the reliability of the person performing the procedure.

Erroneous conclusions may be drawn about location of response. For example, methacholine produces minimal changes in FEV_1 but produces striking changes in SGaw in hay fever subjects [211]. Although one might infer that methacholine has a preferential effect on large airways in hay fever subjects, this need not be true. Neither cited test accurately measures small-airway obstruction, and a maximum inspiration can abolish the methacholine-induced obstruction in hay fever patients (or normal subjects) yet have little effect on or even accentuate the bronchospasm in asthmatic subjects [211–213].

The timing of the measurements is important. Certain physiological events such as mediator release or irritant receptor stimulation occur quickly. If both spirometry and body plethysmography are desired, it may be technically difficult to perform all maneuvers in an ideal time. Even under the best of circumstances the test maneuvers may influence the results.

For diagnostic purposes, a pulmonary function test must be relatively sensitive and specific. Thus, the change in SGaw during a methacholine challenge may be five times greater than the change in FEV_1, but the SGaw need not, therefore, be more sensitive [211]. Any relatively large change must be considered in relation to the wide variability of the test, that is, the standard error (*t*-test). Although SGaw may appear to be more sensitive, it is also quite variable and cumbersome. One cigarette can decrease SGaw more than 35% in normal subjects, and certain asthmatic patients may have a 35% (or greater) fall with just the suggestion that they may experience bronchial obstruction [21].

Although various standardization panels have advocated a minimum acceptable change in FEV_1 of 20% and in SGaw of 35%, these levels are arbitrary. In fact, Fish and Kelly [211], using limited data on intraindividual variability of these measurements, suggested that a fall of 35% in SGaw (PD_{35} SGaw) is more likely to correspond to a 13% fall in FEV_1.

Perhaps more interesting clinically is the lack of specificity of SGaw for differentiating hay fever patients from asthmatic patients in methacholine response. Hay fever patients have a considerable overlap with asthmatics in their PD FEV_1 response [211,22]. With antigen challenge, PD FEV_1 is also less variable from day to day than PD_{35} SGaw. Even normal subjects show a substantial (50%) increase in SGaw after an aerosolized bronchodilator is given. However, in normal subjects, unlike asthmatics, simultaneously measured functional residual capacity usually remains unchanged after the bronchodilator is given. A statistically significant difference from normal is usually defined as a value that would be expected in fewer than 5% of normal subjects. The changes observed should exceed two standard deviations for repeated measures before statistical significance exists. With a gaussian distribution this represents values more than 1.65 times the coefficient of variation below or above the mean. Thus, these values should help clarify whether as true improvement or a deterioration has occurred. Ideally, coefficients of variation should be done for many measurements within a day as well as week to week.

Table 4 Suggested Minimal Changes in Pulmonary Function After Bronchial Inhalation Challenge

Pulmonary function test	Percent change from baseline
Vital Capacity	−10
FEV_1	−20
Maximal midexpiratory flow rate ($FEF_{25\text{–}75\%}$ or $Vmax_{50}$)	−25
Peak expiratory flow rate	−25
Specific airway resistance	+35 to +40
Specific airway conductance	−35 to −40
Functional residual capacity	+25

FEV_1 = forced expired volume in 1 second.

Pennock and co-workers [214] suggested that a significant change in expiratory volume or flow after administration of a bronchodilator is one standard deviation outside the limits of normal in intertrial variability. Thus, a significant change would be greater than 5% for FEV_1 and FVC, and greater than 13% for mean forced expiratory flow during the middle half of the FVC ($FEF_{25\text{–}75\%}$) in normal persons, and greater than 13% for FEV_1, greater than 11% for FVC, and greater than 23% for $FEF_{25\text{–}75\%}$ in obstructed persons. Mean increases in SGaw, although relatively large, are associated with wide variability, so that the statistical significance of SGaw response may be less than that of other tests of forced expiration such as FEV_1.

My recommendations (Table 4) for criteria for a significant change in pulmonary function are based on many of the above considerations. Hruby and Butler [215] concluded that FEV_1 is superior to other commonly used tests of airway obstruction for bronchodilator effect. It has minimum variability compared with plethysmography and $FEF_{25\text{–}75\%}$. The FEV_1, even with its limitations, should be included as one of the measurements of a bronchoconstrictor response to agents such as antigens, methacholine, and histamine. Other pulmonary function measurements can be added, depending on their availability and the need for other information about the bronchoconstrictive response. Chapter 16 should be consulted for further details.

XIII. BRONCHIAL INHALATION CHALLENGE WITH NEUTRAL SUBSTANCES

It is important that the vehicle or diluent in which the allergenic substance is dissolved does not cause bronchial obstruction. If it does, the subject must be tested on another day. The phenomenon of diluent bronchoconstriction was acknowledged by the panel from the Asthma and Allergic Disease Centers of the National Institutes of Health. We advocated excluding from the standardized bronchial challenge persons who had a greater-than-10% fall in FEV_1 ten minutes following inhalation of five breaths of diluent [216]. Mechanisms behind such a response have not been thoroughly studied. The method of delivery, pH, and osmolarity may be important. Preservatives in a diluent, such as glycerol, can cause bronchial obstruction [217].

XIV. INTERPRETATION AND EXPRESSION OF RESULTS

The most popular way of expressing data on bronchoconstrictive substances, including antigens, is calculation of cumulative doses. This procedure assumes that the dose generated is retained and accumulated. In reality this is not true, since part of the generated dose is exhaled, lost in equipment, metabolized, or removed from the site of distribution. Although the clinical effect of an antigen inhalation and, to a small degree, a methacholine challenge is cumulative, histamine inhalations appear to have a short-lived, noncumulative effect. Nevertheless, accumulation of doses is now the most accepted way of expressing data (Table 5).

Patients should be asymptomatic, and medication should be withheld. Baseline FEV_1 should be 80% or more of the previously observed highest value, or approximately 75% or more of the predicted value. A diluent (e.g., saline) should

Table 5 Cumulative Doses for Bronchial Inhalation Challenge with Allergen at Five Breaths per Dilution

Allergen concentration (w/v)[a]	Inhalation units/5 breaths[b]	Cumulative units/5 breaths
1:1,000,000	0.025	0.025
1:500,000	0.05	0.075
1:100,000	0.25	0.325
1:50,000	0.5	0.825
1:10,000	2.5	3.32
1:5,000	5.0	8.32
1:1,000	25.0	33.3
1:500	50.0	83.3
1:100	250.0	300.3

[a]At concentrations of antigens of 1:100 and above, the clinical meaning is unclear.

[b]One inhalation unit = one breath 1:500 w/v dilution.

w/v = weight per volume.

be given first. The diluent value is the control, and if the FEV_1 is not reduced 10% from the baseline, the patient enters the study. Five successive breaths of the bronchoconstrictive substance are given (Table 5). A positive result is a 3-min sustained fall in FEV_1 of 20% or more from the control FEV_1 value. If the test result is negative, five breaths of the next dilution are given; if the result is borderline, fewer than five breaths of the next dilution may be given.

The results are expressed by a dose–response curve using a semilogarithmic plot (Fig. 1). On the logarithmic abscissa the cumulative dose is plotted, and on the linearly expressed ordinate the response as measured by percent of the diluent control aerosol is plotted. A line of best fit is determined, preferably using parabolic, logarithmic, or exponent regression equations. The cumulative dose at which lung function has deteriorated by at least two standard deviations below control values is considered the PD. When asthmatics are compared with normal subjects, two responses below the PD should be recorded to assure that the observed reaction is sustained. When the challenge has provoked a mean reduction of two standard deviations in lung function, the next dose (if given) should be small, that is, no larger than the last dose. This will avoid excessive deteriorations in lung function and distressing symptoms. The antigen (methacholine or hista-

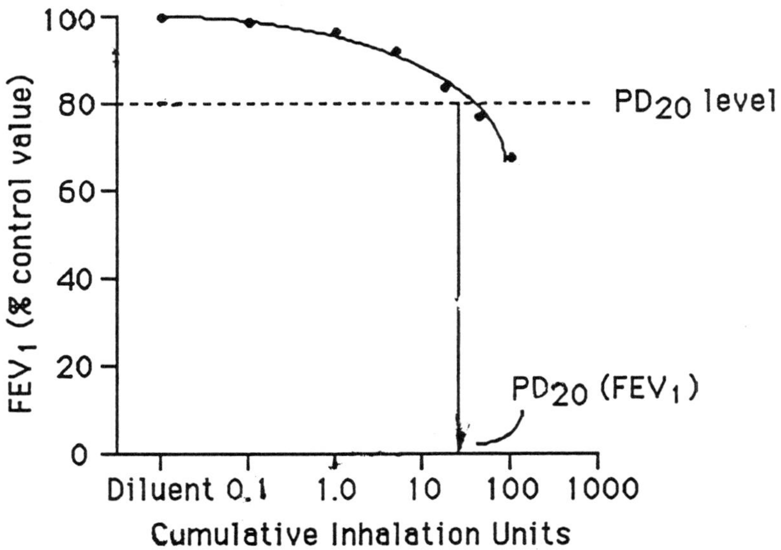

Figure 1 Cumulative dose of a bronchoconstrictive agent such as allergen (abscissa) vs. response expressed as percent of diluent control aerosol (ordinate). The PD_{20} (FEV_1) is the cumulative dose of bronchoconstrictor that corresponds to a 20% fall in forced expired volume in 1 second.

mine) concentration multiplied by the number of breaths (usually five) equals the accumulated dose for each exposure, unless fewer breaths have been used.

Ryan et al. [218] calculated the percent fall in FEV_1 after a bronchoconstrictive substance:

$$\frac{(\text{Lowest FEV}_1 \text{ after saline}) - (\text{Lowest FEV}_1 \text{ after allergen}) \times 100}{\text{Lowest FEV}_1 \text{ after saline}}$$
$$= \text{the fall in FEV}_1$$

Their PD_{20} is obtained from the log dose–response curve by linear interpolation of the last two points. The abscissa is not expressed in cumulative units, and the ordinate plots percent fall in FEV_1 to demonstrate sensitivity and reactivity. Sensitivity is determined by the PD itself, while reactivity is determined by the slope [219]. Abbreviated protocols, as mentioned by Chatham and associates [220], such as using only two or three doses of a bronchoconstrictive agent, can save time but can be more dangerous. In addition, results may not be completely reproducible, since the effect of methacholine or antigens accumulates. Although the dose–response plot is the most common way to express data, other methods have been advocated. The area under the dose–response curve may be more reliable in defining the degree of sensitivity; it is calculated by integrating the best-fit parabola of, for example, the allergen dose–response curve.

REFERENCES

1. Busse, W. W., Respiratory infections: their role in airway responsiveness and the pathogenesis of asthma, *J. Allergy Clin. Immunol.*, *85*, 671–688 (1990).
2. Lee, T. H., Austen, K. F., Leitch, A. G., Israel, E., Robinson, D. R., Lewis, R. A., Corey, E. J., and Drason, J. M., The effects of a fish oil enriched diet on pulmonary mechanics during anaphylaxis, *Am. Rev. Respir. Dis.*, *132*, 1204–1209 (1985).
3. Turkeltaub, P. C., The allergy unit—clinical relevance: issues in allergen standardization, in *Allergen Immunotherapy* (F. Lockey and S. C. Bukanz, eds.), Marcel Dekker, New York, 1991.
4. Gleich, G. J., Larson, J. B., Jones, R. T., and Baer, H., Measurement of the potency of allergy extracts by their inhibitory capacity in the radioallergosorbent test, *J. Allergy Clin. Immunol.*, *53*, 158 (1974).
5. Baer, H., Godfrey, H., Maloney, C. J., Norman, P. S., and Lichtenstein, L. M., The potency and antigen E content of commercially prepared ragweed extracts, *J. Allergy*, *45*, 347 (1970).
6. Jaeger, D., Kleinhans, D., Czuppon, A. B., and Baur, X., Latex-specific proteins causing immediate-type cutaneous, nasal, bronchial, and systemic reactions, *J. Allergy Clin. Immunol.*, *89*, 759–768 (1992).
7. Suphioglu, C., Singh, M. B., Taylor, P., Bellomo, R., et al., Mechanism of grass-pollen-induced asthma, *Lancet*, *339*, 569–572 (1992).
8. Nelson, H. S., The effect of preservatives and dilution on the deterioration of

Russian thistle (*Salsola perifer*), a pollen extract, *J. Allergy Clin. Immunol.*, *63*, 417 (1979).
9. Norman, P. S., and Marsh, D. G., Human serum albumin and Tween 80 as stabilizers of allergen solutions, *J. Allergy Clin. Immunol.*, *62*, 314 (1978).
10. Cockcroft, D. W., Bronchial inhalation tests II, *Ann. Allergy*, *59*, 89–99 (1987).
11. Aas, K., *The Bronchial Provocation Test*, Charles C. Thomas, Springfield, Illinois, 1975.
12. Spector, S. L., Bronchial provocation tests, in *Bronchial Asthma: Mechanisms and Therapeutics*, 2nd Ed. (E. B. Weiss, M. S. Segal, and M. Stein, eds.), Little, Brown, and Company, Boston, 1985, pp. 360–379.
13. Spector, S. L., and Farr, R. S., Bronchial inhalation procedures in asthmatics, *Med. Clin. North Am.*, *58*, 71–84 (1974).
14. Patterson, R., Suszko, I. M., and Zeiss, C. R., Jr., Reactions of primate respiratory mast cells, *J. Allergy Clin. Immunol.*, *50*, 7 (1972).
15. Patterson, R., Talbot, C. H., and Brandfonbrener, M., The use of IgE-mediated responses as a pharmacologic test system: the effect of disodium cromoglycate in respiratory and cutaneous reactions and on the electrocardiograms of rhesus monkeys, *Int. Arch. Allergy*, *41*, 592 (1971).
16. May, C. D., and Williams, C. S., Further studies concerning the fluctuating insensitivity of peripheral leukocytes to unrelated allergens and the meaning of nonspecific "desensitization," *Clin. Allergy*, *3*, 319 (1973).
17. Huggins, K. G., and Brostoff, J., Local production of specific IgE antibodies in allergic rhinitis patients with negative skin tests, *Lancet*, *2*, 148 (1975).
18. Leonardi, A., Fregona, I. A., Gismondi, M., Daniotti, E., et al., Correlation between conjunctival provocation test and systemic allergometric tests in allergic conjunctivitis, *Eye*, 760–764 (1990).
19. Fish, J. D., Rosenthal, R. R., Lichtenstein, L. M., et al., Airway responses to methacholine in allergic and nonallergic subjects, *Am. Rev. Respir. Dis.*, *113*, 579 (1976).
20. Bruce, C. A., Rosenthal, R. R., Lichtenstein, L. M., et al., Quantitative inhalation bronchial challenge in ragweed hay fever patients. A comparison with ragweed-allergic asthmatics, *J. Allergy Clin. Immunol.*, *56*, 331 (1975).
21. Spector, S. L., Luparello, T. J., Kopetzky, M. T., et al., Response of asthmatics to methacholine challenges and suggestion, *Am. Rev. Respir. Dis.*, *113*, 43–50 (1976).
22. Townley, R. G., Dennis, M., and Itkin, I. H., Comparative action of acetyl-beta-methacholine, histamine, and pollen antigens in subjects with hay fever and patients with bronchial asthma, *J. Allergy*, *36*, 121 (1965).
23. Cavanaugh, M. J., Bronsky, E. A., and Buckley, J. M., Clinical value of bronchial provocation testing in childhood asthma, *J. Allergy Clin. Immunol.*, 59–41 (1977).
24. Spector, S. L., and Farr, R. S., Bronchial provocation tests, in *Bronchial asthma: mechanisms and therapeutics* (E. B. Weiss and M. S. Segal, eds.), Little, Brown, and Company, Boston, 1976, pp. 639–647.
25. Killian, D., Cockcroft, D. W., Hargreave, F. E., et al., Factors in allergen-induced asthma: relevance of the intensity of the airways, allergic reaction, and nonspecific bronchial reactivity, *Clin. Allergy*, *6*, 219 (1976).

26. Cockcroft, D. W., Ruffin, R. E., Frith, P. A., et al., Determinants of allergen-induced asthma: Dose of allergen, circulating IgE antibody concentration, and bronchial responsiveness to inhaled histamine, *Am. Rev. Respir. Dis.*, *120*, 1053 (1979).
27. Spector, S. L., and Farr, R. S., Bronchial inhalation challenge with antigen, *J. Allergy Clin. Immunol.*, *64*, 580–586 (1979).
28. Cockcroft, D. W., Ruffin, R. E., Frith, P. A., et al., Determinants of allergen induced asthma: dose of allergen, circulating IgE antibody concentration, and bronchial responsiveness to inhaled histamine, *Am. Rev. Respir. Dis.*, *120*, 1053 (1979).
29. Nathan, R. A., Kinsman, R. A., Spector, S. L., et al., Relationship between airways response to allergens and nonspecific bronchial reactivity, *J. Allergy Clin. Immunol.*, *63*, 150 (1979).
30. Hill, D. J., Shelton, M. J., and Osking, C. S., Predicting the results of allergen bronchial challenge by simple clinical methods, *Clin. Allergy*, *12*, 195 (1982).
31. Bhat, K. N., Arroyave, C. M., Manney, S. M., Jr., et al., Plasma histamine changes during provoked bronchospasm in asthmatic patients, *J. Allergy Clin. Immunol.*, *58*, 647 (1976).
32. Deal, E. C., Jr., Wassermann, S. I., Soder, N. A., et al., Evaluation of role played by mediators of immediate hypersensitivity in exercise-induced asthma, *J. Clin. Invest.*, *65*, 659 (1980).
33. Atkins, P. C., Norman, M., and Zweiman, B., Antigen-induced neutrophil chemotactic activity during immediate hypersensitivity reactions in humans, *Ann. Intern. Med.*, *86*, 415 (1977).
34. Ahmed, T., et al., Abnormal mucociliary transport in allergic patients with antigen-induced bronchospasm: role of slow reacting substance of anaphylaxis, *Am. Rev. Respir. Dis.*, *124*, 110 (1981).
35. Marom, Z., et al., Slow reacting substances, leukotrienes C_4 and D_4 increase the release of mucus from human airways in vitro, *Am. Rev. Respir. Dis.*, *126*, 449 (1982).
36. Kumlin, M., Dahlen, B., Bjorck, T., Zetterstrom, O., et al., Urinary excretion of leukotriene E4 and 11-dihydro-thromboxane B2 in response to bronchial provocations with allergen, *Am. Rev. Respir. Dis.*, *146*, 96–103 (1992).
37. Hsieh, K. H., Effects of PAF antagonist, BN52021, on the PAF-, methacholine-, and allergen-induced bronchoconstriction in asthmatic children, *Chest*, *99*, 877–882 (1991).
38. Maestrelli, P., Boschetto, P., Zocca, E., Crescioli, S., et al., Venous blood platelets decrease during allergen-induced asthmatic reactions, *Clin. Exp. Allergy*, *20*, 267–372 (1990).
39. Hemmendinger, S., Pauli, G., Tenabene, A., Pujol, J. L., et al., Platelet function: aggregation by PAF or sequestration in lung is not modified during immediate or late allergen-induced bronchospasm in man, *J. Allergy Clin. Immunol.*, *83*, 990–996 (1989).
40. Wenzel, S. E., Westcott, J. Y., and Larsen, G. L., Bronchoalveolar lavage fluid mediator levels five minutes after allergen challenge in atopic subjects with asthma:

relationship to the development of late asthmatic responses, *J. Allergy Clin. Immunol.*, *87*, 540–548 (1991).
41. Wenzel, S. E., Larson, G. L., Johnston, K., Voelkel, N. F., and Westcott, J. Y., Elevated levels of leukotriene C4 in bronchoalveolar lavage fluid from atopic asthmatics after endobronchial allergen challenge, *Am. Rev. Respir. Dis.*, *142*, 112–119 (1990).
42. Schwartz, L. B., Metcalfe, D. D., Miller, J. S., et al., Tryptase levels as an indicator of mast cell activation in systemic anaphylaxis and mastocytosis, *N. Engl. J. Med.*, *316*, 1622 (1987).
43. Calhoun, W. J., Reed, H. E., Moest, D. R., and Stevens, C. A., Enhanced superoxide production by alveolar macrophages and airspace cells, airway inflammation, and alveolar macrophage density changes after segmental antigen bronchoprovocation in allergic subjects, *Am. Rev. Respir. Dis.*, *145*, 317–325 (1992).
44. Diaz, P., Gonzalez, M. C., Galleguillos, F. R., Ancic, P., et al., Leukocytes and mediators in bronchoalveolar lavage during allergen-induced late-phase asthmatic reactions, *Am. Rev. Respir. Dis.*, *139*, 1383–1389 (1989).
45. Mengelers, H. J., Maikoe, T., Hooibrink, B., Kuypers, T. W., et al., Down modulation of L-Selectin expression on eosinophils recovered from bronchoalveolar lavage fluid after allergen provocation, *Clin. Exp. Allergy*, *23*, 196–204 (1993).
46. Dorsch, W., et al., Mediator studies in skin blister fluid from patients with dual skin reactions after intradermal allergen injection, *J. Allergy Clin. Immunol.*, *70*, 236 (1982).
47. Christiansen, S. C., Proud, D., Sarnoff, R. B., Juergens, U., et al., Elevation of tissue kallikrein and kinin in the airways of asthmatic subjects after endobronchial allergen challenge, *Am. Rev. Respir. Dis.*, *145*, 900–905 (1992).
48. Knauer, K. A., Lichtenstein, L. M., Adkinson, N. F., Jr., et al., Platelet activation during antigen induced airway reactions in asthmatic subjects, *N. Engl. J. Med.*, *23*, 1404 (1981).
49. Arroyave, C. M., Stevenson, D. D., Vaughan, J. H., et al., Plasma complement challenges during bronchospasm provoked in asthmatic patients, *Clin. Allergy*, *7*, 173 (1977).
50. Pryjma, J., et al., Decrease of complement hemolytic activity after an allergen house-dust bronchial-provocation test, *J. Allergy Clin. Immunol.*, *70*, 306 (1982).
51. Castro, F. F., Schmitz-Schumann, M., Rother, U., and Kirschfink, M., Complement activation by house dust: reduced reactivity of serum complement in patients with bronchial asthma, *Int. Arch. Allergy Appl. Immunol.*, *96*, 305–310 (1991).
52. Deal, E. C., Jr., Wasserman, S. I., Soter, N. A., et al., Evaluation of role played by mediators of immediate hypersensitivity in exercise-induced asthma, *J. Clin. Invest.*, *65*, 659 (1980).
53. Weiler-Ravell, D., and Godfrey, S., Do exercise- and antigen-induced asthma utilize the same pathways? *J. Allergy Clin. Immunol.*, *67*, 391 (1981).
54. Boulet, L. P., Corbeil, F., and Turcotte, H., Influence of a single antigenic challenge on the pattern of airway response to exercise in asthma, *Ann. Allergy*, *68*, 363–370 (1992).
55. Miller, M. M., and Patterson, R., Differential airway reactivity to carbachol and

physostigmine sulfate in rhesus monkeys with and without reagin-mediated respiratory responses, *Int. Arch. Allergy Appl. Immunol.*, *53*, 349 (1977).

56. Miller, M. M., Fish, J. E., and Patterson, R., Methacholine and physostigmine airway reactivity in asthmatic and nonasthmatic subjects, *J. Allergy Clin. Immunol.*, *60*, 116 (1977).
57. Perper, R. J., Sanda, M., and Lichtenstein, L. M., The relationship of in vitro and in vivo allergen histamine release: inhibition in primates by cAMP active agents, *Int. Arch. Allergy Appl. Immunol.*, *43*, 837 (1972).
58. Imbeau, S. A., Harruff, R., Hirscher, M., and Reed, C. E., Terbutaline's effects on the allergy skin test, *J. Allergy Clin. Immunol.*, *62*, 193 (1978).
59. Chipps, B. E., Teet, K. C., Saunders, J. P., et al., The effects of oral theophylline and terbutaline on skin tests and histamine release (abstr.), *J. Allergy Clin. Immunol.*, *61*, 171 (1978).
60. Spector, S. L., Effect of a selective β_2 adrenergic agonist and theophylline on skin test reactivity and cardiovascular parameters, *J. Allergy Clin. Immunol.*, *64*, 23 (1979).
61. Muttari, A., Ahonen, A., Kellomaki, L., et al., The effect of ICI 74,917 on asthma and bronchial provocation tests, *Clin. Allergy*, *8*, 281 (1978).
62. Tiffeneau, R., Amples variations du degré de l'allergie pulmonaire produites par administration d'allergènes par voie respiratoire, *Int. Arch. Allergy*, *17*, 193 (1960).
63. Herxheimer, H., Bronchial hypersensitization and hyposensitization in man, *Int. Arch. Allergy*, *2*, 40 (1951).
64. Moshkevich, V. S., Local immunotherapy for chronic respiratory allergic pathology with allergen aerosols. II. Treatment of bronchial asthma, *Allergol. Immunopathol.*, *13*, 317–321 (1985).
65. Moshkevich, V. S., Tsarevskaya, L. A., Nurpeisov, T. N., et al., Local immunotherapy in chronic allergic rhinitis and bronchial asthma with allergen aerosols. III. Dynamics of some sensitization, *Allergol. Immunopathol.*, *14*, 277–285 (1986).
66. Assem, E. S. K., and McAllen, M. D., Changes in challenge tests following hyposensitization with mite extract, *Clin. Allergy*, *3*, 161 (1973).
67. Price, J. F., Warner, J. O., Hey, E. N., et al., A controlled trial of hyposensitization with absorbed tyrosine Dermatophagoides pteronyssinus antigen in childhood asthma: in vivo aspects, *Clin. Allergy*, *14*, 209–219 (1984).
68. Ohman, J. L., Findlay, S. R., and Leitermann, K. M., Immunotherapy in cat-induced asthma: double-blind trial with evaluation of in vivo and in vitro responses, *J. Allergy Clin. Immunol.*, *74*, 230–239 (1984).
69. Olive, J. R., Jr., and Hyatt, R. E., Maximal expiratory flow and total respiratory resistance during induced bronchoconstriction in asthmatic subjects, *Am. Rev. Respir. Dis.*, *106*, 366 (1972).
70. Ahmed, T., Fernandez, R. J., and Wanner, A., Airway responses to antigen challenge and allergic rhinitis and allergic asthma, *J. Allergy Clin. Immunol.*, *67*, 135 (1981).
71. Olgiati, R., Birch, S., Rao, A., et al., Differential effects of methacholine and antigen challenge on gas exchange in allergic subjects, *J. Allergy Clin. Immunol.*, *67*, 325 (1981).

72. Dorsch, W., Late phase reactions, in *Highlights in Asthmology* (F. B. Michael, J. Bousquet, and P. Goddard, eds.), Springer-Verlag, Berlin, 1987, p. 237.
73. Pelikan, Z., Pelikan-Filipek, M., and Remeijer, L., Effects of disodium chromoglycate and beclomethasone dipropionate on the asthmatic response to allergen challenge: II. Late response (LAR), *Ann. Allergy*, *60*, 217–225 (1988).
74. Lemanske, R. F., Jr., and Kaliner, M., Late phase IgE mediated reactions, *J. Clin. Immunol.*, *8*, 1–13 (1988).
75. Frlund, L., Madsen, F., Scharling, B., Heinig, J. H., and Svendsen, U. G., Bronchial allergen challenge: dose versus concentration, *Clin. Exp. Allergy*, *22*, 219–225 (1992).
76. Lai, C. K., Twentyman, O. P., and Holgate, S. T., The effect of an increase in inhaled allergen dose after rimiterol hydrobromide on the occurrence and magnitude of the late asthmatic response and the associated change in nonspecific bronchial responsiveness, *Am. Rev. Respir. Dis.*, *140*, 917–923 (1989).
77. Machado, L., and St. Alenheim, G., Factors influencing the occurrence of late bronchial reactions after allergen challenge, *Allergy*, *45*, 268–274 (1990).
78. Warner, J. O., Price, J. F., Soothill, J. F., et al., Controlled trial of hyposensitization to *Dermatophagoides pteronyssinus* in children with asthma, *Lancet*, *2*, 912–915 (1978).
79. Robertson, D., Kerigan, A. T., Hargeave, F. E., et al., Late asthmatic responses induced by ragweed pollen allergen, *J. Allergy Clin. Immunol.*, *54*, 244 (1974).
80. Paggiaro, P. L., and Chan-Yeung, M., Pattern of specific airway response in asthma due to Western red cedar (Thuja plicata): relationship with length of exposure and lung function measurements, *Clin. Allergy*, *17*, 333–339 (1987).
81. Paggiaro, P. L., Innocenti, A., Bacci, E., et al., Specific bronchial reactivity to toluene diisocyanate (TDI): relationship with baseline clinical findings, *Thorax*, *41*, 279–282 (1986).
82. O'Brien, M., Harries, M. G., Berg, P. S., et al., Toluene diisocyanate induced asthma: I. Reaction to TDI, MDI, HDI, and histamine, *Clin. Allergy*, *9*, 1–6 (1979).
83. Booij-Noord, H., DeVries, K., Sluiter, H. J., et al., Late bronchial obstructive reaction to experimental inhalation of house dust extract, *Clin. Allergy*, *2*, 43–61 (1972).
84. Kim, C.-J., The bronchial provocation test: its clinical evaluation and the course of induced asthma, *J. Allergy*, *36*, 353–361 (1965).
85. Bronsky, E. A., and Ellis, E. F., Inhalation bronchial challenge testing in asthmatic children, *Ped. Clin. North Am.*, *16*, 85 (1969).
86. Bundgaard, A., and Boudet, L., Reproducibility of the late asthmatic response, *Eur. J. Respir. Dis.*, *68*, 41–43 (1986).
87. Ihre, E. W., Axelsson, I. G. K., and Zetterstrom, O., Late asthmatic reactions and bronchial variability after challenge with low doses of allergen, *Clin. Allergy*, *18*, 557–567 (1988).
88. Atkins, P. C., Martin, G. L., Yost, R., et al., Late onset reactions in humans: correlation between skin and bronchial reactivity, *Ann. Allergy*, *60*, 27–30 (1988).
89. Cockcroft, D. W., Murdock, K. Y., Kirby, J., et al., Prediction of airway responsive-

ness to allergen from skin sensitivity to allergen and airway responsiveness to histamine, *Am. Rev. Respir. Dis.*, *135*, 264–267 (1987).
90. Cockcroft, D. W., Ruffin, R. E., Dolovich, J., and Hargreave, F. E., Allergen induced increase in nonallergic bronchial reactivity, *Clin. Allergy*, *7*, 503–513 (1977).
91. Cartier, A., Thompson, N. C., Frith, P. A., et al., Allergen induced increase in bronchial responsiveness to histamines: relationship to the late asthmatic response and the change in airway caliber, *J. Allergy Clin. Immunol.*, *70*, 170–172 (1982).
92. Boulet, L. P., Cartier, A., Thompson, N. C., et al., Asthma and increases in nonallergic bronchial responsiveness from seasonal pollen exposure, *J. Allergy Clin. Immunol.*, *71*, 399–406 (1983).
93. Machado, L., Increased bronchial hypersensitivity after early and late bronchial reactions provoked by allergen inhalation, *Allergy*, *40*, 580–585 (1985).
94. Violante, B., Pellegrino, R., Crimi, E,. and Brusasco, V., Increase in airway responsiveness and effect of deep inhalation on airway caliber in allergen-induced asthma—relationship to the late-phase response, *Am. Rev. Respir. Dis.*, *46*, 127–131 (1992).
95. Cockcroft, D. W., Murdock, K. Y., Changes in bronchial responsiveness to histamine at intervals after allergen challenge, *Thorax*, *42*, 302–308 (1987).
96. Durham, S. R., Carol, M., Lee, T. H., et al., Mechanisms of early and late asthmatic reactions, in *Proceedings XII International Congress of Allergology and Clinical Immunology* (C. E. Reed, ed.), CV Mosby, St. Louis, 1986, pp. 229–236.
97. Platts-Mills, T. A., Mitchell, E. B., Nock, P., et al., Reduction of bronchial hyperreactivity during prolonged allergen avoidance, *Lancet*, *2*, 675–678 (1982).
98. Metzger, W. J., Donnelly, A., and Richerson, H. B., Modification of late asthmatic responses during immunotherapy for Alternaria-induced asthma (abstr.), *J. Allergy Clin. Immunol.*, *74*, 121A (1983).
99. Murray, A. B., Furguson, A. C., and Morrison, B. J., Nonallergic hyperreactivity in asthmatic children decreases with age and increases with mite immunotherapy, *Ann. Allergy*, *54*, 541–544 (1985).
100. Nagy, L., Lee, T. H., and Kay, A. B., Neutrophil chemotactic factor activity in antigen induced late asthmatic reactions, *N. Engl. J. Med.*, *306*, 497–501 (1982).
101. Howarth, P. H., Durham, S. R., Kay, A. B., and Holgate, S. T., The relationship between mast cell mediator release and bronchial reactivity in allergic asthma, *J. Allergy Clin. Immunol.*, *80*, 703–711 (1987).
102. Murray, J. J., Tonnel, A. B., Brash, A. R., et al., Release of prostaglandin D_2 into human airways during acute antigen challenge, *N. Engl. J. Med.*, *315*, 800–804 (1986).
103. Goetzl, E. J., and Pickett, W. C., Novel structural determinants of the human neutrophil chemotactic activity of leukotriene, *Br. J. Exp. Med.*, *153*, 482–487 (1981).
104. Abraham, W. M., The importance of lipoxygenase products of arachidonic acid in allergen-induced late responses, *Am. Rev. Respir. Dis.*, *135*, S49–S53 (1987).
105. Nakamura, T., Morita, Y., Kuriyama, M., et al., Platelet activating factor in late asthmatic response, *Int. Arch. Allergy Appl. Immunol.*, *82*, 57–61 (1987).

106. Ito, K., Kudo, K., Okudaira, H., et al., IgG1 antibodies to house dust mite (*Dermatophagoides farinae*) and late asthmatic response, *Int. Arch. Allergy Appl. Immunol.*, *82*, 57–61 (1987).
107. Gonzalez, M. C., Diaz, P., Galleguillos, F. R., et al., Allergen induced recruitment of bronchoalveolar helper (OKT_4) and suppressor (OKT_8) T cells in asthma, *Am. Rev. Respir. Dis.*, *136*, 600–604 (1987).
108. Metzger, W. J., Zavala, D., Richerson, H. B., et al., Local allergen challenge and bronchoalveolar lavage of allergic asthmatic lungs: description of the model and local airway inflammation, *Am. Rev. Respir. Dis.*, *135*, 433–449 (1987).
109. Gratziou, C., Carroll, M., Walls, A., Howarth, P. H., and Holgate, S. T., Early changes in T lymphocytes recovered by bronchoalveolar lavage after local allergen challenge of asthmatic airways, *Am. Rev. Respir. Dis.*, *145*, 1259–1264 (1992).
110. Rossi, G. A., Crimi, E., Lantero, S., Gianiorio, P., et al., Late-phase asthmatic reaction to inhaled allergen is associated with early recruitment of eosinophils in the airways, *Am. Rev. Respir. Dis.*, *144*, 379–383 (1991).
111. Cookson, W. O., Craddock, C. F., Benson, M. K., and Durham, S. R., Falls in peripheral eosinophil counts parallel the late asthmatic response, *Am. Rev. Respir. Dis.*, *139*, 458–462 (1989).
112. Frick, W. E., Sedgwick, J. B., and Busse, W. W., The appearance of hypodense eosinophils in antigen-dependent late-phase asthma, *Am. Rev. Respir. Dis.*, *139*, 1401–1406 (1989).
113. Delehunt, J. C., Yerger, L., Ahmed, T., et al., Inhibition of antigen-induced bronchoconstriction by methylprednisolone succinate, *J. Allergy Clin. Immunol.*, *73*, 479–483 (1984).
114. Martin, G. L., Atkins, P. C., Dunsky, E. H., et al., The effects of theophylline, terbutaline, and prednisone on antigen-induced bronchospasm and mediator release, *J. Allergy Clin. Immunol.*, *66*, 204–212 (1980).
115. Boschetto, P., Fabbri, L. M., Zocca, E., et al., Prednisone inhibits late asthmatic reactions and airway inflammation induced by toluene diisocyanate in sensitized subjects, *J. Allergy Clin. Immunol.*, *80*, 261–267 (1987).
116. Burge, P. S., Efthimou, J., Turner-Warwick, M., et al., Double blind trials of inhaled beclomethasone dipropionate and fluocortin butyl ester in allergen induced immediate and late asthmatic reactions, *Clin. Allergy*, *12*, 523–531 (1982).
117. Mattoli, S., Foresi, A., Corbo, G. M., et al., The effects of two doses of cromolyn on allergen-induced asthmatic response and increased responsiveness, *J. Allergy Clin. Immunol.*, *79*, 747–754 (1987).
118. Pelikan, Z., Pelikan-Filipek, M., Shoemaker, M. C., et al., Effects of disodium cromoglycate and beclomethasone dipropionate on the asthma response to allergen challenge. I. Immediate response (IAR), *Ann. Allergy*, *60*, 211–216 (1988).
119. Mapp, C., Boschetto, P., Dal Vecchio, L., et al., Protective effect of antiasthma drugs on late asthmatic reactions and increased airway responsiveness induced by toluene diisocyanate in sensitized subjects, *Am. Rev. Respir. Dis.*, *136*, 1403–1407 (1987).
120. Pauwels, R., Van Renterghem, D., Van Der Straeten, M., et al., The effect of

theophylline and enprofylline on allergen-induced bronchoconstriction, *J. Allergy Clin. Immunol.*, *76*, 583–590 (1985).

121. Pauwels, R., The effects of theophylline on airway inflammation, *Chest*, *92*, 32A–37S (1987).
122. Bonifazi, F., Antonicelli, L., Pieretti, C., et al., Double-blind, cross-over trial to compare the activity of nedocromil sodium and placebo in antigen challenge, *Allergol. Immunopathol.*, *15*, 151–153 (1987).
123. Abraham, W. M., Stevenson, J. S., Champman, G. A., et al., The effect of nedocromil sodium and cromolyn sodium on antigen-induced responses in allergic sheep in vivo and in vitro, *Chest*, *92*, 913–917 (1987).
124. Howarth, P. H., Durham, S. R., Lee, T. H., et al., Influence of albuterol, cromolyn sodium, and ipratropium bromide on the airway and circulating mediator responses to allergen bronchial provocation in asthma, *Am. Rev. Respir. Dis.*, *132*, 986–992 (1985).
125. Guinot, P., Brambilla, C., Duchier, J., et al., Effect of BN52063, a specific PAF acether antagonist, on bronchial provocation tests to allergens in asthmatic patients: a preliminary study, *Prostaglandins*, *34*, 723–731 (1987).
126. Fairfax, A. J., Inhibition of the late asthmatic response to house dust mite by nonsteroidal anti-inflammatory drugs, *Prostaglandins Leukotrienes Med.*, *8*, 239–248 (1982).
127. Joubert, J. R., Sheppard, E., Mouton, W., et al., Nonsteroidal anti-inflammatory drugs in asthma: dangerous or useful therapy? *Allergy*, *40*, 202–207 (1985).
128. Smith, R. M., and Richerson, H. B., A longitudinal study of airway responsiveness to methacholine in ragweed hay-fever patients (abstr.), *Am. Rev. Respir. Dis.*, *137*, 284 (1988).
129. Machado, L., Increased bronchial hypersensitivity after early and late bronchial reactions provoked by allergen inhalation, *Allergy*, *40*, 580–585 (1985).
130. Fairfax, A. J., Inhibition of the late asthmatic response to house dust mite by nonsteroidal anti-inflammatory drugs, *Prostaglandins Leukotrienes Med.*, *8*, 239–248 (1982).
131. Joubert, J. R., Shephard, E., Mouton, W., et al., Non-steroidal anti-inflammatory drugs in asthma: Dangerous or useful therapy? *Allergy*, *40*, 202–207 (1985).
132. Lee, T. H., Austen, K. F., Leitch, A. G., Israel, E., Robinson, D. R., Lewis, R. A., Corey, E. J., and Drazen, J. M. L., The effects of a fish-oil enriched diet on pulmonary mechanics during anaphylaxis, *Am. Rev. Respir. Dis.*, *132*, 1204–1209 (1985).
133. Horton, D. G., et al., Bronchoconstrictive suggestion in asthma: a role for airways, hyperreactivity, and emotions, *Am. Rev. Respir. Dis.*, *117*, 1029 (1978).
134. Melillo, G., Aas, K., Cartier, A., Davies, R. J., Debelic, M., Dreborg, S., Kerrebijn K. F., Lassen, A., Mendes, J. P., Rizzo, A., Rosenthal, R. R., Teishi, S., and Corsico, R., Guidelines for the standardization of bronchial provocation tests with allergens, *Allergy*, *46*, 321–329 (1991).
135. Dahl, R., and Johansson, S. A., The importance of duration of treatment with inhaled budesonide on immediate and late reactions, *Eur. J. Respir. Dis.*, *63*(122), 82–83 (1982).

136. Cockcroft, D. W., and Murdock, K. Y., Comparative effects of inhaled salbutamol, sodium chromoglycate, and beclomethosone dipropionate on allergen induced early asthmatic responses, late asthmatic responses, and increased bronchial responsiveness to histamine, *J. Allergy Clin. Immunol.*, *79*, 734–740 (1987).
137. Herxheimer, H., Bronchial hypersensitization and hyposensitization in man, *Int. Arch. Allergy*, *2*, 40 (1951).
138. Tiffeneau, R., Amples variations du degré de l'allergie pulmonaire produites par administration d'allergènes par voie respiratoire, *Int. Arch. Allergy*, *17*, 193 (1960).
139. Connell, J. T., Quantitative intranasal pollen challenges III. The priming effect on allergic rhinitis, *J. Allergy*, *43*, 33 (1969).
140. Zwick, H., Popp, W., Budik, G., Wanke, T., and Rauscher, H., Increased sensitization to aeroallergens in competitive swimmers, *Lung*, *168*, 111–115 (1990).
141. Molfino, M. A., Wright, S. C., Katz, I., Tarlo, S., et al., Effect of low concentrations of ozone on inhaled allergen responses in asthmatic subjects, *Lancet*, *338*, 199–203 (1991).
142. Young, S., Le Souef, P. N., Geelhoed, G. C., Stick, S. M., et al., The influence of a family history of asthma and parental smoking on airway responsiveness in early infancy, *N. Engl. J. Med.*, *324*, 1168–1173 (1991).
143. Rosenthal, R. R., Norman, P. S., and Summer, W. R., Bronchoprovocation: effect on priming and desensitization phenomenon in the lung, *J. Allergy Clin. Immunol.*, *56*, 338 (1975).
144. Kelly, J. F., Fish, J. E., and Peterman, V. I., Effect of environmental exposure on bronchial sensitivity to antigen, *Int. Arch. Allergy Appl. Immunol.*, *59*, 130 (1979).
145. Hume, K. M., and Gandevia, B., Forced expiratory volume before and after isoprenaline, *Thorax*, *12*, 276 (1957).
146. Goldberg, I., and Cherniack, R. M., The effect of nebulized bronchodilator delivered with and without IPPB on ventilatory function in chronic obstructive emphysema, *Am. Rev. Respir. Dis.*, *91*, 13 (1965).
147. Barbato, A., Pisetta, F., Ragusa, M. S., et al., Modification of bronchial hyperreactivity during pollen season in children allergic to grass, *Ann. Allergy*, *58*, 121–124 (1987).
148. Vedal, S., Enarson, D. A., Chan, H., Ochino, J., Tse, K. S., and Chan-Yeung, M., A longitudinal study of the occurrence of bronchial hyperresponsiveness in Western red cedar workers, *Am. Rev. Respir. Dis.*, *27*, 651–655 (1988).
149. Vincent, N. J., et al., Factors influencing pulmonary resistance, *J. Appl. Physiol.*, *29*, 236 (1970).
150. Orehek, J., et al., Effect of maximal respiratory maneuvers on bronchial sensitivity of asthmatic patients as compared to normal people, *Br. Med. J.*, *1*, 123 (1975).
151. Orehek, J., et al., Bronchomotor effect of bronchoconstriction-induced deep aspirations in asthmatics, *Am. Rev. Respir. Dis.*, *121*, 297 (1980).
152. Dubois, A. B., Botelho, S. Y., and Comroe, J. H., Jr., A new method for measuring airway resistance in man using a body plethysmograph: values in normal subjects and in patients with respiratory disease, *J. Clin. Invest.*, *35*, 227 (1956).
153. Green, M., and Mead, J., Time dependence of flow volume curves, *J. Appl. Physiol.*, *37*, 793 (1974).

154. Nadel, J. A., and Tierney, D. F., Effect of a previous deep inspiration on airway resistance in man, *J. Appl. Physiol.*, *16*, 717 (1961).
155. Orehek, J., et al., Influence of the previous deep inspiration on the spirometric measurement of provoked bronchoconstriction in asthma, *Am. Rev. Respir. Dis.*, *123*, 269 (1981).
156. Gimeno, F., et al., Spirometry-induced bronchial obstruction, *Am. Rev. Respir. Dis.*, *105*, 66 (1972).
157. Gayrard, P., et al., Bronchoconstrictor effects of a deep inspiration in patients with asthma, *Am. Rev. Respir. Dis.*, *111*, 433 (1975).
158. Ingram, R. H., Jr., and McFadden, E. R., Jr., Localization and mechanisms of airway responses, *N. Engl. J. Med.*, *297*, 596 (1977).
159. Ingram, R. H., Jr., et al., Relative contributions of large and small airways to flow limitation in normal subjects before and after atropine and isoproterinol, *J. Clin. Invest.*, *49*, 696 (1977).
160. Spector, S. L., and Souhrada, J. F., Maximal mid-expiratory flow as an index of acute airway changes, *Chest*, *68*, 851 (1975).
161. Gervais, P., Reinberg, A., Gervais, C., et al., Twenty-four-hour rhythm in the bronchial hyperreactivity to house dust in asthmatics, *J. Allergy Clin. Immunol.*, *59*, 207 (1977).
162. Smolensky, M,. Reinberg, A., and Queng, J. T., The chronobiology and chronopharmacology of allergy, *Ann. Allergy*, *47*, 234 (1981).
163. Pipkorn, U., Pharmacological influence of antiallergic medication on in vivo allergen testing, *Allergy*, *43*, 81–86 (1988).
164. Yu, D. T. C., Galant, S. P., and Gold, W. M., Inhibition of antigen-induced bronchoconstriction by atropine in asthmatic patients, *J. Appl. Physiol.*, *32*, 823 (1972).
165. Rosenthal, R. R., Norman, P. S., Summer, W. R., et al., Role of the parasympathetic system in antigen induced bronchospasm, *J. Appl. Physiol.*, *42*, 600 (1977).
166. Fish, J. E., Rosenthal, R. R., Summer, W. R., et al., The effect of atropine on acute antigen-mediated airway constriction in subjects with allergic asthma, *Am. Rev. Respir. Dis.*, *115*, 371 (1977).
167. Irkin, I. H., and Anand, S. C.,The role of atropine as a mediator blocker of induced bronchial obstruction, *J. Allergy*, *45*, 178 (1970).
168. Drazen, J. M., and Austin, K. F., Atropine modification of the pulmonary effects of chemical mediators in the guinea pig, *J. Appl. Physiol.*, *38*, 834 (1975).
169. Bryant, D. H., and Burns, M. W. S., Bronchial histamine reactivity: its relationship to the reactivity of the bronchi to allergens, *Clin. Allergy*, *6*, 523 (1976).
170. Casterline, C. L., Evans, R., and Ward, G. W., The effect of atropine and albuterol aerosols on the human bronchial response to histamine, *J. Allergy Clin. Immunol.*, *58*, 607 (1976).
171. Schiller, I. W., and Lowell, F. C., The effect of drugs in modifying the response of asthmatic subjects to inhalation of pollen extracts determined by vital capacity measurement, *Ann. Allergy*, *5*, 564 (1947).
172. Herxheimer, H., Antihistamines in bronchial asthma, *Br. Med. J.*, *4*, 901 (1949).
173. Popa, V. T., Effect of an H_1 blocker, chlorpheniramine, on inhalation tests with histamine and allergen in allergic asthma, *Chest*, *78*, 442 (1980).

174. Booij-Noord, H., et al., Protection tests on bronchial allergen challenge with disodium chromoglycate and thiazinamium, *J. Allergy*, *46*, 1 (1979).
175. Booij-Noord, H., et al., The influence of various drugs on the vital capacity of asthmatics, *Int. Arch. Allergy*, *10*, 321 (1957).
176. Redier, H., Chanez, P., De Vos, C., Rifai, N., et al., Inhibitory effect of cetirizine on the bronchial eosinophil recruitment induced by allergen inhalation challenge in allergic patients with asthma, *J. Allergy Clin. Immunol.*, *90*, 215–224 (1992).
177. Gong, H., Jr., Tashkin, D. P., Dauphinee, B., Djahed, B., and Wu, T. C., Effects of oral cetirizine, a selective H1 antagonist, on allergen- and exercise-induced bronchoconstriction in subjects with asthma, *J. Allergy Clin. Immunol.*, *85*, 632–641 (1990).
178. Hamid, M., Rafferty, O., and Holgate, S. T., The inhibitory effect of terfenadine and flurbiprofen on early- and late-phase bronchoconstriction following allergen challenge in atopic asthma, *Clin. Exp. Allergy*, *20*, 261–267 (1990).
179. Town, G. I., and Holgate, S. T., Comparison of the effect of loratadine on the airway and skin responses to histamine, methacholine, and allergen in subjects with asthma, *J. Allergy Clin. Immunol.*, *86*, 886–893 (1990).
180. Patek, K. R., et al., The effect of thymoxamine and cromolyn sodium on postexercise bronchoconstriction in asthma, *J. Allergy Clin. Immunol.*, *57*, 285 (1976).
181. Warren, J. B., McCusker, M, and Fuller, R. W., Systemic adrenalin attenuates skin response to antigen and histamine, *Clin. Allergy*, *18*, 197–199 (1988).
182. Booij-Noord, H., Quanjer, P. H., and deVries, K., Protektive Wirkung von Berotec bei Provokations-testen mit spezifischer Allergen Inhalation und Histamin, *Int. J. Clin. Pharmacol.*, *6* (4), 69 (1972).
183. Jorde, W., Smidt, V., and Worth, G., Protective Wirkung von Berotek bei Allergen Inhalation, *Int. J. Clin. Pharmacol.*, *6*, 73 (1972).
184. Martin, G. L., Atkins, P. C., Dunsky, E. H., et al., Effects of theophylline, terbutaline, and prednisone on antigen-induced bronchospasm and mediator release, *J. Allergy Clin. Immunol.*, *66*, 204 (1980).
185. Falliers, C. J., Assessment of oral antiasthmatic drugs by inhalation challenge, *J. Allergy Clin. Immunol.*, *64*, 685 (1979).
186. Taylor, I. K., O'Shaughnessy, K. M., Choudry, N. B., Adachi, M., et al., A comparative study in atopic subjects with asthma of the effects of salmeterol and salbutamol on allergen-induced bronchoconstriction, increase in airway reactivity, and increase in urinary leukotriene E4 excretion, *J. Allergy Clin. Immunol.*, *89*, 575–583 (1992).
187. Twentyman, O. P., Finnerty, J. P., and Holgate, S. T., The inhibitory effect of nebulized albuterol on the early and late asthmatic reactions and increase in airway responsiveness provoked by inhaled allergen in asthma, *Am. Rev. Respir. Dis.*, *144*, 782–787 (1991).
188. Larsson, K., Martinsson, A., and Hjemdhl, P., Influence of β-adrenergic receptor function during terbutaline treatment on allergen sensitivity and bronchodilator response to terbutaline in asthmatic subjects, *Chest*, *101*, 953–960 (1992).
189. Engstrom, I., and Vejinolova, J., The effect of disodium chromoglycate on allergen challenge in children with bronchial asthma, *Acta Allergol.*, *25*, 382 (1970).

190. Herxheimer, H. G. J., and Brewersdorff, H., Disodium chromoglycate in the prevention of induced asthma, *Br. Med. J.*, *2*, 220 (1969).
191. Frith, P. A., Ruffin, R. E., Juniper, E. F., Dolovich, E. F., Jr., and Hargreave, F. E., Inhibition of allergen-induced asthma by three forms of sodium chromoglycate, *Clin. Allergy*, *11*, 67 (1981).
192. Nakazawa, T., Toyoda, T., Furukawa, M., et al., Inhibitory effects of various drugs on dual asthmatic responses in wheat-flour sensitive subjects, *J. Allergy Clin. Immunol.*, *58*, 1 (1976).
193. Pepys, J., et al., The effect of inhaled beclomethasone dipropionate (Becotide) and sodium chromoglycate on asthmatic reactions to provocation tests, *Clin. Allergy*, *4*, 12 (1974).
194. Aalbers, R., Kauffman, H. F., Groen, H., Koeter, G. H., and de Monchv, J. G., The effect of nedocromil sodium on the early and late reaction and allergen-induced bronchial hyperresponsiveness, *J. Allergy Clin. Immunol.*, *87*, 993–1001 (1991).
195. Kopferschmitt-Kubler, M. C., Hutt, N., Bigot, H., Bessot, J. C., and Pauli, G., Protective effect of nedocromil sodium on the dual asthmatic response to bronchial antigen challenge, *Respiration*, *60*, 21–26 (1993).
196. Booij-Noord, H., Orle, N. G. M., and deVries, K., Immediate and late bronchial obstructive reactions to inhalation of house dust and protective effects of disodium chromoglycate and prednisone, *J. Allergy Clin. Immunol.*, *48*, 344 (1971).
197. Cresioli, S., Spinazzi, A., Plebani, M., Pozzani, M., et al., Theophylline inhibits early and late asthmatic reactions induced by allergens in asthmatic subjects, *Ann. Allergy*, *66*, 245–251 (1991).
198. Cockcroft, D. W., Murdock, K. Y., Gore, B. P., O'Byrne, P. M., and Manning, P., Theophylline does not inhibit allergen-induced increase in airway responsiveness to methacholine, *J. Allergy Clin. Immunol.*, *83*, 913–920 (1989).
199. Fish, J. E., et al., Indomethacin modification of immediate-type immunologic airway responses in allergic asthmatic and non-asthmatic subjects, *Am. Rev. Respir. Dis.*, *123*, 609 (1981).
200. Sladek, K., Dworski, R., Fitzgerald, G. A., Buitkus, K. L., et al., Allergen-stimulated release of thromboxane A2 and leukotriene E4 in humans. Effect of indomethacin, *Am. Rev. Respir. Dis.*, *141*, 1441–1445 (1990).
201. Manning, P. J., Stevens, W. H., Cockcroft, D. W., and O'Byrne, P. M., The role of thromboxane in allergen-induced asthmatic responses, *Eur. Respir. J.*, *4*, 667–672 (1991).
202. Taylor, I. K., O'Shaughnessy, K. M., Fuller, R. W., and Dollery, C. T., Effect of cysteinyl-leukotriene receptor antagonist ICI204,219 on allergen-induced bronchoconstriction and airway hyperreactivity in atopic subjects, *Lancet*, *337*, 690–694 (1991).
203. Verdiani, P., Di Carlo, S., Baronti, A., and Bianco, S., Effect of inhaled frusemide on the early response to antigen and subsequent change in airway reactivity in atopic patients, *Thorax*, *45*, 377–381 (1990).
204. Pavord, I. D., Wong, C. S., Williams, J., and Tattersfield, A. E., Effect of inhaled prostaglandin E2 on allergen-induced asthma, *Am. Rev. Respir. Dis.*, *148*, 87–90 (1993).

205. Hoppe, M., Harman, E., and Hendales, L., The effect of inhaled gallopamil, a potent calcium-channel blocker, on the late-phase response in subjects with allergic asthma, *J. Allergy Clin. Immunol.*, *89*, 688–695 (1992).
206. Ahmed, T., Russi, E., Kim, C. S., and Danta, I., Comparative effects of oral and inhaled verapamil on antigen-induced bronchoconstriction, *Chest*, *88*, 176–180 (1985).
207. Arm, J. P., Horton, C. E., Spur, B. W., Mencia-Huerta, J. M., and Lee, T. H., The effects of dietary supplementation with fish oil lipids on the airways response to inhaled allergen in bronchial asthma, *Am. Rev. Respir. Dis.*, *139*, 1395–1400 (1989).
208. Kopferschmitt-Kubler, M. C., Bigot, H., and Pauli, G., Allergen bronchial challenge tests: variability and reproducibility of the early response, *J. Allergy Clin. Immunol.*, *80*, 730–740 (1987).
209. Tiffeneau, R., Hypersensibilité cholinergo-histaminique pulmonaire de l'asthmatique, *Acta Allergol.*, *13*, 187 (1958).
210. Frolund, L., Svendsen, U. G., Neisen, N. H., et al., Bronchial allergen challenge: comparison between two different methods of provocation, *Clin. Allergy*, *17*, 439–338 (1987).
211. Fish, J. E., and Kelly, J. F., Measurements of responsiveness in bronchoprovocation testing, *J. Allergy Clin. Immunol.*, *64*, 592 (1979).
212. Ankin, M. G., Peterman, V. I., and Fish, J. E., Effect of lung inflation on maximum flow responses to methacholine and antigen in hay fever and asthma subjects, *Am. Rev. Respir. Dis.*, 55 (1979).
213. Fish, J. E., Peterman, V. I., and Cugell, D. W., Effect of deep inspiration on airway conductance in subjects with allergic rhinitis and allergic asthma, *J. Allergy Clin. Immunol.*, *60*, 41 (1977).
214. Pennock, B. E., et al., Letter to the editor, *Chest*, *81*, 5 (1982).
215. Hruby, J., and Butler, J., Variability of routine pulmonary function tests, *Thorax*, *30*, 548 (1975).
216. Chai, H., et al., Standardization of bronchial inhalation challenge procedures, *J. Allergy Clin. Immunol.*, *56*, 323 (1975).
217. Haahtela, T., and Lahdensuo, A., Nonspecific reactions caused by dilutents containing glycerol in nasal and bronchial challenge tests, *Clin. Allergy*, *9*, 225 (1979).
218. Ryan, G., et al., Standardization of inhalation provocation tests: inhalation of nebulizer output particle size and method of inhalation, *J. Allergy Clin. Immunol.*, *78*, 156 (1981).
219. Orehek, J., et al., Airway response to carbachol in normal and asthmatic subjects, *Am. Rev. Respir. Dis.*, *115*, 937 (1977).
220. Chatham, M., et al., A screening test for airway reactivity: an abbreviated methacholine inhalation challenge, *Chest*, *82*, 1 (1982).

14

Environmental Challenges to Animal Allergens

Robert A. Wood and Peyton A. Eggleston

The Johns Hopkins University School of Medicine
Baltimore, Maryland

I. INTRODUCTION

Although at times difficult and cumbersome, provocative challenges to naturally occurring allergens offer a number of distinct advantages over standard allergen challenge procedures. Most important, they are intended to mimic more closely the exposures that may occur in a natural setting. They allow for the simultaneous exposure of both the upper and the lower airways and provide for exposure to airborne allergen particles that will be most similar to those encountered in natural environments. Thus, as opposed to the typical allergen challenge that may employ a nebulized allergen delivered solely to the lower airways, environmental exposure challenges use naturally generated allergen delivered to the eyes, nose, and lungs. We have been working with such challenges to cat and rat allergens, and here we will describe the systems that we have developed to perform such challenges, as well as their specific advantages and disadvantages.

II. BACKGROUND

The concept of environmental challenges is certainly not new, as they have been used extensively in the assessment of occupational asthma over the past two decades [1–4]. The simplest occupational challenges involve the monitoring of peak flow rates in and out of the work setting, a technique that can be very helpful in establishing a diagnosis of occupationally induced asthma. In addition to this basic model, more elaborate systems for the laboratory assessment of many occupational agents have now been developed, using both exposure chambers and nebulized aerosols [5]. By controlling the type and level of exposure and carefully monitoring the subject's responses, these methods allow for a more accurate assessment of the specific agents in question, including the levels of exposure that may be capable of inducing symptoms.

We have been interested in applying the principles of occupational challenges to naturally occurring allergens. While there has been extensive experience with laboratory challenge models using a variety of allergens, studies in the "real world" are more limited, particularly with regard to actual challenge systems. Most studies have focused on natural pollen exposure and the effects of various treatment modalities. There has also been a growing interest in the relationship of asthma to dust mite exposure, although most of this work has concentrated on the effects of allergen avoidance or the importance of long-term mite exposure. No studies have examined the effects of short-term mite exposure in a natural setting. To our knowledge, only two American investigators have actually created challenge systems using naturally generated allergens. Ohman and colleagues exposed cat-allergic subjects in a cat-containing apartment to assess the effects of cat immunotherapy [6], and Van Metre et al. developed a more formal cat challenge model, which was used to study both asthmatic responses to cat allergen and the efficacy of cat immunotherapy [7,8].

Ohman and colleagues used an apartment containing two cats to challenge subjects before and after immunotherapy. They monitored nasal, ocular, and pulmonary symptoms as well as peak flow measurements during a 90-min exposure. Airborne *Fel d* I was not measured during challenges, although in a separate study it was reported that levels in the apartment ranged from 0.0001 to 0.00046 FDA units per liter of air (0.4–1.86 ng/m^3) [9]. With this model, they demonstrated a delay in the onset of ocular and pulmonary symptoms in the subjects receiving active immunotherapy.

Van Metre et al. took this concept a step further with the development of a more sophisticated cat challenge system. They created a cat exposure room that was explicitly designed to produce high levels of airborne cat allergen. The room was characterized in detail, and while it was intended to mimic a natural cat environment, the procedure eventually included three low-velocity fans and one high-velocity fan (a leaf blower) to disturb allergen and maintain high airborne-allergen levels. Airborne cat allergen was collected with lapel filters at a flow rate of 30 L/min and measured with a radioimmunoassay. In addition, a Durham gravity sampler and an Anderson sampler were used to study particle counts and particle size distribution. Symptom scores were monitored every minute during the 2-h challenge, and pulmonary function tests were performed every 5 min. The challenge was terminated when subjects experienced a 20% fall in their forced expired volume in 1 second (FEV_1).

With this model, Van Metre et al. estimated that a 20% fall in FEV_1 occurred after a median *Fel d* I exposure of −2.74 log FDA units. They compared these results with a standard inhalation challenge with cat allergen and found that there was an excellent correlation between the two methods ($p < 0.01$), although this study was undertaken only for those subjects who had experienced a 20% fall in FEV_1 in the cat room. This study was extremely useful in proving that a model of "natural" exposure could be developed and that challenge results obtained with this model were comparable to those of standard bronchoprovocation tests. It was limited, however, by the artificial conditions that were created by the use of multiple fans during challenges and by limited study of upper airway responses. Furthermore, the use of a high-flow system for the collection of samples via a lapel filter may not be ideal, in that the actual inhaled dose of allergen may be underestimated when high flow rates are used [10].

We have been working on two different challenge systems involving the study of naturally generated animal allergens. In one, we have performed detailed studies on human responses to rat allergen in an occupational setting. In the second, we have established a cat challenge facility similar to that of Van Metre et al. in an effort to expand their studies on allergic responses to cat allergen. The first is therefore essentially an occupational challenge, while the second is designed to study an important nonoccupational allergen.

III. METHODS

The basic idea is very simple. First, an environment must be identified or created that is rich in the allergen of interest but very low in all others. Second, the means to collect air samples and quantitate the relevant allergen(s) must be established. And third, objective measures to assess the subjects' response to exposure must be designed and implemented.

The first condition may require some creativity, but it is absolutely critical that a proper environment for the challenges be found or established. Again, the basic requirement is a high level of the relevant allergen with insignificant levels of other allergens. We have approached this problem very differently for the study of rat and cat allergens. For rats, we have used existing animal vivaria, while for cats a facility was established for the sole purpose of performing environmental challenges. However, the means used to collect samples, measure allergens, and assess response were quite similar for the two challenge systems.

A. Occupational Exposure Challenges to Rat Allergen

The development of the challenge model began with a detailed study of airborne allergen exposure in laboratory workers performing different tasks with rats [11]. Samples were collected with personal air-sampling devices that were worn by laboratory workers while they performed various tasks, including feeding, cage cleaning, handling, injection, surgery, and sacrifice. These studies demonstrated that exposure varied significantly with these different tasks, airborne-allergen levels encountered during feeding, cleaning, injection, and handling being significantly higher than those associated with surgery or sacrifice. Median *Rat n* I levels ranged from 21 ng/m^3 during cleaning or feeding to 13 ng/m^3 with injection or handling and 3.1 ng/m^3 during surgery or sacrifice. These data were then used in the design of actual challenge procedures in rat vivaria.

The next series of experiments involved the intentional exposure of rat-allergic persons to varying concentrations of rat allergen in the laboratory environment [12]. Subjects were recruited and characterized before challenge with regard to skin test reactivity to rat pelt and other inhalant allergens, serum immunoglobulin E (IgE) levels in response to rat allergen, and methacholine responsiveness. Those with a history of rat-induced respiratory symptoms and a positive skin test to rat allergen, as well as a group of non–rat allergic atopic control subjects, where then invited to undergo a rat exposure challenge.

Before challenge, medications were withheld as follows: antihistamines for 2 days, theophylline, cromolyn, and oral beta-adrenergic agonists for 12 h, and inhaled β-adrenergic agonists and corticosteroids for 4 h. The challenge consisted of standing in a rat-holding room for up to 1 h while airborne *Rat n* I concentrations, symptoms, nasal lavage mediators, and spirometry were measured. Challenges were conducted either during cage cleaning (high-dose exposure) or without cage cleaning (low-dose exposure).

During all challenges, air samples were collected with a battery-powered sampling pump calibrated at a flow rate of about 4 L/min (Gilian Instrument Corporation, Wayne, New Jersey, and E. I. Dupont Corporation, Wilmington, Delaware). The pump was worn at the waist and attached by plastic tubing to a plastic cassette that contained a 25-mm glass-fiber filter (Millipore Corp., Bedford, Massachusetts). The cassette was attached to the subject's lapel in such a way that the sample would most accurately reflect the subject's exposure, referred to as the personal breathing zone. Low flow rates are used for sampling because they have been shown to estimate natural exposure most accurately [10]. After the challenge, the filter was stored in the cassette at −20°C until extraction. The *Rat n* I concentration of the aqueous extract was determined by an inhibition radioimmunoassay. The airborne allergen concentration was then derived from the immunoassay result as follows: antigen concentration times extraction volume (3 ml) divided by the volume of air sampled (flow rate × sampling time), with results expressed as nanograms of allergen per cubic meter of sampled air.

Before the challenge, baseline nasal lavages and spirometry were obtained in an adjacent hallway. It is important to realize that most areas near a vivarium will be contaminated by allergen so that some exposure may occur while these baseline studies are performed. The subject is therefore kept away from the area until immediately before challenge. Nasal lavages were performed according to the technique of Naclerio et al. [13], and lavage samples were analyzed for histamine [14] and TAME-esterase [15] content. Spirometry was measured on a Stead-Wells instrument (Eagle II, Warren E. Collins, Inc.) and compared with published norms. The challenge was not conducted if the baseline FEV_1 was <70% of the predicted value.

During the challenge, upper and lower respiratory symptoms were graded every 2–5 min on an arbitrary point scale of 0–3. Nasal symptoms were divided into congestion, rhinorrhea, and pruritus, and a separate score was assigned for each. Similarly, individual scores were assigned every 2–5 min for chest tightness and wheezing. All coughs and sneezes were counted. Every 15 min, subjects were taken out into the hallway, where the nasal lavage and spirometry were repeated. The challenges were performed for 1 h, unless symptoms became severe or the FEV_1 fell by more than 50% from baseline.

A representative challenge is illustrated in Fig. 1. Overall, 12 rat-allergic subjects underwent challenge, and all experienced nasal symptoms and had an increase in their nasal lavage histamine level and/or TAME-esterase activity. Nasal symptoms and mediator levels tended to be highest at 15 min and then to plateau. The median fall in FEV_1 was 8%, with five subjects having a fall of more than 10% and only one having a fall of more than 20%. Maximum pulmonary responses tended to occur late in the challenge. Of the five non-rat-allergic controls, two had a small change in nasal TAME-esterase activity, but none had fall in FEV_1 of 10% or more.

Airborne *Rat n* I concentrations ranged from <1.5 to 310 ng/m^3. A dose–response relation was noted between the allergen concentrations and the intensity of the nasal response. An absolute threshold for response could not be determined, however. Overall, this challenge procedure proved to be a useful method to assess respiratory responses to an important occupational allergen.

B. The Cat Exposure Facility

We have attempted to use the methods developed in the rat exposure challenges to expand on Van Metre and colleagues' studies of the allergic response to intentional cat exposure. For these challenges, a new cat exposure facility was established at the Johns Hopkins Asthma and Allergy Center. This facility consists of two adjacent rooms: the first room contains two cats and is used for the actual exposure challenges, while the second is free of cat antigen and contains a spirometer, sampling equipment, and medications.

The cat exposure room is 91 inches long and 86.5 inches wide and has a ceiling height of 106 inches (room volume = 13.7 cubic meters) (Fig. 2) [16]. The room has cinder-block walls, a cement floor, and a plaster ceiling. The walls and floor are painted with an epoxy-based paint and the ceiling is painted with a flat enamel

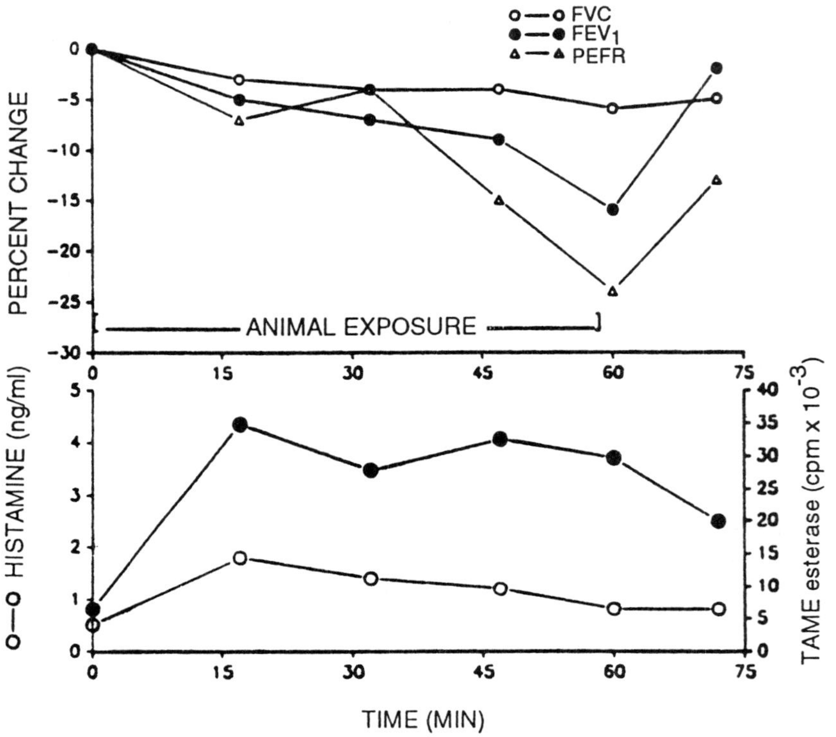

Figure 1 A representative airway response to an occupational exposure challenge to rat allergen in a single volunteer. Pulmonary function test results are plotted in the upper panel as a percent change from baseline. Mediator concentrations in nasal lavage fluids are plotted in the lower panel.

paint. Two adult female cats live in the room at all times. They are free to move about the room except during challenges, when they are placed in a wire holding cage in the room. The room is furnished with a bed, an upholstered chair, and a small carpet. The bed mattress is encased in a plastic cover. The bed sheet is changed weekly, and the room is cleaned by damp mopping every 2 weeks.

The room has been extensively characterized with regard to ventilation, airborne allergen levels, and *Fel d* I particle size distribution. Pressure in the room is negative with respect to the corridor. An exhaust duct is located in the ceiling just inside the door, and the supply grill is located in the ceiling near the wall opposite the door. Ventilation in the room can be controlled by turning the exhaust fan on and off. The room is currently ventilated at a rate of 15 air changes per hour with the fan on and six air changes per hour with the fan off. If both ducts are

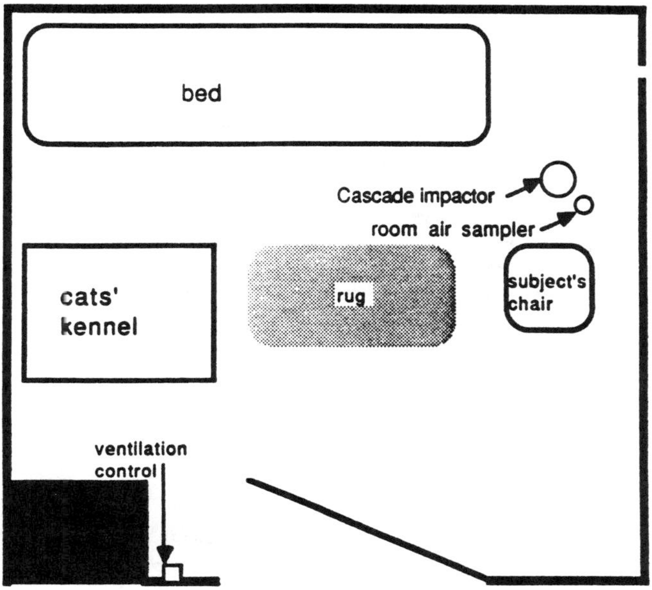

Figure 2 A schematic diagram of the cat challenge room. The room is 91 inches long, 86.5 inches wide, and 106 inches high. Two adult cats live in the room at all times. The room contains a bed, chair, rug, and wire holding cage. The room's ventilation can be controlled by turning off the exhaust fan and blocking the air ducts.

physically blocked, the ventilation can be reduced to less than one air change per hour.

There was no detectable cat or dust mite allergen in dust or air samples when the room was first established. Airborne *Fel d* I levels then began to rise, and this trend continued over the next 2 years (Fig. 3) [16]. *Fel d* I levels have now generally plateaued, with typical levels after disturbance ranging from 1000 to 10,000 ng/m^3, although levels in excess 30,000 ng/m^3 have been detected. This remarkable rise in airborne allergen is most likely the result of a gradual saturation of the reservoirs within the room with cat allergen. These reservoirs include not just the furniture and carpet but also the wall and ceiling surfaces [17]. This phenomenon must be carefully considered in the development of any similar challenge systems, in that initial challenges may be dramatically different from those performed a year or two later.

Extensive studies were also undertaken to characterize airborne *Fel d* I levels and particle size distribution under different conditions of ventilation and disturbance. Particle size determinations were made with an Anderson cascade impactor (Anderson Instruments, Atlanta, Georgia) run at a flow rate of 3.0–3.4 L/min. We

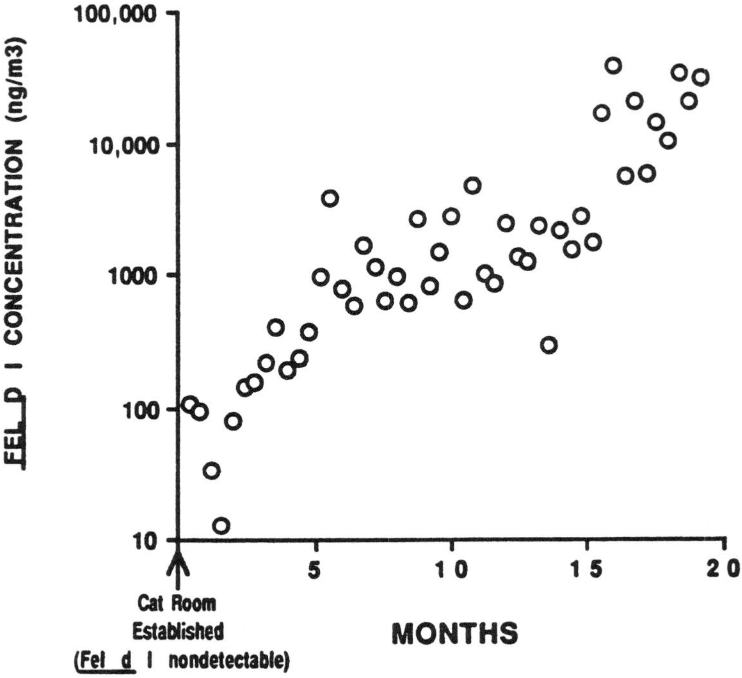

Figure 3 Total airborne *Fel d* I levels, all collected after disturbance and at a ventilation rate of 8 air changes/h, in the first 20 months after the cat room was established. While there was no detectable *Fel d* I in the room before its establishment, antigen levels then rose steadily.

found that both total airborne-allergen levels and *Fel d* I particle size distribution were similar under the different ventilation rates [16]. Under all conditions, at least 50% of the *Fel d* I was detected on particles greater than 17 μm in mean aerodynamic diameter, while no more than 10% was found on particles of less than 4 μm (Fig. 4). Consistent with the preponderance of large particles, *Fel d* I concentrations were found to fall quickly after disturbance, with at least 90% having been cleared within 45 min of disturbance.

C. Cat Exposure Challenges

The challenges are conducted as follows. First, cat-allergic subjects are recruited and characterized by history, skin tests, end-point titration skin tests to cat allergen, measurement of cat-specific IgE, and methacholine challenge. Medications are withheld before challenge in the same fashion as described above for rat challenges.

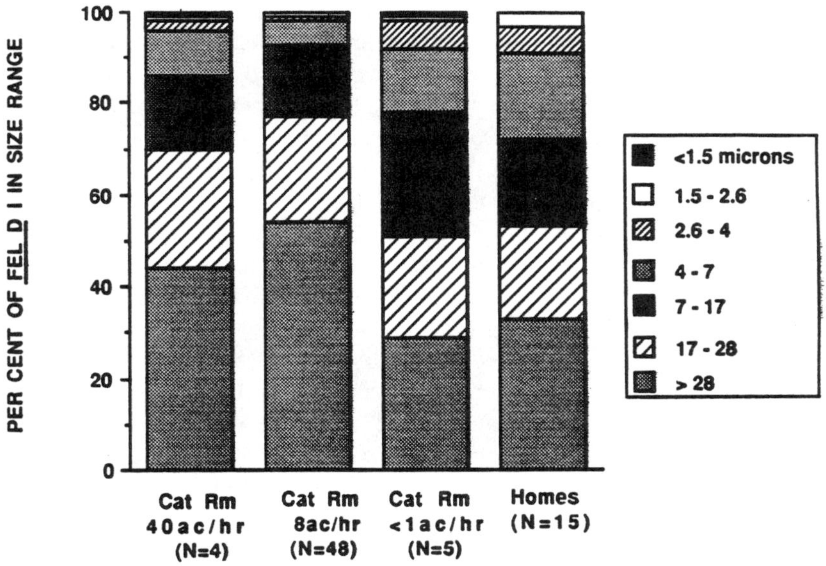

Figure 4 *Fel d* I particle size distribution in the cat room and home environments was studied with an Anderson cascade impactor. Median values of the percent of *Fel d* I detected on each stage are represented here. Under all conditions a majority of the *Fel d* I was found on particles > 17 μm in mean aerodynamic diameter, while < 15% was on particles < 4 μm.

Before challenges, the cats are put in their cage, the room ventilation is turned off, and bedding is shaken to disturb allergen. Baseline spirometry (Eagle II, Warren Collins, Inc.), peak flow, and nasal lavage are performed in the clean room, and the subject then enters the cat room for a 1-h exposure. During the challenge, upper respiratory (congestion, rhinorrhea, and pruritus) and lower respiratory (chest tightness, wheezing) symptoms are graded every 2 min on an arbitrary scale of 0–3 and coughs and sneezes are counted. Every 15 min the subject goes to the clean room, where spirometry and nasal lavage are repeated. The bedding is shaken each time the subject leaves the room, to maintain consistently high allergen levels. After the challenge, peak flow rates and symptom scores are monitored every 1–2 h for 12 h to assess late-phase responses. Challenges are stopped before the 1-h limit if the subject becomes too uncomfortable or if the FEV_1 falls by more than 50%. All challenges are directly supervised by a physician.

Allergen exposure during the challenges is monitored by measuring levels of airborne *Fel d* I with a personal monitor that employs a lapel filter and a pump with a flow rate of about 4 L/min (exactly as in the rat exposure challenges). In addition, an area sample is obtained by mounting an identical filter at a height of 1 m near the rear corner of the room. The area sample is also collected at a flow rate of about 4 L/min. Although there is a significant correlation between the personal and area samples ($R_s = 0.6$, $p < 0.001$), the room samples are consistently higher. These differences are most likely due to the placement of the area sampler near the bed, a major reservoir of allergen in the room. These differences confirm the value of the personal monitor in making the most accurate assessment of exposure.

Air samples are extracted in PIPES/Tween, and *Fel d* I is quantitated by a monoclonal ELISA, with results expressed as nanograms of *Fel d* I per cubic meter of sampled air [16,18]. The nasal lavage fluid is analyzed for histamine and TAME-esterase content as described previously [13–14].

Our initial challenge studies were designed to study both upper and lower respiratory responses to cat exposure and to determine what factors are most important in predicting these responses [19–20]. In our first 52 challenges, all subjects complained of upper respiratory symptoms, and 41 of the 52 experienced lower respiratory symptoms. Twenty-two of the 52 had a fall in FEV_1 of more than 15%, with 17 experiencing a change of more than 20%. Challenges have been performed over a wide range of exposure, with airborne *Fel d* I levels ranging from 13.1 ng/m^3 to 31,381 ng/m^3, and aside from a weak correlation between the antigen level and the number of sneezes ($R_s = 0.34$, $p < 0.05$), no relationship was detected between the *Fel d* I level and any of the outcome variables. Neither skin test reactivity nor cat-specific serum IgE levels helped to predict upper airway responses, although both measures of sensitivity were correlated with lower respiratory responses ($p < 0.05$ for ΔFEV_1, total coughs, and lower respiratory symptoms). Methacholine reactivity was found to be the best predictor of an asthmatic response ($R_s = 0.69$, $p < 0.001$), although three of 22 subjects with negative methacholine challenges had a fall in their FEV_1 of >15%, and 11 of 30 with positive methacholine challenges had no significant change (< 15%) in their FEV_1.

The cat challenge model has subsequently been used in a study of the effects of intranasal steroids on allergic reactions to cat exposure [21]. Similar studies are currently under way with other therapeutic interventions. In addition to these studies, we are working to correlate these data from the cat room with home environments. We have found airborne *Fel d* I levels in cat-containing homes ranging from 2 to 469 ng/m^3 [16]. Most important, the *Fel d* I particle size distribution in homes is very similar to that found in the cat room (Fig. 4). Although the exposure in the cat room is by and large higher than that seen in home environments, 18 of the 52 challenges that have been performed to date were done at allergen levels below 500 ng/m^3, and significant upper and lower respiratory responses were seen at these levels. We therefore feel that challenges at these lower levels are a reasonable approximation of natural exposure in home environments.

IV. ENVIRONMENTAL CHALLENGES: ADVANTAGES

The environmental challenge systems that have been developed offer several major advantages over most conventional challenge methods. First, as opposed to typical bronchial, nasal, or conjunctival challenges, these challenges provide for the simultaneous exposure of both the upper and the lower airways, a situation that more closely mimics the exposure that would occur in natural settings. It is therefore possible to study the interaction of nasal and pulmonary responses and to assess more accurately the effects of various therapeutic interventions on both the nose and the lung.

The second major advantage of environmental challenges is that they provide for exposure to naturally generated airborne allergens. Most challenge methods deliver allergens in an artificial manner, as with a nebulizer in bronchoprovocation challenges, and may therefore not be an accurate representation of natural allergen exposure. This difference can be of critical importance with regard to an allergen's aerodynamic characteristics, particularly its particle size distribution, and therefore its deposition in the respiratory tract.

Finally, the use of naturally generated allergens allows for the study of environmental manipulations designed to reduce allergen exposure. For example, air cleaners, ventilation systems, masks, and other interventions can be studied and the results applied to similar systems in home environments. Critical data regarding allergen thresholds for the induction of symptoms can be obtained with these models.

V. ENVIRONMENTAL CHALLENGES: DISADVANTAGES

These challenges are associated with a number of significant disadvantages that must be recognized and, if possible, overcome. First, it may be difficult or costly to establish the appropriate environment for such challenges. An appropriate facility must be identified, the allergen source must be provided, and the means to disturb allergen in a relevant manner must be determined. While these obstacles can be overcome, they will certainly limit the use of such challenges in any widespread fashion. In addition, even when a suitable environment is established, the procedure is very cumbersome with regard to the need for air pumps and other monitoring equipment and very labor-intensive in the establishment of reliable assays, the handling of samples, the measurement of the allergens, and the supervision of challenges.

As evidenced by our data on the rise in allergens levels in the cat room over time, significant problems may be encountered with variability in allergen exposure. Over time these levels tend to stabilize, but even then tenfold variations in airborne *Fed d* I levels are routinely encountered. These fluctuations must be dealt with in protocol design, and allergen levels must be measured for each challenge.

Once all the logistical problems have been dealt with, these challenges face a significant scientific disadvantage in that it may be difficult or even impossible to blind the exposure. We have the ability to significantly alter allergen levels for cat and rat challenges, but that is as close to blinding as we can come. This leaves open the very real possibility of a significant placebo effect in some subjects, with the mere thought of being near a cat inducing a reaction. Furthermore, it is also possible that some people with highly reactive airways but no animal sensitivity will react to the noxious stimuli of the animal quarters themselves. We are in the process of sorting out these important issues in more detail and will attempt to provide suitable solutions.

VI. SUMMARY

Environmental challenges offer a unique opportunity to study a variety of responses to naturally occurring allergens. They are cumbersome and labor-intensive but offer significant rewards, particularly with regard to the study of potential treatment modalities and their effects on both the upper and the lower airways.

REFERENCES

1. Davies, R. J., Hendrick, D. J., and Pepys, J., Asthma due to inhaled chemical agents: ampicillin, benzyl penicillin, 6 amino penicillanic acid and related substances, *Clin. Allergy*, *4*, 227 (1974).
2. Hendrick, D. J., Davies, R. J., and Pepys, J., Bakers' asthma, *Clin. Allergy*, *6*, 241 (1976).
3. Burge, P. S., O'Brien, I. M., and Harries, M. G., Peak flow records in the diagnosis of occupational asthma due to colophony, *Thorax*, *34*, 308 (1979).
4. Burge, P. S., O'Brien, I. M., and Harries, M. G., Peak flow records in the diagnosis of occupational asthma due to isocyanates, *Thorax*, *34*, 317 (1979).
5. Hammad, Y., Rando, P., and Abdel-Kader, H., Considerations in the design and use of human inhalation challenge delivery systems, *Folia Allergol. Immunol. Clin.*, *321*, 37 (1985).
6. Ohman, J. L., Findlay, S. R., and Leiterman, K., Immunotherapy in cat-induced asthma: double-blind trial with evaluation of in vivo and in vitro responses, *J. Allergy Clin. Immunol.*, *74*, 230 (1984).
7. Van Metre, T. E., Marsh, D. G., Adkinson, N. F., Fish, J. E., Kagey-Sobotka, A., Norman, P. S., Radden, E. B., and Rosenberg, G. L., Dose of cat (*Felis domesticus*) allergen 1 (*Fel d* I) that induces asthma, *J. Allergy Clin. Immunol.*, *78*, 62 (1986).
8. Van Metre, T. E., Marsh, D. G., Adkinson, N. F., Kagey-Sobotka, A., Khattignavong, A., Norman, P. S., and Rosenberg, G.L., Immunotherapy for cat asthma, *J. Allergy Clin. Immunol.*, *82*, 1055 (1988).
9. Findlay, S. R., Stotsky, K., Leiterman, K., Hemady, Z., and Ohman, J. L., Allergens

detected in association with airborne particles capable of penetrating into the peripheral lung, *Am. Rev. Respir. Dis.*, *128*, 1008 (1983).

10. Corn, M., Koegel, A., Hall, T., Scott, A., Newill, C., and Evans, R., Characteristics of airborne particles associated with animal allergy in laboratory workers, *Ann. Occup. Hyg.*, *32* (suppl. 1), 435 (1988).
11. Eggleston, P. A., Newill, C. A., Ansari, A. A., Pustelnick, A., Lou, S.-R., Evans, R. E., Marsh, D. G., and Longbottom, J. L., Task-related variation in airborne concentrations of laboratory animal allergens: studies with *Rat n* I, *J. Allergy Clin. Immunol.*, *84*, 347 (1989).
12. Eggleston, P. A., Ansari, A. A., Zeiman, B., Adkinson, N. F., and Corn, M., Occupational challenge studies with laboratory workers allergic to rats, *J. Allergy Clin. Immunol.*, *86*, 63 (1990).
13. Naclerio, R. M., Proud, D., Togias, A. G., et al., Inflammation mediators in the late antigen-induced rhinitis, *N. Engl. J. Med.*, *313*, 258 (1985).
14. Siraganian, R., An automated continuous flow system for the extraction and fluorometric analysis of histamine, *Anal. Biochem.*, *57*, 283 (1974).
15. Imanari, T., Kaizu, T., Yoshida, H., Yates, H., Pierce, J. V, and Pisano, J. J., Radiochemical assays for human urinary, salivary, and plasma kallikreins, in *Chemistry and Biology of the Kallikrein–Kinin System in Health and Disease* (J. J. Pisano and K. F. Austen, eds.), Washington, D.C., DHEW Publication No. 76-791, 1976,pp. 205–213.
16. Wood, R. A., Ellis, C. A., and Eggleston, P. A., The aerodynamic characteristics of cat allergen, *Clin. Exp. Allergy*, *23*, 733–739 (1993).
17. Wood, R. A., Mudd, K. E., and Eggleston, P. A., The distribution of cat and dust mite allergens on wall surfaces, *J. Allergy Clin. Immunol.*, *89*, 126–130 (1992).
18. Chapman, M. D., Aalberse, R. C., Brown, M. J., and Platts-Mills, T. A. E., Monoclonal antibodies to the major feline allergen *Fel d* I. II. Single step affinity purification of *Fel d* I, N-terminal sequence analysis, and development of a sensitive two-site immunoassay to assess *Fel d* I exposure, *J. Immunol.*, *140*, 812–818 (1988).
19. Wood, R. A., Trent, P. A., Mudd, K. S., Bowes, S. B., and Eggleston, P. A., Determinants of upper and lower airway responses to cat exposure (abstr.), *J. Allergy Clin. Immunol.*, *87*, 169 (1991).
20. Wood, R. A., Jones, L. T., and Eggleston, P. A., Determinants of acute and late-phase pulmonary responses to cat exposure (abstr.), *Am. Rev. Respir. Dis.*, *145*, A692 (1992).
21. Wood, R. A., and Eggleston, P. A., The modification of upper and lower airway responses to cat exposure by intranasal steroids, *J. Allergy Clin. Immunol.*, *91*, 250 (1993).

15

Genetic Aspects of Asthma and Bronchial Hyperresponsiveness

Robert G. Townley, Russell J. Hopp, A. K. Bewtra, and Nicki M. Nair

Creighton University School of Medicine
Omaha, Nebraska

I. INTRODUCTION AND HISTORICAL PERSPECTIVE

Asthma is a well-recognized and common condition. Nearly all asthmatics demonstrate recurrent episodes of shortness of breath, wheezing, and coughing. Asthmatics generally respond to bronchodilator medication. All asthmatics demonstrate a marked sensitivity to inhaled methacholine and histamine [1], termed nonspecific bronchial (airway) hyperresponsiveness (BHR). Airway hyperresponsiveness is a characteristic not only of asthmatics, but can be found in many persons with allergic rhinitis [1] and members of asthmatics' families [2]. A recent report suggests that the presence of BHR usually precedes the development of clinically identifiable asthma [3].

Asthma has for centuries been associated with familial/genetic factors, and extensive reviews of the pertinent literature have recently been published [2,4]. Of historical interest is a report of family histories of 504 allergic subjects [5]. Nearly 50% had positive family histories, as compared with fewer than 15% of the 76 normal subjects. The concept that allergic and nonallergic triggers could be involved with asthma was proposed in the early 20th century [6]. Bray [7] reviewed the literature up to 1930 and suggested that the tendency to develop asthma was inherited. This is similar to our present concept that bronchial reactivity has a genetic basis [8], while the clinical condition of asthma is a complex interaction of genetic and environmental components.

Asthma is characterized by a constellation of biochemical, hematological, and

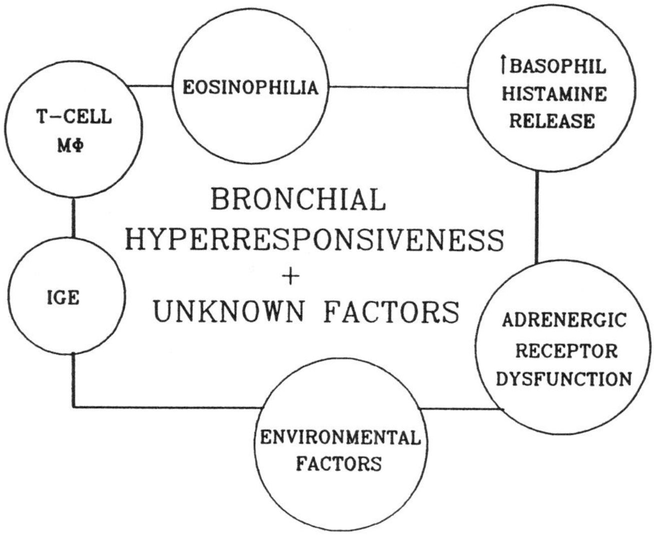

Figure 1 These characteristics encompass the pathogenesis of asthma and need to be included in any theory regarding it. MΦ = macrophage.

pharmacological abnormalities. A role for both genetic and environmental influences is generally accepted. Figure 1 shows the characteristics of asthma that will be reviewed for their genetic basis. These characteristics will be discussed in relation to humans with asthma and the various well-recognized animal experimental models of asthma [9–12].

II. BRONCHIAL HYPERRESPONSIVENESS

Viral infections, industrial pollutants, and exposure to allergens can all increase airway hyperresponsiveness and induce inflammation. In recent years there has been an emphasis on inflammation, including hyperresponsiveness. However, these factors increase airway hyperresponsiveness by a magnitude of only threefold, whereas the hyperresponsiveness of the asthmatic is increased at least three log, or 1000-fold, compared with normal subjects. Even when doses of 256 mg/ml of methacholine are used, a 20% fall in forced expired volume in 1 second (FEV_1) is not obtained in many normal subjects. However, the real question is not why asthmatics respond, but why normal subjects do not. If the airway is taken out and put in a muscle bath, specimens from normal subjects respond very effectively to histamine or methacholine at very low concentrations [13,14]. In fact, several investigators have reported that there really is no difference in vitro between normal subjects and asthmatics in terms of methacholine or histamine sensitivity [14,15]. This suggests the possibility of some basic defect, perhaps one that could be hereditary.

There is a strong correlation between the degree of airway hyperresponsiveness and the severity of asthma [16,17]: the more severe the asthma, the greater the airway hyperresponsiveness. The slope of the dose–response curve is steeper and the degree of response greater, with the maximum fall being obviously larger, in patients with severe asthma than in those with milder asthma (Fig. 2). Several subjects may achieve a 20% fall in FEV_1, but with increasing concentrations of methacholine they reach a plateau and do not have a further drop in FEV_1. This plateau phenomenon is commonly seen in allergic rhinitis subjects (Fig. 2) [16]. In normal subjects, isoproterenol can return the FEV_1 to baseline following a methacholine challenge. Although some former asthmatics show a plateau phenomenon, the majority have a steep response. Former asthmatics as a group are about one-tenth as sensitive as current asthmatics [16]. We have previously compared the bronchodilating response to isoproterenol in former asthmatics with

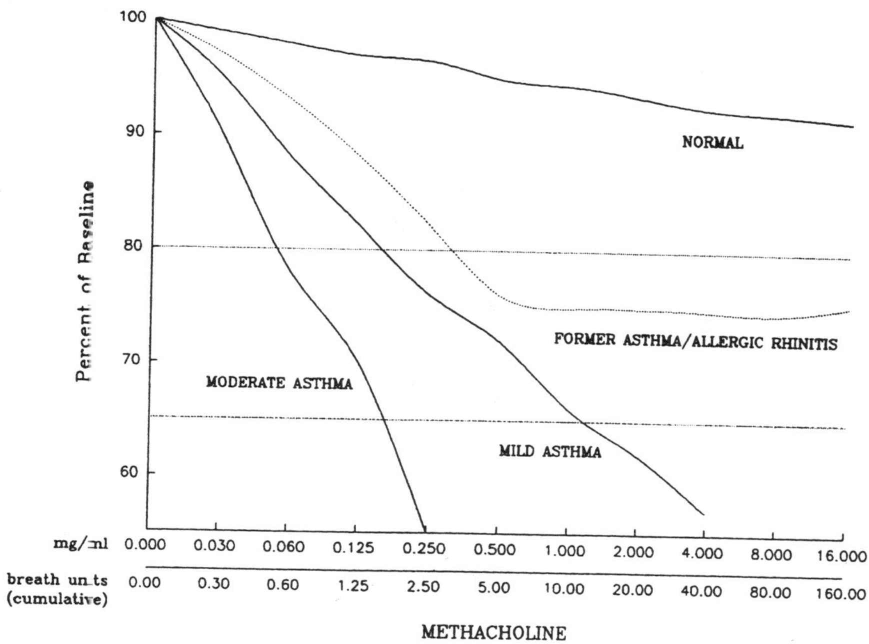

Figure 2 Typical dose–response curves to methacholine in subjects with moderate and mild asthma, in subjects with past asthma (no wheezing for at least 12 months) or allergic rhinitis, and in a normal subject.

that of normal subjects [16]. The former asthmatics have a greater response to methacholine, even though the methacholine dose is much lower in this group. However, isoproterenol is considerably less effective in counteracting bronchoconstriction [16]. The effect of a bronchodilator as a physiological antagonist seems to relate to the degree of bronchoconstriction rather than the amount of methacholine administered.

A. Genetic Studies Using Measurement of Airway Hyperresponsiveness

1. Family Studies

A number of studies, both of families and of twins, have used measures of bronchial hyperresponsiveness to help establish a genetic link to asthma. Rachelefsky et al. [17] have previously reported HLA associations in subjects who respond to a bronchodilator. A positive response was considered an indicator of increased bronchial responsiveness. In their report, there was not an HLA association in families in which the child with asthma was also allergic, but there was an association between HLA antigen and increased bronchial responsiveness.

To determine whether methacholine sensitivity could be used as a potential genetic marker, we studied 750 subjects from 53 asthma families and 26 control families [18,19]. The asthma families were defined as having a proband with current bronchial asthma between the ages of 6 and 25. Both parents had to participate in the testing, and there had to be a minimum of seven family members to qualify for the study. The control families were usually neighbors of the asthma families and were of the same age group and had no atopic disease, atopic eczema, allergic rhinitis, or bronchial asthma for three generations. Probands from both groups of families were removed from the analysis. We measured the area under the dose–response curve using the best-fit parabolic curve [20]. Subjects who had a highly positive response were very sensitive to methacholine and had a small area under the parabolic dose–response curve. We used a 35% fall in FEV_1 as an end point to take into consideration the plateau phenomenon that occurs in some allergic rhinitis subjects. Thus, if the test was stopped at the 20% fall in FEV_1, it would be clearly recorded as a strongly positive reaction. When plateau responders inhaled more methacholine, however, their fall in FEV_1 stabilized and did not fall any farther. This allowed us to separate those subjects from current asthmatics, who do not show a plateau phenomenon. A negative study was defined as one having less than a 20% fall in FEV_1 after 800 cumulative breath units of methacholine. Table 1 compares area and cumulative dose in breath units. A subject who had a 20% fall in FEV_1 with 50 breath units or less would have a maximum area of 306, whereas one with a medium response, with a 20% fall in FEV_1 at 200 breath units or less, would have an area of up to 1225. The standard diagnostic method goes up to only 200 cumulative breath units [21,22].

Table 1 Characterization of Methacholine Inhalation Response

Category	% Drop in FEV_1	Cumulative dose	Area under the curve
High	⩾20%	0–5	0–306
Medium	⩾20%	51–200	306–1225
Low	⩾20%	201–800	1225–4000
Negative	<20%	>800	4000–5600

FEV_1 = forced expired volume in 1 second.

Most children with asthma in our family study responded to 50 breath units or less (Fig. 3). The few nonresponders were former asthmatics, who by definition had been free of all symptoms for at least a year. The preponderance of normal children from the normal families failed to react, even at 800 breath units.

If we analyze the pediatric population from these families, the best sensitivity and specificity was found at about 100 breath units [23]. However, if we look at the total population, the best sensitivity and specificity is at 200 breath units [18]. This

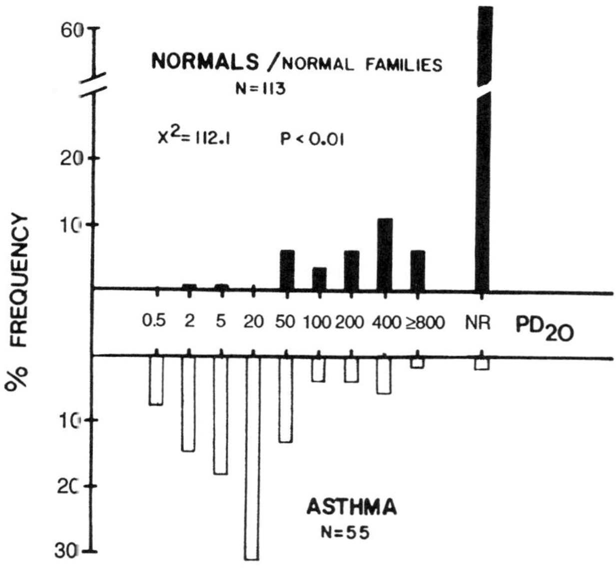

Figure 3 Frequency plot of methacholine sensitivity in normal subjects from the nonatopic families versus asthmatic subjects from the asthma families. The PD_{20} is the provocative dose of methacholine in breath units.

difference in sensitivity and specificity illustrates that normal young children have greater bronchial reactivity [24–26].

Data for the whole population studied are shown in Fig. 4 [18]. The asthmatics, for the most part, reacted by 50 breath units or less, but some asthmatics did not react until 200 breath units. Only 6% of the allergic rhinitis subjects show a high positive response, but about 30% of them would overlap with asthmatics in that they reacted with 200 breath units or less. There is a group of nonatopic subjects from asthma families who responded by 200 breath units, but there was a significantly lower percentage from normal families [18].

Results for the normal nonatopic subjects from the asthma families vs. the normal subjects from the nonatopic families are shown in Fig. 5. This shows a subgroup of subjects from asthma families who respond to methacholine and who are siblings of asthmatics [18,27]. These responders are perhaps at greater risk for subsequent development of asthma. The normal subjects from normal families show a unimodal distribution. However, the normal subjects from the asthma families clearly show a bimodal response. When we compared the characteristics

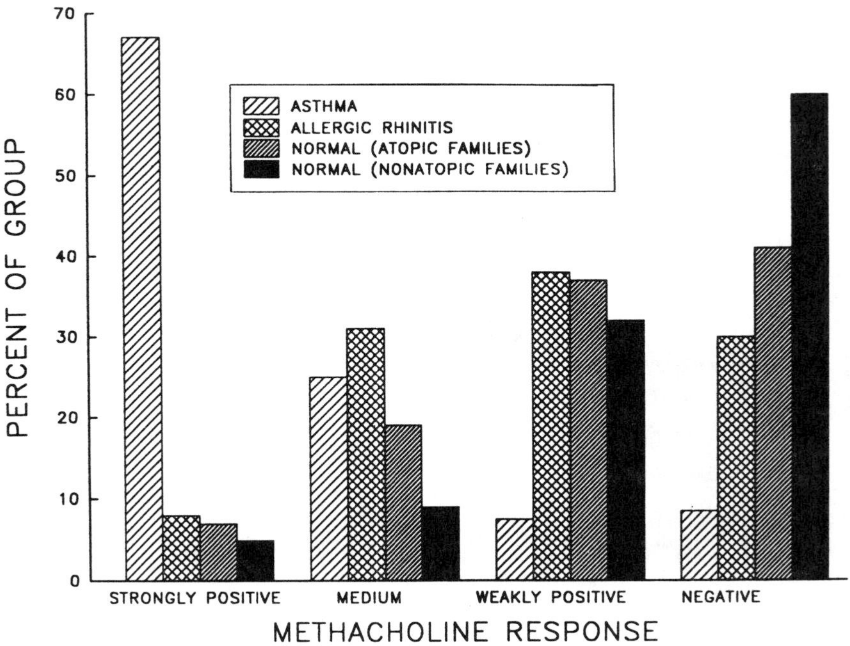

Figure 4 Frequency of high, medium, low, and negative response to methacholine in subjects with asthma or allergic rhinitis and their normal relatives. Matched normal subjects are shown for comparison.

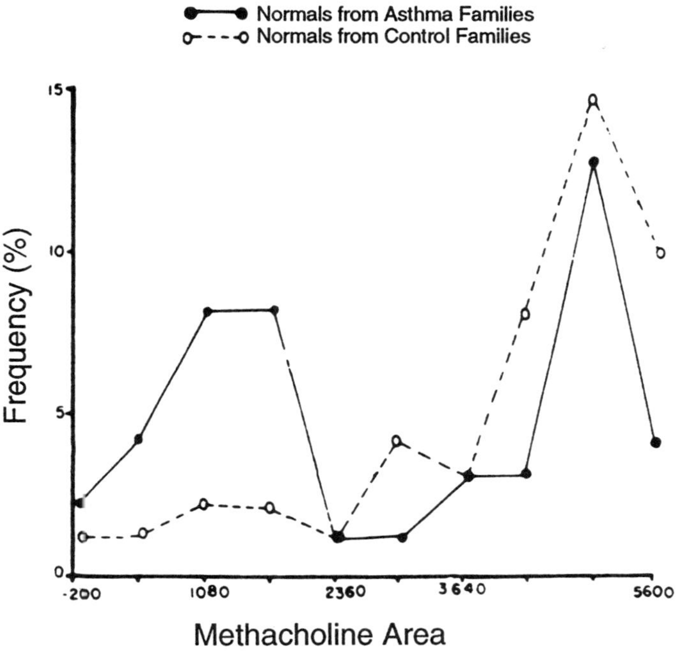

Figure 5 Frequency plot of age-correlated area under dose–response curves for methacholine in normal subjects from both asthmatic and control families. Left-hand mode shows excess number of positive responders from asthmatic families.

of the responders and the nonresponders, there was no difference in the sex distribution, mean age, or serum IgE. There was a slight difference in the total intradermal skin test score, and although this was statistically significant, these scores are small compared with the scores of subjects with known atopic disease.

Data for the parents of the normal children from the nonatopic families and the parents of the children with asthma are shown in Fig. 6 [28,29]. All asthmatic subjects were eliminated for the purpose of comparison. The parents of the normal children from the normal families demonstrate a unimodal distribution. The figure clearly shows a bimodal distribution of the parents of the asthma families. When we compared these groups, there was no difference in sex distribution, age, or serum IgE, but again there was a slight but significant difference in the total skin test score [29]. The parents of asthmatics who did respond had a somewhat greater total intradermal skin test score. This bimodal distribution of airway reactivity in the nonatopic siblings of asthmatics and in nonatopic parents of asthmatic children would suggest a single physiological or perhaps a single genetic abnormality. Consistent with these results is the report by Longo et al. [30], who also found

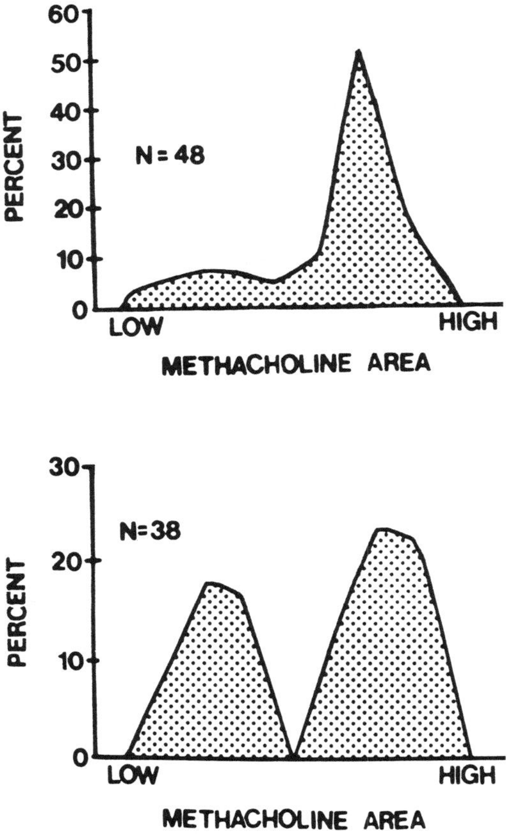

Figure 6 Distribution of methacholine area responses in the subjects studied. The four categories of responses were arbitrarily determined: marked bronchial responsiveness, up to 80 breath units (BU); moderate, up to 340 (BU); minimal, up to 800 (BU); negative, not more than a 19.9% fall in FEV_1 by 800 (BU). (Adapted from Ref. 29 and Townley, R. G., Hopp, R. J., Bewtra, A. K., and Nair, N. M., Airway reactivity in asthmatic families and twins, in *Provocative Challenge Procedures: Background and Methodology* [S. L. Spector, ed.], Futura Publishing, Mount Kisco, NY, 1989.)

bimodal distribution of airway reactivity in parents of asthmatic children but not in control parents. In our study, however, a simple genetic effect was not evident, because segregation analysis of these families excluded a single-gene mechanism [19,27]. However, we could not exclude a strictly environmental effect either. Airway reactivity appears to be determined by both genetic and environmental factors. It is our conclusion that its inheritance is due to a polygenetic mechanism.

After the publication of Townley et al. [19], a reanalysis of the asthma and nonasthma families was performed in late 1990 by Drs. Alex Wilson and Robert Elston at Louisiana State University. New asthma families, studied from 1985 to 1990 and not included in the original segregation analysis [19], were included in the reanalysis. The reanalysis was performed under Bonney's class A regressive model [31]. This model allows for a certain amount of environmental correlation and multifactorial transmission from one generation to the next. The results showed that the phenotype of the offspring (increased BHR) depends to some extent on the parental phenotype. These dependencies cannot be completely accounted for by a single major locus. There may be more than one major locus, polygenic inheritance, a culturally transmitted environmental effect, or perhaps a mixture of these mechanisms.

A recent report further confirms that familial aggregation of increased nonspecific bronchial responsiveness, Clifford et al. [32] studied 50 children who had one parent with asthma. These children had a 50% increase in respiratory symptoms of cough, wheeze, and shortness of breath when compared with control subjects. Over 90% of the asthmatic parents responded to methacholine with a 20% fall in FEV_1 by 6.4 μmol, while 45% of the children had similar responses.

Although methacholine and histamine challenges are the most sensitive indicators of nonspecific bronchial reactivity, other tests are available. Exercise challenges have been used to determine the degree of bronchial lability in relatives of asthmatics. Konig and Godfrey [33] reported exercise challenge and skin test results in 65 first-degree relatives of 12 children with asthma. A positive index for enhanced bronchial lability was obtained for 10 of the 12 asthmatic children, 50% of family members with a current history of asthma, 33% of the family members with a past history of asthma, 40% of those with hay fever, and 32% of the healthy relatives, while 48% of subjects with at least one positive skin test responded. Overall, 28 of the 65 family members responded. Although a control group was not included, it is impressive that many nonasthmatic subjects responded to a challenge that generally is considered not to be as sensitive as methacholine.

In a review of autonomic abnormalities of cystic fibrosis, Davis [34] mentioned that the cholinergic dysfunction seen in asthmatics is also seen in healthy first-degree relatives of cystic fibrosis patients. These abnormal findings include pupillary dysfunction in response to carbachol and increased nonspecific bronchial reactivity. Although not yet investigated in detail, this would suggest a genetic basis for the autonomic abnormalities seen in these two diseases.

2. Twin Studies

Although there are limitations in using the twin model to examine the influence of heredity, genetic analysis of twins remains an accessible and practical method of estimating the weight of genetic influence on clinically measurable parameters. This is true because members of a monozygous pair share a genotype and a relatively similar environment. By comparing clinical or laboratory parameters of a disease condition in monozygous (MZ) twins and dizygous (DZ) twins, it is possible to provide evidence for the genetic determination of those parameters, under reasonable assumptions [35].

The comparison of intrapair correlation coefficients (*r*) provides an indicator of the role of heredity as a clinical marker of atopic disease or bronchial hyperresponsiveness. An estimate of heritability (H), 2 (*r*MZ−*r*DZ), has been used [36]. It provides an estimation of the contribution of heredity to the variance of the measured trait or marker. When H equals 1, the variance of the measurement is due completely to heredity. As H approaches zero, the variance of the measurement is presumed to be determined by environmental factors. In addition, pair- and casewise (proband) concordance rates are commonly used to express the results of twin data [37]

Measurements of bronchial reactivity can be compared in twins. At the Children's Asthma Research Institute, a twin study by Falliers et al. [38] reported that in the decade from 1960 to 1970, 11 asthmatics had an unaffected fraternal twin at home. During the same period, three identical twin pairs were seen, all with asthma. An additional two pairs of identical twins were found to be discordant for asthma diagnosis. Both pairs were atopic and had similar IgE levels. Only the asthmatic twins responded to an exercise challenge. Both asthmatics responded to methacholine, as expected. Neither of the nonasthmatic twins had a methacholine response. The authors suggested that longitudinal studies of identical twins discordant for asthma diagnosis would be valuable.

Konig and Godfrey [39] used a standardized exercise challenge to compare eight identical (five male pairs) and seven nonidentical twin pairs (five male–female, one male–male and one female–female). They found that six pairs of the MZ twins were concordant for exercise lability, while only one of the DZ pairs was concordant.

In our twin studies (Fig. 7a,b), the correlation of methacholine area in 61 pairs of MZ and 47 pairs of DZ twins were determined. Methacholine challenge in the study, as in our family study, is presented using an area under the best-fit parabolic curve [20]. The end point is a 35% fall in the FEV_1. The cumulative dose of methacholine is 800 breath units. All subjects have a quantitative value for their challenge, even if there was a 0% change by the last step [20]. We examined these 108 pairs of twins and observed a significantly greater correlation coefficient of methacholine sensitivity in the MZ twins (0.67) than in the DZ twins (0.34) [40].

We also compared serum IgE levels in the MZ and the DZ twins and found a higher correlation coefficient in the MZ twins. The heritability estimate for IgE was 0.61, and for methacholine sensitivity it was 0.66 [40]. If the variance in these measurements were strictly genetic, this heritability estimate ought to be 1.0. If it were strictly environmental, the heritability estimate would be zero. Thus, our results suggest that there is an important inherited component to both airway reactivity and serum IgE levels.

A study by Zamel [41] of 10 pairs of MZ and 10 pairs of DZ twins did not find a major genetic influence on nonspecific bronchial reactivity. The author had no explanation as to why there was not a better correlation in MZ twins as compared with DZ twins. He suggested that a larger group of twins needed to be studied with his methodology before definitive conclusions are drawn. This study was performed on healthy adults, in contrast to the larger group of twins studied by Hopp et al. [40], who had asthmatic, allergic, and normal histories. This difference in populations may account for the disparity of the reported results.

A recent report provides a unique insight into the genetic contribution to pulmonary function as reflected in twin studies. Ackerman et al. [42] investigated 39 twin pairs at a mean age of 11.4 months. Included were 25 MZ and 14 DZ pairs. A positive family history of asthma was found in 30% of the infants. Pulmonary function in the infants was determined in a sleep state, and the measurements of maximal expiratory functional residual capacity (FRC) were performed with rapid chest compression. There was greater intrapair variation in pulmonary measurements between DZ twins than between MZ twins. Similar findings had previously been reported for a large population of adult twins in a study using standard pulmonary function testing [43].

Bronchial hyperresponsiveness is not only a characteristic of asthma, as it is often found in allergic rhinitis subjects [1] and in some nonasthmatic members of asthmatics' families [44]. A strong association between atopic dermatitis and bronchial hyperresponsiveness has been observed [45]. These investigators observed that 18 of 22 children with atopic dermatitis who never had asthma achieved a PD_{20} to histamine, with a median PD_{20} of 0.22μmol. A recent report suggests the presence of BHR usually precedes the development of clinically identifiable asthma [3].

3. Effect of Age on Bronchial Hyperresponsiveness

It is probable that all humans have increased BHR at birth. Recent evidence suggests that infants and very young children, nearly universally, will demonstrate an exaggerated response to inhaled bronchoconstrictor [46,47]. This response diminishes with advancing age [24,46]. It is our hypothesis that a factor or factors, probably genetic existing within asthma families, slow or halt this "natural" reduction in BHR.

We have investigated this effect of age on methacholine sensitivity in a population study of over 750 subjects [24]. When methacholine responsiveness is plotted against age (Fig. 8) for subjects who have no history of asthma, it can be very easily appreciated that the younger and older subjects have significantly increased bronchial responsiveness. If this factor is not taken into account in clinical practice, there could be a tendency to suggest falsely the presence of hyperresponsive airways in these populations. Dave et al. [48] have shown that allergic nonasthmatic children have increased nonspecific bronchial responsiveness and that this increased bronchial responsiveness persists over time. They

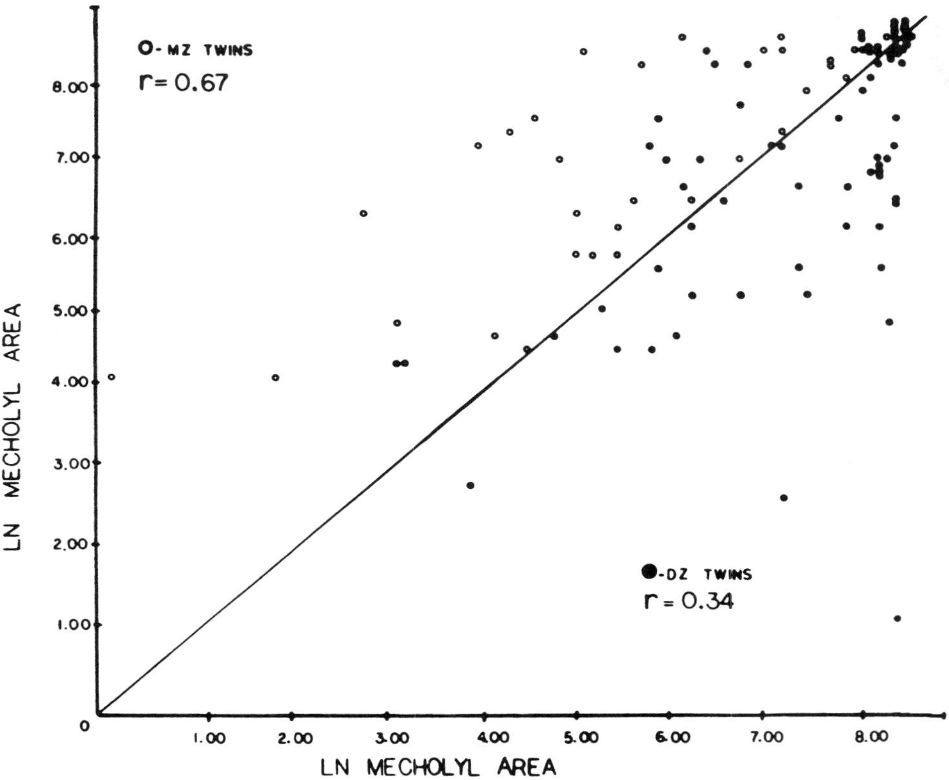

(a)

Figure 7 **(a)** Intrapair correlation of methacholine (metholyl) sensitivity as determined by the area under the dose–response curve. Methacholine area expressed as the natural log shows a correlation coefficient of 0.67 in monozygous (MZ) twins and 0.34 in dizygous (DZ) twins. **(b)** Intrapair correlation of serum immunoglobulin E (IgE) expressed as the natural log. Serum IgE shows a correlation coefficient of 0.825 in the MZ twins and 0.52 in the DZ twins. (From Ref. 29.)

postulate that it is possible that persons with allergies and family members of asthmatic subjects "retain" this enhanced bronchial responsiveness, thus increasing their chance of developing asthma. This would require that increased bronchial responsiveness precede the development of asthma symptoms. Very few large or small prospective studies have been undertaken to date to evaluate this. Hopp and colleagues [3] evaluated 20 children with increased bronchial reactivity over several years and were able to show that 17 of them went on to develop symptoms of asthma years later. However, they also found three subjects in their population

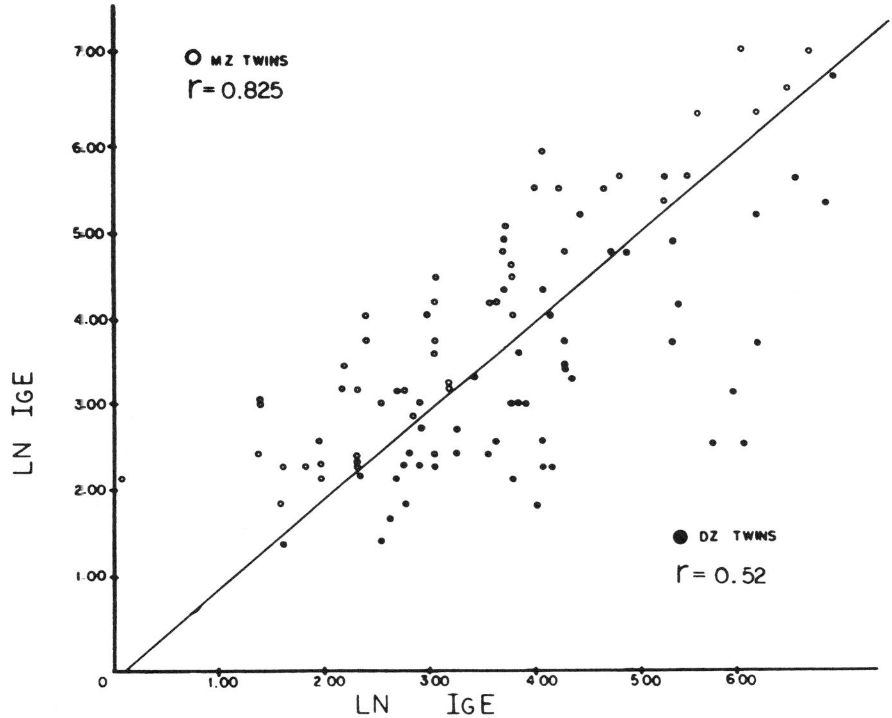

(b)

studies who developed asthma but had had a completely normal methacholine response before the development of symptoms. Sears and colleagues [49] have also been able to show that increased airway responsiveness preexisted in children who later became clinically asthmatic. Although not conclusive, these studies suggest that airway hyperresponsiveness may be genetically determined.

4. Studies in Animals: Dogs, Guinea Pigs and Mice

Animal models of asthma have demonstrated increased nonspecific bronchial responsiveness. Basenjii-greyhound (BG) crosses have proved a valuable animal model. Each breed has minimal or no BHR inherently, but the BG dog does have inherent BHR [50]. The basenjii dog and the BG dog often have atopic dermatitis, although nonatopic BG dogs can have BHR. This suggests an epistatic interaction between at least two genes. Neither a recessive, dominant, nor polygenic model is sufficient. The simplest hypothesis is a dominant mode of inheritance but with penetrance as a function of genetic background.

Studies using mice have shown that specific strains have an increased airway

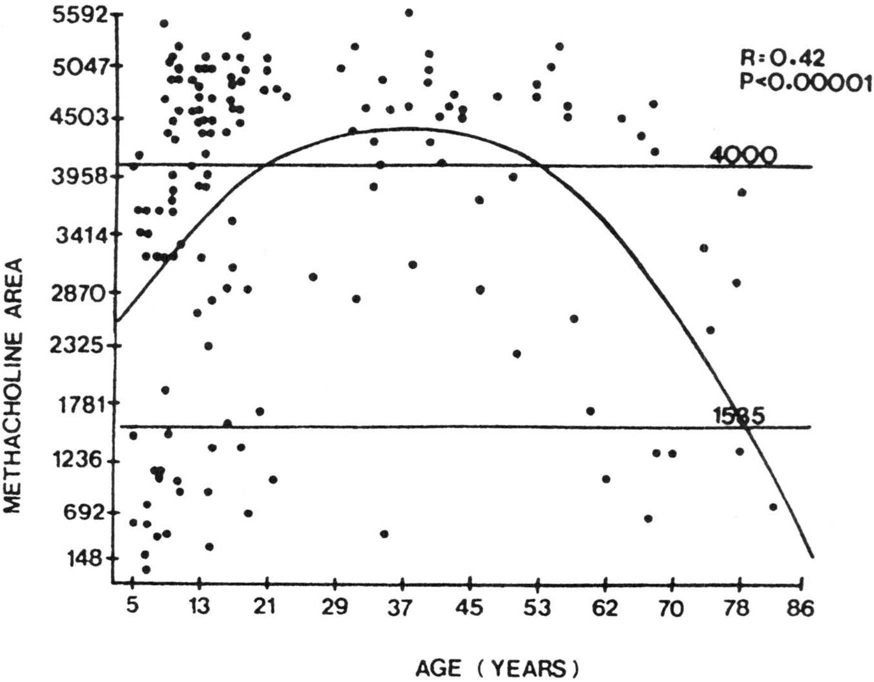

Figure 8 Methacholine responses of subjects studied. Results ≥4000 indicate normal responses. Values ≤1535 indicate values that are ≤200 bu breath units of methacholine. The best-fitting curve is superimposed. (Adapted from Ref. 24.)

response to histamine and serotonin, and that others are totally unresponsive. Experiments with breeding between strains have shown a genetic susceptibility to BHR in mice [9] that is not associated with atopy. Nevertheless, marked strain differences in sensitivity to histamine, serotonin, and methacholine exist in mice and guinea pigs [10,11]. Furthermore, the ability to induce sensitivity to antigens or to pharmacological mediators following various biological manipulations, as with pertussis toxin or β-adrenergic blocking agents, is also under genetic control [10,11].

Guinea pig models are similar to human asthmatic patients, with airways that are sensitive to histamine, methacholine, and serotonin. This sensitivity can be enhanced with β-adrenergic blockade. In strains resistant to airway β-blockade, combining β-blockade with an α-agonist can overcome resistance [51]. Two strains of guinea pig, the Hartley strain and the Trapani–Campbell strain, show airway responsiveness to serotonin, histamine, or methacholine.

In tests with the Hartley guinea pig (Fig. 9), the time to onset of severe dyspnea

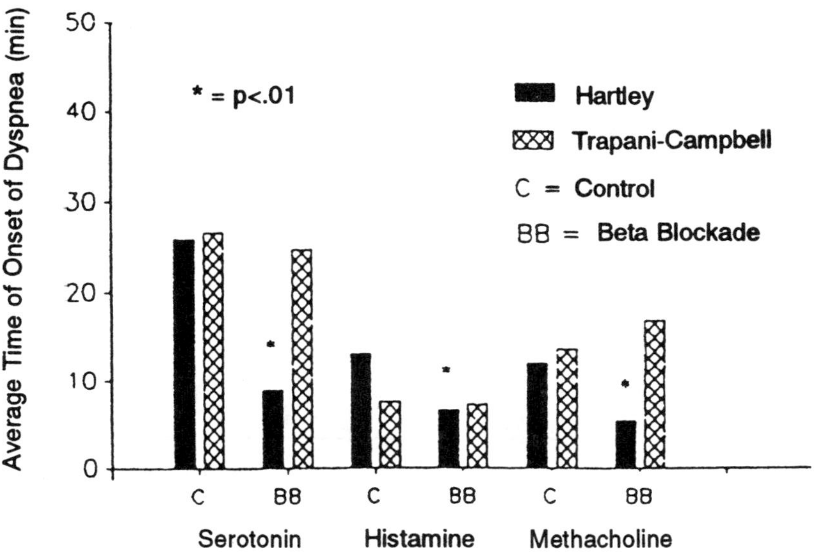

Figure 9 Bronchial sensitivity to serotonin, histamine, and methacholine in β-adrenergically blocked guinea pigs.

after inhalation of serotonin, histamine, or methacholine was significantly decreased when this strain was pretreated with a β-adrenergic blocking agent. This is analogous to the effect of β-adrenergic blocking agents in asthmatics [52]. In the Trapani–Campbell strain, however, the β-blocker alone did not induce significant increased reactivity to serotonin, histamine, or to methacholine.

Townley et al. [12,51] investigated the sensitivity of different mice strains to histamine. In the CFW mouse strain, sensitization by pertussis toxin or with a low dose of the β-blocker sotalol (Mj 1999) followed by histamine challenge resulted in the death of all the mice. In contrast, in CF_1 mice, a strain resistant to pertussis toxin, the same low dose of β-blocker was not lethal. With a high dose, however, resistance to histamine is overcome and there is a mortality rate of 80% (Fig. 10). The obese hyperglycemic mouse, a genetic strain that has been used to study type II diabetes, is resistant to sensitivity to histamine induced by a high dose of β-adrenergic blocker. In contrast, normal littermates of these obese hyperglycemic mice (Fig. 10) are sensitive to histamine following a high dose of β-adrenergic blocker.

Animal strain or breed selectivity makes it difficult to extrapolate to humans evidence from an animal model of a strict genetic basis for BHR [8]. The wide variety of (direct) pharmacological (e.g., histamine) and (indirect) physical stimuli (e.g., distilled water) used in humans and animals to evoke bronchocon-

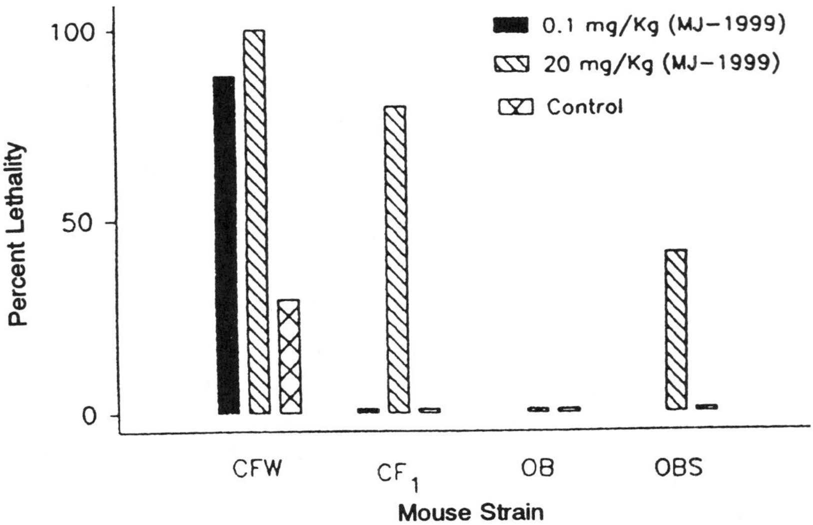

Figure 10 The effect of the obese-hyperglycemic syndrome on the histamine-sensitizing activity of β-adrenergic blockade in mice of different strains. OB is the obese strain, OBS their nonobese littermates.

striction does not clarify our understanding of genetic mechanisms responsible for BHR. Animal models and human studies all strongly suggest the hypothesis of genetic control of BHR. The pattern of inheritance is unclear, and it is unlikely that epidemiological studies will resolve the issues. Linkage analysis performed under a variety of genetic hypotheses is the necessary next step. Since the evidence is strong that BHR is somehow associated with asthma, it is essential to gain understanding of the sources of variation of BHR. Well-designed experiments might then target the full asthma phenotype.

III. GENETICS OF IMMUNOGLOBULIN E AND CYTOKINES

A. Specific Immunoglobulin E (Atopy)

The majority of pediatric-age asthmatics are concomitantly atopic. In the United States, upward of 75% of asthmatics will develop their initial symptoms before age 20. The presence of an atopic disease, such as allergic rhinitis, has a strong genetic determination [53,54]. The ability to generate an IgE response to a specific antigen has been conclusively shown to be associated with specific HLA loci [55].

In two reports [56,57], subjects in nuclear and extended families were labeled as atopic if the subject had an IgE level greater than 2 standard deviations above the mean, if they had one or more positive skin tests, or if they had one or more positive radioallergosorbent IgE tests (RAST). The analysis suggested that the inclination to develop atopy is inherited as an autosomal dominant trait, and in seven families the transmission of atopy was linked to a specific DNA polymorphism (p lambda MS.51, D11S97) assigned to chromosome 11q. Two recent reports [58,59] were *not* able to confirm the linkage between D11s97 of chromosome 11q and atopy. Bronchial hyperreactivity was not linked to 11q in the report by Lympany et al. [58], in which families failed to conform to the dominant model (segregation analysis by SAGE). However, Cookson et al. [60] have recently analyzed maternally derived alleles from 155 sibling pairs affected by atopy to seek evidence of linkage between the gene predisposing to atopy and other markers on chromosome 11q13. They found that the β subunit of the high-affinity receptor for IgE (FcξRI-β) also lies on chromosome 11q13, and that it is in close genetic linkage with the gene for atopy. The known roles of FcξRI in antigen-induced mast cell degranulation and in the release of cytokines that enhance IgE production make the gene for its β subunit a candidate for the chromosome 11 atopy locus. The localization of the atopy locus, under a model of maternal inheritance, included the markers cCI11-319, a cosmid clone, CD20, a lymphocyte surface marker, and FcξRI-β, but excluded DIIS97 (pms51), with which linkage to atopy was originally described. These investigators also found that paternal transmission of atopy does not occur at the chromosome 11q13 locus. At present, the exact localization of gene(s) for the predilection to be atopic (IgE) is in question. The original observation linking atopy with chromosome 11 needs further investigation.

B. Cytokines, Immunoglobulin E, and Atopy

In subjects with genetic inclination to be atopic, serum IgE levels are regulated by a complex interaction of CD4+ and CD8+ lymphocytes. CD4+ lymphocytes release interleukin-4 (IL-4) which induces isotope switching in B lymphocytes to produce IgE antibodies [61]. Interleukin-4 is necessary for human IgE production but requires an additional signal [62]. In humans, a variety of second IgE-inducing signals have been isolated, which work in concert with IL-4 in the induction of IgE synthesis. Second signals include cognate T/B cell interaction, EBV, and hydrocortisone.

Mouse strains have been shown to have a T-helper population (TH_2) preferentially producing cytokines (IL-4 and IL-5) that induce a response to parasites [63]. A recent study in human atopic asthmatics showed significant increases in TH_2-like bronchoalveolar lavage fluid cytokines, in comparison with normal subjects, including IL-4, IL-5, and granulocyte-macrophage colony-stimulating factor (GM-CSF) [64]. The presence of specific phenotypically different human CD4+

T cells has not been clearly established to date, although T cell clones from mite-sensitive subjects produce IL-4 and IL-5 on exposure to mite allergen [65]. These clones provide B cell help for IgE production. Exogenous IL-4 added to TH_1 (non-IL-4/5 clones) induces these clones to produce IL-4. In humans, the genetic drive to produce a TH_2-like cytokine pool (IL-4, IL-5, IL-3, GM-CSF) in response to allergen exposure is highly probable. However, Marsh et al. [66] reported that in 77 unrelated Caucasians there was no association between the total serum IgE level and the repeat sequence within intron 2 of the IL-4 gene (chromosome 5q). It is possible that another gene(s) controls the output (suppression or augmentation) of the IL-4 (and IL-5) gene region.

The onset of asthma in adults has often been linked to intrinsic, presumably nonatopic, factors. Two recent reports [67,68] from a large epidemiological study suggested that IgE levels have a highly significant association with, and are even a risk factor in, adult-onset asthma, despite the absence of positive skin tests in adult asthmatics. Both extrinsic and intrinsic asthmatics have IL-5, IL-3, and GM-CSF in increased amounts in their sera, at concentrations that increase eosinophil survival in vitro [69]. The measurement of cytokine levels from intrinsic and extrinsic asthmatics showed elevated levels of IL-4 and IL-5 in extrinsic asthmatics, and of IL-2 and IL-5 in intrinsic asthmatics [70]. These data would suggest an immunological difference between extrinsic and intrinsic asthma. The mechanism could involve a combination of genetic, autoimmune, allergic, and environmental factors.

The presence of biochemical markers of increased specific or total IgE appears to be intimately associated with the clinical condition of extrinsic asthma. The regulation of IgE response and its association with the asthmatic phenotype is critical.

IV. INCREASED BASOPHIL (MAST CELL) HISTAMINE RELEASE

The principles important to basophil histamine release may not directly relate to mast cells, although the concepts have general applicability. Mast cells are considered to play a critical role in the IgE-mediated early-phase response to allergens, and, equally important, basophils play a role in the late-phase response in asthma and other atopic diseases [71]. The histamine-containing cells in the late asthmatic, nasal, and skin responses contain CD18, a leukocyte antigen, indicating that they are basophils. Basophil releasability suggests that, in addition to IgE, other events affect the ability of basophils (and mast cells) to release mediators in response to stimuli [72]. The basophils found during the late phase appear; to be "activated," and their spontaneous histamine release is enhanced.

A study of basophil histamine releasibility in twins found a significant intrapair correlation in identical twins, but not in nonidentical twins, suggesting a genetic influence [73]. The intrinsic releasability of basophils appears to be enhanced by IL-3 and mononuclear cell–derived peptides termed histamine-releasing factor (HRF). This is especially seen in atopic subjects [74]. The action of HRF is dependent on surface IgE [75]. Histamine-Releasing Inhibitor Factors (HRIF) are mononuclear cell–derived products that turn off histamine and mediator release from basophils [74]. Diminished production of these inhibitors would enhance the atopic (and potentially asthmatic) state.

V. EOSINOPHILIA

Increased peripheral blood eosinophilia and the presence of sputum eosinophilia is a common clinical observation in both intrinsic and extrinsic asthma, and atopic (nonasthmatic) subjects generally have elevated blood eosinophilia. In asthma, the eosinophils are attracted to the target organ (lungs) through a complicated interaction of mediators released during the early- and late-phase pulmonary response to allergen (extrinsic asthma). The presence of eosinophils in subjects with asthma but without atopic triggers (intrinsic) is not totally understood, but potentially suggests a genetic predilection in factors responsible for eosinophil regulation. Eosinophil progenitors in the bone marrow are regulated by cytokines (IL-5, IL-3 and GM-CSF) released by lymphocytes (TH_2) from asthmatics [69]. T cell–derived lymphokines extend the half-life of eosinophils in both intrinsic and extrinsic asthmatics [67,70]. The regulation of eosinophils by lymphocyte-derived cytokines has been extensively investigated in the mouse, utilizing different genetic strains [63].

Bronchial biopsies of asthmatics demonstrate CD4+ cells, and studies of these lymphocytes, utilizing in situ hybridization techniques, demonstrate mRNA for IL-5 [76]. The CD4+ lymphocytes, presumably of the TH_2 subtype, play a focal role in the generation and potentiation of certain recognized characteristics of asthma (e.g., eosinophilia, specific IgE, and increased basophil releasibility).

The presence of sputum and blood eosinophilia in essentially all asthmatics, especially adults, and the diagnostic importance of eosinophilia in distinguishing between chronic obstructive pulmonary disease and asthma in adults, adds to the relevance of the genetic control of the lymphocyte cell subtype and cytokines responsible for eosinophil regulation.

VI. T CELLS AND MACROPHAGES

As discussed above, the T lymphocyte, particularly the CD4+ T cell, has a focal prominence in the regulation of the characteristics seen in asthma and of the cells responsible for the inflammatory component of asthma [64]. Chronic asthma has been termed "chronic eosinophilic bronchitis," and appears to represent a "delayed-type" hypersensitivity, with (sensitized) lymphocytes regulating eosinophil traffic (extrinsic and intrinsic asthma) and IgE production (extrinsic and possibly intrinsic asthma). Of critical importance are the potential genetic differences in the pro-atopy (proinflammatory) cytokine profile (IL-3, IL-4, IL-5, and GM-CSF; IL-2 in intrinsic asthma) in asthmatics and its genetic regulation.

In severely atopic subjects there is an increased percentage of monocytes and macrophages that have surface IgE Fc positivity. Macrophages reside at the critical air–surface interface, and the presence of IgE on macrophage surfaces may be critical in asthma. Macrophages have the ability to release LTB_4 and platelet activating factor, both eosinophil chemo-attractants. Interferon-γ alters macrophage function. This lymphokine, as well as IL-4, may regulate IgE receptor density on lung macrophages [77].

VII. ADRENERGIC RECEPTOR DYSFUNCTION AND PHOSPHODIESTERASE

β-adrenergic hyporesponsiveness has been demonstrated in allergic subjects without asthma and in asthmatics off medication. This could be due to either a decrease in the density of β-adrenoceptors or a defect at a postreceptor site, or both. Exogenous β-agonists or endogenous catecholamines may further down-regulate these receptors. It has been suggested that this refractoriness is a general defect in atopy, and both pre–adenylate cyclase and post–adenylate cyclase factors may be involved. Recent work has shown both salbutamol (homologous) and prostaglandin E (heterologous) stimulation of cAMP production in asthmatics is deficient, suggesting a non-β_2-receptor defect [78]. Since "β-receptor hyporesponsiveness" is probably not directly caused by intrinsic defect(s) in the β-receptor itself, it would suggest potential defects in the signal transduction pathway involving guanine nucleotide regulatory protein, adenylate cyclase enzyme, or even phosphodiesterase (PDE). The basenji-greyhound dog model demonstrates a role for PDE levels in the pathogenesis of the atopic phenotype of this animal [79]. Phosphodiesterase levels are increased in the cross-breed, intermediate in the basenji, and low in the greyhound. Increased PDE activity has been demonstrated in atopic dermatitis and allergic rhinitis subjects [80].

Phosphodiesterase inhibitors are under clinical investigation in asthma [81]. Five isoenzyme types of PDE are recognized, with PDE_4 having the highest affinity for cAMP. Studies of PDE_4 levels in basal U-937 cells showed that exogenous β-agonists increased PDE_4 levels in a time- and dose-dependent manner [82]. This suggests an important functional link between β-agonists and the PDE_4 level. The five isoenzymes are coded by distinct but probably related genes. The genetic profile for PDE in asthmatics or allergic subjects is yet unknown.

VIII. OTHER GENETIC FACTORS

Other genetic associations have been seen in asthma and may play a potential role. Biochemical markers have been studied to determine their connection with asthma. Mano et al. [83] investigated the association of 13 protein and blood enzyme markers in 127 asthmatic subjects and controls. There was a statistical difference in the distribution of α-antitrypsin types (more MS in the asthmatics) and the 6-PGD levels (approaching significance). An increase in bronchial hyperresponsiveness in MS but not in MM or MZ subjects from both asthma families and normal nonatopic families was found by Southard et al. [84]. Mano et al. [83] also found a possible difference in adenosine deaminase (ADA) levels between the two groups. A more definitive study with regard to ADA was subsequently reported [85]. The authors demonstrated the frequency of ADA phenotype 2-1 (random population frequency: 1-1 = 83%, 2-2 = 0.5%, 2-1 = 16%) is significantly reduced in "wheezers" as compared with controls. In a study of children with asthma, patients with increased asthma severity had diminished levels of the enzyme PAF-acetylhydrolase, and the family pedigree analysis suggested an autosomal recessive inheritance [86].

A review of HLA markers in asthma has recently been published [4]. A recent report [87] demonstrated an HLA association of DR3 with mite-sensitive asthmatics, and HLA-DPB1*040 provided protection against the development of asthma. However, further studies are necessary for confirmation.

IX. ENVIRONMENTAL FACTORS

Two factors commonly associated with onset of asthma include viral illness and exposure to tobacco smoke. Many asthmatics, especially children, have the onset of disease in association with viral illness. The roles of exposure to allergens and to viral illness in the development of asthma may have a common basis. It has been suggested [88,89] that in dogs and mice, simultaneous exposure to an allergen and a viral illness (adjuvant) is necessary to reduce immunological tolerance and promote IgE antibodies and clinical disease. A similar hypothesis has been proposed for humans [90]. Several respiratory viruses have been shown to induce an IgE response, including respiratory syncytial virus and parainfluenza virus.

Exposure to tobacco smoke has been shown to increase by twofold the risk for development asthma in children [67]. Although the mechanism is unknown, tobacco smoke exposure is known to increase IgE levels, although the effect of passive smoke exposure on IgE levels is controversial.

Other environmental factors of potential importance are socioeconomic factors, ozone exposure, and nonviral illnesses including chlamydiosis. Diesel particulates have been shown to act as an adjuvant agent for IgE production in mice. Inner city living conditions would also increase the exposure to animal and insect allergens, especially cockroach allergens.

X. CONCLUSION

On the basis of the information presented in this chapter, the following can be concluded:

1. Methacholine can determine the degree of bronchial reactivity, which is certainly a hallmark of asthma.
2. Just coming from an asthma family is a risk factor in terms of subsequent development of asthma and increased airway reactivity.
3. The parent data suggest that airway reactivity is transmitted to succeeding generations.
4. Studies of twins have revealed that the concordance of asthma is higher in monozygotic than in dizygotic twins, but environmental factors are at least as important as genetic factors.
5. Animal models of asthma comparing genetic strains can provide an important link between airway hyperresponsiveness and the allergic response.
6. The inheritance of asthma fits a polygenetic pattern rather than a single-gene pattern.

REFERENCES

1. Townley, R., and Hopp, R., Measurement and interpretation of nonspecific bronchial reactivity (editorial), *Chest*, *94*, 452–453 (1988).
2. Hopp, R., Bewtra, A., Nair, N., and Townley, R., Genetic aspects of bronchial hyperreactivity, in *Genetic and Environmental Factors in Clinical Allergy* (D. G. Marsh and M. Blumenthal, eds.), University of Minnesota Press, Minneapolis, 1990, pp. 143–152.
3. Hopp, R., Townley, R., Biven, R., Bewtra, A., and Nair, N., The presence of airway reactivity before the development of asthma, *Am Rev. Respir Dis.*, *141*, 2–8 (1990).
4. Hopp, R., and Townley, R., Genetics of asthma, in *Asthma as an Inflammatory Disease* (P. O'Byrne, ed.), Marcel Dekker, New York, 1990, pp. 49–70.
5. Cooke, R., and Vander Veer, A., Human sensitization, *J. Immunol.*, *1*, 201–305 (1916).
6. Rackemann, F., Studies in asthma, *Arch. Intern. Med.*, *41*, 346–369 (1928).
7. Bray, G., The hereditary factor in asthma and other allergies, *Br. Med. J.*, *1*, 384–387 (1930).
8. Townley, R., Bewtra, A., Nair, N., Brodkey, F., Watt, G., and Burke, K., Methacholine inhalation challenge studies, *J. Allergy Clin. Immunol.*, *64*(6 part 2), 569–574 (1979).
9. Wanner, A., Abraham, W., Douglas, J., Drazen, J., Richerson, H., and Sri Ram, J., Models of airway hyperresponsiveness, *Am. Rev. Respir. Dis.*, *141*, 253–257 (1990).
10. Levitt, R., Mitzner, W., and Kleeberger, S., A genetic approach to the study of lung

physiology: understanding biological variability in airway responsiveness, *Am. J. Physiol.*, *258*, L157–L164 (1990).
11. Townley, R., Trapani, I., and Szentivanyi, A., Sensitization to anaphylaxis and to some of its pharmacological mediators by blockade of the beta adrenergic receptors, *J. Allergy Clin. Immunol.*, *39*, 177–197 (1967).
12. Townley, R., Daley, D., and Selenke, W., The effect of agents used in the treatment of bronchial asthma on carbohydrate metabolism and histamine sensitivity after beta-adrenergic blockade, *J. Allergy Clin. Immunol.*, *45*, 71–86 (1970).
13. Adolphson, R., and Townley, R., A comparison of the beta-blocking activities of practolol, sotalol, and propranolol in human and guinea pig tracheal smooth muscle, *J. Allergy Clin. Immunol.*, *58*, 683–690 (1976).
14. Paterson, J., Lulich, K., and Goldie, R., The role of beta-adrenoceptors in bronchial hyperreactivity, in *Bronchial Reactivity* (J. Morley, ed.), Academic Press, New York, 1982, pp. 19–37.
15. Vincenc, K., Black, J., Yan, K., Armour, C., Donnelly, P., and Woolcock, A., Comparison of in vivo responses to histamine in human airways, *Am. Rev. Respir. Dis.*, *128*, 875–879 (1983).
16. Townley, R., Ryo, U., Kolotkin, B., and Kang, B., Bronchial sensitivity to methacholine in current and former asthmatic and allergic rhinitis patients and control subjects, *J. Allergy Clin. Immunol.*, *56*, 429–442 (1975).
17. Rachelefsky, G., Park, M., Siegels, S., Terasaki, P., Katz, R., and Saito, S., Strong association between β-lymphocyte group-2 specificity and asthma, *Lancet*, *ii*, 1042–1044 (1976).
18. Townley, R. G., and Bewtra, A. K., Airway reactivity to methacholine in asthma family members and twins, in *Provocative Challenge Procedures: Bronchial, Oral, Nasal, and Exercise* (S. Spector, ed.), CRC Press, Boca Raton, Florida, 1983, pp. 177–185.
19. Townley, R., Bewtra, A., Wilson, A., Hopp, R., Elston, R., Nair, N., and Watt, G. Segregation analysis of bronchial response to methacholine inhalation challenge in families with and without asthma, *J. Allergy Clin. Immunol.*, *77*, 101–107 (1986).
20. Hopp, R., Weiss, S., Nair, N., Bewtra, A., and Townley, R., Interpretation of the results of methacholine inhalation challenge tests, *J. Allergy Clin. Immunol.*, *80*, 821–824 (1987).
21. Chai, H., Farr, R., Froehlich, L., Mathison, D., McLean, J., Rosenthal, R., Seffer, A., Spector, S., and Townley, R., Standardization of bronchial inhalation challenge procedures, *J. Allergy Clin. Immunol.*, *58*, 323 (1975).
22. LaBraico, J., Reed, C., Rosenthal, R., Shapiro, G., Spector, S., and Townley, R., Multicenter evaluation of airways hyperreactivity using a standardized methacholine challenge, *J. Allergy Clin. Immunol.*, *73*, 124 (1984).
23. Hopp, R., Bewtra, A., Nair, N., Watt, G., and Townley, R., Methacholine inhalation challenge studies in a selected pediatric population, *Am. Rev. Respir. Dis.*, *134*, 994–998 (1986).
24. Hopp, R., Bewtra, A., Nair, N., and Townley, R., The effect of age on methacholine response, *J. Allergy Clin. Immunol.*, *76*, 609–613 (1985).
25. Flaherty, D., Geller, M., Surfus, J., Leo, G., Rankin, J., and Reed, C., HLA antigen

frequencies and natural history in Alternaria-sensitive and perennial nonallergic asthmatics, *J. Allergy Clin. Immunol.*, *66*, 408–416 (1980).
26. Tepper, R., Airway reactivity in infants: a positive response to methacholine and metaproterenol, *J. Appl. Physiol.*, *62*, 1155–1159 (1987).
27. Reed, C., and Townley, R., Asthma: classification and pathogenesis, in *Allergy: Principles and Practice*, 2nd Ed. (E. Middleton, C. Reed, and E. Ellis, eds.), C.V. Mosby, St. Louis, 1983, pp. 811–832.
28. Hopp, R., and Townley, R., Evidence that bronchial reactivity may be inherited, *Pediatr. Res.*, *19*(2), 248a (1985).
29. Hopp, R., Bewtra, A., Nair, N., and Townley, R., Bronchial reactivity patterns in nonasthmatic parents of asthmatics, *Ann. Allergy*, *61*, 184–186 (1988).
30. Longo, G., Strinati, R., Poli, F., and Fumi, F., Genetic factors in nonspecific bronchial hyperreactivity, *AJDC*, *141*, 331–334 (1987).
31. Bonney, A., On the statistical determination of major gene mechanisms in continuous human traits: regressive models, *Am. J. Med. Genet.*, *18*, 731–749 (1984).
32. Clifford, R., Pugsley, A., Radford, M., and Holgate, S., Symptoms, atopy, and bronchial response to methacholine in parents with asthma and their children, *Arch. Dis. Child.*, *62*, 66–73 (1987).
33. Konig, P., and Godfrey, S., Prevalence of exercise-induced bronchial lability in families of children with asthma, *Arch. Dis. Child.*, *48*, 513–518 (1973).
34. Davis, P., Physiological implications of the automatic aberrations in cystic fibrosis, *Horm. Metabol. Res.*, *18*, 217–220 (1986).
35. Haseman, J., and Elston, R., An estimation of genetic variance from twin data, *Behav. Genet.*, *1*, 11–19 (1970).
36. Woolf, C., *Principles of Biometry*, D. Van Nostrand, Princeton, New Jersey, 1968, pp. 230–231.
37. Allen, G., Harvald, B., and Sheilds, J., Measures of twin concordance, *Acta Genet. (Basel)*, *17*, 475–481 (1967).
38. Falliers, C., de A Cardoso, R., Bane, H., Coffey, R., and Middleton, E., Jr., Discordant allergic manifestations in monozygotic twins: genetic identity versus clinical, physiologic and biochemical differences, *J. Allergy*, *47*, 207–219 (1971).
39. Konig, P., and Godrey, S., Exercise-induced bronchial lability in monozygotic (identical) and dizygotic (nonidentical) twins, *J. Allergy Clin. Immunol.*, *54*, 280–287 (1974).
40. Hopp, R., Bewtra, A., Watt, G., Nair, N., and Townley, R., Genetic analysis of allergic disease in twins, *J. Allergy Clin. Immunol.*, *73*, 265–270 (1984).
41. Zamel, N., Leroux, M., and Vanderdoelen, J., Airway response to inhaled methacholine in healthy nonsmoking twins, *J. Appl. Physiol.*, *56*, 936–939 (1984).
42. Ackerman, V., Long, V., Hui, C., Eigen, H., and Tepper, R., Evaluation of pulmonary function in twin infants, *Am. Rev. Respir. Dis.*, *137*, 406 (1988).
43. Redline, S., Tishler, P., Lewitter, F., Tager, I., Munoz, A., and Speizer, F., Assessment of genetic and nongenetic influences in pulmonary function, *Am. Rev. Respir. Dis.*, *135*, 217–222 (1987).
44. Hopp, R., Bewtra, A., Nair, N., Biven, R., and Townley, R., Pattern of methacholine-

induced bronchial reactivity in siblings of asthmatic subjects, *Pediatr. Asthma Allergy Immunol.*, *1*, 103–109 (1987).
45. Salob, S., Laverty, A., and Atherton, D., Bronchial hyperresponsiveness in children with atopic dermatitis, *Pediatrics*, *91*, 13–16 (1993).
46. Montgomery, G., and Tepper, R., Changes in airway reactivity with age in normal infants and young children, *Am. Rev. Respir. Dis.*, *142*, 1372–1376 (1990).
47. Le Souef, P., Collis, G., Young, S., Arnott, J., Stick, S., and Landau, L., Bronchial responsiveness through the first year of life after correction for air entrainment, *Am. Rev. Respir. Dis.*, *143*(4), A23 (1991).
48. Dave, N., Hopp, R., Biven, R., Bewtra, A., and Townley, R., Persistence of increased nonspecific bronchial reactivity in allergic children and adolescents, *J. Allergy Clin. Immunol.*, *86*, 147 (1990).
49. Sears, M., Holdaway, M., Hewitt, C., and Silva, P., Bronchial reactivity in children without asthma (abstract), *Aust. NZ J. Med.*, *14*, 542 (1984).
50. Hirshman, C., Downes, H., and Veith, L., Airway responses in offspring of dogs with and without airway hyperreactivity, *J. Appl. Physiol.*, *56*, 1272–1277 (1984).
51. Townley, R., Trapani, I., and Szentivanyi, A., Sensitization to anaphylaxis and to some of its pharmacological mediators by blockade of the beta adrenergic receptors, *J. Allergy Clin. Immunol.*, *39*, 177–197 (1967).
52. Ryo, U., and Townley, R., Comparison of respiratory and cardiovascular effects of isoproterenol, propranolol, and practolol in asthmatic and normal subjects, *J. Allergy Clin. Immunol.*, *57*, 12–24 (1976).
53. Marsh, D., Bias, W., and Ishizaka, K., Genetic control of basal serum immunoglobin E level and its effect on specific sensitivity, *Proc. Natl. Acad. Sci.*, *71*, 3588–3592 (1974).
54. Gerrard, J., Rao, D., and Morton, N., A genetic study of immunoglobulin E, *Am. J. Hum. Genet.*, *30*, 46–58 (1978).
55. Marsh, D., Immunogenetics of allergic disease, in *Allergy, Principles and Practice* (E. Middleton, C. Reed, E. Ellis, N. Adkinson, and J. Yunginger, eds.), St. Louis, C. V. Mosby, 1988, pp. 94–105.
56. Cookson, W., Faux, J., Sharp, P., and Hopkin, J., Linkage between immunoglobulin E responses underlying asthma and rhinitis and chromosome 11q, *Lancet*, *i*, 1292–1295 (1989).
57. Cookson, W., and Hopkin, J., Dominant inheritance of atopic immunoglobulin-E responsiveness, *Lancet*, *336*, 86–88 (1988).
58. Lympany, P., Welsh, K., MacCochrane, G., Kemeny, D., and Lee, T., Genetic analysis using DNA polymorphism and the linkage between chromosome 11q13 and atopy and bronchial hyperresponsiveness to methacholine, *J. Allergy Clin. Immunol.*, *89*, 619–628 (1992).
59. Roitman-Johnson, B., Rich, S., Greenberg, B., Moberg, D., Roberts, S., and Blumenthal, M., Genetics of atopy, *J. Allergy Clin. Immunol.*, *89*(2), 267 (1992).
60. Cookson, W., Young, R. Sandford, A., Moffatt, M., Shirakawa, T., Sharp, P., Faux, J. Julier, C., Le Souef, P., Nakumura, Y., Lathrop, G., and Hopkin, J., Maternal inheritance of atopic IgE responsiveness on chromosome 11q, *Lancet*, *340*, 342–344 (1992).

61. Zhang, X., Werner-Favre, C., Tang, H., Brouwers, N., Bonnefoy, J., and Zubler, R., Il-4 dependent IgE switch in membrane IgA-positive human B cells, *J. Immunol.*, *147*, 3001–3004 (1991).
62. Vercelli, D., and Geha, R., Regulation of IgE synthesis in humans: a tale of two signals, *J. Immunol.*, *88*, 285–295 (1991).
63. Coffman, R., Seymour, B., Hudak, S., Jackson, J., and Rennick, D., Antibody to interleukin-5 inhibits helminth-induced eosinophilia in mice, *Science*, *245*, 308–310 (1989).
64. Robinson, D., Hamid, Q., Ying, S., Tsicopoulos, A., Barkans, J., Bentley, A., Corrigan, C., Duham, S., and Kay, A., Predominant TH_2-like bronchoalveolar T-lymphocyte population in atopic asthma, *N. Engl. J. Med.*, *326*, 298–304 (1992).
65. Romagnani, S., Cytokine profile of T cell clones in allergy, American Academy of Allergy and Immunology: Cytokine Symposium, Orlando, Florida, March 11, 1992.
66. Marsh, D., Krishnaswamy, K., Perry, M., Kautzky, E., Bias, W., and Ghosh, B., Genetic polymorphism in the interleukin 4 gene sequence: relation to total IgE, *J. Allergy Clin. Immunol.*, *89*(2), 219 (1992).
67. Burrows, B., Martinez, F., Halonen, M., Barbee, R., and Cline, M., Association of asthma with serum IgE levels and skin-test reactivity to allergens, *N. Engl. J. Med.*, *320*, 271–277 (1989).
68. Burrows, B., Lebowitz, M., Barbee, R., and Cline, M., Findings before diagnoses of asthma among the elderly in a longitudinal study of a general population, *J. Allergy Clin. Immunol.*, *88*, 870–877 (1991).
69. Walker, C., Virchow, J., Bruijnzeel, P., and Blaser, K., T cell subsets and their soluble products regulate eosinophilia in allergic and nonallergic asthma, *J. Immunol.*, *146*, 1829–1835 (1991).
70. Walker, C., Bode, E., Boer, L., Hansel, T., Blaser, K., and Virchow, J., Allergic and nonallergic asthmatics have distinct patterns of T-cell activation and cytokine production in peripheral blood and bronchoalveolar lavage, *Am. Rev. Respir. Dis.*, *146*, 109–115 (1992).
71. Schleimer, R. P., Fox, C. C., Naclerio, R. M., Plaut, M., Creticos, P., Togias, A., Warner, J., Kogey-Sabotka, A., and Lichtenstein, L., Role of human basophils and mast cells in the pathogenesis of allergic disease, *J. Allergy Clin. Immunol.*, *76*, 369–374 (1985).
72. Akagi, K., and Townley, R., Spontaneous histamine release and histamine content in normal subjects and subjects with asthma, *J. Allergy Clin. Immunol.*, *83*, 742–749 (1989).
73. Marone, G., Poto, S., Celestino, D., and Bonini, S., Human basophil releasibility. III. Genetic control of human basophil releasibility, *J. Immunol.*, *137*, 3588–3592 (1986).
74. Grant, J., Alam, R., and Lett-Brown, M., Histamine-releasing factors and inhibitors: historical perspectives and possible implications in human illness, *J. Allergy Clin. Immunol.*, *88*, 683–693 (1991).
75. MacDonald, S., Lichtenstein, L., Proud, D., Plaut, M., Naclerio, R. M., MacGlashan, D. W., and Kagey-Sobotka, A., Studies of IgE-dependent histamine-releasing factors: heterogeneity of IgE, *J. Immunol.*, *139*, 506–512 (1987).

76. Ying, S., Hamid, Q., Wardlaw, A., Azzawi, M,. Mogbel, R., Corrigan, C., Bradley, B., Durham, S., Collins, J., and Jeffrey, P. Expression of mRNA for IL-5 in mucosal bronchial biopsies for asthma, *J. Clin. Invest.*, *87*, 1541–1546 (1991).
77. Lee, T., and Lane, S., The role of macrophages in the mechanisms of airway inflammation in asthma, *Am. Rev. Respir. Dis.*, *145* (2), S27–S30 (1992).
78. Bachelet, M., Vincent, D., Havet, N., Marrash-Chala, R., Pradalier, A., Dry, J., and Varaftig, R., Reduced responsiveness of adenylate cyclase in alveolar macrophages from patients with asthma, *J. Allergy Clin. Immunol.*, *88*, 322–328 (1991).
79. Hirshman, C., Leu, D., Austin, D., Chan, S., Veith, L., and Hanifan, J., Elevated mononuclear leukocyte phosphodiesterase in allergic macrophages from patients with asthma, *J. Allergy Clin. Immunol.*, *798*, 46–53 (1987).
80. Grewe, S., Chan, S., and Hanifin, J., Elevated leukocyte cyclic AMP–phosphodiesterase in atopic disease: a possible mechanism for cyclic AMP agonist hyporesponsiveness, *J. Allergy Clin. Immunol.*, *70*, 452 (1982).
81. Torphy, T., and Undem, B., Phosphodiesterase inhibitors: new opportunities for the treatment of asthma, *Thorax*, *46*, 512 (1991).
82. Torphy, T., Zhou, H., Foley, J., and Sarau, H., Elevation of cAMP content increases the activity of the cAMP specific phosphodiesterase (PDE-IV) in U-937 cells, *J. Pharmacol. Exp. Ther.*, *263*, 1195–1205 (1992).
83. Mano, K., Harada, S., Miyahara, H., Miyamoto, T., and Horiuchi, Y., The distribution of polymorphic traits in atopic asthmatic patients, *Acta Allergol. (Copenhagen)*, *30*, 80–88 (1975).
84. Southard, J., Radford, P., Hopp, R., Bewtra, A., Nair, N., Ford, L., Elston, R., and Townley, R., Association of MS PI-type with airway hyperresponsiveness, *Chest*, *98*, 594–599 (1990).
85. Ronchetti, R., Lucarini, N., Lucarelli, P., Martinez, F., Macri, F., Carapella, E., and Bottini, E., A genetic basis for heterogeneity of asthma syndrome in pediatric ages: adenosine deaminase phenotypes, *J. Allergy Clin. Immunol.*, *74*, 81–84 (1984).
86. Miwa, M., Miyake, T., Yamanaka, T., Sugatani, J., Suzuki, Y., Sakata, S., Araki, Y., and Matsumoto, M., Characterization of serum platelet activating factor (PAF) acetylhydrolase, *J. Clin. Invest.*, *82*, 1983–1991 (1988).
87. Caraballo, L., Marrugo, J., and Jimenez, S., Role of human major histocompatibility complex (HLA) in the genetics of allergic asthma, *J. Allergy Clin. Immunol.*, *89* (2), 234 (1992).
88. Frick, O., and Brooks, D., IgE antibodies to pollens augmented in dogs by virus vaccines, *Am. J. Vet. Res.*, *44*, 440 (1983).
89. Holt, P., Lines, J., and Bilyk, N., Effect of influenza virus infection in allergen sensitization to inhaled allergen in mice, *Int. Arch. Allergy Appl. Immunol.*, *86*, 121–123 (1988).
90. Frick, O., German, D., and Mills, J., Development of allergy in children: in association with virus infections, *J. Allergy Clin. Immunol.*, *63*, 228–235 (1979).

16

Protective Effect of Inhaled Loop Diuretics on Experimentally Induced Bronchoconstriction

S. Bianco

Ospedale S. Raffaele, Milan, Italy

M. G. Pieroni, R. M. Refini, and P. Sestini

University of Siena, Siena, Italy

M. Robuschi

University of Milan, Milan, Italy

A. Vaghi

Ospedale di Garbagnate, Milan, Italy

I. INTRODUCTION

Bronchoconstriction is induced in asthmatic patients by a variety of stimuli that affect the osmolarity of the bronchial environment, indicating that the control of bronchial tone is affected by the physicochemical characteristics of the airway lining fluid in these patients [1]. The osmotic characteristics of the bronchial lining fluid are largely under the control of ion transport pathways in the airway epithelium [2,3]. The original idea behind a series of acute studies of the effect of furosemide on bronchial reactivity was that, since loop diuretics inhibit basolateral $Na^+/Cl^-/K^+$ cotransport in epithelial cells [4,5], this effect could change the bronchial response to osmolar stimuli. Unexpectedly, these experiments demonstrated that inhaled furosemide is a very effective bronchoprotective agent and hence a potential antiasthmatic drug, through a mechanism of action that is probably not correlated to a direct effect on bronchial osmolarity. The aim of this chapter is to summarize the results obtained using inhaled furosemide and other loop diuretics against a variety of bronchoconstrictor stimuli in asthmatic patients, and to examine the possible mechanism of action of the bronchial protective effect of these drugs. We will also discuss some technical aspects of the administration of furosemide and other loop diuretics by inhalation in asthmatic patients.

II. EFFECT OF INHALED FUROSEMIDE ON EXPERIMENTALLY INDUCED BRONCHOCONSTRICTION

According to the original hypothesis, osmolar stimuli were the first bronchoconstrictor agents against which the effect of inhaled furosemide was tested. In a series of controlled studies, it was found that inhalation of 40 mg furosemide inhibited the bronchoconstrictor response to ultrasonically nebulized water (UNW) [6,7], exercise [8], and hypertonic solutions of NaCl [9]. Under the same experimental conditions, oral furosemide was ineffective, suggesting that this protective effect was due to a direct effect of inhaled furosemide on the bronchial mucosa (Fig. 1). Inhaled furosemide has also been shown to protect asthmatic patients against cold air and hypertonic KCl-induced bronchoconstriction [10,11], and against blood gas changes induced by UNW [12]. The fact that significant protection has been observed against both hypo- and hyperosmotic stimuli suggests that inhaled furosemide does not counteract the osmotic changes directly,

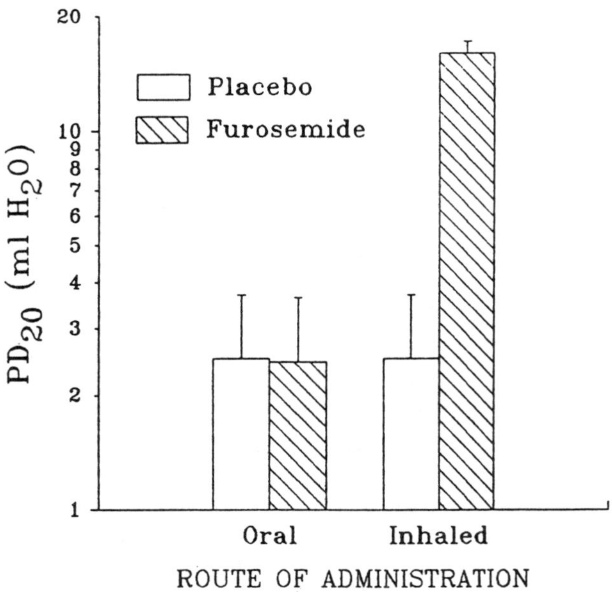

Figure 1 Protective effect of oral and inhaled furosemide on the bronchial obstructive response to ultrasonically nebulized water in a group of nine asthmatic patients. Bars represent mean ± SE. (Modified from Ref. 6.)

but probably interferes with mechanisms activated by these changes, such as stimulation of sensory receptors and/or release of mediators from superficial airway mast cells [13].

To verify whether inhaled furosemide could be acting with a mechanism different from that initially supposed, we investigated the effect of this treatment on the asthmatic response to allergen challenge, which is considered to be mediated by the release of preformed and newly generated mediators from superficial bronchial mastocytes and other inflammatory cells [14]. In controlled studies, inhaled furosemide protected asthmatic subjects from the early and late responses to allergen challenge [15–19] but not from the increase in bronchial reactivity following the late reaction [18]. Inhaled furosemide was also found to reverse the early response when administered after allergen challenge [18]. The observed protective effect against the late response [19] was also of interest, because the time of its occurrence, 4–8 h after the challenge, is beyond the estimated duration of action of inhaled furosemide, which, according to preliminary studies on the UNW-induced airway response, is most active in the first hour after administration [20]. We speculated that furosemide probably exerts its protective activity during the early phase of the reaction, by inhibiting the release of inflammatory mediators necessary for the development of the late response. This hypothesis is supported by preliminary data indicating that inhaled furosemide markedly inhibits the increase in urinary leukotriene E_4 (LTE_4) that follows the early asthmatic reaction [21]. By contrast, in aspirin-sensitive asthmatics challenged with inhaled lysine acetylsalicylate, which causes a slow-onset asthmatic response reaching the maximum intensity 2 h after challenge, we observed that furosemide provided a protective effect limited to the first hour of the reaction, with no differences observed at later time points as compared with placebo [22].

In patients with allergic rhinitis, inhaled furosemide was also shown to prevent the development of bronchial hyperresponsiveness to methacholine induced by the early asthmatic response [17], a finding we were unable to confirm in a subsequent study in asthmatic patients [22]. In animal models, inhaled furosemide protected actively sensitized guinea pigs [16] and dogs [23] against bronchoconstriction induced by antigen inhalation but not against that induced by nonspecific stimuli. In the guinea pig, intravenous infusion of furosemide was ineffective, suggesting that in this model the drug acts via a local mechanism [16].

Furosemide was also found to give significant protection against challenge with other stimuli such as sodium metabisulfite, adenosine, and LTD_4 [24–27], whereas no effect has been observed upon specific challenge in patients sensitive to toluene diisocyanate [28]. In some controlled studies, inhaled furosemide did not protect against methacholine in asthmatic patients [10,24,29], whereas in others a mild protective effect was observed, especially in normal subjects [30,31]. Similarly, furosemide caused minimal [32] or no [25,27] protection against histamine-induced bronchoconstriction and had no effect on the bronchial response to prostaglandin $F_{2\alpha}$ ($PGF_{2\alpha}$) [33].

In addition to the protective activity against bronchoconstriction induced by various stimuli, furosemide has been found to protect against the tussive response to low chloride solutions [34,35] and $PGF_{2\alpha}$ [33]. In contrast, it was ineffective against cough induced by citric acid [36], capsaicin [34], and sodium metabisulfite [37]. Interestingly, the bronchoconstrictor effect of sodium metabisulfite is inhibited by furosemide [24,25,37], but that of $PGF_{2\alpha}$ is not [33], a finding opposite to the results obtained for cough induced by the same stimuli.

III. POSSIBLE MECHANISM OF ACTION

A number of other drugs affecting ion transport have been investigated to provide further information on the mechanism of action of furosemide in asthma. Bumetanide and piretanide are loop diuretics of higher potency than furosemide, as far as inhibition of $Na^+/K^+/Cl^-$ cotransport and natriuretic activity are concerned [38]. These drugs are also more potent than furosemide in inhibiting ion transport in the dog tracheal epithelium [4] and electrically induced contraction of guinea pig bronchial strips in vitro [39]. However, when administered by inhalation to asthmatic subjects at doses with equivalent diuretic activity, bumetanide provided significantly lower protection than furosemide against exercise-induced [40] and adenosine-induced [25] bronchoconstriction, and it had no effect against sodium metabisulfite [25]. Under similar experimental conditions, piretanide showed little protection against UNW-induced [41] and metabisulfite-induced bronchoconstriction [41]. At higher doses, however, piretanide caused significant dose-related protection against UNW and was roughly equivalent to an equimolar dose of furosemide [42]. A newer loop diuretic, torasemide, also had little effect against UNW-induced bronchoconstriction [43].

The reason for the dissociation between the diuretic and the bronchoprotective activities of loop diuretics is not known. The bronchoprotective activity may be mediated by a mechanism different from the $Na^+/K^+/Cl^-$ cotransport inhibition responsible for the diuretic activity, or alternatively, the kinetics of furosemide in the airways may be different from those of other diuretics, resulting in stronger or longer local activity.

Increasing information is available on the bronchial effects of drugs acting on different ion transport mechanisms. Inhalation of the Na^+/K^+-ATPase blocker ouabain does not alter the bronchial responses to exercise or histamine [1] in asthmatic patients. The Na^+ channel blocker amiloride has been reported to slightly reduce bronchoconstriction, but not cough, induced by UNW, and to have no significant effect on bronchoconstriction induced by exercise, sodium metabisulfite, methacholine, or cold air [44–47]. The carbonic anhydrase inhibitor acetazolamide has been shown to reduce the bronchial response to sodium metabisulfite [48] and cold air [49]. Finally, it is interesting to note that sodium cromoglycate, an antiasthmatic drug with a spectrum of activities very similar to that of furosemide, has recently been shown to be a potent Cl^- channel inhibitor in a mast cell–derived tumor line [50].

These findings confirm that drugs affecting ion transport mechanisms participate in the control of bronchial reactivity in asthma, but they do not provide sufficient information to determine the exact mechanism(s) involved. Ion transport pathways are present in virtually every cell type, and all the cells suspected of being involved in the pathogenesis of bronchial hyperreactivity in asthma are potential targets for the action of furosemide. Although smooth muscle cell functions are affected by furosemide [51], an effect on these cells appears unlikely, since in asthmatics furosemide has little protective activity against bronchoconstrictor stimuli acting directly on smooth muscle, such as methacholine or histamine. The effects of loop diuretics and allergen challenge on ion transport in the airways have mostly been investigated in the tracheal epithelium of experimental animals [4,5,52]. In humans, conflicting results have been reported concerning the effect of furosemide on human nasal epithelium in vivo [24,53]. The response of nasal epithelium, however, may not be representative of the action of furosemide at the bronchial level, as we failed to observe consistent protection from nasal allergen challenge following furosemide inhalation in patients with allergic rhinitis (unpublished results). Furosemide has been shown to inhibit allergen-induced histamine release from rat peritoneal mast cells [54] and human blood cells [55] and to inhibit the release of histamine and leukotrienes from human lung fragments sensitized in vitro [56]. Other cells that have been reported to be affected by furosemide include guinea pig eosinophils [57] and human neutrophils [58,59], alveolar macrophages [60,61], and bronchial epithelial cells [61]. In the guinea pig, furosemide and bumetanide inhibit both cholinergic and noncholinergic neurally mediated bronchoconstriction in vitro, through a mechanism not influenced by the presence of the epithelium and which appears to be mediated by inhibition of $Na^+/K^+/Cl^-$ cotransport [39]. No information is available on the effect of loop diuretics on these phenomena in human airways.

The possibility that the protective activity of furosemide on bronchial reactions is mediated by prostaglandins has been investigated with cyclooxygenase inhibitors. In a recent study, the effect of furosemide on exercise-induced bronchoconstriction was reversed by oral indomethacin treatment [62], whereas we found no effect in a previous study with a similar protocol [63]. In another study, oral flurbiprofen failed to affect the protective activity of furosemide on the response to sodium metabisulfite [64]. We have recently observed that inhalation of lysine acetylsalicylate (LASA) strongly potentiates the protective activity of furosemide against UNW-induced responses [65], and it has an additive effect against allergen-induced bronchoconstriction [22]. Inhaled sodium salicylate does not potentiate the activity of furosemide, suggesting that the effect of LASA is due to prostaglandin inhibition [65]. Surprisingly, the protective effect of furosemide on exercise-induced reactions also appears to be further increased by inhaled LASA [66]. Thus, local delivery of cyclooxygenase blockers does not result in inhibition of the protective activity of furosemide.

IV. PRACTICAL ASPECTS OF FUROSEMIDE INHALATION

Furosemide is highly soluble in methanol and in alkaline solutions. The most convenient source for human studies is the standard preparation available for e.v. use (Lasix, Hoechst AG, Frankfurt am Main, Germany). This usually consists of vials containing 20 mg furosemide in 2 ml water, with NaOH added to increase the pH to 8.8. We found that complete nebulization of two vials (40 mg) is well tolerated and optimally effective in most patients. Using a standard jet nebulizer, inhalation of this dose requires 15–20 min, resulting in the delivery of about 28 mg furosemide during inspiration.

We estimate that in our system only about 150 μl of the aerosol, or about 10% of the amount nebulized during inspiration reaches the first 10 bronchial generations [67]. The total amount of periciliary fluid in these bronchi has been estimated to be nearly 1 ml (as discussed in Ref. 68), to which an equal amount of mucus has to be added [69]. Thus we can estimate that the highest concentration of furosemide reached locally during our experiments lies between 0.25 and 1 mg/ml (roughly 10^{-3} M). This is also in agreement with experiments conducted with [^{14}C]amiloride, indicating that the drug nebulized in the airways is diluted about 50-fold with respect to a starting solution of 3.5 ml [70].

The protective effect of furosemide is present at the end of the aerosol, and lasts for at least 1 h [20,31]. At these doses, furosemide did not cause bronchodilatation in any of the studies detailed above. Furthermore, we did not observe any effect of furosemide on specific airway resistance or forced expired volume in 1 second in a group of patients with airway obstruction highly reversible after inhalation of fenoterol (Fig. 2), up to 5 h after inhalation [71]. Furthermore, furosemide does not interact with salbutamol-induced bronchodilatation [72]. However, in a recent study using a dose of 80 mg of furosemide, a small but significant bronchodilator effect was observed [49].

During nebulization, a considerable amount of the drug is likely to deposit in the mouth and to be ingested. Since furosemide is an effective diuretic when administered by the oral route, the ingested drug may cause increased diuresis and vasodilation. When it was used as described, none of our patients has ever noticed increased diuresis or hypotension. When urine was collected after treatment, a statistically significant increase was observed in comparison with placebo during the first 2 h, although the actual difference, an average of 50 ml, was too small to be noticed. This effect must be considered, however, if an higher dose of the drug has to be given. Furthermore, other loop diuretics, such as piretanide,

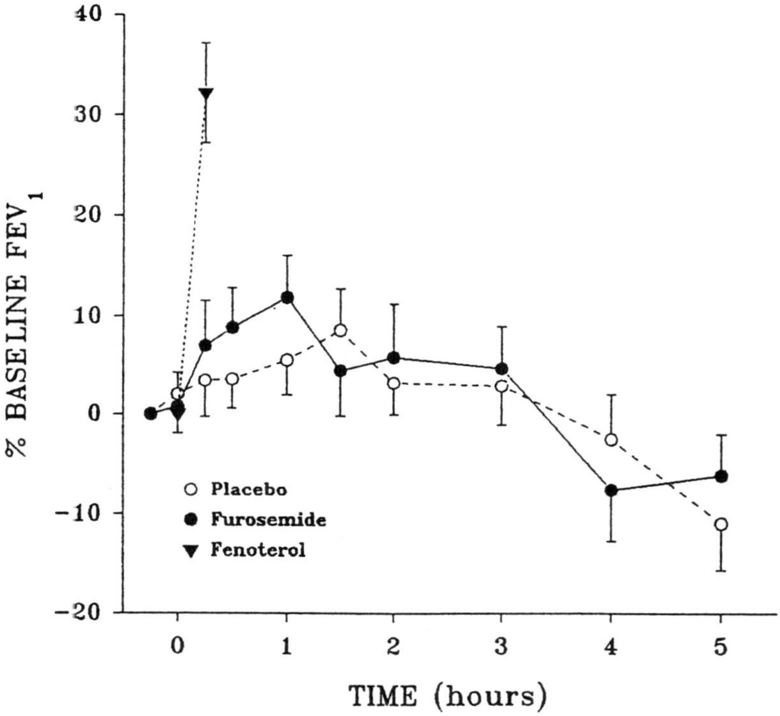

Figure 2 Effect of 40 mg inhaled furosemide or placebo on forced expired volume in 1 second (FEV_1) in a group of eight patients with reversible airway obstruction. The response of the same patients 20 min after inhalation of 400 μg fenoterol (triangles) is reported for comparison. (Modified from Ref. 67.)

bumetanide, or torasemide, given by inhalation, have been observed to cause much more marked diuretic activity, which may result in severe hypotension.

Although adequate for most experimental studies, administration through a jet nebulizer is time-consuming and impractical. A metered dose inhaler has recently been developed by Hoechst AG, delivering 5 mg furosemide/puff in a highly bioavailable form. When the inhalation was optimized using a spacer device, we found that two puffs (10 mg) afforded a degree of protection against UNW-induced bronchoconstriction (Fig. 3) that was not significantly different from that of 40 mg administered with a jet nebulizer [73]. Similar results have been observed for the response to sodium metabisulfite [37]. This inhaler is currently being used in a clinical trial to evaluate the clinical effectiveness of inhaled furosemide in asthma. This method of administration, by restricting the nebulization to the inspiratory phase, is also likely to further reduce the diuretic effect of the drug.

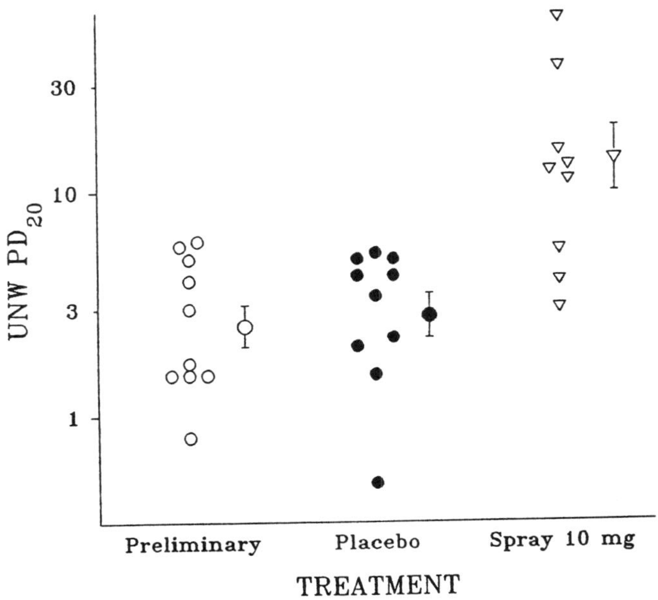

Figure 3 Protective effect of inhaled furosemide, administered through a pressurized metered dose inhaler and a spacer device (Volumatic, Glaxo S.p.A., Verona, Italy), on the bronchial obstructive response to ultrasonically nebulized water (UNW) in a group of asthmatic patients. Symbols with error bars represent the mean and SE of each treatment group. After furosemide, the provocative dose of UNW required to produce a 20% fall in forced expired volume in 1 second (UNW PD_{20}) in this group was increased by 7 ± 2 times compared with placebo, corresponding to an increase of 2.0 ± 0.3 doubling doses.

Taken together, these experimental studies indicate that furosemide has a wide spectrum of activities not confined to epithelial cells but extending to other cell types, including neutrophils, eosinophils, macrophages, and nerve fibers, all of which are involved in the pathogenesis of asthma. These observations suggest that furosemide might provide a novel approach to the treatment of asthma, or might constitute a starting point for the development of new antiasthma drugs. Although inhaled furosemide does not cause bronchodilation, a beneficial effect could be expected in patients with bronchial hyperreactivity, as a result of the prevention of bronchoconstriction. This possibility is speculative at present, and controlled clinical studies to verify the hypothesis are currently under way.

REFERENCES

1. Bianco, S., Robuschi, M., Sestini, P., Vaghi, A., Refini, R. M., Pieroni, M. G., Gambaro, G., Spagnotto, S. Rossoni, G., Berti, F., and Pasargiklian, M., Osmolarity,

bronchial reactivity, and the protective effect of loop diuretics, in *Respiratory Allergy* (G. Melillo, P. S. Norman, and G. Marone, eds.), BC Decker, Toronto, 1990, pp. 119–130.

2. Al-Bazzaz, F. J., Regulation of salt and water transport across airway mucosa, *Clin. Chest Med.*, *7*, 259–272 (1986).
3. Welsh, M. J., Mechanisms of airway epithelial ion transport, *Clin. Chest Med.*, *7*, 273–293 (1986).
4. Widdicombe, J. H., Nathanson, I. T., and Higland, E., Effect of "loop" diuretics on ion transport by dog tracheal epithelium, *Am. J. Physiol.*, *245* (Cell Physiol. 14), C388–C396 (1983).
5. Welsh, M. J., Inhibition of chloride secretion by furosemide in canine tracheal epithelium, *J. Membr. Biol.*, *71*, 219–226 (1983).
6. Robuschi, M., Gambaro, G., Spagnotto, S., Vaghi, A., and Bianco, S., Inhaled furosemide (F) is highly effective in preventing ultrasonically nebulized water (UNH_2O) bronchoconstriction, *Pulm. Pharmacol.*, *1*, 187–191 (1989).
7. Bianco, S., Vaghi, A., and Robuschi, M, Furosemide: a "new" antireactive agent. It works only by inhalation, *Eur. Respir. J.*, *1*, 2s (1988).
8. Bianco, S., Vaghi, A., Robuschi, M., and Pasargiklian, M., Prevention of exercise-induced bronchoconstriction by inhaled fursemide, *Lancet*, *2*, 252–255 (1988).
9. Robuschi, M., Vaghi, A., Gambaro, G., Spagnotto, S., and Bianco, S. Inhaled furosemide (F) is effective in preventing ultrasonically nebulized 5.8% NaCl broncho-constriction, *Eur. Respir. J.*, *1* (suppl 1), 193s (1988).
10. Grubbe, R. E., Hopp, R., Dave, N. K., Brennan, B., Bewtra, A., and Townley, R., Effect of inhaled furosemide on the bronchial response to methacholine and cold-air hyperventilation challenges, *J. Allergy Clin. Immunol.*, *85*, 881–884 (1990).
11. Magyar, P., Debreczeni, L. A., Zsamboki, G., and Gyor, Z., Protective effect of inhaled furosemide on KCl induced bronchospasm, *Eur. Respir. J.*, *4*, 605s (1991).
12. Cogo, A., Dal Negro, R., Clini, E., Turco, P., and Allegra, Protective effect of inhaled furosemide (F) against VA/QC disturbances induced by ultrasonically nebulized distilled water (UNDW) in asthmatics, *Eur. Respir. J.*, *4*, 606s (1991).
13. Moscato, G., Dellabianca, A., Falagiani, P., Mistrello, G., Rossi, G. L., and Rampulla, C., Inhaled furosemide prevents both the bronchoconstriction and the increase in neutrophil chemotactic activity induced by ultrasonic "fog" of distilled water in asthmatics, *Am. Rev. Respir. Dis.*, *143*, 561–566 (1991).
14. O'Byrne, P. M., Dolovich, J., and Hargreave, F. E. Late asthmatic responses, *Am. Rev. Respir. Dis.*, *136*, 740–751 (1987).
15. Bianco, S., Pieroni, M., Refini, M., Sturman, A., and Robuschi, M., Inhaled furosemide (F) prevents allergen induced bronchoconstriction in atopic asthmatics (abstr.), *Am. Rev. Respir. Dis.*, *137*, 27 (1988).
16. Robuschi, M., Pieroni, M., Refini, M., Bianco, S., Rossoni, G., Magni, F., and Berti, F., Prevention of antigen induced early obstructive reaction by inhaled furosemide in (atopic) asthmatics and (actively sensitized) guinea pigs, *J. Allergy Clin. Immunol.*, *85*, 10–16 (1990).
17. Verdiani, P., DiCarlo, S., Baronti, A., and Bianco, S., Effect of inhaled furosemide on the early response to antigen and subsequent change in airway reactivity in atopic patients, *Thorax*, *45*, 377–381 (1990).

18. Bianco, S., Pieroni, M. G., Refini, R. M., Ferretti, B., Beltrami, V., Civai, R., and Sestini, P., Attenuation of the bronchial response to allergen by inhalation of furosemide after allergen challenge, *Am. Rev. Respir. Dis.*, *141*, A474 (1990).
19. Bianco, S., Pieroni, M., Refini, M., Rottoli, L., and Sestini, P., Protective effect of inhaled furosemide on allergen-induced early and late asthmatic reactions, *N. Engl. J. Med.*, *321*, 1069–1073 (1989).
20. Sestini, P., Vaghi, A., Pieroni, M. G., Refini, M., Vagliasindi, M., and Bianco, S., Time course of the protective effect of inhaled furosemide on UNH$_2$O-induced bronchoconstriction, *Eur. Respir. J.*, *3*, 237s (1991).
21. Bianco, S., Sala, A., Robuschi, M., Lupi, S., Sestini, P., and Folco, G., Effects of inhaled furosemide on urinary leukotriene E_4 in allergen induced early asthmatic reactions, *Pharmacol. Res.*, *26*, 36s (1992).
22. Sestini, P., Refini, R. M., Pieroni, M. G., Ferretti, B., Vagliasindi, M., and Bianco, S., Protective effect of inhaled furosemide and lysine acetylsalicylate on allergen-induced bronchial hyperreactivity, *Am. Rev. Respir. Dis.*, *145*, A728 (1992).
23. Wooley, M. J., Matsui, S., Karlsson, J. A., and O'Byrne, P. M., Effect of inhaled furosemide on allergen-induced airway hyperresponsiveness and inflammation in dogs, *Am. Rev. Respir. Dis.*, *141*, A363 (1990).
24. Nichol, G. N., Alton, E. W. F. W., Nix, A., Geddes, D. M., Chung, K. F., and Barnes, P. J., Effect of inhaled furosemide on metabisulfite- and methacholine-induced broncho-constriction and nasal potential difference in asthmatic subjects, *Am. Rev. Respir. Dis.*, *142*, 576–580 (1990).
25. O'Connor, B. J., Chung, K. F., Chen-Wordell, Y. M., Fuller, R. W., and Barnes, P. J., Effect of inhaled fursemide and bumetanide on adenosine 5-monophosphate and metabisulphite-induced bronchoconstriction in asthmatics, *Am. Rev. Respir. Dis.*, *143*, 1329–1334 (1991).
26. Polosa, R., Leu, L. C., and Holgate, S. T., Inhibition of adenosine 5′-monophosphate- and methacholine-induced bronchoconstriction in asthma by inhaled furosemide, *Eur. Respir. J.*, *3*, 665–672 (1990).
27. Cheung, D., Bel, E. H., van der Veen, H., Dijkman, J. H., and Sterk, P. J., The effect of inhaled frusemide on histamine and leukotriene D4–induced airway narrowing in asthmatic subjects, *Eur. Respir. J.*, *4*, 605s (1990).
28. Moscato, G., Dellabianca, A., Lodigiani, L., Marraccini, P., and Vinci, G., Inhaled furosemide does not inhibit the airway response to toluene diisocyanate (TDI), *Am. Rev. Respir. Dis.*, *143*, A437 (1991).
29. Vaghi, A., Robuschi, M., Chilaris, N., and Bianco, S., Inhaled furosemide (F) does not attenuate the bronchial response to methacholine (M) in asthmatics, *Eur. Respir. J.*, *1*, 85s (1988).
30. Polosa, R., Rajakulasingan, K., Gratziou, C., and Holgate, S. T., Inhaled loop diuretics attenuate bronchial responsiveness to methacholine in normal subjects, *Eur. Respir. J.*, *14*, 605s (1991).
31. Fujimura, M., Sakamoto, S., and Kamio, Y., Effect of inhaled furosemide on bronchial responsiveness to methacholine, *N. Engl. J. Med.*, *322*, 935–936 (1990).
32. Vaghi, A., Robuschi, M., Berni, F., and Bianco, S., Effect of inhaled furosemide (F) on bronchial response to histamine (H) in asthmatics, *Eur. Respir. J.*, *1*, 406s (1988).

33. Stone, R. A., Yeo, T. C., Barnes, P. J., and Chung, K. F., Frusemide inhibits cough but not bronchoconstriction to prostaglandin $PGF_2\alpha$ in patients with asthma, *Am. Rev. Respir. Dis.*, *143*, A548 (1991).
34. Ventresca, P. G., Nichol, G. M., Barnes, P. J., and Chung, K. F., Inhaled frusemide inhibits cough induced by low chloride solutions but not by capsaicin, *Am. Rev. Respir. Dis.*, *142*, 143–146 (1990).
35. Stone, R. A., Barnes, P. J., and Chung, K. F., Frusemide and cough induced by low-chloride-content solution: duration of action, *Thorax*, *46*, 280P–281P (1991).
36. Robuschi, M., Vaghi, A., Gambaro, G., Spagnotto, S., Petrigni, G., Sestini, P., and Bianco, S., Effect of inhaled furosemide on cough response to citric acid in normal subjects, *Prog. Respir. Res.*, *24*, 117–121 (1990).
37. O'Connor, B. J., Chen-Worsdell, Y. M., Ylmaz, G., Barnes, P. J., and Chung, K. F., Furosemide via a metered dose inhaler (MDI): dose-dependent inhibition of bronchoconstriction but not cough responses to sodium metabisulphite (MBS) in asthma, *Am. Rev. Respir. Dis.*, *145*, A733 (1992).
38. Lant, A., Diuretics: clinical pharmacology and therapeutical use (part I), *Drugs*, *29*, 57–87 (1985).
39. Elwood, W., Lotvall, J. O., Barnes, P., and Chung, K. F., Loop diuretics inhibit cholinergic and noncholinergic nerves in guinea pig, *Am. Rev. Respir. Dis.*, *143*, (1991).
40. Vaghi, A., Robuschi, M., Sestini, P., Gambaro, G., Spagnotto, S., and Bianco, S., Comparison of inhaled frusemide and bumetanide in preventing ultrasonically nebulized water bronchoconstriction, *Eur. Respir. J.*, *3*, 93s (1990).
41. Yeo, C. T., O'Connor, B. J., Chen-Worsdell, M., Barnes, P. J., and Chung, K. F., Protective effect of loop diuretics, piretanide and frusemide, against metabisulphite induced bronchoconstriction in asthma, *Eur. Respir. J.*, *5*, 1184–1188 (1992).
42. Bianco, S., Robuschi, M., Vaghi, A., Pieroni, M. G., Refini, R. M., and Sestini, P., Protective effect of inhaled piretanide on the bronchial obstructive response to ultrasonically nebulized H_2O: a dose response study, *Chest*, *1993* (in press).
43. Foresi, A., Pelucchi, A., Mastropasqua, B., Cavigioli, G., Carlesi, R. M., and Marazzini, L., Effect of inhaled furosemide and torasemide on bronchial obstructive response to ultrasonically nebulized distilled water in asthmatic subjects, *Am. Rev. Respir. Dis.*, *146*, 364–368 (1992).
44. Knox, A. J., Britton, J. R., and Tattersfield, A. E., Effect of sodium-transport inhibitors on bronchial reactivity in vivo, *Clin. Sci.*, *79*, 325–330 (1990).
45. Wood, A. M., Lowry, R. H., and Higenbottam, T. W., Differential effects of inhaled frusemide and amiloride on airway responsiveness to water and exercise in asthma, *Am. Rev. Respir. Dis.*, *141*, A478 (1990).
46. Netzel, M. A., Hopp, R., Buzzas, R., Palmeiro, E., and Dowling, P., Effect of inhaled amiloride on cold air (CACH) and methacholine challenges (MC), *Ann. Allergy*, *66*, 82 (1991).
47. Badwin, D. R., Grange, K. L., Pavord, I., and Knox, A. J., The effect of amiloride on the airway response to metabisulphite in asthma: a negative report, *Eur. Respir. J.*, *5*, 1189–1192 (1992).
48. O'Connor, B. J., Yeo, C. T., Chen-Worrsdell, Y. M., Barnes, P. J., and Chung, K. F.,

Airway responses to sodium metabisulphite are inhibited by inhaled acetazolamide but not by amiloride, *Eur. Respir. J.*, *4*, 377s (1991).
49. O'Donnell, W. J., Rosenberg, M., Niven, R. W., Drazen, J. M., and Israel, E., Acetazolamide and furosemide attenuate asthma induced by hyperventilation of cold, dry air, *Am. Rev. Respir. Dis.*, *146*, 1518–1523 (1992).
50. Romanin, C. H. R., Reinsprecht, M., Pecht, I., and Schinder, H., The antiallergic drug cromolyn is a potent blocker of Cl^- channel activity in rat mucosal mast cells (RBL-2H3 line), *Naunyn Schmiedebergs Arch. Pharmacol.*, *343*, 313 (1991).
51. Sourhada, M., and Sourhada, J. F., Sodium and calcium influx induced by phorbol esters in airway smooth muscle cells, *Am. Rev. Respir. Dis.*, *139*, 927–932 (1989).
52. Sestini, P., Bienenstock, J., Crowe, S. E., Marshall, J. S., Stead, R. H., Kakuta, Y., and Perdue, M. H., Ion transport in rat epithelium in vitro: role of capsaicin-sensitive nerves in allergic reactions, *Am. Rev. Respir. Dis.*, 393–397 (1990).
53. Wood, A. M., Dinh Xuan, A. T., Higenbottam, T. W., Cremona, G., and Lockart, A., Metoxamine and frusemide inhibit nasal transepithelial potential difference—a possible protective mechanism in the prevention of exercise-induced asthma, *Am. Rev. Respir. Dis.*, *139*, A478 (1989).
54. Berti, F., Rossoni, G., Buschi, A., Zuccari, G., and Villa, L. M., Inhaled furosemide prevents immunological respiratory changes and mediator release in guinea-pig, *Eur. Respir. J.*, *4*, 445s (1991).
55. Gato, J. J., Croce, M., Costa-Manso, E., Senz, M., Oehling, A., *Allergy*, *47*(suppl), 141 (1992).
56. Anderson, S. D., Wei, H., and Temple, D. M., Inhibition of furosemide of inflammatory mediators from lung fragments, *N. Engl. J. Med.*, *324*, 131 (1991).
57. Perkins, R. A., Dent, G., Chung, K. F., and Barnes, P. J., Effects of anion transport inhibitors and choride ions on eosinophil respiratory burst activity, *Am. Rev. Respir. Dis.*, *143*, A331 (1991).
58. Rottoli, L., Rottoli, P., Sparnacci, F., and Bianco, S., In vitro effect of furosemide on O^2 production, *Eur. Respir. J.*, *2*(suppl 8), 861s (1989).
59. Sestini, P., Renzoni, E., Vagliasindi, M., and Bianco, S., Inhibitory effect of furosemide on FMLP-induced chemotaxis of human granulocytes in vitro, *Eur. Respir. J.*, *3*, 348s (1990).
60. Rottoli, P., Rottoli, L., Marino, M., Sparnacci, F., Vagliasindi, M., and Bianco, S., Effect of furosemide on lysosomal enzyme secretion by alveolar macrophages, *Eur. Respir. J.*, *3*, 307–308s (1990).
61. Scoloperto, M., Marini, M., Brasca, C., Fasoli, A., and Mattoli, S., The protective effect of furosemide on the generation of superoxyde anions by human bronchial epithelial cells and pulmonary macrophages in vivo, *Pulmon. Pharmacol.*, *4*, 80–84 (1991).
62. Pavord, I. D., Wisniewski, A., and Tattersfield, A. E., Inhaled frusemide and exercise-induced asthma: evidence of a role for inhibiting prostanoids, *Thorax*, *47*, 797–800 (1992).
63. Vaghi, A., Berni, F., Robuschi, M., Sestini, P., and Bianco, S., Indomethacin (I) does not influence the protective effect of furosemide (F) against exercise-induced bronchoconstriction, *Eur. Respir. J.*, *2* (suppl 8), 790 (1989).

64. O'Connor, B. J., Ridge, S. M., Barnes, P. J., and Chung, K. F., The role of cyclooxygenase products in the inhibition of sodium metabisulphite–induced bronchoconstriction by furosemide in asthma, *Am. Rev. Respir. Dis.*, *143*, A210 (1991).
65. Bianco, S., Vaghi, A., Pieroni, M. G., Robuschi, M., Refini, R. M., Berni, F., and Sestini, P., Potentiation of the antireactive–antiasthmatic effect of inhaled furosemide by inhaled lysine acetylsalicylate, *Allergy*, 1993 (in press).
66. Robuschi, M., Scuri, M., Vaghi, A., Spagnotto, S., Gambaro, G., Fai, V., Sestini, P., and Bianco, S., Inhaled acetylsalicylic acid enhances the protective effect of furosemide against exercise-induced bronchoconstriction, *Am. Rev. Respir. Dis.*, *145*, A729 (1992).
67. Newman, S. P., in *Aerosols and the Lung* (S. W. Clarke and D. Pavia, eds.), Butterworths, London, 1984, pp. 197–224.
68. Smith, C. M., and Anderson, S. D., A comparison between the airway response to isocapnic hyperventilation and hypertonic saline in subjects with asthma, *Eur. Respir. J.*, *2*, 36–43 (1989).
69. Wanner, A., Upper airways, *Clin. Chest Med.*, *7*, 247–258 (1986).
70. Waltner, W. E., Church, N. L., Gatzy, R. C., Boucher, R. C., and Knowles, M. R., Deposition, pharmacokinetics, and toxicity of amiloride aerosol in normal and cystic fibrosis (CF) subjects, *Am. Rev. Respir. Dis.*, *135*, A288 (1987).
71. Sestini, P., Pieroni, M. G., Refini, R. M., Civai, R., Beltrami, V., and Bianco, S., Effect of inhaled furosemide on respiratory function parameters of patients with reversible airway obstruction, in *New Trends in Pneumology and Cardiology* (D. Olivieri, ed.), Monduzzi, Bologna, 1990, pp. 55–59.
72. Vaghi, A., Pieroni, M. G., Robuschi, M., Gambaro, G., Sestini, P., Berni, F., and Bianco, S., Preventive effect of furosemide and salbutamol on ultrasonically nebulized water, *Eur. Respir. J.*, *4*, 606s (1991).
73. Sestini, P., Robuschi, M., Vaghi, A., Gambaro, G., Spagnotto, S., Pieroni, M. G., Refini, R. M., and Bianco, S., Protective effect of furosemide, administered using a pressurized metered dose inhaler and a spacer device, on the bronchial obstructive response to ultrasonically nebulized distilled water, in *Asthma Treatment—a Multidisciplinary Approach* (D. Olivieri, P. J. Barnes, and G. Folco, eds.), Plenum Press, New York, 1992, pp. 257–260.

17

Provocative Challenge by Exercise or Hyperventilation

J. F. Souhrada and M. Souhrada

The John B. Pierce Laboratory and Yale School of Medicine
New Haven, Connecticut

I. INTRODUCTION

The first documented observation that physical activity leads to asthma can be found in writings of Aretaeus of Cappadocia, who lived from A.D. 120 to 180. He was a Greek physician in the Roman province of Cappadocia who wrote, "If from running, gymnastic exercises, or any work the breathing becomes difficult, it is called asthma" [1]. In modern times it was Professor Herxheimer [2] who suggested that bronchoconstriction observed after exercise may be related to hyperventilation. Since that time, exercise-induced bronchoconstriction has been studied by many investigators, but the most extensive initial work was done in the years 1971 through 1976 in London by Professor S. Godfrey and his group (Drs. Anderson, Silverman, and Konig). Detailed reviews of this topic were made by Anderson et al. [3,4], Jones et al. [5–7], Cropp [8], Sly [9], McFadden and Ingram [10], McFadden [11], and Godfrey [12].

II. CLINICAL PRESENTATION OF EXERCISE-INDUCED BRONCHOCONSTRICTION

Shortness of breath with exertion occurs in many types of cardiac and pulmonary disease, but the airway bronchoconstriction that can be detected in asthmatics after short-term exercise is a characteristic response. It is known as exercise-induced asthma or exercise-induced bronchoconstriction. There are two reasons why we prefer to call this phenomenon exercise-induced bronchoconstriction. Since this entity is characterized by postexertional bronchoconstriction that can be objectively measured, it is more appropriate to call it exercise-induced bronchoconstriction. A patient with this particular condition has asthma even before exercise. Second, many patients who are uncertain about their physical capabilities may incorrectly conclude from the name "exercise-induced asthma" that physical activity may worsen their asthma. In contrast, submaximal physical exercise of controlled intensity for 3 months produced a significant improvement in fitness and cardiorespiratory performance that should be advantageous to the exercising asthmatic patient [13]. The majority of patients with asthma thus benefit from physical activity.

Exercise-induced bronchoconstriction (EIB) may have only a mild clinical presentation, but sometimes it may be a life-threatening event leading to hospitalization. Its severity is dependent on the nature and duration of exercise [6], and it is significantly affected by the temperature and humidity of inspired air [14] and the underlying reactivity of airways.

Exercise-induced bronchoconstriction occurs more frequently in asthmatic patients than is ordinarily recognized. The incidence among asthmatic and atopic nonasthmatic children is 63% and 41%, respectively [15]. Another study reported that 75% of children with asthma have EIB [7]. Because of a lack of standardization of the workload, duration, and type of exercise and the methodology used to determine the magnitude of airway obstruction caused, our ability to compare data from different investigators is limited. Thus, one may reasonably expect that if EIB is evaluated with pulmonary function tests less dependent on effort than forced expiration, the incidence of EIB may be even higher than previously reported.

In normal, healthy subjects, short-term exercise can induce bronchodilation that can be documented by a prompt rise in specific airway conductance (SGaw) [16]. Mansfield et al. [17] studied normal children during short-term exercise and found an immediate decrease in respiratory resistance followed by its return to baseline levels at the end of exercise. Similarly, Lefcoe observed that exercise improved the pulmonary function of normal subjects [18]. This improvement is probably related to the stimulation of the sympathetic nervous system and the local effect of blood-borne catecholamines. On the other hand, O'Donnell and Fling [19] studied 100 U.S. Air Force members to determine the incidence of airflow obstruction after standardized free-run exercise. Six subjects had significant airway obstruction after exercise. Three of six subjects with abnormal results observed after exercise showed bronchial hyperresponse to methacholine challenge.

In asthmatics, the degree of EIB is generally proportional to the severity and type of exercise, and its duration. The temperature and humidity of inspired air during physical activity are critical. Although there is a wide range of responses to exercise in asthmatics, a typical bronchoconstrictive response is usually detected after exercise, achieving a maximum level at 7–15 min after exercise [3,4]. Respiratory difficulties may include cough, shortness of breath, chest tightness, and wheezing. Only a few patients develop bronchoconstriction during exercise, and in some, continuation of exercise may bring relief of dyspnea as well as bronchoconstriction. In the majority of asthmatics, if postexercise bronchoconstriction is not too severe, a spontaneous recovery from symptoms is usually observed 30–35 min after exercise. The most characteristic change in pulmonary function is a decrease in maximal expiratory flow rates, as measured by spirometry or change in the maximal expiratory flow–volume relationship. In the majority of practitioners' offices a spirometer is available, and bronchoconstriction in the postexercise period can be measured readily by evaluating the decrease in forced expired volume in 1 second (FEV_1), forced vital capacity (FVC), and midexpiratory flow rate ($FEF_{25-75\%}$). A decrease of 15% in FEV_1 as compared with the baseline value signifies the presence of bronchoconstriction. Usually, an increase in static lung volumes, such as residual volume (RV) and functional residual capacity (FRC), is also detected, leading to the increase in resting respiratory position and a significant lung hyperinflation. Lung hyperinflation is determined from an increase of ratios of RV/total lung capacity (TLC) and FRC/TLC. When these ratios are increased 15–20% above the predicted range, a significant lung hyperinflation is present. If the direct measurement of airway resistance (Raw) is available, a significant increase in this value and a decrease in SGaw are also observed. Peak expiratory flow rate is also used by some clinicians to determine bronchoconstriction induced by exercise. We recommend not using this particular variable, since its value depends on effort and thus may rather reflect the strength of expiratory muscles.

There have been reports describing the observation of late-phase-like bronchoconstriction after exercise [20–22]. However, other investigators have failed to observe this occurrence [23,24].

As one would expect, EIB also leads to the alteration of other functional characteristics [25]. The alveolar–arterial oxygen gradient is increased during and after exercise in asthmatics who develop EIB, a finding that suggests a deterioration of the ventilation–perfusion relationship [26]. However, carbon dioxide partial pressure (P_{CO_2}) remains within baseline range during exercise [27], whereas in postexercise period, a deterioration in gas exchange is observed [26], and the pH of arterial blood is usually decreased [27]. This finding may be related to the presence of higher lactate levels in asthmatics at the completion of exercise (see below).

During exercise, the level of minute ventilation (VE) for a given work, as well as oxygen consumption, was found to be significantly increased in asthmatic as compared with normal children [28]. Poor physical fitness in some asthmatic patients may be the cause of this finding. On the other hand, since the level of ventilation during exercise was shown to decrease after upper airway anesthesia, one can speculate that stimulation of rapidly adapting receptors or cold-sensitive receptors in upper airways with relatively cool and dry air may be responsible for stimulation of ventilation [29]. Indeed, upper airway receptors have been implicated in the regulation of breathing [30].

Increased oxygen consumption observed in asthmatics during exercise may be related to greater effort by the respiratory muscles or a decrease in their efficiency. Bevegard et al. [31] observed that children with more severe asthma seem to work with a larger anaerobic component at maximal exercise loads than children with less pronounced asthma.

Both prostaglandin $F_{2\alpha}$ ($PGF_{2\alpha}$) and norepinephrine measured in the plasma of asthmatics during and after exercise were found not to differ from preexercise levels [32,33]. Similarly, other studies failed to show any changes in peripheral blood PGE and $PGF_{2\alpha}$ [34]. With respect to catecholamines, there are reports that show a significant increase in both norepinephrine and epinephrine during exercise in asthmatics [35]. Studies evaluating the effect of exercise on histamine blood levels are controversial. Some investigators found an increase in histamine and some no changes [36–38]. Another study suggested that during exercise both normal and asthmatic subjects have an increase in whole blood levels of histamine, which may be associated with a concomitant increase in the basophil count [39]. In another laboratory, Barboriak et al. [40] have shown that asthmatic patients have higher levels of blood lactate at all tested workloads as compared with normal subjects. In general, the available data do not suggest that a single indicator is responsible for EIB.

In some patients, a short period of exercise can induce not only bronchoconstriction but symptoms of generalized anaphylaxis as well. In these patients exercise may be followed by cholinergic urticaria, angioedema, or cardiac arrhythmias in addition to bronchoconstriction. This is observed in the absence of history of allergy or evidence of an encounter with an environmental source of antigen during the exercise period [41]. On the other hand, Maulitz et al. [42] have reported a case in which they felt a hypersensitivity to oysters and shrimp was a factor in subsequent adverse reactions to strenuous exercise.

As described in the preceding chapters, inhalation challenges are extensively used in assessing nonspecific airway reactivity. These methods employ the inhalation of an increasing concentration of aerosolized histamine or methacholine while airway response is periodically monitored. These are important clinical tests in the evaluation of airway reactivity. In some patients, however, this approach may suffer from several disadvantages. We can assume that airway response is dependent on the actual dose of the inhaled agent at the site of its deposition along the airways [43–45]. Tested agents will be preferentially distributed in airways with a more normal time constant as compared with those that have changes of airway resistance and compliance. Thus, one can speculate that during inhalation challenge with histamine or methacholine, the airway response of relatively normal airways, as compared with airways in which obstruction exists, is tested. It is possible that the inhaled agents in some instances may not reach the obstructed areas. Thus, there is a considerable overlap between the responses to inhalation challenges in normal subjects, patients with chronic rhinitis, and asthmatic patients [46–48]. Furthermore, following histamine and methacholine inhalation challenge, side effects such as flushing, irritation of the throat, tachycardia, and hyperpnea may be observed. One may argue that all of these factors make the bronchial inhalation challenge with histamine or methacholine a less specific test to determine the level of airway reactivity. Some of these issues may be related to a relatively poor correlation between histamine or methacholine inhalation challenge tests and the results of exercise tests. Some patients with bronchial asthma who showed essentially no response to exercise had a highly significantly response to histamine inhalation challenge, and vice versa [49]. In one particular study [50], a relatively good correlation was found between exercise and methacholine inhalation challenge. However, if one examines these data carefully one can see that from 57 patients tested, 45 responded to methacholine challenge and only 33 responded to exercise as measured by a decrease in peak expiratory flow rate. Thus, when the exercise test fails to demonstrate increased airway reactivity, the use of inhalation challenge testing is justified. The explanation of this discrepancy may be that inhalation challenges examine a different component of hyperreactive airways. Thus, Weiller-Rawall and Godfrey [51] exposed 12 asthmatics to both exercise and specific antigen challenge. When the patients were refractory to exercise challenge they were exposed to inhalation antigen challenge. In this refractory state, six patients failed to respond to antigen challenge, suggesting a common pathway for exercise and antigen challenge. Six other patients in the refractory state developed bronchoconstriction after antigen challenge. This observation suggests an alternative pathway or mechanism for bronchoconstriction after antigen challenge. Recently, Godfrey and associates reported that in children only an exercise test, and not methacholine inhalation challenge, can differentiate asthma from chronic lung disease [52].

III. EXERCISE TESTING PROCEDURES

A. Indications for Exercise Testing

The purpose of exercise testing is to determine whether the patient can develop EIB and, by implication, whether he has an increase in nonspecific airway reactivity. The exercise test is thus a "provocative test." The most frequent indications for this type of testing are

1. To assess latent asthma (patient with allergic rhinitis or frequent bronchitis)
2. To evaluate the severity of known EIB

3. To evaluate the effectiveness of acute or chronic medication in the prevention of symptoms of EIB

Some investigators believe that EIB can be used as an "experimental model" that, if understood, may shed light on the mechanism of airway hyperreactivity and possibly on the pathophysiology of bronchial asthma.

In a clinical setting, several different types of exercise can be employed. Free running for about 6 min is one test to detect the presence of EIB. This activity may increase heart rate, measured manually, to 170 beats/min in children and 140 beats/min in adults. Since this type of physical activity is difficult to quantitate and properly reproduce, its use in the physician's office is limited. The most frequent types of exercise testing employ the bicycle and walking or running on the treadmill. The workload during bicycling is relatively simple to measure, which represents an advantage over treadmill exercise. Work on the bicycle is usually expressed as the amount of power in watts that has to be developed to overcome resistance against pedaling. The disadvantage of bicycling tests is poor tolerance (instability, difficulties with pedaling, etc.) experienced in older patients and some youngsters who are not accustomed to this activity. Furthermore, exercise done on a bicycle is not as asthmagenic as the other techniques. Standardization of an exercise test with a bicycle was reported by Anderson and Schoffel [53].

In contrast, walking or running on the treadmill is a physical activity tolerated well by a majority of patients. In most laboratories exercise testing usually involves fast walking (2–3 mph) on the treadmill. The disadvantage of treadmill testing is the difficulty of properly measuring the work rate and the fact that work depends on the weight of the subject. Since treadmill exercise is usually accompanied with a greater level of minute ventilation than bicycling, walking or running on a treadmill represents a greater bronchoconstrictive stimulus in asthmatics than bicycling.

B. Conditions Under Which Testing Should Be Done

1. Adequate medical information about the patient:
   a. No present illness (review of cardiorespiratory and musculoskeletal system).
   b. No findings from the physical examination and medical history that contraindicate exercise testing, i.e., a major cardiovascular illness, status post–myocardial infarction, systemic hypertension, or lung disease that leads to abnormal gas exchange, such as pulmonary hypertension; fever; upper or lower respiratory tract infection.
   c. In general, testing is not done when resting baseline maximal expiratory flow rates, such as FEV_1, are less than 65% of predicted normal value.
2. Adequate equipment, personnel, and medicines:
   a. Monitoring of heart rate during the exercise is mandatory in all patients over 35 years old. In this patient population, a standard electrocardio-

gram (ECG) should be checked before exercise for the presence of ischemic heart disease or significant arrhythmias.

b. An experienced and qualified observer with a stethoscope should always be present during the test.

c. Appropriate medications, oxygen, and a rapid-acting bronchodilator should be available in the testing room if older patients are tested.

3. Medications: The time for withholding specific medications will depend on the purpose of the exercise study. In general this will depend on the individual medicine's duration of action. Certain medications with a long pharmacokinetic or pharmacodynamic half-life may interfere with the exercise test. Inhaled β_2-agonists should be withdrawn 6–8 h before testing; oral bronchodilators, long-acting theophylline, and potent antihistamines should be withheld 24–36 h before exercise. Cromolyn sodium and nedocromyl should be stopped 48 h before exercise. Inhaled steroids seem to have only a small effect in the prevention of EIB. Particularly in comparative studies, it is important to keep the dose of steroids constant.
4. A recent meal and a recent intake of xanthine-containing products (coffee, cola, chocolate, etc.) would disqualify the person to be tested. An exercise test should be done 2–3 h after a major meal.

During exercise testing all patients should wear a noseclip. This causes some discomfort, but two important conditions are established: (1) The type of ventilation during exercise, i.e., nose or mouth, is controlled. Our data suggest that during exercise, in some instances, patients will use a mixed type of breathing (both nose and mouth), and this may influence the outcome of the test (see Fig. 1). (2) We have shown that in asthmatics, mouth breathing during the exercise test will potentiate EIB [54]. Since the goal of exercise testing is to demonstrate the presence of EIB, a more optimal condition, i.e., mouth breathing, should be selected.

C. Exercise Protocol

There have been several attempts to standardize the exercise testing procedure [55–60], but these attempts have been only partially successful. Recent guidelines for the methodology of exercise challenge have been described by the Bronchoprovocation Committee of the American Academy of Allergy and Immunology [61].

Before exercise testing each patient is asked about a history of exercise-induced bronchoconstriction and any previous exercise testing (see Table 1). Before exercise it should be demonstrated that pulmonary function as measured by spirometry is at least 80% of the patient's usual value and that the FEV_1 is greater than 65% of predicted values. Before the test, patients should be asked about their last medication(s) (see above, "Conditions Under Which Testing Should Be Done").

It should be remembered that younger patients are generally afraid of this test.

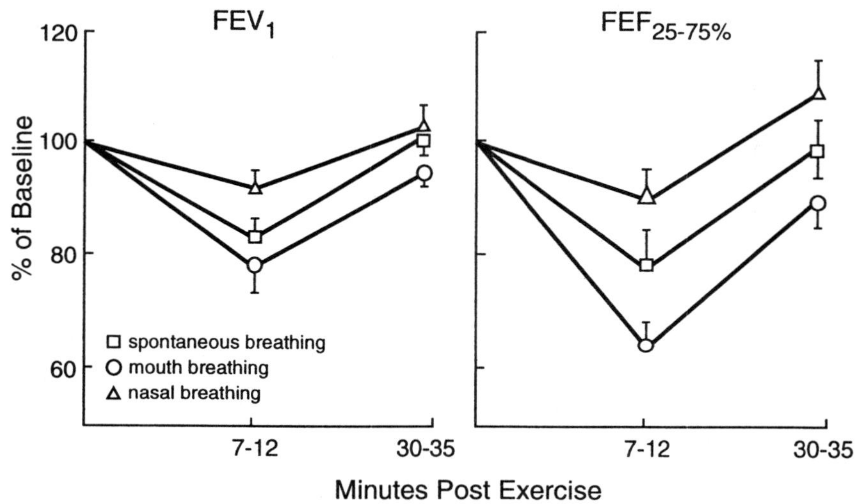

Figure 1 Effect of mouth and nasal breathing on exercise-induced bronchoconstriction in children with asthma. Changes in forced expired volume in 1 second (FEV_1) and midexpiratory flow rate ($FEF_{25-75\%}$) as determined in periods after exercise are shown. In all patients exercise test was done with mouth breathing (circles), nasal breathing (triangles), and spontaneous breathing (squares). Mean ± SE values are shown.

It will help if the purpose of testing is explained and if the patient is shown how to walk on the treadmill, which may include a brief practice. It is advisable to select a low starting speed and to bring the patient up within 2–3 min to the target speed as well as to the target inclination (% grade) of the treadmill.

During exercise, patients should not be allowed to hold on to the treadmill railing. Any support will decrease the workload, which may influence the outcome of testing. Patients should be instructed to support themselves only with one finger, if necessary, on the front railing, alternating hands during the test. This arrangement will make the estimation of treadmill workload more reliable.

When the exercise test is repeated with one patient, it is advisable to do the test at the same time of day for each session. This will minimize variation in baseline pulmonary function and exercise response. An example of the experimental protocol for exercise testing, showing the sequence of different measurements, is given in Fig. 2.

D. Equipment

Equipment needed for exercise testing includes (1) a treadmill (with adjustable grade and speed), (2) an ECG monitoring system, and (3) an emergency set-up (in

Table 1 Example of the Worksheet for Treadmill Exercise Test

Name: Sex: M F Age: Date:
Weight: (kg) Height: (cm)
Time tested:
Noseclip: Yes No
Medication: Off medication:
80% Predicted max. heart rate:

1. Speed (mph)
2. Inclination (% grade)
3. Duration of exercise
4. Total revolutions of treadmill
5. Total distance (m)
6. Total work done (kpm)
7. Power output (kpm/min)
8. Power output (W)
9. Power per body mass (W/kg)
10. Actual max. heart rate

Established pulmonary diagnosis:
History of exercise symptoms:
Reason for study: Diagnostic Drug study Follow-up
Recent URI (colds, flu, etc.):
How patient feels prior to testing:
How patient feels during testing: Wheezing Coughing
Complaints:
How patient feels after the testing:

which fast-acting bronchodilators, oxygen, defibrillator, and other emergency equipment should be present).

E. Selection of Workload and Measurement of Heart Rate

The workload on the treadmill can be selected from two different points of view: the level of the heart rate that should be achieved during exercise and the predicted workload.

During steady-state walking on the treadmill, the tested subject should not reach more than 80% of predicted maximal heart rate. Before the beginning of the exercise test, on the basis of the patient's age, the maximal heart rate is determined from a chart and 80% of this value is recorded on an exercise worksheet (Table 1). The rule is followed that when the patient's heart rate during exercise is higher than 80% of his predicted maximal heart rate, the speed of the treadmill is decreased or exercise is discontinued. Continuous increase of heart rate during exercise toward

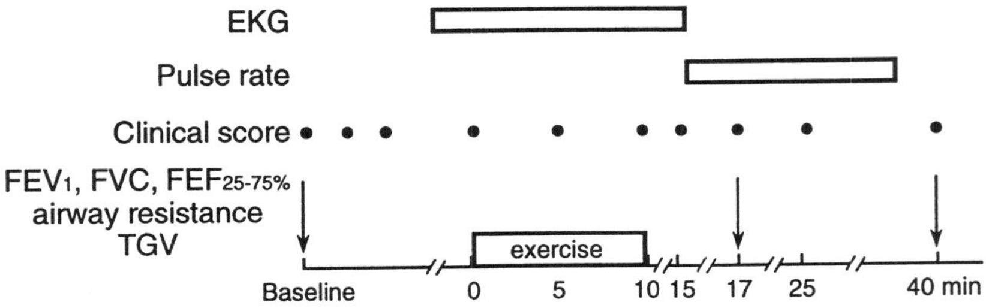

Figure 2 Experimental protocol used in exercise testing, with time sequence of different measurements.

maximum levels, while the patient is performing moderate work, suggests poor fitness of the cardiovascular system and possibly a cardiovascular abnormality.

Usually, three electrodes are required to monitor the heart rate during exercise. The most suitable locations for electrodes are as follows: one electrode on the base of the sternum, a second slightly to the left of and below the left nipple, and the ground electrode placed symmetrically (to the left electrode) on the right side of the chest. All electrodes should be mounted on a bone structure, avoiding any major muscle masses. In order to prevent any loosening of the electrode during exercise, it is recommended that the electrode leads be taped to the body. In order to obtain an adequate ECG signal, the skin should be cleaned with acetone or alcohol. Superficial layers of the skin are removed by scratching the area of skin with a rubber margin located on the electrode, and then the electrodes are attached.

In the majority of tested patients, after 4–5 min of fast walking on the treadmill, at a moderate pace, a steady-state value of the heart rate is usually observed.

The workload on the treadmill also can be judged from the fact that 80% of the maximal heart rate is reached when the subject performs a workload of approximately 2 ± 0.2 W/kg of body weight (BW). Considering this workload and the subject's body weight, one can then estimate the desired speed and grade of the treadmill before the exercise test begins. The relationship of these two variables for different work loads is shown in Fig. 3. It is obvious that the same workload can be done by combining varying speeds and inclinations of the treadmill. Thus, in smaller children a higher workload can be done by increasing the inclination (grade) at a lower speed of the treadmill. A grade of 10% and speed of 5 km/h (3 mph) for 10 min has been found to be sufficient to induce significant bronchoconstriction in both children and adults who have hyperreactive airways.

F. Evaluation of Workload on the Treadmill

After exercise testing, work on the treadmill can be estimated relatively simply if certain conditions are met [62]. As mentioned above, the speed of the treadmill

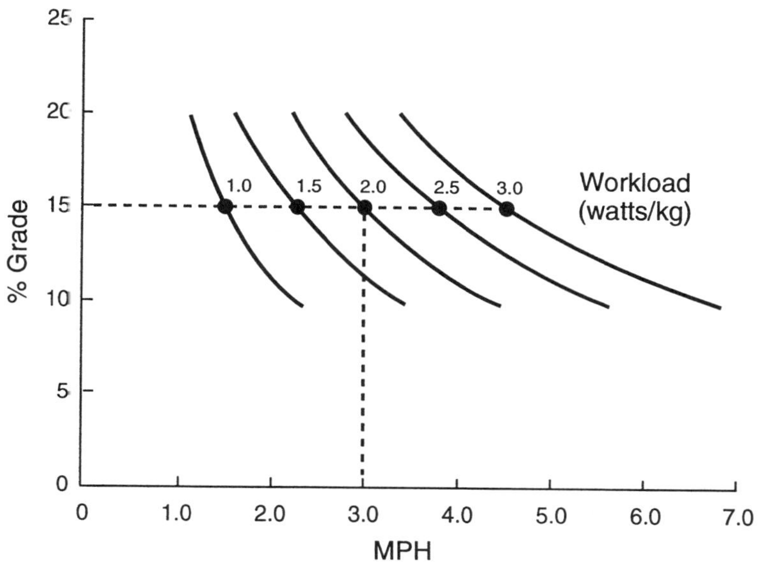

Figure 3 Selection of workload on the treadmill from treadmill speed and elevation.

and percent of the grade (inclination) are first selected and recorded on the worksheet (Table 1, items #1 and #2). To determine total work, all exercise testing is always done with the grade of the treadmill greater than 5%. The duration of the exercise test is usually 6–10 min (#3) and the total revolutions of the treadmill (#4) are recorded at the end of exercise. Revolutions of the treadmill are converted into total distance in meters (#5) using a conversion factor found in a treadmill manual. Total work done (#6) on the treadmill is calculated as follows:

$$\text{Total work (KPM)} = \text{distance (in meters)} \times \frac{\%\ \text{grade} \times \text{kg BW}}{100}$$

To obtain *power output per minute* (#7), this value (#6) is divided by the duration of exercise (#3) in minutes. To obtain *power output* in watts (#8), power output (#7) is divided by 6.12, since 1 W is equal to 6.12 KPM (kilopondmeter). *Power per body mass* (#9) relates power output (#8) to body weight. The metabolic cost of treadmill exercise with respect to oxygen consumption can also be estimated using the Silverman and Anderson diagram [63].

G. Environmental Conditions in the Laboratory

The exercise should be done in a special room with a constant temperature of 19–21°C and a known relative humidity. The room should also have good ventilation and be free of any pollutants or airborne particles and allergens. Exercise testing done in a room with high temperature and humidity of air will attenuate development of EIB.

H. Measurement of Pulmonary Function

Measurement of pulmonary function is done before exercise (baseline) and 7–15 min after exercise. At this time a maximal change in pulmonary function usually occurs. If the efficacy of the specific drug is tested 15–30 min after the agent is administered, the baseline pulmonary function testing is always repeated before the exercise test is done. The patient should be monitored for symptoms throughout the exercise and for 30 min afterward. At this time, in the majority of patients, pulmonary function usually returns to the baseline value.

Utilizing variables such as FEV_1, $FEF_{25-75\%}$, $FEV_1\%$, and FVC, the response to treadmill exercise can be assessed. Response to exercise is usually expressed as a percentage change from baseline. A decrease of 15% in FEV_1 and a fall in midexpiratory flow rate ($FEF_{25-75\%}$) greater than 35% are considered abnormal responses that signify the presence of EIB. Some investigators consider the test

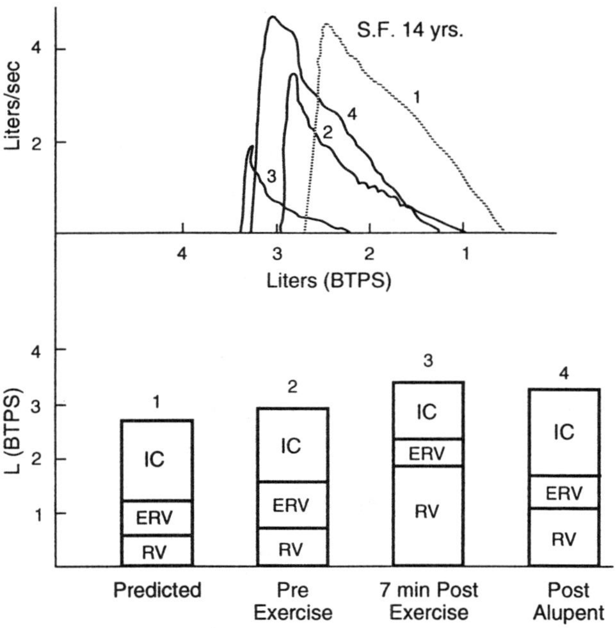

Figure 4 Example of exercise-induced bronchoconstriction as measured by maximal expiratory flow–volume curves (MEFV curve) and static lung volumes in 14-year-old boy with asthma.

positive if FEV_1 is decreased by 10%. It is our experience that the measurement of peak expiratory flow rate is grossly dependent on patient effort and muscle strength and in many instances does not reflect an objective measurement of postexercise airway bronchoconstriction. Preferably, airway response after exercise is simply described by measuring the maximal expiratory flow–volume relationship (MEFV curve), as can be seen in Fig. 4. In this instance, after the exercise test the patient had a dramatic decrease in maximal expiratory flow rates and an increase in RV and FRC. If the measurement of static lung volumes is available (as by using body plethysmography), one should express changes in expiratory flow rates considering the static lung volumes ("isovolume condition"), as seen in Fig. 4. Buckley et al. [56] compared the relative sensitivity of different pulmonary function variables of asthmatic patients in the postexercise period and found that the measurements of Raw and SGaw are most sensitive to describe changes in airway diameter in asthmatics, as compared with other pulmonary function tests. However, these particular tests are available only in the more sophisticated pulmonary function laboratories. Since forced expiration, such as that done during spirometry measurements, may induce bronchoconstriction, determination of airway resistance and thoracic gas volume should always precede spirometry.

IV. HYPERVENTILATION TESTS

The principal stimulus for bronchoconstriction developed after exercise testing is the level of minute ventilation rather than the exercise itself [64]. Exercise is a natural stimulus to increase the minute ventilation and thus in the majority of studies can be an optimal test to assess nonspecific airway reactivity. On the other hand, nonspecific airway reactivity can be assessed with voluntary isocapnic hyperpnea (VIH), i.e., an increase in minute ventilation without exercise [28,65]. As with exercise, this test is more convenient than inhalation challenges, since no administration of agents such as histamine or methacholine is involved. It is easy to employ, and the dose–response-like relationship, i.e., the relationship between the level of minute ventilation and the degree of following bronchoconstriction as measured by pulmonary function testing, can be readily determined [65]. This test is particularly suitable in the testing of asthmatic patients who, for some reason, cannot perform exercise. Similarly, this test may be used in some older patients with chronic bronchitis or patients with chronic obstructive pulmonary disease, in whom an increase in heart rate or oxygen consumption during exercise is not desirable.

Hyperventilation-induced bronchoconstriction has a time course very similar to that of EIB. The level of ventilation achieved during exercise usually induces a similar degree of bronchoconstriction when achieved through voluntary isocapnic hyperventilation [64].

A. Voluntary Isocapnic Hyperpnea (Hyperventilation) Test—Done with "Room-Temperature" Air

In this procedure, each patient voluntarily ventilates for 5 min at three different levels of effort, with 7- to 10-min intervals between ventilatory levels. During the entire procedure the level of patient end-tidal CO_2 is constantly maintained. The experimental setup used in VIH testing is shown in Fig. 5. It consists of a low-resistance two-way breathing valve (Rudolf Co.), of which the inspiratory part is connected to a Fleish #3 pneumotachygraph. The patient inhales a mixture of room air (or compressed air) and CO_2 at a temperature of 20–22°C and a relative humidity of 7–15% (% of humidity if uncompressed air is used) from a gas-mixing chamber. Continuous analysis of expired O_2 and CO_2 can be made using a mass spectrometer or other gas-analyzing system. Values of CO_2 are used to adjust the flow of CO_2 that is added to the gas-mixing chamber. Each person tested can see the display of minute ventilation, tidal volume, and respiratory rate on the monitor and can maintain relatively well the selected level of ventilation. Voluntary isocapnic hyperventilation will induce significant bronchoconstriction of a degree comparable to that expected after moderate exercise [64]. Patients with asthma have a linear relationship between the decrease in SGaw and the level of minute ventilation in the range of tested ventilation, i.e., 25–45 L/min. A similar relationship can exist between the level of VIH and maximal expiratory flow rate determined at 70% of total lung capacity [65].

Pulmonary function tests are determined immediately before and 3–5 min after each VIH test. Within 15 min after VIH tests there is a return of pulmonary function to baseline values. Furthermore, contrary to the exercise test, no refrac-

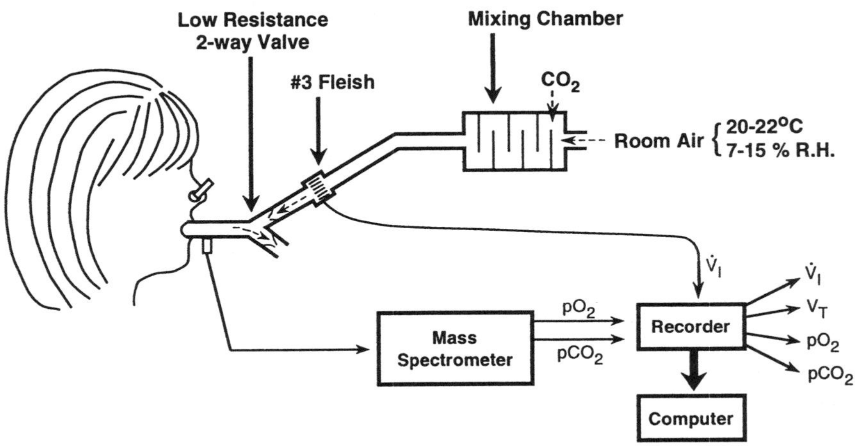

Figure 5 Experimental set-up for voluntary isocapnic hyperventilation.

tory period is observed after the VIH test. Pulmonary function tests may include determination of partial flow–volume curves, maximal expiratory flow–volume curve (MEFV curve), or variables such FEV_1, FVC, or $FEF_{25-75\%}$.

It should be kept in mind that the relative humidity of the inspired air will significantly influence the outcome of this test. The inhalation of dry air (compressed air) may potentiate the development of differentiation-induced bronchoconstriction. If the test is done in a humid environment, a higher level of minute ventilation should be used to induce significant bronchoconstriction in asthmatics.

Voluntary isocapnic hyperventilation is a simple procedure that may be used to evaluate nonspecific airway reactivity. Airway response, as measured by pulmonary function, is proportional to the level of minute ventilation. This test is well tolerated by patients, and the airway response in patients with hyperreactive airways has good reproducibility within 4 days of testing. An obvious disadvantage is the need for several special items, such as low-resistance valves, flowmeter, and gas analyzer (determination of CO_2).

B. Voluntary Isocapnic Hyperpnea (Hyperventilation)—Done with Cool Air

In this test, instead of room-temperature air, VIH is done with cool air (4°C) [66]. Clearly, decreasing temperature (and humidity) of inspired air will potentiate the airway response of asthmatic patients after hyperventilation testing. It is not worth the effort to use subfreezing air. The special heat exchanger that is required to decrease the temperature of inspired air presents an additional expense. A majority of patients with asthma develop bronchoconstriction after isocapnic hyperventilation (~60 L/min) of dry air at room temperature (20–22°C).

V. MECHANISMS OF EXERCISE-INDUCED BRONCHOCONSTRICTION AND HYPERVENTILATION-INDUCED BRONCHOCONSTRICTION

As repeatedly pointed out, normal airways show a measurable airway response, i.e., bronchoconstriction to stimuli such as inhalation of different chemicals, dust inhalation, and mechanical irritation [67]. This is a normal response of airways and is usually explained as a response of epithelial receptors (C-fiber receptors, rapidly adapting receptors, and slowly adapting receptors) to stimulation. Since intervention such as cooling or surgical disruption of the vagus nerve, pharmacological vagal blockade, or local anesthesia could inhibit this response, it is believed that this bronchoconstrictive response is reflex in nature and is probably mediated through the vagus nerve [68–71]. The mechanism of airway stimulation does not seem to be very specific, since a great variety of stimuli as described above can cause this response.

In the airways of patients with bronchial asthma, the exaggerated response to different stimulations is probably based on the damaged airway epithelium and other surrounding cells [72]. The sensory epithelial nerve fibers are probably more accessible to different stimuli. Recently it has also been suggested that the permeability of the tight junctions of the epithelial cells may be changed so that epithelial receptors are more accessible to direct or indirect (mediator) stimulation [73]. Even though nonspecific airway hyperreactivity is a very important clinical phenomenon that seems to reflect a relatively early phase of airway injury and airway inflammation, few studies have examined this problem on the tissue level.

As pointed out by Widdicombe [71], allergens and chemical mediators can also exhibit a "nonvagal" action on airway smooth muscle. This mechanism should also be considered in the evaluation of patients' airway hyperreactivity.

In patients with bronchial asthma, airway hyperreactivity is frequently unchanged even after long-term treatment even though measures of pulmonary function, such as FEV_1, can be within the normal range of predicted values. It is of great interest that adults who had asthma in childhood but are no longer symptomatic still manifested increased airway reactivity. On the other hand, as seen from the study of Empy et al. [74] and Laitinen et al. [75], viral disease–induced airway hyperreactivity was within the normal range 6 weeks after acute viral infections, suggesting that at least in some instances this abnormality is reversible.

A. Heat and Water Exchange in Upper Airways

In humans, one of the most important functions of the nose is to modify inspired air. In addition to removing small particles and some gases (e.g., sulfur dioxide), the nose provides an important place for the adjustment of inspired air to the body temperature and for its humidification. Because the saturation of air with water depends on the temperature, more water vapor is required for maintaining full saturation as the inspired air is warmed to 37°C. This nasal air-conditioning function is highly efficient under resting conditions, when the level of ventilation varies from 8 L/min to 15 L/min. Even during exercise (up to certain ventilatory levels), a subject is normally capable of breathing through the nose, because during exercise a special reflex mechanism constricts vessels in the nose and this in turn decreases resistance to the nasal airflow. As the level of exercise and ventilation increases even more, increasing nasal resistance raises the work of breathing, and then breathing is done through the mouth only. Consequently, the conditioning of inspired air through the nose is eliminated. Under these conditions, air inhaled into the upper airways will be cooler and drier. Thus, during physical work in a particularly cold environment, the temperature and humidity of the upper airways can be compromised. At these higher levels of ventilation a significant cooling and also drying of the mucosa can occur even in more peripheral airways. Pioneering work by McFadden et al. [76–78] has shown that during quick breathing most of the heating of the inspired air took place in the upper airways. However, during hyperventilation and inhalation of subfreezing-temperature air, a temperature decrease could be detected even in small peripheral airways. This finding suggests that the conditioning of inspired air is a continuous process probably involving most of the tracheobronchial tree.

B. Role of Minute Ventilation

Hyperventilation per se has been implicated as a possible causative factor in EIB [2,64]. It has been shown that warm and humid air supplied during exercise to asthmatic patients can prevent the development of EIB [14]. In addition, it has been demonstrated that the severity of EIB is decreased if asthmatic children are instructed to use only nasal breathing during exercise. In contrast, oral breathing during exercise potentiated EIB [54].

In carefully controlled studies, it has been shown that significant bronchoconstriction, comparable in severity to that observed after moderate treadmill exercise, can be induced in asthmatics by VIH of 3-min and 10-min duration. In both hyperventilation and exercise, nasal breathing inhibited bronchoconstriction, whereas mouth breathing potentiated the bronchoconstrictive response. It is of interest that 10 min of VIH did not represent a greater bronchoconstrictive stimulus than did 10 min of exercise or 3 min of isocapnic hyperventilation [64].

The results of our study conclusively demonstrate that hyperventilation can be considered critical in the mechanism of EIB. This and the above studies confirm that the temperature and humidity of inspired air are decisive factors in the development of postexercise or posthyperventilation bronchoconstriction. The immediate consequence of ventilation of relatively dry and cold air will be heat and water loss from airways.

C. Consequence of Heat Loss

It has been well documented that in both asthmatic and nonasthmatic subjects esophageal temperature during exercise decreases significantly [79]. However, no differences were observed in the fall in temperature when normal subjects were compared with asthmatics. These investigators extended their previous conclusions that the magnitude of EIB is directly proportional to the thermal load placed on airways and can be described in terms of respiratory heat exchange [80]. They concluded that asthmatics are apparently more responsive to the effect of cool air. In further studies, McFadden and associates [76–78] directly measured temperature in the tracheobronchial tree in normal subjects during inhalation of air of different temperatures. They observed that as the level of breathing increases, the temperature of the distal airways progressively falls and the thermal burden thus progresses deeper into the periphery of the lung.

In an extension of this work, McFadden and associates [76] determined intraairway thermal profiles of six different points in the tracheobronchial tree during exercise and voluntary hyperventilation. With both exercise and hyperventilation, temperatures fell dramatically to a comparable level in both groups of subjects. These data are compatible with previous results showing that if voluntary hyperventilation is done at the same level of ventilation as observed during exercise, a similar decrease in pulmonary function can be observed [64].

An obvious question that needs to be asked is whether a difference in airway temperature as observed during exercise and hyperventilation can have any physiological effect on structures in the airway wall. In a study using isolated segments of airways, it was found that a decrease in temperature has an important and direct effect on the level of resting membrane potential of airway smooth-muscle cells. The resting membrane potential of airway smooth-muscle cells decreased with decreasing temperature [81]. It was also found that airway smooth-muscle cell Na^+/K^+-ATPase is directly involved in the mechanism of the temperature effect. Furthermore, it was also reported that at lower temperatures, contractile and electrical responses of airway smooth-muscle cells to histamine were significantly potentiated [81].

Similarly, cooling also increased the contractile response of airway smooth muscle to acetylcholine [82] and substance P [83]. Additionally, it was shown that when the segments of isolated airways are suddenly cooled, a significant increase in airway tone can be elicited. In the same study, the authors also found that rapid rewarming of an isolated airway also caused an increase in the airway tone [84]. Other investigators reported similar findings [85,86]. When sensitized rabbits were exposed to cool-air challenge, an amplification of the bronchoconstrictive response in comparison with control animals was detected [87,88]. The same investigators also noticed that cool air potentiates the bronchoconstrictive response of rabbits to inhaled histamine. In contrast, in situ cooling of normal dog airways failed to potentiate acetylcholine-induced contraction. In the same study, cooling potentiated acetylcholine-induced contraction of isolated airway segments [89]. One may speculate that the discrepancy between this study and that done with rabbits [87,88] could be related to species differences.

D. Consequence of Water Loss

Using a highly innovative approach, Anderson and associates [90,91] reported that EIB is caused by water loss from airways rather than by heat loss. According to these authors, the loss of water from the surface of airways may create a hyperosmotic environment around specific cells. In the case of mast cells, this osmotic change will initiate a prompt degranulation and consequent mediator release, leading to responses such as bronchoconstriction, increase in mucus secretion, and development of edema. The same authors also suggested that an increase in the osmolarity of respiratory mucosa may stimulate epithelial receptors

[92], which may lead to the activation of the vagal reflex. The same conclusions were echoed by other investigators [93].

These observations in human studies are supported by data from some animal models. Thus, Freed and associates reported [94] that in normal dogs, cooling of airways actually has an inhibitory effect on the airway tone, while hyperosmotic changes in dog airways lead to bronchoconstriction. Interestingly, in experiments with isolated preconstricted guinea pig tracheas, a hyperosmolar stimulus actually caused relaxation [95]. The same investigators also demonstrated that this relaxation was epithelium-dependent.

It is likely that discussion concerning the relative role of water loss and heat loss in the development of EIB will continue. Experimental evidence suggests that water loss may be a more important factor than heat loss. The temperature and humidity of airway surfaces depends on numerous factors. Some, such as bronchial circulation, were only recently identified as critical. Thus, McFadden speculated [96] that exercise and hyperventilation may lead to the release of mediators and neurotransmitters, resulting in a microvascular response of mucosal and submucosal capillaries. According to this hypothesis, consequent engorgement of these structures may lead to capillary leakage, mucosal edema formation, and development of airway obstruction. However, this hypothesis awaits direct experimental evidence [97]. Another fact that should be taken into consideration is

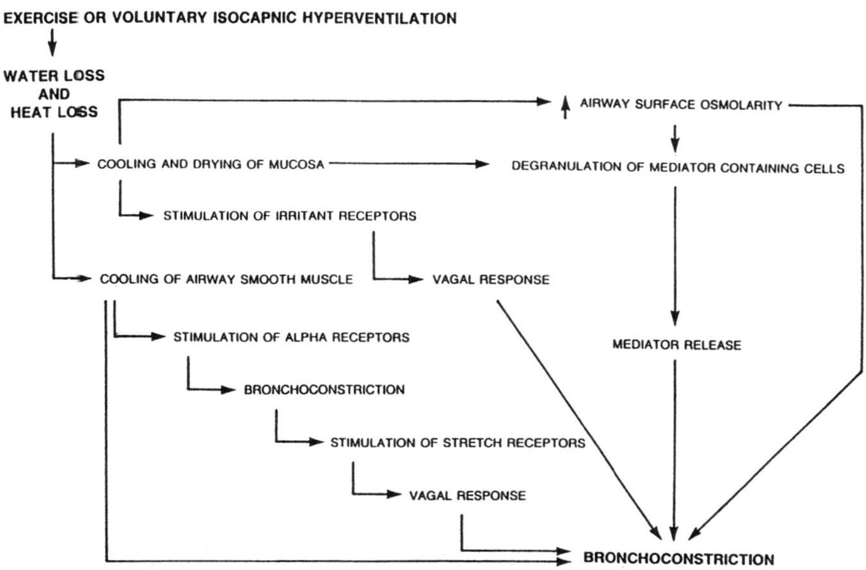

Figure 6 Mechanisms participating in exercise-induced bronchoconstriction.

that cooling and drying of airway surfaces occurs in anatomically compromised airways. An attempt to reconcile both the water-loss and the heat-loss hypotheses in the mechanism of EIB is summarized in Fig. 6.

VI. SUMMARY

The results of clinical studies suggest that EIB is caused by multiple factors that occur in response to the loss of water and heat from the surface of airways. It is likely that the initiating stimuli are water and heat loss, which both lead to the cascade of events culminating in bronchoconstriction. Furthermore, it is possible that in different patients with bronchial asthma, the importance of different pathways that lead to bronchoconstriction may vary.

REFERENCES

1. Cohen, S. G., and Samter, M., eds., *Excerpts from Classics in Allergy*, 2nd Ed., Symposia-Foundation, Carlsbad, California, 1992.
2. Herxheimer, H., Hyperventilation asthma, *Lancet*, *1*, 87–89 (1946).
3. Anderson, S. D., Silverman, M., Konig, P., and Godfrey, S., Exercise-induced asthma, *Br. J. Dis. Chest*, *69*, 1–17 (1975).
4. Anderson, S., Issues in exercise-induced asthma, *J. Allergy Clin. Immunol.*, *76*, 762–722 (1985).
5. Jones, R. S., Buston, M. H., and Wharton, M. J., The effect of exercise on ventilatory function in the child with asthma, *Br. J. Dis. Chest*, *56*, 78–84 (1962).
6. Jones, R. S., Wharton, M. J., and Buston, M. H., The place of physical exercise and bronchodilator drugs in the assessment of the asthmatic child, *Arch. Dis. Child.*, *38*, 539–545 (1963).
7. Jones, R. S., Assessment of respiratory function in the asthmatic child, *Br. Med. J.*, *2*, 972–975 (1966).
8. Cropp, G. J. A., Exercise-induced asthma, *Pediatr. Clin. North Am.*, *22*, 63–76 (1975).
9. Sly, R. M., Exercise-induced asthma, in *Bronchial Asthma, Mechanisms and Therapeutics* (E. B. Weiss and M. S. Segal, eds.), Little, Brown, Boston, 1976, p. 537–546.
10. McFadden E. R., Jr., and Ingram, R. H., Jr., Exercise-induced asthma, *N. Engl. J. Med.*, *301*, 763–769 (1979).
11. McFadden, E. R., Jr., An analysis of exercise as a stimulus for the production of airway obstruction, *Lung*, *159*, 3–11 (1981).
12. Godfrey, S., Exercise testing in children, *Applications in Health and Disease*, W.B. Saunders Corp., Ltd., London, 1974.
13. Cochrane, L. M., and Clark, C. J., Benefits and problems of a physical training program for asthmatic patients, *Thorax*, *45*, 345–351 (1990).
14. Chen, W. Y., and Horton, D. J., Heat and water loss from the airways and exercise-induced asthma, *Respiration*, *34*, 305–313 (1977).

15. Kawabori, S., Pierson, W. E., Conquest, C. W., Incidence of exercise-induced asthma in children, *J. Allergy Clin. Immunol.*, *58*, 447–455 (1976).
16. Kagawa, J., and Kerr, H. D., Effects of brief graded exercise on specific airway conductance in normal subjects, *J. Appl. Physiol.*, *28*, 138–142 (1970).
17. Mansfield, L., McDonnell, J., Morgan, W., and Souhrada, J. F., Airway response in asthmatic children during and after exercise, *Respiration*, *38*, 135–143 (1979).
18. Lefcoe, N. M., The time course of maximum ventilatory performance during and after moderately heavy exercise, *Clin. Sci.*, *36*, 47–52 (1969).
19. O'Donnel, A., and Fling, J., Exercise-induced airflow obstruction in a healthy military population, *Chest*, *103*, 742–744 (1993).
20. Boulet, L. P., Legris, C., Turcotte, H., and Hebert, J., Prevalence and characteristics of late asthmatic response to exercise, *J. Allergy Clin. Immunol.*, *80*, 655–662 (1987).
21. Lee, T. H., and O'Hickey, S. P., Exercise-induced asthma and late phase reactions, *Eur. Respir. J.*, *2*, 195–197 (1989).
22. Speelberg, B., Davis, E. A. H., and Bijl, D., Late asthmatic responses after exercise challenge are reproducible, *J. Allergy Clin. Immunol.*, *87*, 1128–1137 (1991).
23. Rubinstein, I., Levison, H., and Slutsky, A. S., Immediate and delayed bronchoconstriction after exercise in patients with asthma, *N. Engl. J. Med.*, *317*, 482–485 (1987).
24. Karjalainen, J., Exercise response in 404 young men with asthma: no evidence for a late asthmatic reaction, *Thorax*, *46*, 100–104 (1991).
25. Kattan, M., Keens, T. G., Mellis, C. M., and Levison, H., The response to exercise in normal and asthmatic children, *J. Pediatr.*, *92*, 718–721 (1978).
26. Katz, R. M., Whipp, B. J., Heimlich, E. M., and Wasserman, K., Exercise-induced bronchospasm, ventilation and blood gases in asthmatic children, *J. Allergy*, *47*, 148–158 (1971).
27. Vassallo, C. L., Gee, J. B. L., and Domm, B. M., Exercise-induced asthma: observations regarding hypocapnia and acidosis, *Am. Rev. Respir. Dis.*, *105*, 42–49 (1972).
28. Kivity, S., and Souhrada, J. F., Hyperpnea: the common stimulus for bronchospasms in asthma during exercise and voluntary isocapnic hyperpnea, *Respiration*, *40*, 169–177 (1980).
29. Enright, P. L., McNally, J. F., and Souhrada, J. F., Effect of lidocaine on the ventilatory and airway responses to exercise in asthmatics, *Am. Rev. Respir. Dis.*, *122*, 823–828 (1980).
30. Guz, A., Control of ventilation in man with special reference to abnormalities, in *Asthma, Physiology, Immunopharmacology, and Treatment* (L. M. Lichtenstein and K. F. Austen, eds.), Academic Press, New York, 1977, pp. 211–223.
31. Bevegard, S., Eriksson, B. O., Graff-Lonnevig, V., Kraepelien, S., and Saitin, B., Circulatory and respiratory dimensions and functional capacity in boys aged 8–13 years with bronchial asthma, *Acta Paediatr. Scand. Suppl.*, *217*, 86–92 (1971).
32. Anderson, S. D., Poser, R., Smith, I. D., and Temple, D., Exercise-related changes in plasma levels of 15-keto-13,14-dihydro-prostaglandin $F_{2\alpha}$ and noradrenaline in asthmatic and normal subjects, *Scand. J. Respir. Dis.*, *57*, 41–48 (1976).
33. Field, J., Auegria, J., Trauticin, J., Demers, L., Gillin, M., and Zelis, R., Measure-

ment of plasma prostaglandins during exercise-induced bronchospasm, *J. Allergy Clin. Immunol.*, *58*, 581–589 (1976).

34. Chryssanthopoulos, C., Barboriak, J. J., Fink, J. N., Stekiel, W., and Maksud, M. G., Adrenergic responses of asthmatic and normal subjects to submaximal and maximal work levels, *J. Allergy Clin. Immunol.*, *61*, 17–23 (1978).
35. Griffiths, J., Leung, F. Y., Grzybowski, S., and Chan-Yeung, M. M. W., Sequential estimation of plasma catecholamines in exercise-induced asthma, *Chest*, *62*, 527–533 (1972).
36. McFadden, E. R., Jr., and Soter, A., A search for clinical mediators of immediate hyperreactivity and humoral factors in the pathogenesis of exercise-induced asthma, in *Asthma, Physiology, Immunopharmacology, and Treatment* (L. M. Lichtenstein and K. F. Austen, eds.), Academic Press, New York, 1977, pp. 351–366.
37. McFadden, E. R., Jr., Soter, N. A., and Ingram, R. H., Jr., Magnitude and site of airway response to exercise in asthmatics in relation to arterial histamine levels, *J. Allergy Clin. Immunol.*, *66*, 472–477 (1980).
38. Granerus, G., Simonsson, B. G., Skoogh, B.-E., and Wetterqvist, H., Exercise-induced bronchoconstriction and histamine release, *Scand. J. Respir. Dis.*, *52*, 13–19 (1971).
39. Harries, M. G., Burge P. S., O'Brien, I., Cromwell, O., and Pepys, J., Blood histamine levels after exercise testing, *Clin. Allergy*, *9*, 437–442 (1979).
40. Barboriak, J. J., Sosman, A. J., Fink, J. N., Maksud, M. G., McConnell, L. H., and Hamilton, L. H., Metabolic changes in exercise-induced asthma, *Clin. Allergy*, *3*, 83–89 (1973).
41. Shaffer, A. L., and Austen, F., Exercise-induced anaphylaxis, *J. Allergy Clin. Immunol.*, *66*, 106–109 (1980).
42. Maulitz, R. M., Pratt, D. S., and Schocket, A. L., Exercise-induced anaphylactic reaction to shellfish, *J. Allergy Clin. Immunol.*, *63*, 433–439 (1979).
43. Orehek, J., Yatraro, P., Smith, A. P., Grimaud, C., and Charpin, J., Airway response to carbachol in normal and asthmatic subjects. Distribution between bronchial sensitivity and reactivity, *Am. Rev. Respir. Dis.*, *115*, 937–944 (1977).
44. Pavia, D., Thomson, M. L., Clarke, S. W., and Shannon, H. S., Effect of lung function and mode of inhalation on penetration of aerosol into the human lung, *Thorax*, *32*, 194–199 (1977).
45. Thomson, M. L., and Pavia, D., Particle penetration and clearance in the human lung, *Arch. Environ. Health*, *29*, 214–219 (1974).
46. Fish, J. E., Rosenthal, R. R., Batra, G., Menkes, H., Summer, W., Permutt, S., and Norman, P., Airway response to methacholine in allergic and nonallergic subjects, *Am. Rev. Respir. Dis.*, *113*, 519–524 (1976).
47. Permutt, S., Rosenthal, R. R., Norman, P. S., and Menkes, H. A., Bronchial challenge in ragweed-sensitive patients, in *Asthma Physiology, Immunopharmacology, and Treatment* (L. M. Lichtenstein and K. F. Austen, eds.), Academic Press, New York, 1977, pp. 266–281.
48. Juniper, E. F., Frith, P. A., Dunnett, C., Cockcroft, D. W., and Hargreave, F. E., Reproducibility and comparison of responses to inhaled histamine and methacholine, *Thorax*, *33*, 705–712 (1978).

49. Eggleston, P. A., A comparison of the asthmatic response to methacholine and exercise, *J. Allergy Clin. Immunol.*, *63*, 104–109 (1979).
50. Kiviloog, J., Bronchial reactivity to exercise and methacholine in bronchial asthma, *Scand. J. Respir. Dis.*, *54*, 347–357 (1973).
51. Weiler-Rawal, D., and Geoffrey, S., Do exercise- and antigen-induced asthma utilize the same pathways? Antigen provocation in patients rendered refractory to exercise-induced asthma, *J. Allergy Clin. Immunol.*, *67*, 391–397 (1981).
52. Godfrey, S., Springer, C., Noviski, N., Haayan, C. H., and Auital, A., Exercise but not methacholine differentiates asthma from chronic lung disease in children, *Thorax*, *46*, 488–492 (1991).
53. Anderson, S. D., and Schoffel, R. E., Respiratory heat and water loss during exercise in patients with asthma, *Eur. J. Respir. Dis.*, *63*, 472–480 (1982).
54. Shturman-Ellstein, R., Zeballos, R. J., Buckley, J. M., and Souhrada, J. F., The beneficial effect of nasal breathing or exercise-induced bronchoconstriction, *Am. Rev. Respir. Dis.*, *118*, 65–73 (1978).
55. Silverman, M., and Anderson, S. D., Standardization of exercise tests in asthmatic children, *Arch. Dis. Child.*, *47*, 882–889 (1972).
56. Buckley, J. M., Souhrada, J. F., and Kopetzky, M. T., Detection of airway obstruction in exercise induced asthma, *Chest*, *66*, 244–251 (1974).
57. Buckley, J. M., and Souhrada, J. F., A comparison of pulmonary function tests in detecting exercise-induced bronchoconstriction, *Pediatrics*, *56* (suppl 2), 887–889 (1975).
58. Eggleston, P. A., Methods of exercise challenge, *J. Allergy Clin. Immunol.*, *73*, 666–669 (1984).
59. Eggleston, P. A., Exercise challenge: indications, techniques, and data analysis. Laboratory evaluation of exercise-induced asthma: methodologic considerations, *J. Allergy Clin. Immunol.*, *64*, 604–612 (1979).
60. Eggleston, P. A., Rosenthal, R. R., Anderson, S. A., Anderton, R., Bierman, C. W., Bleecker, E. R., Chai, H., Cropp, G. J. A., Johnson, J. D., Konig, P., Morse, J., Smith, L. J., Summers, R. J., and Trauttein, J. J., Guidelines for the methodology of exercise challenge testing of asthmatics, *J. Allergy Clin. Immunol.*, *64*, 642–645 (1979).
61. Bleecker, E. R., Exercise-induced asthma: physiologic and clinical considerations, *Clin. Chest Med.*, *5*, 109–119 (1984).
62. Fisher, H. K., Holton, P., Buxton, R. S. J., and Nadel, J. A., Resistance to breathing during exercise-induced asthma attacks, *Am. Rev. Respir. Dis.*, *101*, 885–892 (1970).
63. Silverman, M., and Anderson, S. D., Metabolic cost of treadmill exercise in children, *J Appl. Physiol.*, *33*, 690–696 (1977).
64. Zeballos, R. J., Shturman-Elistein, R., McNally, J. F., Jr., Hirsch, J. E., and Souhrada, J F., The role of hyperventilation in exercise-induced bronchoconstriction, *Am. Rev. Respir. Dis.*, *118*, 877–884 (1978).
65. Kivity, S., Souhrada, J. F., Metzer, E., A dose–response-like relationship between minute ventilation and exercise-induced bronchoconstriction in young asthmatic patients, *Eur. J. Respir. Dis.*, *61*, 342–346 (1980).
66. Deal, E. C., Jr., McFadden, E. R., Jr., Ingram, R. H., Jr., Breslin, F. J., and Jaeger,

J. J., Airway responsiveness to cold air and hyperpnea in normal subjects and in those with hay fever and asthma, *Am. Rev. Respir. Dis.*, *121*, 621–628 (1980).
67. Nadel, J. A., Neurophysiologic aspects of asthma, in *Asthma, Physiology, Immunopharmacology, and Treatment* (K. F. Austen and L. M. Lichtenstein, eds.), Academic Press, New York, 1973, pp. 29–38.
68. Gold, W. M., Cholinergic pharmacology in asthma, in *Asthma, Physiology, Immunopharmacology, and Treatment* (K. F. Austen and L. M. Lichtenstein, eds.), Academic Press, New York, 1973, pp. 169–184.
69. Simonsson, B. G., Jacobs, F. M., and Nadel, J. A., Role of autonomic nervous system and the cough reflex in the increased responsiveness of airways in patients with obstructive airway disease, *J. Clin. Invest.*, *46*, 1812–1818 (1967).
70. Anderton, R. C., Cuff, M. T., Frith, P. A., Cockcroft, D. W., Morse, J. L. C., Jones, N. L., and Hargreave, F. E., Bronchial responsiveness to inhaled histamine and exercise, *J. Allergy Clin. Immunol.*, *63*, 315–318 (1979).
71. Widdicombe, J. G., Reflex control in tracheobronchial smooth muscle in experimental and human asthma, in *Asthma, Physiology, Immunopharmacology, and Treatment* (L. M. Lichtenstein and K. M. Austen, eds.), Academic Press, New York, 1977, pp. 225–236.
72. Laitinen, L. A., Heino, M., Laitenen, A., Kava, T., Haahzela, T., Damage of the airway epithelium and bronchial reactivity in patients with asthma, *Am. Rev. Respir. Dis.*, *131*, 599–600 (1985).
73. Lozewitz, S., Wells, C., Goméz, E., Ferguson, H., Richman, P., DeValia, J., and Davies, R. J., Morphological integrity of the bronchial epithelium in mild asthma, *Thorax*, *45*, 12–15 (1990).
74. Empey, D. W., Laitienen, L. A., Jacobs, L., Gold, W. M., and Nadel, J. A., Mechanisms of bronchial hyperreactivity in normal subjects following upper respiratory tract infection, *Am. Rev. Respir. Dis.*, *113*, 131–139 (1976).
75. Laitinen, L. A., Elkin, R. B., Empey, D. W., Jacobs, L., Mills, J., and Nadel, J. A., Bronchial hyperresponsiveness in normal subjects during attenuated influenza virus infection, *Am. Rev. Respir. Dis.*, *143*, 358–361 (1991).
76. McFadden, E. R., Jr., and Pichurko, B. M., Intraairway thermal profiles during exercise and hyperventilation in normal man, *J. Clin. Invest.*, *76*, 1007–1010(1985).
77. McFadden, E. R., Jr., Pichurko, B. M., Bowman, H. F., Ingenito, E., Burns, S., Dowling, N., and Solway, J., Thermal mapping of the airways in humans, *J. Appl. Physiol.*, *58*, 564–570 (1985).
78. Gilbert, I. A., Fouke, J. M., and McFadden, E. R., Jr., The effect of repetitive exercise on airway temperature, *Am. Rev. Respir. Dis.*, *142*, 826–831 (1990).
79. Deal, E. C., Jr., McFadden, E. R., Jr., and Ingram, R. H., Jr., Esophageal temperature during exercise in asthmatics and nonasthmatic subjects, *J. Appl. Physiol.*, *46*, 484–490 (1979).
80. Deal, E. C., Jr., McFadden, E. R., Jr., Ingram, R. H., Jr., Strauss, R. H., and Jaeger, J. J., Role of respiratory heat exchange in production of exercise-induced asthma, *J. Appl. Physiol.*, *46*, 467–475 (1979).
81. Souhrada, M., and Souhrada, J. F., The direct effect of temperature on airway smooth muscle, *Respir. Physiol.*, *44*, 311–323 (1981).

82. Ishii, T., and Shimo, Y., Cooling-induced supersensitivity to acetylcholine in the isolated airway smooth muscle of the rat, *Naunyn Schmiedebergs Arch. Pharmacol.*, *329*, 167–175 (1985).
83. Ishii, T., and Shimo, Y., Cooling-induced augmentation of the contractile response of the golden hamster tracheal muscle to substance P in vitro, *J. Pharm. Pharmacol.*, *38*, 403–405 (1985).
84. Souhrada, J. F., Preseley, D., and Souhrada, M., Mechanisms of the temperature effect on airway smooth muscle, *Respir. Physiol.*, *53*, 225–237 (1983).
85. Kolbeck, R. C., Chaudhary, B. A., and Spier, W. A., Jr., Studies of mediator involvement in cooling-induced alteration of guinea pig tracheal smooth muscle contractility, *Proc. Soc. Exp. Biol. Med.*, *187*, 82–88 (1988).
86. Ortiz, J. L., Cortijo, J., Sanz, C., DeDiego, A., Esplugues, J., and Moreillo, E., Cooling-induced contraction of trachea isolated from normal and sensitized guinea pigs, *Nauny Schmiedebergs Arch. Pharmacol.*, *343*, 418–426 (1991).
87. Jammes, Y., Barthelemy, P., Fornaris, M., and Grimaud, C. H., Cold-induced bronchospasm in normal and sensitized rabbits, *Respir. Physiol.*, *63*, 347–360 (1986).
88. Badier, M., Barthelemy, P., Soler, M., and Jammes, Y., In vivo and in vitro studies on cold-induced airway response in normal and sensitized rabbits, *Respir. Physiol.*, *73*, 1–10 (1988).
89. Bethel, R. A., Tanaka, D. T., Mitchell, L. S., Curtis, S. P., Leff, A. R., and Irvin, C. H. G., Effect of cooling on the responsiveness of canine tracheal muscle, *Am. Rev. Respir. Dis.*, *142*, 1402–1406 (1990).
90. Anderson, S., Is there a unifying hypothesis for exercise-induced asthma? *J. Allergy Clin. Immunol.*, *73*, 660–665 (1984).
91. Hahn, A., Anderson, S. D., Morton, A. R., Black, J. L., and Fitch, K. D., A reinterpretation of the effect of temperature and water content of the inspired air in exercise-induced asthma, *Am. Rev. Respir. Dis.*, *130*, 575–579 (1984).
92. Smith, C. M., and Anderson, S. D., A comparison between the airway response to isocapnic hyperventilation and hypertonic saline in subjects with asthma, *Eur. Respir. J.*, *2*, 36–43 (1989).
93. Sheppard, D., and Eschenbacher, W. L., Respiratory water loss as a stimulus to exercise-induced bronchoconstriction, *Am. Rev. Respir. Dis.*, *73*, 640–642 (1984).
94. Freed, A. N., Bromberper-Barnea, B., and Menkes, H. A., Dry air induced constriction in lung periphery: a canine model of exercise-induced asthma, *J. Appl. Physiol.*, *59*, 1986–1990 (1985).
95. Kunakata, M., Kitner, W., and Menkes, H., Osmotic stimuli induce epithelial-dependent relaxation in the guinea pig trachea, *J. Appl. Physiol.*, *64*, 466–471 (1988).
96. McFadden, E. R., Jr., Hypothesis: exercise-induced asthma as a vascular phenomenon, *Lancet*, *335*, 880–882 (1990).
97. Anderson, S. D., and Daviskas, E., The airway microvasculature and exercise-induced asthma, *Thorax*, *47*, 748–752 (1992).

18

Inhalation Bronchoprovocation in Children

Paul V. Williams and Gail Shapiro

University of Washington School of Medicine
Seattle, Washington

I. INTRODUCTION

In children as in adults, airway hyperreactivity is the tendency of airway smooth muscle of patients with asthma to constrict after exposure to stimuli that do not affect the airways of most normal persons. This is a key feature of asthma, the degree of hyperreactivity relating more closely to the severity of asthma than does resting lung function [1,2]. Within a sample of patients with asthma, there is a correlation between reactivity and clinical disease, so that greater airway reactivity is associated with more symptoms, lower morning peak flow rates, greater diurnal variation in peak flow, greater response to bronchoconstricting stimuli, and a more intense level of treatment [3]. In a given population, however, an individual may show extreme nonspecific reactivity but have mild disease, and vice versa [4]. In addition, some patients manifest hyperreactivity, usually to a mild degree, without showing clinical evidence of reactive airway disease. These patients may have residual reactivity years after the cessation of clinical asthma or may have transient reactivity following a respiratory infection or associated with allergic rhinitis [5]. Other pediatric diseases associated with airway hyperreactivity include bronchopulmonary dysplasia and cystic fibrosis, and smoking, both active and passive, also is associated with hyperreactivity [6]. Because of this, hyperreactivity as measured with bronchoprovocative challenges cannot be considered synonymous with asthma. Rather, these challenges are diagnostic techniques used to verify impressions derived from a history and physical examination.

Even in childhood, both genetically determined and acquired factors contribute to airway hyperreactivity. Several population studies [7–10], done with a variety of bronchoprovocation challenges, have demonstrated a unimodal distribution of reactivity, confirming that both genetic and environmental factors play a role. Another indicator of genetic and environmental factors is the fact that reactivity varies in different populations and different environments [11]. In twin studies, concordance for bronchial hyperreactivity is greater for identical than for nonidentical twins. However, concordance is less than 50% [12]. Studies of siblings and parents of asthmatic children demonstrate that 39% have abnormal bronchial lability [13].

Age also appears to be a significant factor in airway reactivity. Several studies [14–16] have noted a high incidence of airway reactivity in infants. Normal healthy patients aged less than 21 years and more than 60 years have higher bronchial reactivity than those aged 21–60 years (Fig. 1) [17].

Environmental factors causing bronchial hyperreactivity include infections and environmental contaminants. A history of croup or more than two lower respiratory infections in early childhood is associated with increased bronchial reactivity as late as 10 years after infection [18,19]. Pertussis may evoke a first episode

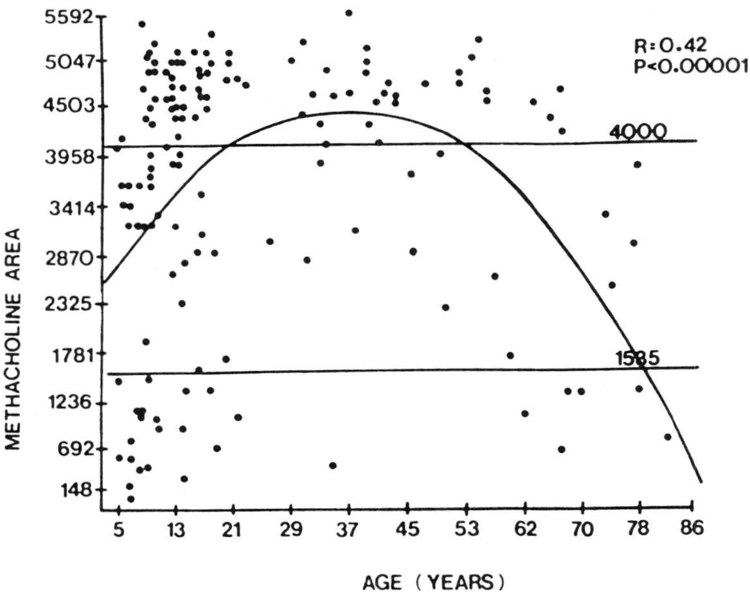

Figure 1 Methacholine responses in unselected patients, showing differences in reactivity with age. Results >4000 indicate normal responses. Values <1535 indicate methacholine responses that are <250 breath units of methacholine. (From Ref.17.)

of bronchospasm in children. Patients recovering from pertussis may have persistent bronchial reactivity for months or years, or permanently [20]. Respiratory syncytial virus (RSV) infection in children may be the precursor of subsequent asthma, children with a history of bronchiolitis in infancy showing a high frequency of abnormal bronchial lability later in childhood [18,21]. Interestingly, Welliver et al. [22] have shown an association between RSV-specific immunoglobulin E (IgE) and histamine release in nasopharyngeal secretions of children with the infection who wheeze. Increased bronchial lability may also be seen after rhinovirus infection [7]. Environmental pollutants such as SO_2, NO_2, and O_3 may transiently enhance bronchial hyperreactivity [23,24]. More persistently harmful are low-molecular-weight chemicals encountered in occupational settings that are not pertinent to airway problems of children.

Although bronchial hyperreactivity is measured in terms of degree of bronchospasm following bronchoprovocation, this depends on innate reactivity of smooth muscle itself and exacerbation due to inflammation in the airway from the factors mentioned above, i.e., infections and environmental influences. These factors may work through injury to the airway epithelium, resulting in release of mediators that are themselves bronchostimulating and also encourage the migration of inflammatory cells, which amplify reactivity.

II. WHY PERFORM BRONCHOPROVOCATION CHALLENGES IN CHILDREN?

The reasons for applying challenge techniques to children differ little from those for adults (Table 1). A variety of methods have been used to determine the presence and severity of airway hyperreactivity. These include both pharmacological (methacholine and histamine) and nonpharmacological (exercise, nonisotonic aerosol, or cold-air hyperventilation) methods. These bronchoprovocative chal-

Table 1 Purposes for Bronchoprovocation Challenges in Children

- To clarify diagnosis of asthma
- To quantify severity of disease
- To determine and compare utility of drugs for asthma control
- To determine and compare duration of action of drugs
- To understand asthma mechanisms
- Epidemiological studies of airway reactivity

Source: Modified from Shapiro, G. G., et al., in *Provocative Challenge Procedures: Background and Methodology* (S. L. Spector, ed.), Futura Publishing Co., New York, 1989, pp. 395–416.

lenges are important clinically as methods to clarify whether symptoms that suggest a diagnosis of airway hyperreactivity are indeed due to this condition. For example, patients sometimes present after having received an assortment of antiasthma medications for cough or recurrent bronchitis, although no physician has ever documented reversibility of obstruction after bronchodilator inhalation. If baseline pulmonary function is normal in the face of such a history, bronchoprovocative challenge may be valuable. At times a challenge test may be used to judge the severity of a patient's asthma. In the research setting, bronchoprovocative challenges provide a method for studying pharmacological modulation of asthma; e.g., the ability of a drug to diminish airway reactivity suggests clinical usefulness. The degree to which this reactivity can be modified can be used as a means to compare the antiasthma characteristics of drugs. Bronchial provocation challenges have also been used in epidemiological studies of large groups of healthy, as well as asthmatic, children. These studies have helped clarify the role of airway reactivity in asthmatic and normal children.

III. PHARMACOLOGICAL CHALLENGES

Bronchoprovocation challenges with the chemicals methacholine and histamine measure smooth muscle reactivity. These chemical challenges depend on the ability of these agents to affect bronchial smooth muscle receptors in such a way as to produce bronchoconstriction in subjects with reactive airways at concentrations that have little or no effect on normal subjects.

Looking at these tests from a historical perspective, in the late 1940s, investigators noted that small amounts of nebulized methacholine caused a striking reduction in vital capacity of asthmatic but not normal subjects [25,26]. Tiffeneau [27] suggested that the response to cholinergic aerosols might be a useful diagnostic test for asthma. Parker et al. [28] simplified a provocative aerosol challenge for clinical use. Along similar lines, Townley et al. [29], Makino [30], and Felarca and Itkin [31] showed a significant reduction of the forced expired volume in 1 second (FEV_1) in asthmatic subjects but in none of a nonatopic control population following methacholine and histamine bronchial inhalation challenge.

Much data of the 1960s and 1970s expounds the usefulness of chemical bronchoprovocation. Both methacholine and histamine emerged as useful agents for eliciting latent bronchial reactivity [31–34], their inhalation in graded doses producing similar dose–response curves capable of sorting subjects with reactive airways from normals subjects. Most of these studies, however, involved patients who were either clearly asthmatic or clearly normal. Several recent epidemiological studies of large numbers of unselected children [10,35–38] have shown that not all asthmatics have positive challenge tests at all times, and that asymptomatic patients may have airway reactivity (Fig. 2). Thus, as we mentioned above, airway reactivity cannot be considered synonymous with asthma, and these challenges

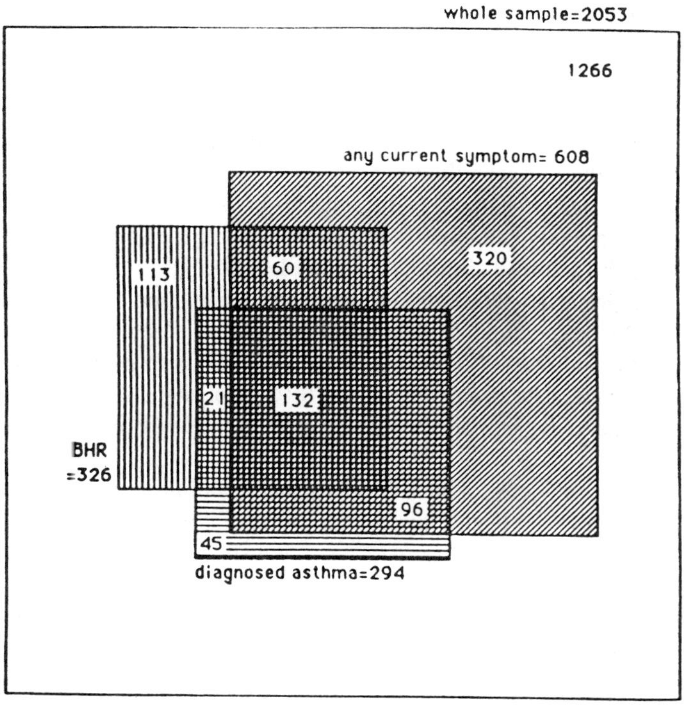

Figure 2 Proportionate Venn diagram showing combined overlap of children with "any current symptom," those with diagnosed asthma, and those with bronchial hyperreactivity (BHR) in a group of 2053 children. Numbers of children in each category are shown. From Ref. 37.)

are not particularly useful as screening tests for asthma in unselected populations of children. The probability of asthma in patients with a positive provocative challenge is largely established by the history, physical examination, and clinical impression of the likelihood of asthma [39,40]. A decrease of FEV_1 of more than 20% is generally accepted as a discriminating end point to separate the normal and hyperreactive groups, the terms PD_{20} and PC_{20}, provocative dose or provocative concentration of test agent causing a 20% decline in FEV_1, being popular bronchoprovocation jargon. Recently, Hopp et al. [41] have suggested that the area under the dose–response curve plotted with methacholine concentration vs. the drop in FEV_1 is a more discriminating measure for quantifying airway reactivity. Other methods of expressing the response to challenge include the slope of the dose–response curve, defined as the percentage fall in FEV_1 at the last dose divided by the total dose administered [10], and the bronchial responsiveness index, defined as the log of the slope of the percent decline from baseline FEV_1 after the last dose per unit dose of methacholine [38]. These two methods may be more useful in epidemiological studies, because a value that relates well to symptom history can be calculated for the entire sample, even if a patient does not experience a 20% drop in FEV_1. For clinical use, however, the PD_{20} or PC_{20} remains the simplest method of recording the response.

Challenge techniques with histamine and methacholine have been well standardized and are easily applied to children. They involve having the subject inhale increasing amounts of drug until the protocol is completed or a drop in FEV_1 of more than 20% has occurred. By 20–30 min following this induction of bronchospasm, there will usually be spontaneous recovery. If the patient is uncomfortable, bronchodilator inhalation will rapidly return pulmonary function to normal. The short duration of bronchoconstriction, the ability to control the dose of bronchoconstrictive stimuli, and the lack of a late-phase response are positive features of these challenges.

The two widely used techniques for administering methacholine and histamine challenges to adults are also applicable to children. One of these involves tidal volume breathing of aerosol that is generated continuously by a nebulizer and delivered directly into a face mask (Fig. 3). This technique has an advantage for the testing of children, since little patient cooperation is required. The second method involves intermittent generation of aerosol by a nebulizer with a mouthpiece connected to a Rosenthal–French dosimeter, a solenoid-valve device that allows aerosol to be generated for a specified time interval. The patient can initiate nebulization by pressing a button or spontaneously with inspiration (Fig. 4).

A number of factors must be standardized to allow for comparison between different challenges of the same subject and for comparisons between different centers. With the continuous-generation method, nebulizer output needs to be regulated. If a Wright nebulizer is used, output should be 0.13–0.16 ml/min. Since Wright nebulizers have at times been difficult to obtain, other nebulizers are often used. Some of these have been characterized so that the output that appears to give results comparable to the Wright standard is known. It is important to use this data or create one's own equivalency data if one is to characterize the patient's sensitivity with relation to scales established with the Wright nebulizer [42]. While the nebulizer output is an important technical variable, it is also important to consider the effect of evaporation on the test parameters. Evaporative losses have been shown to decrease the temperature of the solution up to 11°C, most of the decrease occurring in the first 2 min. There will be a decrease in output with time, and an increase in solute concentration over time [43]. As a consequence, the use of the total output to determine the dose could overestimate the amount of agonist delivered. Also, these findings suggest that the nebulizer solutions should be changed after each test, and that nebulizers should be calibrated under the exact

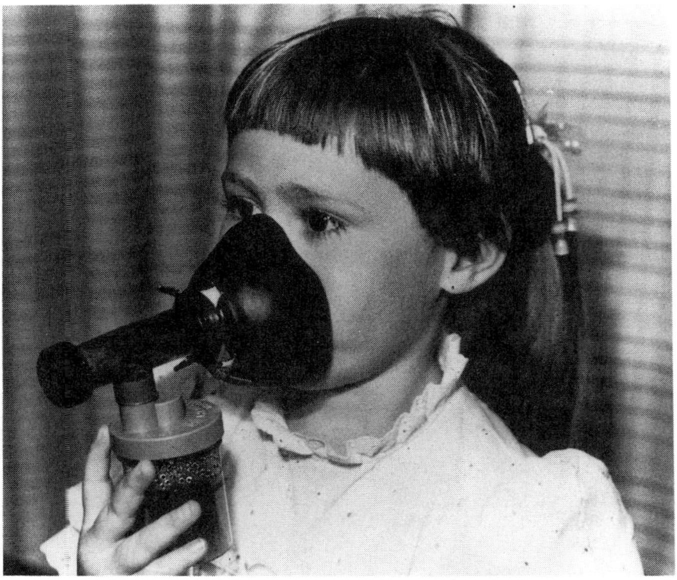

Figure 3 A child breathes a nebulized solution from a face mask during challenge with the continuous method of methacholine generation. (From Shapiro, G. G., et al., in *Provocative Challenge Procedures: Background and Methodology* [S. L. Spector, ed.], Futura Publishing Co., New York. 1989, pp. 395–416.)

parameters of the test. Particle size generated should be between 1 and 4 μm aerodynamic mass median diameter, and time of inhalation must be 2 min.

With the dosimeter method, a De Vilbiss 42 or 646 nebulizer has generally been used. Output per inhalation and the number of inhalations must be standardized. Also, patients must consistently start at the same lung volume, attempt to inhale at the same rate, and hold their breath for the same amount of time with each inspiration. These requirements may be difficult for younger children, in which case the continuous (tidal volume) method should be utilized. When these guidelines have been followed, the continuous method and intermittent method result in similar levels of sensitivity to chemical challenge and good reproducibility [44,45].

To summarize the dosimeter method, compressed air at 20 psi is connected to the input valve of the dosimeter, which is set at 0.6 s per inhalation. A De Vilbiss 42 or 646 nebulizer is also connected to the dosimeter. The patient inhales from a mouthpiece attached to the nebulizer containing the methacholine solution. Each respiration begins from functional residual capacity. With each inspiration, metha-

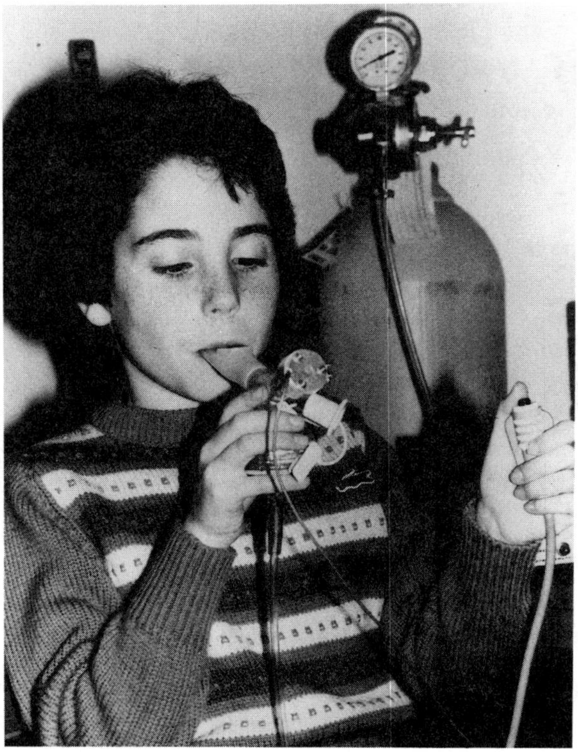

Figure 4 A child depresses the button that triggers nebulization of methacholine during a challenge using the dosimeter method. (From Shapiro, G. G., et al., in *Provocative Challenge Procedures: Background and Methodology* [S. L. Spector, ed.], Futura Publishing Co., New York. 1989, pp. 395–416.)

choline or histamine is delivered for 0.6 s. According to the protocol established by the Bronchoprovocation Committee of the American Academy of Allergy and Immunology in 1975 [46], after an initial inhalation of five breaths of normal saline, five breaths each of nine increasing concentrations of drug are delivered, with no breath-hold between inspirations (9 mg of aerosol being generated per inhalation). The FEV_1 is measured at 1½ and 3 min after each concentration with two expiratory efforts (the best being taken), until the FEV_1 drops by 20% or more or until all nine concentrations have been delivered. Failure to obtain a 20% decline in FEV_1 makes the diagnosis of hyperreactive airways unlikely.

With the continuous-generation method, aerosol is generated by a Wright nebulizer and delivered directly into a face mask. The subject has a nose clip in place and breathes with tidal breathing through the mouth for 2 min. Nebulizer output is kept constant. The subject inhales saline followed by increasing doses of methacholine or histamine. Again, the challenge is discontinued if there is a drop in FEV_1 of 20% or more below the value after saline inhalation.

Since baseline airway caliber can influence methacholine results, and patients with moderate airway obstruction are more susceptible to bronchoconstricting stimuli, it is usually recommended that the FEV_1 be greater than 70% of the predicted value in order to perform the challenge. This can be difficult in moderate to severe asthmatics, who cannot maintain stable airways if they have to stop taking their medications, as is usually recommended. Weiss et al. [47] have devised a three-tiered medication regimen that allows for maintenance of FEV_1 >70% in most asthmatic children and still maintains reproducibility (Table 2). It is unlikely, however, that children with a low FEV_1 would be challenged with methacholine or histamine unless participating in a research protocol. They also noted that methacholine challenge in children is reproducible within one doubling concentration for at least 1 month (Fig. 5).

The dosage schedules often used for methacholine and histamine are, in general, increasing twofold increments (Table 3). Results are expressed in terms of the concentration required to cause a 20% drop in FEV_1 or the number of breath units required, where one breath unit equals one breath of 1 mg/ml of methacholine or histamine. A truncated methacholine protocol (Table 4) has been useful clinically for adults and children, since it decreases the number of inhaled concentrations from nine to five, thus shortening the procedure [48]. This is especially helpful for children, whose attention span may be shorter than one expects for adults. An abbreviated histamine protocol, using fewer doses and a shorter time interval for measuring FEV_1, also compares favorably with the standard protocol (Table 5).

Analysis of the responses in asthmatic as compared with normal subjects has also suggested that the PD_{12} may be sufficient for methacholine challenge [50] and that the PC_{10} or PC_{15} correlates well with the PC_{20} in histamine challenge [51]. One small study suggested that the response that best separates asthmatic from normal subjects may differ for each type of challenge [50]. These findings require further confirmation, but if true they could enable one to shorten the challenges even further.

Methacholine challenge has been applied to the diagnosis of asthma in children under 5 years of age, the production of cough and/or wheezing being the criterion for a positive challenge [52]. This technique may be extremely useful in clinical settings and may be made more objective with the addition of peak flow measurements before challenge and after delivery of each concentration. Avital and coworkers [53] used the production of tracheal wheezing as an end point in defining bronchial hyperresponsiveness in a pediatric sample. Among older children who could perform spirometry, the agreement between the two methods was 80%. They recommended this method as being simpler than and as efficacious as an

Table 2 Medication Protocol as Modified by Weiss and His Group, to Maintain $FEV_1 > 70\%$ of Predicted Value

Regimen 1
- Omit cromolyn inhaler for 24 h before the test.
- Omit theophylline for 12 h before the test.
- Metaproterenol pills may be taken 8 h before the test if needed.
- Metaproterenol or albuterol inhalers may be used once if needed, up to 4 h before the test.
- Steroids (oral or inhaled) may be continued.

Regimen 2
- Omit cromolyn inhaler for 24 h before the test.
- Give theophylline in A.M. as usual on the day of the test.
- Give metaproterenol pills 8 h before the test

  or

- Give metaproterenol or albuterol inhaler 4 h before the test.
- Steroids (oral or inhaled) may be continued.

Regimen 3
- Omit cromolyn inhaler for 24 h before the test.
- Give theophylline in A.M. as usual on the day of the test.
- Give metaproterenol pills 8 h before the test

  or

- Give metaproterenol or albuterol inhaler 4 h before the test.
- Give methylprednisolone pills (0.3 to 0.5 mg/kg) each morning starting 3 days before the test; the last dose should be in the morning on the test day (total, four doses).

alternative method of looking at a drop in transcutaneous oxygen tension, studied by Mochizuki et al. [54] and Murakami et al. [55] (Fig. 6). Computerized lung sound analysis has also been used in histamine challenge in young children and found to be as sensitive as, or more sensitive than, conventional PC_{20} or tracheal auscultation [56].

Histamine and methacholine challenges are tremendously valuable in clinical situations. It has been documented that they are more sensitive than a history and physical examination in the diagnosis of asthma [57]. Cough may be the only manifestation of asthma, and chemical challenge may be uniquely capable of confirming this diagnosis [58]. Shapiro et al. [59] studied 166 children to clarify the etiology of their chronic cough or other undiagnosed pulmonary symptomatology. Methacholine challenge was negative in 58 (35%), and in these children the diagnosis of asthma was therefore improbable. Forty-one patients (25%) had mild methacholine sensitivity, 49 (30%) had moderate sensitivity, and 18 (11%) had

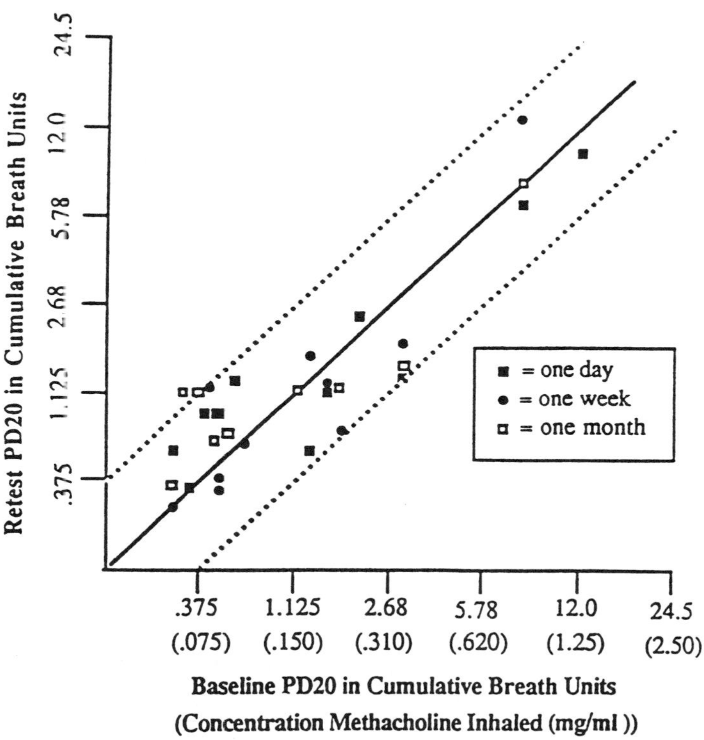

Figure 5 Comparison of responses to inhaled methacholine. Individual data points plotting the FEV_1 in cumulative breath units are shown for the baseline test in comparison with tests done 1 day later ($r = 0.98$, $p < 0.0001$), 1 week later ($r = 0.95$, $p < 0.0001$), and 1 month later ($r = 0.98$, $p < 0.0001$). The inner solid line is the line of identity and the outer dashed lines delimits the region of one doubling concentration difference. The intervals on the x and y axis are doubling cumulative breath units of methacholine. Noncumulative doubling concentrations of inhaled methacholine are also shown in parentheses on the abscissa. (From Ref. 47.)

extreme sensitivity. Many of the patients had chief complaints of cough or bronchitis and did not complain of wheezing. Methacholine challenge helped to clarify appropriate therapy for these children.

Numerous evaluations of pharmacological modulation of asthma include chemical challenge as a means of showing whether a drug can alter airway reactivity. Furukawa and co-workers studied theophylline compared with cromolyn for control of mild to moderate chronic asthma in children [60]. While asthma symptoms and pulmonary function were similar with the two drugs, only cromo-

Table 3 Breath Units for Methacholine and Histamine on a mg/ml Basis[a]

Concentrations (mg/ml)	Cumulative no. breaths	Units/ breath	Units/ 5 breaths	Cumulative units/ 5 breaths[b]
Methacholine				
0.075	5	0.075	0.375	0.375
0.15	10	0.15	0.750	1.125
0.31	15	0.31	1.55	2.68
0.62	20	0.62	3.10	5.78
1.25	25	1.25	6.25	12.0
2.50	30	2.50	12.50	24.5
5.00	35	5.00	25.00	49.5
10.00	40	10.00	50.00	99.5
25.00	45	25.00	125.00	225.00
Histamine base				
0.03	5	0.03	0.15	0.15
0.06	10	0.06	0.30	0.45
0.12	15	0.12	0.60	1.05
0.25	20	0.25	1.25	2.30
0.50	25	0.50	2.50	4.80
1.00	30	1.00	5.00	9.80
2.50	35	2.50	12.50	22.30
5.00	40	5.00	25.00	47.30
10.00	45	10.00	50.00	97.30

[a]One breath unit = 1 inhalation of 1 mg/ml methacholine or histamine base.
[b]If the final FEV_1 test is performed at other than a 5-breath interval, the cumulative units are calculated as follows: for methacholine, at 23 breaths, by adding $3 \times 0.62 = 1.86$ to $5.78 = 7.54$; for histamine, by adding $3 \times 0.25 = 0.75$ to $2.30 = 3.05$.
Source: Ref. 46.

Table 4 Truncated Methacholine Protocol

Methacholine concentrations (mg/ml)	Cumulative breaths	Units/ 5 breaths	Cumulative units/ 5 breaths
0.025	5	0.13	0.13
0.25	10	1.25	1.38
2.50	15	12.50	13.88
10.00	20	50.00	63.88
25.00	25	125.00	188.88

Source: Shapiro, G. G., et al., in *Provocative Challenge Procedures: Background and Methodology* (S. L. Spector, ed.), Futura Publishing Co., New York, 1989, pp. 395–416.

Table 5 Dosing and Cumulative Breath Units for the Standard Histamine Protocol and the Abbreviated Histamine Protocol

Standard histamine protocol			Abbreviated histamine protocol		
Concentration (mg/ml)	Inhalation	Cumulative breath units (mg/ml)	Concentration (mg/ml)	Inhalations	Cumulative breath units (mg/ml)
0.3	5	0.15	.06	1	0.16
0.6	5	0.45	.16	3	0.64
0.12	5	1.05	2.12	1	2.76
0.25	5	2.3	2.12	4	11.24
0.5	5	4.8	10.6	3	43.04
1.0	5	9.8	10.6	4	85.44
2.5	5	22.3			
5.0	5	47.3			
10.0	5	97.3			

Source Ref. 49.

lyn diminished bronchial reactivity measured with methacholine challenge. A pediatric study comparing chronic therapy with the β agonist terbutaline alone, cromolyn alone, or the two combined showed a reduction in methacholine sensitivity with the regimens that included cromolyn and an increase with terbutaline alone [61].

The amount of time that a drug diminishes airway reactivity as measured by chemical challenge is a useful means of establishing duration of action of the drug. Chemical challenges are also used in epidemiological research to define the proportion of subjects with reactive airways as well as to classify their characteristics. Hopp and co-workers [62] compared methacholine sensitivity in a nonatopic pediatric population and a population of current asthmatic children. The best specificity and sensitivity of the challenge occurred at a provocative dose of 100 breath units of methacholine. Challenges may be useful for discerning asthma mechanisms. Bhagat and Grunstein [63] found extreme methacholine sensitivity among patients with extremely labile asthma characterized by rapid deterioration, though this group's histamine sensitivity was not clustered in the extreme range (Figs. 7 and 8). Provocative testing can also be useful in discerning severity of asthma, as a guide to patient management of children and adults [2,63]. Murray et al. [2] evaluated a population of children with asthma who were symptom-free. The correlation between asthma history score and provocative histamine dose was stronger than that between asthma score and any spirometric test, suggesting that the histamine test more accurately assessed the overall severity of the asthma.

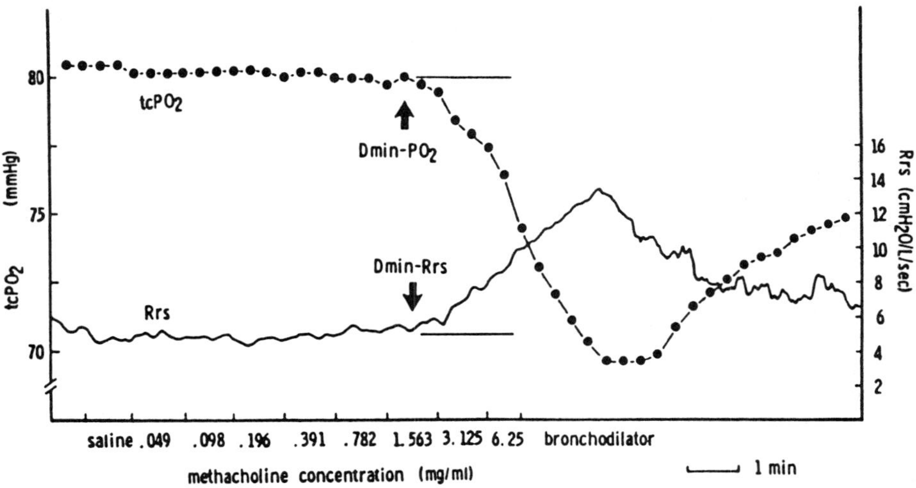

Figure 6 Typical methacholine inhalation challenge with monitoring of respiratory resistance (Rrs) by the oscillation method and transcutaneous oxygen partial pressure (tcPO2). The Dmin-PO2 indicates the inflection point where the tcPO2 changed linearly and denotes the bronchial sensitivity. The Dmin-Rrs indicates the point of change of respiratory resistance. (From Mochizuki, H., et al., *Ann. Allergy*, *60*, 103–106 [188].)

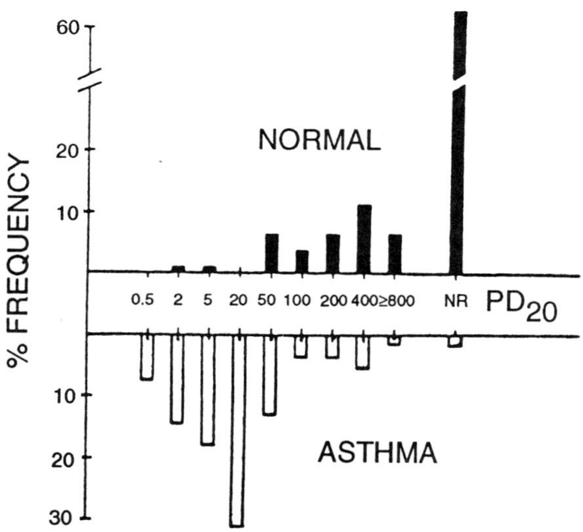

Figure 7 Percent of normal and asthmatic subjects responding at each PD_{20} concentration. (From Ref. 62.)

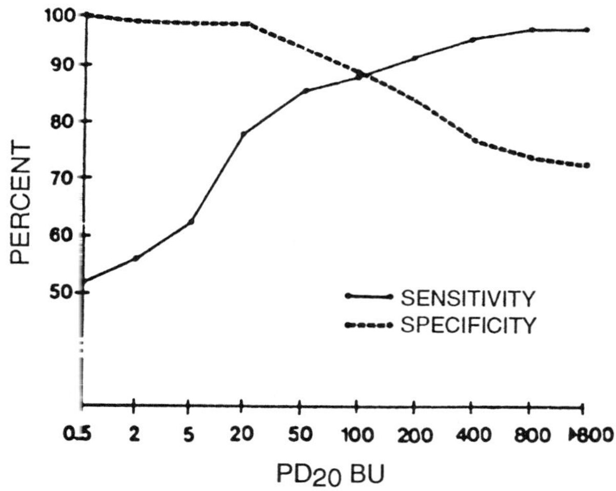

Figure 8 Comparison of the sensitivity and specificity of the PD_{20} response and clinical diagnosis. (From Ref. 62.)

IV. NONPHARMACOLOGICAL CHALLENGES

Bronchoprovocation challenges involving inhalation of cold air, water and saline seem to elicit bronchial hyperreactivity by altering salt and fluid homeostasis in the airways and, thus, changing airway osmolarity. A change in airway osmolarity is also thought to be at least part of the mechanism of exercise-induced asthma [65]. While the response to methacholine and histamine is limited to transient smooth-muscle effects, osmotic challenges can produce sequelae such as a refractory period, late-phase reaction, and heightened reactivity to a subsequent methacholine or histamine challenge. These alterations suggest that in contrast to chemical challenges, which directly and transiently affect smooth muscle, osmotic challenges affect the epithelium and may stimulate nervous and inflammatory excitation that either causes or occurs concurrently with bronchoconstriction.

Cold-air hyperventilation provides an alternative to chemical bronchoprovocation for children, just as it does for adults. While there is the advantage that cold air is a "natural" stimulus, there are disadvantages of this technique compared with chemical challenge. While recent data suggest that there is a dose–response relationship [66] and that a dose–response curve can be plotted by interrupting the cold-air challenge at 1-min intervals and measuring pulmonary function, most studies have used a single period of stimulus delivery after which pulmonary function is measured, precluding the establishment of a dose–response curve. The equipment needed for air cooling and maintaining the patient in a eucapnic state is more expensive than the apparatus for chemical challenge. Lastly, protocols have not been standardized among centers.

The equipment for isocapnic hyperventilation of cold air involves a source of compressed air delivered to a heat exchanger that can bring the temperature to −15°C to −10°C. Most studies have used a 5- to 7-L target balloon as a visual cue to regulate the patient's breathing. The patient is coached to hyperventilate at a minute ventilation of about 25 times FEV_1, which is comparable to that of moderately strenuous activity. The patient can learn to breath at this rate by being required to keep the target balloon inflated while it is evacuated at the necessary rate by a vacuum pump. Alternatively, some protocols provide audible recorded breathing sounds to the subject and train him or her to breathe at this rate. Hypocapnia is avoided by use of a compressed air mixture of 5% CO_2, 21% O_2, and 74% N_2 or by directing a constant stream of 5% CO_2 at 2 L/min into the inspiratory line [67–70]. An example of an apparatus for this procedure appears in Fig. 9.

Hyperventilation has generally been for 4-min period. Spirometry is performed at every few minutes after challenge for 15–20 min, the best of several trial FEV_1s being used. A drop in FEV_1 of 10% or more has been considered positive [68]. It appears that maximal falls in FEV_1 occur at 3–4 min and that recovery to < 10% drop in FEV_1 occurs by 11 min [71]. Reisman et al. [68] suggest spirometry at 4, 6, and 8 min after challenge. Considering a drop in FEV_1 > 10% a positive test, they claim sensitivity of 95% and specificity of 89% for cold-air challenge, results similar to those of methacholine challenge. This differs from earlier work from the

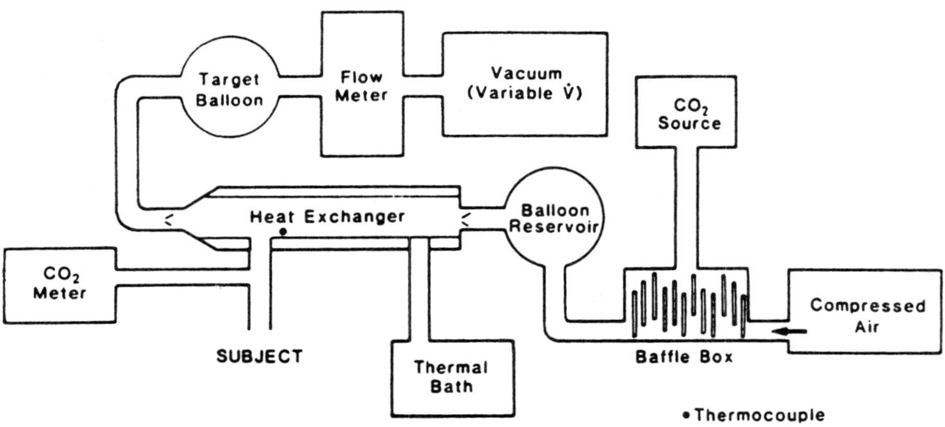

Cold air inhalation challenge apparatus.

Figure 9 Cold air inhalation challenge apparatus. (From Ref. 70.)

same center, in which a somewhat different protocol yielded 100% specificity but only 57% sensitivity [72].

Challenge with ultrasonically nebulized distilled water (UNDW) challenge is another bronchoprovocative technique that lacks a standardized protocol. It appears to be very specific for diagnosing airway hyperreactivity but is much less sensitive than chemical challenge (Table 6). The UNDW challenge requires minimal equipment and little extra effort from the patient, since tidal breathing is used [73]. A dose–response curve is generated, since patients begin by breathing a low dose of water, and this dose is gradually increased.

During a typical procedure, UNDW is generated at a known rate, allowing inspired volume to be recorded. For precision, the delivered dose should be checked by weighing the cannister and tubing before and after each interval of the challenge (Fig. 10) [74]. Hopp et al. [73] have used a system generating approximately 8 ml of water per minute. Subjects inhale nebulized water for 15 s, 15 s, 30 s, 1 min, 2 min, 4 min, and 4 min. For each of these intervals the subject tidal-breathes, with a nose clip in place, through a mouthpiece connected to a Hans-Rudolph nonrebreathing valve (#2700) that is attached to the nebulizer (Fig. 11). Three minutes after each step above, subjects perform two or three forced expiratory maneuvers, the highest being recorded. The test is stopped when the subject's FEV_1 drops 20% or more compared with baseline or the second 4-min step is completed. The UNDW challenge is not a useful screening test for asthma because of its lack of sensitivity, but it remains an interesting research tool. Comparing UNDW challenge with methacholine challenge in children, Galdes-Sebaldt and co-workers found 100% specificity for the former compared with 83% for the latter, but only 71% sensitivity with ultrasonic mist compared with 95% for methacholine [72]. In a study in children by Eichler et al. [75], up to 100% of the patients had significant falls in small-airway function, suggesting a peripheral-airway effect. Eichler et al. suggested that the midexpiratory flow rate at 25% of vital capacity (MEF_{25}) and at 50% of vital capacity (MEF_{50}) might be better variables to evaluate in UNDW challenges. Bronchoconstriction persisted for 10 min after their challenges, so a bronchodilator may be indicated. In addition, UNDW challenges have been associated with increases in bronchial hyperreactivity, and late reactions have been described [76]. This technique has also been used in infants with similar results [77].

Anderson [74] initiated interest in ultrasonic saline as a bronchoprovocative challenge. Patients inspire increasing volumes of 4.5% NaCl, though for patients suspected of being highly sensitive, a solution of 2.7% NaCl is used. Spirometry is performed after incremental volumes of saline are inspired, the challenge being completed when there is a reduction of more than 20% in FEV_1 or a total of 33 ml has been administered. Continued experience with the test suggests that the total volume to be administered can be reduced to as little as 15 ml, with only a minor decrease in sensitivity [78]. Furthermore, since normal patients do not have a

Table 6 Sensitivity of Distilled-Water Challenges in Different Studies

Clinical Studies	Sample size/ age range (y)	Amount inhaled (ml)	Decrease in FEV_1 to define response (%)	Sensitivity to asthma (%)	Type of nebulizer
Galdes-Sebaldt et al.	21/7–16	—	10	71	DeVilbiss model 65
Lemire et al.	11/20–43	44	20	91	DeVilbiss ultra neb 100
Bascom and Bleecker	15/28–40	38	20	53	DeVilbiss model 65
Anderson et al.	55/11–56	33	20	100	Mist 02 Gen EN 143a
Black et al.	12/20–41	33	20	75	Mist 02 Gen EN 143 a
Hopp et al.	66/21–37	82	10	76	DeVilbiss model 646
Epidemiologic study, Frischer et al.	446/7–10	20	10	36	Habel m608

Source: Ref. 9.

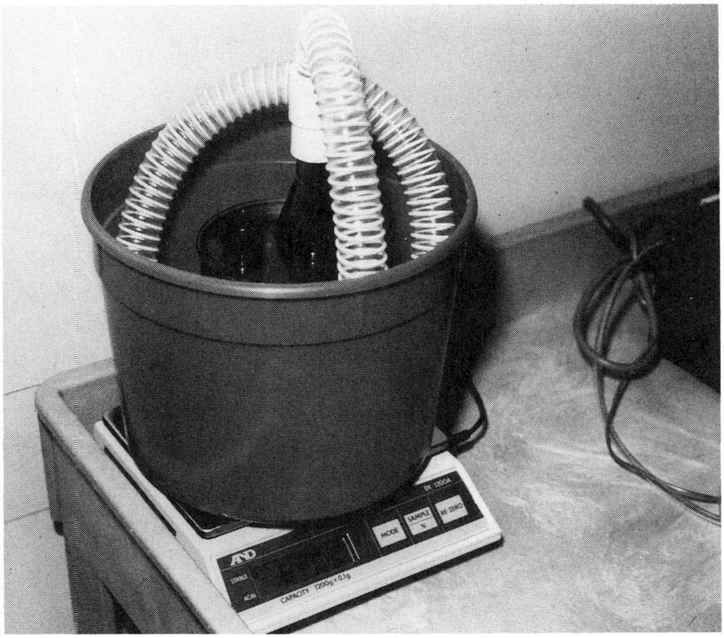

Figure 10 Nebulizer canister and tubing are weighed after each interval of a nonisotonic aerosol challenge. (From Williams, P. V., *Am. J. Asthma Allergy Pediatr.*, *5* (4), 197–202 [1992].)

decrease of FEV_1 of more than 10%, a change in FEV_1 of 15% after hypertonic saline challenge may be sufficient, increasing the sensitivity to over 92% in one study [78]. Fifty percent of asthmatics tested with hypertonic saline have a 20% reduction in FEV_1 after inhaling less than 2 ml. Others have modified this protocol, using water of increasing salinity for 2-min increments and recording pulmonary function after each concentration is inhaled. There is currently no accepted standardized hypertonic-saline protocol. In contrast to UNDW challenges, neither increases in methacholine reactivity nor late responses have been observed after hypertonic saline challenges [79]. Both UNDW and hypertonic-saline challenges are likely to identify asthmatics with moderate to severe airway hyperreactivity, with less sensitivity for identifying subjects with milder asthma. Hypertonic-saline challenges have been shown to be reproducible to within 1.5 doubling volumes over a period of several weeks [78]. Both UNDW and hypertonic-saline challenges have been shown to produce a refractory period [77,80] and, in the case of hypertonic saline, a cross-refractoriness with exercise [80].

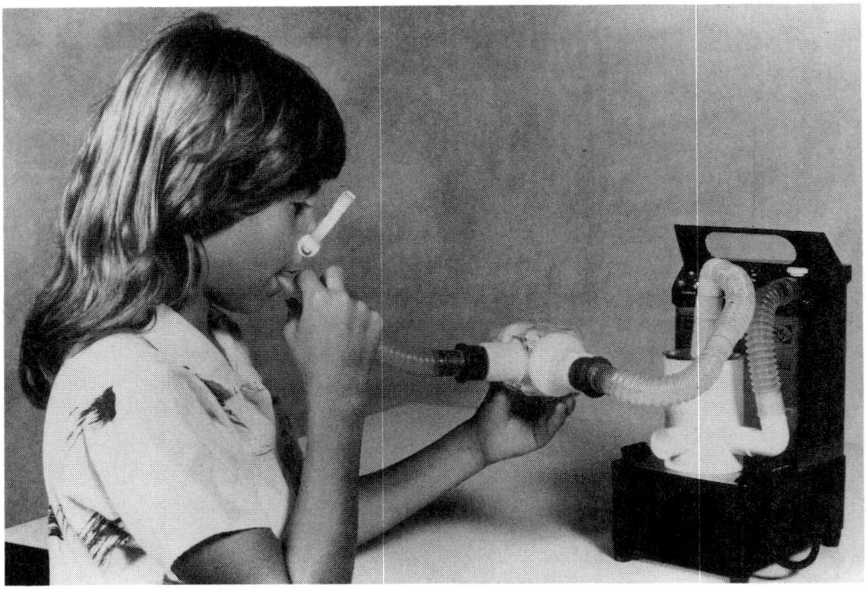

Figure 11 A girl breathes ultrasonic nebulized water through a mouthpiece attached to a Hans-Rudolph nonrebreathing valve. (From Shapiro, G. G., et al., in *Provocative Challenge Procedures: Background and Methodology* [S. L. Spector, ed.], Futura Publishing Co., New York, 1989, pp. 395–416.)

Antigen challenges are infrequently used in children. They are potentially dangerous, since late responses, which may be severe, are common. Also, there is an overlap in response by subjects whose allergic sensitivity to an antigen is manifested clinically as rhinitis only and those who also have bronchospasm. Thus, the occurrence of bronchospasm during a challenge is not specific for clinically significant disease [81].

Antigen provocation can be performed with dust, dust mite, mold, and animal antigens. Lyophilized antigens that have been reconstituted within several days of challenge should be used. Prick testing followed by serial dilutions of intradermal skin testing should be done to establish the initial concentration for challenge, the weakest intradermal-test concentration producing a wheal 5 mm greater than control being a proper starting point. The challenge procedure resembles the dosimeter method of chemical provocation. First five inhalations of saline are delivered, and spirometry is performed. The best of two or three expiratory efforts is taken as baseline. At 10-min intervals, five inhalations of increasingly strong concentrations of antigen are delivered, unless there is a drop of $\geqslant$ 15% in FEV_1. For a decrease of 15–19%, the same dose is repeated, and fewer inhalations may be given at the physician's discretion. The challenge is complete after there has been a decrease of > 20% in FEV_1 or the entire sequence of dilutions is administered. Since late reactions may occur for up to 12 h after challenge, the patient should be studied for hourly intervals, at least with peak flow determinations. Steroid therapy may be necessary to treat the increased bronchial hyperreactivity that may result from a positive challenge [3,67].

V. COMPARISONS OF CHALLENGES

Methacholine and histamine challenges are extremely sensitive indicators of airways hyperreactivity. Their advantage is their diagnostic thoroughness for reactivity. Epidemiological surveys have assessed the methacholine responsiveness of asthmatic and normal children in order to determine a reasonable discriminating point between these groups. When one administers a challenge that incorporates dosing up to 800 breath units (BU) of methacholine, in contrast to the typical challenge of up to 200 BU, a fascinating relationship is revealed. Ninety-eight percent of asthmatic subjects respond with a 20% or greater drop in FEV_1, and 87% have a PD_{20} of 100 BU or less. Among normal subjects, 12% have a PD_{20} under 100 BU, 25% have a PD_{20} over 100 BU, and 63% do not have a fall in FEV_1 of 20%. The best sensitivity and specificity (89% for each) occurs at a PD_{20} of 100 BU. This cut-off gives a false positive rate of 19% and a false negative rate of 6%. Using a cut-off of 200 BU methacholine decreases the false-negative rate to 4%, but the false-positive rate increases to 27% [62]. Backer and co-workers examined the sensitivity and specificity of histamine challenge in an unselected population of children and adolescents and found that the best results occurred at a PC_{20} of <2.4mg/ml [35]. For clinical studies, however, they found that a PC_{20} of <8mg/ml was best, although the positive predictive value was low.

Those patients who are apparently normal but have positive methacholine challenge may be a group earmarked for future reactive-airway disease. A significant number of these patients may develop clinical asthma in subsequent years (Table 7) [82], particularly if they have a positive family history of asthma [83]. Alternatively, they may have residual reactivity that may continue to wane with time, or reactivity that is genetically predetermined but will never be of clinical consequence. Since the future for any particular person is unpredictable, an isolated methacholine challenge that is positive is of no clinical value. Rather, chemical challenges take on validity when they are used to clarify and corroborate information derived from the history and physical examination.

Bronchial responsiveness to histamine and to methacholine correlates fairly well. However, histamine may be less reliable for distinguishing normal from asthmatic subjects, and it may cause headaches and facial flushing at higher concentrations [84,85].

Exercise challenge is less sensitive than chemical challenge and is a poorer

Table 7 Development of Asthma in Asymptomatic Patients with Bronchial Asthma, as it Relates to the Degree of Hyperreactivity[a]

Severity of bronchial hyperresponsiveness	No.	No. of cases of asthma	%
Moderate or severe	1	1	100
Mild	10	4	40
Slight	47	4	8.2
Undetectable	88	2	2.2

[a] $\chi^2 = 18.88$, $p<0.01$
Source: Ref. 82.

screening test for airway hyperreactivity. Chatham et al. noted that 6 of 15 asthmatics did not respond to maximal exercise challenge with a 10% fall in FEV_1, while 1 of 10 normal subjects did. Comparisons of cold-air, ultrasonic-mist, and methacholine inhalation tests in normal and asthmatic children [72] reiterated the increased sensitivity of methacholine, which was 95% vs. 57% for cold air and 71% for UNDW. However, cold-air challenge with 4 min of cold-air hyperventilation at 25 × FEV_1 rather than at 4 levels of ventilation (2,5,10, and 20 × FEV_1) showed similar sensitivity and specificity for methacholine and cold-air challenge in children [68]. Cold-air challenge was equivalent to methacholine in distinguishing adult asthmatics from normal subjects [86].

Smith and Anderson [87] have shown similar responses of asthmatics to isocapnic hyperventilation and ultrasonically nebulized 4.5% NaCl (Table 8). They hypothesized that the parallel PD_{20}s and slopes of water loss compared with drop in FEV_1 attest that airway hyperosmolarity is the mechanism for isocapnic hyperventilation–induced bronchospasm, hypertonic inhalation–induced bronchospasm, and inferentially, exercise-induced bronchospasm.

From these comparisons it appears that methacholine, histamine, and isocapnic hyperventilation of cold air are sensitive indicators of bronchial hyperreactivity. Hypertonic-saline challenge, though less well studied, is also sensitive. Exercise challenge and ultrasonically nebulized hypotonic solutions are less sensitive for separating asthmatic and normal subjects.

The challenge that one chooses will largely depend on one's goals. If one seeks to define a child's level of physical disability from exercise-induced bronchospasm, an exercise challenge will obviously be most helpful. There may on occasion be a need to confirm that a particular antigen is asthma-producing. For most purposes, chemical challenge with methacholine or histamine will be most valuable. These agents promise excellent sensitivity, fairly good specificity, short duration of action, simplicity, and standardized protocols.

Table 8 Specificity, Sensitivity, Positive and Negative Predictive Values, and Accuracy of Bronchial Challenge with 4.5% NaCl, Histamine, and Isocapnic Cold = Air Hyperventilation (ICH)

	ICH (%)	4.5% NaCl (%)	Histamine (%)
Specificity	100	100	92
Sensitivity	58	58	92
Positive predictive value	100	100	92
Negative predictive value	71	71	92
Accuracy	79	79	92

Source: From Araki, et al., *J. Allergy Clin. Immunol.*, *84*, 99–107 (1989).

REFERENCES

1. Juniper E. F., Frith, P. A., and Hargreave, F. E., Airways responsiveness to histamine and methacholine; relationship to minimum treatment to control symptoms of asthma, *Thorax*, *36*, 575–579 (1981).
2. Murray, A. B., Ferguson, A. C., and Morrison, B., Airway responsiveness to histamine as a test for overall severity of asthma in children, *J. Allergy Clin. Immunol.*, *68*, 119 (1981).
3. Hargreave, F. E., Dolovich, J., and Boulet, L. P., Inhalation provocation tests, *Semin. Respir. Med.*, *4*, 224–236 (1983).
4. Chhabra, S. K., Gaur, S. N., and Khanna, A. K., Clinical significance of nonspecific bronchial hyperresponsiveness in asthma, *Chest*, *96*, 596–600 (1989).
5. Boulet, L. P., Cartier, A., Thomson, N. C., Roberts, R. S., Dolovich, J., and Hargreave, F. E., Asthma and increases in nonallergic bronchial responsiveness from seasonal pollen exposures, *J. Allergy Clin. Immunol.*, *71*, 399–406 (1983).
6. Martinez, F. D., Antognoni, G., Macri, F., Bonci, E., Midulla, F., De-Castro, G., and Ronchelli, R., Parental smoking enhances bronchial responsiveness in nine year old children, *Am. Rev. Respir. Dis.*, *138*, 518–523 (1988).
7. Halperin, S. A., Eggleston, P. A., Besley, P., Suratt, P., Hendley, J. O., Groschel, D. H. M., and Gwaltney, J. M., Jr., Exacerbations of asthma in adults during experimental rhinovirus infection, *Am. Rev. Respir. Dis.*, *132*, 976–980 (1985).
8. Backer, V., and Ulrick, C. S., Bronchial responsiveness to exercise in a random sample of 494 children and adolescents from Copenhagen, *Clin. Exp. Allergy*, *22*, 741–747 (1992).
9. Frischer, T., Studnicka, M., Neumann, M., and Gotz, M., Determinants of airway response to challenge with distilled water in a population sample of children aged 7–10 years old, *Chest*, *102*, 764–770 (1992).
10. Peat, J. K., Salome, C. M., Berry, G., and Woolcock, A. J., Relation of dose–

response slope to respiratory symptoms in a population of Australian school children, *Am. Rev. Respir. Dis.*, *144*, 663–667 (1991).

11. Turner, K. J., Dowse, G. K., Stewart, G. A., and Alpers, M. P., Studies on bronchial hyperreactivity, allergic responsiveness and asthma in rural and urban children of the highlands of Papua, New Guinea, *J. Allergy Clin. Immunol.*, *77*, 558–566 (1986).
12. Bias, W. B., The genetic basis of asthma, in *Asthma* (K. F. Austen and L. M. Lichtenstein, eds.), Academic Press, New York, 1973.
13. Godfrey, S., and Konig, P., Exercise-induced bronchial liability in wheezy children and their families, *Pediatrics*, *56* (suppl), 851–855 (1975).
14. LeSouef, P. N., Geelhoed, G. C., Turner, D. J., Morgan, S. E. G., and Landau, L. I., Response of normal infants to inhaled histamine, *Am. Rev. Respir. Dis.*, *139*, 62–66 (1989).
15. Tepper, R. S., Airway reactivity in infants: a positive response to methacholine and metaproterenol, *J. Appl. Physiol.*, *62*, 1155–1159 (1987).
16. Landau, L. I., Stick, S., Turnbull, S., and LeSoeuf, P., Increased bronchial responsiveness in infants compared with children (abstr.), *Am. Rev. Respir. Dis.*, *139* (pt. 2), A128 (1989).
17. Hopp, R. J., Bewtra, A., Nair, N. M., and Townley, R. G., The effect of age on methacholine response, *J. Allergy Clin. Immunol.*, *76*, 609–613 (1985).
18. Pullan, C. R., and Hey, E. N., Wheezing, asthma and pulmonary dysfunction 10 years after infection with respiratory syncytial virus in infancy, *Br. Med. J.*, *284*, 1665 (1982).
19. Weiss, S. T., Tager, I. B., Munoz, A., and Speizer, F. E., The relationship of respiratory infections in early childhood to the occurrence of increased levels of bronchial responsiveness and atopy, *Am. Rev. Respir. Dis.*, *131*, 573 (1985).
20. Ellis, E. F., Acute bronchopulmonary infections, in *Allergic Diseases From Infancy to Adulthood*, 2nd Ed. (C. W. Bierman and D. S. Pearlman, eds.), W.B. Saunders, Philadelphia, 1988, pp. 536–546.
21. McConnochie, K. M., and Roghmann, K. J., Bronchiolitis as a possible cause of wheezing in childhood: new evidence, *Pediatrics*, *74*, 1 (1984).
22. Welliver, R. C., Wong, D. T., Sun, M., Middleton, E., Jr., Vaughan, R. S., and Ogra, P. L., The development of respiratory syncytial virus–specific IgE and the release of histamine in nasopharyngeal secretions after infection, *N. Engl. J. Med.*, *305*, 841 (1981).
23. Hargreave, F. E., Dolovich, J., O'Byrne, P. M., Ramsdale, E. H., and Daniel, E. E., The origin of airway hyperresponsiveness, *J. Allergy Clin. Immunol.*, *78*, 825–832 (1986).
24. Sheppard, D., Mechanisms of acute increases in airway responsiveness caused by environmental chemicals, *J. Allergy Clin. Immunol.*, *81*, 128–132 (1988).
25. Curny, J. J., Comparative action of acetyl-beta-methylcholine and histamine on the respiratory tract in normals, patients with hay fever, and subjects with bronchial asthma, *J. Clin. Invest.*, *26*, 430–438 (1947).
26. Schiller, I. W., and Lowell, F. C., The effect of drugs on modifying the response of asthmatic subjects to inhalation of pollen extracts as determined by vital capacity measurements, *Ann. Allergy*, *5*, 564–566 (1947).

27. Tiffeneau, R., Evaluation of degree of asthma by pharmacologic test: measure of acetylcholine excitability of lung, *Ann. Med.*, *56*, 582–602 (1955).
28. Parker, C. D., Bilbo, R. E., and Reed, C. E., Methacholine aerosol as test for bronchial asthma, *Arch. Intern. Med.*, *115*, 452–458 (1965).
29. Townley, R. G., Dennis, M., and Itkin, I. H., Comparative action of acetyl-beta-methylcholine, histamine and pollen antigens in subjects with hay fever and patients with bronchial asthma, *J. Allergy*, *36*, 121–137 (1965).
30. Makino, S., Clinical significance of bronchial sensitivity to acetylcholine and histamine in bronchial asthma, *J. Allergy*, *38*, 127–142 (1966).
31. Felarca, A. B., and Itkin, I. H., Curve of dose response to acetyl-beta-methylcholine in patients with asthma of known and unknown origin, hay fever subjects, and nonatopic volunteers, *J. Allergy*, *37*, 223–235 (1966).
32. Muittari, A., The value of the methacholine test as a diagnostic method on bronchospastic disorders, *Ann. Med. Inter. Fenn.*, *57*, 197–203 (1968).
33. Townley, R. G., Ryo, U. Y., Kolotkin, B. M., and Kang, B., Bronchial sensitivity to methacholine in current and former asthmatic and allergic rhinitis patients and control subjects, *J. Allergy Clin. Immunol.*, *56*, 429–442 (1975).
34. Fish, J. E., Rosenthal, R. R., Batra, G., Menkes, H., Summer, W., Permutt, S., and Norman, P., Airway responses to methacholine in allergic and nonallergic subjects, *Am. Rev. Respir. Dis.*, *113*, 579–586 (1976).
35. Backer, V., Groth, S., Dirksen, A., Bach-Mortensen, N., Hansen, K. K., Laursen, E. M., and Wendelboe, D. Sensitivity and specificity of the histamine challenge test for the diagnosis of asthma in an unselected sample of children and adolescents, *Eur. Respir. J.*, *4*, 1093–1100 (1991).
36. Backer, V., Dirksen, A., Bach-Mortensen, N., Hansen, K. K., Laursen, E. M., and Wendelboe, D., The distribution of bronchial responsiveness to histamine and exercise in 527 children and adolescents, *J. Allergy Clin. Immunol.*, *88*, 68–76 (1991).
37. Pattemore, P. K., Asher, M. I., Harrison, A. C., Mitchell, E. A., Rea, H. H., and Stewart, A. W., The interrelationships among bronchial hyperresponsiveness, the diagnosis of asthma, and asthma symptoms, *Am. Rev. Respir. Dis.*, *142*, 549–554 (1990).
38. Burrows, B., Sears, M. R., Flannery, E. M., Herbison, G. P., and Holdaway, M. D., Relationships of bronchial responsiveness assessed by methacholine to serum IgE, lung function, symptoms and diagnoses in 11-year-old New Zealand children, *J. Allergy Clin. Immunol.*, *90*, 376–385 (1992).
39. Gilbert, R., and Auchincloss, J. H., Post-test probability of asthma following methacholine challenge, *Chest*, *97*, 562–565 (1990).
40. Palmeiro, E. M., Hopp, R. J., Biven, R. E., Bewtra, A. K., Nair, N. N., and Townley, R. G., Probability of asthma based on methacholine challenge, *Chest*, *101*, 630–633 (1992).
41. Hopp, R. J., Weiss, S. J., Nair, M. N., Bewtra, A. K., and Townley, R. G., Interpretation of the results of methacholine inhalation challenge tests, *J. Allergy Clin. Immunol.*, *80*, 821–830 (1987).
42. Juniper, E. F., and Hargreave, F. E., Airway responsiveness by aerosol inhalation

tests: variability in results due to unexpected differences between calibrated nebulizers (abstr.), *Bull. Eur. Physiopathol. Respir.*, *22*, 165S (1986).

43. Cockcroft, D. W., Hurst, T. S., and Gore, B. P., Importance of evaporative losses during standardized nebulized inhalation provocation tests, *Chest*, *96*, 505–508 (1989).
44. Ryan, G., Dolovich, M. B., Obminski, G., Cockcroft, D. W., Juniper, E., Hargreave, F. E., and Newhouse, M. T., Standardization of inhalation provocation tests: influence of nebulizer output, particle size and method of inhalation, *J. Allergy Clin. Immunol.*, *67*, 156–161 (1981).
45. Ryan, G., Dolovich, M. B., Roberts, R. S., Frith, P. A., Juniper, E. F., Hargreave, F. E., and Newhouse, M. T., Standardization of inhalation provocation tests: two techniques of aerosol generation and inhalation compared, *Am. Rev. Respir. Dis.*, *123*, 195–199 (1981).
46. Chai, H., Farr, R. S., Roehlich, L. A., Mathison, D. A., McLean, J. A., Rosenthal, R. R., Sheffer, A. L., Spector, S. L., and Townley, R. G., Standardization of bronchial inhalation challenge procedures, *J. Allergy Clin. Immunol.*, *56*, 323–327 (1975).
47. Weiss, M. E., Wheeler, B., Eggleston, P., and Adkinson, N. F., A protocol for performing reproducible methacholine inhalation tests in children with moderate to severe asthma, *Am. Rev. Respir. Dis.*, *139*, 67–72 (1989).
48. LaBraico, J. M., Reed, C. E., Rosenthal, R. R., Shapiro, G. G., Spector, S. L., and Townley, R. G., Multicenter evaluation of airways hyperreactivity using a standardized methacholine challenge (abstr.), *J. Allergy Clin. Immunol.*, *73*, 124 (1984).
49. Schmidt, L. E., Thorne, P. S., Watt, J. L., and Schwartz, D. A., Is an abbreviated bronchial challenge with histamine valid? *Chest*, *101*, 141–145 (1992).
50. Eliasson, A. H., Phillips, Y. Y., Rajagopal, K. R., and Howard, R. S., Sensitivity and specificity of bronchial provocation testing. An evaluation of four techniques in exercise-induced bronchospasm, *Chest*, *102*, 347–355 (1992).
51. Van Aalderen, W. M. C., Gerritsen, J., Koeter, G. H., van der Weele, L. T., Postma, D. S., and Knol, K., The reproducibility and agreement of three indices of airway responsiveness to histamine in asthmatic children, *Pediatr. Pulmonol.*, *6*, 113–117 (1989).
52. Adinoff, A., and Strunk, R., Methacholine inhalation challenge (MC) in young children: results of testing and follow up (abstr.), *J. Allergy Clin. Immunol.*, *73*, 124 (1984).
53. Avital, A., Bar-Yishay, E., Springer, C., and Godfrey, S., Bronchial provocation tests in young children using tracheal auscultation, *J. Pediatr.*, *112*, 591–594 (1988).
54. Muchizuki, H., Mitsuhashi, M., Tokuyame, K., Tajima, K., Morikawa, A., and Kuroume, T., A new method of estimating bronchial hyperresponsiveness in younger children, *Ann. Allergy*, *55*, 162 (1985).
55. Murakami, G., Igarashi, T., Adachi, Y., Matsuno, M., Adachi, Y., Sawai, M., Yoshizumi, A., and Okada, T., Measurement of bronchial hyperreactivity in infants and preschool children using a new method, *Ann. Allergy*, *64*, 383–387 (1990).
56. Beck, R., Dickson, U., Montgomery, M. D., and Mitchell, I., Histamine challenge in young children using computerized lung sound analysis, *Chest*, *102*, 759–763 (1992).

57. Pratter, M. R., Hingston, D. M., and Irwin, R. S., Diagnosis of bronchial asthma by clinical evaluation, *Chest*, *84*, 42–47 (1983).
58. Corrao, W. M., Braman, S., and Irwin, S., Chronic cough as the sole presenting manifestation of bronchial asthma, *N. Engl. J. Med.*, *300*, 633–637 (1979).
59. Shapiro, G. G., Furukawa, C. T., Pierson, W. E., and Bierman, C. W., Methacholine bronchial challenge in children, *J. Allergy Clin. Immunol.*, *69*, 365 (1982).
60. Furukawa, C. T., DuHamel, T. R., Weimer, L., Shapiro, G. G., Pierson, W. E., and Bierman, C. W., Cognitive and behavioral findings in children taking theophylline, *J. Allergy Clin. Immunol.*, *81*, 83–88 (1988).
61. Shapiro, G. G., Furukawa, C. T., Pierson, W. E., Sharpe, M. J., Menendez, R., and Bierman, C. W., Double-blind evaluation of nebulized cromolyn, terbutaline and the combination for childhood asthma, *J. Allergy Clin. Immunol.*, *81*, 449–454 (1988).
62. Hoppe, R. J., Bewtra, A. K., Nair, N. M., and Townley, R. G., Specificity and sensitivity of methacholine inhalation challenge in normal and asthmatic children, *J. Allergy Clin. Immunol.*, *74*, 154–158 (1984).
63. Bhagat, R. G., and Grunstein, M. M., Comparison of responsiveness to methacholine, histamine and exercise in subgroups of asthmatic children, *Am. Rev. Respir. Dis.*, *129*, 224–224 (1984).
64. Hargreave, F. E., Ryan, G., Thomson, N. C., O'Byrne, P. M., Latimer, K., Juniper, E. F., and Dolovich, J., Bronchial responsiveness to histamine or methacholine in asthma: measurement and clinical significance, *J. Allergy Clin. Immunol.*, *68*, 347–355 (1981).
65. Anderson, S. D., Issues in exercised-induced asthma, *J. Allergy Clin. Immunol.*, *76*, 763–772 (1985).
66. Zach, M. S., and Polgar, G., Cold air challenge of airway hyperreactivity in children: dose-response interrelation with a reaction plateau, *J. Allergy Clin. Immunol.*, *80*, 9–17 (1987).
67. Townley, R. J., and Hopp, R. J., Inhalation methods for the study of airway responsiveness, *J. Allergy Clin. Immunol.*, *80*, 111–124 (1987).
68. Reisman, J., Mappa, L., de Benedictis, F., McLaughlin, J., and Levison, H., Cold air challenge in children with asthma, *Pediatr. Pulmonol.*, *3*, 251–254 (1987).
69. Heaton, R. W., Henderson, A. F., and Costello, J. F., Cold air as a bronchial provocation technique, *Chest*, *86*, 810–814 (1984).
70. McLaughlin, F. J., and Dozor, A. J., Cold air inhalation challenge in the diagnosis of asthma in children, *Pediatrics*, *72*, 503–509 (1983).
71. Tal, A., Pasterkamp, H., Serrette, C., Leahy, F., and Chernick, V., Response to cold air hyperventilation in normal and in asthmatic children, *J. Pediatr.*, *104*, 516–521 (1984).
72. Galdes-Sebaldt, M., McLaughlin, F. J., and Levison, H., Comparison of cold air ultrasonic mist and methacholine inhalation as tests of bronchial reactivity in normal and asthmatic children, *J. Pediatr.*, *107*, 526–530 (1985).
73. Hopp, R. J., Christy, J., Brewtra, A., Nair, N. M., and Townley, R. G., Incorporation and analysis of ultrasonically nebulized distilled water challenges in an epidemiologic study of asthma and bronchial reactivity, *Ann. Allergy*, *60*, 129–133 (1988).

74. Anderson, S. D., Bronchial challenge by ultrasonically nebulized aerosols, *Clin. Rev. Allergy*, *3*, 427–439 (1985).
75. Eichler, I., Gotz, M., Zarbovic, J. J., and Kofinger, A., Distilled water challenges in asthmatic children: comparison of different protocols, *Chest*, *102*, 753–758 (1992).
76. Mattioli, S., Foresi, A., Corbo, G. M., Valente, S., Patalano, F., and Clappi, G., Increase in bronchial responsiveness to methacholine and late response after the inhalation of ultrasonically nebulized distilled water, *Chest*, *90*, 726–732 (1986).
77. O'Callaghan, C., Milner, A. D., and Swarbick, A., Nebulized water as a bronchoconstricting challenge in infancy, *Arch. Dis. Child.*, *66*, 948–951 (1991).
78. Smith, C. M., and Anderson, S. D., Inhalation challenges using hypertonic saline in asthmatic subjects: a comparison with responses to hyperpnea, methacholine and water, *Eur. Respir. J.*, *3*, 144–151 (1990).
79. Smith, C. M., Anderson, S. D., and Black, J. L., Methacholine responsiveness increases after ultrasonically nebulized water but not after ultrasonically nebulized hypertonic saline in patients with asthma, *J. Allergy Clin. Immunol.*, *79*, 85–92 (1987).
80. Belcher, N. G., Rees, P. J., Clark, T. J. H., and Lee, T. H., A comparison of the refractory periods induced by hypertonic airway challenge and exercise in bronchial asthma, *Am. Rev. Respir. Dis.*, *135*, 822–825 (1987).
81. Bruce, C. A., Rosenthal, R. R., Lichtenstein, L. M., and Norman, P. S., Quantitative inhalation bronchial challenge in ragweed hay fever patients: a comparison with ragweed-allergic asthmatics, *J. Allergy Clin. Immunol.*, *56*, 331 (1975).
82. Zhong, N. S., Chen, R. C., Yang, M. O., Wu, Z. Y., Zheng, J. P., and Li, Y. F., Is asymptomatic bronchial hyperresponsiveness an indication of potential asthma? A two year follow up of young students with bronchial hyperresponsiveness, *Chest*, *102*, 1104–1109 (1992).
83. Townley, R. G., Hopp, R. J., Bewtra, A. K., and Nair, N. M., Predictive value of airway reactivity, *J. Allergy Clin. Immunol.*, *86*, 650–652 (1990).
84. Chatham, M., Bleecker, E. R., Smith, P. L., Rosenthal, R. R., Mason, P., and Norman, P. S., A comparison of histamine, methacholine, and exercise airway reactivity in normal and asthmatic subjects, *Am. Rev. Respir. Dis.*, *126*, 235–240 (1982).
85. Hargreave, F. E., Dolovich, J., O'Byrne, P., Ramsdale, E. H., and Daniel, E. E., The origin of airway hyperresponsiveness, *J. Allergy Clin. Immunol.*, *78*, 825–832 (1986).
86. O'Byrne, P. M., Ryan, G., Morris, M., McCormach, D., Jones, N. L., Morse, J. L., and Hargreave, F. E., Asthma induced by cold air and its relation to nonspecific bronchial responsiveness to methacholine, *Am. Rev. Respir. Dis.*, *125*, 281–285 (1982).
87. Smith, C. M., and Anderson, S. D., Hyperosmolarity as the stimulus to asthma induced by hyperventilation? *J. Allergy Clin. Immunol.*, *77*, 729–736 (1986).

19

Use of Inhalation Bronchial Challenge for Occupational Diseases

David J. Hendrick

University of Newcastle upon Tyne
Newcastle, England

John E. Salvaggio

Tulane University Medical Center
New Orleans, Louisiana

I. INTRODUCTION

Occupational disorders of the lung are conveniently considered in three major categories: (1) acute toxic reactions, (2) chronic inflammatory/fibrotic disorders and disorders of long latency such as industrial bronchitis, pneumoconiosis, and cancer, and (3) hypersensitivity disorders.

Toxic agents induce acute inflammatory reactions in all exposed workers, the severity of the response depending on the degree of the exposure rather than on individual susceptibility or reactivity. Symptoms develop within minutes (or occasionally hours) of exposure to the appropriate concentration of the agent concerned, irrespective of any earlier exposures, and full recovery is generally observed in those who survive. Occupational agents that induce such responses are quickly recognized, and there is rarely diagnostic uncertainty when working populations or isolated individuals become affected by them. In any event, diagnostic uncertainty cannot be resolved by inhalation challenge tests, since similar levels of exposure can be expected to produce similar responses in all of us.

With industrial bronchitis, pneumoconiosis, and occupational lung cancer, the situation is rather different. Although these responses are closely related to exposure doses, many years of occupational exposure to the provoking agent are required before disease becomes apparent, and no clinical response can be detected following a single challenge exposure.

It is for the third category of occupational disorders of the lung that inhalation challenge tests may be of value, namely, the "hypersensitivity" disorders, asthma and hypersensitivity pneumonitis. In some countries the latter is known more commonly as extrinsic allergic alveolitis to emphasize that extrinsic allergens rather than autoallergens are involved and that the alveoli are dominantly affected. These disorders result from exposure to a number of common environmental agents as well as to occupational agents, and so they occur in the general population as well as in occupational populations. More important, they affect a minority of those exposed to the particular inducing agent, and it is usually months (occasionally years) after exposure begins that symptoms first develop.

These features suggest that allergic mechanisms are responsible for the inflammatory response, and much evidence has accrued in support of this. Indeed, specific immunoglobulin E (IgE) antibody responses have been demonstrated against a wide variety of relevant (i.e., asthmagenic) organic dusts and simple chemicals present in respirable form in multiple workplace environments. Exposure to these stimuli causes acute bronchoconstriction and, if they are repetitive, chronic inflammation. They induce a complex series of biochemical events that result in the release of a wide variety of mast cell mediators [1]. Among these are histamine, leukotrienes B_4, C_4, D_4, and E_4, prostaglandins D and $F_{2\alpha}$, thromboxane, platelet activating factor, and chemotactic factors for neutrophils and eosinophils. This mediator response can profoundly constrict the airway smooth muscle, stimulate mucus secretion, increase vascular permeability, and result in the influx of large numbers of inflammatory cells, particularly eosinophils, lymphocytes, and neutrophils. These effects in turn are important in causing chronic inflammatory changes, "late-phase" reactions, and increases in airway responsiveness [2,3]. It is also possible that genetically determined idiosyncrasies play a role in some cases. With hypersensitivity pneumonitis, pathogenic mechanisms are less certain, but immunological sensitization is fundamental, and tissue injury is associated with T cell activation and immune-complex deposition.

The salient points for the present discussion are first, that characteristic acute exacerbations may be readily provoked by further challenge exposure to the responsible agent; and second, that such responses are not provoked in previously unexposed (or exposed but unaffected) workers. The mechanism is not therefore one of direct toxicity. Inhalation challenge tests with the causative agent may in these circumstances be definitive in establishing a specific etiological diagnosis.

Inhalation challenge tests of a different type may help establish a diagnosis of asthma in a manner that is etiologically nonspecific. As described in other chapters, a fundamental feature of asthma is undue responsiveness of the airways to a number of relatively nonspecific inhaled stimuli. These include histamine, cholinergic agents, and a number of irritants, as well as exercise and cold-air hyperventilation. Standardized inhalation challenge tests with aerosols of histamine or methacholine may be of considerable value when a primary diagnosis of asthma is itself in question, a not uncommon event when occupational exposure ceases and symptoms regress. The greater the degree of airway responsiveness observed to any of these stimuli, the greater the likelihood that asthma has indeed developed. This hyperresponsiveness may, however, regress within a few weeks after occupational exposure ceases, and so it should be interpreted simply as a reflection of contemporary asthmatic activity.

The nonspecific pulmonary response to inhaled histamine or methacholine is immediate. That is, diffuse airway obstruction develops within a few minutes of the challenge exposure and resolves spontaneously within an hour or two. Once an unequivocal response has been provoked, it may be reversed speedily with a bronchodilator. If any particular challenge dose fails to produce a significant response, the next incremental dose may be administered within minutes. The whole study can usually be completed conveniently in an hour and carries negligible risk if supervised adequately.

By contrast, challenge tests with specific occupational agents often provoke late rather than immediate responses in subjects with occupational asthma (though both immediate and late, i.e., dual, reactions may occur), and they provoke late responses only in patients with hypersensitivity pneumonitis. In our experience, the onset of such late responses may be delayed from 1 to 18 h after the onset of exposure, though most begin after 3–9 h. The ideal challenge exposure involves a dose that is just sufficient to provoke an unequivocally positive response. With such a dose, late reactions usually resolve spontaneously within 24 h. Following higher challenge exposures, full spontaneous recovery may require days or even weeks. In the case of late asthmatic reactions, a distinctive pattern of recurrent nocturnal exacerbations may be induced, their severity usually diminishing slowly over a period of several days. With hypersensitivity pneumonitis, no obvious circadian rhythm is seen. The late asthmatic reaction is generally less readily reversed than the immediate one, and with late reactions at both airway and parenchymal levels, corticosteroids may be required to speed recovery. This implies that a further period of some 4–6 h can be expected before any beneficial clinical effect is apparent.

These features of specific inhalation challenge tests impose certain constraints on their use. Only one test should be performed on any one day, and medical supervision is required for prolonged periods. In many cases, hospital admission may be necessary, which itself imposes further constraints. A series of challenges using steadily increasing exposure doses is necessary if any particular agent is to be proved irrelevant to the disorder under investigation. Safe incremental increases are on the order of two to five times, and so four or more "antigen" challenges may be required, together with one or more control tests. The use of specific inhalation challenge tests is consequently time-consuming, expensive, and not without risk. They are best limited to institutions with special interest and expertise in the field. Their use in epidemiological investigations of large populations is not feasible, while their use in the management of individuals may be limited by the suitability and compliance of the individual concerned. He or she should give informed consent, and should understand not only the rationale and risks, but also the demands the tests will have on his or her time if they are to be completed satisfactorily. Boredom may prove to be the greatest problem, and compliance may be improved by offering flexibility in the investigation schedule.

II. INDICATIONS

A. Inhalation Tests to Measure (Nonspecific) Airway Responsiveness

Measurements of airway responsiveness to histamine, methacholine and other "nonspecific" stimuli are not perfectly correlated, reflecting the different mechanisms by which they provoke bronchoconstriction [4]. All do, nevertheless, provide close quantitative measures of asthmatic activity. In this sense these stimuli can be considered to be "nonspecific" triggering factors in asthma that are unrelated to immunological sensitization. The mechanisms involved are actually quite specific, and so the term "nonspecific bronchial responsiveness" has been losing its popularity in recent years in favor of "airway responsiveness to [for example] methacholine." We shall follow this recent trend in this chapter, using "airway responsiveness" to imply responsiveness provoked by any of these nonallergic mechanisms. In fact, our references to airway responsiveness generally involve methacholine, which is the most commonly used bronchoconstrictor agent for such tests. Since a full discussion of airway responsiveness is presented in another chapter, we shall concentrate here on its relevance to the use of inhalation tests in occupational diseases of the lungs.

A further realization over recent years has concerned the unimodal (not bimodal) distribution of airway responsiveness in the population at large. The threshold point at which the level of airway responsiveness is said to be increased or undue (i.e., at which there is hyperresponsiveness) is consequently arbitrary and of limited value. It depends crucially on the method used for measurement. With the popular Wright nebulizer and tidal-breathing method, symptomatic asthma is generally recognized with PC_{20} values (provocative concentrations of methacholine responsible for a 20% decrement in forced expired volume in 1 second [FEV_1]) up to 8 mg/ml [5]. This is equivalent to a PD_{20} (cumulative provocative dose of methacholine responsible for a 20% decrement in FEV_1) on the order 800–1000 μg when measured by a dosimeter method [6].

An important additional variable to consider is the subjective awareness of bronchoconstriction. Some subjects describe appreciable discomfort following FEV_1 decrements of less than 20%, while others barely notice decrements exceeding 20%. Such variability will inevitably exert an influence on the threshold measurement of airway responsiveness that distinguishes clinical asthma from apparent normality.

1. When There Is No Other Objective Evidence for Asthma

A major role for inhalation challenge tests that measure airway responsiveness lies with the investigation of subjects with suspected occupational asthma in whom little or no objective evidence of disease persists by the time of referral. This is not an infrequent situation when asthma is truly occupational in origin, for once suspicion arises, exposure tends to diminish or cease. In a medicolegal setting where compensation is an issue, it may not be possible for the subject to return to his working environment. It is precisely in such a setting that objective evidence is most needed to evaluate what may be a biased or distorted clinical history.

The increase in airway responsiveness that normally follows viral infections or exposure to certain air pollutants lasts for relatively brief periods, and the magnitude of the increase is rarely such that clinically significant airway obstruction results, unless the subject already suffers from asthma. With symptomatic occupational asthma, airway hyperresponsiveness usually persists a good deal longer once exposure ceases. The work of Chan-Yeung and colleagues concerning the fate of cedar asthma in 75 retired workers (none had asthma before cedar exposure, and all were proved to be reactive by specific challenge tests) showed that only 51% were asymptomatic 1–9 years after exposure ceased (mean 3.5 years), and that even in these, airway hyperresponsiveness persisted in the majority [7]. Data from our own studies of workers from a variety of industries are in agreement with these findings, and similar experience has been reported by numerous other investigators. It is unlikely, then, that a worker previously affected by occupational asthma will fail to show airway hyperresponsiveness if he or she is tested within a few weeks following relevant exposure. When much longer periods elapse, the significance of a negative histamine or methacholine test is less certain. A positive test, on the other hand, merely indicates that the subject has hyperresponsive airways consistent with active asthma. It in no way implies an occupational origin, unless by some chance airway hyperresponsiveness was known to be absent immediately before the occupational environment was entered.

2. As a Possible Screening Test

There is speculation that preexisting airway hyperresponsiveness is a risk factor for the development of occupational asthma, and so a further possible (but unproved) role for its measurement lies with screening examinations of potential new employees. However, in some occupational environments the prevalence of asthma (and hence airway hyperresponsiveness) has substantially exceeded the usual prevalence of airway hyperresponsiveness in the population at large. Until longitudinal use of airway responsiveness measurements provides evidence to the contrary, it must consequently be assumed that in many, and probably most, instances, airway hyperresponsiveness was a direct consequence of the occupational exposure rather than a predisposing cause of the occupational asthma.

3. To Detect Change

If certain occupational exposures induce asthma, they must also increase airway responsiveness. Such a phenomenon may be readily recognized if airway responsiveness is measured before and after inhalation tests with relevant occupational agents that provoke late asthmatic reactions. Methacholine (and histamine) tests may consequently provide a useful supplementary means of monitoring challenge tests with occupational agents, in addition to measurements of ventilatory function. The combination of a late (rather than early) asthmatic reaction with increasing airway responsiveness is particularly valuable in distinguishing an occupational environment likely to play an inducing (i.e., causative) role in occupational asthma from one that merely triggers asthmatic reactions through irritant mechanisms in subjects already suffering coincidentally from asthma. In the latter circumstances, only an immediate asthmatic reaction is to be expected, without change in airway responsiveness.

Where challenge tests with occupational agents are not easily arranged, serial measurements of airway responsiveness may be used to detect worsening levels at work succeeded by improving levels following vacations or secondments to different jobs with lesser degrees of exposure. This alone may provide convincing evidence for asthma of occupational origin, or even of occupational asthma during its emergent phase. The ability to detect emerging occupational asthma before there is the fear of permanent disability could be particularly valuable in managing at-risk populations.

The ability to detect improvement in airway responsiveness in individuals or populations could also provide invaluable insight regarding the effectiveness of hygiene improvements within the workplace, changes in production, or personal use of respirators or medication. Critical to any serial use of airway responsiveness measurement is, however, the ability to define the precision of the test method and hence its limits of repeatability. At best, coefficients of repeatability from groups of individuals have been reported to be on the order of 2–3. That is to say, the 95% confidence interval for the results of a repeated PD_{20} (or PC_{20}) measurement should, when expressed arithmetically, lie between one-half or one-third of the first measurement at one extreme and two or three times the first measurement at the other, if no significant change in airway responsiveness has occurred in the interim [6]. Significant change is therefore implied if the second measurement lies outside this range, an increase in PD_{20} indicating an improvement in airway responsiveness and a decrease in PD_{20} indicating a deterioration. Individuals within a study group may show greater or lesser degrees of variability, and if change in a particular individual is sought it is best to obtain personal confidence intervals from repeated baseline measurements. With methacholine, refractoriness to repeated tests may last up to 24 h (with histamine it is much less prolonged), and there is suspicion of a circadian rhythm. Tests should therefore be repeated at much the same time of day and after minimum intervals of 48 h.

It is now clear that the degree of any asthmatic response to an inhaled allergen depends not only on the dose inhaled and the degree of sensitization to it, but also on the degree of airway responsiveness. Chester and colleagues made the interesting observation that in some cases toluene diisocyanate challenge tests provoked asthma only during periods of convalescence from viral infections, i.e., at times of heightened airway responsiveness [8]. Such an interaction between occupational and nonoccupational factors may also have been responsible for an undue frequency of acute attacks of "bronchitis" associated with wheezing that occurred in workers exposed to formaldehyde [9].

The measurement of airway responsiveness is consequently a useful preliminary to conducting inhalation challenge tests with specific occupational agents suspected of causing asthma, not only to provide an additional method of monitoring the response but to assist in choosing a suitable initial challenge dose. If marked airway responsiveness is demonstrated, greater caution should be exercised. With hypersensitivity pneumonitis no comparable "third factor" has been recognized, and the strength of any response to inhalation challenge appears to depend only on the test subject's level of sensitivity and the challenge dose.

B. Inhalation Challenge Tests with Specific Occupational Agents

The chief purpose in carrying out inhalation tests with specific occupational agents are, of course, to establish whether specific sensitization exists and whether exposure at realistic dose levels does provoke responses characteristic of asthma or hypersensitivity pneumonitis. The tests may consequently focus primarily on the agent (is it really a cause of occupational lung disease?) or the test subject (is he or she really affected?). Additional benefits may include objective evaluation of threshold levels and dose–response relationships, the effects of management interventions (e.g., respiratory protection devices, drugs, physical changes in the agent's dispersal), and natural history. The last requires serial investigations. The chief indications for such tests are consequently diagnostic and can usefully be considered under the headings of diagnostic uncertainty, diagnostic dispute, and research.

1. Diagnostic Uncertainty

The most potent indication for challenge tests with specific occupational agents arises when the responsible physician is uncertain of their etiologic relevance, and the worker concerned wishes to continue with his or her occupation. A number of questions need to be considered in these circumstances. What are the risks if the current occupation is pursued? Would it be more prudent to find a new job? Could compensation properly be expected, especially if a new job is less remunerative or a new job is unobtainable?

Chan-Yeung and colleagues suggest that with cedar asthma, the longer the periods of exposure before and after the onset of symptoms, the less favorable is the long-term outlook [7]. Comparable data from other investigators, or from groups of workers affected by other occupational agents, are limited, but it is clear that unless exposure ceases within a few months (and certainly within 1–2 years) of the first appearance of symptoms, there is a considerable risk of persisting active asthma irrespective of whether exposure to the causative agent does eventually cease. The responsible physician cannot be complacent with advice to the asthmatic patient who works with industrial gases, vapors, or dusts, particularly if symptoms first arose after the onset of such exposures.

With hypersensitivity pneumonitis, too, there is evidence that in some subjects, continuing exposure can lead to progressive irreversible pulmonary fibrosis, though this is not necessarily of a disabling degree and does not occur in all affected persons. Braun and colleagues found radiographic evidence of fibrosis in 39% of 92 subjects restudied 15 years after they presented with the acute form of farmer's lung [10]. During this period, 70% had continued to live on farms. An accurate and confident diagnosis is consequently critical to the management of both occupational asthma and occupational hypersensitivity pneumonitis.

Diagnostic uncertainty may arise for a number of reasons. The subject may be a poor historian, or the relationship between symptoms and occupation may be unclear, particularly when the immediate type of reaction is not involved and disease is chronically active. There may also be confounding factors. In some cases, true occupational asthma may become symptomatic only following colds, while in others, airway hyperresponsiveness induced occupationally may lead to asthmatic reactions from nonoccupational triggers. When a strongly suggestive history is obtained, the working environment may contain no obvious respirable agent of relevance. Conversely, there may be several possible etiological agents in both the working environment and the domestic environment.

Serum antibody titers tend to reflect exposure rather than disease and are of limited diagnostic value [11,12]. Indeed, for several occupational agents responsible for asthma or hypersensitivity pneumonitis, an antibody response has not been consistently demonstrated. Increasing numbers of respirable occupational agents, particularly chemicals, are being recognized as inducing asthma (and, to a much lesser extent, hypersensitivity pneumonitis), as might be expected from the rapid growth of the chemical industry. Inevitably, then, workers will present from occupational environments not previously associated with respiratory hazards. A careful clinical history, including an inquiry about the health of current and former workmates, is of crucial importance in recognizing that the cause may be occupational.

Commonly, no clinical evidence of asthma or pneumonitis persists at the time definitive advice is sought, particularly if the initially consulted family physician or general internist has referred the individual worker to a specialized center. Inhalation challenge tests with the suspected etiological agent may be particularly valuable in these circumstances, since they can be expected to reproduce acutely the clinical features of the disease and to confirm the etiological significance of the specific provoking agent.

2. Diagnostic Dispute

At times, the responsible physician may feel confident that asthma or pneumonitis can be attributed to a certain occupational agent but find that this opinion is not universally accepted. Although the physician may not require the definitive evidence of formal inhalation challenge tests, these may nevertheless become desirable if the subject concerned or his or her employer (or the latter's attorney), family, insurance company, or other medical advisors are to be equally satisfied.

3. Research

Much of our knowledge of occupational asthma and hypersensitivity pneumonitis has been gained, at least partly, through inhalation challenge tests. Their continuing use in a research setting can be expected to increase our understanding of both diseases, our ability to evaluate newer therapeutic approaches (e.g., pharmaceutical agents, respirators, even hyposensitization), and our ability to define previously unrecognized causative agents. An expanding use of both specific and nonspecific inhalation challenge tests is to be encouraged in the investigation of the fate of occupational asthma, because of the concern that active disease may persist after exposure to the initial inducing agent ceases, and the fear that continuing airway hyperresponsiveness, even when not associated with respiratory symptoms, may imply a persisting undue susceptibility.

III. CONTRAINDICATIONS

The use of inhalation challenge tests designed to reduce lung function in subjects already affected by lung disease is limited by two major considerations, aside from the willingness of the subjects to cooperate and the presence or absence of other serious diseases. These are the potential hazards of inducing a significant decrement in lung function, and the need for continuing medications that might affect the validity of the tests.

A final consideration is whether a positive response could provoke a permanent decrement in lung function. Extensive experience with asthma has thus far failed to show confirmatory evidence of this, while the limited studies involving hypersensitivity pneumonitis have produced equally reassuring results [13]. This is not surprising, since test subjects have generally submitted themselves already to numerous "natural" exposures in the workplace. Against these, the additional doses used in challenge tests contribute trivially to the overall cumulative level of exposure.

A. In Asthma

1. Hazard of Reducing Lung Function

Test-provoked decrements in FEV_1 that exceed 30% of the baseline (prechallenge) values can generally be avoided by careful choice of (1) the initial challenge exposure dose and (2) the magnitude of any subsequent increment. If baseline values of FEV_1 are not less than 70% of the predicted value, the minimal level at the height of a positive response will not fall below 50% of the predicted value. Reduction to such a level is safe, providing there is no complicating cardiac disease, in particular severe coronary artery disease. Life-threatening asthma is characterized by FEV_1 values as low as 10–20% of predicted values and by poor responsiveness to bronchodilator therapy. Fortunately, severe immediate reactions to inhalation challenge procedures (which may cause considerable alarm because of their rapid development) are usually readily reversed. Late reactions, by contrast, are often poorly responsive to bronchodilators. However, several hours are usually required for the peak of a late response to be reached, and so it is usually possible to modify the ultimate severity by treatment with corticosteroids as soon as an unequivocally positive response gives rise to concern.

When baseline values of FEV_1 are less than 70% of predicted, the risks of inhalation challenge tests increase, and individual judgment has to be exercised in deciding whether the benefits of the tests outweigh the risks. With close medical supervision and the use of small increments in challenge exposure dose (not more than twofold), the risks are likely to be relatively small in patients whose baseline FEV_1 lies in the range of 60–70% of the predicted normal value. When the baseline FEV_1 is 50–60% of the predicted value, challenge tests are rarely justified; and only exceptional circumstances should allow them to be considered when baseline FEV_1 is less than 50% of the predicted value.

2. Need for Continuing Medication

A continuing need for regular medication is a less serious drawback to the use of inhalation challenge tests. Ideally, test subjects should cease occupational exposure for 1 or even 2 weeks before the tests, thereby diminishing the need for such therapy. Medication during this period, particularly corticosteroids, should be reduced to the minimum level compatible with reasonable comfort and adequate baseline lung function. When possible, inhaled short-acting bronchodilators and short-acting anticholinergic agents should be discontinued for at least 12 h before challenge testing, and inhaled long-acting β-agonists, long-acting anticholinergic preparations, cromoglycate, and nedocromil, together with oral medications, should be discontinued for at least 24 h.

In circumstances where medication can not be discontinued but the minimum levels necessary have been determined, challenge tests with the relevant occupational agent can still be expected to demonstrate significant changes in lung function when compared with control tests carried out under the same conditions. It is crucial, however, that medications be taken at precisely standardized dose levels and times, and that active and control challenges be similarly administered at identical times on the separate study days. It is fortunate that corticosteroids appear to exert little, if any, inhibitory effect on immediate asthmatic reactions, while their effect on late reactions is closely dose-dependent.

B. In Hypersensitivity Pneumonitis

With hypersensitivity pneumonitis, it is fortunate that mild reactions following challenge exposures near the threshold of responsiveness are characterized more by a systemic influenzalike illness than by respiratory symptoms with derangements in lung function. The risk of a life-threatening or even distressing reduction in respiratory function is consequently remote, even when baseline levels are seriously impaired, provided challenge exposure is not excessive. However, the flulike symptoms induced are often more distressing than an exacerbation of asthma, and there is much to recommend the routine use of corticosteroids once a positive parenchymal response is evident, particularly if baseline lung function is appreciably impaired. The latter situation may well pertain in the more chronic form of hypersensitivity pneumonitis, the form in which an etiological diagnosis is less easily established. Fortunately, subjects affected in this way usually do respond in the typically acute fashion when challenged with sufficiently high doses of the appropriate occupational agent. They may also produce obstructive responses in the airways (i.e., asthmatic responses) in addition to parenchymal responses, and so the safety guidelines suggested for asthma are broadly applicable to hypersensitivity pneumonitis as well. In the absence of asthmatic reactions, however, somewhat lower levels of baseline FEV_1 are acceptable. Both FEV_1 and forced vital capacity (FVC) should ideally be above 60% of the predicted level, but when there is particular need to conduct inhalation provocation tests, baseline levels of FEV_1, FVC, and gas transfer of 50–60% of predicted values are acceptable.

IV. METHODS

A. Airway Responsiveness

Of the two measurement methods that are currently most popular, that using the Wright jet nebulizer has become conventional throughout much of Canada, Australasia, and Europe [5]. Aerosol is generated continuously over successive periods of 2 min from doubling concentrations of methacholine (or histamine) and is inhaled by the test subject during tidal breathing. The dose delivered consequently depends on tidal volume and ventilatory frequency as well as on aerosol output, and so it is not readily quantified—though it may be closely repeatable for the individual subject. Continuous nebulization may also cause an appreciable increase in solute concentration because of evaporation (jet nebulizers release vapor as well as aerosol), which further complicates the task of calculating dose output [14]. As a result, airway responsiveness is expressed by the provocative concentration of methacholine (rather than the delivered dose) that is estimated to induce a 20% decrement in FEV_1—i.e., PC_{20}. The alternative method, which is currently popular in the United States and some European countries, uses a "dosimeter" and attempts to deliver a precise dose of methacholine during part of a single inspiratory maneuver [15]. This allows airway responsiveness to be expressed by the actual dose provoking a 20% decrement in FEV_1 (PD_{20}).

This method has been developed in Newcastle by means of a microcomputer-controlled dosimeter that nebulizes 10 μl of true challenge solution per inhalation and delivers sequential doubling cumulative doses of methacholine over a range of 3.125–6400 μg at 5-min intervals. We have compared it with the conventional Wright nebulizer method by duplicating tests with both methods in the same subjects [6]. Precision (coefficient of repeatability) was significantly better for the dosimeter method, but the technique for quantifying FEV_1 at each time point (mean of the best three of six measurements vs. the lower of two measurements) contributed more to this than did the technique for delivering methacholine. A PC_{20} of 1 mg/ml proved to be equivalent to a PD_{20} of 103 μg. In the continuing absence of a universally accepted method for measuring airway responsiveness, it is important that estimates of precision and equivalence be similarly provided for every reported method.

B. Asthma

1. Challenge Exposure

Workplace Challenge. By far the most convenient method of reproducing the circumstances of occupational exposure is for the subject to return to his or her normal working activities. Ventilatory function is monitored by the subject with a device measuring peak expiratory flow (PEF), and any changes that occur are compared against corresponding data obtained during control days spent away from the working environment. This simple but very effective approach has been ably championed by Burge and colleagues, and two of their studies are illustrated in Figs. 1 and 2 [16,17]. Figure 1 records hourly PEF rates during waking hours. The decline noted on the Monday and Friday is convincingly different from the minimal circadian change noted on the Sunday away from work. It can reasonably be attributed to the occupational environment, which in this case contained a respirable agent known to induce asthma (colophony fumes). Figure 2 illustrates

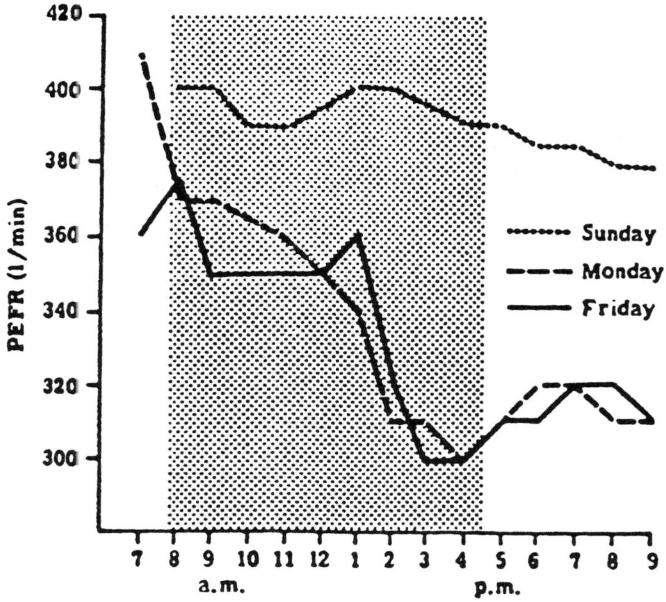

Figure 1 Hourly peak expiratory flow rate (PEFR) of an electronics factory supervisor exposed to colophony fumes. The shaded zone indicates the work period on Monday and Friday. (From Ref. 16.)

the use of PEF measurements over a much longer period, only the maximum, minimum, and mean values being plotted each day. In this particular case, 2–3 weeks were required for full recovery after a prolonged period at work. No significant improvement was observed when occupational exposure to isocyanate vapor was briefly discontinued, and a change in work shift had no effect.

This approach has obvious advantages. There is minimal danger, since the challenge exposure involved has been encountered safely many times previously. This reduces the need for and expense of close medical supervision and possible hospital admission. The use of an inexpensive peak flow meter by the unsupervised subject eliminates the need for sophisticated lung function equipment and the services of laboratory personnel. Finally, an unequivocally positive response generated in the workplace itself may, for some, provide more convincing evidence of occupational asthma than a response generated artificially in the laboratory.

The disadvantages of this technique are equally obvious. Peak expiratory flow provides a relatively imprecise measure of ventilatory function, and recordings are made by the test subject without supervision. Although this may satisfy the responsible physician, it may not be acceptable when a novel and potentially

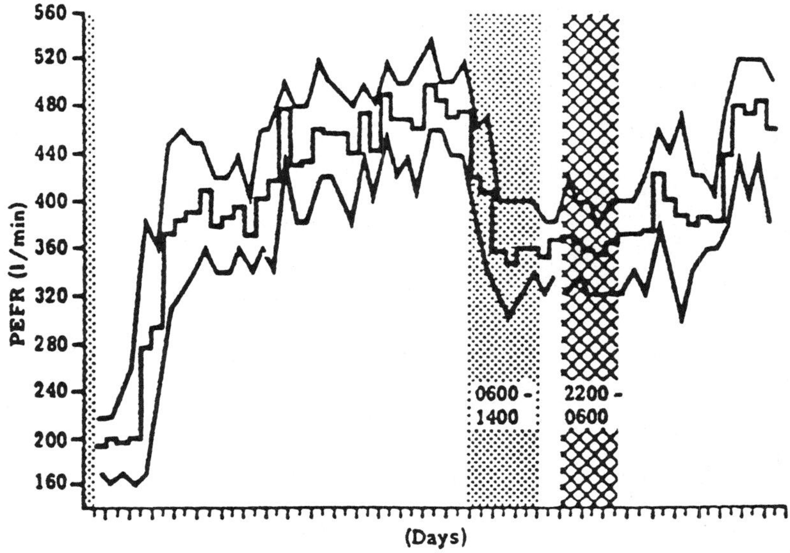

Figure 2 Daily peak expiratory flow rate (PEFR) of a printer exposed to isocyanate vapor. The shaded and cross-hatched zones indicate work days. The record begins after a prolonged period at work. Upper line = maximum PEFR daily; middle line = mean PEFR daily: lower line = minimum PEFR daily. (From Ref. 17.)

important cause of occupational asthma is under investigation, and it may not be satisfactory in litigious or research settings. Criticism could also be directed to the lack of "blinding" in the test protocol, since the off-work control days are clearly indistinguishable from the challenge days at work.

It is conceivable that asthmatic responses triggered at work could result from factors that are not strictly occupational. Specific common antigens and nonspecific irritants such as smoke, cold air, or air pollutants may be encountered intermittently anywhere away from the home; and asthma-provoking analgesics (for headaches or arthritis) or tartrazine (in foods and beverages from the workplace canteen) may be taken in greater quantity on workdays than on days of leisure. Similarly, exercise may be of greater degree at work. The return-to-work method of challenge is thus nonspecific. It tests the entire work-related environment rather than any single specific occupational agent.

Laboratory Challenge with Dusts. When challenge tests are carried out in the laboratory, reliable measurements of lung function are more readily obtained, and control-day studies can often be performed under the same blinded conditions as studies with specific occupational agents. Workplace exposures to particulates (dusts) can still be closely simulated if challenge exposures are of the type

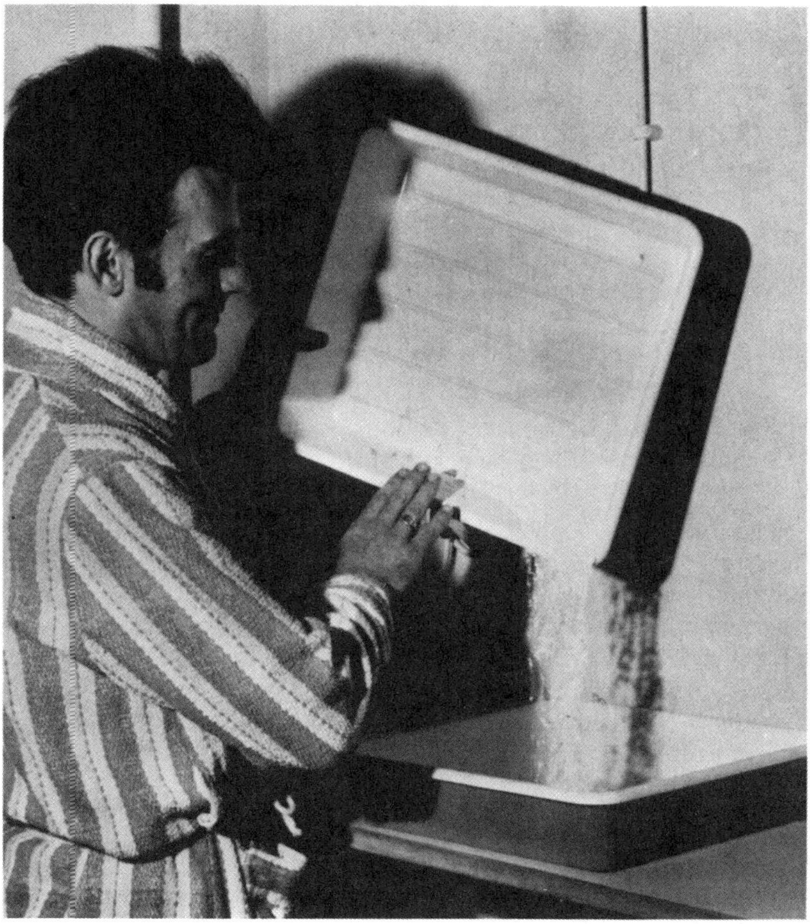

Figure 3 Laboratory challenge with chemical dust. (From Ref. 19.).

advocated by Pepys and colleagues [18]. Figure 3 shows a worker tipping finely powdered dry lactose to and fro between container trays [19]. Appropriate quantities of a test dust of occupational origin (in this case piperazine) may be added to a given amount of lactose so that the dusty occupational atmosphere is simulated when tipping begins. As lactose alone can be used for control tests, the challenge procedure can be carried out in a single- or even double-blind fashion—providing the test agent does not need to be added in such high concentration that it becomes detectable by its color, odor, taste, or texture. Even then, masking agents can often be added to prevent the test agent from being recognized.

This technique was used extensively in the investigation of occupational asthma in workers engaged in the manufacture of ampicillin from benzyl penicillin [20]. Challenge concentrations were steadily increased from 1 mg antibiotic in 250 gm of lactose, and typical late asthmatic reactions were observed in a number of affected workers when challenge mixtures containing 1–10 g of antibiotic were used over periods of 30–60 min.

Considerable differences have been noted in potency between the various agents found thus far to be associated with occupational asthma, as illustrated in Fig. 4 [20,21]. Immediate, late, and dual asthmatic responses were provoked following dust challenges with ammonium hexachlorplatinate (10 mg in 250 g lactose), purified ampicillin (10 g in 250 g lactose), and flour alone (250 g), respectively. For these three particular agents, potency appeared to vary 25,000-fold—though with flour it is quite possible, if not probable, that the specific provoking agent was a contaminating mold, mite, weevil, or even pesticide of considerably greater potency than the crude flour itself. Much care is consequently required in choosing the concentration for the initial challenge when a previously untested occupational agent is first used.

Laboratory Challenge Using a Nebulizer. A more sophisticated method of laboratory challenge and the most convenient technique for conducting challenge

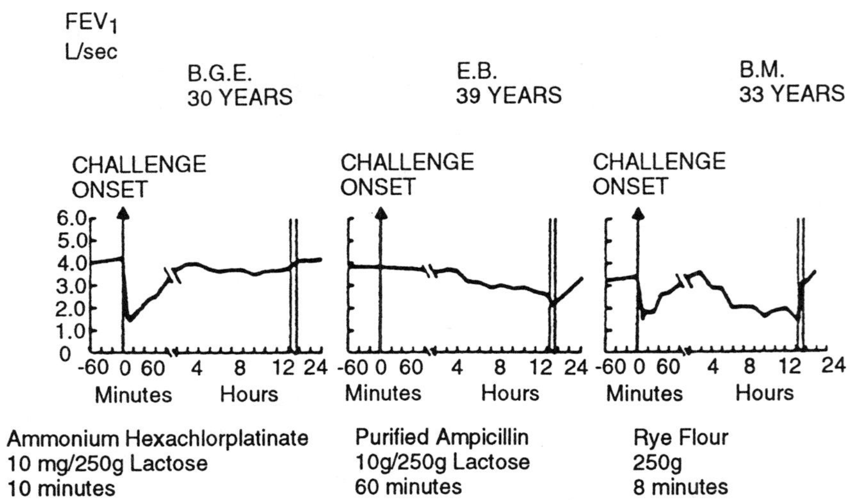

Figure 4 Immediate, late, and dual asthmatic reactions to challenge with different quantities of ammonium hexachlorplatinate, ampicillin, and rye flour. FEV_1 = forced expired volume in 1 second.

tests with soluble (or liquid) agents is to generate respirable aerosols of appropriate solutions. The jet nebulizers used for methacholine or histamine tests are equally suited to tests of this nature, though dosimeters delivering known challenge doses are preferable to nebulizers that release aerosol continuously. The great advantage of this method (and of most methods generating vapors and gases) is that control and "antigen" challenges are not readily distinguishable, providing the latter have no characteristic color, odor, or taste. When this is the case, the addition of a little coloring matter or phenol (0.4%) to all challenge fluids usually masks any differences.

Atmospheric measurements in the workplace of cumulative daily exposures provide the best guide to the choice of challenge dose range. Initial doses should ideally simulate minimal exposures encountered naturally in the workplace, while maximum doses (often the statutory workplace exposure limit) should just exceed the maximum likely to have been experienced. This implies a sequence of incremental challenges (one test per day), a protocol that is not always practical. When experience has been gained with a particular agent, a good deal of protocol shortening may be allowable, but until this has been achieved safety considerations must dominate. Where the minimum daily dose can be estimated only crudely, safety may require that challenge testing begin with a tenth or even a hundredth of this. It is not known whether identical daily cumulative doses administered over the brief seconds or minutes of a conventional aerosol challenge test give results similar to those of a natural exposure over 8 h in the workplace, though some evidence suggests that stronger reactions may follow such peak levels of exposure. A negative test with the maximum dose should consequently suffice to exclude asthmatic sensitivity in the test subject.

Once minimum and maximum dose levels have been chosen, the investigator must select a suitable dose increment for sequential tests. Increments of two- to fivefold have generally proved satisfactory, our own usual choice being $\sqrt{10}$ (i.e., 3.2-fold). This allows a convenient and safe dose sequence of 1, 3.2, 10, 32, 100 . . . units. A seven-dose sequence consequently encompasses a 1000-fold dose range, and a nine-dose sequence a 10,000-fold dose range. These should be more than adequate for most purposes and may allow threshold levels and dose–response characteristics to be defined [22]. The insertion of control challenges at random points in the sequence allows the challenges to be blinded and introduces great diagnostic power to the protocol. This may be increased if the physician immediately supervising the tests is also blinded to the nature of the test agents. If, finally, any positive reaction is shown to be repeatable, the diagnostic value of such a protocol becomes formidable. It can, of course, be applied equally successfully to other methods of challenge exposure.

Laboratory Challenge Using an Exposure Chamber. Aerosols may be generated openly in the laboratory or in an exposure chamber, which in addition provides the most suitable method of controlling challenges with gases, vapors, or fumes. Initially, human exposure chambers were designed simply to confine atmospheric dispersal of the challenge agents, thereby preventing contamination of the laboratory and protecting the staff. Evolution brought the ability to measure atmospheric concentrations and hence to evaluate dose–response relationships. More recent innovations include continuously ventilated chambers with selected levels of temperature and humidity, and constant generation of the challenge agent. Challenge environments can therefore be closely controlled in a dynamic equilibrium, and precise exposure levels can be maintained over periods of many hours. Thus, the exposures of whole working shifts may be closely simulated. The larger the chamber and the more comfortable its fittings (armchairs, television, video), the more readily can long periods of challenge exposure be investigated.

In practice, the desired cumulative doses of exposure are more conveniently administered at higher concentration levels but over rather shorter periods—usually a matter of 10–60 min. Further convenience may be achieved by testing several subjects simultaneously, providing the chamber is sufficiently large. With large chambers the technical problems of maintaining a chosen atmospheric environment with precision over long periods are reduced, but expense is necessarily increased and may be unrealistic for some investigators.

A novel alternative is the recently described small external mixing chamber, from which the challenge atmosphere can be sampled by test subjects via its access ports [23]. Again, there is a dynamic equilibrium, as air and the test agent are fed continuously under controlled conditions into the mixing chamber. Concentrations within the chamber are monitored throughout and adjusted when necessary, and the test subject breathes the test atmosphere from a mouthpiece or face mask. Depending on the number of ports and the flow rates into the chamber, it may be possible to test more than one subject at a time using such a system. Some environmental leakage into the laboratory is likely, however, unless the test subject exhales into a closed and exhausted breathing circuit, and there may be greater difficulty in controlling exposure concentrations. The system is also less suited to long periods of challenge exposure, but it offers an admirable alternative when the use of whole-body exposure chambers is unrealistic.

Whether an occupational agent of possible relevance to asthma is encountered as a vapor or as an aerosol may have important practical implications, since these different physical forms may lead to different patterns of deposition within the respiratory tract. The more peripherally asthma-provoking agents are deposited, the higher is the dose required to trigger a reaction. In the case of methylene diphenylisocyanate (MDI), sampling impingers that measure ambient concentrations assuming it to be vapor grossly underestimate its true concentration in milligrams per cubic meter if it is predominantly in aerosol form [24]. Polyurethane spraying operations that use MDI may in fact generate appreciable airborne concentrations of MDI aerosol, while the mixing of MDI with polyols in a container (to produce insulating material for underground telephone cables, for example) is more likely to release MDI vapor, particularly in hot ambient environments. However, MDI has low volatility, and laboratory attempts to generate meaningful amounts of vapor by heating may be foiled because of an increased risk of oxidation [25].

Problems of this sort can be overcome by the use of special equipment, and controlled chamber exposures of known physical and chemical composition can now be generated for a number of occupational chemicals known to induce asthma [26,27]. This is not to say that sophisticated equipment is always mandatory. Asthma from occupational exposure to the vapor/gas of toluene diisocyanate (TDI) and formaldehyde has been simply confirmed by affected subjects' "painting" the test agents onto cardboard within an exposure chamber, using mixtures of polyurethane varnish plus activator (TDI) for the one and solutions of formaldehyde in water (formalin) for the other [9,28].

Recent advances in laboratory challenge methods with vapors and gases are illustrated by the exposure chamber system at Tulane Medical Center for Bioenvironmental Research [25]. The system consists of three components: a source of clean breathing air, an agent-generation system, and a delivery system. The challenge chamber is composed of a 4-foot-wide, 6.2-foot-high, 7.2-foot-long stainless steel chamber with an observation window through which the test subject can be observed during exposure. Room air enters the chamber through high-efficiency particulate and charcoal filters and is blended with the test agent in a narrow throat to ensure complete mixing. The mixture then enters the chamber through air-splitter veins and diffusion screens. It then flows around the entire chamber and is exhausted through another set of veins and screens by a blower. An even distribution of the agent is ensured throughout the chamber, which is maintained at the slightly negative pressure (0.5–1.5 inches of water) to prevent leakage. The test subject enters the chamber through a special air lock that minimizes any change in agent concentration. Other access ports in the chamber can be used to monitor such parameters as blood, vital sings, and pulmonary function while the subject is inside the chamber. Exposure monitoring instruments can be placed in the chamber or can be used to examine atmospheric samples drawn through the access ports. Figure 5 illustrates the chamber in outline. We have used this system for challenges with many vapors and gases, including formaldehyde, TDI and diphenyl methane diisocyanate.

Figure 6 illustrates separate exposure profiles in the chamber with formaldehyde and TDI. It shows both the target concentration (T) and the average concentration (A), plus the standard deviation [25]. In the case of formaldehyde, for example, the particular protocol employed required exposure at 0.3 parts per million (ppm) for 10 min followed by 1.0 ppm for 10 min and then 3.0 ppm for 60 min. It can be seen that the system was able to generate formaldehyde concentrations that were extremely close to the desired target concentrations. In the case of TDI, the challenge was with 20 parts per billion for 4 h. The average concentra-

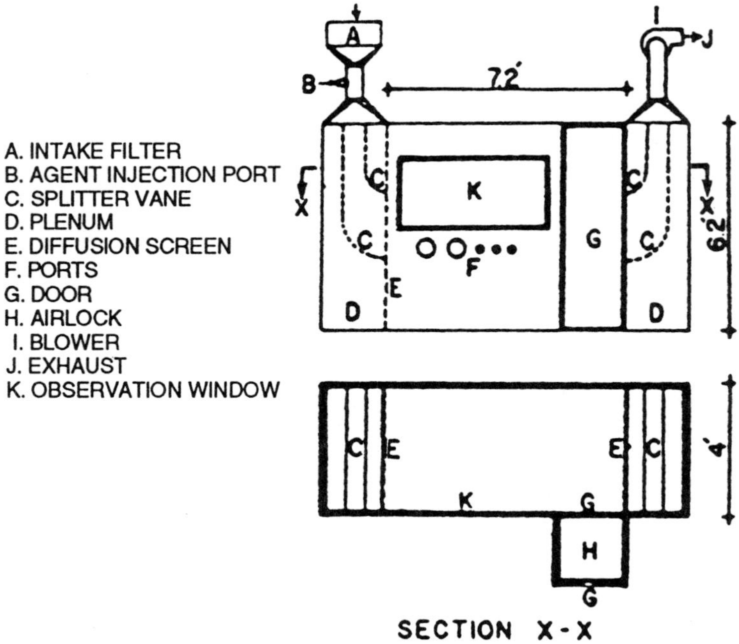

Figure 5 Schematic diagram of the Tulane human exposure chamber. (From Ref. 25.)

tion of TDI was within 0.5% of the target concentration, and fluctuations during the 4-h period remained within 5%.

2. Monitoring Investigations

The relative merits of the various lung-function tests used to monitor asthma need not be discussed at length. Although somewhat insensitive, the conventional FEV_1 remains the most useful because of its reproducibility, simplicity, and ready availability. Airway resistance, specific conductance, and expiratory flow at low lung volumes are sometimes used when more sensitive indices of response are desired, but greater measurement variability coupled with the greater cost and complexity of these lung-function tests makes them much less satisfactory than FEV_1 in monitoring prolonged asthmatic reactions. Peak expiratory flow offers a convenient alternative when the test subject monitors his or her own ventilatory function from unsupervised measurements outside the laboratory.

The importance of precision in measuring ventilatory function at any given time point is matched by the importance of obtaining frequent measurements during waking hours and of establishing the usual pattern of hour-to-hour and day-to-day variability. Unless "normal" changes can be quantified, significant change

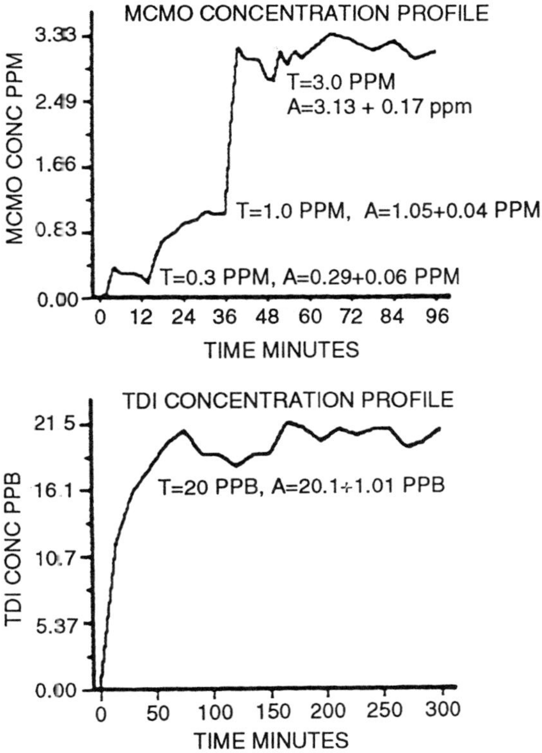

Figure 6 Profiles of atmospheric concentrations of formaldehyde (HCHO) and toluene diisocyanate (TDI) in exposure chamber showing both target concentration (T) and average concentration (A) with standard deviation. (From Ref. 25.)

attributable to the challenge exposure cannot be identified with any confidence. A late reaction may be particularly difficult to identify, since circadian change in ventilatory function is a common characteristic of asthma in general. This is well illustrated in Fig. 7. In this instance, sequential daily challenges with increasing exposures to formaldehyde at the same time of day gave apparently positive late-phase reactions in a pathologist who had had atopic asthma in childhood [29]. Persisting airway disease in adult life had been attributed to smoker's bronchitis until the possibility of occupational formaldehyde asthma was raised. The circadian changes observed following sequential challenges with formaldehyde were not affected by exposure dose, nor were they different from the changes noted on a control day without formaldehyde exposure. A diagnosis of formaldehyde asthma was therefore excluded. In this particular case there was a marked circadian rhythm, but the pattern was very similar from day to day.

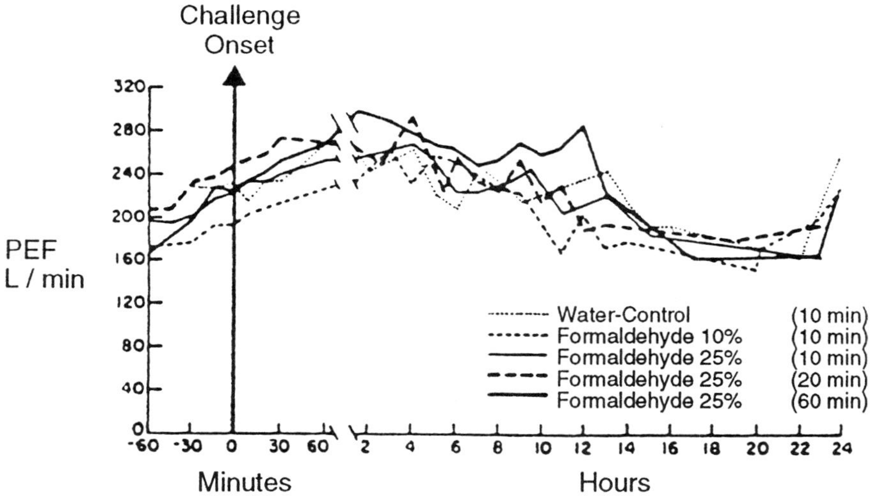

Figure 7 Marked circadian change in peak expiratory flow (PEF) rate in a pathologist exposed to formaldehyde. Maximally concentrated solutions of formaldehyde in water (formalin) were diluted with water and "painted" onto cardboard in an exposure chamber. (From Ref. 29.)

In Fig. 8 we illustrate a converse picture. Again the subject had active asthma, and an occupational cause was suspected. The figure displays time-matched peak expiratory flow measurements on three separate control days during which there was no occupational exposure. A circadian rhythm was much less striking, but there was moderate variability in measurement from hour to hour, and rather more variability from day to day. Had day 1 been used alone to provide "control" data, the measurements obtained on both day 2 and day 3 might have been interpreted as showing late asthmatic reactions—there were sustained late decrements of 15% or more in relation to baseline measurements and to time-matched control measurements. When the control data from all three days were considered together, however, it was possible to determine 95% confidence limits against which statistically significant changes could subsequently be recognized. Unfortunately, 3 days of control data represent the minimum from which meaningful confidence limits can be derived, thereby adding further complexity and effort if challenge tests are to be carried out under ideal standardized circumstances.

These difficulties have greatly influenced the evolution of the full protocol currently used in our laboratory. It is demanding and time-consuming and might be considered idealized to a degree that is often impractical. It does, nevertheless, provide a useful standard, and it gives a test methodology of high sensitivity and specificity—valuable properties if a novel but strategically important industrial

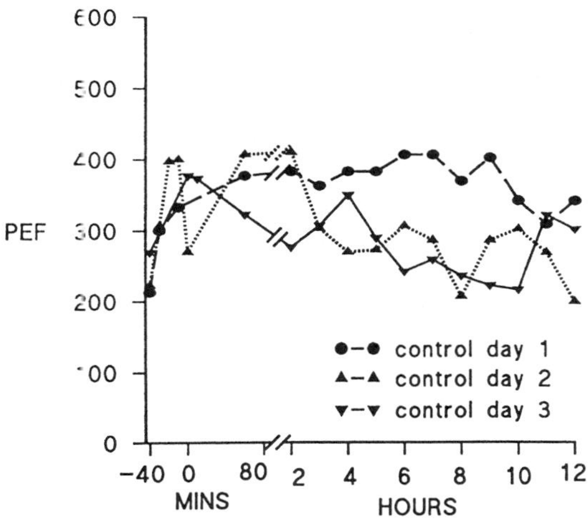

Figure 8 Variability in peak expiratory flow (PEF) rate during 3 control days in a subject with suspected occupational asthma.

agent is under investigation [22]. During a 1- to 2-week period away from work, the test subject undergoes (if necessary) a carefully supervised reduction in medication to the minimum level required for comfort and safety. One or two methacholine tests are then performed to quantify airway responsiveness, and control measurements of FEV_1 are obtained over 3 days at standardized times. The latter are determined according to the mutually convenient standardized "start time" that is chosen to commence challenge exposures (usually 1000 h). The FEV_1 is measured at 10-min intervals for 40 min before and 80 min after the start time, which allows any immediate reaction to be detected. Subsequent measurements are obtained hourly from 2–12 and 22–24 h after the start time, which provides adequate data to recognize a late reaction. We do not wake subjects routinely, but additional nocturnal measurements are sometimes useful when a late reaction peaks during the night 12–22 h after the start time. In practice, however, the period 2–12 h after challenge is almost always sufficient to demonstrate a late reaction.

The FEV_1 is determined as the mean of the three best of six measurements at each time point, a procedure that minimizes variability. Expiratory maneuvers are, however, terminated after 1 s, which usefully minimizes fatigue and improves compliance. Whenever possible, a double-blind technique is achieved by the random insertion of indistinguishable control challenges in the test sequence, and doses are increased by increments of $\sqrt{10}$ (i.e., 3.2)-fold. When a positive result is observed, its repeatability is tested.

While immediate reactions may reasonably be diagnosed by FEV_1 decrements of 15–20% of baseline within 80 min of the start time, two statistical techniques are used to distinguish late reactions from spontaneous hour-to-hour and day-to-day variability. A single area-under-the-curve measure (usually the 2–12 h area decrement) is used to quantify cumulatively any "late" decrement in FEV_1 and is illustrated in Fig. 9. The 95% confidence interval derived from the 3 control days (Student's *t*-test) allows any significant increase in this area decrement to be recognized. Figure 10 shows the results of such investigation in a worker with suspected occupational asthma due to a newly developed detergent ingredient, sodium isononanoyl oxybenzene sulfonate (SINOS) [22]. The second statistical technique is illustrated in Fig. 11 from the same investigation of the SINOS worker. Using a pooled standard deviation of the 11 hourly measurements of FEV_1 2–12 hours after the start time, the figure gives a "lower boundary" (similar to a lower 95% confidence limit) below the mean FEV_1 measurements obtained from the 3 control days. Measurements of FEV_1 that broached this boundary following the SINOS challenge indicate the period(s) during which significant late decrements occurred. Although a single excursion below the boundary can be considered significant in a statistical sense, we would regard a late reaction to have occurred only when two consecutive hourly measurements fall below the boundary.

Not only do statistical analyses offer greater confidence in interpreting results, but they allow the recognition of reactions that are relatively small but nevertheless real. Unnecessarily high challenge doses can consequently be avoided in a planned

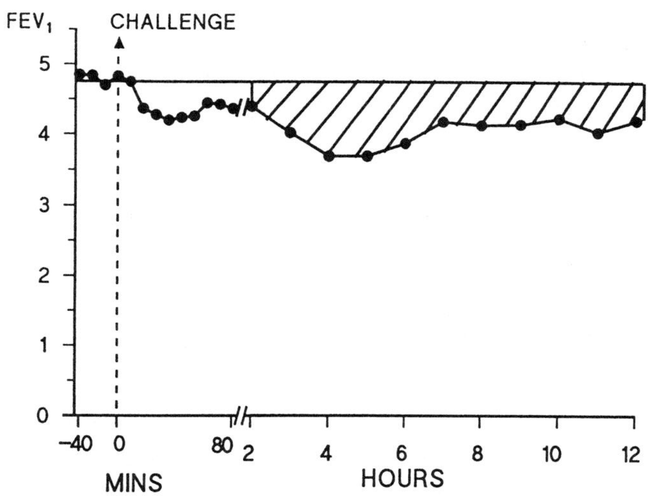

Figure 9 The forced expired volume in 1 second (FEV_1) area decrement 2–12 h after challenge (i.e., the 2–12 h area decrement).

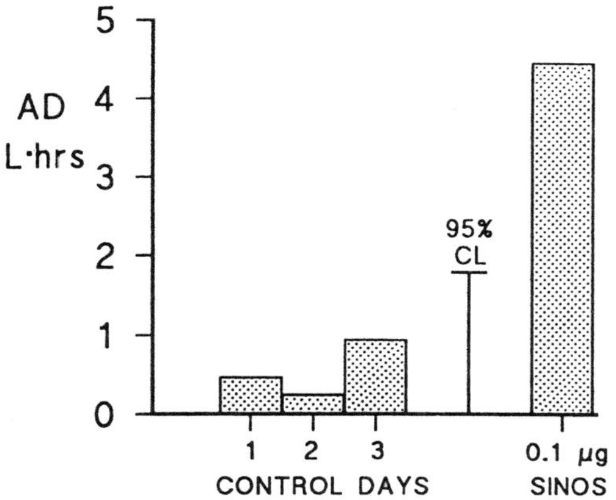

Figure 10 The 2–12 h area decrements (AD) in forced expired volume in 1 second (FEV_1) measured in liter·hours (L·hrs) on 3 control days and following challenge with sodium isononanoyl oxybenzene sulfonate (SINOS) 0.1 μg.

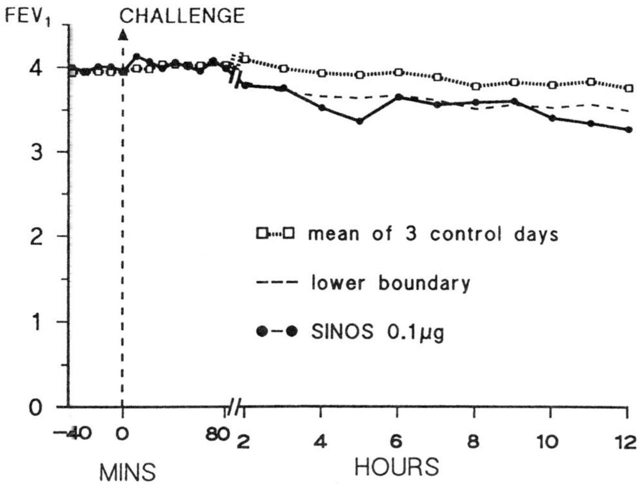

Figure 11 Mean control values for forced expired volume in 1 second (FEV_1), lower boundary (lower 95% confidence limit), and excursions following challenge with sodium isononanoyl oxybenzene sulfonate (SINOS) 0.1 μg.

sequence of incremental challenge doses. This improves safety and minimizes discomfort, investigation time, and cost.

While a positive result using both the above analytical methods indicates that there has been a statistically significant late fall in ventilatory function (we would take a conservative stance if the two statistical techniques give discordant results, and would deem the outcome to be "equivocal"), this does not prove it is a consequence of the challenge exposure. Other factors, either exogenous or endogenous, could conceivably be responsible, and the investigator should consider whether the FEV_1 measurements are likely to have been reliable and whether the outcome noted is plausible. In this respect, the use of a double-blind protocol is most helpful, as is the demonstration that the late reaction is repeatable. Finally, the methacholine test should be repeated after the challenge series is complete, a significant increase in airway responsiveness providing invaluable supportive evidence of asthmatic sensitivity to the challenge agent.

An eosinophil leukocyte response is commonly associated with late asthmatic reactions to challenge, possibly because of the release of eosinophil chemotactic factor of anaphylaxis following macrophage activation or the activation of complement by the alternative pathway. It may be recognized in both circulating blood and bronchial secretions, though in practice samples of the latter are not readily obtained for examination. We have sometimes found it useful, as a monitoring test, to draw blood samples approximately 8 and 24 h after the start time in addition to a sample drawn immediately beforehand. A doubling of the eosinophil count is commonly observed with late reactions, and absolute eosinophilia is often generated if it was not already present.

C. Hypersensitivity Pneumonitis

1. Challenge Exposure

The methods of challenge exposure used in the investigation of occupational asthma are equally appropriate to hypersensitivity pneumonitis. In general, parenchymal responses are provoked by organic dusts and contaminating microbial antigens, though a few cases have been reported in which chemicals appeared to be responsible. The potency of these organic dusts is usually of a lesser order of magnitude than that of the chemical agents responsible for occupational asthma. Laboratory dust challenges that simulate natural occupational exposure often require "undiluted" samples of the etiological agent (e.g., moldy straw, hay, barley, grain), and so the ability to administer the challenge exposure in a blinded fashion may be no greater than in a return-to-work study. The dispersion of the etiological dust in large volumes of air in the workplace may, however, produce comparatively low levels of exposure, while occupational-type dust challenges in a laboratory exposure chamber may produce unnaturally high concentrations. Such challenge exposures can be difficult to control and occasionally result in quite severe reactions. Prior sampling of the occupational and challenge environments is of some value, but facilities for this are not commonly available. Furthermore, the precise etiological agent, which could be derived from any one of a number of contaminating microorganisms, may not be entirely clear.

Occupational-type dust challenge in the laboratory and return-to-work challenges are convenient methods of investigating the acute form of hypersensitivity pneumonitis but are less suited to the chronic form. The latter, under natural conditions, requires periods of weeks, months, or more for significant changes to become apparent—both of recovery following cessation of exposure, and of relapse following recommencement of regular exposure. Furthermore, the investigator could not be confident that full recovery would follow such a prolonged period of challenge test exposure. Fortunately, most (but not all) subjects with the chronic form of hypersensitivity pneumonitis appear to react in the typical acute fashion if exposed to appropriately large doses [13,30]. For such exposure, aerosol challenge from nebulized solutions of antigen is often the best approach. It is also suitable for investigation of the acute form of the disease and allows the challenge test to be conducted in a blinded fashion. The exposure level at which a negative response can be deemed to exclude hypersensitivity is, however, difficult to establish, and must depend on wide experience with both affected and control subjects. The recommendations of the American Thoracic Society regarding antigen challenge in the investigation of asthma provide some useful guidelines [31].

2. Monitoring Investigations

A characteristic feature of acute reactions in subjects with hypersensitivity pneumonitis is a systemic influenzalike illness comprising malaise, widespread aches and pains, headache, tiredness, fever, and anorexia [13,30,32,33]. This usually dominates respiratory symptoms, particularly after exposures near the threshold of responsiveness. With high levels of exposure, pulmonary effects become more prominent. Undue shortness of breath on exercise is the earliest and most sensitive pulmonary symptom, which may be followed by cough (usually dry), chest discomfort (often described as difficulty in taking a deep, satisfying breath), and shortness of breath at rest. When the last is present, it is usually possible to show several abnormalities of lung function: restricted ventilation (though residual volume is often increased), diminished diffusing capacity and compliance, and hypocapnia (indicating hyperventilation). There may also be auscultatory crackles and radiographic infiltrates. Following massive natural exposures, pulmonary failure and life-threatening hypoxia may occur, although a fatal outcome is exceedingly rare.

In general, symptoms have proved to be more sensitive than monitoring tests that measure objective changes, and the systemic flu-like response has proved to be more sensitive than the pulmonary response. It is not surprising, then, that many investigators have experienced difficulty in demonstrating significant changes in lung function in association with apparently positive (though not severe) reactions. As a result, such responses have been considered "confirmed" by fever or leukocytosis alone. This approach is vulnerable to two criticisms: (1) a systemic response, even if specific, could be unrelated to a "coexisting" pulmonary disease; and (2) the systemic response may not be specific, since the challenge material is likely to have been derived from material contaminated with microbial toxins, animal serum, or other substances that could activate the alternative pathway of complement or induce nonspecific inflammation by other mechanisms.

Any rebuttal to such criticisms must depend on careful measurements of lung function coupled with critical use of control challenge tests, i.e., control challenges in the same subjects and antigen challenges in control subjects. Our own experience with 144 control and antigen tests in 29 subjects with suspected farmer's lung, mushroom worker's lung, and bird fancier's lung, and two control subjects, strongly supports the validity and usefulness of challenge tests in the investigation of hypersensitivity pneumonitis [13]. Twenty-three positive reactions were observed in 18 subjects. No reactions were observed in the two control subjects or in 11 other nonreactors, and so toxic mechanisms are unlikely to have been relevant. On the other hand, all of six subjects considered to have convincing evidence of hypersensitivity pneumonitis before undergoing challenge tests proved to be reactors. Parenchymal reactions were reproducible and characteristic, irrespective of the antigen involved or its means of delivery. All followed antigen rather than control challenges, and all were confidently recognized by the subjects concerned despite the use of a single-blind method of challenge in most cases. Although systemic flulike disturbances did dominate the clinical picture, significant changes in lung function were recorded. Furthermore, the responses produced closely simulated the acute diseases with which the farm workers and pigeon workers had presented initially.

Four subjective and six objective features proved to be useful in characterizing the reactions provoked by near-threshold challenge exposures. Table 1 records the distribution of the subjective features (symptoms and clinical signs corresponding to a flulike illness and undue respiratory effort on exercise), according to the results of each test. The result category was defined at the time before any analysis was made of the monitoring data. When both subject and investigator were convinced that a reaction had been provoked, the results were considered positive. When either party was suspicious but not convinced, the results were defined as equivocal, and when neither party was suspicious, the results were considered to be negative.

The objective features are given in Table 2. All showed changes of a statistically significant degree, and all were of diagnostic value retrospectively in identifying positive reactions. Diagnostic end points were chosen to produce specificities of approximately 95%. As a result, sensitivities of 48–85% were

Table 1 Challenge Tests in the Investigation of Hypersensitivity Pneumonitis: Distribution of Symptoms and Clinical Signs Developing During the 36 Hours Following Challenge

		Number of tests associated with			
		Symptoms		Clinical Signs	
Result category	Tests (n)[a]	"Flulike" (n)	Dyspnea (n)	Appearance (n)	Breathing (n)
Reactors (n = 18)					
Antigen tests					
Positive	23	22/22	23	16/20	18/18
Equivocal	14	11	12	3/13	3/10
Negative	25	0	1	0	0
Control tests	24	0	2	0/23	0/23
Nonreactors (n = 13)					
Antigen tests	49	0	3	0	1
Control tests	9	0	0	0	0

[a]Tests were excluded from table whenever the records were incomplete.
Source: Ref. 13.

obtained for these six simple and readily available monitoring tests. Measurement of exercise minute ventilation (treadmill test at a comfortable work rate) proved to be the most useful, as illustrated in Fig. 12. Auscultation, measurement of diffusing capacity, lung volume subdivisions, minute ventilation/respiratory frequency at rest, and chest radiography proved to be much less sensitive and gave significant changes only with the most severe reactions. It is possible of course that more sophisticated tests of lung function could have been more sensitive, but the more sophisticated the test, the less widely available it is. The above monitoring tests were all easily performed, with the possible exception of the exercise test, and in combination they proved to be very sensitive. The use of six objective monitoring tests was, however, time-consuming, and it is questionable whether the routine use of all six was cost-effective. Over 90% of the positive tests were associated with a maximum body temperature exceeding 37.2°C or a rise in circulating neutrophils of at least 2500/mm^3. In practice, these two tests are likely to suffice.

V. CONCLUSIONS

A great deal of experience has now been accumulated from the use of specific and nonspecific inhalation challenge tests in the investigation of occupational asthma.

Table 2 Challenge Tests in the Investigation of Hypersensitivity Pneumonitis: Mean Maximal Changes of Objective Monitoring Tests During the 36 Hours Following Challenge

	Tests (n)	Body temperature (°C)	Leukocyte counts/mm³		Exercise 5 min (%)		FVC	
			Neutrophils	Lymphocytes[a]	Minute volume	Respiratory frequency	%	l
Reactors (n = 18)								
Antigen tests								
Positive	23	+1.4	+5405	−351	+32	+40	−20	(−0.61)
Equivocal	14	+0.3	+1446	−46	+7	+6	−11	(−0.36)
Negative	25	+0.2	+625	+346	+0	+1	−5	(−0.16)
Control tests	24	+0.2	−412	+704	−3	0	−7	(−0.22)
Nonreactors (n = 13)								
Antigen tests	49	+0.4	+404	+444	+1	+2	−5	(−0.19)
Control tests	9	+0.4	−234	−268	−5	+3	−6	(−0.19)
Statistical comparisons								
Reactors (positive vs. control tests)	p<	0.01	0.01	0.01	0.01	0.01	0.05	
Antigen tests (reactors vs. nonreactors)	p<	0.01	0.01	0.01	0.01	0.01	0.01	
Diagnostic end point		>37.2	⩾+2500	⩾−500[b]	⩾+15	⩾+25	⩾−15	
Specificity		95%	96%	97%	95%	94%	97%	
Sensitivity		78%	68%	52%	85%	64%	48%	

[a]From morning to evening.
[b]With lymphopenia.
FVC = forced vital capacity.
Source: Ref. 13.

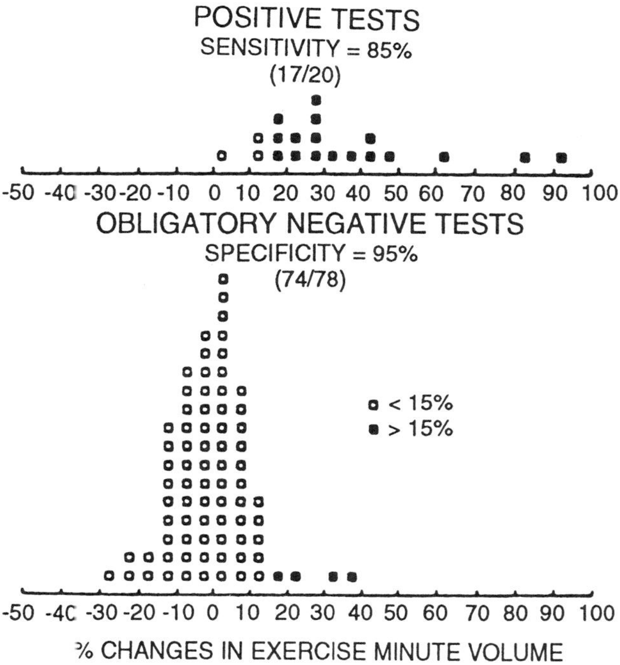

Figure 12 Challenge tests in the investigation of hypersensitivity pneumonitis in 31 subjects: distributions of maximal changes in exercise minute ventilation during 36 h after challenge. (From Ref. 13.)

By comparison, the use of challenge tests in the investigation of hypersensitivity pneumonitis is in its infancy, partly because of the difficulties in evaluating parenchymal responses, and partly because occupational hypersensitivity pneumonitis is far less common than occupational asthma. Nevertheless, these tests can be of great value for both diseases, and their use is likely to continue to increase. They may be very time-consuming, however, and they are not without risk. Furthermore, the results are not always easy to interpret. They are tools that are best left to investigators prepared to use them regularly.

REFERENCES

1. Ishizaka, T., White, J. R., and Saito, H., Activation of basophils and mast cells for mediator release, *Int. Arch. Allergy Appl. Immunol.*, *82*, 327–332 (1987).
2. Kaliner, M., Hypothesis on the contribution of late phase allergic response to the understanding and treatment of allergic disease, *J. Allergy Clin. Immunol.*, *73*, 311–315 (1984).

3. Lemanske, R. F., and Kaliner, M., Mast cell dependent late phase reactions, *Clin. Immunol. Rev.*, *1*, 547–580 (1982).
4. Connolly, M. J., Avery, A. J., Walters, E. H., and Hendrick, D. J., The relationship between bronchial responsiveness to methacholine and bronchial responsiveness to histamine in asthmatic subjects, *Pulmon. Pharmacol.*, *1*, 53–58 (1988).
5. Juniper, E. F., Frith, P. A., Dunnett, C., Cockroft, D. W., and Hargreave, F. E., Reproducibility and comparison of responses to inhaled histamine and methacholine, *Thorax*, *33*, 705–710 (1978).
6. Beach, J. R., Young, C. L., Avery, A. J., Stenton, S. C., Dennis, J. H., Walters, E. H., and Hendrick, D. J., Measurement of airway responsiveness to methacholine: relative importance of the precision of drug delivery and the method of assessing response, *Thorax*, *48*, 239–243 (1993).
7. Chan-Yeung, M., Lam, S., and Koerner, S., Clinical features and natural history of occupational asthma due to western red cedar (Thuja plicata), *Am. J. Med.*, *72*, 411 (1982).
8. Chester, E. H., Martinez-Catinchi, F. L., Schwartz, H. J., et al., Patterns of airway reactivity to asthma produced by exposure to toluene di-isocyanate, *Chest*, *75* (suppl), 229 (1979).
9. Hendrick, D. J., and Lane, D. J., Occupational formalin asthma, *Br. J. Industr. Med.*, *34*, 11 (1977).
10. Braun, S. R., doPico, G. A., Tsiatis, A., et al., Farmer's lung disease: longterm clinical and physiologic outcome, *Am. Rev. Respir. Dis.*, *119*, 185 (1979).
11. Fink, J. N., Schlueter, D. P., Sosman, A. J., et al., Clinical survey of pigeon breeders, *Chest*, *62*, 277 (1972).
12. Salvaggio, J. E., Diagnostic significance of serum precipitins in hypersensitivity pneumonitis (editorial), *Chest*, *62*, 242 (1972).
13. Hendrick, D. J., Marshall, R. Faux, J. A., et al., Positive "alveolar" responses to antigen inhalation provocation tests: their validity and recognition, *Thorax*, *35*, 415 (1980).
14. Dennis, J. H., Stenton, S. C., Beach, J. R., Avery, A. J., Walters, E. H., and Hendrick, D. J., Jet and ultrasonic nebuliser output: use of a new method for direct measurement of aerosol output, *Thorax*, *45*, 728–732 (1990).
15. Chai, H., Farr, R. S., Froehlich, L. A., Mathison, D. A., Mclean, J. A., Rosenthal, R. R., Sheffer, A. L., Spector, S. L., and Townley, R. G., Standardization of bronchial inhalation challenge procedures, *J. Allergy Clin. Immunol.*, *56*, 323–327 (1975).
16. Burge, P. S., O'Brien, I. M., and Harries, M. G., Peak flow rate records in the diagnosis of occupational asthma due to colophony, *Thorax*, *34*, 308 (1979).
17. Burge, P. S., O'Brien, I. M., and Harries, M. G., Peak flow rate records in the diagnosis of occupational asthma due to isocyanates, *Thorax*, *34*, 317 (1979).
18. Pepys, J., and Hutchcroft, J. J., Bronchial provocation tests in etiologic diagnosis and analysis of asthma, *Am. Rev. Respir. Dis.*, *112*, 829 (1975).
19. Pepys, J., Pickering, C. A. C., and Loudon, H. W. G., Asthma due to inhaled chemical agents—piperazine dihydrochloride, *Clin. Allergy*, *2*, 189 (1972).
20. Davies, R. J., Hendrick, D. J., and Pepys, J., Asthma due to inhaled chemical agents: ampicillin, benzyl penicillin, 6 amino penicillanic acid and related substances, *Clin. Allergy*, *4*, 227 (1974).

21. Hendrick, D. J., Davies, R. J., and Pepys, J., Bakers' asthma, *Clin. Allergy*, *6*, 241 (1976).
22. Stenton, S. C., Dennis, J. H., Walters, E. H., and Hendrick, D. J., The asthmagenic properties of a newly developed detergent ingredient—sodium iso-nonanoyl oxybenzene sulphonate, *Br. J. Industr. Med.*, *47*, 405–410 (1990).
23. Cloutier, Y., Lagier, F., Cartier, A., and Malo, J.-L., Validation of an exposure system to particles for the diagnosis of occupational asthma, *Chest*, *102*, 402–407 (1992).
24. Dharmarajan, V., and Weill, H., Physical state of airborne p,p′-diphenylmethane diisocyanate (MDI) and its measurement, *Am. Ind. Hyg. Assoc. J.*, *39*, 737 (1978).
25. Hammad, Y., Rando, P., and Abdel-Kader, H., Considerations in design and use of human inhalation challenge delivery systems, *Folia Allergol. Immunol. Clin.*, *32*, 37–44 (1985).
26. Butcher, B. T., Karr, R. M., O'Neil, C. E., et al., Inhalation challenge and pharmacologic studies of toluene diisocyanate (TDI) sensitive workers, *J. Allergy Clin. Immunol.*, *64*, 146 (1979).
27. Gerblich, A. A., Horowitz, J., Chester, E. H., et al., A proposed standardized method for bronchoprovocation tests in toluene diisocyanate–induced asthma, *J. Allergy Clin. Immunol.*, *64*, 658 (1979).
28. Pepys, J., Pickering, C. A. C., and Therry, K. J., Asthma due to inhaled chemical agents—toluene diisocyanate, *Clin. Allergy*, *2*, 225 (1972).
29. Hendrick, D. J., and Lane, D. J., Formalin asthma in hospital staff, *Br. Med. J.*, *1*, 607 (1975).
30. Hargreave, F. E., and Pepys, J., Allergic respiratory reactions in bird fanciers provoked by allergen inhalation tests: relation to clinical features and allergic mechanism, *J. Allergy Clin. Immunol.*, *50*, 157 (1972).
31. American Thoracic Society, Guidelines for bronchial inhalation challenges with pharmacologic and antigenic agents, ATS News, April 11, 1980.
32. Reed, C. E., Sosman, A., and Barbee, R. A., Pigeon breeders' lung, *JAMA*, *193*, 261 (1965).
33. Warren, W. P., Hypersensitivity pneumonitis due to exposure to budgerigars, *Chest*, *62*, 170 (1972).

20

Measurement and Significance of the Bronchodilator Response: Bronchodilation and Inhibition of Bronchoprovocation

Donald P. Tashkin

UCLA Medical Center
Los Angeles, California

I. INTRODUCTION

Bronchodilator challenges are performed for a variety of reasons. They are often used to assess the presence and degree of reversible airflow obstruction (1) in *individual patients*, to aid in diagnosis and treatment; (2) in participants in single- and multidose *clinical trials*, to evaluate the effectiveness of investigational or established agents alone or in combination; or, less frequently, (3) in *general populations* participating in epidemiological studies, to evaluate the prevalence of airway reactivity to a bronchodilator and its value in predicting the course of obstructive airway disease. They are also commonly performed to monitor the clinical effectiveness of bronchodilator therapy over time in acutely and chronically ill patients with reversible airflow obstruction. The response to a bronchodilator is most often determined by measurement of pulmonary function before and at various times after bronchodilator administration. The efficacy of a bronchodilator may also be judged by its protective effect against bronchospasm provoked by a variety of specific and nonspecific stimuli, its impact on objectively measured exercise performance, or its influence on respiratory symptoms, sleep, and the frequency and severity of episodic bronchospasm.

Several factors influence the response to a bronchodilator measured in terms of either improvement in indices of airway caliber or inhibition of bronchoprovocation, thus potentially confounding interpretation. These factors include (1) baseline airway caliber; (2) the baseline level of bronchial hyperresponsiveness (BHR);

(3) the class of bronchodilator agent being evaluated (β_2-adrenergic, methylxanthine, or anticholinergic); (4) the dose administered; (5) the route of administration and, for the inhaled route, the method of aerosol generation and technique of inhalation; (6) the timing of the test in relation to the peak action of the drug; (7) possible residual effects of previously administered bronchodilator drugs that have not yet "washed out"; (8) the tests used for measuring the response; and (9) effects of long-term bronchodilator therapy (tachyphylaxis, changes in airways responsiveness).

Once the response to a bronchodilator has been measured, it needs to be interpreted. This interpretation is influenced by the factors noted above as well as the intertrial variability of the test, the method of expressing the response in quantitative terms, the question of what constitutes a "significant" response, and the related problem of differentiating between statistically and clinically "significant" responses.

In this chapter we will discuss the methods of evaluating a bronchodilator response, the various factors influencing the response, methods of quantitatively expressing the response, and the interpretation of "significance."

II. METHODS OF EVALUATING BRONCHODILATOR RESPONSE

A. Response Measures

1. Tests of Forced Exhalation—Timed Spirometry and Maximal Expiratory Flow–Volume Curves

Most commonly, the response to a bronchodilator is measured by performing pulmonary function tests before and after bronchodilator administration. A test of forced exhalation is most commonly employed. Following inhalation to total lung capacity (TLC), the subject performs a maximally forced complete exhalation down to residual volume (RV) into a volumetric or flow-sensing spirometer. The spirometer generates a forced expired volume–time curve (spirogram) or maximal expiratory flow–volume (MEFV) curve. From the spirogram, the forced vital capacity (FVC), or total volume expired, and the forced expired volume in 1 second (FEV_1) are determined, and forced expiratory flow (FEF) is calculated over different portions of the curve, such as the middle half ($FEF_{25-75\%}$) (Fig. 1). Vital capacity (VC) can also be determined from a slow (or unforced) complete exhalation from TLC to RV. From the MEFV curve peak expiratory flow is easily determined and FEF (or $\dot{V}max$) is calculated at different instants corresponding to different percentages of the FVC, such as 25%, 50%, and 75% below TLC ($FEF_{25,50 \text{ or } 75\%}$ or $\dot{V}max_{25,\ 50 \text{ or } 75\%}$) (Fig. 2). Peak expiratory flow rate (PEFR) can be read off the peak of the MEFV curve, or it can be determined separately with a simple, portable, hand-held spring-loaded rotary-vane device, or peak flow meter (Wright and McKerrow, 1959). Recommendations have been published for stan-

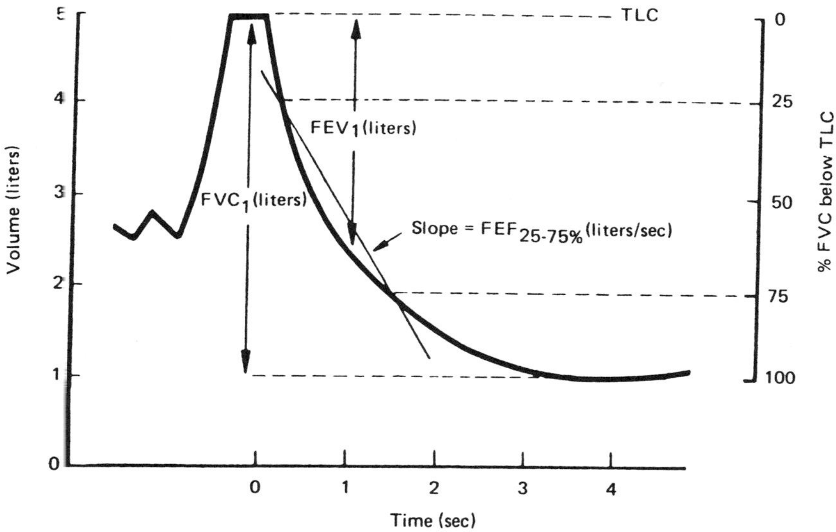

Figure 1 Forced expired volumes and flow rates derived from the forced expiratory volume–time curve. $FEF_{25-75\%}$ is the mean forced expiratory flow over the middle portion of the vital capacity.

dardization of spirometric equipment and testing procedures (American Thoracic Society, 1987). It is crucially important to adhere to these standards in order to achieve accurate and reproducible results that can be reliably compared before and after challenge with a bronchodilator.

2. Partial Flow–Volume Curves

The partial flow–volume technique (Fig. 3) can be used to obviate possible effects of the deep inspiration to TLC just before forced exhalation. The maximal inspiratory maneuver can cause either transient bronchoconstriction (Lloyd, 1963) or bronchodilation (Vincent et al., 1970; Green and Mead, 1974), which will affect FEF ($\dot{V}$max) during the immediately subsequent forced exhalation (see below). A partial flow–volume curve is obtained after a partial, rather than deep, inspiratory maneuver, followed by a maximally forced exhalation to RV; from RV the subject then inhales fully to TLC, from which he performs a maximally forced exhalation to RV. The full inspiratory maneuver establishes TLC as a reference point for calculating $\dot{V}$max from the corresponding partial expiratory flow–volume curve at a fixed percentage of the FVC from TLC.

3. Airway Resistance and Thoracic Gas Volume

The response to a bronchodilator is sometimes assessed by whole-body plethysmographic measurement of changes in airway resistance (Raw) and thoracic gas

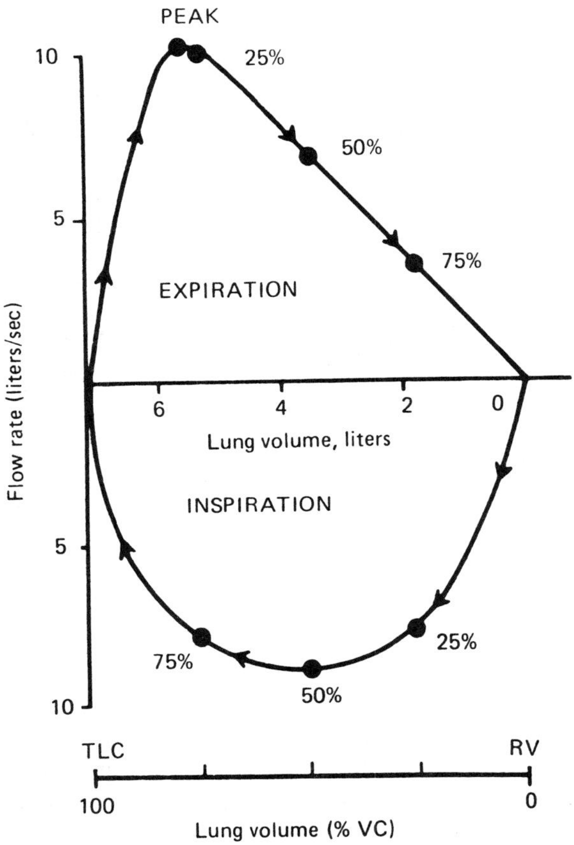

Figure 2 Maximal expiratory and inspiratory flow–volume curves. Instantaneous forced expiratory and inspiratory flow rates can be readily determined at 25%, 50%, and 75% of the expiratory and inspiratory vital capacity, respectively.

volume (Vtg) at functional residual capacity (FRC). The other subdivisions of lung volume (e.g., TLC and RV) can be calculated from plethysmographically determined FRC and measurements derived from an accompanying slow vital capacity maneuver. This technique provides a rapid means of assessing changes in static lung volumes in response to bronchodilator therapy, in contrast to the more time-consuming methods of determining lung volume using inert gas distribution or dilution. Plethysmographic measurements of Raw and FRC are generally carried out with a technique of rapid, shallow panting (2/s), which maximizes the glottic opening, thereby minimizing laryngeal resistance (DuBois et al., 1956a,b), although the tests can also be performed during slow tidal breathing (Miller and

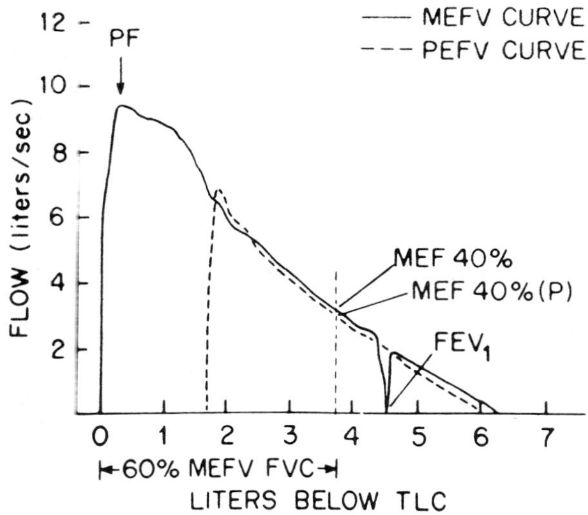

Figure 3 Maximal (solid line) and partial (dashed line) expiratory flow–volume curves. The MEF 40% is the flow rate measured at a lung volume 60% of the forced vital capacity below total lung capacity. From the partial expiratory flow–volume curve, MEF 40% (P) is the flow rate measured at the same lung volume as the MEF 40%. (From Littner et al., 1979.)

Simi, 1976). The tests are performed in a whole-body plethysmograph either of constant volume "pressure" box) (DuBois et al., 1956a,b) or with an attached spirometer or pneumotachygraph at an outlet in the wall of the box ("volume" or "flow" box) (Mead, 1960; Bouhuys, 1969; Leith and Mead, 1974).

Another clinically useful method of measuring resistance to breathing that does not require a body plethysmograph or esophageal balloon catheter uses a modification of the technique of forced oscillation originally described by DuBois et al. (1956c), which estimates total respiratory flow resistance (Rrs). This technique can be used as a practical alternative to body plethysmography to assess the effect of a bronchodilator (or bronchoconstrictor) on flow resistance. Advantages of this technique are that it does not require bulky equipment, causes minimal subject inconvenience (a mouthpiece and nose clip), and requires little subject cooperation.

4. Inhalation Challenges with Bronchoconstrictor Stimuli

Bronchodilator drugs afford variable protection against bronchoconstriction experimentally induced by methacholine, histamine, exercise, eucapnic hyperventilation with cold, dry air, ultrasonically nebulized distilled water, antigen, inflammatory mediators, or other stimuli. Therefore, bronchial inhalation challenge studies can be used to evaluate the effectiveness of different doses of a bronchodilator (compared with placebo or another bronchodilator) in preventing induced bronchospasm. Such studies provide another means of evaluating the response to a bronchodilator for assessing clinical effectiveness and studying the pathophysiology of asthma. The methodology of bronchial challenge procedures has been reviewed elsewhere (Spector, 1989).

5. Respiratory Symptoms

In clinical trials of bronchodilator therapy, various approaches have been used to score respiratory symptoms (daytime and/or nocturnal wheeze, cough, sputum, chest tightness, dyspnea), asthma "attacks" or exacerbations of chronic obstructive pulmonary disease (COPD), nocturnal awakenings due to respiratory symptoms, and use of comedication for as-needed symptomatic relief. An asthma attack or COPD exacerbation may be defined as an acute increase over and above an individual patient's baseline level of symptoms. Symptoms can be scored individually and the score summated, or an overall symptom evaluation can be performed by the patient, using multipoint scales: e.g., 0–3, in which 0 = none (no symptoms), 1 = mild (symptoms present but not bothersome), 2 = moderate (symptoms bothersome and may interfere with some activities), and 3 = severe (symptoms are present at rest and interfere with routine activities). Quality-of-life data can also be assessed with a formal questionnaire, e.g., the IUATLD bronchial symptoms questionnaire (Burney et al., 1989) or the questionnaire developed by Guyatt (1986), or a determination of time lost from work or school or limitation of specific activities because of asthma or COPD. Comedication use can be analyzed by summing the number of doses of an inhaled bronchodilator (e.g., two puffs from a metered-dose inhaler [MDI] = one dose) and equating one dose of a long-acting theophylline preparation to two doses of an inhaled bronchodilator. Symptoms and comedication can be combined to establish whether treatment with a bronchodilator (or placebo) is successful, a failure, or indeterminate, according to the following:

		Comedication		
		↓	→	↑
	↓	Success	Success	Indeterminate
Symptoms	→	Success	No change	Failure
	↑	Indeterminate	Failure	Failure

6. Measures of Exercise Performance

In long-term bronchodilator therapy, a dissociation has been noted between improvement in pulmonary function tests and symptomatic benefit (McGavin et al., 1976, 1978; Alexander et al., 1980; Eaton et al., 1982). A closer parallel has been noted between subjective improvement and better performance on exercise tests such as incremental cycloergometry or the 12-min walk (12MW). A 12MW is performed by instructing patients to walk on level ground (e.g., in a hospital corridor) for a 12-min period at a pace of their own choice. The total distance covered in the 12 min is noted. For more severely disabled subjects, a 6-min walk can be substituted. Subjective reporting of the level of daily physical activities can be related to oxygen consumption by the oxygen-cost diagram. In this diagram, everyday activities are ranked along a 100-mm vertical scale that indicates the oxygen consumption corresponding to any given activity. Patients are asked to mark the line at the point best describing their activity capabilities at the present time. The 12MW and the oxygen-cost diagram can be used as objective or semiquantitative subjective indicators of exercise performance and activity tolerance for assessing the impact of a bronchodilator therapeutic regimen in patients with disabling chronic airflow obstruction due to asthma or chronic bronchitis and emphysema with a reversible component (Alexander et al., 1980).

B. Bronchodilator Administration

For diagnostic evaluation, the bronchodilator usually administered is a β-adrenergic agonist aerosol inhaled via a freon-propelled MDI or a compressed gas–powered Venturi-type nebulizer. The advantages of an inhaled over an oral bronchodilator for routine assessment of acute bronchodilator responsiveness are mainly the faster onset of action, shorter time to peak bronchodilation, and lower incidence of unwanted side effects associated with the inhaled route. Although increasing attention is being paid to anticholinergic compounds, a β-agonist aerosol is still generally preferable for diagnostic purposes because of the shorter interval before maximal bronchodilation, which may be delayed for as long as 60–90 min following inhalation of an anticholinergic aerosol, in contrast to 15–30 min for the most commonly used β-adrenergic aerosols. However, there may be special circumstances in which evaluation of the bronchodilator response specifically to an anticholinergic compound can be useful (see below).

III. FACTORS INFLUENCING THE RESPONSE TO A BRONCHODILATOR

A. Responsiveness of Airway Smooth Muscle

The responsiveness of airway smooth muscle (ASM) is related to the presence and degree of increased smooth muscle tone and the ability of the contracted smooth muscle to relax in response to pharmacological manipulation (stimulation of membrane β-adrenoceptors, inhibition of muscarinic receptors, calcium antagonism). It is the responsiveness of ASM that we are attempting to measure by quantitating the acute response to a bronchodilator, assuming that all other factors influencing bronchodilator effects are controlled. Responsiveness to a *bronchodilator* bears some relation to bronchial responsiveness to nonspecific constrictor stimuli, which is increased in both asthma and COPD (O'Connor et al., 1989), although generally to a lesser degree in the latter (Brand et al., 1991). Nonspecific bronchial hyperresponsiveness (BHR) may be due to a number of factors, including (1) abnormal autonomic control of ASM (increased cholinergic and α-adrenergic responsiveness, decreased β-adrenergic responsiveness) (Szentivanyi, 1968; Tattersfield et al., 1973; Coleridge et al., 1976; Simonsson et al., 1967; Holtzman et al., 1980); (2) increased contractile responsiveness of the smooth muscle itself unrelated to specific pharmacoreceptor activity (Boushey et al., 1980; Kepron et al., 1977; Anthonisen et al., 1980; Souhrada and Dickey, 1976); (3) reduced airway caliber (Yan et al., 1985); (4) increased thickness of the airway wall on either the luminal or the adventitial side of ASM (Moreno et al., 1986); (5) alterations in forces opposing bronchoconstriction ("preload"), e.g., lung elastic recoil, tracheobronchial cartilaginous support (Moreno et al., 1986; Freedman, 1972; Thurlbeck et al., 1974); and (6) bronchial inflammation (Barnes, 1989; Laitinen and Laitinen, 1988). A bronchodilator could relax contracted ASM by counteracting defects in the activity of cell-surface autonomic receptors, in the smooth muscle cell's intrinsic electromechanical contractility, or in other non-receptor-mediated contractile mechanisms.

B. Baseline Airway Caliber

Normal subjects show little improvement in FEV_1 or FVC when given bronchodilators (Watanabe et al., 1974; Lorber et al., 1978; Dales et al., 1988). Asthmatics with no or only mild airflow obstruction at baseline exhibit a greater increase in FEV_1 or FVC than do healthy subjects, but the improvement, if detectable, is generally relatively modest, since they have little room for improvement in these parameters. As their airflow obstruction increases, so does their spirometric response to bronchodilator therapy, reflecting their greater degree of possible functional improvement, in addition to functional geometric factors that amplify the effect on airway resistance of relatively small changes in the caliber of narrowed airways, particularly ones with increased wall thickness (see below). On the other hand, when obstruction becomes severe, response is again diminished, most likely because of factors other than bronchospasm (secretions, edema, inflammation) that are not readily reversible, as well as excessive central deposition of the bronchodilator aerosol with impaired peripheral penetration. Thus, as noted by Hume and Gandevia (1957), the curve relating FEV_1 responses to varying baseline FEV_1 values is bell-shaped, the response being smallest when obstruction is very mild or very severe and greatest when obstruction is moderate.

Similar considerations apply in evaluating the inhibitory effect of a bronchodilator on experimentally induced bronchoconstriction. A significant, although relatively weak, negative correlation has been noted between baseline lung function and bronchial hyperreactivity in both asthma (Hargreave et al., 1981; Greenspon and Morrissey, 1986; Cockcroft et al., 1977; Ryan et al., 1985; Dutoit et al., 1987; Chung et al., 1982) and COPD (Bahous et al., 1985; Yan et al., 1985; Barter and Campbell, 1976; Greenspon and Parrish, 1988; Tashkin et al., 1992), in which BHR has been noted to increase progressively as the percent predicted FEV_1 or FEV_1/FVC ratio declines. Several mechanisms have been proposed to account for this association between BHR and baseline airway caliber. These include (1) well-described geometric principles of aerodynamics (Poisseuille's law), whereby the same absolute degree of ASM contraction in response to a constrictor stimulus causes a disproportionately greater increase in Raw in a narrowed than in a normal-sized airway (Boushey et al., 1980); (2) a decrease in preload on ASM by reduced elastic recoil or cartilaginous softening, lessening the opposition to airway constriction (Moreno et al., 1986); (3) increased baseline tone or contractile strength due to hyperplastic, hypertrophic ASM (Freedman, 1972); and (4) airway wall thickening or secretions that magnify the narrowing of the airway lumen for a given degree of ASM shortening (Moreno et al., 1986; Wiggs et al., 1992). Since baseline airway function correlates somewhat with airway reactivity, the inhibitory effect of a bronchodilator could be due, at least in part, to a change in resting airway caliber. Clearly, however, other mechanisms must account for the protective effect of a bronchodilator against induced bronchoconstriction, since a dissociation between the magnitude of bronchodilation and the degree of inhibition of airway reactivity has frequently been noted (Greenspon and Morrissey, 1986; Chung et al., 1982; Sheppard et al., 1984; Ahrens et al., 1984; Cockcroft and Murdock, 1977; Britton et al., 1988).

C. Baseline Level of Airway Reactivity

In asthmatic subjects, but not in normal subjects, a significant negative correlation between the baseline level of nonspecific airway hyperresponsiveness and inhibition of methacholine-induced bronchoconstriction by isoproterenol has been observed (Greenspon and Morrissey, 1986). A significant negative correlation between airway reactivity and the inhibitory effect of a bronchodilator has also been noted in patients with COPD (Greenspon and Parrish, 1988); in the latter group, however, only those subjects with severe airflow obstruction ($FEV_1 < 50\%$ predicted) demonstrated both hyperresponsiveness to methacholine and protection by isoproterenol. Since hyperresponsiveness to nonspecific bronchoconstrictor agents is a highly characteristic feature of asthma, less prominent in COPD, and encountered only infrequently and to a lesser extent in normal subjects, it is not surprising that the degree of inhibition of inducible bronchoconstriction via a bronchodilator is most striking among asthmatics, less so among chronic bronchitics, and least apparently in healthy subjects (Fig. 4). These observations imply that studies evaluating inhibition of airway reactivity need to take into account the population tested, baseline lung function, and the baseline level of airway reactivity.

D. Type of Bronchodilator(s) Used

The presence and degree of bronchodilator response in any individual patient may depend on the class of bronchodilator used and the mechanism(s) of reversible airflow obstruction in that particular patient. For example, patients with chronic

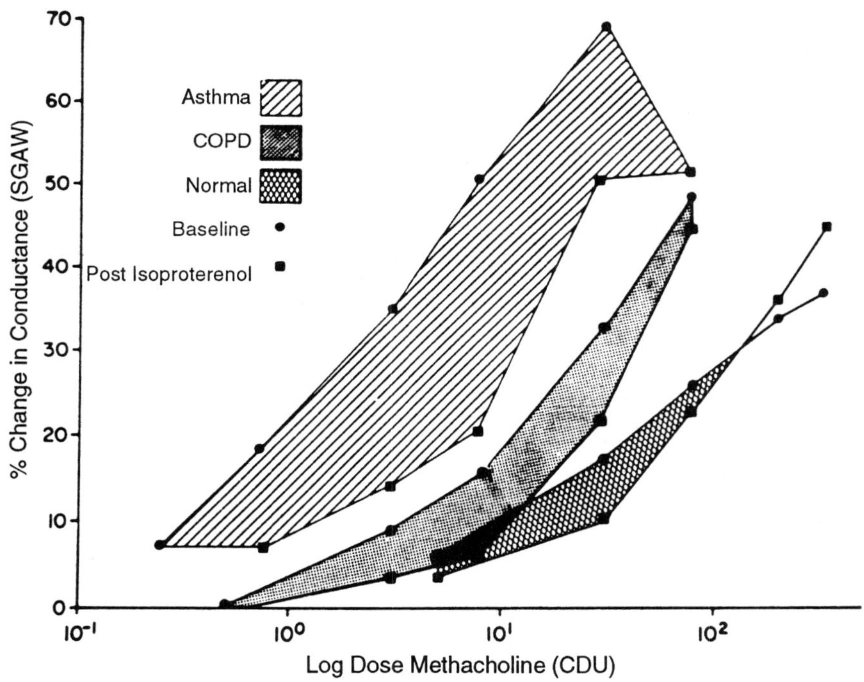

Figure 4 Methacholine dose–response curves for normal subjects, patients with chronic obstructive pulmonary disease (CODP), and asthmatics. Percent change in specific airway conductance is plotted against the cumulative dose units of methacholine inhaled. Closed circles represent baseline studies; closed squares represent studies repeated after isoproterenol. The shaded area represents the shift in the dose–response curve after isoproterenol. Note the greater rightward shift of the mean dose–response curve after isoproterenol compared with the baseline curve in the groups with the greater degree of baseline reactivity (i.e., with the more leftward position of the baseline dose–response curve). (From Greenspon and Parrish, 1988.)

bronchitis generally exhibit a greater magnitude and duration of response to anticholinergic than to β-adrenergic bronchodilators (Tashkin et al., 1986; Braun, 1991), while some respond well to anticholinergic agents but not at all to β-adrenergic agonists (Klock et al,. 1975; Marini and Lakshminarayan, 1980), implying that cholinergic influences may play a more important role than adrenergic factors in the pathophysiology of reversible airflow obstruction in patients with chronic bronchitis. Therefore, inaccurate conclusions could be drawn regarding the presence or absence of a reversible bronchospastic component in such subjects if the bronchomotor response were assessed only in relation to a β-adrenergic agonist. In contrast, asthmatic subjects tend to exhibit a greater peak magnitude of response to a β-agonist than to anticholinergic medication (Bruderman et al., 1983; Elwood and Abboud, 1982; Ruffin et al., 1982), suggesting that in asthma adrenergic influences may be more important pathogenetically than cholinergic mechanisms. On the other hand, some asthmatics who respond poorly to an adrenergic bronchodilator respond well to an anticholinergic, possibly reflecting β-adrenergic tolerance (Burge et al., 1980).

Additive bronchodilation has been noted when bronchodilator compounds of different classes are administered together. For example, in asthmatic patients the combination of theophylline with either an oral (Wolfe et al., 1978) or an inhaled (Smith et al., 1980) β-agonist has been found to produce greater *acute* bronchodilation than that achieved with either agent alone, even when both compounds were administered in high doses (Wolfe et al., 1978). On the other hand, others have failed to observe additive *long-term* benefit of combined therapy with a long-acting oral theophylline preparation and regularly scheduled therapy with an inhaled β-agonist in the management of chronic asthma (Joad, 1987) or short-term benefit when intravenous theophylline was added to a nebulized β-agonist in the treatment of severe acute asthma (Fanta et al., 1986; Littenberg, 1988). In some studies (Casali, 1979; Lees et al., 1980; Leitch et al., 1978; Petrie and Palmer, 1975; Lightbody et al., 1978), but not all (Easton et al., 1985; Lloberes et al., 1988), the combination of anticholinergic and β-adrenergic agents has been shown to produce additive bronchodilation in patients with asthma or chronic bronchitis. For example, in asthmatics, Ullah et al. (1981) found that the addition of either inhaled albuterol or ipratropium after maximal bronchodilation had been produced by the other agent caused a further increase in FEV_1. Douglas and associates (1979) reported similar results in patients with severe bronchitis. These findings suggest that the results of bronchodilator challenge studies employing a single agent, even when administered in maximally effective doses, can underestimate the presence or degree of airway responsiveness.

Different classes of bronchodilators show varying *protective efficacy* against different bronchospastic stimuli, as indicated in Table 1 for inhaled β-agonist and anticholinergic drugs. Moreover, Cockcroft et al. (1977) have shown that in comparable therapeutic doses, inhaled β-agonists are more effective inhibitors of

Table 1 Summary of Comparative Efficacy of Anticholinergic and β-Adrenergic Bronchodilators Against Different Bronchospastic Stimuli

Stimulus	Efficacy of anticholinergic agents	Efficacy of adrenergic agents relative to anticholinergic agents
Cholinergic agents	Fully protective	
Histamine	Partially protective at most	More effective
Various mediators, $PGF_{2\alpha}$, serotonin, bradykinin	Partially protective at most	
Beta-blockade	Effective reversal	Much less effective
Gases, dust, irritants	Variable, usually some protection	
Antigens	Variable, from none to excellent	More effective
Exercise, hyperventilation, cold air	Moderately effectively, possibly more so in large doses	Invariably more effective
Psychogenic factors	Good protection	Probably less effective

Source: Gross and Skorodin, 1984.

histamine-induced bronchoconstriction (12-fold increase in PC_{20} or 3.5 doubling doses) than inhaled anticholinergic agents, theophylline, or β-agonists administered in oral form (2.1- to 2.8-fold increases in PC_{20} or 1–1.5 doubling doses) (Fig. 5). In addition, aerosolized β-agonists afford better protection than anticholinergic bronchodilators against the early phase of antigen-induced bronchospasm (Gross and Skorodin, 1984), as well as against exercise-induced asthma (Tashkin et al., 1977; Borut et al., 1977), while the inhibitory effect of theophylline against these bronchoprovocative stimuli has generally been found to be relatively weak (Ellis, 1984; Pauwels et al., 1985), although not insignificant (Crescioli et al., 1988; Magnussen et al., 1988). In contrast, β-agonists of intermediate duration of action (3–6 h) do not appear to have a significant inhibitory influence on the late response to antigen when inhaled before challenge (Cockcroft and Murdock, 1987), whereas theophylline (Dutoit et al., 1987) and ultra-long-acting inhaled β-agonists (e.g., salmeterol and formoterol) (Twentyman et al., 1990a,b; Wong et al., 1992) do exert a protective effect. This protective effect is believed to be due to functional antagonism of the action of late-phase mediators of bronchoconstriction (Wong et al., 1992) (Fig. 6), rather than prevention of the inflammatory changes responsible for the late-phase reaction. β-agonist and anticholinergic aerosols have comparable effectiveness against methacholine-induced bronchospasm (Gross and Skorodin, 1984), while oral bronchodilators (β-agonist, theophylline) generally cause less inhibition

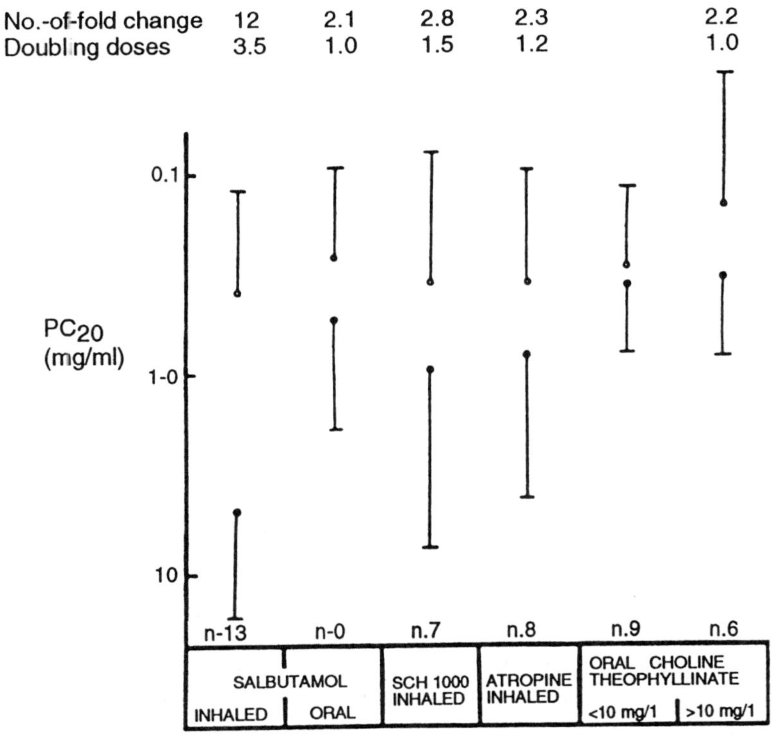

Figure 5 Geometric mean PD_{20} FEV_1 (mg/ml) for histamine with and without pretreatment with various inhaled or oral bronchodilators. Open circles represent control values, closed circles represent values after administration of noted drugs, and vertical bars represent 1 geometric standard deviation. The degree of protection afforded by each bronchodilator against induced bronchospasm is indicated at the top of the figure by the no.-of-fold change or the number of doubling doses of histamine required to produce a 20% decline in FEV_1 after administration of the bronchodilator as compared with the control condition. (Adapted from Cockcroft et al., 1977.)

(Cockcroft and Murdock, 1977; Spector, 1978; Decotiis et al., 1980; McWilliams et al., 1984; Magnussen et al., 1987). The marked differences in degree of inhibition of bronchial reactivity by different classes of bronchodilators (and different routes of administration of the same bronchodilator) contrast with the frequent similarity in the magnitude of bronchodilation produced by these agents. These contrasting effects on airway dilation and reactivity suggest different mechanisms by which bronchodilators antagonize spontaneous and induced bronchoconstriction and underscore the importance of factors other than change in airway caliber as determinants of the inhibitory action of a bronchodilator on reactivity.

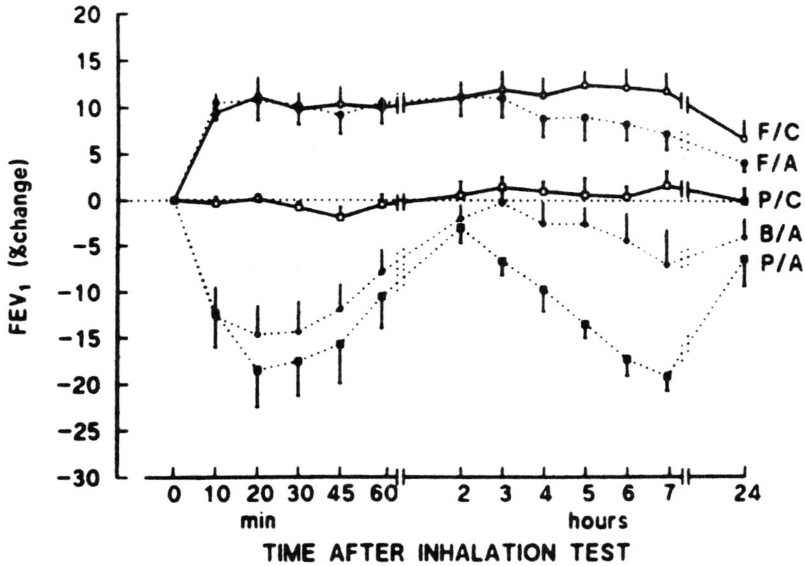

Figure 6 Mean ± SEM changes in FEV_1 from baseline (%) after control (C) or allergen (A) inhalation preceded by placebo (P), formoterol (F), or beclomethasone (B). Formoterol caused bronchodilation and inhibited the late asthmatic response. This inhibition, however, is likely due, at least partly, to functional antagonism, since FEV_1 values 3–24 h after antigen challenge preceded by formoterol (F/A) are significantly lower than those after formoterol followed by placebo challenge (F/C). (From Wong et al., *Am Rev Respir Dis* 1992.)

E. Doses of the Bronchodilator Administered

The bronchodilator response to a pharmacological agent is dependent on the dose given, the relationship between ASM relaxation and dose (or serum concentration) being log linear (Nelson et al., 1983; Mitenko and Ogilvie, 1973). The dose chosen for clinical purposes is generally adjusted to produce maximal bronchodilation and minimal unwanted physiological effects and varies with the route of administration (see below). While the inhaled route is generally preferred for β-adrenergic and anticholinergic bronchodilators, there is disagreement as to the optimal dose of these agents (Nelson et al., 1983; Gross, 1975; Wood and Paterson, 1975; Simonsson et al., 1975; Kamburoff and Gunther, 1975; Ferguson and Cherniak, 1993). For MDIs, two inhalations are commonly administered as a standard "dose" both for therapy and for formal measurement of bronchodilator response. This practice is supported by the results of several investigators who have failed to demonstrate progressively greater bronchodilation with higher metered doses of either a β-agonist (Alliott et al., 1972; Ruffin et al., 1978; Heimer et al., 1980; Williams and Kane, 1975) or ipratropium, an anticholinergic bronchodilator (Gross, 1975; Yeager et al., 1976; Storms et al., 1975; Baigelman and Chodosh, 1977; Newcomb et al., 1985). On the other hand, others (Nelson et al., 1983) have shown a linear relationship between the increase in FEV_1 and the log dose of albuterol delivered via MDI in doses of from one to eight inhalations; the response to four to six inhalations was significantly greater than that of one inhalation ($p < 0.05$), and that to eight inhalations was significantly greater than the response to one or two inhalations ($p < 0.01$) (Fig. 7). For ipratropium

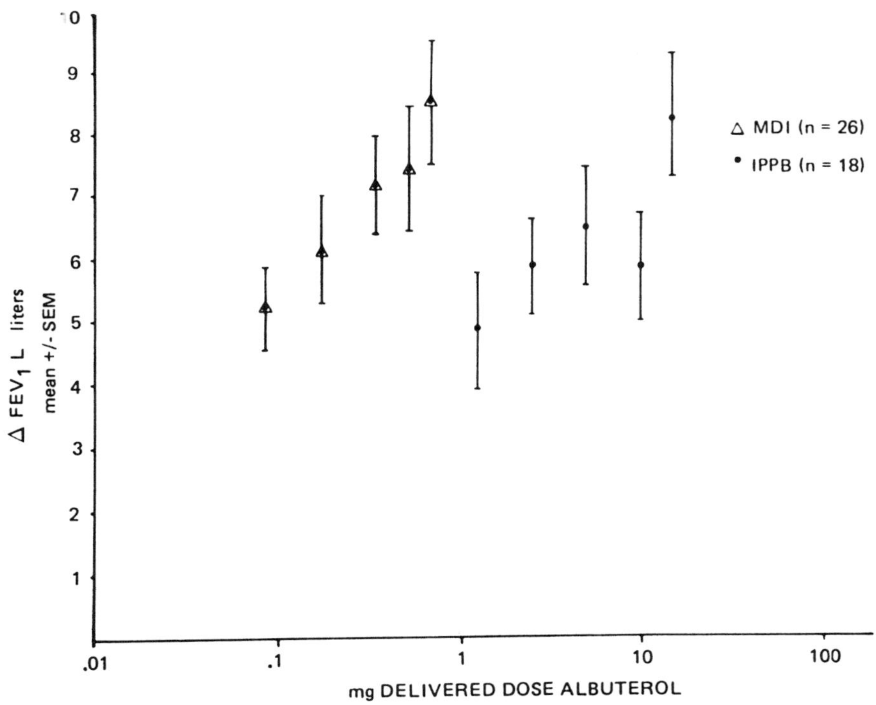

Figure 7 Maximum increases in FEV_1 are plotted against an aerosolized dose of albuterol by metered dose inhaler (MDI) (26 patients) and intermittent positive-pressure breathing (IPPB) (18 patients). The correlation by each mode of administration between the log of the dose of albuterol and absolute improvement in FEV_1 is significant. The response to the highest three doses by MDI is significantly greater than that to the lowest dose ($p < 0.05$), whereas the response to the highest dose by IPPB is significantly greater than that to any other dose ($p < 0.05$) (Note: the "delivered dose" from IPPB was the dose placed in the nebulizer.) (From Nelson et al., 1983.)

delivered by MDI, some authors have demonstrated increasing bronchodilation up to a dose of 60–80 μg (three or four puffs) (Wood and Paterson, 1975; Newcomb et al., 1985; Millar et al., 1990). Nelson et al. (1983) showed that, in *stable asthmatics*, the response to 15 mg of isoproterenol administered by intermittent positive-pressure breathing (IPPB) exceeded that to a standard therapeutic dose of isoproterenol of 1.25 mg ($p < 0.01$), as well as that to 2.5, 5, and 10 mg ($p < 0.05$) also administered by IPPB. These findings suggest, particularly for inhaled β-agonists, that the customarily administered "therapeutic dose" of two inhalations from an MDI or 1.25 mg isoproterenol (or the equivalent of other β-agonist solutions) via a compressed gas–driven nebulizer may elicit less than a maximally attainable bronchodilator response and thus may underestimate the presence or degree of bronchodilator responsiveness. Dose requirements for inhaled bronchodilators in *severe acute asthma* are generally considerably higher than for stable asthma because of increased central deposition of the aerosolized drug at sites of exaggerated narrowing, with impaired delivery to peripheral airways, and because of greater requirements for functional antagonism of the action of increased levels of inflammatory mediators (Tashkin, 1991).

Several studies show a relationship between bronchodilator dose and the degree of inhibition of reactivity. For example, Britton et al. (1988) found that doubling doses for PD_{20} FEV_1 histamine increased nearly linearly to a maximum of 2.87 in proportion to an exponential increase in the dose of inhaled albuterol from 5 to 1000 μg (Fig. 8). Moreover, Sheppard et al. (1984) noted that while an eightfold

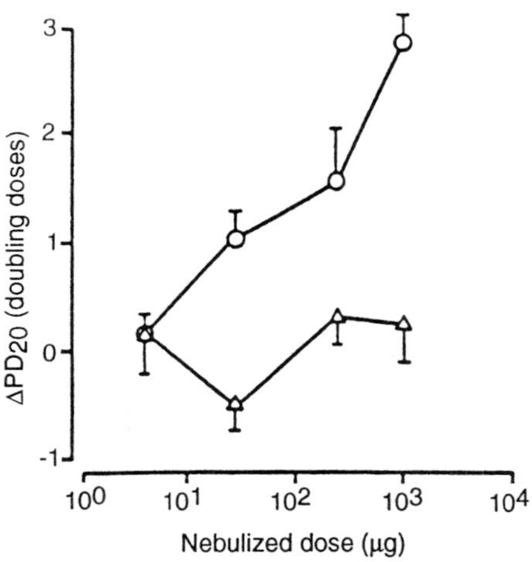

Figure 8 Change in histamine PD_{20} FEV_1 (expressed as doubling doses) with increasing dose (in μg) of albuterol (open circles) and ipratropium (triangles) in six mild asthmatics. (From Britton et al., 1988.)

increase in the dose of nebulized atropine sulfate (from 0.26 to 2.08 mg) had little impact on the degree of bronchodilation, it doubled the protection against methacholine-induced bronchoconstriction from approximately 1.25 to 2.5 doubling doses. Magnussen et al. (1987, 1988) observed dose-related effects of theophylline on airway responses to inhaled histamine and methacholine, as well as on protection against bronchoconstriction induced by exercise during cold-air breathing. These observations imply that bronchodilator dose must be taken into account in comparisons of the inhibitory effects of different bronchodilators on airway reactivity, and that the dose producing maximum bronchodilation is not necessarily equivalent to the dose required for maximum protection against induced bronchoconstriction.

F. Route of Administration

The onset, magnitude, and duration of bronchodilation or protection against induced bronchospasm are influenced by the route of bronchodilator administration and, for inhaled agents, by the method of drug delivery.

1. Aerosol Route

β-Adrenergic agonists and anticholinergic bronchodilators are most commonly administered as aerosols. The effectiveness of these aerosols in reducing bronchomotor tone is dependent on the actual dose of the drug delivered to the lung, the site(s) of deposition within the lung (tracheobronchial, alveolar), and the degree of dispersion throughout the surface of the lower airways. These factors, in turn, are influenced by the following: (1) the aerodynamic properties of the nebulized particles, which are determined, in part, by the type of aerosol delivery device, its output characteristics, and the method used to operate the device (Newman, 1991); (2) the pattern of inhalation of the aerosol, including the inspiratory flow rate, lung volume over which the aerosol is inhaled, and breath-holding time at end-inspiration; (3) the geometry of the airways; and (4) the time sequence of aerosol administration.

Bronchodilator aerosols are most often generated by either cartridge-type MDIs containing freon propellants or jet-type nebulizers powered by compressed air (motor-driven compressor or IPPB device) (Newman, 1991). With the impending ban on chlorofluorocarbon production, future devices for delivery of these aerosols will probably consist of either MDIs with alternative propellants (e.g., hydrofluoroalkanes) or breath-activated finely micronized dry powder inhalers. Aerosols generated by currently used devices are polydispersed through a broad range of particle sizes, the larger particles (> 10 μm) being trapped in the jet-type nebulizer or the actuator of the MDI. Only about 10% of the solution aerosolized by the jet-type device ever leaves the nebulizer, as opposed to approximately 85% of the aerosol generated by an MDI. Consequently, the dose of a β-agonist that must be added to a "wet" nebulizer can be as much as 10 times the metered-dose output of an MDI producing an equivalent degree of bronchodilation (Nelson et al., 1983) (Fig. 8). Depending on the method of aerosol generation and delivery, the dose efficiency ratio for producing similar degrees of bronchodilation via an MDI vs. a solution nebulizer has varied quite widely, from approximately 2:1 to 12:1 (Lewis, 1984).

Aerosol particles deposit in the respiratory tract by three mechanisms: inertial impaction, gravitational sedimentation, and brownian diffusion. Most particles > 5–10 μm are deposited by inertial impaction in the upper airway, where the linear velocities of flow are highest, whereas particles 0.5–1 μm in size are mostly deposited by gravitational sedimentation and brownian diffusion in peripheral airways, where flow velocities are low. The breathing pattern also influences the site of deposition of an inhaled aerosol. A rapid breathing pattern with a high inspiratory flow rate favors deposition by impaction in the upper and central airways, whereas lower inspiratory flow rates and longer transit times through any segment of the airway favor deposition by gravitational sedimentation at more peripheral sites within the lung (Landahl et al., 1951). A longer breath-hold at end-inspiration also favors greater retention of very small particles in the lung by allowing more time for flow velocities to diminish sufficiently for such particles to settle out by gravity, thus reducing loss of inhaled particles in the exhaled air. Using submicronic aerosols labeled with ^{99m}Tc and comparable aerodynamically to bronchodilator aerosols generated by MDIs, Newman and co-workers (1982) found that a larger fraction of the particles (14%) deposited in the lung when patients with asthma or bronchitis inhaled the aerosol at low inspiratory flow rates (0.5 L/s) with a long breath-holding time (10 s) than when inhaled flow rates were faster (1.33–1.5 L/s) or breath-holding time was shorter (4 s). Each of the latter breathing patterns effectively halved the bronchial deposition rate to 7% (Fig. 9). For all breathing patterns, > 70% of the aerosol was deposited in the oropharynx.

A number of subjects have evaluated the possible advantages of extension-tube or aerosol-chamber attachments to MDIs in enhancing particle deposition in the lungs and improving the efficacy of bronchodilator aerosols (Morgan et al., 1982; Fuglsang et al., 1986; Gervais and Begin, 1987; Turner et al., 1988). Theoretically, these attachment devices should improve aerosol delivery to the lung by allowing a longer time and distance before the aerosol reaches the mouth for the aerosol velocity to slow and particle size to diminish by evaporation. The slower velocity and smaller particle size of the aerosol entering the mouth should lessen the likelihood of inertial impaction on the oropharynx and favor penetration into the lower respiratory tract. Using radiolabeled particles, Newman et al. (1981) demonstrated that extension devices (10-cm cylindrical tube, 22-cm cone) do increase deposition in the lung while decreasing deposition in the oropharynx because, in part, of trapping of larger particles in the device. However, greater aerosol penetration of the lung with use of spacer attachments may not necessarily translate into superior bronchodilation. The results of several studies in asthmatics

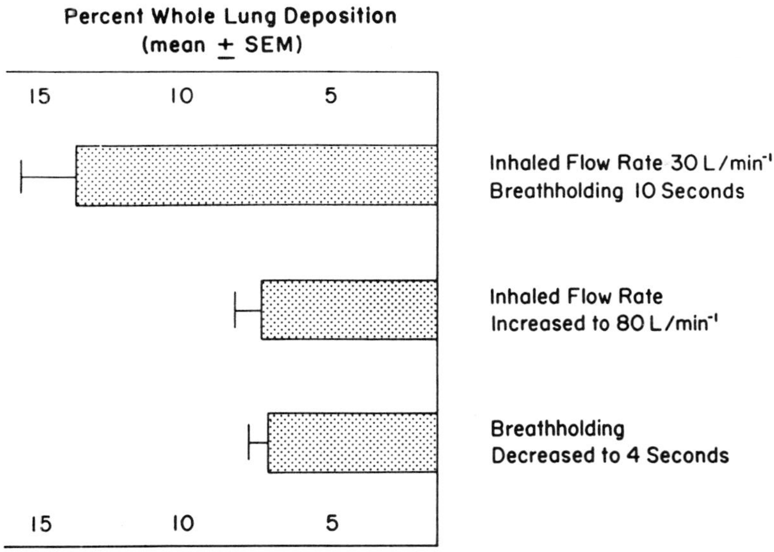

Figure 9 Effect of inhalation mode on the deposition of a pressurized suspension aerosol in the lungs. A mean 14% of the dose reached the lung when the aerosol was inhaled slowly (30 L/min) followed by 10-s breath holding. Deposition was reduced when the inhaled flow rate was increased to 80/L/min, or when breath holding was reduced to 4 s. (From Newman et al., 1982.)

with mild to marked airflow obstruction do not demonstrate consistently significant differences in magnitude or duration of bronchodilation when MDIs with and without spacer attachments were compared (Lindgren et al., 1980; Bloomfield et al., 1979; Godden and Crompton, 1981; Spicer et al., 1980; Poppius, 1980; Gomm et al., 1980; Dolovich et al., 1983). Nonetheless, one of the advantages of an extension tube or aerosol reservoir attached to an MDI is to compensate partially for an uncoordinated technique of MDI use, leading to improved aerosol delivery and bronchodilation in some subjects.

With respect to the relative efficacy of different methods of bronchodilator aerosol generation (MDI, compressor-driven nebulizer, IPPB), no difference has been noted in the effectiveness of inhaled β-adrenergic bronchodilators delivered via an MDI with an aerochamber extender (Monaghan) or an expandable bag reservoir (Inspirease) versus a hand-held compressed gas–driven nebulizer in patients treated in the hospital or emergency room for acute bronchospastic disease (Berenberg et al., 1985; Turner et al., 1988; Idriss et al., 1993). Other studies have failed to demonstrate any differences in the effectiveness of aerosolized bronchodilators delivered by continuous pressure–driven nebulizers and

IPPB (Loren et al., 1977; Smelzer and Barnett, 1973; Chang and Levison, 1972; Intermittent Positive Pressure Breathing Trial Group, 1983). Blake et al. (1992) compared the relative effects of albuterol delivered by an MDI attached to an Inspirease device and by an updraft nebulizer on the provocative concentration of histamine required to produce a 20% fall in FEV_1 as a bioassay method for assessing the relative amounts of the aerosolized bronchodilator delivered to the lung by these two methods. They estimated that ten puffs from the MDI (0.9 mg) delivered about the same amount of albuterol to the lung as 2.5 mg of the nebulizer solution.

The predominant site of deposition of nebulized particles is also dependent on the geometry of the airways. In the normal tracheobronchial tree, small-size aerosols (< 2 μm) inhaled during slow breathing deposit mainly in the small nonciliated airways in the lung periphery (Taplin et al., 1977). On the other hand, under pathological conditions in which bronchospasm, inflammation, and increased secretions cause irregular narrowing of the larger airways, even submicronic aerosols can deposit preferentially at these sites of narrowing in the central airways, with reduced peripheral penetration (Taplin et al., 1977; Stuart, 1973). Theoretically, the preferred sites of deposition of a bronchodilator aerosol are those airways that are most narrowed by bronchospasm and thus are probably most responsive to the bronchodilator action of the locally deposited drug. On the other hand, deposition of the aerosol at sites of narrowing due to excessive retained mucus may not lead to any beneficial action in these areas while retarding penetration of the drug to more peripheral airways that may be narrowed by bronchospasm. While excessive central deposition of submicronic aerosols has been noted in patients with obstructive airway disease, nonetheless sufficient peripheral penetration of bronchodilator aerosols does occur in patients with bronchospastic disease to cause dilation of smaller airways (Ingram et al., 1977a,b; Fairshter and Wilson, 1980; Pierce et al., 1981).

The response to inhalation of a bronchodilator from an MDI is also influenced by the sequential timing of the inhalations. Heimer et al. (1980) showed that three puffs from a metaproterenol MDI (0.6 mg per puff) inhaled in rapid sequence were significantly less effective than the same three puffs inhaled in a sequence of one puff every 10 min. These findings may result from greater penetration of the more slowly sequenced aerosol into airways already partially dilated by each previous inhalation of the aerosol, which has had sufficient time to peak or near-peak levels of bronchodilation before the next dose. These findings imply that in cumulative dose–response studies of aerosolized bronchodilators, effects that some have attributed to higher cumulative doses of the drug (Nelson et al., 1983) may be due, instead or in part, to the sequential method of administering the drug. The benefits of delaying the second (or third) puff of a metered-dose bronchodilator to achieve greater overall bronchodilation must be weighed against the inconvenience of these delays and the possibility of forgetting to take the subsequent puff(s), causing reduced effectiveness.

In the management of *severe acute asthma* in children, after an initial treatment with nebulized albuterol 0.15 mg/kg (maximum dose 5 mg), Robertson et al. (1985) compared the efficacy of this same dose of nebulized albuterol administered at hourly intervals with divided doses of albuterol (0.05 mg/kg, maximum dose 1.7 mg) administered every 20 min for a total of 2½ h. These authors found (Fig. 10) a smooth, progressive improvement in FEV_1 in the group treated at 20-min intervals, in contrast to deterioration before the next scheduled dose in the group treated at hourly intervals and a diminished overall response to the dose administered hourly. They attributed the superior results with the regimen of more

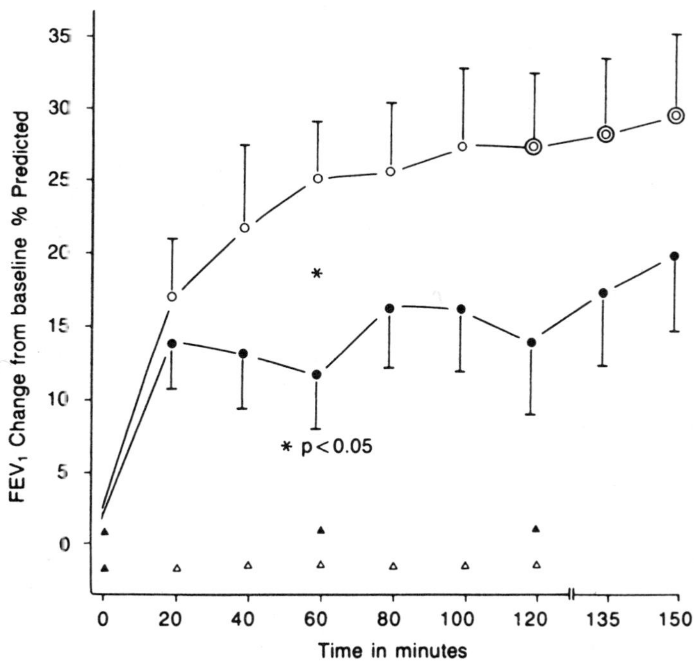

Figure 10 Change in percent predicted FEV_1 from baseline at 20-min intervals in pediatric patients with acute severe asthma receiving nebulized albuterol (○ = 0.05 mg/kg every 20 min; ● = 0.15 mg/kg every hour). Following the first dose of medication, note the greater and more sustained improvement in FEV_1 in the patients receiving nebulized albuterol every 20 min, in contrast to the tendency for the improvement to diminish between successive doses in the group receiving nebulized treatments every hour. (From Robertson et al., 1985.)

frequently administered aerosol treatments to the following: Because the duration of bronchodilator response in severe acute asthma is frequently very short, airflow obstruction is more likely to worsen before the next scheduled nebulizer treatment in the hourly than in the thrice-hourly regimen. As a result, the response to the hourly treatments is likely to be less successful because of poorer peripheral penetration of the aerosolized medication into airways that had been permitted to narrow before the next scheduled treatment. These findings indicate that small frequent doses of an aerosolized β-agonist can have a greater overall therapeutic effect in acute severe asthma than larger, less frequently administered doses.

2. Oral Route

Oral bronchodilators include methylxanthines and β-adrenergic stimulants. In comparison with topically administered β-adrenergic aerosols, especially those generated by MDIs, the oral β-agonists (which are delivered to airway smooth muscle indirectly via the circulation) must be given in much larger doses to achieve a comparable peak bronchodilator effect. The aerosol and oral routes also differ with respect to the time of onset and peak magnitude of bronchodilation. The onset of bronchodilation is generally rapid (from less than 1 to 5 min) following most β-agonist aerosols, slightly slower after anticholinergic aerosols, such as ipratropium, and slower still (approximately 30 min) after ingestion of an oral β-agonist, because of delay in gastrointestinal absorption. Oral methylxanthines have a variable onset of action that depends on the absorption and release characteristics of the preparation, being most rapid (15–30 min) for hydroalcoholic solutions, other liquid preparations, and fast-acting tablet formulations and slowest (1–2 h) for slow-release preparations. Furthermore, food may slow the absorption of all oral bronchodilators. *Peak* bronchodilation also begins sooner after a β-agonist aerosol (approximately 5–30 min) than after an anticholinergic agent (> 60 min), an oral β-agonist (2–4 hours), or methylxanthine (2 h, 4–6h, and 8–12 h after short-, intermediate-, and long-acting preparations, respectively).

Duration of action is highly variable, irrespective of the route of bronchodilator administration. The duration of action of the catecholamine aerosols (epinephrine, isoproterenol, and isoethrine; 1–3 h) is shorter than that of the newer noncatecholamine β-agonist aerosols (metaproterenol, albuterol, terbutaline, bitolterol, fenoterol, and pirbuterol; 4–6 h). The duration of effectiveness of oral preparations of the latter compounds is comparable to their duration of action when they are given by inhalation. Recently, highly lipophilic, ultra-long-acting β-agonist aerosols (salmeterol and formoterol) with a duration of action of ⩾ 12 h have become available (Ullman and Svedmyr, 1988; Maesens, 1990). The length of action of theophylline compounds is quite variable and is a function not only of the absorption and release characteristics of the compound but also of metabolic clearance and the achievement of a "relatively steady" plasma concentration with multiple dosing following initiation of therapy. Bronchodilation lasts about 4–6 h after shorter-acting theophylline compounds and approximately 8–24 h following longer-acting sustained-release preparations.

Inhaled β-agonists afford essentially complete protection against exercise-induced bronchospasm, while the same compounds administered orally in equivalent bronchodilator doses have only a negligible protective effect (Anderson et al., 1976; Konig et al., 1981). Similarly, inhaled β-adrenergic stimulants are far more effective than the oral formulations against histamine- and methacholine-induced bronchoconstriction (Cockcroft et al., 1977; Salome et al., 1981) (Fig. 11). These differences between the protective effects of the aerosol and oral forms of a

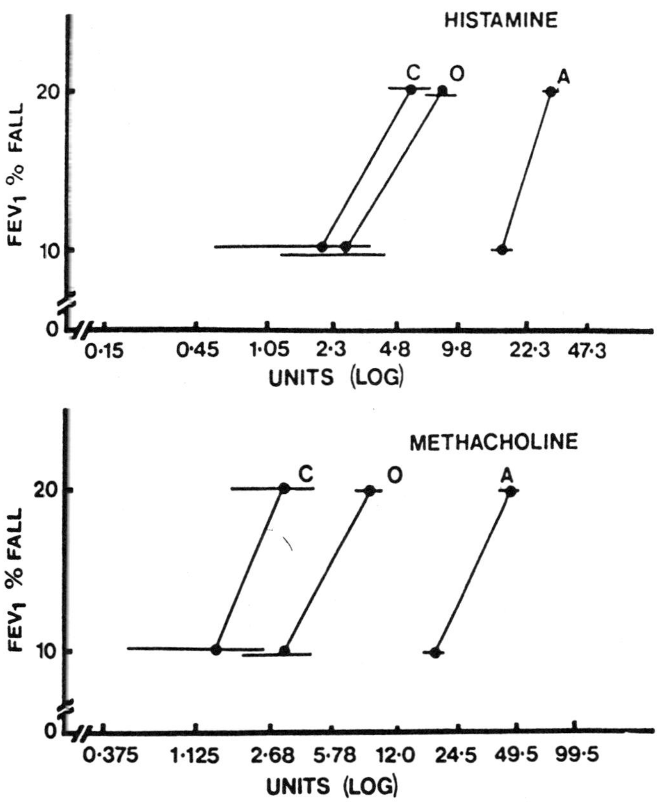

Figure 11 Mean geometric PD_{10} FEV_1 and PD_{20} FEV_1 (± standard error) during histamine and methacholine challenge in atopic asthmatics under control conditions (challenge alone), 90 min after pretreatment with 5 mg oral fenoterol (O) or 15 min after 400 μg aerosol fenoterol (A). (From Salome et al., 1981.)

β-agonist could reflect differences in local concentrations of the drug delivered either to airway smooth muscle in central vs. peripheral sites in the respiratory tract or to the epithelial surface of the airway, where protective action may be more critical because of effects on a number of surface structures (afferent nerve endings, epithelial cells, intraepithelial junctions, intraepithelial inflammatory cells, etc.) that may mediate bronchial hyperresponsiveness.

3. Subcutaneous and Intravenous Routes

Bronchodilators are sometimes given subcutaneously (epinephrine, terbutaline) or by slow intravenous infusion (aminophylline, albuterol, terbutaline, isoproterenol) to patients with severe asthma whose response to inhaled drugs is unsatisfactory. In these patients, the parenteral route may have the advantage of delivering the bronchodilator via the systemic circulation to sites in the airways distal to occlusive plugs and thus inaccessible to the aerosol. Despite this theoretical advantage, most studies comparing β-agonists given parenterally with large doses of the same agents administered by inhalation in severe acute asthma fail to demonstrate a clear-cut advantage of the parenteral route, as reviewed by Jenne and Tashkin (1993).

G. Timing of the Test in Relation to the Peak Action of the Drug

Bronchodilator responsiveness is often assessed by performing measurements at only one time following administration of a bronchodilator rather than attempting to characterize the entire time course of the response. In the former circumstance, it is necessary to perform the postbronchodilator measurements at or close to the expected time of peak action; otherwise, the degree of responsiveness may be underestimated or its presence masked. In view of the longer delay before the appearance of peak bronchodilation after inhalation of some of the longer-acting β-agonist aerosols (as long as 30–45 min) in comparison with isoproterenol (about 5 min), the common practice of waiting only 5 min following inhalation of the aerosol before performance of the postbronchodilator measurement could lead to false conclusions concerning true bronchodilator responsiveness. Similarly, the even longer time lag before peak bronchodilation after inhaled anticholinergic medication ($\geq$60 min) requires a correspondingly longer delay in the postbronchodilator measurement for accurate assessment of response to this class of bronchodilators.

Ahrens and coworkers (1984) have shown a dichotomy between the *duration* of bronchodilation and that of inhibition of airway responsiveness to methacholine following administration of an aerosolized bronchodilator in asthmatic subjects. While inhaled metaproterenol produced persistent bronchodilation for 4 h, its inhibiting effect on airway responsiveness decreased by 50% 2.25 h after dosing (compared with the degree of inhibition at 0.75 h) and had disappeared by 4 h. Comparable findings were noted by Salome et al. (1983) with aerosolized fenoterol, which produced a maximal increase in histamine PD_{20} at 0.25–1 h, followed by a progressive decline in PD_{20} to the initial control value over the ensuing 4 h (Fig. 12), despite little change in FEV_1 over the same period. A similar diminution in the protective effect of a β-agonist aerosol against exercise-induced bronchospasm over a period of 4 h has been noted despite persistent bronchodila-

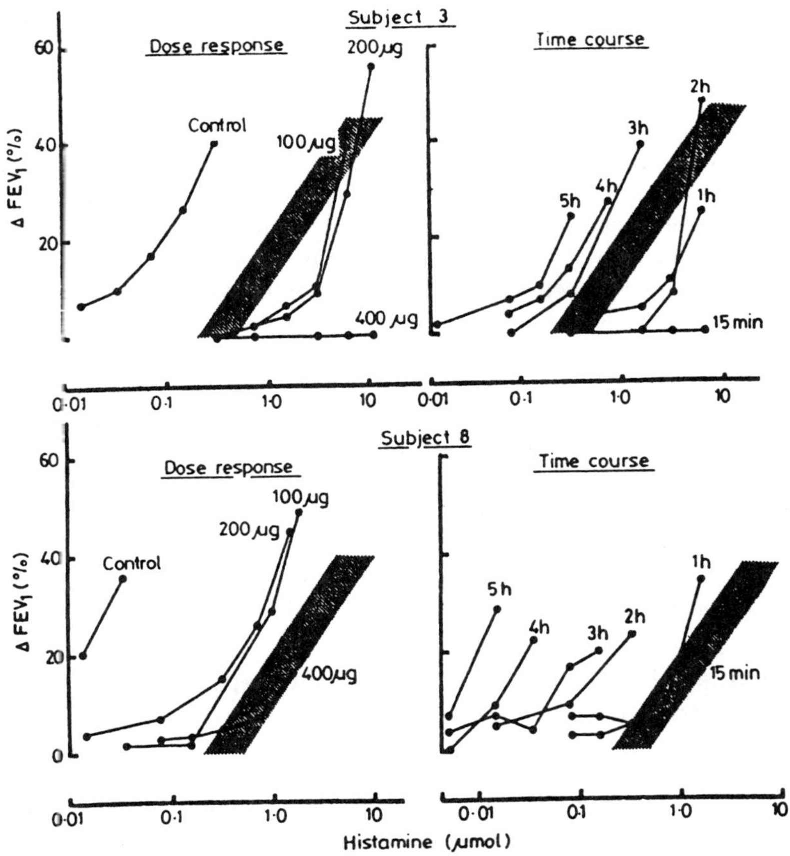

Figure 12 Histamine dose–response curves in two asthmatic subjects under control conditions (histamine challenge only) and 15 min following pretreatment with different doses of aerosolized fenoterol (left-hand panel) and at hourly intervals after 400 µg fenoterol (right-hand panel). Note the progressive leftward shift of the histamine dose–response curve toward the control level of reactivity from 1 to 5 h after administration of the highest dose of fenoterol. (From Salome et al., 1983.)

tion (Konig et al., 1984). These differences in the time course between bronchodilation and inhibition of induced bronchospasm could reflect differences in the mechanism for these two β_2-adrenergic actions. Alternatively, Ahrens and coworkers (1984) have suggested that this dichotomy could be due to differences in the potency of the bronchoconstrictor stimulus involved. Bronchodilation may involve counteracting a relatively mild bronchoconstrictive stimulus responsible for the baseline or spontaneous level of airflow obstruction, while inhibition of bronchoconstriction may require a substantially greater action to counteract a more potent constrictor stimulus that induces additional bronchoconstriction over and above the bronchospasm that was present spontaneously. Thus, a larger concentration of a β-agonist may be required to oppose the latter type of stimulus as compared with the relatively modest level of bronchospasm present at baseline. The administered dose of a β-agonist aerosol may readily exceed that required for maximal inhibition of the spontaneous level of bronchospasm. Therefore, a diminution in the retained dose of bronchodilator over time may not affect the degree of bronchodilation but would result in progressively reduced effectiveness in counteracting the more potent bronchoconstriction induced by the provocative challenge. The relatively short duration of protection afforded by inhaled β-agonists against histamine-, methacholine-, and exercise-induced bronchospasm in relation to their more prolonged bronchodilator action has important implications for asthma management. Current dosing recommendations for inhaled β-agonists, which are based on their duration of bronchodilation, may have to be revised if the aim of therapy is not only to reverse existing bronchospasm but also to protect against naturally occurring bronchoprovocative stimuli. On the other hand, newer aerosolized β-agonists with high lipophilicity and exceptionally tenacious binding to the β-adrenoceptor in the ASM cell membrane (salmeterol, formoterol) appear to provide a particularly long duration of protection against nonspecifically induced bronchospasm ($\geqslant$ 12 h) that is comparable to their exceptionally long duration of bronchodilation (Becker and Simons, 1989; Twentyman et al., 1990).

H. Residual Effects of Previously Administered Bronchodilators

If some residual bronchodilation from previous bronchodilator administration is present at baseline, the measured acute response to an administered bronchodilator is likely to underestimate the magnitude of possible response, since the airways are already partially bronchodilated. For patients receiving oral and/or inhaled β-agonists, a wash-out period of approximately 8–12 h may be sufficient before a diagnostic bronchodilator challenge to avoid the confounding influence of residual drug-related bronchodilation. A longer washout period of 18–24 h is needed after the last dose of salmeterol or formoterol, while a 24 to 48 h washout is required for serum theophylline levels to decline to subtherapeutic levels following the last dose of a twice- or once-daily theophylline preparation, respectively. Care must also be taken to avoid consumption of caffeine-containing beverages within several hours before testing to avoid confounding by caffeine-related bronchodilation (Gong et al., 1986).

I. Residual Effects of Previous Bronchial Challenges

Repeated bronchial challenges are sometimes performed to evaluate the inhibitory effect of a bronchodilator in comparison with placebo, another bronchodilator, or the same bronchodilator in different doses. Short- or long-term effects of previous challenges on subsequent bronchial reactivity could confound the interpretation of such studies. For example, exercise-induced bronchospasm is followed by a refractory period lasting up to 2–3 h during which the bronchoconstrictor response to repeated exercise is blunted (McNeill et al., 1966; Edmunds et al., 1978). Similar refractoriness following analogous challenges, including eucapnic hyperventilation with cold air (Bar-Yishay et al., 1983) and ultrasonically nebulized distilled water (Anderson et al., 1983), has been reported. Some workers (Magnussen et al., 1987; Manning and O'Byrne, 1988) have found a modest degree of tachyphylaxis to consecutive challenges with histamine, but not with a cholinergic agonist, repeated at 1-h intervals on a single day, while others (Ruffin et al., 1981) failed to find any change in sensitivity to inhaled histamine with repeated testing at 30-, 60-, or 120-min intervals. Intraindividual responses to both histamine and methacholine on separate days are highly reproducible (Juniper et al., 1978). On the other hand, allergen-induced late asthmatic responses are associated with an increase in nonspecific airway responsiveness, the magnitude and duration of which correlate with the magnitude of the late asthmatic response (Cartier et al., 1982). Such allergen-related increases in airway responsiveness not infrequently last up to 2 weeks and can even persist for as long as 10 or more weeks (Cartier et al., 1982). Increases in nonspecific BHR have also been noted following exposure to certain occupational agents (Lam et al., 1979; Mapp et al., 1986), oxidizing pollutants (Golden et al., 1978; Dimeo et al., 1983; Orehek et al., 1976), and viral respiratory tract infection (Empey et al., 1978). The enhancement of nonspecific airway responsiveness by experimental or natural exposure to allergens or other asthmagenic stimuli needs to be taken into account in studies of the inhibitory effects of drugs on airway reactivity.

J. Effects of Long-Term Bronchodilator Therapy

If diminished responsiveness (tachyphylaxis) to the acute relaxant effect of a bronchodilator on ASM developed after multiple dosing, then the measured short-term airway response to a bronchodilator would be affected by long-term therapy. However, no decline in acute bronchodilator responsiveness to theophylline or anticholinergic bronchodilators has been demonstrated after long-term treatment with these agents (Klaustermeyer et al., 1989). Moreover, although tachyphylaxis to the bronchodilator effect of β-agonists is readily evident in *normal* subjects, it has not been shown consistently in *asthmatic* subjects, as reviewed by Tattersfield (1985) and Jenne et al. (1993). In contrast, β-receptor down-regulation in leukocyte membranes (Tashkin et al., 1977) and tachyphylaxis to other *systemic* effects of β-agonists on heart rate, tremor, and blood glucose and serum potassium concentration have been well documented.

Despite the lack of consistent evidence of significant tachyphylaxis to β-agonist–induced *bronchodilation* in asthmatics, several studies have demonstrated a temporary, small but statistically significant increase in reactivity to histamine or methacholine in the range of approximately 0.5–1.5 doubling doses after withdrawal of long-term therapy with an inhaled β-agonist (Kerrebijn et al., 1987; Kraan et al., 1985; Van Schyack et al., 1990; Vathenen et al., 1988). It is possible that this increase in nonspecific BHR after long-term β-agonist therapy represents a more subtle indication of subsensitivity of β-receptors on ASM than can be gleaned from measures of bronchodilation. This possibility is supported by several studies demonstrating tolerance to the protective effect of a β-agonist against bronchoconstriction induced by histamine (Vathenen et al., 1988), methacholine (O'Connor et al., 1992; Cheung et al., 1992) or adenosine monophosphate (AMP) (O'Connor et al., 1992). Tolerance to these *nonbronchodilator* effects of β-agonist therapy has been suggested as a possible explanation for the recent observations that regular use of β-agonists, even in conventional doses, worsens asthma control, possibly contributing to the increased mortality and morbidity from asthma in recent decades (Sears et al., 1990).

On the basis of their observations that β-agonists produced greater protection against bronchoconstriction induced by AMP (an important stimulus of mast-cell mediator release) than that induced by methacholine (an ASM constrictor agonist), O'Connor et al. (1992) speculated that β-receptor function might be more important for protection against stimuli of mediator release than against agonists that directly provoke bronchoconstriction. These authors also showed that regular dosing with a β-agonist produced more tolerance against AMP-induced than against methacholine-induced bronchoconstriction, suggesting down-regulation of mast-cell β receptors (Fig. 13). Recently, Cockcroft et al. (1993) have shown that 2 weeks of regularly scheduled treatment with conventional metered doses of albuterol increased baseline airway responsiveness to allergen and produced tolerance to the protective effect of albuterol against allergen-induced (as well as methacholine-induced) bronchoconstriction (Fig. 14). They interpreted these findings as also suggesting the development of β-agonist–induced down-regulation of β receptors on mast cells. They suggested, further, that such downregulation, leading to increased allergen responsiveness in asthmatics, could predispose to late-phase reactions to allergen inhalation and thus greater airway inflammation, possibly accounting for the increase in airway responsiveness to histamine and methacholine noted after regular use of β-agonists.

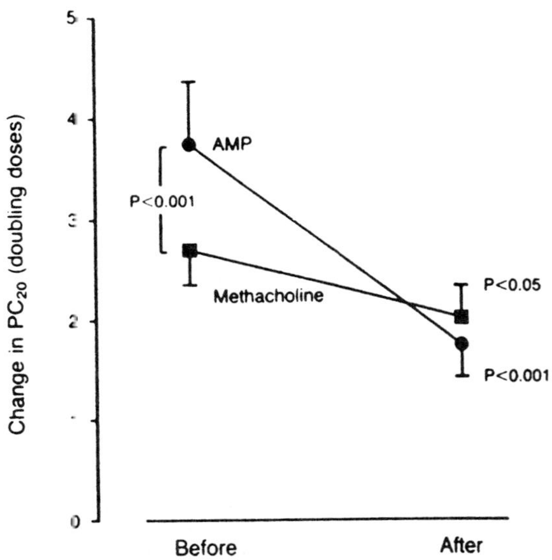

Figure 13 Effect of a single 500-μg inhalation of terbutaline on airway responsiveness to methacholine and adenosine monophosphate (AMP). The effect is shown as the mean (± SEM) change in PC_{20}, expressed in doubling doses, after the inhalation of terbutaline as compared with placebo, before and after 7 days of treatment with terbutaline. After the 7-day period, there was significantly reduced protection against AMP ($p < 0.001$) and methacholine ($p < 0.05$) as compared with the values before treatment. The difference in the changes in PC_{20} for AMP and methacholine was significant before treatment ($p < 0.001$), but was abolished after treatment. These findings indicate a greater loss of protective efficacy of the β-agonist against bronchospasm induced by AMP (the action of which is mediated by mast cells) than against bronchospasm induced by methacholine (which acts directly on airway smooth muscle). (From O'Connor et al., 1992.)

K. The Tests Used to Measure a Bronchodilator Response

The measured bronchodilator response is dependent on (1) the very tests used to measure the response and the maneuvers required in performing these tests (which may themselves alter airway physiology, depending on the nature of the underlying disease), (2) host factors (such as effort, motivation, learning, and the nature and severity of the underlying pulmonary disease process), and (3) normal intertrial test variability.

1. Forced Expiratory Flow

Forced expiratory flow may be reduced in asthma or COPD for any one or more of the following reasons: (1) reduced lung recoil due to reversible or irreversible loss of lung stiffness, (2) increased airway resistance due to narrowing by inflammatory edema, mucous secretions, fibrosis, and/or bronchospasm, (3) increased

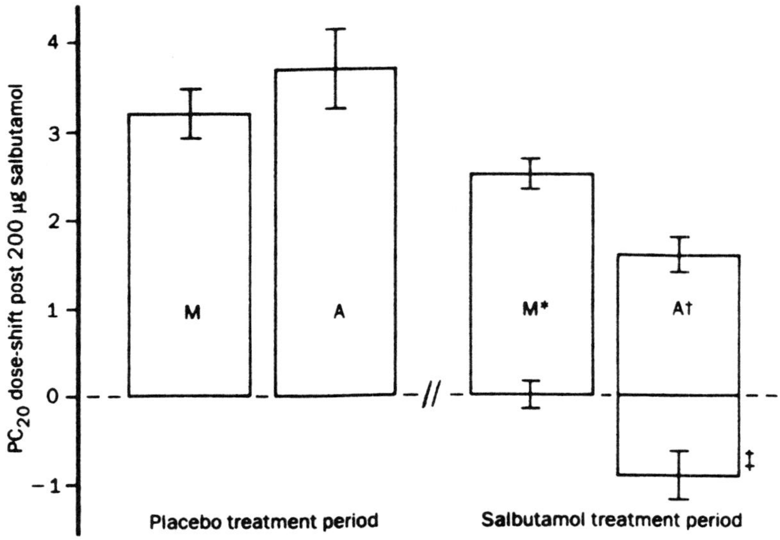

Figure 14 Dose-shift in methacholine PC_{20} and allergen PC_{20} with vs. without pretreatment with 200 μg salbutamol during two 2-week treatment periods during which subjects used two inhalations of either placebo metered-dose inhaler (MDI) or salbutamol MDI four times daily. Results (n = 12) are expressed as the dose shift (mean ± SEM) calculated as $\Delta \log_{10} PC_{20} \div 0.3$. Baseline PC_{20} values during placebo treatment period are arbitrarily defined as 0. The SE bars at the bottom of the two salbutamol treatment period bars represent dose-shift in baseline level of reactivity compared with placebo period (methacholine 0 [0.18], allergen, 0.91 [0.20]). M = methacholine; A = allergen; $*p = 0.026$; $\dagger p=0.025$; $\ddagger p=0.0009$. These results indicate that regular use of salbutamol MDI for 2 weeks leads to a loss of protection by the β-agonist against both methacholine- and antigen-induced bronchospasm, as well as an increase in the baseline degree of reactivity to antigen, reflected by the decrease in baseline PC_{20} for antigen. (From Cockcroft et al., 1993.)

compliance of airway walls due partly to the relaxing effect of bronchodilators on airway smooth muscle or to cartilaginous damage (as in emphysema), and (4) decreased effort due to muscle fatigue, lack of motivation, or other factors. The effect of a bronchodilator on forced expiratory flow is the net outcome of effects on each of the above-mentioned determinants of flow. For example, although bronchodilators can increase resting airway caliber by relaxing airway smooth muscle, at the same time they can increase airway wall compliance by reducing myogenic tone (Stamm et al., 1976; Bouhuys and van de Woestijne, 1971; Lonky and Tisi, 1980), and β-adrenergic bronchodilators can decrease lung elastic recoil (McFadden et al., 1970; Ayres et al., 1974), possibly as a result of a relaxant effect on contractile elements in alveolar ducts and air spaces in the lung (Colebatch, 1970;

Laitinen et al., 1976). An increase in airway wall compliance predisposes to dynamic compression of airways downstream from equal pressure points by the high pleural pressures generated during a forced expiratory maneuver that are applied to the lateral walls of the airways. At the same time, a reduced recoil pressure lowers the driving pressure for forced expiratory flow and decreases the tethering effect that helps hold airways open. Thus, the effects of a bronchodilator on airway wall compliance and lung recoil can negate or blunt its beneficial effect on airway resistance, resulting in no or relatively little net increase in forced expiratory flow.

2. Volume-Dependence of Forced Expiratory Flow Rates

Forced expiratory flow is determined largely by lung elastic recoil pressure (Pel) and airflow resistance. Both Pel and airflow resistance are related to lung volume (Pel decreases and resistance increases as lung volume diminishes). Forced expiratory flow is therefore dependent on the volume at which it is measured. Consequently, in comparing pre- and postbronchodilator values of FEF it is important to use an isovolume technique, i.e., to calculate forced expiratory flow at the same volume or over the same volume range from the pre- and postbronchodilator flow–volume or volume–time curves. Vital capacity is often increased by a bronchodilator as result of a reduction in RV due to lessening of air trapping, whereas TLC is generally not altered (Paré et al., 1983; McFadden et al., 1970). Therefore, the volume corresponding to any given percentage of the postbronchodilator FVC will represent a lower percentage of TLC, i.e., a lower absolute lung volume, than the volume corresponding to the same percentage of the prebronchodilator FVC. Similarly, the middle range of the postbronchodilator FVC may also span a lower range of absolute lung volume than the middle range of the prebronchodilator FVC. The isovolume method is easily accomplished by matching the pre- and postbronchodilator curves at the same volume or over the same range of volume as that used for calculating flow rates from the prebronchodilator curve (Sherter et al., 1978; Boggs et al., 1982) (Fig. 15). Failure to use the isovolume method can result in an underestimation of any improvement in FEF after bronchodilator therapy. Use of FEV_1 to assess bronchodilator responsiveness avoids this problem because FEV_1 is always measured from the same absolute lung volume, namely TLC.

3. Influence of Test Maneuvers on Airway Physiology

The single deep inspiration required for measurement of forced expiratory volumes and flow rates causes a transient increase in airway resistance and decrease in maximal expiratory flow in most asthmatics (Gayrard et al., 1975; Zamel et al., 1983), which can be partially or completely blocked by anticholinergic or β-agonist bronchodilators, implying a reflex mechanism. In contrast, normal subjects (Nadel and Tierney, 1961; Fish et al., 1981) and a few asthmatics (Zamel

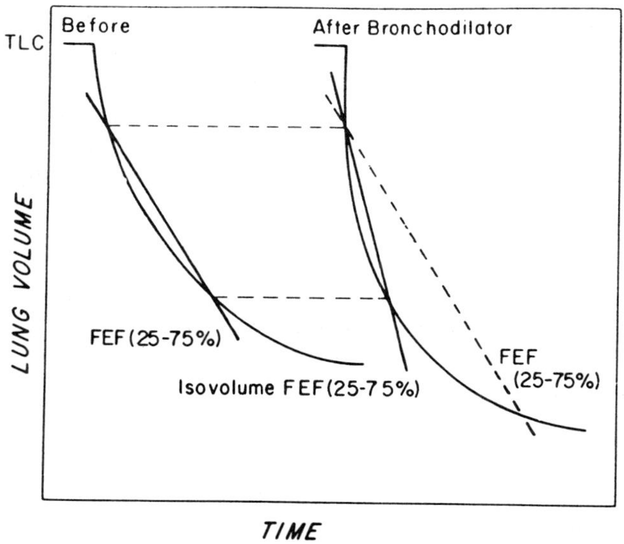

Figure 15 Isovolume maximal midexpiratory flow ($FEF_{25-75\%}$) is measured by matching maximal inspiratory points of tracings before and after bronchodilator therapy. Points at 25% and 75% of curves after bronchodilator therapy are matched to those measured on tracing before bronchodilator therapy. Thus, on tracing after bronchodilator therapy, one is not measuring flow in middle 50% of that breath, but during same segment of volume as on forced expiration before bronchodilator therapy. (From Sherter et al., 1978.)

et al., 1983) exhibit a transient decrease in airway resistance and increase in maximal flow rates after a deep inspiration, especially following pharmacological induction of bronchoconstriction, possibly because of stress relaxation of airway smooth muscle that may be augmented in the contracted state. Interestingly, many asthmatics with postinspiration bronchoconstriction respond to pharmacologically induced bronchospasm by losing the bronchoconstrictor response to deep inspiration and, in some instances, even acquiring a further dilator response (Zamel et al., 1983). The presence and degree of spirometrically measured inhibition of induced bronchoconstriction by a bronchodilator may be confounded by a complex interaction between the effects of the bronchodilator and that of the single deep inhalation preceding forced exhalation on the contractile state of the airways. These confounding effects can be obviated by methods of assessing change in airway caliber that do not require a deep inspiration, such as whole-body plethysmography (DuBois et al., 1956a), forced oscillation (DuBois et al., 1956b) or partial flow–volume curves (Littner et al., 1979). On the other hand, while some studies have suggested that plethysmographic measurements of airway resistance and specific airway conductance are more sensitive than spirometry in detecting changes in airway caliber (Anthonisen et al., 1986; Lloyd, 1963; Watanabe et al., 1974), Light et al. (1977) found the FEV_1 to be superior to airway resistance in detecting a statistically significant bronchodilator response in asthmatics, because of less test variability. In healthy subjects who are relatively unresponsive to airway constrictors, Littner and co-workers (1979) have shown partial flow–volume curves to be a sensitive technique for detecting dose-related decreases in flow rates after challenge with histamine and methacholine, as well as pharmacological augmentation and inhibition of the constrictor response.

4. Airway Resistance

Plethysmographic airway resistance (Raw) reflects resistance to air flow generally at or near FRC and at flow rates of $\pm$ 0.5 L/s. Resistance measured by the forced oscillation technique also reflects mainly the resistance of the airways plus the additional resistance of the lung tissue and chest wall. Airway resistance measurements are not affected by the turbulence generated by high linear velocities of flow, by convective acceleration, or by dynamic airway compression, which influence flow resistance during forced expiratory maneuvers. Of 51 patients with a clinical diagnosis of emphysema studied by Gimeno et al. (1993), 10% exhibited significant reversibility by Raw (decrease from baseline of $>$ 28%) but not by spirometry (increases in FEV_1 and inspiratory vital capacity of $\leqslant$ 23% and $\leqslant$ 13%, respectively, from baseline), while an additional 39% showed significant reversibility by both spirometric and plethysmographic measurements and another 22% by inspiratory vital capacity (IVC) alone. The cut points selected for determination of significant changes in Raw, FEV_1, and IVC were equivalent to the mean coefficients of variation + 2 SD for these measures, derived from repeated daily measurements over 10 days in a subset of the subjects tested. These findings suggest that measurement of Raw is a useful addition to spirometry in identifying reversibility of airway obstruction in patients with emphysema.

5. Functional Residual Capacity

Thoracic gas volume at FRC is the resting volume of the respiratory system; it is normally determined by the relative recoil properties of the lung and chest wall which, at FRC, are equal and opposite in sense. When lung recoil is reduced, as in emphysema or asthma, FRC increases, as a new equilibrium between lung and chest wall recoil is established at a higher lung volume. In obstructive lung diseases, FRC may also be increased as a consequence of gas-trapping behind airways that are functionally closed in the normal FRC range. The latter mechanism probably contributes substantially to the hyperinflation of asthma, since bronchodilation very often is associated with a reduction in FRC, presumably because of a lessening of air trapping rather than an increase in lung recoil. In fact, the effect of a bronchodilator on the static elastic properties of the lung is, if anything, to reduce recoil in the FRC range (McFadden et al., 1970; McCarthy and Sigurdson, 1980).

The plethysmographic assessment of changes in lung volumes in asthma can be erroneous because of nonhomogeneous swings in alveolar pressure, which are likely to be greater in regions supplied by closed airways; as a result, alveolar pressure swings measured at the mouth are underestimated, leading to an overestimation of thoracic gas volume. This source of error could account for an exaggerated apparent increase in lung volume during acute exacerbations of asthma and a reciprocal exaggerated reduction in lung volumes when severe bronchospasm is relieved by bronchodilator therapy (Brown et al., 1978). Rodenstein et al. (1981) found an apparent link between the error in plethysmographic measurement of lung volume and the severity of obstruction and noted errors as large as 1.9 L. They conclude that the plethysmographic method is unsuitable for measuring lung volume in patients with airway obstruction, particularly when the obstruction is severe.

6. Vital Capacity: Isolated or Predominant Volume Responses to Bronchodilator Therapy

When the flow response to a bronchodilator is blunted by the factors noted previously, the vital capacity can still improve if the peripheral airways are dilated. This improvement is due to relief of air trapping and reduction in residual volume. Since the relaxed peripheral airways are likely to be located upstream from equal pressure points, they are not susceptible to dynamic airway compression by the positive pleural pressure generated during exhalation to residual volume. Acute reductions in FRC are also common following bronchodilator therapy; the decreases in FRC are probably secondary to relief of air trapping in the tidal volume range.

Ramsdell and Tisi (1979) noted an isolated volume response to a bronchodilator in a large proportion of patients with chronic airflow obstruction. Of 129 patients who exhibited a "significant" fall (mean 27%) in Raw 10 min after inhalation of 2.25 mg isoproterenol, 46 (41%) had a "significant" increase in VC (mean 15%) and a "significant" decline in plethysmographically determined FRC (mean 13%), without any change in forced expiratory flow. Interestingly, those patients with an isolated volume response to the bronchodilator showed a mean reduction in Raw similar to that noted in the patients whose forced expiratory flow increased following the bronchodilator. However, the isolated volume responders had a more marked degree of airway obstruction and hyperinflation compared with the flow responders, consistent with a decreased Pel in the former. The decreased Pel in these patients could have reduced the tethering support of their intrapulmonary airways, thereby predisposing them to more dynamic airway compression during a forced expiratory maneuver. This effect could be exaggerated by bronchodilator therapy if the latter is associated with a further reduction in Pel, as well as an increase in airway wall compliance due to a reduction in myogenic tone.

Girard and Light (1983) studied 17 patients with moderate to severe chronic airflow obstruction who exhibited sizable increases in FVC (27% ± 8%) after a bronchodilator with little or no increase in FEV_1 (3.6% ± 3.8%). They noted two different types of response accounting for the increase in FVC. One was characterized by associated increases in FEV_3 and FEV_6 (seven patients), which they attributed to true bronchodilation involving peripheral airways that contribute to the latter portion of the timed spirogram. The other type of response was associated with no increase in FEV_3 or FEV_6 (10 patients); in these patients the improvement in FVC was attributed simply to an increase in the duration of expiration after bronchodilator administration, possibly due to learning to blow out longer after repetitive maneuvers. However, the possibility that the latter response also represents a bronchodilator effect cannot be excluded.

Ayres and coworkers (1974) noted a variable spirometric and plethysmographic response to isoproterenol in 134 patients with COPD. Over 90% of the patients showed a significant (> 15%) decrease in Raw (mean decrease approximately 40%), approximately 25% showed a significantly increased VC (mean increase 22%), and a partially overlapping 25% showed an increase in forced expiratory flow (mean increase in peak expiratory flow rate 36%). Thus, nearly all patients with chronic airflow obstruction examined appeared to respond to bronchodilator administration by reducing bronchomotor tone, while fewer than half responded by increasing VC and/or forced expiratory flow. The authors concluded that failure of forced expiratory flow to increase after inhalation of a β-agonist should not be interpreted as evidence of an unresponsive airway. In the absence of measurements of airway resistance and FRC, an increase in VC may be the only indication of bronchodilator responsiveness.

L. Test Validity and Reliability

The validity of assessments of bronchodilator response using tests of forced exhalation depends on the accuracy of measurements of forced expiratory volumes and flow rates. The latter, in turn, depends on the performance characteristics of the measuring instrument, the effort and cooperation of the patient, and the technical skill of the person performing the tests, including the ability to motivate the patient to perform maximally. It is clearly important that equipment be properly calibrated, that subjects be adequately instructed in the testing procedures, and that results be accurately calibrated and transcribed. The reader is referred elsewhere for a detailed discussion of pulmonary function testing methodology and quality control (Clausen, 1980; Intermountain Thoracic Society Pulmonary Function Task Force, 1984; American Thoracic Society Statement, 1987).

M. Test Variability

Assessment of the response to a bronchodilator is affected by the intraindividual variability of the tests used to measure the response. Test variability is dependent on the particular type of measurement being performed, equipment accuracy, technical skill, and a number of factors relating to the subject performing the test. The latter include effort, ability to perform the test properly, level of pretest physical activity, diurnal variability, prior exposure to bronchodilator or constrictor influences (e.g., medication, methylxanthine-containing food or beverages, aeroallergens, cigarette smoke, air pollution, viral respiratory tract infection), and the presence or absence and magnitude of ventilatory abnormality. Diurnal variability in measures of airways obstruction can be particularly marked in asthmatic subjects (Hetzel and Clark, 1980; Barnes, 1985) and needs to be taken into consideration when responses to a bronchodilator are measured over several hours. Comparison with responses to placebo on a separate day and administration of the test agent at the same time of day will control for this source of variability.

Pennock et al. (1981) performed spirometry on 20 asthmatic subjects nine times daily and found an individual within-day coefficient of variation (SD/mean) of 6.7%, 8.1%, and 14% for FVC, FEV_1, AND $FEF_{25-75\%}$, respectively. Assuming that a Gaussian distribution was applicable, they suggested that these values might be used to assess the significance of changes in spirometric indices after a bronchodilator. Since values more than 1.65 times the coefficient of variation would be expected in $< 5\%$ of the population as a result of "normal" variability, a significant change in FVC, FEV_1, and $FEF_{25-75\%}$ within a day's time in an asthmatic subject would be one that was greater than 11%, 13%, and 23%, respectively. Similar cut points could be used to assess the significance of short-term changes in these spirometric indices after administration of a bronchodilator to obstructed subjects. Since larger individual week-to-week coefficients of variation were observed, even greater changes in FVC, FEV_1 and $FEF_{25-75\%}$ (21%, 23%, and 30%, respectively, in asthmatic subjects) would have to occur 1 or more weeks following the initiation of a bronchodilator program before such changes could be considered significant.

Tweeddale et al. (1984, 1987) also used short-term variability in FEV_1 and VC to define statistically significant changes for assessing acute bronchodilator responsiveness. In normal subjects and a small group of patients with restrictive ventilatory abnormality, they found that natural short-term variability in FEV_1 was constant over a wide range of FEV_1 values; on the basis of these results they suggested that the criterion of a true bronchodilator response should be an absolute change in FEV_1 of $\geqslant$ 190 ml. More recently, the same authors determined short-term variability in FEV_1 and VC and bronchodilator responses in 150 consecutive patients with varying degrees of airways obstruction who were referred for bronchodilator testing (Tweeddale et al., 1987). They divided their patients into three groups depending on the severity of their obstructive defect, as defined by their baseline FEV_1. The natural variability in FEV_1 and VC over a 20-min interval in the three groups is shown in Table 2a. No significant differences in natural variability of *absolute* changes in FEV_1 were found between the groups, but variability in *percent* changes increased as baseline airways obstruction increased. The *absolute* increases in FEV_1 and VC needed to distinguish a true bronchodilator response from natural variability in these patients were 160 ml and 330 ml, respectively. Because the *percent* normal variability in FEV_1 differed between groups, a single *percent* change in FEV_1 that would separate a bronchodilator response from spontaneous variability could not be defined.

The number (percentage) of patients in each of the above groups with a significant FEV_1 response to two inhalations of albuterol or terbutaline MDI defined by an absolute increase of 160 ml or an arbitrarily defined percent increase of 10% or 15% is shown in Table 2b. The *proportion* of patients with a significant *absolute* response to the bronchodilator declined as the baseline FEV_1 fell, but the *magnitude* of the FEV_1 response was similar across groups. In contrast, the

Table 2a Natural Variability in FEV_1 and Vital Capacity Over 20-Min Time Interval[a]

	Group A	Group B	Group C
No. of patients	72	51	27
FEV_1			
Range (1, BTPS)	0.50–1.10	1.15–2.40	2.45–4.70
AC (ml)			
Mean	3	19	21
SD	96	100	84
PC (%)			
Mean	−0.1	−1.6	−0.7
SD	12.4	6.5	3.0
Vital capacity			
Range (1, BTPS)	0.55–4.10	1.95–4.95	3.40–6.80
AC (ml)			
Mean	48	43	−46
SD	211	189	181
PC (%)			
Mean	2.6	1.3	−1.2
SD	12.5	6.6	4.3

[a]Groups A, B and C are defined by the level of airways obstruction FEV_1 = forced expired volume in 1 second; BTPS = ; AC = absolute change; PC = percentage change.
Source: Tweeddale et al., 1987.

Table 2b Number of Patients with FEV_1 Response to Bronchodilator

	Group A	Group B	Group C	All patients
No. of patients	72	51	27	150
FEV_1 Range (1, BTPS)	0.5–1.1	1.15–2.4	2.45–4.7	0.5–4.7
AC responders (% of group)	17 (24)	23 (45)	18 (66)	58 (39)
PC 15% responders (% of group)	23 (31)	15 (29)	2 (7)	39 (26)
PC 10% responders (% of group)	36 (50)	22 (43)	11 (41)	69 (46)

AC responders = patients showing an absolute increase of > 160 ml in forced expired volume in 1 second (FEV_1); PC 15% responders = patients showing a percentage increase > 15% in FEV_1; PC 10% responders = patients showing a percentage increase of > 10% in FEV_1.
Source: Tweeddale et al., 1987.

proportion with a significant *percent* response rose with increasing airways obstruction by the 15% criterion and did not change when the 10% criterion was used, and the *magnitude* of the percent response was significantly higher in the most obstructed patients. These findings underscore the difficulties in applying uniform criteria to define bronchodilator responsiveness in patients with a broad range of initial airway obstruction.

Sourk and Nugent (1983) used a slightly different approach to define confidence intervals for assessing statistically significant responses to an inhaled bronchodilator. They measured changes in spirometry following double-blind inhalation of a placebo aerosol in 40 patients referred to the pulmonary function laboratory for routine evaluation. Two-tailed 95% confidence intervals were then derived for *percent changes* in PEFR, FVC, FEV_1, FEV_1/FVC ratio, and $FEF_{25-75\%}$ from the baseline preplacebo values and for *absolute changes* in these indices from baseline. Table 3 shows the mean percent and absolute changes in spirometry after placebo inhalation as well as the upper 95% confidence limits for a two-tailed population, defined as the mean plus 2 SD of the mean, which would exclude 2.5% of normal responses to placebo. The upper limits of normal variability for FVC and FEV_1 are similar to those noted by Pennock et al. (1981), but the variation in $FEF_{25-75\%}$ is about twice as large.

Differing variability among the various physiological measures of a bronchodilator response will affect the sensitivity of these measures in detecting a true response (in comparison with placebo) and in distinguishing statistically between the responses to different bronchodilator agents. Light et al. (1977) analyzed the

Table 3 Mean Percent and Absolute Changes in Spirometric Indices After Placebo Inhalations in Asthmatic Subjects

Index	Mean % change	SD	Upper confidence limit[a]
PEFR[b]	−7.50	39.2%	71.7%
FVC	1.27	6.7%	14.9%
FEV_1	0.97	5.6%	12.3%
$FEF_{25-75\%}$	−0.14	22.4%	45.1%
	Absolute mean difference	SD	Upper confidence limit[a]
PEFR	−7.6 L/s	32.9 L/s	58.9 L/s
FVC	0.025 L	0.156 L	0.340 L
FEV_1	0.011 L	0.083 L	0.178 L
$FEF_{25-75\%}$[c]	−0.039 L/s	—	

[a]Ninety-five percent of the population is defined by the mean ± 2.02 standard deviations of the mean.
[b]Not a normal distribution in form of percent change. Range: −28.2–37.9%. Confidence limits calculated by logirithmic transformation and then converted back to percent change form.
[c]Not a normal distribution. Range: −2.04 to +0.39 L/s.
PEFR = peak expiratory flow rate; FVC = forced vital capacity; FEV_1 = forced expired volume in 1 second; $FEF_{25-75\%}$ = maximal midexpiratory flow.
Source: Sourk and Nugent, 1983.

acute effect of different bronchodilator regimens on several tests of lung function (SGaw, Raw, FVC, FEV_1, FEV_1/FVC%, and $FEF_{25-75\%}$) in 20 asthmatic subjects. They noted a disparity between the *magnitude* of improvement in lung function, expressed as percent change from baseline, and the *level of significance* of the difference in improvement between different drug regimens, expressed as the F value derived from analysis of variance (ANOVA) (Fig. 16). The F value is a measure of the ratio of between-group separation to within-group variation and thus takes into account the inherent variability of the test. For example, although both SGaw and $FEF_{25-75\%}$ showed a greater mean percent improvement following the active bronchodilator agents than did FEV_1, the latter measure yielded the highest F value of ANOVA and detected the largest number of statistically significant differences in pairwise comparisons of the various drug regimens. These findings suggest that the FEV_1 may be superior to plethysmographic airway resistance and other measures derived from spirometry in detecting a true bronchodilator response. In contrast, the FEV_1/FVC ratio yielded the lowest F value, indicating that it is a poor index of bronchodilator responsiveness. This

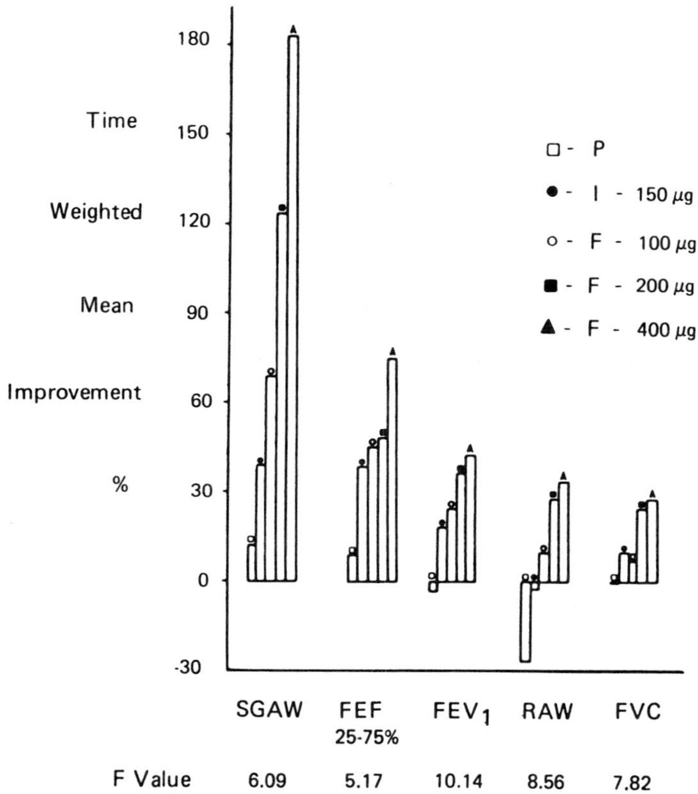

Figure 16 The mean time-weighted percent improvements after placebo (P), isoproterenol (I), and varying dosages of fenoterol (F) for the various tests and the associated F values. While the percentage of improvement after each drug is greatest when measured by airway resistance (Raw) the F value is greatest for forced expired volume in 1 second (FEV_1). (From Light et al., 1977.) SGaw = specific airway conductance; $FEF_{25-75\%}$ = maximal midexpiratory flow; FVC = forced vital capacity.

finding is not surprising, since the FVC often improves along with the FEV_1 in response to a bronchodilator, thus minimizing any change in FEV_1/FVC ratio.

In contrast to the above findings in patients with reversible airways obstruction, Watanabe et al. (1974) found that in 75 *normal* subjects of varying size the only measures that improved significantly in response to a bronchodilator aerosol were plethysmographic indices (SGaw, Raw, Gaw) ($p < 0.001$) and $FEF_{25-75\%}$ ($p < 0.02$); FVC and FEV_1 showed no significant change (Table 4). Bouhuys and van de Woestijne (1971) and McFadden et al. (1970) also noted much greater changes in SGaw than in forced expiratory flow rates in normal subjects after bronchodilator

Table 4 Mean Plethysmographic and Spirometric Values Before and After Bronchodilator in 75 Normal Subjects

	Before bronchodilator (mean ± SD)	After bronchodilator (mean ± SD)	Percent change (mean ± SD)	p
Raw	1.393 (0.368)	1.125 (0.270)	−18.4 (9.5)	< 0.0001
Gaw	0.762 (0.180)	0.938 (0.220)	+24.3 (14.8)	< 0.0001
Vtg	3059 (753)	3069 (743)	+0.3 (11.3)	NS
SGaw	0.257 (0.065)	0.317 (0.083)	+23.6 (13.6)	< 0.0001
FVC	4521 (1051)	4528 (1047)	+0.2 (2.5)	NS
FEV_1	3610 (856)	3692 (861)	+2.5 (3.9)	NS
$FEF_{25-75\%}$	3.78 (1.33)	4.37 (161)	+16.2 (16.4)	< 0.02

Raw = airway resistance (cm H_2O/L/s); Gaw = conductance = 1 R_{aw} (L/s/cm H_2O); Vtg = thoracic gas volume (ml); SGaw = specific airway conductance = G/Vtg (L/s/cm H_2O/L); FVC = forced vital capacity (ml); FEV_1 = forced expired volume in 1 second (ml); $FEF_{25-75\%}$ = maximal midexpiratory flow (L/min). NS = statistically not significant ($p >$ 0.05).

Source Watanabe et al., 1974.

administration. This disparity between plethysmographic and spirometric responses to a bronchodilator challenge in normal subjects may be due to factors already mentioned that affect the spirometric response. The significant improvement in some measures following administration of a bronchodilator to healthy subjects reflects the bronchomotor tone that is normally present. The large standard deviations of the percent increases in some of these indices (Table 4) suggest that there is wide variation in resting bronchomotor tone among normal persons.

N. Variability in Underlying Airway Responsiveness

Intraindividual variability in airway reactivity over time could lead to misinterpretation of inhibition by a bronchodilator. A number of factors can affect the reactive state of the airways, including previous environmental exposure (relevant antigens, atmospheric and occupational pollutants, viral infection, etc.) and treatment (and withdrawal of treatment) with β-agonists (Kerrebijn et al., 1987; Kraan et al., 1985; Van Schayck, 1990; Vathenen et al., 1988) or anti-inflammatory drugs (Clarke, 1982; Jenkins and Breslin, 1987; Kerrebijn et al., 1987; Dutoit et al., 1987; Haahtela et al., 1991; Waalkens et al., 1993). In addition, residual inhibition by recent treatment with a bronchodilator (especially a long-acting theophylline) or a mediator antagonist (such as an H_1-antihistamine) could exert a confounding effect. In the absence of such confounding influences, airways responsiveness to histamine and methacholine is highly reproducible within the same individual from day to day (Juniper et al., 1978), while reproducibility of exercise-induced bronchoconstriction in individual patients on separate days within 1 week is good, provided the exercise test is standardized (Silverman and Anderson, 1972; Godfrey et al., 1973). Within-day reproducibility, after the acutely induced bronchoconstriction has worn off, is excellent for methacholine (Magnussen et al., 1987) but affected by refractoriness to sequential exercise (McNeill et al., 1966; Edmunds et al., 1978; Silverman and Anderson, 1972; Godfrey et al., 1973) or nebulized hypotonic solutions (Anderson et al., 1983) and mild tachyphylaxis to serial challenges with histamine (Magnussen et al., 1987; Manning and O'Byrne, 1988). Unfortunately, the reproducibility of repeated antigen challenges, even on separate days, is undermined by the increase in nonspecific airway responsiveness attending the late inflammatory reaction to antigen, which can persist for 1–2 weeks and sometimes much longer (Cartier et al., 1982). Reproducibility of the inhibitory effect of a β-agonist against bronchospasm induced by methacholine (O'Connor et al., 1992; Cheung et al., 1992), histamine (Vathenen et al., 1988), exercise (Gibson et al., 1978; Peel and Gibson, 1980) or antigen (Cockcroft et al., 1993) also appears to be affected by tachyphylaxis resulting from long-term β-agonist therapy.

IV. EXPRESSING THE RESULTS

A. Bronchodilator Responses

The method of expressing the bronchodilator response in quantitative terms can influence interpretation of the statistical as well as clinical "significance" of the response. The three most common methods of expression are (1) percent improvement of baseline ([postbronchodilator − prebronchodilator]/prebronchodilator × 100, %), (2) absolute improvement (postbronchodilator value − prebronchodilator value), and (3) absolute improvement expressed as percent of the predicted value ([postbronchodilator value − prebronchodilator value]/predicted value × 100, %). A fourth method of expression that has been proposed is the percent of maximal achievable improvement ([postbronchodilator value − prebronchodilator value]/[best value ever recorded − prebronchodilator value], × 100, %), in which the "predicted value" may be substituted for the "best value ever recorded." Use of each of these methods can lead to problems in interpretation. Fig. 17 graphically illustrates the percent improvement of the initial baseline value of FEV_1 (A), percent of achievable improvement (B), absolute improvement (C), and percent improvement of the predicted value (D) of a hypothetical patient studied on seven different occasions, during which the baseline FEV_1 varied from 0.51 to 3.5 L, predicted being 4.0 L. Curve C illustrates a parabolic relationship between absolute response to a bronchodilator and baseline lung function, as previously

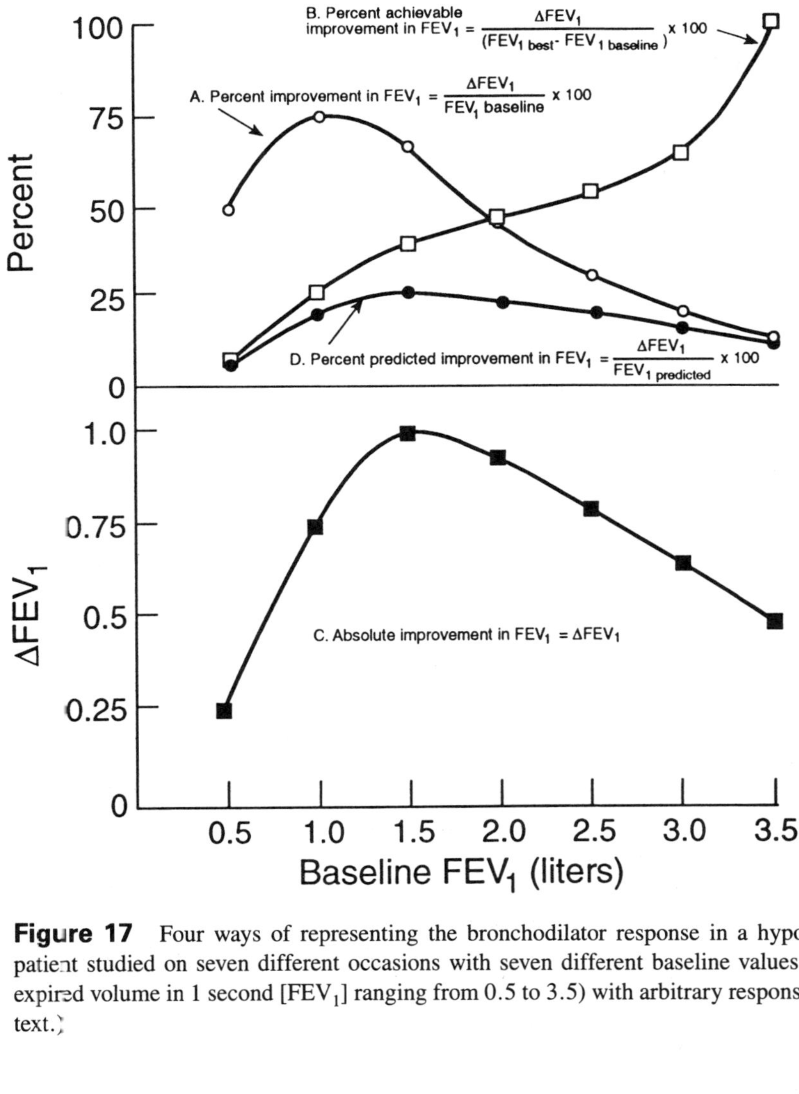

Figure 17 Four ways of representing the bronchodilator response in a hypothetical patient studied on seven different occasions with seven different baseline values (forced expired volume in 1 second [FEV_1] ranging from 0.5 to 3.5) with arbitrary responses. (See text.)

noted by Hume and Gandevia (1957) in six asthmatic patients studied on numerous occasions. When lung function is near normal, relatively little absolute improvement is possible. As obstruction increases, more reversible bronchospasm is present and improvement is greater. With more severe obstruction, however, acute bronchodilator responses decrease because of less readily reversible bronchial pathology, including secretions, inflammation, and edema. The small bronchodilator response noted when obstruction is severe (low baseline FEV_1) is indicated by the sloping down of *all* the curves on the left side of the figure. On the other hand, when obstruction is mild and there is relatively little room for improvement, full achievement of the small degree of possible improvement is reflected by an aberrantly high level of percent achievable improvement (curve B), an intermediate level of absolute improvement (curve C), and a strikingly low level of percent improvement (curve A). The minimal percent improvement results from dividing a relatively small absolute change by a high baseline value. Curve A appears to be the most misleading way of representing a bronchodilator response, since it is most dependent on baseline lung function; for example, it overestimates the bronchodilator response when initial FEV_1 values are low (Brand et al., 1990). In contrast, curve D shows fairly comparable levels of improvement in relation to the predicted value for all absolute degrees of improvement, except during severe obstruction, when absolute improvement is smallest. For this reason, expressing the change in FEV_1 as a percent of the predicted FEV_1 may have advantages over the other methods, as suggested by some authors (Brand et al., 1990; Weir et al., 1991). For example, in 121 patients with COPD with a mean baseline FEV_1 of 1.8 L (43.9% predicted) who were administered bronchodilator doses expected to elicit maximal responses (a combination of 500 μg ipratropium and 10 mg albuterol by nebulization), the change in FEV_1 expressed as a percentage of either the prebronchodilator value or of the maximal possible increase was correlated with the baseline FEV_1, while the response expressed as a percentage of the patient's predicted FEV_1 was least dependent on the starting value (Weir et al., 1991). On the other hand, Hansen et al. (1993) found that use of the latter method of expression underestimated responsiveness in severely obstructed subjects. None of the methods of expressing a bronchodilator response completely eliminates the confounding effect of the level of baseline lung function on the response. Therefore, in comparative studies of bronchodilator drugs or different dosages of the same agent, it is important that each subject have fairly comparable baseline lung function at each testing session. Subjects should not be tested unless the prebronchodilator FEV_1 values fall within a predetermined range, usually within 20% of each other.

Obtaining measurements at serial times after a bronchodilator is administered permits determination of the time of onset, peak magnitude, and duration of bronchodilation, as well as the time to peak action. The latter is an important consideration when postbronchodilator measurements are obtained at only one time point. The duration of bronchodilation is also important, since it determines the frequency of regularly scheduled dosing that is required to prevent "breakthrough" bronchospasm when the bronchodilator effect has worn off. Furthermore, tachyphylaxis to a β-agonist may be manifested more by reduction in the duration than in the peak magnitude of bronchodilation (Plummer, 1978). Postbronchodilator measurements over time can be analyzed by calculating the area under the response–time curve by the trapezoidal method. The areas obtained with one drug can then be compared with those obtained with other active agents or placebo.

B. Inhibition of Airways Reactivity by a Bronchodilator

The protective effect of a bronchodilator against bronchoconstriction induced by inhalation of a constrictor aerosol can be quantitated by measuring the change in the provocative dose (PD) or concentration (PC) of the constrictor agent after, compared with before, bronchodilator pretreatment. This comparison is usually expressed as a number-of-fold change ($PD_{bronchodilator}/PD_{control}$), a change in the log PD or PC, or the number of doubling provocative doses (Tattersfield, 1987). Thus, if the PD of a constrictor stimulus were 0.5 units before and 5 units after pretreatment, the bronchodilator would have decreased reactivity 10-fold, a shift of one log to the right or 3.2 doubling doses.

Protection against exercise-induced bronchospasm is often measured in terms of a protective index, calculated as 1 minus the ratio of the postexercise percent fall in FEV_1 (or specific airway conductance) after pretreatment to that without pretreatment, expressed as a percent. Care must be taken to calculate the percent fall from the postbronchodilator baseline just before exercise rather than the prebronchodilator baseline; otherwise the protective effect of the bronchodilator on exercise-induced bronchospasm will be overestimated. Even so, the increase in airway caliber caused by a bronchodilator will, in and of itself, magnify the protective index compared with the effect of a prophylactic agent (such as cromolyn) without any bronchodilator properties. This magnifying influence is due to at least two factors: (1) geometric aerodynamic considerations (see above); and (2) a calculation artifact caused by the larger denominator for calculation of the exercise-induced percent fall in FEV_1 (or SGaw) after as compared with before the bronchodilator, thus tending to minimize the postbronchodilator *percent* decline in FEV_1 (or SGaw) with exercise. Similar considerations apply to interpreting the protective effect of a bronchodilator against bronchospasm induced by eucapnic cold-air hyperventilation or by constrictor aerosols.

V. DEFINING A SIGNIFICANT RESPONSE TO A BRONCHODILATOR

The significance of a bronchodilator response can be defined by the test(s) performed to quantitate the response and the variability of the particular tests used. The various confounding factors that can influence a bronchodilator response (discussed above) need to be taken into consideration. Since some tests are inherently more variable than others, a greater degree of improvement is required for the response to be considered significant. Moreover, because test variability is affected by the presence or absence and degree of baseline dysfunction, obstructed subjects tend to show more variable responses than do healthy people, although patients with the most severe obstruction have the lowest *absolute* variability (Hansen et al., 1993). Furthermore, intertrial variability in test results increases over time, so that tests separated by a week or a month will require a larger change than tests performed only minutes apart for differences in these results to be considered significant. For example, in the average obstructed patient, the FEV_1 or FVC would have to increase by ≥12% within the same day to be considered significant, while an improvement of 20–25% would be necessary if results a week or month apart were being compared (Pennock et al., 1981).

There is no complete agreement on the recommended criteria for judging a short-term response to a bronchodilator to be "significant," partly because of the lack of consensus concerning how the bronchodilator response should be expressed (American Thoracic Society, 1991). Published criteria for assessing bronchodilator responsiveness are shown in Table 5, adapted from Hansen et al. (1993). The criteria listed are based on the measured short- and long-term variability of FEV_1 and VC in selected populations of obstructed subjects or on short-term responses of healthy or obstructed persons to active bronchodilators or placebo. According to these criteria, clinically meaningful or significant FEV_1

Table 5 Published Criteria to Assess Bronchodilator Response

First author	FEV_1	VC
Percentage of improvement over baseline required		
Lorber (1978)	8%	10%
Dales (1988)	9%	
Dawson (1966)	10%	10%
Reis (1982)		10%
Pennock (1981)	12%	12%
Intermountain Thoracic Society (1984)	12%	15%
Berger (1988); Snider, ACCP (1974)	15%	15%
Rozas (1982)	17%	15%
Dull (1984)	25%	
Absolute improvement required		
Tweeddale (1987)	160 ml	330 ml
Both percentage of and absolute improvement required		
Sourk (1983)	15% and 180 ml	15% and 340 ml
American Thoracic Society (1991)	12% and 200 ml	12% and 200 ml
Reis (1982)	15% and 200 ml	
Other suggestions		
Anthonisen (1986); Eliasson (1985)	Percent improvement of predicted FEV_1	

FEV_1 = forced expired volume in 1 second; VC = vital capacity.
Source: Hansen et al., 1993.

responses vary from 8% to 25% (when expressed as percent increases from baseline) and/or 160 to 200 ml (when expressed as absolute changes). FEV_1 and VC responses to a bronchodilator are generally calculated by using the single *best* values obtained from a series of three or more spirometric maneuvers that meet American Thoracic Society (1987) criteria for acceptability and reproducibility *both* before and after administration of the bronchodilator. Recently, Hansen and colleagues have recommended using the variability in each individual patient's spirometric values obtained repeatedly (from five "adequate" maneuvers) both before and after bronchodilator administration to ascertain whether a statistically significant bronchodilator response occurred. Statistical significance was determined using the nonparametric Mann–Whitney rank sum statistic comparing the five values obtained before and after the bronchodilator. Because of the fatiguing effect of multiple repeated *full* forced expiratory maneuvers that are required to measure VC or FVC and the dependence of the latter measures on the time of exhalation, these authors assessed FEV_1 and forced expired volume in 3 s (FEV_3), instead of FEV_1 and VC. They defined *responders* as those with statistically significant changes in both FEV_1 *and* FEV_3 5–10 min after four inhalations of nebulized albuterol (5 mg/ml).

Of 50 consecutive adult patients with airways obstruction ($FEV_1/VC \leq 70\%$) of minimal to very marked severity (FEV_1 21–100% predicted) referred for routine lung function testing, Hansen and colleagues (1993) found 36 (72%) to be responders. In comparing their findings with previously published criteria for defining bronchodilator responsiveness (Table 5), the greatest agreement was found using the 8–10% FEV_1 criterion (Lorber et al., 1978; Dales et al., 1988; Dawson, 1966) and the least using criteria that required an absolute increase and/or a larger percentage increase (Berger and Smith, 1988; Snider, 1974; Rozas and Goldman, 1982; Dull and Alexander, 1984; Tweeddale et al., 1987; Sourk and Nugent, 1983; American Thoracic Society, 1991; Reis, 1982). The six "responders" with very severe obstruction (FEV_1 21–38% predicted) were not identified by most published criteria. Since patients with more severe obstruction were noted to have lower *absolute* variability for FEV_1 at the same time that the severely obstructed "responders" tended to show a greater *percentage* response to the bronchodilator, criteria requiring an absolute volume change were found to exclude many severely obstructed patients with statistically significant bronchodilator responses. Moreover, while most "responders" with mild to moderately severe obstruction were identified by criteria requiring an 8–12% response, about two-thirds of the "responders" with only minimal obstruction were missed by the latter criterion. Furthermore, even when responsiveness was expressed as a percentage change from *predicted* rather than *measured* values, as recommended by some authorities (American Thoracic Society, 1991; Anthonisen et al., 1986; Eliasson and DeGraff, 1985; Weir et al., 1991), Hansen and colleagues noted that statistically significant bronchodilator responses in patients with moderate to very severe obstruction were often not recognized by such criteria. The authors concluded that published criteria that are largely based on population variability rather than the variability of the individual patient undergoing testing tend to identify mainly responders with mild to moderately severe obstruction but often do not identify responders with either very severe obstruction or only minimal obstruction.

When the response to a bronchodilator is measured in a particular patient to assess its therapeutic effectiveness, the question often arises of the clinical significance of the results. Statistically significant responses are not necessarily clinically important for a given patient, nor does the absence of a statistically significant response during any single testing session exclude the possibility of clinical effectiveness of bronchodilator therapy in the subject being tested, since the measured response to a bronchodilator may vary considerably from one session to another (Guyatt et al., 1988). Moreover, a patient may respond to long-term bronchodilator therapy even though a statistically significant bronchodilator response is not apparent in any single test session (American Thoracic Society, 1991). Clinical decisions concerning the appropriateness of bronchodilator therapy in any given patient must therefore be based not only on the results of the measured response to a bronchodilator in the laboratory, but also on complete clinical information, including the underlying disease process, symptoms, drug toxicity, tolerance of side effects, medication cost, cooperation, and adherence to the physician's prescribing recommendations.

In examining responses to a bronchodilator in a *group* of subjects rather than an individual patient, statistical tests can be applied to determine whether a significant change in the mean group value has occurred after a bronchodilator and whether this change is statistically greater than that found after placebo. The confidence interval usually selected is 95% for a one-tailed test of significance or 97.5% for a two-tailed test. However, as already noted, statistically significant responses to a bronchodilator do not necessarily imply clinical effectiveness. A bronchodilator response may be statistically significant and yet not be important clinically, and vice versa. For this reason, in clinical trials, as well as in individual patients, other indices of effectiveness are often sought, such as improvement in symptoms and exercise tolerance. Adverse side effects also need to be considered in evaluating the overall benefit of bronchodilator therapy.

REFERENCES

Ahrens, R. C., Bonhan, A. C., Maxwell, G. A., and Weinberger, M. M. (1984), A method for comparing the peak intensity and duration of action of aerosolized bronchodilators using bronchoprovocation with methacholine, *Am. Rev. Respir. Dis.*, *129*, 903–906.

Alexander, M. R., Dull, W. L., and Kasik, J. E. (1980), Treatment of chronic obstructive pulmonary disease with orally administered theophylline, *JAMA*, *244*, 2286–2290.

Alliott, R. J., Lang, B. D., Rawson, D. R. W., and Leckie, W. J. H. (1972), Effects of salbutamol and isoprenaline/phenylephrine in reversible airways obstruction, *Br. Med. J.*, *1*, 539–542.

American Thoracic Society Statement (1987), Standardization of spirometry—1987 update, *Am. Rev. Respir. Dis.*, *136*, 1285–1298.

American Thoracic Society (1991), Lung function testing: selection of reference values and interpretative strategies, *Am. Rev. Respir. Dis.*, *144*, 1202–1218.

Anderson, S. D., Seale, J. P., Rozea, P., Bandler, L., Theobald, G., and Lindsay, D. A. (1976), Inhaled and oral salbutamol in exercise-induced asthma, *Am. Rev. Respir. Dis.*, *114*, 493–500.

Anderson, S. D., Schoeffel, R. E., and Finney, M. (1983), Evaluation of ultrasonically nebulized solution for provocation testing in patients with asthma, *Thorax*, *38*, 284–291.

Anthonisen, L. A. Mitchell, R. W., Kroeger, E. A., Kepron, W., Stephens, N. L., and Bergen, J. (1980), Histamine pharmacology in airway smooth muscle from a canine model of asthma, *J. Pharmacol. Exp. Ther.*, *213*, 150–155.

Anthonisen, N. R., Wright, E. C., and the IPPB Trial Group (1986), Bronchodilator response in chronic obstructive pulmonary disease, *Am. Rev. Respir. Dis.*, *133*, 814–819.

Ayres, S. M., Griesbach, S. J., Reimold, F., and Evans, R. G. (1974), Bronchial component in chronic obstructive lung disease, *Am. J. Med.*, *57*, 183–191.

Bahous, J., Cartier, A., Ouimet, G., et al. (1984), Nonallergic bronchial hyperexcitability in chronic bronchitis, *Am. Rev. Respir. Dis.*, *129*, 216–220.

Baigelman, W., and Chodosh, S. (1977), Bronchodilator action of the anticholinergic drug, ipratropium bromide (Sch 1000), as an aerosol in chronic bronchitis and asthma, *Chest*, *71*, 324–328.

Barnes, P. J. (1985), Circadian variation in airway function, *Am. J. Med.*, *79*, Suppl. 6A, 5–9.

Barnes, P. J. (1989), New concepts in the pathogenesis of bronchial hyperresponsiveness and asthma, *J. Allergy Clin. Immunol.*, *83*, 1013–26.

Barnes, P. J. (1990), Effect of corticosteroids on airway hyperresponsiveness, *Am. Rev. Respir. Dis.*, *141*, S70–S76.

Barter, C. E., and Campbell, A. H. (1976), Relationship of constitutional factors and cigarette smoking to decrease in 1-second forced expiratory volume, *Am. Rev. Respir. Dis.*, *113*, 305–314.

Bar-Yishay, E., Ben-Dov, I., and Godfrey, S. (1983), Respiratory period following hyperventilation-induced asthma, *Am. Rev. Respir. Dis.*, *127*, 572–580.

Becker, A. B., and Simons, F. E. R. (1989), Formoterol, a new long-acting selective beta$_2$-adrenergic receptor agonist: double blind comparison with salbutamol and placebo in children with asthma, *J. Allergy Clin. Immunol.*, *84*, 891–895.

Benson, M. K. (1975), Bronchial hyperreactivity, *Br. J. Dis. Chest*, *69*, 227–239.

Benson, M. K. (1978), Bronchial responsiveness to inhaled histamine and isoprenaline in patients with airways obstruction, *Thorax*, *33*, 211–213.

Berenberg, M. J., Baigelman, W., Cupples, L. A., and Pearce, L. (1985), Comparison of updraft nebulizer versus metered dose inhaler attached to an aerochamber for the administration of metaproterenol to hospitalized patients (abstr.), *Am. Rev. Respir. Dis.*, *131*, A95.

Berger, R., and Smith, D. (1988), Acute postbronchodilator changes in pulmonary function parameters in patients with chronic airways obstruction, *Chest*, *93*, 541–546.

Blake, K. V., Hoppe, M., Harman, E., et al. (1992), Relative amount of albulterol delivered to lung receptors from a metered-dose inhaler and nebulizer solution. Bioassay by histamine bronchoprovocation, *Chest*, *101*, 209–215.

Bloomfield, P., Crompton, G. K., and Winsley, N. J. P. (1979), A tube spacer to improve inhalation of drugs from pressurized aerosols, *Br. Med. J.*, *2*, 1479.

Boggs, P. B., Phat, K. D., Vekovius, W. A., et al. (1982), The clinical significance of volume-adjusted maximal midexpiratory flow (iso-volume $FEF_{25-75\%}$) in assessing airway responsiveness to inhaled bronchodilator in asthmatics, *Ann. Allergy*, *48*, 139–142.

Borut, T. C., Tashkin, D. P., Fischer, T. J., Katz, R. M., Rachelefsky, G. S., and Siegel, S. C. (1977), Comparison of aerosolized atropine sulfate and SCH-1000 on exercise-induced bronchospasm in children, *J. Allergy Clin. Immunol.*, *60*, 127–133.

Bouhuys, A. (1969), Recent applications of volume displacement body plethysmographs, *Prog. Respir. Res.*, *4*, 24–38.

Bouhuys, H. A. and van de Woestijne, K. P. (1971), Mechanical consequences of airway smooth muscle relaxation, *J. Appl. Physiol.*, *30*, 670–676.

Boushey, H. A., Holtzman, M. J., Sheller, J. R., and Nadel, J. A. (1980), Bronchial hyperreactivity, *Am. Rev. Respir. Dis.*, *121*, 389–413.

Brand, P. L. P., Quanjer, P. H., Postma, D. S., et al. (1990). A comparison of different ways to express bronchodilator response, *Am. Rev. Respir. Dis.*, *141* (part 2), A20.

Brand, P. L. P., Postma, D. S., Kerstijens, H. A. M., et al. (1991), Relationship of airway hyperresponsiveness to respiratory symptoms and diurnal peak flow variation in patients with obstructive lung disease, *Am. Rev. Respir. Dis.*, *143*, 916–921.

Braun, S. R., McKensie, W. N., Copeland, C., et al. (1989), A comparison of the effect of ipratropium and albuterol in the treatment of chronic obstructive airway disease, *Arch. Intern. Med.*, *149*, 544–547.

Britton, J., Hanley, S. P., Garrett, H. V., Hadfield, J. W., and Tattersfield, A. E. (1988), Dose-related effects of salbutamol and ipratropium bromide on airway calibre and reactivity in subjects with asthma, *Thorax*, *43*, 300–305.

Brown, R., Ingram, R. H., Jr., and McFadden, E. R., Jr. (1978), Problems in the plethysmographic assessment of changes in total lung capacity in asthma, *Am. Rev. Respir. Dis.*, *118*, 685–692.

Bruderman, I., Cohen-Aronovski, R., and Smorzik, J. (1983), A comparative study of various combinations of ipratropium bromide and metaproterenol in allergic asthmatic patients, *Chest*, *83*, 208–210.

Burge, P. S., Harries, M. G., and I'Anson, E. (1980), Comparison of atropine with ipratropium bromide in patients with reversible airways obstruction unresponsive to salbutamol, *Br. J. Dis. Chest*, *74*, 259–262.

Burney, P. G. J., Laitinen, L. A., Perdrizet, S., et al. (1989), Validity and repeatability of the IUATLD (1984) bronchial symptoms questionnaire: an international comparison, *Eur. Respir. J.*, *2*, 940–945.

Cartier, A., Thomson, N. C., Frith, P. A., Roberts, R., and Hargreave, F. E. (1982), Allergen-induced increase in bronchial responsiveness to histamine: relationship to the late asthmatic response and change in airway caliber, *J. Allergy Clin. Immunol.*, *70*, 170–177.

Casali, L., Grassi, C., Rampulla, C., et al. (1979), Clinical pharmacology of a combination of bronchodilators, *Int. J. Clin. Pharmacol. Biopharm.*, *17*, 277–280.

Chang, N., and Levison, H. (1972). The effect of a nebulized bronchodilator administered with or without intermittent positive pressure breathing on ventilatory function in children with cystic fibrosis and asthma, *Am. Rev. Respir. Dis.*, *106*, 867–872.

Cheung, D., Timmers, M. C., Zwinderman, A. H., et al. (1992), Long-term effects of a long-acting β_2-adrenoceptor agonist, salmeterol, on airway hyperresponsiveness in patients with mild asthma, *N. Engl. J. Med.*, *327*, 1198–1203.

Chung, K. F., Keyes, S. J., and Snashall, P. D. (1982), Histamine dose–response relationships in normals and asthmatic subjects. The importance of starting caliber, *Am. Rev. Respir. Dis.*, *126*, 849–854.

Clarke, P. S. (1982), The effect of beclomethosone dipropionate on bronchial hyperreactivity, *J. Asthma*, *19*, 91–93.

Clausen, J. L., ed. (1982), *Pulmonary Function Testing Guidelines and Controversies, Equipment, Methods and Normal Values*, Academic Press, New York.

Cockcroft, D. W., Killian, D. N., Mellon, J. J., and Hargreave, F. E. (1977), Protective effect of drugs on histamine-induced asthma, *Thorax*, *32*, 429–437.

Cockcroft, D. W., and Murdock, K. Y. (1987), Comparative effects of inhaled salbutamol, sodium cromoglycate, and beclomethasone dipropionate on allergen-induced early asthmatic response, late asthmatic responses, and increased bronchial responsiveness to histamine, *J. Allergy Clin. Immunol.*, *79*, 734–740.

Cockcroft, D. W., McParland, C. P., Britto, S. A., et al. (1993), Regular inhaled salbutamol and airway responsiveness to allergen, *Lancet*, *342*, 833–837.

Colebatch, H. J. H. (1970). The humoral regulation of alveolar ducts. In *Airway Dynamics, Physiology and Pharmacology* (A. Bouhuys, ed.), Springfield, Illinois, Charles C. Thomas, pp. 169–189.

Coleridge, H. M., Coleridge, J. C. G., Ginzel, K. H., Baker, D. G., Banzett, R. B., and Morrison, M. A. (1976), Stimulation of "irritant" receptors and afferent C-fibres in the lungs of prostaglandins, *Nature (Lond.)*, *264*, 451–453.

Crescioli, S., Spinazzi, A., Paleari, D., Pozzan, M., Mapp, C. E., and Fabbri, L. M. (1988), Theophylline inhibits early and late asthmatic reactions induced by allergens in atopic subjects with asthma (abstr.), *Am. Rev. Respir. Dis.*, *137* (part 2), 35.

Dales, R. E., Spitzer, W. O., Tousignant, P., et al. (1988), Clinical interpretation of airway response to a bronchodilator, *Am. Rev. Respir. Dis.*, *138*, 317–320.

Dawson, A. (1966), Reproducibility of spirometric measurements in normal subjects, *Am. Rev. Respir. Dis.*, *93*, 264–268.

DeCotiis, B. A., Braman, S. S., and Corrao, W. M. (1980), The protective effect of theophylline and terbutaline on a methacholine inhalation challenge (abstr.), *Am. Rev. Respir. Dis.*, *121*, 125.

Dimeo, M. J., Glenn, M. G., Holtzman, M. J., Sheller, J. R., Nadel, J. A., and Boushey, H. A. (1983), Threshold concentration of ozone causing an increase in bronchial reactivity in humans and adaptation with repeated exposures, *Am. Rev. Respir. Dis.*, *124*, 245–248.

Dolovich, M., Eng, P., Ruffin, R., Corr, D., and Newhouse, M. T. (1983), Clinical evaluation of a simple demand inhalation MDI aerosol delivery service, *Chest*, *84*, 36–41.

Douglas, N. J., Davidson, I., Sudlow, M. F., and Flenley, D. C. (1979), Bronchodilation and the site of airway resistance in severe chronic bronchitis, *Thorax*, *34*, 51–56.

DuBois, A. B., Botelho, S. Y., Bedell, G. N., Marshall, R., and Comroe, J. H., Jr. (1956a), A rapid plethysmographic method for measuring thoracic gas volume: a comparison with a nitrogen washout method for measuring functional residual capacity in normal subjects, *J. Clin. Invest.*, *35*, 322–326.

DuBois, A. B., Botelho, S. Y., and Comroe, J. H., Jr. (1956b). A new method for measuring airway resistance in man using a body plethysmograph: values in normal subjects and in patients with respiratory disease, *J. Clin. Invest.*, *35*, 327–335.

DuBois, A. B., Brody, A. W., Lewis, D. H., and Burgess, B. F., Jr. (1956c), Oscillation mechanics of lung and chest in man, *J. Appl. Physiol.*, *8*, 587–594.

Dull, W. L., and Alexander, M. R. (1984), Theophylline in stable chronic airflow obstruction: a reappraisal, *Arch. Intern. Med.*, *144*, 2399–2401.

Dutoit, J. I., Salome, M., and Woolcock, A. J. (1987), Inhaled corticosteroids reduce the severity of bronchial hyperresponsiveness in asthma but oral theophylline does not, *Am. Rev. Respir. Dis.*, *136*, 1174–1178.

Easton, J. G. (1981), Effect of an inhaled corticosteroid on methacholine airway reactivity, *J. Allergy Clin. Immunol.*, *67*, 388–390.

Easton, P. A., Jadue, C., Dhingra, S., et al. (1986), A comparison of the bronchodilating effects of a beta-2-adrenergic agent (albuterol) and an anticholinergic agent (ipratropium bromide) given by aerosol alone or in sequence, *N. Engl. J. Med.*, *315*, 735–739.

Eaton, M. L., MacDonald, F. M., Church, T. R., and Niewoehner, D. E. (1982), Effects of theophylline on breathlessness and exercise tolerance in patients with chronic airflow obstruction, *Chest*, *82*, 538–542.

Edmunds, A. T., Tooley, M., and Godfrey, S. (1978), The refractory period after exercise-induced asthma: its duration and relation to the severity of exercise, *Am. Rev. Respir. Dis.*, *117*, 247–254.

Eliasson, O., and DeGraff, A. C., Jr. (1985), The use of criteria for reversibility and obstruction to define patient groups for bronchodilator trials, *Am. Rev. Respir. Dis.*, *132*, 858–864.

Ellis, E. F. (1984), Inhibition of exercise-induced asthma by theophylline, *J. Allergy Clin. Immunol.*, *73*, 690–692.

Elwood, R. K., and Abboud, R. T. (1982), The short-term bronchodilator effects of fenoterol and ipratropium in asthma, *J. Allergy Clin. Immunol.*, *69*, 467–473.

Empey, D. W., Laitenen, L. A., Jacobs, L., Gold, W. M., and Nadel, J. A. (1978), Mechanisms of bronchial hyperreactivity in normal subjects following upper respiratory tract infection, *Am. Rev. Respir. Dis.*, *118*, 287–294.

Fairshter, R. D., and Wilson, A. F. (1980), Relationship between the site of airflow limitation and localization of the bronchodilator response in asthma, *Am. Rev. Respir. Dis.*, *122*, 27–32.

Fanta, C. H., Rossing, T. H., and McFadden, E. R., Jr. (1986), Treatment of acute asthma.

Is combination therapy with sympathomimetics and methylxanthines indicated? *Am. J. Med.*, *80*, 5–10.

Ferguson, G. T., and Cherniak, R. M. (1993), Management of chronic obstructive pulmonary disease, *N. Engl. J. Med.*, *328*, 1017–1022.

Fish, J. E., Ankin, M. G., Kelly, J. F., and Peterman, V. (1981), Regulation of bronchomotor tone by lung inflation in asthmatic and nonasthmatic subjects, *J. Appl. Physiol.*, *50*, 1079–1086.

Freedman, B. J. (1972), The functional geometry of the bronchi, *Bull. Physiopathol. Respir.*, *8*, 545–551.

Fuglsang, G., and Pedersen, S. (1986), Comparison of Nebuhaler and nebulizer treatment of acute severe asthma in children, *Eur. J. Respir. Dis.*, *69*, 109–113.

Gayrard, P., Orehek, J., Grimaud, C., and Charpin, J. (1975), Bronchoconstrictor effects of a deep inspiration in patients with asthma, *Am. Rev. Respir. Dis.*, *111*, 433–439.

Gervais, A., and Begin, P. (1987). Bronchodilation with a metered-dose inhaler plus an extension, using tidal breathing versus jet nebulization, *Chest*, *92*, 822–824.

Gibson, G. J., Greenacre, J. K., Konig, P., et al. (1978), Use of exercise challenge to investigate possible tolerance to beta-adrenoceptor stimulation in asthma, *Br. J. Dis. Chest*, *72*, 199–206.

Gimeno, F., Postma, D. S., and van Altena, R. (1993), Plethysmographic parameters in the assessment of reversibility of airways obstruction in patients with clinical emphysema, *Chest*, *104*, 467–470.

Girard, W. M., and Light, R. W. (1983), Should the FVC be considered in evaluating response to bronchodilator? *Chest*, *84*, 87–89.

Godden, D. J., and Crompton, G. K. (1981), An objective assessment of the tube spacer in patients unable to use a conventional pressurized aerosol efficiently, *Br. J. Dis. Chest*, *75*, 165–168.

Godfrey, S., Silverman, M., and Anderson, S. (1973), Problems of interpreting exercise-induced asthma, *J. Allergy Clin. Immunol.*, *52*, 199–209.

Golden, J. A., Nadel, J. A., and Boushey, H. A. (1978), Bronchial hyperreactivity in healthy subjects after exposure to ozone, *Am. Rev. Respir. Dis.*, *118*, 287–294.

Gomm, S. A., Keaney, N. P., Winsey, N. J. P., and Stretton, T. B. (1980), Effect of an extension tube on the bronchodilator efficacy of terbutaline delivered from a metered dose inhaler, *Thorax*, *35*, 552–556.

Gong, H., Jr., Simmons, M. S., Tashkin, D. P., et al. (1986), Bronchodilator effects of caffeine in coffee. A dose–response study of asthmatic subjects, *Chest*, *89*, 335–342.

Green, M., and Mead, J. (1974), Time dependence of flow–volume curves, *J. Appl. Physiol.*, *37*, 793–797.

Greenspon, L. W., and Parrish, B. (1988), Inhibition of methacholine-induced bronchoconstriction in patients with chronic obstructive pulmonary disease, *Am. Rev. Respir. Dis.*, *137*, 281–285.

Greenspon, L. W., and Morrissey, W. L. (1986), Factors that contribute to methacholine-induced bronchoconstriction, *Am. Rev. Respir. Dis.*, *133*, 735–739.

Gross, N. J. (1975), Sch 1000: A new anticholinergic bronchodilator, *Am. Rev. Respir. Dis.*, *112*, 823–828.

Gross, N. J., and Skorodin, M. S. (1984), Anticholinergic, antimuscarinic, bronchodilators, *Am. Rev. Respir. Dis.*, *129*, 856–870.

Guyatt, G. H., Townsend, M., Nogradi, S., et al. (1988), Acute response to bronchodilator: an imperfect guide for bronchodilator therapy in chronic airflow limitation, *Arch. Intern. Med.*, *148*, 1949–1952.

Guyatt, G. (1986), The chronic respiratory disease index questionnaire, background information and interviewing tips, McMaster University, Hamilton, Ontario, unpublished report, July 1986.

Haahtela, T., Jarvinen, M., Kava, T., et al. (1991), Comparison of a β_2-agonist, terbutaline, with an inhaled corticosteroid, budesonide, in newly detected asthma, *N. Engl. J. Med.*, *325*, 388–392.

Hansen, J. E., Casaburi, R., and Goldberg, A. (1993), A statistical approach for assessment of bronchodilator responsiveness in pulmonary function testing, *Chest*, *104*, 1119–1126.

Hargreave, F. E., Ryan, G., Thomson, N. C., O'Byrne, P. M., Latimer, K., Juniper, E. F., and Dolovich, J. (1981), Bronchial responsiveness to histamine and methacholine in asthma: measurement and clinical significance, *J. Allergy Clin. Immunol.*, *68*, 347–355.

Heimer, D., Shim, C., and Williams, M. H., Jr. (1980), The effect of sequential inhalations of metaproterenol aerosol in asthma, *J. Allergy Clin. Immunol.*, *66*, 75–77.

Hetzel, M. R., and Clark, T. J. H. (1980), Comparison of normal and asthmatic circadian rhythms in peak expiratory flow rate, *Thorax*, *35*, 732–738.

Holtzman, M. J., Sheller, J. R., DiMeo, M., Nadel, J. A., and Boushey, H. A. (1980), Effect of ganglionic blockade reactivity in atopic subjects, *Am. Rev. Respir. Dis.*, *122*, 17–25.

Hume, K. M., and Gandevia, B. (1957), Forced expiratory volume before and after isoprenaline, *Thorax*, *12*, 276–278.

Idris, A. H., McDermott, M. F., Raucci, J. C., et al. (1993), Emergency department treatment of severe asthma. Metered-dose plus holding chamber is equivalent in effectiveness to nebulizer, *Chest*, *103*, 665–672.

Ingram, R. H., Jr., and McFadden, E. R., Jr. (1977a), Localization and mechanisms of airway responses, *N. Engl. J. Med.*, *297*, 596–600.

Ingram, R. H., Jr., Wellman, J. J., McFadden, E. R., Jr., and Mead, J. (1977b). Relative contributions of large and small airways to flow limitation in normal subjects before and after atropine and isoproterenol, *J. Clin. Invest.*, *59*, 696–703.

Intermittent Positive Pressure Breathing Trial Group (1983), Intermittent positive pressure breathing therapy of chronic obstructive pulmonary disease. A clinical trial, *Ann. Intern. Med.*, *99*, 612–620.

Intermountain Thoracic Society Pulmonary Function Task Force (1984), *Clinical Pulmonary Function Testing*, 2nd Ed. (A. H. Morris, R. E. Kanner, R. O. Crapo, and R. M. Gardner, eds.), Intermountain Thoracic Society, Salt Lake City.

Jenkins, C. J., and Breslin, A. B. X. (1987), Long-term study of the effect of sodium cromoglycate on non-specific bronchial hyperresponsiveness, *Thorax*, *42*, 664–669.

Jenne, J. J., and Tashkin, D. P. (1993), Beta-adrenergic agonists, in *Bronchial Asthma: Mechanisms and Therapeutics*, 3rd Ed. (E. R. Weiss and M. Stein, eds.), Little, Brown and Company, Boston, pp. 700–748.

Joad, J., Ahrens, R. C., Lindgren, S. D., et al. (1987), Relative efficacy of maintenance therapy with theophylline, inhaled albuterol and the combination for chronic asthma, *J. Allergy Clin. Immunol.*, *79*, 78–85.

Juniper, E. F., Frith, P. A., Dunnett, C., Cockcroft, D. W., and Hargreave, F. E. (1978), Reproducibility and comparison of responses to inhaled histamine and methacholine, *Thorax*, *33*, 705–710.

Kamburoff, P. L., and Günthner, W. (1975), Dose-dependent effects of Sch 1000 MDI on the airways resistance indices in patients with chronic airways obstruction, *Postgrad. Med. J.*, *51* (suppl 7), 97.

Kepron, W., James, J. M., Kirk, B., Sehon, A. H., and Tse, K. S. (1977), A canine model for reaginic hypersensitivity and allergic bronchoconstriction, *J. Allergy Clin. Immunol.*, *59*, 64–69.

Kerrebijn, K. F., van Essen-Zandvliet, E. E. M., and Neijens, H. J. (1987), Effect of long-term treatment with inhaled corticosteroids and beta-agonists on the bronchial responsiveness in children with asthma, *J. Allergy Clin. Immunol.*, *79*, 653–659.

Klaustermeyer, W. B., Wong, S. C., Kurohara, M. L., Gross, N. J., Braun, S. R., and Hudson, L. D. (1989), Absence of tachyphylaxis to inhaled atropine in patients with chronic obstructive pulmonary disease, *Am. Rev. Respir. Dis.*, *40*, 582–585.

Klock, L. E., Miller, T. D., Morris, A. H., Watanabe, S., and Dickman, M. (1975), A comparative study of atropine sulfate and isoproterenol hydrochloride in chronic bronchitis, *Am. Rev. Respir. Dis.*, *112*, 371–376.

Konig, P., Eggleston, A., and Serby, C. W. (1981), Comparison of oral and inhaled metaproterenol for prevention of exercise-induced asthma, *Clin. Allergy*, *11*, 597–604.

Konig, P., Hordvik, N. L., and Serby, C. W. (1984), Fenoterol in exercise-induced asthma. Effect of dose on efficacy and duration of action, *Chest*, *85*, 462–464.

Kraan, J., Koeter, G. H., v.d. Mark, T. H. W., Sluiter, H. J., and de Vries, K. (1985), Changes in bronchial hyperreactivity induced by 4 weeks of treatment with antiasthmatic drugs in patients with allergic asthma: a comparison between budesonide and terbutaline, *J. Allergy Clin. Immunol.*, *76*, 628–636.

Laitinen, L. A., Empey, D. W., Poppius, H., Lemen, R. J., Gold, W. M., and Nadel, J. A. (1976), Effects of intravenous histamine on static lung compliance and airway resistance in normal man, *Am. Rev. Respir. Dis.*, *114*, 291–295.

Laitinen, L. A., and Laitinen, A. (1988), Mucosal inflammation and bronchial hyperreactivity, *Eur. Respir. J.*, *1*, 488–489.

Lam, S., Wong, R., and Yeung, M. (1979), Nonspecific bronchial reactivity in occupational asthma, *J. Allergy Clin. Immunol.*, *63*, 28–34.

Landahl, H. D., Tracewell, T. N., and Lassen, W. H. (1951), On the retention of air-borne particulates in the human lung. II. *Arch. Indust. Hyg. Occup. Med.*, *3*, 359–366.

Lees, A. W., Allan, G. W., and Smith, J. (1980), Nebulised ipratropium bromide and salbutamol in chronic bronchitis, *Br. J. Clin. Pract.*, *3*, 340–342.

Leitch, A. G., Hopkin, J. M., Ellis, D. A., et al. (1978), The effect of aerosol ipratropium bromide and salbutamol on exercise tolerance in chronic bronchitis, *Thorax*, *33*, 711–713.

Leith, D. E., and Mead, J. (1974), *Principles of Body Plethysmography*, Bethesda, Maryland, National Heart and Lung Institute.

Lewis, R. A. (1984). Inhalation drugs in asthma management: state of the art, factors affecting delivery, and clinical response to inhaled drugs, *NER Allergy Proc.*, *5*, 23–33.

Light, R. W., Conrad, S. A., and George, R. B. (1977), The one best test for evaluating the effects of bronchodilator therapy, *Chest*, *72*, 512–516.

Lightbody, I. M., Ingram, C. G., Legge, J. S., et al. (1978), Ipratropium bromide, salbutamol and prednisolone in bronchial asthma and chronic bronchitis, *Br. J. Dis. Chest*, *72*, 181–186.

Lindgren, S. B., Formgren, H., and Morén, F. (1980), Improved aerosol therapy of asthma: effect of actuator tube size on drug availability, *Eur. J. Respir. Dis.*, *61*, 56–61.

Littenberg, B. (1988), Aminophylline treatment in severe, acute asthma. A meta-analysis, *JAMA*, *259*, 1678–1684.

Littner, M. R., Schacter, E. N., and Bouhuys, A. (1979), Modification of induced airway constriction in healthy subjects, *Ann. Allergy*, *43*, 135–143.

Lloberes, P., Ramis, L., Montserrat, J. M., et al. (1988), Effect of three different bronchodilators during an exacerbation of chronic obstructive pulmonary disease, *Eur. Respir. J.*, *1*, 536–539.

Lloyd, T. C., and Wright, G. W. (1963), Evaluation of methods used in detecting changes in airway resistance in man, *Am. Rev. Respir. Dis.*, *87*, 529–537.

Lloyd, T. C., Jr. (1963), Bronchoconstriction in man following single deep inspirations, *J. Appl. Physiol.*, *18*, 114–116.

Lonky, S. A., and Tisi, G. M. (1980), Determining changes in airway caliber in asthma: the role of submaximal expiratory flow rates, *Chest*, *77*, 741–748.

Lorber, D. B., Kaltenborn, W., and Burrows, B. (1978), Responses to isoproterenol in a general population sample, *Am. Rev. Respir. Dis.*, *118*, 855–861.

Loren, M., Chai, H., Miklich, D., Barwise, G. (1977), Comparison between simple nebulization and intermittent positive-pressure in asthmatic children with severe bronchospasm, *Chest*, *72*, 145–147.

Lowhagen, O., and Rak, S. (1985), Modification of bronchial hyperreactivity after treatment with sodium cromoglycate during pollen season, *J. Allergy Clin. Immunol.*, *75*, 460–467.

Maesens, F. P. V., Smeets, J. J., Gulbelmans, H. L. L., and Zweers, P. G. M. A., (1990), Bronchodilator effect of inhaled formoterol vs. salbutarnol over 12 hours, *Chest*, *97*, 590–594.

Magnussen, H., Reuss, G., and Jorres, R. (1988), Methylxanthines inhibit exercise-induced bronchoconstriction at low serum theophylline concentration and in a dose-dependent fashion, *J. Allergy Clin. Immunol.*, *81*, 531–537.

Magnussen, H., Reuss, G., and Jorres, R. (1987), Theophylline has a dose-related effect on the airway response to inhaled histamine and methacholine in asthmatics, *Am. Rev. Respir. Dis.*, *136*, 1163–1167.

Manning, P. J., and O'Byrne, P. M. (1988). Histamine bronchoconstriction reduces airway responsiveness in asthmatic subjects *Am. Rev. Respir. Dis.*, *137*, 1323–1325.

Mapp, C. E., DiGracomo, G. R., Omni, C., Broseghini, C., and Fabbri, L. M. (1986), Late, but not early, asthma reactions induced by toluene diisocyanate are associated with increased airway responsiveness to methacholine, *Eur. J. Respir. Dis.*, *69*, 276–284.

Mapp, C., Boschetto, P., del Vecchio, L., Crescioli, S., de Marzo, N., Paleari, D., and Fabbri, L. M. (1987), Protective effect of antiasthma drugs on late asthmatic reactions and increased airway responsiveness induced by toluene diisocyanate in sensitized subjects, *Am. Rev. Respir. Dis.*, *136*, 1403–1407.

Marini, J. J., and Lakshminarayan, S. (1980), The effect of atropine inhalation in "irreversible" chronic bronchitis, *Chest*, *77*, 591–596.

McCarthy, D. S., and Sigurdson, M. (1980), Lung elastic recoil and reduced airflow in clinically stable asthma, *Thorax*, *35*, 298–302.

McFadden, E. R., Jr., Newton-Howes, J., and Pride, N. B. (1970), Acute effects of inhaled isoproterenol on the mechanical characteristics of the lungs in normal man, *J. Clin. Invest.*, *49*, 779–790.

McGavin, C. R., Gupta, S. P., and McHardy, G. J. R. (1976), Twelve-minute walking test for assessing disability in chronic bronchitis, *Br. Med. J.*, *1*, 822–823.

McGavin, C. R., Artvinli, M., Naoe, H., and McHardy, G. J. R. (1978), Dyspnoea, disability and distance walked: comparison of estimates of exercise performance in respiratory disease, *Br. Med. J.*, *2*, 241–245.

McNeill, R. S., Nairn, J. R., Millar, J. S., and Ingram, C. G. (1966), Exercise-induced asthma, *Quart. J. Med.*, (new series), *35*, 55–67.

McWilliams, B. C., Menendez, R., Kelly, W. H., and Howick, J. (1984), Effects of theophylline on inhaled methacholine and histamine in asthmatic children, *Am. Rev. Respir. Dis.*, *130*, 193–197.

Mead, J. (1960), Volume displacement body plethysmography for respiratory measurements in human subjects, *J. Appl. Physiol.*, *15*, 736–740.

Millar, A. B., Bush, A., Al-Hillawi, H., et al. (1990), Ipratropium bromide: are patients treated with optimal therapy? *Postgrad. Med. J.*, *66*, 1040–1042.

Miller, W. C., and Simi, W. W. (1976), Clinical application of quiet breathing airway resistance, *J. Asthma Res.*, *13*, 137–141.

Mitenko, P. A., and Ogilvie, R. I. (1973), Rational intravenous doses of theophylline, *N. Engl. J. Med.*, *289*, 600–603.

Moreno, R. H., Hogg, J. C., and Paré, P. D. (1986), Mechanics of airway narrowing in asthma and in chronic obstructive pulmonary disease, *Am. Rev. Respir. Dis.*, *133*, 1171–1180.

Morgan, M. D. L., Singh, B. V., Frame, M. R., et al. (1982), Terbutaline aerosol given through pear shaped spacer in acute severe asthma, *Br. Med. J.*, *285*, 849–850.

Nadel, J. A., and Tierney, D. F. (1961), Effect of a previous deep inspiration on airway resistance in man, *J. Appl. Physiol.*, *16*, 717–719.

Nelson, H. S., Spector, S. L., Whitsett, T. L., George, R. B., and Dwek, J. H. (1983), The bronchodilator response to inhalation of increasing doses of aerosolized albuterol, *J. Allergy Clin. Immunol.*, *72*, 371–375.

Newcomb, R., Tashkin, D. P., Hui, K. K., Conolly, M. E., Lee, E., and Dauphinee, B. (1985), Rebound hyperresponsiveness to muscarinic stimulation after chronic therapy with an inhaled muscarinic antagonist, *Am. Rev. Respir. Dis.*, *132*, 12–15.

Newman, S. P., Morén, F., Pavia, D., Little, F., and Clarke, S. W. (1981), Deposition of pressurized suspension aerosols inhaled through extension devices, *Am. Rev. Respir. Dis.*, *124*, 317–320.

Newman, S. P., Pavia, D., and Clarke, S. W. (1982), Kinetics of the inhaled route, in: *New Concepts in the Topical Treatment of Asthma and Related Disorders*. Cliggot Publishing Company, London, pp. 5–9.

Newman, S. P. (1991), Aerosol generators and delivery systems, *Respiratory Care*, *91*, 939–951.

O'Connor, G. T., Sparrow, D., and Weiss, S. T. (1989), The role of allergy and nonspecific airway hyperresponsiveness in the pathogenesis of chronic obstructive pulmonary disease, *Am. Rev. Respir. Dis.*, *140*, 225–252.

O'Connor, B. J., Aikman, S. L., and Barnes, P. J. (1992), Tolerance to the nonbronchodilator effects of inhaled β_2-agonists in asthma, *N. Engl. J. Med.*, *327*, 1204–1208.

Orehek, J., Mazzari, J. P., Gayrard, J. P., Grimaud, C., and Charpin, J. (1976), Effect of short-term, low-level nitrogen dioxide exposure on bronchial sensitivity of asthmatic patients, *J. Clin. Invest.*, *57*, 301–307.

Paré, P. D., Lawson, L. M., and Brooks, L. A. (1983), Patterns of response to inhaled bronchodilators in asthmatics, *Am. Rev. Respir. Dis.*, *127*, 680–685.

Pauwels, R., Van Renterghem, D., Van der Straeten, M., Johannesson, N., and Persson, C. G. A. (1985), The effect of theophylline and enprofylline on allergen-induced bronchoconstriction, *J. Allergy Clin. Immunol.*, *76*, 583–590.

Peel, E. T., and Gibson, G. J. (1980), Effects of long-term inhaled salbutamol therapy on the provocation of asthma by histamine, *Am. Rev. Respir. Dis.*, *121*, 973–978.

Pennock, B. E., Rogers, R. M., and McCaffree, D. R. (1981), Changes in measured spirometric indices. What is significant? *Chest*, *80*, 97–99.

Petrie, G. R., and Palmer, K. N. V. (1975), Comparison of aerosol ipratropium bromide and salbutamol in chronic bronchitis and asthma, *Br. Med. J.*, *1*, 430–432.

Pierce, R. J., Payne, C. R., Williams, S. J., Denison, D. M., and Clark, T. J. H. (1981), Comparison of intravenous and inhaled terbutaline in the treatment of asthma, *Chest*, *79*, 506–511.

Plummer, A. L. (1978), The development of drug tolerance to beta$_2$-adrenergic agents, *Chest*, *73* (suppl), 949–958.

Poppius, H. (1980), Inhalation of terbutaline spray through an extended mouthpiece, *Respiration*, *40*, 278–283.

Ramsdell, J. W., and Tisi, G. M. (1979), Determination of bronchodilation in the clinical pulmonary function laboratory. Role of changes in static lung volumes, *Chest*, *76*, 622–628.

Ramsdell, J. W., Nachtweg, J. F., and Moser, K. M. (1982), Bronchial hyperreactivity in chronic obstructive bronchitis, *Am. Rev. Respir. Dis.*, *126*, 829–832.

Reis, A. L. (1982), Response to bronchodilators, in *Pulmonary Function Testing: Guidelines and Controversies* (J. L. Clausen, ed.), Academic Press, New York, 1982.

Robertson, C. F., Smith, F., Beck, R., and Levison, H. (1985), Responses to frequent low doses of nebulized salbutamol in acute asthma, *J. Pediatr.*, *106*, 672–674.

Rodenstein, D., Stanescu, D. C., Cauberghs, M., and van de Woestijne, K. P. (1981), Failure of body plethysmography to accurately measure long volume in bronchial obstruction (abstr.), *Am. Rev. Respir. Dis.*, *123*, 88.

Rozas, C. J., and Goldman, A. L. (1982), Daily spirometric variability, *Arch. Intern. Med.*, *142*, 1287–1291.

Ruffin, R. E., Kenworthy, M. C., and Newhouse, M. T. (1978), Response of asthmatic patients to fenoterol inhalation: a method of quantifying the airway bronchodilator dose, *Clin. Pharmacol. Ther.*, *23*, 338–345.

Ruffin, R. E., Alpers, J. H., Crockett, A. J., and Hamilton, R. (1981), Repeated histamine inhalation tests in asthmatic patients, *J. Allergy Clin. Immunol.*, *67*, 285–289.

Ruffin, R. E., McIntyre, E., Crockett, A. J., Zielonka, K., and Alpers, J. H. (1982), Combination therapy in asthma, *J. Allergy Clin. Immunol.*, *69*, 60–65.

Ryan, G., Latimer, K. M., Juniper, E. F., Roberts, R. S., and Hargreaves, F. E. (1985), Effect of beclomethasone diproprionate on bronchial responsiveness to histamine in controlled non-steroid-dependent asthma, *J. Allergy Clin. Immunol.*, *75*, 25–30.

Salome, C. M., Schoeffel, R. E., and Woolcock, A. J. (1981), Effect of aerosol and oral fenoterol on histamine and methacholine challenge in asthmatic subjects, *Thorax*, *36*, 580–584.

Salome, C. M., Schoeffel, R. E., Yan, K., and Woolcock, A. J. (1983), Effect of aerosol fenoterol on the severity of bronchial hyperreactivity in patients with asthma, *Thorax*, *38*, 854–858.

Sears, M. R., Taylor, D. R., Print, C. G., et al. (1990), Regular inhaled beta-agonist treatment in bronchial asthma, *Lancet*, *336*, 1391–1396.

Sheppard, D., Epstein, J., Skoogh, B. E., Bethel, R. A., Nadel, J. A., and Boushey, H. A. (1984), Variable inhibition of histamine-induced bronchoconstriction by atropine in subjects with asthma, *J. Allergy Clin. Immunol.*, *73*, 82–87.

Sherter, C. B., Connolly, J. J., and Schilder, D. P. (1978), The significance of volume-adjusting the maximal midexpiratory flow in assessing the response to a bronchodilator drug, *Chest*, *73*, 568–571.

Silverman, M., and Anderson, S. D. (1972), Standardization of exercise tests in asthmatic children, *Arch. Dis. Child.*, *47*, 882–889.

Simonsson, B. G., Jacobs, F. M., and Nadel, J. A. (1967), Role of autonomic nervous system and the cough reflux in the increased responsiveness of airways in patients with obstructive airway disease, *J. Clin. Invest.*, *46*, 1812–1818.

Simonsson, B. G., Jonson, B., and Ström, B. (1975), Bronchodilatory and circulatory effects of inhaling increasing doses of anti-cholinergic drug, ipratropium bromide (Sch 1000), *Scand. J. Respir. Dis.*, *56*, 138–149.

Smelzer, T. H., and Barnett, T. B. (1973), Bronchodilator aerosol. Comparison of administration methods, *JAMA*, *223*, 844–889.

Smith, J. A., Weber, R. W., and Nelson, H. S. (1980), Theophylline and aerosolized terbutaline in the treatment of bronchial asthma. Double-blind comparison of optimal doses, *Chest*, *78*, 816–818.

Snider, G. L. (1974), Criteria for assessment of reversibility in airways obstruction. Report of the committee on emphysema, American College of Chest Physicians, *Chest*, *65*, 552–553.

Souhrada, J. F., and Dickey, D. W. (1976), Mechanical activities of trachea as measured *in vitro* and *in vivo*, *Respir. Physiol.*, *26*, 27–40.

Sourk, R. L., and Nugent, K. M. (1983), Bronchodilator testing: confidence intervals derived from placebo inhalations, *Am. Rev. Respir. Dis.*, *128*, 153–157.

Spector, S. L. (1978), Effect of beta-adrenergic agents on skin test responses and bronchial challenge responses, *Chest*, *73* (suppl), 976–977.

Spector, S. L., ed. (1989), *Provocative Challenge Procedures: Background and Methodology*, Futura Publishing Co., Mount Kisco, NY, 1989.

Spicer, J. E., Cayton, R. M., Frame, M. H., and Winsey, N. J. P. (1980), Influence of tube-spacer on aerosol efficacy, *Lancet*, *2*, 1248.

Stamm, A. M., Clausen, J. L., and Tisi, G. M. (1976), Effect of aerosolized isoproterenol on resting myogenic tone in normals, *J. Appl. Physiol.*, *40*, 525–532.

Storms, W. W., DoPico, G. A., and Reed, C. E. (1975), Aerosol Sch 1000. An anticholinergic bronchodilator, *Am. Rev. Respir. Dis.*, *111*, 419–422.

Stuart, B. O. (1973), Deposition of inhaled aerosols, *Arch. Intern. Med.*, *131*, 60–73.

Szentivanyi, A. (1968), The beta adrenergic theory of the atopic abnormality in bronchial asthma, *J. Allergy*, *42*, 203–232.

Taplin, G. V., Tashkin, D. P., Chopra, S. K., et al. (1977), Early detection of chronic obstructive pulmonary disease using radionuclide lung imaging procedures, *Chest*, *71*, 567–575.

Tashkin, D. P., Katz, R. M., Kerschnar, H., Rachelefsky, G. S., and Siegel, S. C. (1977), Comparison of aerosolized atropine, isoproterenol, atropine plus isoproterenol, disodium cromoglycate and placebo in the prevention of exercise-induced asthma, *Ann. Allergy*, *39*, 311–318.

Tashkin, D. P., Conolly, M. E., Deutsch, R. I., Hui, K. K., Littner, M., Scarpace, P., and Abrass, I. (1982), Subsensitization of beta-adrenoceptors in airways and lymphocyte of healthy and asthmatic subjects, *Am. Rev. Respir. Dis.*, *125*, 185–193.

Tashkin, D. P., Ashutosh, K., Bleecker, E. R., et al. (1986), Comparison of the anticholinergic bronchodilator ipratropium bromide with metaproterenol in chronic obstructive pulmonary disease: a 90-day multi-center study, *Am. J. Med.*, *81* (suppl 5A), 81–90.

Tashkin, D. P. (1991), Dosing strategies for bronchodilator aerosol delivery, *Respiratory Care*, *36*, 977–987.

Tashkin, D. P., Altose, M. D., Bleecker, E. R., et al. (1992), The Lung Health Study: airway responsiveness to inhaled methacholine in smokers with mild to moderate airflow limitation, *Am. Rev. Respir. Dis.*, *145*, 301–310.

Tattersfield, A. E. (1985), Tolerance to beta-agonists, *Bull. Eur. Physiopathol. Respir.*, *21*, 1s–5s.

Tattersfield, A. E. (1987), Effect of beta-agonists and anticholinergic drugs on bronchial reactivity, *Am. Rev. Respir. Dis.*, *136* (part 2), S64–S68.

Tattersfield, A. E., Leaver, D. G., and Pride, N. B. (1973), Effects of β-adrenergic blockade and stimulation on normal human airways, *J. Appl. Physiol.*, *35*, 613–619.

Thurlbeck, W. M., Pun, R., Toth, J., et al. (1974), Bronchial cartilage in chronic obstructive lung disease, *Am. Rev. Respir. Dis.*, *109*, 73–80.

Turner, J. R., Corkery, K. J., Eckman, D., et al. (1988), Equivalence of continuous flow nebulizer and MDI with reservoir bag for treatment of acute airflow obstruction, *Chest*, *93*, 476–581.

Tweeddale, P. M., Merchant, S., Leslie, M., et al. (1984), Short term variability in FEV_1: relation to pretest activity, level of FEV_1 and smoking habits, *Thorax*, *39*, 928–932.

Tweeddale, P. M., Alexander, F., and McHardy, G. J. R. (1987), Short term variability in FEV_1 and bronchodilator responsiveness in patients with obstructive ventilatory defects, *Thorax*, *42*, 487–490.

Twentyman, O. P., Finnerty, J. P., and Holgate, S. T. (1990), Time course of bronchodilation and functional antagonism of histamine-induced bronchoconstriction after salmeterol, *Thorax*, *45*, 786.

Twentyman, O. P., et al. (1990), Protection against allergen-induced asthma by salmeterol, *Lancet*, *336*, 1338–1342.

Ullah, M. I., Newman, G. B., and Saunders, K. B. (1981), Influence of age on response to ipratropium and salbutamol in asthma, *Thorax*, *36*, 523–529.

Ullman, A., and Svedmyr, N. (1988), Salmeterol, a new long-acting inhaled beta-2 adrenoceptor agonist: comparison with salbutamol in adult asthmatic patients, *Thorax*, *43*, 674–678.

Van Schayck, C. P., Graafsma, S. J., Visch, M. B., et al. (1990), Increased bronchial hyperresponsiveness after inhaling salbutamol during 1 year is not caused by subsensitization to salbutamol, *J. Allergy Clin. Immunol.*, *86*, 793–800.

Vathenen, A. S., Knox, A. J., Higgins, B. G., Britton, J. R., and Tattersfield, A. E. (1988), Rebound increase in bronchial responsiveness after treatment with inhaled terbutaline, *Lancet*, *1*, 554–557.

Vincent, N. J., Knudson, R., Leith, D. E., Macklem, P. T., and Mead, J. (1970), Factors influencing pulmonary resistance, *J. Appl. Physiol.*, *29*, 236–242.

Waalkens, H. J., Van Essen-Zandvliet, E. E., Hughes, M. D. et al. (1993), Cessation of long-term treatment with inhaled corticosteroid (budesonide) in children with asthma results in deterioration, *Am. Rev. Respir. Dis.*, *148*, 1252–1257.

Watanabe, S., Renzetti, A. D., Jr., and Begin, R. (1974), Airway responsiveness to a bronchodilator aerosol, *Am. Rev. Respir. Dis.*, *109*, 530–537.

Weir, D. C., Sherwood Burge, P. (1991), Measures of reversibility in response to bronchodilators in chronic airflow obstruction: relation to airway calibre, *Thorax*, *46*, 43–45.

Wiggs, B. R., Bosken, C., Paré, P. D., et al. (1992), A model of airway narrowing in asthma and in chronic obstructive pulmonary disease, *Am. Rev. Respir. Dis.*, *145*, 1251–1258.

Williams, M. H., Jr., and Kane, C. (1975), Dose response of patients with asthma to inhaled isoproterenol, *Am. Rev. Respir. Dis.*, *111*, 321–324.

Wolfe, J. D., Tashkin, D. P., Calvarese, B., and Simmons, M. (1978), Bronchodilator effects of terbutaline and aminophylline alone and in combination in asthmatic patients, *N. Engl. J. Med.*, *298*, 363–367.

Wong, B. J., Dolovich, J., Ramsdale, E. H., et al. (1992), Formoterol compared with beclomethasone and placebo on allergen-induced asthmatic responses, *Am. Rev. Respir. Dis.*, *146*, 1156–1160.

Wood, M. J., and Paterson, J. W. (1975), Evaluation of cumulative doses of Sch 1000 in asthmatics (abstr.), *Postgrad. Med. J.*, *51* (suppl 7), 100.

Wright, B. M., and McKerrow, C. B. (1959), Maximum forced expiratory flow rate as a measure of ventilatory capacity, *Br. Med. J.*, *2* (2), 1041–1047.

Yan, K., Salome, C. M., and Woolcock, A. J. (1985), Prevalence and nature of bronchial hyperresponsiveness in subjects with chronic obstructive pulmonary disease, *Am. Rev. Respir. Dis.*, *132*, 25–29.

Yeager, H., Jr., Weinberg, R. M., Kaufman, L. V., and Katz, S. (1976), Asthma: comparative bronchodilator effects of ipratropium bromide and isoproterenol, *J. Clin. Pharmacol.*, *16*, 198–204.

Zamel, N., Hughes, D., Levison, H., Fairshter, R. D., and Gelb, A. F. (1983), Partial and complete maximum expiratory flow–volume curves in patients with spontaneous bronchospasm, *Chest*, *83*, 35–39.

21

Airway Hyperresponsiveness in "Irreversible" Chronic Obstructive Pulmonary Disease

Donald P. Tashkin, Murray D. Altose, John E. Connett, Richard E. Kanner, Wondra Wong Lee, Robert Wise, and the Lung Health Study Research Group

UCLA Medical Center
Los Angeles, California

I. INTRODUCTION

Airway hyperresponsiveness (AHR) to a variety of provocative stimuli is a cardinal feature of asthma, in which condition it appears to be due, in large part, to inflammatory changes in the airways that can be modified by anti-inflammatory therapy. Several studies have also demonstrated an association between nonasthmatic chronic obstructive pulmonary disease (COPD) and airway hyperresponsiveness to nonspecific pharmacological constrictor agonists [1–6]. Comparisons of AHR in COPD and asthma reveal significant differences in frequency, extent, and nature, possibly due to differing mechanisms of this phenomenon in these two types of disorder. This chapter briefly reviews the prevalence and severity of AHR in COPD, examines its determinants, and discusses its prognostic and therapeutic implications. In addition, recently published data on methacholine responsiveness in a large sample of smokers with early COPD participating in a nationwide trial of early intervention (the Lung Health Study) are reviewed.

II. PREVALENCE AND SEVERITY OF AHR IN COPD

In relatively small samples (n = 27–59) of smokers or ex-smokers with historical characteristics of COPD (chronic cough and/or breathlessness but no history of asthma or clinical features suggestive of asthma), a higher *prevalence* (46–77%) of AHR to histamine (H) or methacholine (M) ($PD_{20} \leqslant 3.9$ μmol H; $PC_{20} < 16$

mg/ml M) than that expected in healthy subjects has been observed [2–4]. Furthermore, the *degree* of AHR noted in patients with COPD is often in the asthmatic range of sensitivity to histamine or methacholine; for example, 19 of 27 COPD patients studied by Ramsdale et al. [2] had values for $PC_{20} < 8$ mg/ml. On the other hand, the degree of AHR in COPD is generally less than that noted in asthma with respect to both *sensitivity* (i.e., position of the dose–response curve) and *reactivity* (i.e., slope of the linear portion of the dose–response curve). In one series, 27 patients with COPD with a positive reaction to histamine had a mean $PD_{20}FEV_1$ of 1.62 μmol, compared with an average PD_{20} of 0.23 μmol in 17 asthmatics with a comparable prechallenge baseline FEV_1 (Fig. 1). Brand and colleagues [6] also observed a significantly lower $PC_{20}H$ in 81 asthmatics than in 44 COPD patients, all with moderately severe airway obstruction, even when comparisons were made at similar levels of baseline lung function. Furthermore, Bel et al. [7] noted less reactivity to both histamine and methacholine, as indicated by significantly less steep dose–response slopes, in 11 patients with COPD than in 12 asthmatic patients, even though the baseline FEV_1 (as a percent of predicted) was lower in the former patients (Fig. 2).

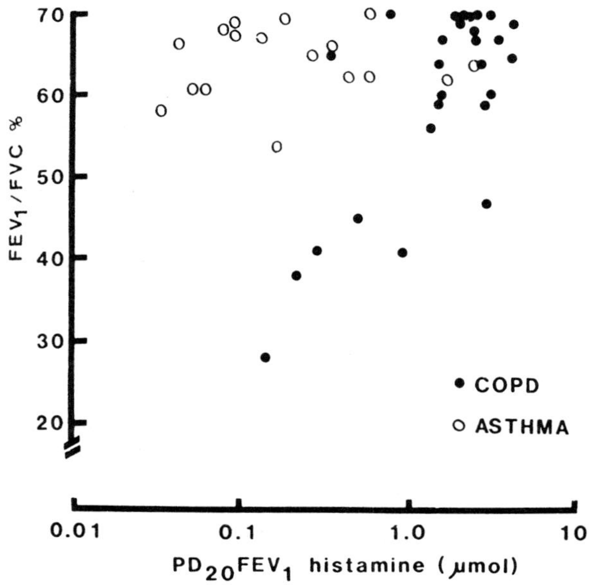

Figure 1 The relationship between FEV_1/FVC and $PD_{20}FEV_1$ values in subjects with chronic obstructive pulmonary disease (COPD) and asthmatic subjects. (From Ref. 4.)

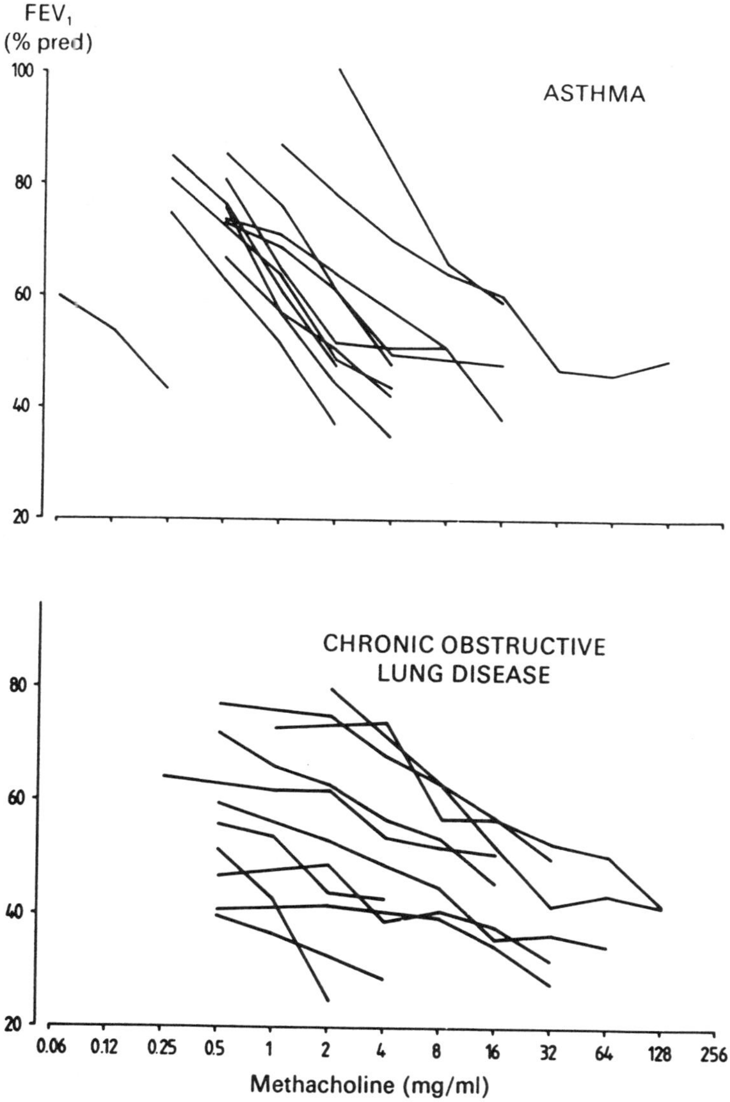

Figure 2 Individual dose–response curves for inhaled methacholine (expressed in FEV_1, % predicted) in 12 asthmatic patients and 11 patients with chronic obstructive pulmonary disease. (From Ref. 7.)

III. DEPENDENCE OF AHR IN COPD ON BASELINE AIRWAY CALIBER

A consistently reported feature of nonspecific AHR in COPD is its dependence on the baseline degree of airway obstruction [1,3–6,8]. Among COPD patients exhibiting a broad range of airway obstruction, strong correlations (r = 0.72–0.86; $p<0.001$) have been noted between sensitivity to histamine or methacholine and the prechallenge FEV_1 or FEV_1/FVC ratio [2,4] (Fig. 2), although no correlation was found in patients with a normal or nearly normal baseline FEV_1 [4]. In contrast, findings in asthmatic subjects have been inconsistent; a significant relationship between the level of AHR and baseline lung function in asthma has been observed by some authors (r = 0.42–0.49; $p<0.02$) [9,10] but not by others [4,11] (Fig. 2). It is also noteworthy that AHR is significantly less common in patients with early COPD and only minimal airway obstruction than in patients with more advanced disease, whereas AHR of varying severity is present in nearly all patients with asthma, including those with normal lung function.

IV. MECHANISMS OF AHR IN COPD

The dependence of AHR on the level of baseline lung function in COPD and its relative independence of starting airway caliber in asthma suggest that differing pathophysiological mechanisms underlie AHR in these two types of obstructive pulmonary disease. The strong influence of the prechallenge FEV_1 on AHR in COPD suggests that functional geometrical factors are probably an important determinant of AHR in this condition, while inflammatory mechanisms play a more critical role in the "true" AHR of asthma. According to well-known geometrical principles of aerodynamics [12,13], airway resistance, and therefore FEV_1, is related to the fourth or fifth power of the airway diameter; consequently, the same absolute degree of airway smooth muscle contraction in response to a constrictor stimulus would lead to a disproportionately greater increase in airway resistance (or decrease in FEV_1) in a narrowed airway as compared with a normal-size airway. Increased thickness of the airway wall and/or increased secretions partially occluding the airway lumen, as found in COPD, can also increase airway reactivity by a functional geometrical mechanism that leads to greater narrowing for a given degree of airway smooth muscle contraction in a thick-walled or partially occluded airway than in a thin-walled, fully patent airway [14,15]. Furthermore, alterations in the amount or stiffness of tracheobronchial cartilage, as has been reported in COPD [8,16], could predispose to AHR by reducing the load on airway smooth muscle that normally opposes smooth muscle shortening in cartilaginous airways. Decreased lung elastic recoil due to emphysema could decrease the tethering effect of lung parenchyma on airways, thus also reducing the load on airway smooth muscle and increasing airway responsiveness [14]. It is also possible that the hypertrophy or hyperplasia of airway smooth muscle described in some patients with COPD or the airway inflammation and epithelial damage due to the disease process itself may be associated with increased bronchomotor tone that could contribute to both reduced baseline lung function and AHR. The positive association between nonspecific AHR and bronchodilator responsiveness noted by some authors [17] is consistent with this possibility. Finally, expressing airway responsiveness in terms of a percent decline in baseline FEV_1 could magnify the level of responsiveness in persons with reduced starting lung function.

Other mechanisms besides alterations in functional geometry due to airway damage and narrowing could also account for the increased prevalence of AHR in COPD. First, *cigarette smoking* itself may have an independent causal effect on both AHR and COPD in persons with initially normal airway responsiveness. Evidence from population studies [12,13,18–20] and small convenience samples of smokers and nonsmokers [21,22] suggests that cigarette smoking itself may have a positive effect on AHR independent of airway obstruction, possibly because of effects on bronchial inflammation, mucosal permeability, immune responses, or airway smooth muscle itself [18]. On the other hand, other studies show either a questionable or an absent relationship between smoking and AHR [19,23–28]. Second, smokers with preexisting AHR due to genetic or environmental factors unrelated to smoking may be more likely to develop COPD, as suggested by Dutch investigators [29,30]. Third, smoking may in some persons cause airway inflammation that in turn leads first to AHR and later to airway damage and narrowing. Additional research is needed to distinguish among these possible mechanisms.

V. DIFFERENCES IN AHR BETWEEN COPD AND ASTHMA

Besides a disparity in prevalence, severity, and relationship to baseline lung function, other differences between the nonspecific AHR of COPD and that of asthma have been noted. Mention has already been made of the differences in *shape* of the histamine or methacholine dose–response curves, patients with asthma exhibiting steeper dose–response slopes than those with COPD. In addition, asthmatic patients characteristically display excessive airway narrowing following increasing doses of histamine or methacholine, in which a *maximal response plateau* usually cannot be demonstrated even after falls in FEV_1 as large as 60% from baseline, in contrast to the reproducible maximal response exhibited by normal subjects at relatively mild degrees of airway narrowing (equivalent to a 15–45% decline in FEV_1) [31,32]. In 14 of 16 smokers with mild COPD (mean FEV_1/FVC 66.9%), Du Toit et al. [33] noted a maximal response plateau after only a 30–50% fall in FEV_1, comparable to findings in normal subjects but less than the maximal declines observed in asthmatic patients with similar histamine sensitivity. On the other hand, Bel and colleagues [7] were able to demonstrate a maximal response plateau to histamine or methacholine in only a minority of patients with either COPD (mean FEV_1 61.6% predicted) (3–4 of 11 patients) or asthma (0–3 of 12 patients), suggesting that excessive airway narrowing may also be a feature of moderately severe COPD.

Another discrepancy between the AHR of COPD and that of asthma is that the hypersensitivity in COPD appears to be limited mainly to nonspecific pharmacological agents, such as histamine and methacholine. Unlike asthmatic patients, in whom methacholine responsiveness correlates with responsiveness to isocapnic hyperventilation of cold air, only a small minority of patients with COPD with AHR to methacholine in the asthmatic range exhibit cold-air responsiveness [2,34] (Fig. 3). These results are consistent with the concept that the apparent hyperresponsiveness of COPD patients to nonspecific pharmacological constrictor agonists is a reflection mainly of decreased airway caliber, and that cold-air hyperventilation (respiratory heat loss), in contrast to methacholine or histamine, does not provoke airway smooth muscle contraction directly, but rather indirectly; for example, through mediators that are more readily released in asthma. On the other hand, a majority of subjects with both COPD and asthma studied by

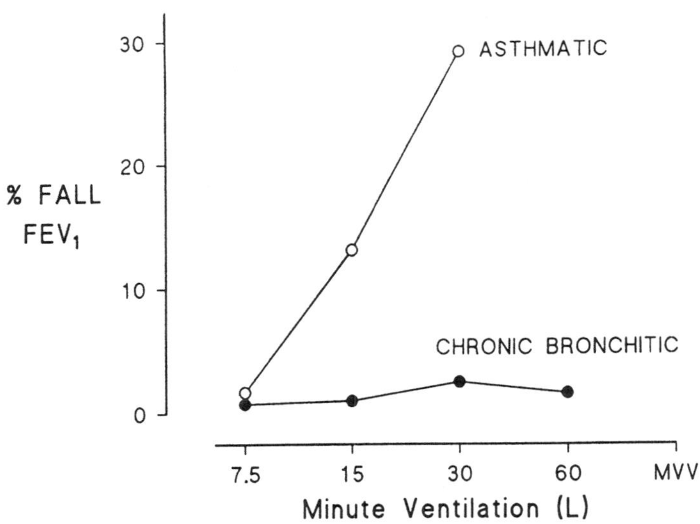

Figure 3 Change in FEV_1 after isocapnic hyperventilation in an asthmatic subject (baseline FEV_1, 2.2 L; methacholine PC_{20}, 0.2 mg/ml) and a subject with chronic obstructive pulmonary disease (COPD) (baseline FEV_1, 2.1 L; methacholine PC_{20}, 0.24 mg/ml). The asthmatic, but not the patient with COPD, developed bronchoconstriction after isocapnic hyperventilation. (From Ref. 3.)

Woolcock et al. [32] responded to an osmotic stimulus (4.5% saline), although the COPD patients required larger provocative doses of hypertonic saline and displayed shallower dose–response slopes than the asthmatics. Asthmatic subjects characteristically develop bronchoconstriction in response to inhaled propranolol [32], whereas only a few patients with COPD do so and normal subjects are not responsive. Finally, smokers with mild COPD, even those with responses to histamine in the asthmatic range, rarely respond to the α-adrenoreceptor stimulant methoxamine [33], in contrast to findings in asthmatic subjects [35], in whom it has been speculated that methoxamine causes bronchoconstriction through the release of humoral mediators.

Patients with COPD and those with asthma also differ with respect to their relative sensitivity to histamine vs. methacholine. Of 26 patients with mild COPD studied by Woolcock et al. [32], 24 were more sensitive to histamine than to equimolar doses of methacholine [32,33] (Fig. 4); similar findings were reported by Bel and colleagues [7]. In contrast, asthmatic subjects typically display similar degrees of sensitivity to histamine and methacholine [7,32,33,36,37] (Fig. 4). The reason for this discrepancy is not known, but it could reflect differing

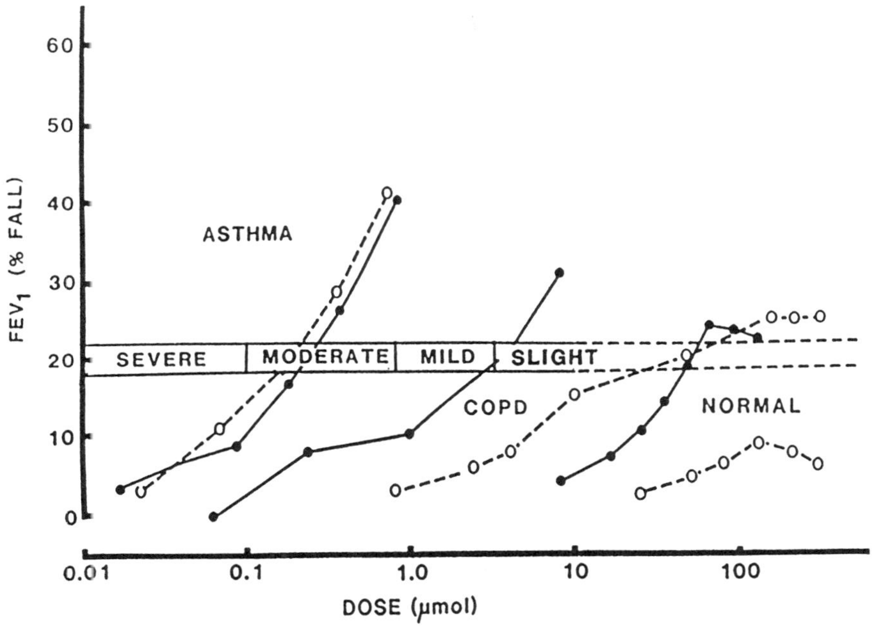

Figure 4 Typical dose–response curves to histamine (solid circles) and methacholine (open circles) in an asthmatic, a subject with chronic obstructive pulmonary disease (COPD), and a normal subject. (From Ref. 32.)

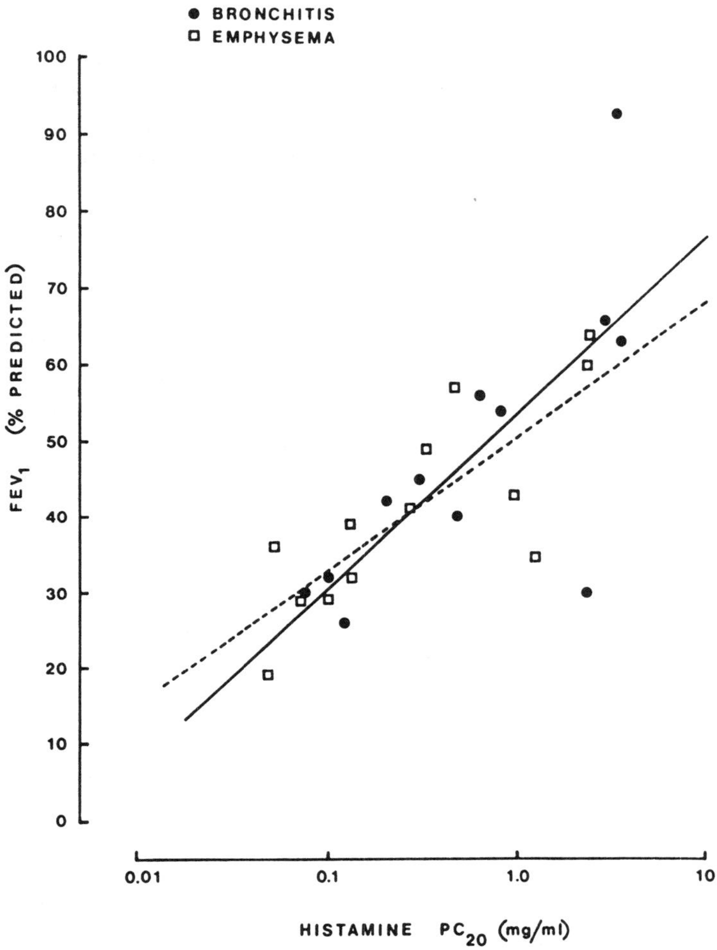

Figure 5 Regression of $\log_{10}$ PC_{20} (mg/ml) on horizontal axis vs. FEV_1 (% predicted) on vertical axis of two groups. Regression lines for emphysema ($y = 17.6x + 50.6$, $r = 0.79$; $p<0.001$) and bronchitis ($y = 23.3x + 53.9$, $r = 0.73$; $p<0.01$) were essentially identical. (From Ref. 5.)

densities and/or agonist affinities of muscarinic vs. histamine receptors in the two types of disorder.

VI. SIMILARITY IN AHR BETWEEN EMPHYSEMA AND CHRONIC OBSTRUCTIVE BRONCHITIS

Verma and co-workers [5] compared AHR to histamine in two types of patient with nonasthmatic COPD: those with nonemphysematous intrinsic airway disease and chronic bronchitis (mucous hypersecretion) vs. those with emphysema predominantly, without chronic bronchitis. The authors hypothesized that bronchitic patients with predominant intrinsic airways disease would be more responsive to a bronchoconstrictor agonist (histamine) than those with mainly emphysema and little bronchitis. However, in these two groups of COPD patients, similar degrees of airway responsiveness to histamine were found, and in each group, the AHR showed similarly strong correlations with the baseline percent predicted FEV_1 (r = 0.73-79) [5] (Fig. 5). These findings provide additional evidence that in COPD, AHR is due mainly to altered airway geometry, and furthermore, that it is independent of whether the major mechanism of the airflow limitation is reduced elastic recoil secondary to parenchymal lung destruction (emphysema) or increased peripheral airway resistance secondary to intrinsic damage to the small airways (chronic obstructive bronchitis).

VII. PROGNOSTIC AND THERAPEUTIC IMPLICATIONS OF AHR IN COPD

As summarized by O'Connor et al. [38], longitudinal studies of persons with [39–41] and without [42–44] established COPD have shown an association between AHR and accelerated rates of decline in lung function, even after adjustment for baseline lung function [40–42]. These findings are consistent with the "Dutch hypothesis" that AHR may be an inherent risk factor that predisposes particularly "susceptible" smokers to the development of progressive COPD [29,30]. The concept that AHR is etiologically important in the development of COPD is supported by a prospective study in which airway obstruction developed more readily in initially hyperresponsive compared with normally responsive iron workers without evidence of airways obstruction initially [45]. On the other hand, it has been suggested that AHR follows, rather than precedes, the development of progressive airway obstruction in the "susceptible" smoker, consistent with the concept that AHR is the *result*, rather than a *cause*, of the airway damage and pathophysiological changes produced by smoking. This possibility is supported by findings from a 4-year prospective study in which AHR progressed in parallel with worsening airway obstruction in 27 continuing smokers, while AHR and airway obstruction both remained stable in 16 ex-smokers who continued to refrain from smoking [46]. Additional prospective epidemiological studies are required, however, to determine whether AHR follows or predates the development of COPD.

If AHR does play a causal role in the evolution of COPD, pharmacological suppression of the hyperreactive state could potentially add to the benefit of other preventive measures, such as smoking cessation, in slowing progression of the disease. This possibility is indirectly supported by findings from two prospective studies demonstrating a slower rate of decline of lung function in those patients with chronic airflow obstruction who were more responsive to a bronchodilator initially and received maintenance bronchodilator therapy [47,48]. In the absence of bronchodilator therapy, on the other hand, bronchodilator responsiveness has been found to be associated with an accelerated annual decline in lung function in patients with chronic bronchitis and/or emphysema [40,41,49]. Since bronchodilator responsiveness also appears to be correlated with methacholine responsiveness [40], these data imply that while heightened responsiveness of the airways to either bronchoconstrictor or bronchodilator compounds predicts an adverse longitudinal decline in lung function, pharmacological modulation of AHR, e.g., by reduction in bronchomotor tone, may be particularly beneficial in persons with COPD and hyperreactive airways. More recent data for patients with COPD, suggesting a favorable effect of corticosteroid therapy on measures of airway inflammation [50] and, when combined with a β-adrenergic bronchodilator, on airways reactivity and the annual decline in FEV_1 [51] are also consistent with this concept.

VIII. THE LUNG HEALTH STUDY

The hypothesis that regular "preventive" therapy with an inhaled bronchodilator may slow the accelerated fall in FEV_1 in smokers with early COPD is currently being tested by the Lung Health Study (LHS). The LHS is a 10-center clinical trial, supported by the National Heart, Lung, and Blood Institute, that is evaluating the impact of early intervention on the annual rate of decline in lung function and on respiratory morbidity in smokers with mild to moderate airflow limitation who are at high risk for developing symptomatic COPD [52]. Nearly 6000 cigarette smokers (63% male) 35–59 years of age (mean 48.5 ± 6.8 years) with an FEV_1/FVC ratio of ≤70% (mean 63.0% ± 5.5%) and an FEV_1 55–90% of predicted who were in good general health were enrolled in the study between November 1986 and January 1989. Enrollment followed a three-stage screening process that included spirometry before and after inhalation of 180 μl isoproterenol from a metered-dose inhaler and, on a separate day, an inhalation challenge with methacholine. Methacholine challenge tests (MCTs) were performed according to an abbreviated modification of the Chai protocol [53] using a manually triggered dosimeter and a DeVilbiss 646 nebulizer powered by compressed air at 20 psi and delivering 0.01054 ± 0.00127 ml per actuation; methacholine solutions were administered in a sequence of 0.0 (diluent), 1.0, 5.0, 10.0, and 25.0 mg/ml, as previously described [54]. If the FEV_1 at the end of the MCT was $\geq$10% below the diluent control value, isoproterenol (0.15μg) was administered.

After completion of the MCT, participants were randomly assigned to receive "usual care" (no intervention) or "special intervention." The latter consisted of a state-of-the-art smoking-cessation and relapse-prevention program with nicotine replacement and maintenance therapy with two inhalations from a metered-dose inhaler containing either placebo or a bronchodilator (ipratropium bromide, 40 μg per inhalation). Assignment to the placebo vs. active bronchodilator was random and double-blind. Following an initial intensive smoking-cessation program, special-intervention participants are followed every 4 months to monitor and reinforce adherence to the intervention measures. All participants are evaluated annually for 5 years with a detailed respiratory questionnaire and spirometry before and after a bronchodilator. Within a month of the fifth annual visit, a second MCT is performed.

Methacholine challenge tests conducted during the third screening visit were successfully completed in 5666 LHS participants. The results permit determination of (1) the feasibility and safety of MCTs in middle-aged smokers with mild to moderate airflow limitation, (2) the prevalence and severity of AHR in a large group of smokers with early COPD, (3) the association between AHR and clinical and physiological variables in this population, (4) the relationship between baseline AHR and subsequent decline in lung function, (5) the impact of smoking cessation and/or maintenance bronchodilator therapy on AHR and the associated age-related decline in lung function, and (6) the influence of baseline AHR on response to smoking cessation and/or bronchodilator treatment. Since only cross-sectional data from the LHS are currently available, only the first three of the above six objectives can be addressed at this time.

A. Feasibility and Safety of Methacholine Challenge Tests

Of 5887 eligible participants with physiological evidence of early COPD, MCTs were successfully completed in more than 96%; 10 refused methacholine challenge testing, and 211 (3.6%) had the MCT prematurely terminated because of symptoms induced by the test, subject refusal to continue, or a spirometer or computer problem. Of the first 4918 MCTs, for which technician-recorded comments on adverse reactions were open-ended, symptoms induced by inhalation of methacholine were recorded in only 246 (5%). Of the last 969 tests, for which technicians were required to answer specific questions regarding the presence and severity of symptomatic reactions to methacholine, one or more specific symptoms were noted in 356 (37%) participants: cough (25%); shortness of breath (21%); wheezing (9.5%); dizziness (6%); headache (2%); other symptoms (5%); any one or more symptoms (37%). The reliability of these results may be questioned, however, since completely uniform or standardized procedures were not used in implementing the symptom checklist, as suggested by the wide variability in the frequency of recorded symptomatic reactions from center to center (7.2–92.7%). Nonetheless, most of the recorded symptoms were mild and transient, and rarely (<1%) was the MCT discontinued because of symptoms. Initially, there had been concern that commencing the test with five inhalations of 1 mg/ml methacholine might induce severe bronchospasm in sensitive subjects, particularly those with moderately reduced starting lung function (minimum baseline FEV_1 48% of predicted; average 74.8% of predicted). However, even though methacholine-induced declines in FEV_1 were as large as 76.2% (average 26.5%) and the FEV_1 after the last dose of methacholine was as low as 16.2% of predicted (average 58.3% of predicted), the test proved to be remarkably safe. These results are in agreement with previous studies demonstrating the safety of MCTs in other populations, including subjects with both healthy and diseased airways (Table 1). Findings from the LHS, as well as those of Ramsdell and coworkers [1], suggest that published guidelines recommending restriction of bronchial challenges with nonspecific pharmacological bronchoconstrictors to subjects with normal or nearly normal lung function [55] may not be applicable to COPD.

B. Prevalence and Severity of AHR in LHS Men and Women

Of the 5666 LHS participants successfully completing the MCT, 412 (7.3%) had physician-diagnosed asthma. Characteristics of the remaining 5264 participants without asthma are listed in Table 2. Among the nonasthmatic subjects with

Table 1 Safety of Methacholine (Mch) Challenge Tests (MCTs)

Townley (1979)	1500 MCTs in normal, rhinitic, and asthmatic subjects
	Effects of MCT short-lived, easily reversed with isopreterenol, never required hospitalization, never delayed in onset
Spector (1989)	2/? asthmatics with Mch-induced bronchospasm resistant to bronchodilator treatment and persisting for hours
Hendrick (1986)	255 healthy polyurethane workers challenged with Mch
	27% complained of symptoms, mainly cough, wheeze or sore throat, regardless whether MCT was + or −
	Symptoms rarely severe, mostly resolved within 5 h
Ramsdell (1982)	MCTs in 22 patients with severe COPD (FEV_1 < 1 L)
	12/22 developed annoying shortness of breath and cough associated with significant bronchospastic responses to Mch
	Symptoms similar to spontaneous exacerbations of COPD
	All symptoms responded promptly to inhaled bronchodilator

COPD = chronic obstructive pulmonary disease.

Table 2 Demographic and Smoking Characteristics and Lung Function of Participants Undergoing Methacholine Challenge Testing (Physician-Confirmed Asthmatics Excluded)

	Total (n = 5254)		Men (n = 3314)		Women (n = 1940)	
	Mean	SD	Mean	SD	Mean	SD
Age (yr)	48.7	6.8	48.6	6.9	48.7	6.5
Height (m)	1.72	0.09	1.77	0.07	1.64	0.06
Cigarettes/day[a]	31.4	12.9	32.7	13.3	29.1	11.8
Years smoked	31.2	7.4	31.5	7.6	30.5	7.0
Pack-years	40.8	19.2	43.2	20.1	36.6	17.0
FEV_1 (% predicted)[b]	75.3	8.8	75.3	8.8	75.2	8.8
FEV_1/FVC (%)[b]	65.7	5.9	65.6	6.0	65.9	5.7

[a]At screening day 1.
[b]At screening day 2, pre-bronchodilator.
FEV_1 = forced expired volume in 1 second; FVC = forced vital capacity.

COPD, a high proportion of men (45.4%) and a significantly higher proportion of women (73.8%) responded to 10 mg/ml of methacholine (Fig. 6). (Positive responses were defined as a ≥20% decline in FEV_1 after inhalation of three to five breaths of either diluent or the designated concentration of methacholine; <1% of participants were diluent responders). Interestingly, nearly 50% of nonasthmatic women and 25% of nonasthmatic men had provocative concentrations of methacholine in the asthmatic range ($PC_{20} \leq 5$ mg/ml). The difference between the proportion of male and female responders was highly significant ($p < 0.001$) and was apparent in all ranges of age and baseline severity of airflow obstruction. Although some studies have shown smoking to be related to AHR independent of baseline lung function [6,12,13,20,22,56,57], the discrepancy between the intensity and duration of smoking between LHS men and women was relatively small (32.7 vs. 29.1 cigarettes/day and 31.5 vs. 30.5 years smoked, respectively) and thereby unlikely to account for the sex-related differences in AHR.

C. Association Between AHR and Physiological Demographic, and Clinical Characteristics

The greater degree of baseline airways obstruction, the higher the proportion of both men and women with positive responses to methacholine (Fig. 7). Among participants with moderate airflow obstruction (FEV_1 approximately 59–65% of predicted), >90% of women and approximately 75% of men had PC_{20} FEV_1 values ≤10 mg/ml. Even among participants with FEV_1 values ≥80% of predicted, a relatively high proportion (approximately 60% of women and nearly 30%

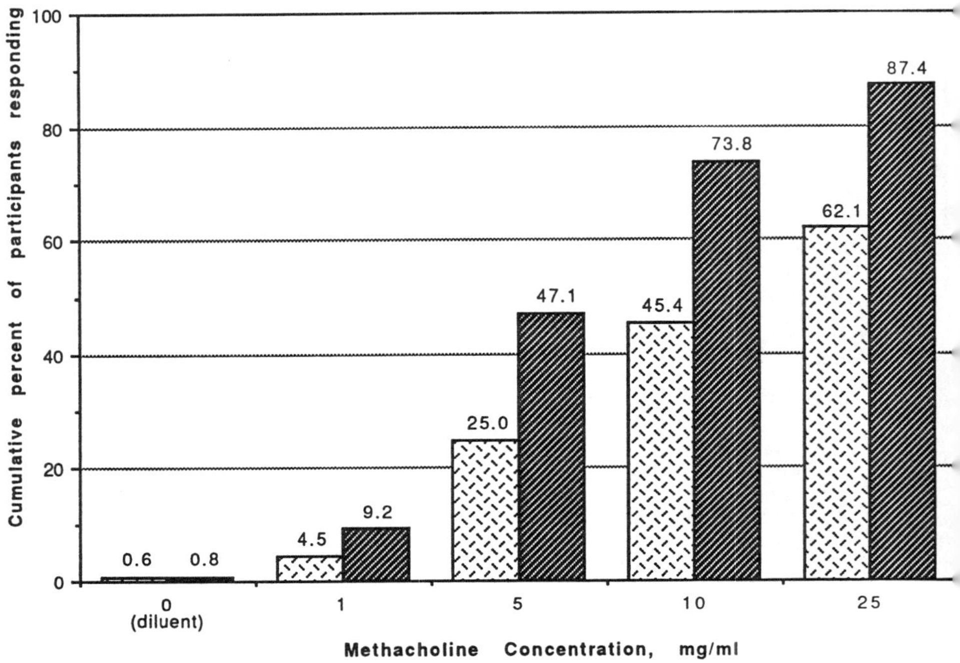

Figure 6 Cumulative percentages of Lung Health Study men (speckled bars, n = 3314) and women (hatched bars, n = 1940) without a physician-confirmed diagnosis of asthma who responded to diluent and 1, 5, 10, and 25 mg/ml of methacholine with a ≥20% decline in FEV_1 from baseline. The baseline value used to calculate the response to diluent was the prediluent FEV_1. The baseline value for calculating the response to each concentration of methacholine was the postdiluent FEV_1.

of men) responded to 10 mg/ml methacholine; however, these subjects had FEV_1/FVC ratios ≤70%, suggesting the presence of obstructive airway disease despite an FEV_1 in the statistically normal range. Moreover, for both men and women, logistic regression showed a strong effect of baseline lung function (p <0.001) on the proportion of responders to ≤10 and ≤5 mg/ml of methacholine. These findings are in agreement with observations by previous investigators of a significant positive relationship between the presence or level of AHR and the degree of obstructive ventilatory impairment in much smaller samples of persons with COPD [3,4,39,58]. Possible mechanisms that might explain the association between AHR and baseline lung function have been discussed previously [14,15,16,59,60] (see above).

Table 3 summarizes the results of logistic regression analyses of the associations between responsiveness to ≤10 mg/ml methacholine and various physiologi-

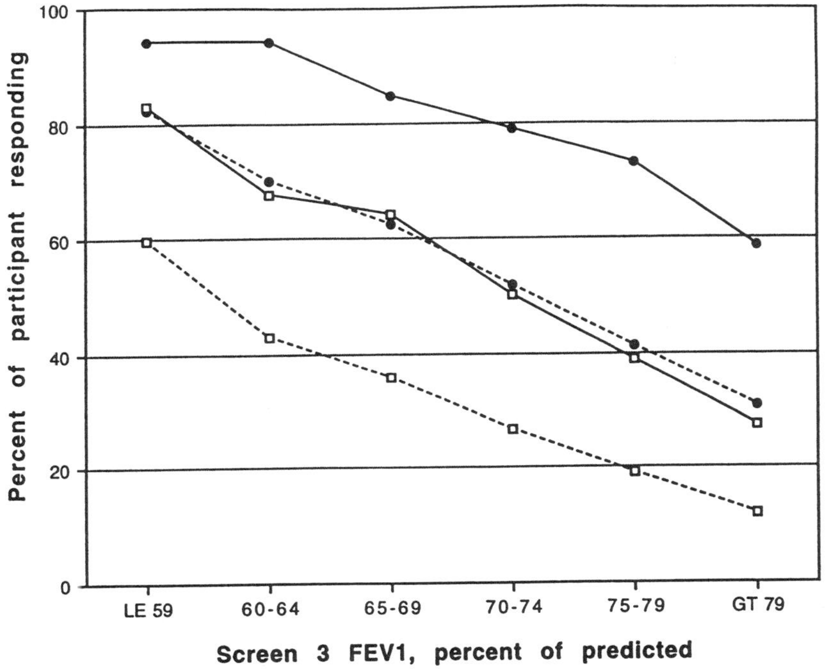

Figure 7 Percentages of Lung Health Study men and women without a physician-confirmed diagnosis of asthma responding to ≤10 and ≤5 mg/ml concentrations of methacholine with a ≥20% decline in FEV_1 from baseline, by baseline FEV_1, % predicted. Solid circles, solid lines = women, 10 mg/ml; open squares, solid lines = men, 10 mg/ml; solid circles, dashed lines = women, 5 mg/ml; open squares, dashed lines = men, 5 mg/ml.

cal and clinical characteristics of LHS participants with COPD who did not have physician-confirmed asthma and were not receiving regular bronchodilator therapy. As already noted, *sex* and *baseline lung function* were strongly associated with AHR. Consequently, analyses were performed for men and women separately, and adjustments were made for baseline FEV_1 and FEV_1/FVC ratio. Neither *age* nor *clinical center* had a significant effect in either sex, but both were included in the model. After adjustment for baseline lung function, age, and clinical center, among men, significant associations were found between AHR and the symptoms of chronic cough and/or phlegm and wheeze and pack-years of cigarette smoking. In women, AHR was associated only with wheeze. In neither men nor women was a significant association noted between AHR and the following: shortness of breath, physician-confirmed hay fever or emphysema, current smoking amount (cigarettes/day), or bronchodilator responsiveness.

Table 3 Odds Ratios of Positive Methacholine Challenge Test Associated with Specified Changes in Predictor Variables and 95% Confidence Intervals, Based on Logistic Regression

		Men		Women	
	Δ[a]	Odds ratio	95% CI	Odds ratio	95% CI
Factors entered in all models					
FEV_1 % predicted at screening day 2	10%	0.52	[0.47, 0.58]S	0.62	[0.53, 0.72]S
FEV_1/FVC at screening day 2	10%	0.47	[0.40, 0.55]S	0.28	[0.21, 0.38]S
Age	10 yr	0.91	[0.82, 1.02]NS	0.86	[0.73, 1.02]NS
Clinical center indicator variables	—	—	—	—	—
Other predictors[b]					
Hay fever, M.D.-confirmed (0–1)[c]	1	1.12	[0.86, 1.46]NS	1.39	[0.94, 2.06]NS
Emphysema, M.D.-confirmed (0–1)[c]	1	0.98	[0.63, 1.53]NS	1.26	[0.60, 2.62]NS
Chronic bronchitis (0–1)[c]	1	1.25	[1.06, 1.48]S	1.00	[0.78, 1.29]NS
Chronic cough (0–1)[c]	1	1.21	[1.04, 1.41]S	1.10	[0.88, 1.38]NS
Chronic phlegm (0–1)[c]	1	1.26	[1.08, 1.47]S	1.04	[0.82, 1.32]NS
Wheezing score (0–3)[d]	3	1.45	[1.19, 1.77]S	1.58	[0.19, 2.10]S
Shortness of breath (0–5)[d]	5	1.54	[0.99, 2.39]NS	1.12	[0.70, 1.79]NS
Cigarettes/day at screening day 1	20	1.11	[0.99, 1.24]NS	1.01	[0.84, 1.21]NS
Pack-years	20	1.09	[1.00, 1.18]S	1.06	[0.92, 1.22]NS
Positive bronchodilator response	10	1.16	[0.99, 1.36]NS	1.12	[0.88, 1.41]NS

[a]Δ = change in variable on which odds ratio computation is based.
[b]Each "other predictor" effect is adjusted for FEV_1 % predicted, max. FEV_1/max. FVC, age, and clinical center.
[c]0 = absent; 1 = present.
[d]See text for definition of score.
FEV_1 = forced expired volume in 1 second; FVC = forced vital capacity; S = statistically significant; NS = not significant.

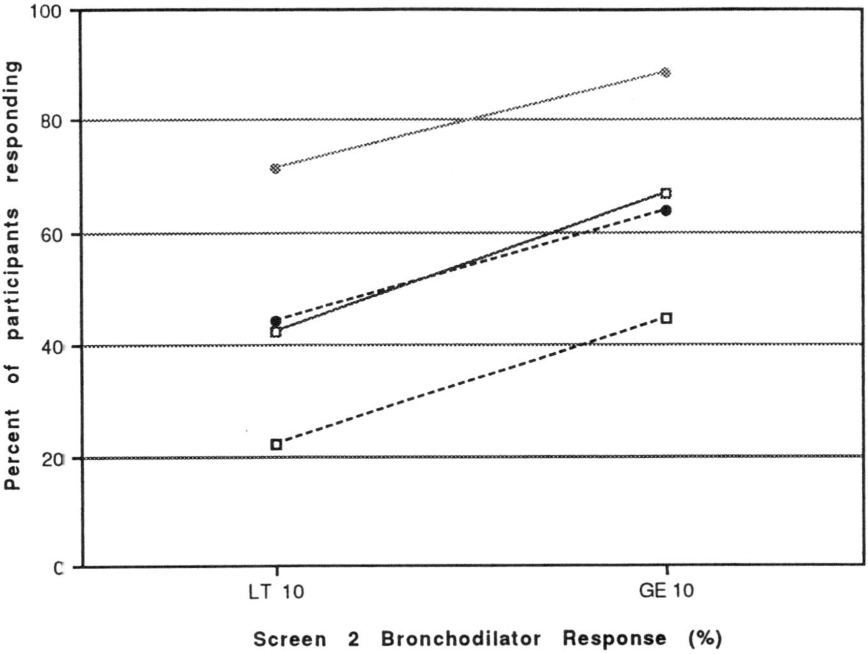

Figure 8 Percentage of Lung Health Study men and women without a physician-confirmed diagnosis of asthma responding to ≤10 and ≤5 mg/ml concentrations of methacholine by bronchodilator response category (<10% or ≥10% improvement in FEV_1 following isoproterenol at the second screening visit). Solid circles, solid lines = women, 10 mg/ml; open squares, solid lines = men, 10 mg/ml; solid circles, dashed lines = women, 5 mg/ml; open squares, dashed lines = men, 5 mg/ml.

Figure 8 illustrates the relationship between AHR and bronchodilator response unadjusted for baseline lung function. While a positive relationship was suggested, it is noteworthy that only a small minority of these subjects with early COPD (10% of men and 12% of women) responded to isoproterenol, with as little as 10% improvement in FEV_1. This finding may have been due to the exclusion of smokers with more severe airways obstruction and those receiving regular therapy with bronchodilators. However, despite these restrictions and in contrast to the low prevalence of bronchodilator responsiveness in this population, a relatively large proportion of participants still responded to methacholine.

It is of interest that *wheeze* was the only chronic respiratory symptom that was strongly associated with AHR in *both* male and female LHS participants; a relationship between wheeze and AHR has been noted previously in more general population studies [19,27,44,61]. These findings are consistent with a possible causal relationship, since nonspecific hyperresponsiveness could lead to symptoms following spontaneous exposures to constrictor stimuli. This possibility was suggested by Ramsdell et al. [1], whose patients with established COPD remarked on the similarity between their spontaneous symptoms and those induced by methacholine.

While findings from several [6,12,13,20–22,56,62] but not all [19,24–28] studies suggest an effect of *cigarette smoking* itself on AHR independent of baseline lung function, an association of AHR only with pack-years, but not with daily frequency, of cigarette smoking was apparent in LHS men, and no association with either current intensity or cumulative lifetime amount of smoking was noted in LHS women (Table 3). These negative findings could be due to the select nature of the LHS population, which was composed mainly of moderately heavy cigarette smokers (>1½ packs/day), thus narrowing the spectrum of cigarette exposure and diminishing the ability to demonstrate a dose–response relationship. In addition, all LHS participants already had airflow obstruction and therefore were more likely to exhibit AHR as either an etiological factor, or a result, of cigarette-related COPD.

The absence of a demonstrable relationship between *age* and AHR in the mostly middle-aged (35–59 years) smokers with early COPD participating in the LHS is consistent with findings from healthy populations of a nearly constant prevalence of AHR over a comparable age range [19,57]. On the other hand, an association with age might be expected in COPD patients in general because of the likely effects on AHR of such age-related factors as a larger cumulative number of pack-years of smoking and a smaller airway caliber in older smokers with COPD. However, because a fixed FEV_1/FVC ratio (rather than one adjusted for age) was a criterion for enrollment in the LHS, a selection bias favored enrolling younger participants with more airflow obstruction relative to age than their older counterparts, thus negating the potentially modifying effects of the above age-related factors on AHR.

One of the most striking observations in the LHS was the apparent relationship between sex and AHR (Figs. 6 and 7). As already noted, the marked difference between the proportions of LHS men and women with AHR could not be attributed to differences in age, degree of baseline airflow obstruction, or cigarette smoking. These findings are in contrast to most population studies, which have failed to find a significant relationship between sex and AHR [12,21,57,61,63]. In a recent study of a Norwegian general population, on the other hand, Bakke et al. [62] also noted a higher prevalence of AHR among women than among men, even though mean baseline FEV_1 % predicted and FEV_1/FVC of men and women were nearly identical. However, when their findings were adjusted for differences in baseline *airway caliber*, as reflected by absolute FEV_1 (significantly smaller in women), the sex-related differences in AHR disappeared in nonsmokers and were actually reversed in smokers and ex-smokers [62].

Lung Health Study data were also analyzed by logistic regression using AHR (defined separately as a PC_{20} either $\leq$5 mg/ml or $\leq$10 mg/ml methacholine) as a dichotomous outcome variable and the following features as dependent variables: sex, age, respiratory diagnoses (including hay fever and emphysema; subjects with asthma were excluded from the analysis), respiratory symptoms (chronic cough and/or phlegm, wheezing, and shortness of breath), pack-years of smoking, and different measures of baseline lung function (absolute FEV_1 alone and together with FEV_1/FVC or FEV_1 % predicted) (Table 4). The results indicate that adjustment for FEV_1 alone abolished or reversed the sex effect for PC_{20} $\leq$10 mg/ml and $\leq$5 mg/ml, respectively, consistent with the observations of Bakke et al. [62] in current and former smokers. However, in the absence of a restrictive ventilatory abnormality, a comparable absolute FEV_1 in a man and a woman of the same height and age implies the presence of obstructive airway disease in the former, probably accounting for the apparent association of AHR with the male sex after adjustment for FEV_1 alone. Therefore, an additional adjustment for FEV_1/FVC or FEV_1 % predicted was made in order to control for the effect of airway disease. These additional adjustments resulted in a restoration of the sex effect for PC_{20} $\leq$10 mg/ml, favoring more AHR in women than men, although the effect favoring women was not as strong as that in the absence of any adjustment for baseline lung function. These findings suggest that AHR is influenced by sex and that this influence is largely, but not completely, explained by male–female differences in baseline airway caliber. Other possible reasons for the sex-related difference in AHR are unclear but could include male–female differences in aspects of airway disease (e.g., inflammation, epithelial damage, or the structural support of the airways) that are not completely reflected in baseline FEV_1.

Table 4 Odds Ratios and 95% Confidence Intervals for Women Being More Likely Than Men to React to Methacholine (Mch), According to Variables Entered into the Model

	Odds ratios (95% CI)	
Variables	$PC_{20} \leq$ 5 mg/ml Mch	$PC_{20} \leq$ 10 mg/ml Mch
Model 1: Age, sex, respiratory diagnosis, symptoms, and packs/day	2.77 (2.44, 3.15)	3.50 (3.08, 3.98)
Model 2: Model 1 plus measured FEV_1	0.71 (0.59, 0.85)	0.89 (0.74, 1.07)
Model 3: Model 2 plus FEV_1/FVC	1.18 (0.97, 1.45)	1.48 (1.21, 1.81)
Model 4: Model 2 plus FEV_1 % predicted	1.26 (0.98, 1.63)	1.78 (1.39, 2.27)

FEV_1 = forced expired volume in 1 second; FVC = forced vital capacity.

In summary, cross-sectional findings from the Lung Health Study indicate that in middle-aged smokers with mild to moderate COPD ($FEV_1/FVC \leqslant 70\%$; $FEV_1 \geqslant 50\%$) (1) methacholine challenge testing using an abbreviated protocol starting with five inhalations of 1 mg/ml methacholine is safe; (2) nearly half of male and three-fourths of female smokers with mild to moderate airflow limitation have nonspecific AHR ($PC_{20} \leqslant 10$ mg/ml); (3) AHR is strongly related to the baseline degree of airflow obstruction but only variably related to respiratory symptoms other than wheeze and unrelated to age or cigarette smoking intensity; (4) despite an apparent association with AHR, bronchodilator responsiveness is far less common than nonspecific AHR to pharmacological constrictor stimuli; and (5) AHR is significantly more common in women than in men. The last sex-related difference is partly, but not completely, explained by the smaller airway caliber in women after adjustment for degree of airflow obstruction. Future analysis of longitudinal data from the LHS should provide a large body of additional data pertaining to the prognostic and therapeutic implications of AHR in COPD. These implications include the relationship between baseline AHR and subsequent decline in FEV_1, as well as the modification of this relationship by smoking cessation or maintenance bronchodilator therapy, and the effect of these interventions, singly and together, on both AHR and the annual decline in lung function.

REFERENCES

1. Ramsdell, J. W., Nachtwey, J., and Moser, K. M., Bronchial hyperreactivity in chronic obstructive bronchitis, *Am. Rev. Respir. Dis.*, *126*, 829–832 (1982).
2. Ramsdale, E. H., Morris, M. M., Roberts, R. S., and Hargreave, F. E., Bronchial responsiveness to methacholine in chronic bronchitis: relationship to airflow obstruction and cold air responsiveness, *Thorax*, *39*, 912–918 (1984).
3. Bahous, J., Cartier, A., Ouimet, G., Pineau, L., and Malo, J.-L., Nonallergic bronchial hyperexcitability in chronic bronchitis, *Am. Rev. Respir. Dis.*, *129*, 218–220 (1984).
4. Yan, K., Salome, C. M., and Woolcock, A. J., Prevalence and nature of bronchial hyperresponsiveness in subjects with chronic obstructive pulmonary disease, *Am. Rev. Respir. Dis.*, *132*, 25–29 (1985).
5. Verma, V. K., Cockroft, D. W., and Dosman, J. A., Airway responsiveness to inhaled histamine in chronic obstructive airways disease, *Chest*, *94*, 457–461 (1988).
6. Brand, P. L. P., Postma, D. S., Kerstjens, H. A. M., Koeter, G. H., and the Dutch CNSLD Study Group, Relationship of airway hyperresponsiveness to respiratory symptoms and diurnal peak flow variation in patients with obstructive lung disease, *Am. Rev. Respir. Dis.*, *143*, 916–921 (1991).
7. Bel, E. H., Zwinderman, A. H., Timmers, M. C., Dijkman, J. H., and Sterk, P. J., The protective effect of a $beta_2$ agonist against excessive airway narrowing in response to bronchoconstrictor stimuli in asthma and chronic obstructive lung disease, *Thorax*, *46*, 9–14 (1991).

8. Muller, J. B., Wiggs, B. R., Wright, J. L., Paré, P. D., and Hogg, J. C., Cartilaginous airway inflammation in smokers (abstr.), *Am. Rev. Respir. Dis.*, *129*, A317 (1984).
9. Cockcroft, D. W., Killian, D. N., Mellon, J. J. A., and Hargreave, F. E., Bronchial reactivity to inhaled histamine: a method and clinical survey, *Clin. Allergy*, *7*, 235–243 (1977).
10. Beaupre, A., and Malo, J. L., Histamine dose-response curves in asthma: relevance of the distinction between PC_{20} and reactivity in characterizing clinical state, *Thorax*, *36*, 731–736 (1981).
11. Rubenfeld, A. R., and Pain, C. F., Relationship between bronchial reactivity, airway caliber, and severity of asthma, *Am. Rev. Respir. Dis.*, *115*, 381–387 (1977).
12. Burney, P. G. J., Britton, J. R., Chinn, S., et al., Descriptive epidemiology of bronchial reactivity in an adult population: results from a community study, *Thorax*, *42*, 38–44 (1987).
13. Welty, C., Weiss, S. T., Tager, I. B., et al., The relationship of airways responsiveness to cold air, cigarette smoking, and atopy to respiratory symptoms and pulmonary function in adults, *Am. Rev. Respir. Dis.*, *130*, 198–203 (1984).
14. Moreno, R. H., Hogg, J. C., and Paré, P. D., Mechanics of airway narrowing, *Am. Rev. Respir. Dis.*, *133*, 1171–1180 (1986).
15. Freedman, B. J., The functional geometry of the bronchi, *Bull. Physiopathol. Respir.*, *8*, 545–551 (1972).
16. Thurlbeck, W. M., Pun, R., Toth, J., and Frazer, R. G., Bronchial cartilage in chronic obstructive lung disease, *Am. Rev. Respir. Dis.*, *109*, 73–80 (1974).
17. Ryan, G., Latimer, K. M., Dolovich, J., and Hargreave, F. E., Bronchial responsiveness to histamine: relationship to diurnal variation of peak flow rate, improvement after bronchodilator, and airway calibre, *Thorax*, *37*, 423–429 (1982).
18. Sparrow, D., O'Connor, G., Colton, T., Barry, C. L., and Weiss, S. T. The relationship of nonspecific bronchial responsiveness to the occurrence of respiratory symptoms and decreased levels of pulmonary function: the normative aging study, *Am. Rev. Respir. Dis.*, *135*, 1255–1260 (1987).
19. Rijcken, B., Schouten, J. P., Weiss, S. T., Speizer, F. E., and Van der Lende, R., The relationship of nonspecific bronchial responsiveness to respiratory symptoms in a random population sample, *Am. Rev. Respir. Dis.*, *136*, 62–68 (1987).
20. Kibiraj, M. U., Simonsson, B. G., Groth, S., Bjorklund, A., Bulow, K., and Lindell, S.-E., Bronchial reactivity, smoking, and alpha$_1$-antitrypsin: a population-based study of middle-aged men, *Am. Rev. Respir. Dis.*, *126*, 864–869 (1982).
21. Malo, J. L., Filiatrault, S., and Martin, R. R., Bronchial responsiveness to inhaled methacholine in young asymptomatic smokers, *J. Appl. Physiol.*, *52*, 1464–1470 (1982).
22. Gerrard, J. W., Cockcroft, D. W., Mink, J. T., Cotton, D. J., Poonawala, R., and Dosman, J. A., Increased nonspecific bronchial reactivity in cigarette smokers with normal lung function, *Am. Rev. Respir. Dis.*, *122*, 577–581 (1980).
23. Sparrow, D., O'Connor, G., and Weiss, S. T., The relation of airway responsiveness and atopy to the development of chronic obstructive lung disease, *Epidemiol. Rev.*, *10*, 29–47 (1988).
24. Brown, N. E., McFadden, E. R., Jr., and Ingram, R. H., Jr., Airway responses to

inhaled histamine in asymptomatic smokers and nonsmokers, *J. Appl. Physiol.*, *42*, 508–513 (1977).

25. Buczko, G. B., Day, A., Vanderdoelen, J. L., et al., Effects of cigarette smoking and short-term smoking cessation on airway responsiveness to inhaled methacholine, *Am. Rev. Respir. Dis.*, *129*, 12–14 (1984).
26. Enarson, D. A., Chan-Yeung, M., Tabona, M., Kus, J., Vedal, S., and Lam, S., Predictors of bronchial hyperexcitability in grain handlers, *Chest*, *85*, 452–455 (1985).
27. Vedal, S., Enarson, D. A., Chan, J., Ochnio, J., Tse, K. S., and Chan-Yeung, M., A longitudinal study of the occurrence of bronchial hyperresponsiveness in Western red cedar workers, *Am. Rev. Respir. Dis.*, *137*, 652–655 (1990).
28. Kennedy, S. M., Elwood, R. K., Wiggs, B. J. R., Paré, P. D., and Hogg, J. C., Increased airway mucosal permeability of smokers: relationship to airway reactivity, *Am. Rev. Respir. Dis.*, *129*, 143–188 (1984).
29. Orie, N. G. M., Sluiter, H. J., de Vries, K., Tammeling, G. J., and Witkop, J., The host factor in bronchitis, *Bronchitis* (N. G. M. Orie and H. J. Sluiter, eds.), Assen, The Netherlands, Royal Vangorcum, 1961, pp. 43–59.
30. Van der Lende, R., de Kroon, J. P. M., Van der Meulen, G. G., et al., Possible indicators of endogenous factors in the development of CNSLD, in *Bronchitis III* (N. G. M. Orie and R. Van der Lende, eds.), Assen, the Netherlands: Royal Vangorcum, 1970, pp. 52–79.
31. Woolcock, A. J., Salome, C. M., and Yan, K., The shape of the dose–response curve to histamine in asthmatic and normal subjects, *Am. Rev. Respir. Dis.*, *130*, 71–75 (1984).
32. Woolcock, A. J., Anderson, S. D., Peat, J. K., Du Toit, J. I., Zhang, Y. G., Smith, C. M., and Salome, C. M., Characteristics of bronchial hyperresponsiveness in chronic obstructive pulmonary disease, *Am. Rev. Respir. Dis.*, *143*, 1438–1443 (1991).
33. Du Toit, J. I., Woolcock, A. J., Salome, C. M., Sundrum, R., and Black, J. L., Characteristics of bronchial hyperresponsiveness in smokers with chronic airflow limitation, *Am. Rev. Respir. Dis.*, *134*, 498–501 (1986).
34. O'Byrne, P. M., Ramsdale, E. H., and Hargreave, F. E., Isocapnic hyperventilation for measuring airway hyperresponsiveness in asthma and in chronic obstructive pulmonary diseases, *Am. Rev. Respir. Dis.*, *143*, 1444–1445 (1991).
35. Black, J. L., Salome, C. M., Yan, K., and Shaw, J., Comparison between airways response to an alpha-adrenoceptor agonist in asthmatic and nonasthmatic subjects, *Br. J. Clin. Pharmacol.*, *14*, 464–465 (1982).
36. Salome, C. M., Schoeffel, R. E., and Woolcock, A. J., Comparison of bronchial reactivity to histamine and methacholine in asthmatics, *Clin. Allergy*, *10*, 541–546 (1980).
37. Juniper, E. F., Frith, P. A., Dunnett, C., Cockcroft, D. W., and Hargreave, F. E., Reproducibility and comparison of responses to inhaled histamine and methacholine, *Thorax*, *33*, 705–710 (1978).
38. O'Connor, G. T., Sparrow, D., and Weiss, S. T., The role of allergy and nonspecific airway hyperresponsiveness in the pathogenesis of chronic obstructive pulmonary disease, *Am. Rev. Respir. Dis.*, *140*, 225–252 (1989).

39. Barter, C. E., and Campbell, A. H., Relationship of constitutional factors and cigarette smoking to decrease in 1-second forced expiratory volume, *Am. Rev. Respir. Dis.*, *113*, 305–314 (1976).
40. Campbell, A. H., Barter, C. E., O'Connell, J. M., and Higgins, R., Factors affecting the decline of ventilatory function in chronic bronchitis, *Thorax*, *40*, 741–748 (1985).
41. Kanner, R. E., The relationship between airways responsiveness and chronic airflow limitation, *Chest*, *86*, 54–57 (1989).
42. Tabona, M., Chan-Yeung, M., Enarson, D., MacLean, L., Dorken, E., and Schulzer, M., Host factors affecting longitudinal decline in lung spirometry among grain elevator workers, *Chest*, *85*, 782–786 (1984).
43. Taylor, R. G., Joyce, H., Gross, E., Holland, F., and Pride, N. B., Bronchial reactivity to inhaled histamine and annual rate of decline in FEV_1 in male smokers and exsmokers, *Thorax*, *40*, 9–16 (1985).
44. Vollmer, W. M., Johnson, L. R., and Buist, A. S., Relationship of response to a bronchodilator and decline in forced expiratory volume in one second in population studies, *Am. Rev. Respir. Dis.*, *132*, 1186–1193 (1985).
45. Pham, W. T., Mur, J. M., Chau, N., Gabiano, M., Henquel, J. C., and Teculescu, D., Prognostic value of acetylcholine challenge test: a prospective study, *Br. J. Indust. Med.*, *41*, 267–271 (1984).
46. Lim, T. K., Taylor, R. G., Watson, A., Joyce, H., and Pride, N. B., Changes in bronchial responsiveness to inhaled histamine over four years in middle aged male smokers and ex-smokers, *Thorax*, *43*, 599–604 (1988).
47. Anthonisen, N. R., Wright, E. C., and the IPPB Trial Group, Bronchodilator response in chronic obstructive pulmonary disease, *Am. Rev. Respir. Dis.*, *133*, 814–819 (1986).
48. Postma, D. S., de Vries, K., Koeter, G. H., and Sluiter, H. J., Independent influence of reversibility of airflow obstruction and nonspecific hyperreactivity on the long-term course of lung function in chronic air-flow obstruction, *Am. Rev. Respir. Dis.*, *134*, 276–280 (1986).
49. Kanner, R. E., Renzetti, A. D., Jr., Klauber, M. R., Smith, C. B., and Golden, C. A., Variables associated with changes in spirometry in patients with obstructive lung diseases, *Am. J. Med.*, *67*, 44–50 (1979).
50. Thompson, A. B., Mueller, M. B., Heires, A. J., et al., Aerosolized beclomethasone in chronic bronchitis, *Am. Rev. Respir. Dis.*, *146*, 389–395 (1992).
51. Kerstjens, H. A. M., Brand, P. L. P., Hughes, M. D., et al., and the Dutch Chronic Non-Specific Lung Disease Study Group, A comparison of bronchodilator therapy with or without inhaled corticosteroid therapy for obstructive airways disease, *N. Engl. J. Med.*, *327*, 1413–1419 (1992).
52. Anthonisen, N. R., Lung health study (editorial), *Am. Rev. Respir. Dis.*, *140*, 871–872 (1989).
53. Chai, H., Farr, R. S., Froelich, L. A., et al., Standardization of bronchial inhalation challenge procedures, *J. Allergy Clin. Immunol.*, *56*, 323–327 (1975).
54. Tashkin, D. P., Altose, M. D., Bleecker, E. R., Connett, J. E., Kanner, R. E., Lee, W. W., Wise, R., and the Lung Health Study Research Group, The Lung Health Study:

airway responsiveness to inhaled methacholine in smokers with mild to moderate airflow limitation, *Am. Rev. Respir. Dis.*, *145*, 301–310 (1992).

55. Eiser, N. M., Kerrebijn, K. F., Quanjer, P. H., et al., and the SEPCR Working Group, Guidelines for standardization of bronchial challenges with (nonspecific) bronchoconstricting agents, *Bull. Eur. Physiopathol. Respir.*, *19*, 495–514 (1983).
56. Sparrow, D., O'Connor, G., Colton, T., Barry, C. L., and Weiss, S. T., The relationship of nonspecific bronchial responsiveness to the occurrence of respiratory symptoms and decreased levels of pulmonary function: the normative aging study, *Am. Rev. Respir. Dis.*, *135*, 1255–1260 (1987).
57. Hopp, R. J., Bewtra, A., Nair, N. M., and Townley, R. G., The effect of age on methacholine response, *J. Allergy Clin. Immunol.*, *76*, 609–613 (1985).
58. Greenspon, L. C., and Parris, B., Inhibition of methacholine-induced bronchoconstriction in patients with chronic obstructive pulmonary disease, *Am. Rev. Respir. Dis.*, *137*, 218–285 (1988).
59. Benson, M. K., Bronchial hyperreactivity, *Br. J. Dis. Chest*, *69*, 227–239 (1975).
60. Boushey, H. A., Holtzman, M. J., Sheller, J. R., and Nadel, J. A., Bronchial hyperreactivity, *Am. Rev. Respir. Dis.*, *121*, 389–413 (1980).
61. Weiss, S. T., Tager, I. B., Weiss, J. W., Munoz, A., Speizer, F. E., and Ingram, R. H., Airways responsiveness in a population sample of adults and children, *Am. Rev. Respir. Dis.*, *129*, 898–902 (1984).
62. Bakke, P. S., Baste, V., and Gulsvik, A., Bronchial responsiveness in a Norwegian community, *Am. Rev. Respir. Dis.*, *143*, 317–322 (1991).
63. Townley, R. G., Bewtra, A. K., Nair, N. M., Brodkey, F. D., Watt, G. D., and Burke, K. M., Methacholine inhalation challenge studies, *J. Allergy Clin. Immunol.*, *64*, 569–574 (1979).

22

Aspirin, Sulfur Dioxide/Sulfite, and Other Chemical Sensitivities and Challenges in Asthmatic Patients

David A. Mathison, Ronald A. Simon, and Donald D. Stevenson

Scripps Clinic & Research Foundation
La Jolla, California

I. INTRODUCTION

A variety of reactions to drugs per se, chemicals added to foods and drugs, and aeropollutants may incite an asthmatic attack or perpetuate chronic asthmatic relapse. Anaphylactic reactions triggered by the interaction of a drug such as penicillin and immunoglobulin E (IgE) antibodies of the susceptible host may include a component of bronchospasm. The pathophysiology of asthma includes a state of relative β_2-adrenergic blockade; therefore, pharmacological agents such as propranolol, used for their β_1-blocking action in the cardiovascular system but also possessing β_2-blocking action, can unmask a latent asthmatic potential, or compound ongoing asthma, and therefore are best avoided in the asthmatic patient. The focus of this chapter is on the roles of idiosyncratic responses to aspirin and aspirinlike nonsteroidal anti-inflammatory drugs (NSAIDs) and reactions to sulfur dioxide/sulfites and other chemicals in asthma.

II. ASPIRIN

Aspirin has been used for over 90 years in the United States as an anti-inflammatory, antipyretic, and analgesic agent, and in recent decades as a platelet-inhibiting agent to prevent thrombotic and embolic disease [see Ref. 1 for overall review]. The average per capita consumption is more than 60 five-grain tablets per year. An asthmatic reaction to aspirin was first reported in 1911 [2]; the intervening history of observations on idiosyncratic sensitivity reactions to aspirin was summarized by VanArsdel [3]. Reactions to aspirin may be anaphylactic-like [4] or manifest by exacerbation of rhinitis–asthma or urticaria–angioedema; only a very few persons have been reported to have both respiratory and cutaneous response to aspirin [5].

A. Spectrum of Reactions

The typical aspirin-sensitive respiratory syndrome [6,7] primarily affects adults [8], though onset may be in childhood [9]. The disease evolves over decades and ordinarily begins with a perennial vasomotor irritant–aggravated type of rhinitis, though half of these patients also have IgE-mediated cutaneous reactions to aeroallergen extracts [8]. Next, an eosinophilic hyperplastic rhinosinusitis with nasal polyps ensues, and not infrequently, this is complicated by bouts of purulent bacterial sinusitis. Asthma then appears and progresses to require treatment with systemic steroids. The hallmark of aspirin sensitivity is the appearance of facial or generalized flush, ocular and nasal congestion and watering, and acute, often severe, asthmatic attack within 30 min to several hours after ingesting an ordinary dose of aspirin or aspirinlike drug. Even though the patient soon learns to avoid aspirin and similar drugs, the underlying respiratory disease continues.

A spectrum of adverse respiratory responses to aspirin in sensitive asthmatic patients extends from the typical upper and lower respiratory response to no response at all [10]. Of 50 consecutive asthmatic patients with a history of aspirin sensitivity challenged with aspirin, 36 demonstrated the typical asthmatic response with a decline of forced expired volume in 1 second (FEV_1) of more than 20% from baseline; six patients developed acute rhinoconjunctivitis without asthmatic response; and eight patients had no adverse response. Furthermore, of 28 patients who underwent multiple challenges at intervals of weeks to years, seven showed different responses on repeated challenges. We classify aspirin reactions as "typical" or "classical" when nasal, ocular, and asthmatic response occurs; "purely asthmatic" when there is asthmatic response without nasal–ocular symptoms; "partial asthmatic" when there is a fall of FEV_1 in the 15–20% range with or without nasal-ocular symptoms; and "nasal–ocular" for reaction without a 15% change in FEV_1 values.

The prevalence of aspirin sensitivity in patients with asthma varies according to the population studied and the methods used to detect the sensitivity. Falliers [11] noted a history of aspirin reaction in fewer than 2% of nearly 1300 asthmatic children surveyed. Giraldo et al. [12] found that 3–5% of hospitalized adult asthmatic patients had a history of reaction to aspirin. At Scripps Clinic, an asthma and allergic diseases center, we found that about 10% of our asthmatic population was aspirin-sensitive [8]. At the National Jewish Center, where an even more highly selective group of severely asthmatic patients was studied, 19% were found by oral challenges to react to aspirin [13]. Of asthmatic patients with pansinusitis and nasal polyps, 30–40% are aspirin-sensitive [14].

B. Cross-Sensitivity to Other Nonsteroidal Anti-Inflammatory Drugs

The Nobel Prize in Medicine in 1982 was awarded to Dr. Sune Bergström, Dr. Bengt Samuelsson, and Dr. John Vane for their studies of the metabolism of arachidonic acid and the generation of eicosanoids (Fig. 1) [15,16]. Dr. Vane identified as a mechanism of action of aspirin the inhibition of prostaglandin synthesis from the cyclooxygenase pathway of arachidonate metabolism [17].

Other NSAIDs that inhibit this pathway also can provoke respiratory reaction in aspirin-sensitive asthmatic subjects [5,13,18]. As shown in Table 1, cross-reactivity correlates with the effectiveness of cyclooxygenase inhibition. Potent inhibitors of the cyclooxygenase enzyme show a very high degree of cross-reactivity in aspirin-sensitive patients; agents such as acetaminophen [19] and salsalate [20], which are weak inhibitors even at high concentrations, have a low incidence of cross-reactivity even with high doses; nonacetylated salicylates [21], analgesics, and inhibitors of platelet aggregation that do not act through cyclooxygenase inhibition have not been shown to be cross-reactive. Ophthalmic indomethacin has been reported to incite asthmatic attack [22], and ophthalmic ketorolac (Acular), diclofenac (Voltarin), profenol (Suprofen), and flurbiprofen (Ocufen) might also be expected to do so in the aspirin-sensitive patient.

C. Mechanism of Reaction

The mechanism of reactivity to aspirin has not been fully elucidated [23–25]. Figure 1 indicates the site of action of aspirin/NSAIDs in the generation of eicosanoids. Goetzl et al. [26] found a greater ratio of leukotriene D_4 (LTD_4) to prostaglandin E_2 (PGE_2) generation in response to aspirin by basophil-containing leukocytes of aspirin-sensitive patients than in those of control asthmatic and rhinitic patients. Ferrari et al. [27] found increasing levels of LTC_4 in nasal secretions of aspirin-sensitive patients during reaction to aspirin, whereas subjects desensitized to aspirin, non-aspirin-sensitive asthmatics, and normal subjects did not have change in LTC_4 in nasal lavage fluids before and after administration of 650-mg doses of aspirin; however, PGE_2 levels became undetectable in all groups. Picado et al. [28] and Kowalski et al. [29] have reported similar leukotriene responses in aspirin-sensitive asthmatic patients. Several groups [30–33] have reported increases of urinary LTE_4 after aspirin challenge in aspirin-sensitive asthmatic subjects; airway responsiveness to LTE_4 is increased in those subjects [34]; and, following desensitization to aspirin, urinary LTE_4 decreased with continued treatment with aspirin in one patient [33]. Juergens et al. [35] found that monocytes of aspirin-sensitive asthmatics released more thromboxane B_2 (TXB_2)

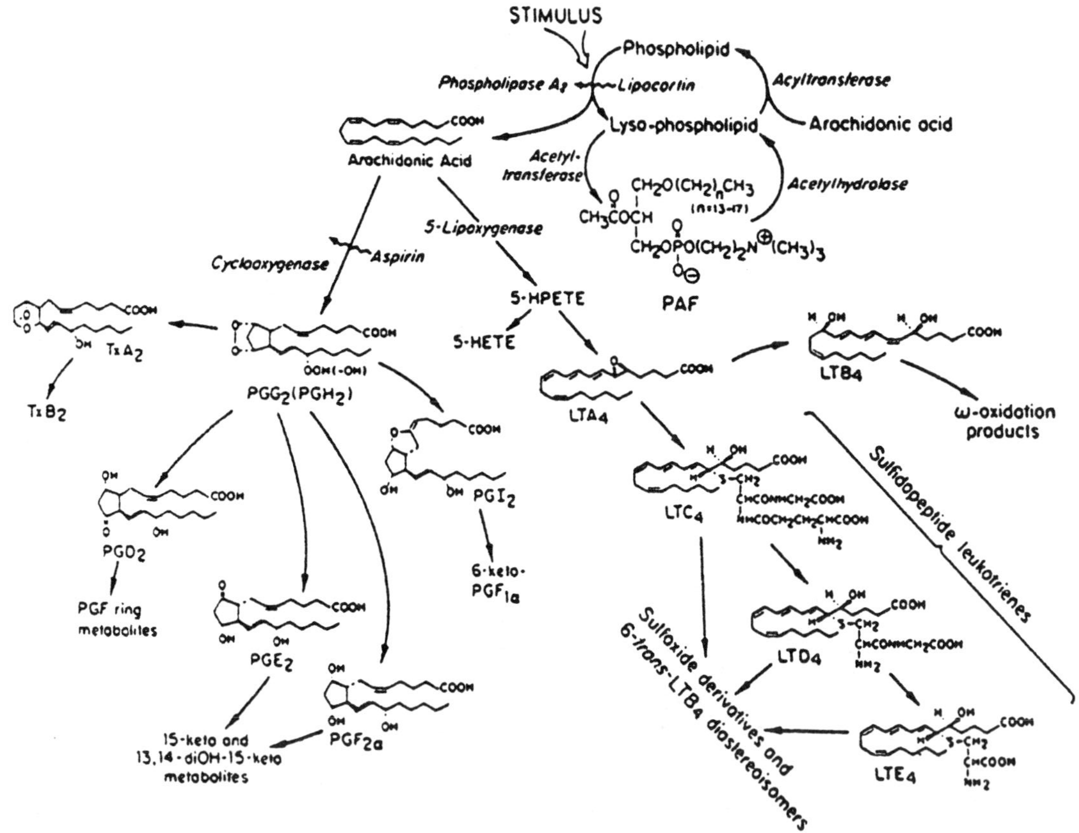

Figure 1 Phospholipid–arachidonic acid metabolic pathways. Aspirin and NSAIDs inhibit (wavy lines) cyclooxygenase and generation of prostaglandins. (From Henderson WR, *J. Allergy Clin. Immunol.*, *79*, 545 [1987].)

Table 1 Cross-Reactivity Between Aspirin and Nonsteroidal Anti-Inflammatory Drugs in Aspirin-Sensitive Asthmatics

Cyclooxygenase inhibition		Cross-Reactivity
Strong inhibitors		
Indomethacin	(Indocin)	High, ≥90%
Meclofenamate	(Meclomen)	
Mefenamic acid	(Ponstel)	
Naproxen	(Anaprox, Naprosyn)	
Ibuprofen	(Advil, Haltran, Medipren, Motrin, Nuprin, Rufen)	
Fenoprofen	(Nalfon)	
Diflunisal	(Dolobid)	
Ketoprofen	(Orudis)	
Piroxicam	(Feldene)	
Sulindac	(Cilnoril)	
Tolmetin	(Tolectin)	
Diclofenac	(Voltaren)	
Flurbiprofen	(Ansaid)	
Ketorolac	(Toradol)	
Etodolac	(Lodine)	
Nabumetone	(Relafen)	
Oxaprozin	(Daypro)	
Weak inhibitors		
Acetaminophen	(Datril, Tylenol)	Low, ≤20%
Phenylbutazone	(Butazolidin)	
Salicylsalicylic acid, salsalate	(Disalcid, Salflex)	
Choline, magnesium, sodium salicylate	(Trilisate, Doan's, Magan)	
Noninhibitors/analgesics/platelet inhibitors		
Propoxyphene	(Darvon)	None, or rare cases reported
Dipyridamole	(Persantine)	
Hydroxychloroquine	(Plaquenil)	
Ticlopidine	(Ticlid)	

to calcium ionophore and that this release decreased more following aspirin administration than did releases by monocytes from normal subjects. The leukotriene antagonist SK&F 104353 inhibits aspirin-induced asthma [36].

Elevation of serum mast cell tryptase [37] and neutrophil chemotactic activity [38] consistent with mast cell activation, cleavage of high-molecular-weight kininogen [39], enhanced basophil histamine release by platelet activating factor [40], elevation of plasma $PGF_{2\alpha}$ [41], and activation of fibrinolysis [42] have all been noted during reaction to aspirin. Abnormalities of platelets from aspirin-sensitive asthmatics have been reported by some [43–45], but not by others [46–48]. The relevance of these findings to the occurrence of respiratory response is uncertain. Complement activation [49], IgE antibodies [50], or other immunological responses to aspirin have not been consistently identified. Inhaled furosemide blocks inhaled lysine aspirin–induced bronchoconstriction in aspirin-sensitive asthmatics [51].

About 10% of aspirin-sensitive asthmatic subjects have been reported to experience significant initial bronchoconstrictor response to intravenously administered hydrocortisone or methylprednisolone succinate but not to the phosphate salts [52,53]. There is a significant difference in the incidence of HLA-DR3 between aspirin-sensitive and aspirin-tolerant asthmatic subjects [54].

D. Indications for Challenges

Since aspirin sensitivity may appear only after years of progression of respiratory disorder and vary in its expression, and since some asthmatic patients can avoid aspirin and NSAIDs, the most conservative approach is to advise avoidance of these drugs by substituting 325- to 500-mg (but not 1000-mg) doses of acetaminophen or using another analgesic, anti-inflammatory, or platelet-inhibitor drug that does not cross-react with aspirin (Table 1). Asthmatic patients who have recently tolerated aspirin or NSAIDs and for whom aspirin or an NSAID is indicated may elect to use these drugs but should be made aware of the potential risk of developing sensitivity. However, patients who have a high potential for aspirin sensitivity (i.e., pansinusitis with polyps and asthma necessitating corticosteroid treatment) or have a history of aspirin-sensitivity respiratory reactions, and who also have headache or rheumatic, cardiovascular, or diabetic disease for which aspirin is indicated, or for whom aspirin desensitization followed by continued treatment with aspirin for the respiratory disease per se (see below) has been recommended, can safely undergo challenges—desensitization with incremental doses of aspirin or an aspirinlike drug followed by daily administration of aspirin [55].

E. Methods for Challenges

Currently there has been no organized attempt to standardize methodology for challenges with aspirin/NSAIDs. Investigators have reported challenges with bronchial inhalation [33,56,57] and nasal insufflation [58] of lysine acetylsalicylate and with intravenous indomethacin [59], and oral challenges with aspirin and aspirinlike NSAIDs [55,60].

Challenges and desensitizations must be performed using a number of safety practices. At Scripps Clinic, we perform challenges within the hospital, where emergency resuscitative equipment, an intensive care unit, and trained personnel are readily available. Challenges are always started in the morning so that optimal time and staff for treatment are available to ensure ease of recovery from the reaction. Patients are challenged at a time when their asthma is in remission; if need be, we administer additional corticosteroid for several days to a week before challenge to ensure that there is full remission. To proceed with the challenge, the patient must have an FEV_1 greater than 70% of the predicted value or his best previously recorded value, and in absolute numbers, this must be greater than 1.5 L.

Patients are instructed to continue theophylline and steroid medications and to suspend anticholinergics, antihistamines, cromolyn [61], acetaminophen, non-aspirin salicylates [62], and, if feasible, inhaled adrenergic bronchodilator medications for 24 h before challenge. We recognize that continuation of medications may counter a mild reaction and thereby lead to a false-negative result, and that withholding of medications may allow for spontaneous deterioration of asthma during the challenge, which could lead to a false conclusion of reactivity. Blinded challenge with placebo or non-aspirinlike drug over one day with repeated spirometric measurements as planned during aspirin challenge can be helpful in identifying subjects likely to have false-positive responses.

Patients with mild asthma for whom the history does not suggest a likelihood of aspirin reactivity (no rhinosinusitis or nasal polyps and previous recent ingestion of aspirin without apparent reaction) can be challenged over a half-day with 30, 150, 325, and 650 mg doses of aspirin (or 5%, 10%, 50%, and 100% of the usual therapeutic dose of another NSAID) administered at hourly intervals, with spirometric measurements also performed hourly and continued for 2 h after the last dose. This is equivalent to the "test dose" method used for other medications when an adverse reaction is judged to be unlikely.

Asthmatic patients with moderate asthma but without rhinosinusitis–polyps who have not ingested aspirin or NSAIDs for months or years may undergo a 1-day challenge. Aspirin doses of 30, 60, and 150 mg are administered hourly, and then doses of 325 and 650 mg at 2-h intervals (5%, 10%, and 20%, then 50% and 100% of the usual dose for another NSAID), with spirometry measurements at hourly intervals continued for 3 h after the last dose. This is a more conservative "test dose" method when an adverse response is not expected.

Asthmatic patients with history of adverse respiratory response to aspirin/NSAIDs or those with severe disease, including rhinosinusitis with nasal polyps and remote history of aspirin ingestion, undergo challenges over a 2-day interval with an initial dose of 3, 15, or 30 mg followed by 60 and 100 mg on the first day at 3-h intervals and then 150, 325, and 650 mg at 3-h intervals on the second day (1.5% or 5%, 10% and 20%, then 30%, 50%, and 100% of the usual dose for another NSAID), with spirometric measurements recorded hourly and continued for 3 h after the last dose on both days. A 2-day challenge is not initiated until a full-day placebo challenge has confirmed stable lung function.

For any patient, if ocular, nasal, or asthmatic symptoms appear, or if there is a fall in FEV_1 of more than 20%, no additional doses are administered, and the patient is treated with inhalations of an adrenergic bronchodilator (albuterol or terbutaline) delivered by nebulized aerosol and repeated at 10- to 20-min intervals until improvement occurs. If no response appears after the initial treatment, 200–300 μg of epinephrine is also administered subcutaneously; and if there is no response, intravenous corticosteroid and aminophylline and oxygen are initiated, and preparations for transfer to intensive care, including intubation and mechanical ventilation, are made. Ordinarily, there is gradual recovery from the reaction over several hours coincident to treatment; slower recovery over 24 h is not unusual.

Challenge response is interpreted as being "negative" if no symptoms and less than a 15% fall in FEV_1 occur during the entire period of observation. Patients with "negative" challenge are instructed to proceed with the indicated drug in ordinary therapeutic dosages. However, if there is a history suggestive of previous reaction, they are also cautioned that they may redevelop reactivity to aspirin/NSAIDs if they omit the treatment for a day or more and must continue to be cautious regarding the use of aspirin/NSAIDs.

Challenge response is interpreted as being "asthmatic" if the fall in FEV_1 exceeds 20% and if on another day blinded similar challenge with a placebo or non-aspirinlike drug produces a fall in FEV_1 of less than 15% and no symptoms. Asthmatic reactions are judged to be "typical-classic" or "purely asthmatic" if no nasal–ocular symptoms occur. Response is judged to be "partial-asthmatic" if FEV_1 falls 15–20% or "nasal–ocular" if nasal–ocular symptoms occur without asthmatic symptoms or signs.

Patients with reaction for whom aspirin or an NSAID is indicated for ongoing treatment are subject to desensitization [55]. Desensitization is accomplished by repeated daily challenges, providing the criteria for initial challenge are met, beginning with the dose that provoked reaction on the previous day and continuing upward until 650 mg (100% of the usual dose of another NSAID) is achieved without reaction. Figure 2 shows an example of desensitization.

F. Desensitization and Treatment

In 1922, Widal et al. [63] reported treating a patient who had reacted to 100 mg aspirin with increasing doses of aspirin over a 7-day interval until the patient could tolerate 600 mg without manifesting sensitivity. In 1976, Zeiss and Lockey [64] reported the serendipitous discovery of a 72-h refractory period to the adverse effects of indomethacin and aspirin during a double-blind protocol study of graded doses of aspirin in an aspirin-sensitive asthmatic patient. Subsequently, Bianco et al. [56] reported that inhalations of lysine acetylsalicylate provoked bronchoconstriction but that administration of inhaled or ingested aspirin immediately thereafter did not evoke further reaction.

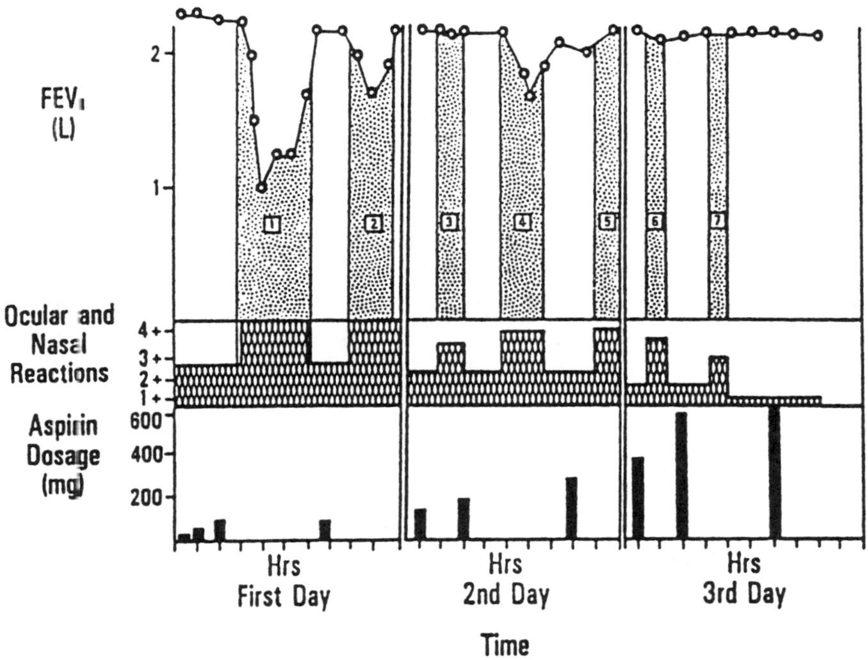

Figure 2 Aspirin challenges—desensitization in an aspirin-sensitive asthmatic patient; seven (numbers in boxes, stippled and hatched areas) nasal-ocular reactions, some (1,2,4) with asthmatic reaction as well, occurred before 650-mg dose on third day was tolerated without reaction, indicating desensitized state.

In 1979, we found two aspirin-sensitive asthmatic patients to be refractory to further adverse effects of aspirin following "typical-classical" respiratory reactions to challenge, and on continued daily aspirin treatment, both of these patients showed improvement of their respiratory disorder [65]. We subsequently have successfully desensitized over 100 aspirin-sensitive asthmatic patients by repeated incremental oral aspirin challenges, as noted above, until each patient was able to ingest 650 mg of aspirin without response. In some patients, up to eight or more aspirin-provoked asthmatic attacks were required before a desensitized state was achieved. Sensitization will recur from 1 to 5 days after the interruption of aspirin therapy; for this reason, it is imperative that the patient continue taking aspirin/NSAID on a daily basis if continuous treatment with aspirin is the objective [55].

We further studied the efficacy of treatment with aspirin in 25 aspirin-sensitive asthmatic patients in a 7-month, randomized, placebo-controlled, double-blind, crossover trial [66]. Significant improvement in rhinosinusitis occurred in two-thirds of the patients during aspirin treatment as compared with the placebo, and a majority of these patients had improvement in their asthma, though five of the patients had greater respiratory symptoms while taking aspirin as compared with the placebo.

As of 1990, 65 patients, from over 100 patients with aspirin sensitivity confirmed at Scripps Clinic or oral aspirin challenge, elected to be desensitized and to continue open trials of aspirin treatment, at dosages from 320 mg daily up to 650 mg four times daily, for periods of up to 8 years. Half of these patients continue aspirin treatment and have had significant improvement in symptom scores, reduced numbers of emergency visits or hospitalizations, and decrease of systemic and inhaled (but not nasal–insufflated) steroid dose as compared with the pretreatment period and with a control group of aspirin-sensitive patients not treated with aspirin. The half who discontinued treatment did so primarily because of alimentary side effects; respiratory disease, though improved during aspirin treatment, tended to revert toward pretreatment status after discontinuation of aspirin [67,68].

In separate studies, we have desensitized–treated aspirin-sensitive patients with chronic rhinosinusitis without asthma and have shown favorable response in blinded studies in the majority of these patients [69].

Other reports of aspirin desensitization and treatment in both aspirin-sensitive and tolerant asthmatic patients have been published and generally support the efficacy of this treatment regimen [70–78].

III. SULFUR DIOXIDE/SULFITES

In A.D. 79, the respiratory death of Pliny the Elder was attributed to the sulfur dioxide (SO_2)-rich gases emanating from the eruption of Mount Vesuvius. Sulfur oxides, including SO_2 and particulate sulfuric acid (H_2SO_4), are generated from the combustion of sulfur-containing fossil fuels and may be significant aeropollutants for asthmatic persons [79,80]. Plumes of exhaust fumes in the vicinity of power plants and smelters reach concentration peaks of 0.5–1 ppm SO_2 for 5- to 10-min intervals yet do not exceed the National Ambient Air Quality standard of 0.14 ppm average for 24 h [81].

Sulfur dioxide gas inhalation challenges in asthmatic subjects induce bronchoconstriction dependent on the concentration of SO_2 [82,83], the minute ventilation at which it is inhaled [84], and the severity of asthma as measured by nonspecific bronchial hyperreactivity to histamine or methacholine [82]. The response occurs more readily with oral than with nasal breathing [85] and is mitigated during breathing at high-temperature, high-humidity as compared with low-temperature, low-humidity conditions [86]. The maximal bronchoconstrictor response occurs over 5–10 minutes, and if not sufficient to produce symptoms necessitating bronchodilator treatment, it does not progress over ensuing hours of continued exposure. Eucapnic hyperventilation or moderate exercise while breathing SO_2 at 0.5–1 ppm has produced clinically significant bronchoconstriction in most asthmatics studied [81,83,85–88]; at 0.25 ppm the effect is small [89].

Likewise, sulfuric acid aerosols at a concentration of 1000 μg/m³, the threshold limit value of the Environmental Protection Agency for occupational exposure, produce significant declines of FEV_1 in asthmatic subjects [90], whereas aerosols at 100 μg/M³, the "worst case" for ambient exposure, do so only in asthmatic subjects during exercise [91–93]. The prevalence of persistent cough and phlegm is significantly higher among adults living in a Utah community near a smelter, with exposure at the 100 μg/M³ mean annual level, than among subjects in communities with exposure at one-third of that level or less [94].

The effects, if any, on the induction or maintenance of bronchial hyperreactivity of lesser concentrations of SO_2 and sulfuric acid particles—for example, the annual averages in urban Southern California are in the range of 0.001 to 0.01 ppm SO_2—singly or in combination with other aeropollutants or other factors associated with asthma, such as atopic state and viral respiratory infection, have not yet been clearly elucidated.

Sulfur dioxide, potassium metabisulfite ($K_2S_2O_5$), potassium bisulfite ($KHSO_3$), sodium sulfite (Na_2SO_4), sodium bisulfite ($NaHSO_3$), and sodium metabisulfite ($Na_2S_2O_5$) have been used for centuries as preservatives, sanitizing agents for food containers, selective inhibitors of growth of microorganisms in the fermentation industries, and inhibitors of enzyme-catalyzed oxidative discoloration and nonenzyme browning during the preparation, storage, distribution, and presentation of foods and beverages.

Sulfur dioxide–sulfite equilibrium (Fig. 3) at physiological or slightly acidic pH, as in the respiratory tract [84], favors bisulfite formation. Bisulfite can bind to sulfur-containing amino acids/proteins or, by sulfitolysis, disrupt disulfide bonds; sulfited moieties may be converted by sulfite oxidase to sulfates, which, unlike sulfites, are excretable by the kidneys.

Up to the late 1970s, sulfites were generally regarded as safe, in that healthy young adults could ingest gram amounts without apparent ill effect. In Table 2 are listed the sulfite contents, expressed as ppm SO_2 equivalents (mg sulfite/kg or 0.3 mg sulfite/ounce) for various foods, beverages, and drugs; also tabulated are the potentials for bisulfite and SO_2 liberation and thus clinical reaction in asthmatic subjects. At the top of the list are sulfite-freshened vegetables and fruits, previously encountered at restaurant salad bars in the late 1970s and early 1980s, followed by sulfur dioxide–preserved packaged fruits such as apples, apricots, and white raisins, sulfite-preserved wines, seafood, and potatoes, and other sulfite-preserved packaged foods. Drugs preserved with sulfites [95] included inhaled bronchodilators such as isoetharine (Bronkosol) and isoproterenol (Isuprel) and injectables including epinephrine, some parenteral corticosteroids, and local anesthetics with epinephrine.

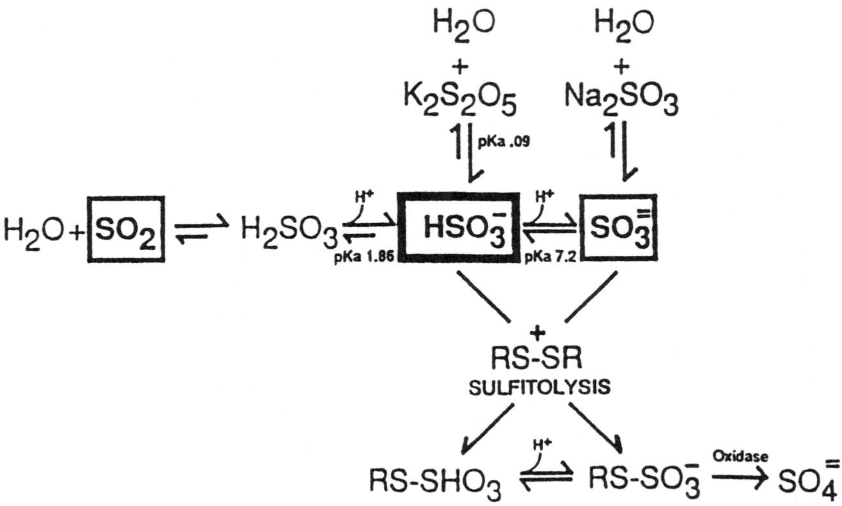

Figure 3 Equilibrium distribution of sulfur dioxide (SO_2), potassium metabisulfite ($K_2S_2O_5$), and sodium sulfite (Na_2SO_3), and interrelationships of bisulfite (HSO_3^-) and sulfite ($SO_3^=$) with proteins (RS-SR) and sulfate ($SO_4^=$). At physiological pH in aqueous solution, bisulfite (HSO_3^-) dominates.

Table 2 SO_2/Sulfites in Preserved Foods, Beverages, and Drugs

	ppm SO_2/sulfite equivalents (mg/kg or 0.03 mg/ounce)	Potential for SO_2/sulfite liberation–clinical reaction
Foods and beverages		
Sulfite-"freshened" salads and vegetables[a]	100 to ≥3,500	High
SO_2-dried fruits (apples, apricots, etc.)	275–3,000	High
Sulfite-preserved wine (labeled "sulfite added")	100–150	Moderate
Sulfite-preserved seafood and "fresh" potatoes	15–600	Low
All other sulfite-preserved (labeled "sulfite added")	10 to ≥10,000	Very low to high if label not heeded
Drugs		
Sulfite-preserved inhalants	0.5–1.5	High-rare[b]
Sulfite-preserved subcutaneous injectants	0.3–10	Very low
Sulfite-preserved intravenous injectants	0.3–10	Low

[a]FDA-prohibited, 8/86.
[b]Rare bronchoconstriction but (?) no bronchodilation.

A. Spectrum of Reactions to Sulfur Dioxide/Sulfites

In 1976, Prenner and Stevens [96] reported the case of a 50-year-old man who developed urticaria, swelling of the tongue, and chest tightness minutes after eating a green salad at a restaurant; he had wheal-flare cutaneous reaction to prick test with sodium bisulfate 10 mg/ml; his serum passively transferred this reaction in classical Prausnitz–Küstner testing; and ingestion of 10 mg of the sodium bisulfite solution reproduced the reaction. There have since been reported a handful of cases suggestive of anaphylactic sensitivity to ingested sulfites [97–99], including one to wine [100], and there are additional reports of cutaneous wheal-flare reactivity to test with sulfites [101,102]; however, rigorous proof of the presence of IgE antibody specific to sulfite as a hapten to account for reaction has not been achieved, and the question of true anaphylactic sensitivity remains open.

Asthmatic response to sulfites was first suggested by Kochen, who reported a child with repeated episodes after ingestion of dried fruits that had been treated with sulfur dioxide [103]. In 1981, Stevenson and Simon [104] reported four asthmatic patients who had moderate to severe exacerbations of bronchospasm while ingesting food or drink in restaurants, and showed in blinded challenge that ingestion of 5–10 mg of potassium metabisulfite in capsules reproduced the asthmatic reaction. They theorized that heterozygous sulfite oxidase deficiency might account for these reactions [105,106]. A report of blocking reaction with cyanocobalamin in four of five sulfite-reactive children is consistent with this hypothesis [107].

Subsequently, a series of reports [108,109] confirmed acute asthmatic distress with ingestion of meals likely to contain relatively high quantities of bisulfites and/or SO_2 and with inhalation treatment with sulfite-preserved bronchodilators [110]. Over the next few years, 17 deaths reported to the Food and Drug Administration (FDA) were linked to sulfites; this led in 1986 to a federal ban on the use of sulfiting agents on raw fruits and vegetables and a requirement for labeling of packaged foods containing 10 or more ppm SO_2 equivalents [111]. In addition, sometimes seemingly conflicting reports were published concerning the prevalence of reactions in various asthmatic populations challenged with sulfites in solution, swished, gargled, and swallowed or expectorated, or inhaled or injected [reviewed in Ref. 112].

Oral challenges with sulfites in doses up to 200 mg in solution have provoked bronchoconstriction in 3–20% of various asthmatic populations [82,84,112]. Graded inhalation challenges with metabisulfite in doses from 0.1 to 12.8 μmol provoke bronchoconstrictive responses in all asthmatics tested [113]. Pretreatment with ipatropium, furosemide, and budesonide significantly protects against metabisulfite-induced bronchospasm [114,115]. Metabisulfite-induced bronchoconstriction may involve bradykinin B_2 receptors, with subsequent activation of cholinergic mechanisms [116]. These results are consistent with the probability that reactivity to SO_2/sulfites is yet another measure of nonspecific bronchial hyperreactivity in asthma, though there is no direct correlation between metabisulfite and histamine or methacholine reactivity for individual subjects [117].

From a practical viewpoint, the risk of sulfite reactions among asthmatics now appears to be reduced in the United States. Reactions occur only in those with markedly hyperactive airways, especially those who require systemic corticosteroids for control of their disease; in those who attempt to ingest SO_2-treated dried fruit, relatively large amounts of sulfites in wines [118,119], or labeled processed packaged foods [120] or perhaps sulfite-preserved shrimp or processed potatoes [121]; in those who receive sulfite-containing bronchodilators by inhalation (but even so they may not have bronchoconstriction but merely lack pharmacological dilation); and in those who receive intravenous sulfite [108,110]. The risk of asthmatic reaction to subcutaneous injection of sulfites, including sulfite antioxidant in epinephrine, is virtually nil [122].

B. Indications and Methods for Challenges

From the late 1980s, the indications for challenges with SO_2, sulfite, and sulfurous acid particles have become limited to scientific investigation and very occasional clinical purposes.

Challenges for investigation of the environmental and occupational hazards of SO_2 and sulfuric acid exposures include epidemiological studies and studies of asthmatic populations aimed at better drawing the lines for regulating emissions of these chemicals [79]. Likewise, scientific investigations aimed at better understanding the bronchial hyperreactivity associated with asthma may employ SO_2 or sulfite challenges akin to histamine, methacholine, exercise, water, osmolar, allergen, mediator, and pharmacological challenges outlined in other chapters in this text.

For clinical purposes, when an asthmatic patient recognizes reactivity to SO_2/sulfite, as is most likely to occur with exposure-ingestion of dried fruits or wine, he can avoid these sulfite sources and is further protected by regulations of the FDA requiring labeling of processed food containing more than 10 ppm SO_2 equivalents. If there is suspicion, particularly if there is uncertainty regarding reaction to dried fruits, wine, processed potatoes, or shrimp, or when an asthmatic patient must be reassured that he is not relevantly sensitive to sulfites, oral challenge with the suspected food or beverage [121] or capsule doses of sulfite under single-blind, and if the result is apparently positive, then double-blind conditions, is appropriate.

At Scripps Clinic, we use the following protocol for sulfite capsule challenges: patients are challenged at a time when their asthma is in remission as documented by FEV_1 greater than 70% of the predicted or best previously observed value and at least 1.5 L absolute. Inhaled cromolyn [123] and anticholinergic [124], antihistamine [124], and adrenergic bronchodilator medications are withheld on the day of challenge; other medications are continued. Open oral challenges with capsule doses of 5, 25, 50, 100, and 200 mg of potassium metabisulfite at 30-min intervals are administered, and spirometric measurements are performed before each dose. If there is a fall of FEV$_1$ of 20% or more, the challenge is suspended, and obstruction is reversed with inhalations of adrenergic bronchodilator. Apparent reactions need be verified with double-blind, placebo-controlled challenges.

IV. OTHER CHEMICALS

A. Tartrazine

Tartrazine (FD&C yellow no. 5), a coal tar–derived azo dye, has been reported to provoke asthmatic reaction by several authors; however, virtually all of the reports do not include blinded and placebo-controlled challenges [125]. Since 1970 at Scripps Clinic, we have performed over 230 single-blind challenges of asthmatic patients with tartrazine by mouth, in doses up to 75 mg (10 times the "worst case" ordinary ingestion) and identified seven patients with apparent reactivity; however, of the six of these who returned at a later date for double-blind, placebo-controlled challenges, none was confirmed to be tartrazine-sensitive [126].

B. Monosodium Glutamate

Ingestion of gram amounts of the flavor-enhancer monosodium glutamate produces over a period of 30 min, in susceptible persons, the "Chinese restaurant syndrome" of facial–generalized burning flush sensation and sweating, with or without nausea, chest tightness, or pulsatile headache [127]. Several reports have suggested asthmatic response, with or without "Chinese restaurant syndrome," occurring over a period of several hours or 6–12 h after ingestion of monosodium glutamate [128–130]; however, blinding of challenges is difficult because of the flush response, and late-occurring asthma may reflect withholding of medications or unstable asthma. Monosodium glutamate challenges can be performed under conditions as outlined for aspirin and sulfite challenges, with capsules containing doses of 0.25, 0.5, 1, and then 2 g doses given at 30-min intervals (or longer if the history suggests late reaction), with spirometric measurements performed before each dose; apparent reaction needs to be verified by double-blinded, placebo-controlled challenges. We have not confirmed asthmatic reaction to monosodium glutamate among patients seen at Scripps Clinic in the past 25 years.

C. Benzalkonium Chloride

Paradoxical responses to nebulized ipatropium bromide [131] and beclomethasone dipropionate [132] led to the discovery that the antibacterial preservative benzalkonium chloride causes bronchoconstriction in about 60% of asthmatic subjects; the characteristics of the responses—rapid onset with slow recovery over 60 min, and inhibition by cromolyn but not ipatropium—suggest a mechanism of action via release of mediators [133]. The benzalkonium chloride concentration in commercial nebulizer solutions has been reduced so that only the rare patient with apparent immunological sensitivity will now react [134].

D. Others

Though concern has been raised through reports of asthma apparently aggravated by ingestion of sodium benzoate, parahydroxybenzoic acid, parabens, other azo and non-azo dyes (amaranth, ponceau, sunset yellow, brilliant blue, erythrocene, and indigotin), butylated hydroxyanisole (BHA), butylated hydroxytoluene (BHT), or potassium sorbate, when double-blinded, placebo-controlled challenges have been performed with these agents, confirmation of such sensitivity has not been obtained [135–137]. When the question arises of reactivity to these substances, challenge is indicated. Challenges may be accomplished according to the methods outlined for aspirin and sulfites, with 10%, 20%, 50%, 100%, and 200% of the usually ingested amounts given at 30-min intervals, with spirometric and clinical monitoring; should there be a suggestion of reaction, repeat challenges by double-blinded, placebo-controlled methods are indicated.

The flavors spearmint (*Mentha spicata*), peppermint (*Mentha piperita*), and menthol (*Mentha labiateae*), used in chewing gum and toothpaste, have been confirmed by challenges in two cases to have triggered asthma [138,139].

ACKNOWLEDGMENTS

Supported by grants AI 32834 and M01 RR00833 from the National Institutes of Health.

This is publication number 8004-MEM from the Scripps Research Institute, La Jolla, California.

REFERENCES

1. Brooks, P. M., and Day, R. O., Nonsteroidal antiinflammatory drugs—differences and similarities, *N. Engl. J. Med.*, *324*, 1716–1725 (1991).
2. Gilbert, G. B., Unusual idiosyncracy to aspirin, *JAMA*, *56*, 1262 (1911).
3. VanArsdel, P. P., Aspirin idiosyncracy and tolerance, *J. Allergy Clin. Immunol.*, *73*, 431–434 (1984).
4. Manning, M. E., Stevenson, D. D., and Mathison, D. A., Reactions to aspirin and other nonsteroidal anti-inflammatory drugs, *Immunol. Allergy Clin. North Am.*, *12*, 611–631 (1992).

5. Szczeklik, A., Gryglewski, R. J., and Czernigwska-Mysik, G., Clinical patterns of hypersensitivity to nonsteroidal anti-inflammatory drugs and their pathogenesis, *J. Allergy Clin. Immunol.*, *60*, 276–284 (1977).
6. Szczeklik, A., Aspirin-induced asthma: pathogenesis and clinical presentation, *Allergy Proc.*, *13*, 163–173 (1992).
7. Manning, M. E., and Stevenson, D. D., Pseudoallergic drug reactions. Aspirin, nonsteroidal antiinflammatory drugs, dyes, additives, and preservatives, *Immunol. Allergy Clin. North Am.*, *11*, 659–678 (1991).
8. McDonald, J. R., Mathison, D. A., and Stevenson, D. D., Aspirin intolerance in asthma, detection by oral challenge, *J. Allergy Clin. Immunol.*, *50*, 198–207 (1972).
9. Tan, Y., and Collins-Williams, C., Aspirin-induced asthma in children, *Ann. Allergy*, *48*, 1 (1982).
10. Pleskow, W. W., Stevenson, D. D., Mathison, D. A., et al., Aspirin-sensitive rhinosinusitis/asthma: spectrum of adverse reactions to aspirin, *J. Allergy Clin. Immunol.*, *71*, 574–579 (1983).
11. Falliers, C. J., Aspirin and subtypes of asthma: risk factor analysis, *J. Allergy Clin. Immunol.*, *52*, 141–147 (1973).
12. Giraldo, B., Blumenthal, M. N., and Spink, W. W., Aspirin intolerance and asthma: a clinical and immunological study, *Ann. Intern. Med.*, *71*, 479–496 (1969).
13. Spector, S. L., Wangaard, C. H., and Farr, R. S., Aspirin and concomitant idiosyncrasies in adult asthmatic patient, *J. Allergy Clin. Immunol.*, *64*, 500–506 (1979).
14. Stevenson, D. D., Mathison, D. A., Tan, E. M., and Vaughan, J. H., Provoking factors in bronchial asthma, *Arch. Intern. Med.*, *135*, 777–783 (1975).
15. Samuelsson, B., Leukotrienes: mediators of immediate hypersensitivity reactions and inflammation, *Science*, *220*, 568–575 (1983).
16. Lewis, R. A., Austen, K. F, and Soberman, R. J., Leukotrienes and other products of the 5-lipoxygenase pathway, *N. Engl. J. Med.*, *323*, 645–655 (1990).
17. Vane, J. R., Inhibition of prostaglandin synthesis as a mechanism of action for aspirin-like drugs, *Nature*, *231*, 232–235 (1971).
18. Vicks, S. D., Dean, R. J., and Tenholder, M. F., Ketorolac induced respiratory failure in an aspirin sensitive asthmatic, *Immunol. Allergy Prac.*, *13*, 23–25 (1991).
19. Settipane, R. A., and Stevenson, D. D., Cross-sensitivity with acetaminophen in ASA-sensitive asthmatics (abstr.), *J. Allergy Clin. Immunol.*, *81*, 180 (1988).
20. Stevenson, D. D., Hougham, A. J., Schrank, P. J., et al., Salsalate cross-sensitivity in aspirin-sensitive asthmatic patients, *J. Allergy Clin. Immunol.*, *86*, 749–758 (1990).
21. Szczeklik, A., Dworski, R., and Nizankowska, E., Choline magnesium trisalicylate in patients with aspirin-induced asthma (abstr.), *J. Allergy Clin. Immunol.*, *83*, 178 (1989).
22. Sheehan, G. J., Kutzner, M. R., Chin, W. D., Acute asthma attack due to ophthalmic indomethacin, *Ann. Intern. Med.*, *111*, 337–338 (1989).
23. Stevenson, D. D., and Lewis, R., Proposed mechanisms of aspirin sensitivity reactions, *J. Allergy Clin. Immunol.*, *80*, 788–790 (1987).
24. Ameisen, J. C., and Capron, A., Aspirin-sensitive asthma, *Clin. Exp. Allergy*, *20*, 127–129 (1990).

25. Lee, T. H., Smith, C. M., Arm, J. P., and Christie, P. E., Mediator release in aspirin-induced reactions, *J. Allergy Clin. Immunol.*, *88*, 827–829 (1991).
26. Goetzl, E. J., Valacer, D. J., Payan, D. G., et al., Abnormal responses to aspirin of leukocyte oxygenation of arachidonic acid in adults with aspirin intolerance, *J. Allergy Clin. Immunol.*, *77*, 693–698 (1986).
27. Ferreri, N. R., Howland, W. C., Stevenson, D. D., and Spiegelberg, H. L., Release of leukotrienes, prostaglandins, and histamine into nasal secretions of aspirin-sensitive asthmatics during reactions to aspirin, *Am. Rev. Respir. Dis.*, *137*, 847–854 (1988).
28. Picado, C., Ramis, I., Rosellò, J., Prat, J., Bulbena, O., Plaza, V., Montserrat, J. M., and Gelpí, E., Release of peptide leukotriene into nasal secretions after local instillation of aspirin in aspirin-sensitive asthmatic patients, *Am. Rev. Respir. Dis.*, *145*, 65–69 (1992).
29. Kowalski, M. L., Sliwinska-Kowalska, M., Igarashi, Y., White, M. V., Wojciechowksa, B., Brayton, P., Kaulbach, H., Rozniecki, J., and Kaliner, M. A., Nasal secretions in response to acetylsalicylic acid, *J. Allergy Clin. Immunol.*, *91*, 580–598 (1993).
30. Christie, P. E., Tagari, P., Ford-Hutchinson, A. W., Charlesson, S., Chee, P., Arm, J. P., and Lee, T. H., Urinary leukotriene E_4 concentrations increase after aspirin challenge in aspirin-sensitive asthmatic subjects, *Am. Rev. Respir. Dis.*, *143*, 1025–1029 (1991).
31. Christie, P. E., Tagari, P., Ford-Hutchinson, A. W., Black, C., Markendorf, A., Schmitz-Schumann, M., and Lee, T. H., Urinary leukotriene E_4 after lysine-aspirin inhalation in asthmatic subjects, *Am. Rev. Respir. Dis.*, *146*, 1531–1534 (1992).
32. Knapp, H. R., Sladek, K., and Fitzgerald, G. A., Increased excretion of leukotriene E_4 during aspirin induced asthma, *J. Lab. Clin. Invest.*, *119*, 48–51 (1992).
33. Kumlin, M., Dahlen, B., Bjorck, T., Zetterstrom, O., Granstrom, E., and Dahlen, S. E., Urinary excretion of leukotriene E4 and 11-dehydro-thromboxane B2 in response to bronchial provocations with allergen, aspirin, leukotriene D4, and histamine in asthmatics, *Am. Rev. Respir. Dis.*, *146*, 96–103 (1992).
34. Arm, J. P., O'Hickey, S. P., Spur, B. W., and Lee, T. H., Airway responsiveness to histamine and leukotriene E_4 in subjects with aspirin-induced asthma, *Am. Rev. Respir. Dis.*, *140*, 148–155 (1989).
35. Juergens, U. R., Christiansen, S. C., Stevenson, D. D., and Zuraw, B. L., Arachidonic acid metabolism in monocytes of aspirin-sensitive patients before and after oral aspirin challenge, *J. Allergy Clin. Immunol.*, *90*, 636–645 (1992).
36. Christie, P. E., Smith, C. M., and Lee, T. H., The potent and selective sulfidopeptide leukotriene antagonist, SK&F 104353, inhibits aspirin-induced asthma, *Am. Rev. Respir. Dis.*, *144*, 957–958 (1991).
37. Bosso, J. V., Schwartz, L. B., and Stevenson, D. D., Tryptase and histamine release during aspirin-induced respiratory reactions, *J. Allergy Clin. Immunol.*, *88*, 830–837 (1991).
38. Hollingsworth, H. M., Downing, E. T., Braman, S. S., et al., Identification and characterization of neutrophil chemotactic activity in aspirin-induced asthma, *Am. Rev. Respir. Dis.*, *130*, 373 (1984).

39. Lang, D. M., Christiansen, S. C., Stevenson, D. D., et al., Plasma high molecular weight kiningen (HMWK) is cleaved in aspirin (ASA) sensitive asthmatic patients during aspirin challenge, *J. Allergy Clin. Immunol.*, *81*, 192 (1988).
40. Okuda, Y., Hattori, H., Takashima, T., Miyatake, A., Yamatodani, A., Tsuyuguchi, I., and Kishimoto, S., Basophil histamine release by platelet-activating factor in aspirin-sensitive subjects with asthma, *J. Allergy Clin. Immunol.*, *86*, 558–553 (1990).
41. Williams, W. R., Pawlowicz, A., and Davies, B. H., Aspirin sensitive asthma: significance of the cyclooxygenase inhibiting and protein binding properties of the analgesic drugs, *Int. Arch. Allergy Appl. Immunol.*, *95*, 303–308 (1991).
42. Kowalski, M. L., Grzelewska-Rzymowski, I., Szmidt, M., et al., Fibrinolysis blood coagulation and platelet function during aspirin-induced bronchoconstriction in aspirin-intolerant asthmatics, *Ann. Allergy*, *58*, 367 (1987).
43. Ameisen, J. C., Capron, A., Joseph, M., et al., Aspirin-sensitive asthma: abnormal platelet response to drugs inducing asthmatic attacks, *Int. Arch. Allergy Appl. Immunol.*, *78*, 438–448 (1985).
44. Lassalle, P., Joseph, M., Ramon, P., Dracon, M., Tonnel, A., and Capron, A. Plasmapheresis in a patient with severe asthma associated with auto-antibodies to platelets, *Clin. Exp. Allergy*, *20*, 707–712 (1990).
45. Pearson, D. J., Suarez-Mendez, V. J., Day, J. P., and Miller, P. F., Selenium status in relation to reduced glutathione peroxidase activity in aspirin sensitive asthma, *Clin. Exp. Allergy*, *21*, 203–208 (1991).
46. Williams, W. R., Pawlowicz, A., and Davies, B. H., In vitro tests for the diagnosis of aspirin-sensitive asthma, *J. Allergy Clin. Immunol.*, *86*, 445–451 (1990).
47. Guez, S., Gualde, N., Bezian, J. H., and Cabanieu, G., *In vitro* study of platelets and circulating mononuclear cells of subjects presenting an intolerance to aspirin, *Int. Arch. Allergy Appl. Immunol.*, *97*, 233–236 (1992).
48. Plaza, V., Casals, F., Alonso, A., and Picado, C., Platelet kinetics in asthmatic patients with and without aspirin intolerance, *Thorax*, *47*, 533–536 (1992).
49. Pleskow, W. W., Chenoweth, D. E., Simon, R. A., Stevenson, D. D., and Curd, J. G., The absence of complement activation in aspirin sensitive asthmatic patients during aspirin challenge, *J. Allergy Clin. Immunol.*, *72*, 462–468 (1983).
50. Zhu, D., Becker, W.-M., Schulz, K.-H., Schubeler, K., and Schlaak, M., The presence of specific IgE to salicyloyl and O-methylsalicyloyl in aspirin sensitive patients, *Asian Pac. J. Allergy Immunol.*, *10*, 25–32 (1992).
51. Vargas, F. S., Croce, M., Teixeira, L. R., Terra-Filho, M., Cukier, A., and Light, R. W., Effect of inhaled furosemide on the bronchial response to lysine-aspirin inhalation in asthmatic subjects, *Chest*, *102*, 408–411 (1992).
52. Szczeklik, A., Nizankowska, E., Czerniawska-Mysik, G., and Sek, S., Hydrocortisone and airflow impairment in aspirin-induced asthma, *J. Allergy Clin. Immunol.*, *76*, 530–536 (1985).
53. Taniguchi, M., and Sato, A., Aspirin-induced asthmatics (AIA) have cross-sensitivity with the steroid succinate esters (abstr.), *NER Allergy Proc.*, *9*, 388 (1988).
54. Lympany, P., Welsh, K. I., Christie, P., Schmitz, M., and Lee, T. H., Genetic

analysis of the linkage between aspirin-induced asthma and antigens of the major histocompatibility complex (abstr.), *J. Allergy Clin. Immunol.*, *89*, 234 (1992).
55. Pleskow, W. W., Stevenson, D. D., Mathison, D. A., Simon, R. A., Zieger, R., and Schatz, M., Aspirin desensitization in aspirin-sensitive asthmatic patients: clinical manifestations and characterization of the refractory period, *J. Allergy Clin. Immunol.*, *69*, 11–19 (1982).
56. Bianco, S., Robuschi, M, and Petrigini, G., Aspirin-induced tolerance in aspirin-asthma detected by a new challenge test, *IRCS J. Med. Sci.*, *5*, 129 (1977).
57. Phillips, G. D., Foord, R., and Holgate, S. T., Inhaled lysine-aspirin as a bronchoprovocation procedure in aspirin-sensitive asthma: its repeatability, absence of a late-phase reaction, and the role of histamine, *J. Allergy Clin. Immunol.*, *84*, 232–241 (1989).
58. Pawlowicz, A., Williams, W. R., and Davies, B H., Inhalation and nasal challenge in the diagnosis of aspirin induced asthma, *Allergy*, *46*, 405–409 (1991).
59. Martelli, N. A., Bronchial and intravenous provocation tests with indomethacin in aspirin-sensitive asthmatics, *Am. Rev. Respir. Dis.*, *120*, 1073–1079 (1979).
60. Stevenson, D. D., and Simon, R. A., Sensitivity to aspirin and nonsteroidal antiinflammatory drugs, in: *Allergy Principles and Practice* (E. Middleton, et al., eds.), Mosby Year Book, St. Louis, 1993, pp. 1747–1765.
61. Stevenson, D. D., Simon, R. A., and Mathison, D. A., Cromolyn pretreatment delays onset of aspirin (ASA) induced asthmatic reactions, *J. Allergy Clin. Immunol.*, *73*, 162 (1984).
62. Nizankowska, E., Dworski, R., Soja, J., and Szczeklik, A., Salicylate pretreatment attenuates intensity of bronchial and nasal symptoms precipitated by aspirin in aspirin intolerant patients, *Clin. Exp. Allergy*, *20*, 646–652 (1990).
63. Widal, M. F., Abramin, P., and Lermoyez, J., Anaphylaxie et idiosyncrasie, *Presse Med.*, *30*, 189 (1922).
64. Zeiss, C. R., and Lockey, R. F., Refractory period to aspirin in a patient with aspirin-induced asthma, *J. Allergy Clin. Immunol.*, *57*, 440–448 (1976).
65. Stevenson, D. D., Simon, R. A., and Mathison, D. A., Aspirin sensitive asthma: tolerance to aspirin after positive oral aspirin challenges, *J. Allergy Clin. Immunol.*, *66*, 82–85 (1980).
66. Stevenson, D. D., Pleskow, W. W., Simon, R. A., Mathison, D. A., Lumry, W. R., Schatz, N., and Zeiger, R. S., Aspirin-sensitive rhinosinusitis asthma: a double-blind crossover study of treatment with aspirin, *J. Allergy Clin. Immunol.*, *73*, 500–507 (1984).
67. Sweet, J. M., Stevenson, D. D., Simon, R. A., and Mathison, D. A., Long-term effects of aspirin desensitization—Treatment for aspirin-sensitive rhinosinusitis-asthma, *J. Allergy Clin. Immunol.*, *85*, 59–65 (1990).
68. Stevenson, D. D., Commentary: the American experience with aspirin desensitization for aspirin-sensitive rhinosinusitis and asthma, *Allergy Proc.*, *13*, 185–192 (1992).
69. Lumry, W. R., Curd, J. G., Zeiger, R. S., Pleskow, W. W., and Stevenson, D. D., Aspirin sensitive rhinosinusitis: the clinical syndrome and effects of aspirin administration, *J. Allergy Clin. Immunol.*, *71*, 580–587 (1983).

70. Chu, J. T., Improvement in aspirin-sensitive asthmatic subjects after rapid desensitization and aspirin maintenance (ADAM) treatment, *J. Allergy Clin. Immunol.*, *71*, 560–567 (1983).
71. Donker, R. E., and Wedner, H. J., Aspirin-desensitization in aspirin-sensitive asthma: failure to maintain a desensitized state during prolonged therapy, *Am. Rev. Respir. Dis.*, *128*, 953–955 (1983).
72. Asad, S. I., Kemeny, D. M., Youlton, L. J., et al., Effect of aspirin in "aspirin sensitive" patients, *Br. Med. J.*, *288*, 745–748 (1984).
73. Kowalski, M. L., et al., Clinical efficacy of aspirin in "desensitised" aspirin-sensitive asthmatics, *Eur. J. Respir. Dis.*, *69*, 219–225 (1986).
74. Kowalski, M. L., Management of aspirin-sensitive rhinosinusitis–asthma syndrome: what role for aspirin desensitization? *Allergy Proc.*, *13*, 175–183 (1992).
75. Kordansky, D., Adkinson, F., Jr., Norman, P. S., and Rosenthal, R. R., Asthma improved by nonsteroidal anti-inflammatory drugs, *Ann. Intern. Med.*, *88*, 508–511 (1978).
76. Szczeklik, A., and Nizankowska, E., Asthma improved by aspirin-like drugs, *Br. J. Dis. Chest*, *77*, 153–158 (1983).
77. Nelson, R. P., Stablein, J. J., and Lockey, R. F., Asthma improved by acetylsalicylic acid and other nonsteroidal anti-inflammatory agents, *NER Allergy Proc.*, *7*, 117–121 (1986).
78. Fernandez-Rivas, M., Cesar, J. M., and Losada, E., Asthma relieved by aspirin: clinical studies, platelet function, and arachidonate metabolism, *J. Allergy Clin. Immunol.*, *89*, 141–143 (1992).
79. Boushey, H., Asthma, sulfur dioxide and the Clean Air Act. Medical staff conference, University of California, San Francisco, *West. J. Med.*, *136*, 129–135 (1982).
80. Sheppard, D., Sulfur dioxide and asthma—a double-edged sword? *J. Allergy Clin. Immunol.*, *82*, 961–964 (1988).
81. Balmes, J. R., Fine, J. M., and Sheppard, D. Symptomatic bronchoconstriction after short term inhalation of sulfur dioxide, *Am. Rev. Respir. Dis.*, *136*, 1117–1121 (1987).
82. Sheppard, D., Wong, W. S., Uehara, C. F., Nadel, J. A., and Boushey, H. A., Lower threshold and greater bronchomotor responsiveness of asthmatic subjects to sulfur dioxide, *Am. Rev. Respir. Dis.*, *122*, 873–878 (1980).
83. Fine, J. M., Gordon, T., and Sheppard, D., The roles of pH and ionic species in sulfur dioxide– and sulfite-induced bronchoconstriction, *Am. Rev. Respir. Dis.*, *136*, 1122–1126 (1987).
84. Linn, W. S., Avol, E. L., Peng, R. C., et al., Replicated dose–response study of sulfur dioxide effects in normal, atopic and asthmatic volunteers, *Am. Rev. Respir. Dis.*, *136*, 1127–1134 (1987).
85. Bethel, R. A., Erle, D. J., Epstein, J., et al., Effect of exercise rate and route of inhalation on sulfur dioxide–induced bronchoconstriction in asthmatic subjects, *Am. Rev. Respir. Dis.*, *128*, 592–596 (1983).
86. Linn, W. S., Shamoo, D. A., Anderson, D. R., et al., Effects of heat and humidity on the response of exercising asthmatics to sulfur dioxide exposure, *Am. Rev. Respir. Dis.*, *131*, 221–225 (1985).

87. Linn, W. S., Venet, T. G., Shamoo, D. A., et al., Respiratory effects of sulfur dioxide in heavily exercising asthmatics, *Am. Rev. Respir. Dis.*, *127*, 278–283 (1983).
88. Bethel, R. A., Epstein, J., Sheppard, D., et al., Sulkfur dioxide–induced bronchoconstriction in freely breathing, exercising, asthmatic subjects, *Am. Rev. Respir. Dis.*, *128*, 987–990 (1983).
89. Bethel, R. A., Sheppard, D., Geffroy, B., et al., Effect of 0.25 ppm sulfur dioxide on airway resistance in freely breathing, heavily exercising, asthmatic subjects, *Am. Rev. Respir. Dis.*, *131*, 659–661 (1985).
90. Utell, M. J., Morrow, P. E., Speers, D. M., et al., Airway response to sulfite and sulfuric acid aerosols in asthmatics, *Am. Rev. Respir. Dis.*, *128*, 444–450 (1983).
91. Koenig, J. Q., Pierson, W. E., and Horike, M., The effect of inhaled sulfuric acid on pulmonary function in adolescent asthmatics, *Am. Rev. Respir. Dis.*, *128*, 221–225 (1983).
92. Utell, M. J., Frampton, M. W., and Morrow, P. E., Air pollution and asthma: clinical studies with sulfuric acid aerosols, *Allergy Proc.*, *12*, 385–388 (1991).
93. Hanley, Q. S., Koenig, J. Q., Larson, T. V., Anderson, T. L., Van Belle, G., Rebolledo, V., Covert, D. S., and Pierson, W. E., Response of young asthmatic patients to inhaled sulfuric acid, *Am. Rev. Respir. Dis.*, *145*, 326–331 (1992).
94. Chapman, R. S., Calafiore, D. C., and Hassiblad, V., Prevalence of persistent cough and phlegm in young adults in relation to long-term ambient sulfur oxide exposure, *Am. Rev. Respir. Dis.*, *132*, 261–267 (1985).
95. Settipane, G. A., Sulfites in drugs: a new comprehensive list, *NER Allergy Proc.*, *7*, 543–545 (1986).
96. Prenner, B. M., and Stevens, J. J., Anaphylaxis after ingestion of sodium bisulfite, *Ann. Allergy*, *37*, 180–182 (1976).
97. Schwartz, H. J., Sensitivity to ingested metabisulfite: variations in clinical presentation, *J. Allergy Clin. Immunol.*, *71*, 487–489 (1983).
98. Hobenicht, H. A., Preuss, L., and Lovell, R. G., Sensitivity to ingested metabisulfites: cause of bronchoconstriction and urticaria, *Immunol. Allergy Pract.*, *5*, 243–245 (1983).
99. Yang, W. H., Purchase, E. C. R., and Rivington, R. N., Positive Prausnitz-Küstner reaction in metabisulfite subjects, *J. Allergy Clin. Immunol.*, *75*, 198 (1985).
100. Clayton, D. E., and Busse, W., Anaphylaxis to wine, *Clin. Allergy*, *10*, 341–343 (1980).
101. Selner, J., Bush, R., Nordlee, J., et al., Skin reactivity to sulfite and sensitivity to sulfited foods in a sulfite-sensitive asthmatic (abstr.), *J. Allergy Clin. Immunol.*, *79*, 241 (1987).
102. Wells, J. H., Metabisulfite (MBS) skin testing in 2000 allergy clinic patients, *J. Allergy Clin. Immunol.*, *81*, 220 (1988).
103. Kochen, J., Sulfur dioxide, a respiratory tract irritant even if ingested, *Pediatrics*, *52*, 145–146 (1973).
104. Stevenson, D. D., and Simon, R. A., Sensitivity to ingested metabisulfites in asthmatic subjects, *J. Allergy Clin. Immunol.*, *68*, 26–32 (1981).
105. Jacobsen, D. W., Simon, R. A., and Singh, M., Sulfite oxidase deficiency and cobalamin protection in sulfite-sensitive asthmatics, *J. Allergy Clin. Immunol.*, *73*, 135 (1984).

106. Stevenson, D. D., and Simon, R. A., Sulfites and asthma, *J. Allergy Clin. Immunol.*, *74*, 469–472 (1984).
107. Añíbarro, B., Caballero, M. T., García-Ara, M. C., Díaz-Pena, J. M., and Ojeda, J. A., Asthma with sulfite intolerance in children: a blocking study with cyanocobalamin, *J. Allergy Clin. Immunol.*, *90*, 103–109 (1992).
108. Baker, G. J., Collett, P., and Allen, D. H., Bronchospasm induced by metabisulphite-containing foods and drugs, *Med. J. Australia*, *2*, 614–617 (1981).
109. Schwartz, H. J., and Chester, E., Bronchospastic responses to aerosolized metabisulfite in asthmatic subjects: potential mechanisms and clinical implications, *J. Allergy Clin. Immunol.*, *74*, 511–513 (1984).
110. Twarog, F. J., and Leung, D. Y. M., Anaphylaxis to a component of isoetharine (sodium bisulfite), *JAMA*, *248*, 2030–2032 (1982).
111. FDA Drug Bulletin, 1988, pp. 8À.
112. Bush, R. K., Taylor, S. L., and Busse, W., A critical evaluation of trials in reactions to sulfites, *J. Allergy Clin. Immunol.*, *78*, 191–202 (1986).
113. Wright, W., Zhang, Y. G., Salome, C. M., and Woolcock, A. J., Effect of inhaled preservatives on asthmatic subjects. I. Sodium metabisulfite, *Am. Rev. Respir. Dis.*, *141*, 1400–1404 (1990).
114. Bellingan, G. J., Dixon, C. M. S., and Ind, P. W., Inhibition of inhaled metabisulphite induced bronchoconstriction by inhaled furosemide and ipratropium bromide, *Br. J. Clin. Pharmacol.*, *34*, 71–74 (1992).
115. O'Connor, B. J., Ridge, S. M., Barnes, P. J., and Fuller, R. W., Greater effect of inhaled budesonide on adenosine 5′-monophosphate–induced than on sodium-metabisulfite–induced bronchoconstriction in asthma, *Am. Rev. Respir. Dis.*, *146*, 560–564 (1992).
116. Mansour, E., Ahmed, A., Cortes, A., Caplan, J., Burch, R. M., and Abraham, W. M., Mechanisms of metabisulfite-induced bronchoconstriction: evidence for bradykinin B_2-receptor stimulation, *J. Appl. Physiol.*, *72*, 1831–1837 (1992).
117. Magnussen, H., Jörres, R., Wagner, H. M., and Nieding, G., Relationship between the airway response to inhaled sulfur dioxide, isocapnic hyperventilation, and histamine in asthmatic subjects, *Int. Arch. Occup. Environ. Health.*, *62*, 485–491 (1990).
118. Gershwin, M. E., Ough, C., Bock, A., et al., Grand rounds: adverse reactions to wine, *J. Allergy Clin. Immunol.*, *75*, 411–420 (1985).
119. Dahl, R., Henriksen, J. M., and Harving, H., Red wine asthma: a controlled challenge study, *J. Allergy Clin. Immunol.*, *78*, 1126–1129 (1986).
120. Nagy, S. M., Teuber, S. S., Murphy, P., and Loscutoff, S. M., Adverse reactions to a salsa containing high levels of sulfites (abstr.), *J. Allergy Clin. Immunol.*, *91*, 150 (1993).
121. Taylor, S. L., Bush, R. K., Selner, J. C., et al., Sensitivity to sulfited foods among sulfite-sensitive subjects with asthma, *J. Allergy Clin. Immunol.*, *81*, 1159–1167 (1988).
122. Simon, R. A., Adverse reactions to drug additives, *J. Allergy Clin. Immunol.*, *74*, 623–630 (1984).
123. Koenig, J. Q., Marshall, S. G., Van Belle, G., et al., Therapeutic range cromolyn dose–response inhibition and complete obliteration of SO_2-induced bronchoconstriction on atopic adolescents, *J. Allergy Clin. Immunol.*, *81*, 897–901 (1988).

124. Simon, R. A., Goldfarb, G., and Jacobsen, D. W., Blocking studies in sulfite-sensitive asthmatics, *J. Allergy Clin. Immunol.*, *73*, 136 (1984).
125. Stevenson, D. D., Simon, R. A., Lumry, W. R., and Mathison, D. A., Adverse reactions to tartrazine, *J. Allergy Clin. Immunol.*, *78*, 182–191 (1986).
126. Stevenson, D. D., Simon, R. A., Lumry, W. R., and Mathison, D. A., Pulmonary reactions to tartrazine, *Pediatr. Allergy Immunol.*, *3*, 222–227 (1992).
127. Wilkin, J. K., Flushing reactions: consequences and mechanisms, *Ann. Intern. Med.*, *95*, 468–476 (1981).
128. Allen, D. H., and Baker, G. J., Chinese restaurant asthma, *N. Engl. J. Med.*, *305*, 1154–1155 (1981).
129. Koepke, J. W., and Selner, J. C., Combined monosodium glutamate (MSG)/ metabisulfite (MBS) induced asthma, *J. Allergy Clin. Immunol.*, *77*, 158 (1986).
130. Allen, D. H., Delohery, J., and Baker, G., Monosodium L-glutamate–induced asthma, *J. Allergy Clin. Immunol.*, *80*, 530–537 (1987).
131. Beasley, C. R. W., Rafferty, P., and Holgate, S. T., Bronchoconstrictor properties of preservatives in ipratropium bromide (Atrovent) nebuliser solution, *Br. Med. J.*, *294*, 1197–1198 (1987).
132. Clark, R. J., Exacerbation of asthma after nebulised beclomethasone diproprionate, *Lancet*, 574 (1986).
133. Zhang, Y. G., Wright, W. J., Tam, W. K., Nguyen-Dang, T. H., Salome, C. M., and Woolcock, A. J., Effect of inhaled preservatives on asthmatic subjects. II. Benzalkonium chloride, *Am. Rev. Respir. Dis.*, *141*, 1405–1408 (1990).
134. Ponder, R. D., and Wray, B. B., A case report: sensitivity to benzalkonium chloride, *J. Asthma*, *30*, 229–231 (1993).
135. Weber, R. W., Hoffman, M., Raine, D. A., and Nelson, H. S., Incidence of bronchoconstriction due to aspirin, azo dyes, non-azo dyes, and preservatives in a population of perennial asthmatics, *J. Allergy Clin. Immunol.*, *64*, 32–37 (1979).
136. Rosenhall, L., Evaluation of intolerance to analgesics, preservatives and food colorants with challenge tests, *Eur. J. Respir. Dis.*, *63*, 410–419 (1982).
137. Simon, R. A., Adverse reactions to food additives, *NER Allergy Proc.*, *7*, 533–542 (1986).
138. Spurlock, B. W., and Dailey, T. M., Shortness of (fresh) breath–toothpaste-induced bronchospasm (letter), *N. Engl. J. Med.*, *323*, 1845–1846 (1990).
139. Subiza, J., Subiza, J. L., Valdivieso, R., Escribano, P. M., Garcia, R., Jerez, M., and Subiza, E., Toothpaste flavor–induced asthma, *J. Allergy Clin. Immunol.*, *90*, 1004–1006 (1992).

23

Diagnosing Food Allergy

Hugh A. Sampson

The Johns Hopkins University School of Medicine
Baltimore, Maryland

I. INTRODUCTION

The term "food allergy" is frequently used to denote any "adverse food reaction" a misnomer that has led to substantial confusion in this field. In addition, the "perceived" prevalence of food allergy is far greater than the "actual" prevalence. Household surveys suggest that approximately one-third of American families alter their eating patterns because one family members is believed to be food-"allergic" [1]. In this chapter, the recognition and diagnosis of well-characterized food-allergic reactions will be discussed.

"Adverse food reaction" is a generic term referring to any untoward event resulting from the ingestion of a food [2]. It may be the result of a *food hypersensitivity*, i.e., an adverse immunological reaction, or a *food intolerance*, i.e., an adverse physiological reaction. Food intolerances probably constitute the majority of adverse food reactions and are secondary to toxic or pharmacological substances found in some foods, such as chemical or microbial contaminants, or to metabolic disorders of the host (e.g., lactose intolerance). *Food aversions* may mimic adverse food reactions, but they cannot be reproduced when the patient ingests the food unknowingly or in a blinded challenge.

The prevalence of food allergies in the general population is unknown. Bock followed 480 babies in a general pediatric practice from birth until their third birthday. Parents suspected adverse food reactions in 28% of the infants, but only 38 children (or 8% overall) had symptoms confirmed by oral food challenge [3]. In a study of 1759 Danish infants, the prevalence of cow's milk allergy was found to be 2.2% [4]. A similar study of infants on the Isle of Wight reported a 2.5% prevalence of cow's milk allergy [5]. The majority of food allergies are manifested in the first year of life, but only a minority persist beyond a child's third birthday (about 15% in the Danish study). Although no comprehensive epidemiological studies are available, the prevalence of *true food allergy* is probably 3% to 4% among young children and 1% to 2% among adults.

The gastrointestinal tract has two main functions: to process ingested food into forms that can be absorbed and utilized for energy and cell growth, and to prevent intact foreign antigens from gaining access to the body. Although more than 98% of ingested antigens are blocked by this gastrointestinal barrier, minute amounts of intact food antigens are absorbed and transported throughout the body [6]. Antigenically intact food proteins entering the circulation do not normally cause adverse reactions, because most people develop *tolerance* to ingested food antigens. However, a breakdown of or failure to develop oral tolerance may result in a variety of hypersensitivity responses to ingested food antigens.

Immunoglobulin E (IgE)-mediated food hypersensitivity reactions are probably the best understood [7]. Food-specific IgE antibodies bind high-affinity $Fc_{\epsilon}RI$ receptors on mast cells and basophils as well as low-affinity $Fc_{\epsilon}RII$ receptors on macrophages, monocytes, lymphocytes, eosinophils, and platelets. Food allergens penetrating mucosal barriers circulate and may contact IgE-bearing cells, activating them to generate a variety of mediators and cytokines. With repeated ingestion of food allergens, mononuclear cells may be stimulated to secrete "histamine-releasing factors," some of which interact with IgE molecules bound to the surface of basophils (and perhaps mast cells), increasing their "releasability" [8].

Cell-mediated hypersensitivity is generally implicated in food-allergic disorders in which symptoms develop several hours after the ingestion of a suspected food allergen and no evidence of food-specific IgE antibodies can be demonstrated [7]. Although this mechanism may contribute to several forms of adverse food reaction, no clear example of a cell-mediated food hypersensitivity disorder has been substantiated.

II. CLINICAL MANIFESTATIONS OF FOOD HYPERSENSITIVITY

When attempting to diagnose food-allergic disorders, it is most useful to determine whether the suspected reaction is consistent with one of the many well-characterized food hypersensitivity disorders previously described. A brief description of the various disorders follows:

A. Immunoglobulin E–Mediated Reactions

1. Gastrointestinal Food Hypersensitivity

A number of gastrointestinal syndromes associated with food-induced IgE-mediated food allergy have been reported in humans, including the oral allergy syndrome, gastrointestinal anaphylaxis, and a subgroup of allergic eosinophilic gastroenteritis and infantile colic.

Oral Allergy Syndrome. Symptoms confined to pruritus and edema of the lips, tongue, palate, and throat constitute the oral allergy syndrome and may be considered analogous to a contact urticaria of the oral mucosa and tongue. However, these symptoms also may be seen in the initial phase of a generalized food-allergic reaction. The oral allergy syndrome generally occurs in patients with allergic rhinitis following the ingestion of various fresh fruits and raw vegetables [9]. Oral symptoms following the ingestion of bananas and melons (watermelon, cantaloupe, honeydew, etc.) are frequently associated with ragweed pollinosis, and those following the ingestion of raw carrots, celery, potatoes, apples, and hazelnuts are associated with birch pollen allergy. The responsible cross-reacting allergens appear to be heat-labile, since these patients generally can ingest these foods in their cooked form without symptoms.

Gastrointestinal Anaphylaxis. Symptoms secondary to food-induced, IgE-mediated reactions develop within minutes to 2 h of ingesting a food allergen and consist of nausea, abdominal pain, cramps, vomiting, and, less frequently, diarrhea [10]. Interestingly, the frequent ingestion of a food allergen by some allergic persons appears to induce partial desensitization of gastrointestinal mast cells, resulting in subclinical symptoms such as poor appetite, periodic abdominal pain, and poor weight gain. Moderate malabsorption has been demonstrated with various absorption markers (e.g., lactulose, mannitol, polyethylene glycol). Elimination of the responsible food allergen often is followed by improved appetite and weight gain.

Allergic Eosinophilic Gastroenteropathy. Immunoglobulin E–mediated food allergy is responsible for symptoms in a subset of patients with allergic eosinophilic gastroenteropathy syndrome. Patients with this syndrome commonly present with postprandial nausea and vomiting, abdominal pain, diarrhea (occasionally steatorrhea), and weight loss, or, in young infants, with failure to thrive [11]. Patients with food-induced symptoms generally have other atopic disorders, elevated serum IgE levels, positive prick skin tests to a variety of foods and inhalants, peripheral blood eosinophilia, iron deficiency anemia, and hypoalbuminemia. In some infants, generalized edema occurs secondary to marked protein-losing enteropathy and hypoalbuminemia, often in the presence of minimal gastrointestinal symptoms [12]. Rarely, pyloric stenosis with outlet obstruction has been shown to be secondary to allergic eosinophilic gastroenteropathy [13]. Elimination of the responsible food allergen from the diet for up to 12 weeks may be necessary to bring about resolution of symptoms and normalization of intestinal histology.

Infantile Colic. Paroxysmal fussiness with "inconsolable crying," drawing up of the legs, abdominal distention, and excessive gas are the hallmarks of infantile colic. Symptoms generally develop in the first month of life and persist through the third to fourth month of life. Double-blind, crossover trials have implicated IgE-mediated hypersensitivity as a pathogenic factor in a selected group of infants with colic. However, this mechanism probably accounts for only about 15% of cases of infantile colic [14].

2. Respiratory Food Hypersensitivity Reactions

Both upper and lower respiratory reactions have been provoked during double-blind, placebo-controlled oral food challenges (DBPCFCs). Although isolated airway symptoms are rare [15], respiratory symptoms not uncommonly accompany allergic reactions involving the skin and gastrointestinal tract. Within minutes to 2 h of ingestion, food allergens may induce typical signs and symptoms of rhinoconjunctivitis, laryngeal edema, and asthma.

Allergic Rhinoconjunctivitis. Symptoms of food-induced rhinoconjunctivitis include periocular pruritus and erythema, and tearing; and nasal congestion, pruritus, sneezing, and rhinorrhea. In children with atopic dermatitis undergoing DBPCFC, nasal lavage fluid histamine levels were found to increase significantly with the onset of nasal symptoms, strongly implicating a pathogenic role for nasal mast cell activation [16]. Similarly, pulmonary function studies during DBPCFCs have demonstrated significant drops in forced vital capacity (FVC), forced expired volume in 1 second (FEV_1), and maximal midexpiratory flow (MMEF) in patients experiencing a positive food challenge [17]. More recently, changes in airway reactivity following positive DBPCFCs have been demonstrated by pre- and postchallenge methacholine inhalation studies [18].

Consumption of food allergens is rarely the main aggravating factor in chronic rhinoconjunctivitis and asthma. Two studies indicated that food allergens may play a major pathogenic role in 6–8% of pediatric patients with asthma followed in pulmonary clinics [19,20] or in 16% referred to an allergy specialty center [21]. Interestingly, nearly all asthmatic children with food-induced wheezing had either atopic dermatitis or a history of eczema.

3. Cutaneous Reactions

The skin may be the most common target organ in IgE-mediated food hypersensitivity. Ingestion of food allergens may provoke the rapid onset of cutaneous symptoms or aggravate more chronic conditions.

Urticaria/Angioedema. Acute urticaria and angioedema are among the most common symptoms of food-allergic reactions, but the exact prevalence of these reactions is unknown. Most patients with acute food induced urticaria/angioedema do not seek medical assistance or even report the reaction. The onset of hives or swelling occurs within minutes of ingesting the responsible food allergen, making the cause-and-effect nature of the reaction obvious to the patient. In children, eggs, milk, peanuts, and nuts are most frequently implicated, and in adults, fish, shellfish, nuts, and peanuts are most commonly responsible. Acute contact urticaria may result from contact with raw meats, fish, vegetables, and fruits [22]. Food hypersensitivity is occasionally incriminated in chronic urticaria and angioedema (symptoms lasting longer than 6 weeks). In one series of 163 children with chronic or recurrent urticaria, food allergy was implicated in only 10% of patients [23].

Atopic Dermatitis. The pathogenic role of food hypersensitivity in atopic dermatitis is most important in the pediatric population. In a series of children referred to a university dermatology and allergy clinic for evaluation of atopic dermatitis, IgE-mediated food allergy affected about 30% of patients [24]. In general, a single ingestion of food allergen does not provoke obvious cutaneous symptoms, but the repeated ingestion of food allergen leads to chronic inflammation and the typical eczematous lesions.

Of 320 patients with chronic, severe atopic dermatitis, about 60% were found to have food hypersensitivity [25]. Patients were evaluated for food allergy by DBPCFCs after clearing of their skin lesions, in a research unit setting. Symptoms provoked by food challenges developed within minutes to 2 h, leading to cutaneous reactions in 74% of positive challenges. During the initial evaluation, skin symptoms generally consisted of the abrupt onset of a markedly pruritic, erythematous, morbilliform rash in predilection sites for atopic dermatitis. Urticarial lesions were rare. Plasma histamine concentration rose significantly in conjunction with positive DBPCFCs, with no evidence of immediate activation of circulating basophils [26]. Approximately 4–8 h following initial skin symptoms, patients often developed diffuse pruritus, and less frequently, an erythematous macular rash. Biopsies obtained 8–14 h after a positive challenge demonstrated an eosinophilic infiltration of lesional skin [25].

Although gastrointestinal complaints are rarely elicited, 53% of patients developed gastrointestinal symptoms including nausea, abdominal cramping, and vomiting and/or diarrhea. Upper respiratory symptoms, especially laryngeal edema (sensation of itching and tightness in the throat, persistent throat clearing with dry hacking cough, and hoarseness), were seen in approximately 40% of the challenges and wheezing in about 10% of challenges.

Continuous ingestion of food allergens appears to provoke the spontaneous production of histamine-releasing factor (HRF) from mononuclear cells in vitro, and most likely in vivo [8]. The generation of HRF is associated with increased spontaneous release of histamine from basophils in vitro and increased cutaneous hyperirritability (state of increased reactivity of the skin to a variety of minor nonspecific stimuli, e.g., heat, cold, detergents, etc.). Removal of incriminated food allergens from the diet results in normalization of spontaneous generation of

HRF over a 6- to 9-month period, normalization of spontaneous basophil histamine release, and marked decrease of cutaneous hyperirritability. In addition, nearly one-third of symptomatic food allergies were lost after 1–2 years of dietary allergen elimination. The probability of developing tolerance appeared to depend on the degree of dietary compliance and the food allergen responsible for the reaction.

Generalized Anaphylaxis. The prevalence of food-induced anaphylaxis is unknown, although Bock estimates at least 1000 emergency room visits for food-induced anaphylaxis each year in the United States [27]. Yunginger et al. reported seven food-induced anaphylactic deaths reviewed over a period of 14 months [28]. More recently, six fatal and seven near-fatal food-induced anaphylactic reactions in children (aged 2–17 years) were reviewed [29]. All the children had asthma and had suffered a previous allergic reaction to the incriminated food. About half the patients experienced biphasic or protracted anaphylaxis. No patients in either series who had a fatal reaction received epinephrine immediately. However, four patients with near-fatal reactions did receive epinephrine 5–55 min before developing severe symptoms, but still went on to develop respiratory collapse and hypotension.

B. Non-IgE-Mediated Food Hypersensitivity

1. Gastrointestinal Food Hypersensitivity

A number of gastrointestinal syndromes are believed to be secondary to adverse immunological reactions, but the exact mechanisms are unknown.

Food-induced Enterocolitis Syndrome. Cow's milk– and soy protein–induced enterocolitis frequently presents in infants between 1 and 3 months of age with protracted vomiting and diarrhea, not infrequently resulting in dehydration [30,31]. It is occasionally seen in breast-fed infants as a result of antigen passed in maternal milk. Similar symptoms have been reported in older children in reaction to eggs, rice, wheat, and peanuts. Occult blood, eosinophils, and polymorphonuclear neutrophils are generally present in the stools. Prick skin tests and radioallergosorbent tests (RASTs) with the responsible food allergen are negative. Jejunal biopsies reveal patches of flattened villi, edema, and increased numbers of lymphocytes, eosinophils, and mast cells. Dietary elimination of the responsible food generally leads to resolution of symptoms within 72 h. The diagnosis is established by oral food challenge. Once diagnosed, children should be given a hypoallergenic formula (Alimentum, Nutramigen, or Pregestimil) until about 9–12 months of age, since about 50% will develop a similar sensitivity to soy if given a soy-based formula. Most children with food-induced enterocolitis "outgrow" their hypersensitivity by their second or third birthday.

Food-Induced Colitis. Food-induced colitis also presents in the first few months of life and is generally secondary to cow's milk or soy protein hypersensitivity, but it also may occur in exclusively breast-fed infants [32,33]. Unlike infants with food-induced enterocolitis, these children generally appear healthy, and colitis is discovered only because of the presence of gross or occult blood in their stool. Sigmoidoscopic findings are variable but range from areas of patchy mucosal injection to severe friability with small aphthoid ulcerations and bleeding. Mucosal edema and a prominent eosinophilic infiltrate in the crypt epithelium and lamina propria are seen on biopsy. Blood in the stools generally clears within 72 h of appropriate food allergen elimination, but resolution of the mucosal lesions may take several weeks. Reintroduction of the responsible food leads to resumption of symptoms within several hours to days. Infants with food-induced colitis can generally tolerate the responsible allergen after 6 months to 2 years of allergen avoidance.

Malabsorption Syndromes. Diarrhea and weight loss or poor weight gain may be secondary to hypersensitivity to a variety of food proteins including cow's milk, soy, wheat and other cereal grains, and egg [33,34]. Symptoms may include protracted diarrhea, vomiting, and failure to thrive, with increased fecal fat and secondary carbohydrate malabsorption. Cow's milk sensitivity appears to be the most frequent cause of this syndrome in young infants. Eliminating the responsible food from the diet brings about resolution of symptoms, but this may require several days to weeks. A patchy villous atrophy similar to that of celiac disease but generally less severe is seen on endoscopy, and biopsy reveals a prominent mononuclear round cell infiltrate of the epithelium and lamina propria, with a small number of eosinophils. Complete resolution of the intestinal lesions may require 6–18 weeks of food allergen avoidance. The natural history of this disorder has not been well studied.

Celiac disease is a severe form of the malabsorption syndrome [35]. Total villous atrophy and extensive cellular infiltrate are associated with hypersensitivity to gliadin, a component of gluten found in wheat, oats, rye, and barley. Patients often present with diarrhea or frank steatorrhea, abdominal distension and flatulence, weight loss, and rarely nausea and vomiting. Although some patients reportedly are able to tolerate small amounts of gluten, lifelong elimination of gluten-containing foods is necessary to avoid the increased risk of gastrointestinal malignancy and lymphoma.

2. Cutaneous Food Hypersensitivity

Although some investigators suggest that eczematous lesions are secondary to a food-induced cell-mediated reaction, there is little evidence to exclude an IgE-mediated component.

Dermatitis Herpetiformis. This disorder is occasionally mistaken for atopic dermatitis and is characterized by a chronic, intensely pruritic, papulovesicular rash symmetrically distributed over the extensor surfaces of the extremities and buttocks. About 85% of patients have gluten-sensitive enteropathy [36]. Both involved and uninvolved skin are infiltrated with neutrophils and contain deposits of IgA and C3 in the dermoepidermal junction. The histology of the intestinal lesion is virtually identical to that seen in celiac disease, although villous atrophy and inflammatory infiltrates are milder. The diagnosis of dermatitis herpetiformis is established by the presence of the characteristic skin lesions and the demonstration of IgA deposition in the skin. Sulfones are the mainstay of therapy and lead to rapid resolution of pruritus within 24–72 h, but they have virtually no effect on intestinal symptoms. Elimination of gluten from the diet often leads to a gradual resolution of skin symptoms over several weeks to months and normalization of intestinal findings over several months.

3. Respiratory Food Hypersensitivity

A rare form of pulmonary hemosiderosis is believed to be secondary to a non-IgE-mediated hypersensitivity.

Heiner's Syndrome. This rare form of pulmonary hemosiderosis is characterized by recurrent episodes of pneumonia associated with pulmonary infiltrates, hemosiderosis, gastrointestinal blood loss, and iron deficiency anemia, and failure to thrive has rarely been reported in young infants [37,38]. Hemosiderin-laden macrophages may be found in gastric aspirates or in biopsy specimens of the lung. Although peripheral blood eosinophilia and multiple serum precipitins to cow's milk are a relatively constant feature, the immunological mechanisms responsible for this disorder are not known. Egg and pork also have been implicated in this disorder. Resolution of symptoms with elimination of the implicated food from the diet is considered diagnostic. Challenges are not recommended, since allergen ingestion can induce a fatal pulmonary bleed.

C. Other Food-Induced Hypersensitivity Reactions

A large number of subjective symptoms have been attributed to food allergic reactions, but DBPCFCs generally fail to confirm a cause-and-effect relationship [39–41].

1. Arthritis

Although there has been considerable interest in the potential role of food hypersensitivity in arthritis, the literature contains only one well-documented case in which exacerbations of joint symptoms were associated by DBPCFC with ingestion of a specific food [42].

2. Migraine Headaches

Both food intolerance and food allergies have been implicated in the pathogenesis of migraine headaches. A double-blind, placebo-controlled study in adults implicated non-IgE-mediated food-induced symptoms in 15% of 104 adults with migraine headaches [43].

III. DIAGNOSING ADVERSE FOOD REACTIONS

As outlined in Fig. 1, the evaluation of a patient for suspected adverse food reactions involves a thorough history, physical examination, and laboratory tests. With the history, an attempt is made to establish whether the patient is suffering from an intolerance or a hypersensitivity reaction, and if the latter, whether a non-IgE-mediated or IgE-mediated mechanism is involved. In IgE-mediated syndromes, the clinical impression may be reenforced by skin tests or in vitro diagnostic tests. Diets *completely* eliminating suspected food allergens are used both in the initial evaluation and in subsequent therapy for food allergy.

A. History

Although critical to the evaluation of food hypersensitivity, the patient (or parent) history may be misleading because of public misperceptions about these disorders. In most series involving DBPCFCs, historical reports of adverse food reactions are verified about 30–40% of the time [44]. Nevertheless, several historical points must be established if possible: (1) the identity and quantity of the food allergen suspected of provoking the reaction, (2) the time elapsed between the ingestion of the suspected food and the onset of symptoms, (3) a complete description of the symptoms elicited and the duration of the reaction, (4) whether similar symptoms have occurred in the past when the food was eaten, and the therapeutic measures taken, and (5) whether other factors (e.g., exercise) appear necessary for the development of symptoms. Reactions that occur within minutes to hours of ingesting a specific food and conform to a pattern of signs and symptoms outlined above are more likely to represent a food hypersensitivity. In general, the history is used in an effort to exclude a number of disorders that may mimic food-allergic reactions (Table 1) and to determine which laboratory studies would be worthwhile (e.g., skin tests, IgA antigliadin antibody, etc.).

Diet diaries are sometimes used as an adjunct to the history. Patients (or parents) are asked to keep a chronological record of all items ingested over a set period of time, generally no longer than a week, and any symptoms occurring during this time. The diary is reviewed in an effort to correlate ingestion of specific foods with the development of symptoms, but in this era of processed foods and prepackaged meals, this is generally a futile exercise.

B. Skin Testing

If an IgE-mediated food sensitivity is suspected, skin testing with food extracts by the prick or puncture method may be helpful [45–47]. Routine intradermal skin tests with food extracts are too sensitive (excessive false-positive tests) and are not indicated. *A positive skin test indicates the presence of allergen-specific IgE antibodies on cutaneous mast cells; it does not mean the patient will develop*

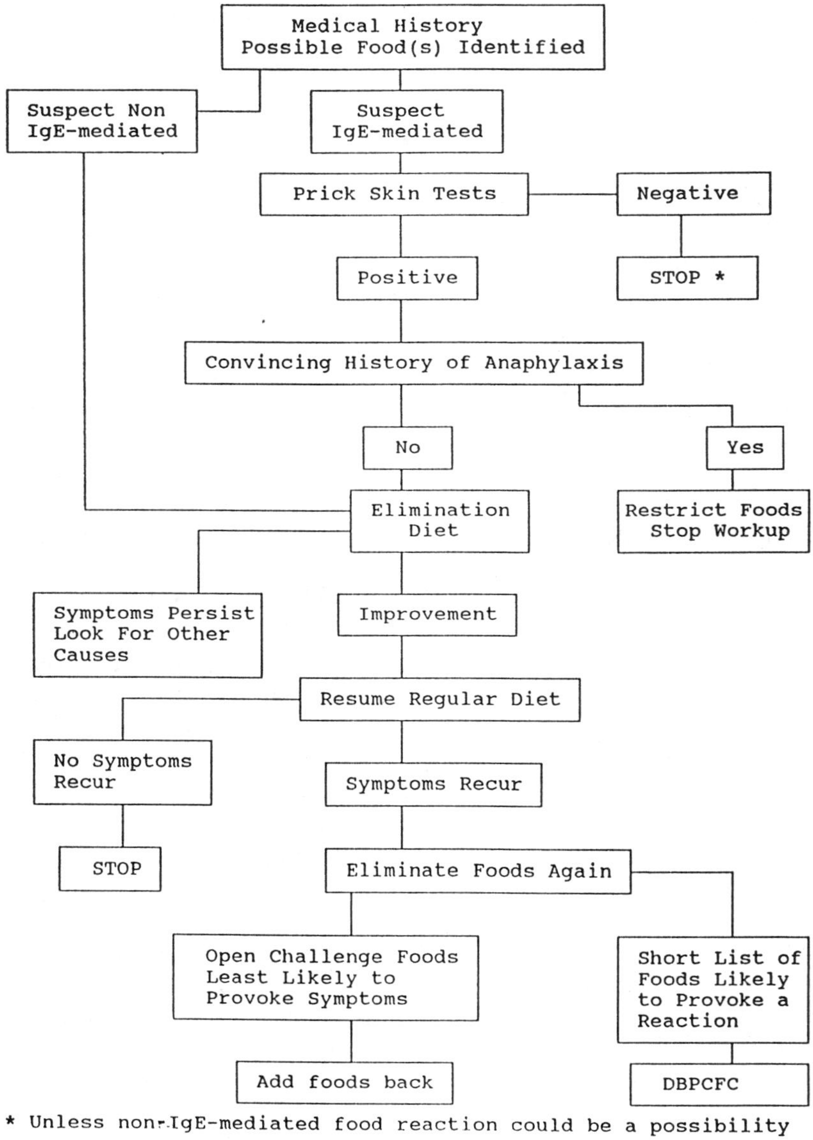

Figure 1 Diagnosing food hypersensitivity. (From James, J. M., and Sampson, H. A., *Pediatr. Allergy Immunol.*, *3*, 67–78 [1992].)

Table 1 Differential Diagnosis of Adverse Food Reactions

- Gastrointestinal disorders (vomiting and/or diarrhea)
  - Structural abnormalities
    - Hiatal hernia
    - Pyloric stenosis
    - Hirschsprung's disease
    - Tracheosophageal fistula
  - Enzyme deficiencies (primary vs. secondary)
    - Disaccharidase deficiency (lactase, sucrase–isomaltase, glucose–galactose)
    - Galactosemia
    - Phenylketonuria
  - Malignancy
  - Other
    - Pancreatic insufficiency (cystic fibrosis, Schwachman–Diamond syndrome)
    - Gallbladder disease
    - Peptic ulcer disease
- Contaminants and additives
  - Flavorings and preservatives
    - Sodium metabisulfite
    - Monosodium glutamate
  - Dyes
    - Tartrazine, (?) other azo dyes
  - Toxins
    - Bacterial (*Clostridium botulinum*, *Staphylococcus aureus*)
    - Fungal (aflatoxins, trichothecenes, ergot)
    - Seafood-associated
      - Scrombroid poisoning (tuna, mackerel)
      - Ciguatera poisoning (grouper, snapper, barracuda)
      - Saxitoxin (shellfish)
  - Infectious organisms
    - Bacteria (*Salmonella*, *Shigella*, *Escherichia coli*, *Yersinia*, Campylobacter)
    - Parasites (*Giardia*, Trichinella)
    - Viruses (hepatitis, rotavirus, enterovirus)
  - Mold antigens (?)
  - Accidental contaminants
    - Heavy metals (mercury, copper)
    - Pesticides
    - Antibiotics (penicillin)
- Pharmacological agents
  - Caffeine (coffee, soft drinks)
  - Histamine (fish, sauerkraut)
  - Serotonin (banana, tomato)
  - Tyramine (cheeses, pickled herring)
  - Glycosidal alkaloid solanine (potatoes)
  - Alcohol
  - Theobromine (chocolate, tea)
  - Tryptamine (tomato, plum)
  - Phenylethylamine (chocolate)
- Psychological reactions

Source: Adapted from Sampson, H. A., *J. Allergy Clin. Immunol.*, *78*, 212–219 (1986).

symptoms when ingesting the specific food. In fact, the positive predictive values of most prick skin tests are less than 50%. In contrast, the negative predictive accuracies are excellent, and IgE-mediated allergic reactions are extremely rare in the face of negative skin tests.

Food extracts for skin testing may be purchased from a number of companies (weight:volume = 1:20), but extract quality varies somewhat from one company to another [47]. Wheals 3 mm or more larger than the negative control wheal are seen in virtually all patients with IgE-mediated allergic reactions to foods. However, in evaluating sensitivity to many fruits and vegetables, especially with the oral allergy syndrome, prick skin testing ("prick + prick") must be performed with fresh fruits and vegetables to exclude IgE-mediated food hypersensitivity.

C. In Vitro Tests of Food-Specific IgE Antibodies

Skin testing is not feasible or recommended in some clinical situations: patients with extensive skin disease, significant and prolonged dermatographism, or a history of exquisite sensitivity (i.e., exposure to minute quantities of a specific food resulted in a life-threatening reaction). In addition, the increased use of long-acting antihistamines (e.g., astemizole) often makes skin testing impractical. In such cases, in vitro diagnostic tests are used to demonstrate food allergen–specific IgE antibodies.

1. Radioallergosorbent Test

The RAST has been the standard in vitro test for demonstrating allergen-specific IgE antibodies [46,48]. A number of similar tests utilizing enzyme-linked or fluorescein-linked antibodies are also available. These tests are slightly less sensitive than skin testing in the evaluation of allergic reactions to foods. The Pharmacia CAP System appears to provide improved sensitivity as compared with the RAST and an increased dynamic range. Preliminary studies suggest that it may have better positive predictive values for some food allergens (e.g., egg, milk, peanut) (unpublished data).

2. Basophil Degranulation Tests

Recently, commercial assays have become available to measure the amount of histamine released by basophils in response to a food allergen. In addition, some commercial laboratories perform this assay, claiming increased diagnostic predictability. To date, the diagnostic value of basophil degranulation tests for distinguishing symptomatic food allergy has not been demonstrated.

D. Elimination Diets

If the history or preliminary laboratory studies suggest certain foods may be provoking symptoms in a patient, it is useful to eliminate those foods (and all "hidden" sources of that food) totally from the patient's diet for a period of 1–2 weeks. If symptoms clear *completely*, further characterization of the sensitivity should be pursued (e.g., endoscopy and biopsy, blinded challenge, etc.). Prick skin testing should be performed if it was not done before initiating the elimination diet. The presence or absence of food allergen–specific IgE antibodies is useful for counseling the patient about the potential danger of accidental food ingestion and, for young children, the likelihood of "outgrowing" the sensitivity and that of developing other food sensitivities [4]. In some chronic disorders such as atopic dermatitis, asthma, or chronic diarrhea, factors in addition to the food sensitivity may be triggering symptoms, so failure to see resolution of symptoms does *not* necessarily rule out a food hypersensitivity.

In cases where food hypersensitivity or intolerance is suspected but no specific foods can be incriminated, a brief trial (i.e., 2–4 weeks) of an oligoantigenic diet may be helpful. In young infants (< 4 months of age), this would consist of providing only an extensively hydrolyzed casein formula (Alimentum, Nutramigen, or Pregestimil) or an amino acid–derived formula (Neocate). The following diets may be used for older children: 4–8 months of age: infant diet + rice cereal + pears; 9–24 months of age: 4–8 month diet + rice + squash + lamb; > 24 months of age: 9–24 month diet + fresh lettuce + potato + safflower oil + tea + sugar; or elemental formulas may be tried (e.g., Vivonex T.E.N. or Tolerex with flavor packs).

E. Double-Blind, Placebo-Controlled Food Challenge

The DBPCFC is the "gold standard" for diagnosing food allergies [49] and has been used successfully in both children and adults for examining a variety of food-related complaints [50]. The choice of foods used in DBPCFCs is based on history, skin test (or RAST) results, and/or foods suspected on the basis of elimination diets. In the practice setting, open or single-blind oral food challenges may be used to screen for food-allergic reactions. However, in cases where multiple food allergies are diagnosed, positive responses should be confirmed by DBPCFC. Some investigators believe it is unnecessary to blind challenges in very young infants. It must be remembered that an infant or young child forced to drink or ingest something he or she does not want often becomes very irritable and upset, which may lead to cutaneous erythema, a morbilliform rash and/or scratching, and occasionally wheezing and emesis. Failure to use appropriate placebo controls and blinding may lead to misinterpretation of such challenges.

In order to maximize the positive predictive value of DBPCFCs, suspect foods should be eliminated for 10–14 days, and for up to 1 month in some gastrointestinal disorders. Optimally, all medication should be discontinued. Antihistamines should be discontinued for a sufficient time to allow return of a normal histamine skin test; e.g., a diphenhydramine for 3–6 days, hydroxyzine for 7–14 days, astemizole for 4–8 weeks. Systemic corticosteroids should be discontinued for 4–8 weeks before admission, inhaled corticosteroids and cromolyn for at least

12 h, oral theophylline for 8 h, and inhaled β-adrenergic medications for at least 6–8 h before the beginning of all DBPCFCs [50]. In patients with unstable asthma or chronic urticaria, it is not always possible to discontinue medications, but every effort should be made to minimize drugs to levels sufficient to prevent breakthrough of acute symptoms. When challenges were performed in patients taking antihistamines, skin symptoms were partially masked, but there appeared to be little effect on gastrointestinal or respiratory symptoms (personal communication, C. Bindslev-Jensen). In patients with asthma and food hypersensitivity, inhaled beclomethasone or sodium cromoglycate did not prevent wheezing or changes in airway hyperreactivity in many patients (manuscripts submitted).

In order to optimize the probability that the food challenge will provide a definitive outcome, the patient's symptoms must be stabilized before the challenge is initiated. For example, patients with atopic dermatitis or unstable asthma may require aggressive topical therapy in the hospital to obtain a stable baseline with minimal symptoms. Performing challenges on patients with active symptoms is

Table 2 Potential Sources of Food for Use in the Administration of Double-Blind, Placebo-Controlled Food Challenges

Food	Challenge substances[a]
Egg	Dehydrated whole egg
Milk	Dry skim milk powder
Wheat	Whole wheat or cake flour[b]
Soy	Soy flour
Peanut	Peanut flour, peanut butter, or crushed peanut (food processor or mortar and pestle)
Fish	16 g raw fish
Barley	Barley flour
Rye	Rye flour
Corn	Corn meal or corn flour
Oat	Oat flour
Rice	Brown rice flour
Potato	Potato flour, instant potato flour
Nuts	Nut butter, crushed nut
Meats	16 g baby food, chicken, turkey, ham, lamb, beef

[a]Except where specified use 10 grams of the substance. Read labels ensuring that all ingredients are appropriate.

[b]Some cake flours are 100% wheat, while others contain barley/malt. The flours are available in health food stores. Purchase flours prepackaged rather than from bulk bins, where cross contamination of the bins is likely to occur. A bakery supplier is your best bet for finding dehydrated whole eggs. It must be 100% egg with nothing added. The dry skim milk powder and baby food meats may be purchased from a grocery store. Fresh fish may be purchased from a grocery store or market.

not only an exercise in frustration; it may place a patient at increased risk of a severe reaction, since early mild symptoms may be overlooked.

The food challenge should be administered in the fasting state, starting with a dose unlikely to provoke symptoms [25–500 mg of lyophilized food in liquid or capsules). Table 2 lists sources of food for use in challenges, and Table 3 lists several vehicles for administering the test food in noncapsular form. The dose is generally doubled every 15–60 min, depending on the type of reaction suspected. During the challenge, activities (e.g., games, videos, television) should be available so that the patient does not focus on symptoms. With young children, it is generally very useful to observe their activity level; they will often become quiet and withdrawn when symptoms start to develop. Early symptoms may include pruritus or tingling of the tongue or palate, itching or tightness in the throat (sometimes inducing a sensation of itching in the inner ear), nausea, and abdominal cramps.

If a patient suspected of IgE-mediated hypersensitivity tolerates 10 g of lyophilized food, clinical reactivity is generally ruled out. However, *all negative blinded challenges must be followed by an open feeding of the food in usual*

Table 3 Vehicles for Use in Double-Blind, Placebo-Controlled Food Challenges (DBPCFCs)

Fruit juices

Fruit juices, because they are rapidly absorbed, are the vehicles of choice when administering DBPCFCs. Apple, fruit punch, orange, cranberry, and grape are juices commonly selected by patients; however, cominations of these, or other juice combinations, have been requested.

Tolerex/Vivonex T.E.N.

Flavored Tolerex/Vivonex T.E.N. masks the test of challenge substances. The palatable Vivonex flavor packets (Vanilla, cherry/vanilla, raspberry, orange/pineapple, lemon/lime), combined with the hypoallergenicity of Tolerex/Vivonex T.E.N., makes it an excellent vehicle.

Baby fruits

Baby applesauce, bananas, pears, peaches, plums, or other tolerable baby food fruits can be used as a vehicle for administering DBPCFCs.

Hot cereals

Instant grits, oatmeal, cream of wheat, and cream of rice cereals are prepared following package directions. This is the most acceptable way to administer nut challenges.

Making Good Challenges

One of the difficulties of administering challenges in noncapsular form is the offensive odors and tastes of liquid preparations. Preparing challenges ahead of time and chilling them will cut down on the smell and taste. Taking time to prepare the challenges and mixing them thoroughly are also important for acceptability.

quantities under observation to rule out the rare false-negative challenge. Although the DBPCFC is considered highly sensitive and specific, false-positive and false-negative results occur, as with any diagnostic test (see Table 4). Some foods are affected by the freeze-drying process. In a study of fish-allergic patients [51], approximately one-third of patients tolerating a fish species in the blinded challenge developed allergic symptoms when fed the fish openly in a usual fashion.

Challenges must be randomized, and an equal number of placebo and food antigen challenges must be administered, to control adequately for potential confounding factors, such as variability in symptoms of chronic diseases, temporal effects, psychogenic factors, patient or observer bias, etc. The appearance, taste, and volume of the challenge and placebo should be similar. Challenges should be randomized by a third party not involved in scoring the challenges. A standardized scoring system should be used for all challenges [44,49]. When a suspected immediate food hypersensitivity is being evaluated, administration of test foods should be separated by an observation period of 24 h; longer periods are required for "delayed" or "late" reactions. The "timing" of the reaction should be based on the time elapsed since the last challenge dose given and the onset of the first objective symptoms.

The diagnosis of food-induced enterocolitis syndrome generally is established with an open oral food challenge, which consists of administering 0.4–0.6 g/kg body weight of the suspected protein allergen [30]. A positive challenge results in vomiting and diarrhea within 1–6 h and occasionally (in about 15% of challenges) may be accompanied by hypotension. A positive challenge is accompanied by a rise in the absolute neutrophil count (> 3500 cells/mm^3) 4–6 h after symptoms develop, and neutrophils, eosinophils, and occasionally red blood cells are generally seen in the stools.

Food-induced colitis syndrome is diagnosed by demonstrating the characteristic mucosal findings on sigmoidoscopy and biopsy. The specific food allergen responsible for the disorder is established by administering 0.4–0.6 g/kg body

Table 4 Diagnostic Accuracy of Double-Blind, Placebo-Controlled Oral Food Challenges (DPPCFCs)

	False-negative	False-positive
Bock	12/257 (4.6%)	8/831 (0.9%)
Burks	1/19 (0.5%)	3/196 (1.5%)
	[Fish* 3/11 (27%)]	
Sampson	5/280 (1.8%)	4/805 (0.5%)
	[Fish* 7/33 (21%)]	

[a]DPPCFCs to fish species considered separately; see text.

weight of the suspected protein allergen in an open oral food challenge. Gross or occult blood should appear in the stools within 24–48 h [32].

Quantitation of IgA antigliadin and of IgA antiendomysial antibodies appear promising as screening tests for celiac disease [52]. However, the diagnosis is dependent on demonstrating biopsy evidence of villous atrophy and inflammatory infiltrate while the patient is ingesting gluten, resolution of biopsy findings after 6–12 weeks of gluten elimination, and recurrence of biopsy changes following reinstitution of gluten [53].

The observation period following a challenge depends on the type of reaction being investigated. For example, 2-h follow-up generally is sufficient for IgE-mediated reactions, whereas 4–8 h may be necessary in cases of milk-induced enterocolitis. In general, DBPCFCs should be conducted in a clinical or hospital setting, especially if an IgE-mediated reaction is suspected, and trained personnel and equipment should be available for treating systemic anaphylaxis [54]. Emergency medications should be at hand and the appropriate doses calculated (Table 5). Normally, challenges should not be performed to a food suspected of causing a life-threatening anaphylactic reaction, especially if the presence of IgE specific antibodies is confirmed. However, in cases where the causative antigen cannot be conclusively determined by history, a challenge should be conducted in the intensive care unit of a center that frequently deals with food-allergic reactions.

Evaluation of largely subjective complaints, such as chronic abdominal pain, recurrent headaches, or behavioral problems, may be carried out safely on an outpatient basis. Often such symptoms are said to require several ingestions of the responsible food to reproduce the complaint. With such subjective symptoms, it is generally necessary to perform three placebo-controlled challenges to rule out random chance, i.e., $p < 0.05$. Patients are given weekly supplies of capsules or liquid challenges that have been randomized to provide three sets of test food and placebo, and they are required to record all symptoms in a daily diary. At the end of the 6-week period, the diary is reviewed to determine whether symptoms occurred during the active or placebo arms of the challenge series. A cause-and-effect relationship can be inferred only if there are no responses to placebo and repeated responses to the food allergen.

The diagnosis of food allergy is a clinical exercise that requires a careful history, selective skin tests or RASTs in cases of suspected IgE-mediated disorders, appropriate exclusion diets, and blinded provocation challenges. At the present time, there is no evidence of diagnostic utility for the following assays: quantitation of food-specific IgG or IgG_4 antibodies or food antigen–antibody complexes, evidence of lymphocyte activation (^3H uptake, interleukin-2 production, leukocyte inhibitory factor production, etc.), or sublingual or intracutaneous provocation. In gastrointestinal disorders for which pre- and postchallenge biopsy studies are required for diagnosis (e.g., malabsorption syndromes, including celiac disease), the challenge may not require blinding.

Table 5 Pharmacological Treatment of Systemic Anaphylaxis

Agents	Indications	Dosages
Airway or cutaneous reactions		
Initial Therapy		
Epinephrine	Bronchospasm, laryngeal edema, urticaria, angiodema	0.3–0.5 ml of 1:1000 dilution (0.3–0.[illegible] mg) subcutaneously every 10–20 min (children: 0.01 mg/kg/dose)
Oxygen	Hypoxemia	40–100%
Metaproterenol[a]	Bronchospasm	0.3 ml (5% solution) in 2.5 ml of saline, inhaled through nebulizer
Secondary Therapy[b]		
Racemic Epinephrine	Throat tightness	Metered dose inhaler 2–4 puffs every 10–15 min
Aminophylline	Bronchospasm	Loading dose if necessary (6 mg/kg intravenously over a 30-min period); 0.3–0.9 mg/kg/h intravenously as maintenance dose[c]
Corticosteroids	Bronchospasm	250 mg of hydrocortisone or 50 mg of methylprednisolone intravenously every 6 h for 2–4 doses (children: hydrocortisone 5–8 mg/kg/dose; methylprednisolone 1–2 mg/kg/dose)
Antihistamines	Urticaria	25–50 mg of hydroxyzine or diphenhydramine intramuscularly or orally every 6–8 h as needed (children: hydroxyzine 1 mg/kg/dose; diphenhydramine 1–1.5 mg/kg/dose) 300 mg of cimetidine intravenously or orally every 6 h (children: 5–10 mg/kg/dose every 6 h)
Cardiovascular reactions		
Initial Therapy		
Intravenous fluids (saline, colloid)	Hypotension	1 L every 20–30 min as needed (children: 10 ml/kg)
Epinephrine	Hypotension	1 ml of 1:1000 dilution in 500 ml of distilled water intravenously at a rate of 0.5–5 μg/min (0.25–2.5 ml)/min (children: 0.1–1 μg/min)
Secondary Therapy		
Norepinephrine	Hypotension	4 mg in 1 L of distilled water intravenously at a rate of 2–12 μg (0.5–3 ml)/min

able 5 Continued

gents	Indications	Dosages
Antihistamines	Hypotension	25–50 mg of hydroxyzine or diphenhydramine intramuscularly or orally every 6–8 h as needed 300 mg of cimetidine intravenously or orally every 6 h
Glucagon[d]	Refractory hypotension	1 mg in 1 L of distilled water intravenously at a rate of 5–15 μg (5–15 ml)/min

lbuterol (0.5 ml of the 0.5% solution in 2.5 ml of saline) or isoetharine (0.5 ml of the 1% solution in 2 ml of line) can also be used.

hese agents have little or no efficacy during the acute anaphylactic reaction; they may reduce or prevent recurrent prolonged reactions.

ower rates are suggested for older patients, those taking medications that reduce metabolism, those with hepatic sfunction, and those with congestive heart failure; higher rates should be used for younger persons or cigarette nokers.

lay be particularly useful in patients taking β-adrenergic blockers, since its ability to stimulate both inotropic nd chronotropic cardiac function may be unaltered by β-adrenergic blockade.

IV. THERAPY FOR FOOD-ALLERGIC DISORDERS

Once the diagnosis of food hypersensitivity is established, strict *elimination* of the offending allergen is the only proven therapy. Clinical reactivity to food allergens is generally very specific, and patients rarely react to more than one member of a botanical or animal family. Prescribing an elimination diet is no different from prescribing any medication or treatment modality; both have definite benefits and risks and may have unwanted side effects. Elimination diets may lead to malnutrition, especially if they exclude a large number of foods or are used for extended periods of time. Eating disorders, adverse family psychosocial interactions, and other psychological problems may be exacerbated by implementation of restricted diets.

One of the most common failures in the treatment of food-allergic disorders is to educate patients properly in the avoidance of all "hidden" sources of a food [55]. Unless one is willing to provide careful counseling on how to recognize label ingredients that indicate the presence of a particular food (e.g., sodium caseinate, whey, or lactoglobulin for milk), to watch for hidden sources of food antigens (e.g., casein in canned tuna fish, whey in "nondairy" creamer), and to substitute "safe" foods for allergenic foods, the patient will not be able or willing to comply. A dietitian knowledgeable in food-allergy diets can ensure a nutritionally balanced diet, provide appropriate substitutes for specific food allergens, and anticipate any potential dietary deficiencies (e.g., of calcium on a milk-free diet). The Food

Allergy Network (4744 Holly Avenue, Fairfax, VA 22030) provides invaluable material to assist patients in complying with allergen elimination diets.

Several *drugs* have been used in an attempt to protect patients with food hypersensitivity. H_1 and H_2 antihistamines, ketotifin, and corticosteroids may modify symptoms to food allergens, but overall they have minimal efficacy or unacceptable side effects. Oral cromolyn sodium has been extensively studied, and although results are conflicting, most well-controlled studies have failed to demonstrate efficacy. To date, appropriately designed trials have *never* demonstrated efficacy for the use of *oral desensitization*, *injection immunotherapy*, or *subcutaneous provocation and neutralization*.

Patients must be prepared for inadvertent ingestion of a food allergen. In one study of children with peanut allergy, about one-half of the children had experienced an accidental ingestion within 1 year of the follow-up interview [56]. The treatment of food-allergic symptoms is similar to that for allergic symptoms provoked by other factors. Laryngeal or pulmonary symptoms following an inadvertent food exposure should be treated immediately with epinephrine, inhaled bronchodilators, or both. The treatment of food-induced anaphylaxis requires subcutaneous or intravenous epinephrine, H_1 and H_2 antihistamines, aggressive volume expansion, bronchodilators, oxygen, and possibly other vasopressors (Table 4). Current data suggest that the early administration of epinephrine may abort an anaphylactic reaction. Consequently, a patient with an IgE-mediated food allergy, especially one with asthma, a history of a previous severe allergic reaction, or sensitivity to peanuts, nuts, fish, or shellfish, should be taught how to self-administer epinephrine. Injectable epinephrine (AnaGuard or EpiPen) and an antihistamine (liquid diphenhydramine [1.25–1.5 mg/kg]) should be prescribed and available to the patient at all times. For children, day-care centers and schools should have a list of emergency telephone numbers with backups. Caregivers should be warned that a patient may experience only mild symptoms in the first few minutes after ingesting a food to which he or she is allergic, and then develop severe respiratory distress and hypotension 10–120 min later. Following self-medication for systemic reactions, the patient should immediately seek medical attention. *All patients with IgE-mediated food allergy, especially those children with asthma*, should be warned about the possibility of developing a severe anaphylactic reaction and should be educated in the appropriate treatment measures to be taken in case of an accidental ingestion.

Food-allergic disorders affect 1–2% of the population. Although much remains to be learned about the immunopathogenesis of these disorders, many of the syndromes have been well characterized and can be accurately diagnosed with the appropriate studies. It is clear that the allergist cannot rely solely on tests of food-specific IgE antibodies to diagnose food hypersensitivities, because many patients with IgE antibodies to food do not experience any untoward reaction when ingesting the food, and several food hypersensitivities are not IgE-mediated. Oral food challenges are essential for establishing the correct diagnosis and for monitoring the natural history of the food hypersensitivity. Although loss of reactivity to peanuts, tree nuts, fish, and shellfish is extremely unlikely, many children and adults will lose their symptomatic hypersensitivity to other foods after maintaining a strict allergen-elimination diet for several years [56–58]. In addition to developing more practical diagnostic tests for food hypersensitivities, future efforts in this field need to clarify the basic immunopathogenetic mechanisms at work in these disorders and to unravel the mysteries of tolerance induction.

ACKNOWLEDGMENTS

Supported in part by grant AI24439 from the National Institute of Allergy and Infectious Diseases and grant RR00052 from the General Clinical Research Center Program, DRR.

REFERENCES

1. Sloan, A. E., and Powers, M. E., A perspective on popular perceptions of adverse reactions to foods, *J. Allergy Clin. Immunol.*, *78*, 127–133 (1986).
2. American Academy of Allergy and Immunology/National Institute of Allergy and Infectious Diseases, *Adverse Reactions to Foods* (J. A. Anderson and D. D. Sogn, eds.), NIH Publication # 84-2442, 1984, pp. 1–6.
3. Bock, S. A., Prospective appraisal of complaints of adverse reaction to foods in children during the first 3 years of life, *Pediatrics*, *79*, 683–688 (1987).
4. Host, A., and Halken, S., A prospective study of cow milk allergy in Danish infants during the first 3 years of life, *Allergy*, *45*, 587–596 (1990).
5. Hide, D. W., and Guyer, B. M., Cows milk intolerance in Isle of Wight infants, *Br. J. Clin. Pract.*, *37*, 285–287 (1983).
6. Wilson, S. J., and Walzer, M., Absorption of undigested proteins in human beings. IV. Absorption of unaltered egg protein in infants, *Am. J. Dis. Child.*, *50*, 49–54 (1935).
7. Sampson, H. A., Immunologic mechanisms in adverse reactions to foods, *Immunol. Allergy Clin. North Am.*, *11*, 701–716 (1991).
8. Sampson, H. A., Broadbent, K. R., and Bernhisel-Broadbent, J., Spontaneous release of histamine from basophils and histamine-releasing factor in patients with atopic dermatitis and food hypersensitivity, *N. Engl. J. Med.*, *321*, 228–232 (1989).
9. Ortaloni, C., Ispano, M., Pastorello, E. A., Ansaloni, R., and Magri, G. C., Comparison of results of skin prick tests (with fresh foods and commercial food extracts) and RAST in 100 patients with oral allergy syndrome, *J. Allergy Clin. Immunol.*, *83*, 683–690 (1989).
10. Sampson, H. A., Food Allergies, in *Gastrointestinal Disease* (M. H. Sleisinger, J. S. Fordtran, B. F., Scharschmidt, and M. Feldman, eds.), W.B. Saunders, Philadelphia, 1993, pp. 1233–1240.

11. Min, K., and Metcalfe, D. D., Eosinophilic gastroenteritis, *Immunol. Allergy Clin. North Am.*, *11*, 799–814 (1991).
12. Waldman, T. A., Wochner, R. D,. Laster, R. D., and Gordon, R. S., Allergic gastroenteropathy. A cause of excessive gastrointestinal protein loss, *N. Engl. J. Med.*, *276*, 761–769 (1967).
13. Snyder, J. D., Rosenblum, N., Wershil, B., et al., Pyloric stenosis and eosinophilic gastroenteritis in infants, *J. Pediatr. Gastroenterol. Nutr.*, *6*, 543–547.
14. Sampson, H. A., Infantile colic and food allergy: fact or fiction? *J. Pediatr.*, *115*, 583–584 (1989).
15. Bock, S. A., and Atkins, F. M., Patterns of food hypersensitivity during sixteen years of double-blind placebo-controlled food challenges, *J. Pediatr.*, *117*, 561–567 (1990).
16. Sampson, H. A., and Metcalfe, D. D., Immediate reactions to foods, in *Adverse Reactions to Foods and Food Additives* (D. D. Metcalfe, H. A. Sampson, and R. A. Simon, eds.), Blackwell Scientific Publications, Oxford, 1991, pp. 99–112.
17. James, J. M., Bernhisel-Broadbent, J., and Sampson, H. A., Respiratory reactions provoked by double-blind food challenges in children, *Am. J. Resp. Crit. Care Med.*, *149*, 59–64 (1994).
18. James, J. M., Eggleston, P. A., and Sampson, H. A., Food allergy increases airway reactivity (abstr.), *J. Allergy Clin. Immunol.*, *91*, 344.
19. Oehling, A., and Cagnani, C. E. B., Food allergy and child asthma, *Allergol. Immunopathol.*, *8*, 7–14 (1980).
20. Novembre, E., de Martino, M., and Vierucci, A., Foods and respiratory allergy, *J. Allergy Clin. Immunol.*, *81*, 1059–1065 (1988).
21. Bock, S. A., Respiratory reactions induced by food challenges in children with pulmonary disease, *J. Pediatr. Allergy Immunol.*, *3*, 188–194 (1992).
22. Winton, G. B., and Lewis, C. W., Contact urticaria, *Int. J. Dermatol.*, *21*, 573–578 (1982).
23. Kauppinen, K., Juntunen, K., and Lanki, H., Urticaria in children, *Allergy*, *39*, 469–472 (1984).
24. Burks, A. W., Mallory, S. B., Williams, L. W., and Shirrell, M. A., Atopic dermatitis: clinical relevance of food hypersensitivity reactions, *J. Pediatr.*, *113*, 447–451 (1988).
25. Sampson, H. A., Immunopathogenic role of food hypersensitivity in atopic dermatitis, *Acta Dermato-Venereologica*, *176* (suppl), 34–37 (1992).
26. Sampson, H. A., and Jolie, P. L., Increased plasma histamine concentrations after food challenges in children with atopic dermatitis, *N. Engl. J. Med.*, *321*, 228–232 (1984).
27. Bock, S. A., The incidence of severe adverse reactions to food in Colorado, *J. Allergy Clin. Immunol.*, *90*, 683–685 (1992).
28. Yunginger, J. W., Sweeney, K. G., Sturner, W. Q., et al., Fatal food-induced anaphylaxis, *JAMA*, *260*, 1450–1452 (1988).
29. Sampson, H. A., Mendelson, L., and Rosen, J. P., Fatal and near-fatal food-induced anaphylaxis in children, *N. Engl. J. Med.*, *327*, 380–384 (1992).
30. Powell, G. K., Milk and soy induced enterocolitis of infancy: clinical features and standardization of challenge, *J. Pediatr.*, *93*, 553–560 (1978).

31. Katz, A. J., Twarog, F. J., Zeiger, R. S., and Falchuk, Z. M., Milk-sensitive and eosinophilic gastroenteropathy: similar clinical features with contrasting mechanisms and clinical course, *J. Allergy Clin. Immunol.*, *74*, 72–78 (1984).
32. Gryboski, J. D., Gastrointestinal milk allergy in infants, *Pediatrics*, *40*, 354–362 (1967).
33. Goldman, H., and Proujansky, R., Allergic proctitis and gastroenteritis in children, *Am. J. Surg. Pathol.*, *10*, 75–86 (1986).
34. Kuitunen, P., Visakorpi, J. K., Savilahti, E., et al., Malabsorption syndrome with cow's milk intolerance: clinical findings and course in 54 cases, *Arch. Dis. Child.*, *50*, 351–356 (1975).
35. Trier, J. S., Celiac sprue, in *Gastrointestinal Disease* (M. H. Sleisinger, J. S. Fordtran, B. F., Scharschmidt, and M. Feldman, eds.), W.B. Saunders, Philadelphia, 1993, pp. 1078–1096.
36. Hall, R. P., The pathogenesis of dermatitis herpetiformis: recent advances, *J. Am. Acad. Dermatol.*, *16*, 1129–1144 (1987).
37. Heiner, D. C., and Sears, J. W., Chronic respiratory disease associated with multiple circulating precipitins to cow's milk, *Am. J. Dis. Child.*, *100*, 500–502 (1960).
38. Boat, T. F., Polmar, S. H., Whitman, V., et al., Hyperreactivity to cow milk in young children with pulmonary hemosiderosis and cor pulmonale secondary to nasopharyngeal obstruction, *J. Pediatr.*, *87*, 23–29 (1975).
39. Rix, K. J. B., Pearson, D. J., and Bentley, S. J., A psychiatric study of patients with supposed food allergy, *Br. J. Psychiatry*, *145*, 121–126 (1984).
40. Parker, A. L., Leznoff, A., Sussman, G. L., Tarlo, A. M., and Krondl, M., Characteristics of patients with food-related complaints, *J. Allergy Clin. Immunol.*, *86*, 503–511 (1990).
41. Selner, J. C., and Staudenmayer, H., Food allergy: psychological considerations, in *Food Allergy: Adverse Reactions to Foods and Food Additives* (D. D. Metcalfe, H. A. Sampson, and R. A. Simon, eds.), Blackwell Scientific Publications, Boston, 1991, pp. 370–381.
42. Panush, R. S., Stroud, R. M., and Webster, E. M., Food-induced (allergic) arthritis, *Arthritis Rhum.*, *29*, 220–226 (1986).
43. Weber, R. F., and Vaughan, T. R., Food and migraine headache, *Immunol. Allergy Clin. North Am.*, *11*, 831–841 (1991).
44. Bock, S. A., Sampson, H. A., Atkins, F. M., et al., Double-blind placebo-controlled food challenge as an office procedure: a manual, *J. Allergy Clin. Immunol.*, *82*, 986–997 (1988).
45. Bock, S. A., Buckley, J., Holst, A., and May, C. D., Proper use of skin tests with food extracts in diagnosis of food hypersensitivity, *Clin. Allergy*, *8*, 559–564 (1978).
46. Sampson, H. A., and Albergo, R., Comparison of results of skin tests, RAST, and double-blind placebo-controlled food challenges in children with atopic dermatitis, *J. Allergy Clin. Immunol.*, *74*, 26–33 (1984).
47. Sampson, H. A., Comparative study of commercial food antigen extracts for the diagnosis of food hypersensitivity, *J. Allergy Clin. Immunol.*, *82*, 718–726 (1988).
48. Ownby, D. R., In vitro assays for the evaluation of immunologic reactions to foods, *Immunol. Allergy Clin. North Am.*, *11*, 851–862 (1991).

49. Sampson, H. A., Immunologically mediated food allergy: the importance of food challenge procedures, *Ann. Allergy*, *60*, 262–269 (1988).
50. Metcalfe, D. D., and Sampson, H. A., Workshop on experimental methodology for clinical studies of adverse reactions to foods and food additives, *J. Allergy Clin. Immunol.*, *86*, 421–442 (1990).
51. Bernhisel-Broadbent, J., and Sampson, H. A., Fish hypersensitivity. II. Clinical relevance of altered fish allergenicity secondary to various preparation methods, *J. Allergy Clin. Immunol.*, *90*, 622–629 (1992).
52. Tucker, N. T., Barghuthy, F. S., Prihoda, T. J., et al., Antigliadin antibodies detected by enzyme-linked immunosorbent assay as a marker of childhood celiac disease, *J. Pediatr.*, *113*, 286–289 (1988).
53. McNeish, A. S., Harms, H. K., Rey, T., et al., The diagnosis of coeliac disease, *Arch. Dis. Child.*, *54*, 783–786 (1979).
54. Executive Committee of the Academy of Allergy and Immunology, Personnel and equipment to treat systemic reactions caused by immunotherapy with allergic extracts (position statement), *J. Allergy Clin. Immunol.*, *77*, 271–273 (1986).
55. Barnes-Koerner, C., and Sampson, H. A., Diets and nutrition, in *Food Allergy: Adverse Reactions to Foods and Food Additives* (D. D. Metcalfe, H. A. Sampson, and R. Simon, eds.), Blackwell Scientific Publications, Boston, 1991, pp. 332–354.
56. Bock, S. A., The natural history of food sensitivity, *J. Allergy Clin. Immunol.*, *69*, 173–177 (1982).
57. Sampson, H. A., and Scanlon, S. M., Natural history of food hypersensitivity in children with atopic dermatitis, *J. Pediatr.*, *115*, 23–27 (1989).
58. Pastorello, E. A., Stocchi, L., Pravettoni, V., et al., Role of the elimination diet in adults with food allergy, *J. Allergy Clin. Immunol.*, *84*, 475–483 (1989).

24

Nasal Provocative Testing

William R. Solomon

University of Michigan Hospitals
Ann Arbor, Michigan

I. INTRODUCTION

The observation, made almost 150 years ago, that direct intranasal placement of grass pollen reproduced the hay fever syndrome established pollinosis as a credible entity and, incidentally, demonstrated the utility of upper-airway provocation. In the century that followed, technically simple, direct exposure of the nose to allergens was increasingly attempted. The nasal membranes offered a readily accessible test organ and responses that, when marked, were easily recognized. In addition, nasal challenge often was possible with materials in forms typical of natural exposure but inappropriate for lower airway use.

More recent inquiries into upper airway function also have exploited direct nasal testing. When correlated with lower-airway data, this experience indicates that nasal and bronchial reactions of a single subject to pharmacological agents and irritant aerosols may differ. However, depending on the stimuli employed, reactivity to test allergens also may be expressed by both the nose and the bronchi [1]. Accordingly, cautious inferences regarding lower-airway response have been attempted on the basis of nasal provocation.

Since testing data often provide a persuasive indicator of nasal reactivity, interest in upper-airway provocation has continued to grow. Once involved, each investigator must soon recognize that methods for eliciting and recording upper-airway response are diverse, and that bases for their technical comparison and standardization remain tenuous. These realities currently preclude any single, "standard" technique of nasal challenge and interpretation. Instead, this section will outline currently useful modalities of nasal study, criteria for choice among these, and manifest sources of error.

II. THE ANATOMICAL AND FUNCTIONAL SUBSTRATE OF NASAL CHALLENGE

A. The Mucus Blanket

By contrast with deeper respiratory levels, the nasal passages are narrow and tortuous flow channels designed to control airway access, facilitate olfaction, and optimize respiratory heat and moisture flux. In the mucosa, goblets cells and complex glands, capable of voluminous secretion, commonly maintain a shallow (approximately 0.5 mm deep) mucus layer. Coordinated ciliary action moves this blanket, with entrapped materials, along somewhat irregular and broadly curved pathways. Except for the most anterior portions of the septum and turbinates, mucus flow normally is toward the nasopharynx [2]. Slower clearance of materials follows deposition at mucosal sites where cilia have been lost or on the nonciliated squamous epithelium of the nasal vestibule. Ciliary function may be affected adversely by chemical agents including, especially, locally applied vasoconstrictor substances [2,3]. The effects of many air-quality variables on cilia remain controversial, although in normal subjects working at low humidity, activity has been unimpaired [4]. However, a reversible shedding of ciliated cells is well documented during virus attack [5] and may be a feature of allergic inflammation [6]. Ciliary loss (possibly leading to squamous metaplasia) also has occurred with nasal suppuration [7] and exposure to industrial irritants [8] and at impingement points of forcefully directed air currents within the nose [2]. When nasal mucociliary clearance is unimpaired, translocation rates of markers may average 5 mm/min; however, depending on the site and methods employed, values from 0 to >10 mm/min are recorded [9]. Since mucus flow potentially affects both the distribution and the time course of local effects for challenge materials, this function deserves renewed attention.

B. Entrance and Penetration of Aerosols

In adults especially, the vibrissae (vestibular hairs) form an incomplete barrier that intercepts particles of increasing size with progressively higher efficiency. However, even without this coarse filter, aerosol penetration into the upper airway would be limited by the predominantly downward (rather than forward) disposition of the human nares, which is observed despite racial variations [10]. To enter the nose, most horizontal, ambient air currents must follow a sharply curved path during natural inspiration. While quite small particles (e.g., <3 μm) easily respond to the necessary angular accelerations, larger ones often do not and tend to impact on surfaces at the nasal verge. The extent of such losses has not been estimated but should increase with both particle size and ambient wind speed [11]. Their effect is to render the human nose less than 100% efficient as a "particle collector" with ambient aerosols.

Challenge materials introduced within the nasal vestibule avoid the vibrissae and adverse entrance effects. However, all aerosols undergo depletion while traversing the narrow, tortuous nasal passages. Deposition of materials is largely by impaction and, accordingly, increases with particle size and with the speed of inhaled (or insufflated) air. Although minute aerosols (i.e., $\leqslant 5\ \mu m$) may pass through the nasal cavities with relative ease, the removal of larger types can be remarkably efficient; only 5–10% of inhaled pollens, for example, reaches the nasopharynx [12]. Sniffing tends to divert the airstream upward toward the olfactory cleft [13] and augments particle impaction on presenting surfaces of the vestibule, turbinate tips, and deeper passages. Similarly, challenge materials introduced forcefully may achieve only limited airway penetration, most being intercepted by these same superficial baffles—especially if aerosol injection and inhalation are not synchronized. Materials deposited in the nasal vestibule undergo little or no mucociliary transport and may remain in situ for prolonged periods [14] or drip from the open nostrils. Water-soluble gases (e.g., SO_2, NH_3) diffuse readily and are taken up by moist nasal surfaces, exerting their effects largely in the upper airway [15]. By contrast, hydrophobic agents (e.g., ozone), which tend to bypass the upper airway, can reach and preferentially affect deeper respiratory levels.

C. The Airway as a Variable Flow Channel

1. Structural Features of Mucosal Blood Vessels

Nasal modulation of airflow, which facilitates its air-conditioning and olfactory functions, involves both anatomically fixed and variable resistance components. The latter deserve special attention for the marked, short-period airway changes they produce. In turn, these luminal events provide widely valuable indications of nasal reactivity (as well as significant artifacts) related to the challenge process. Since the determinants of nasal patency also critically affect strategies of provocation and indicators of response, they will be considered in some detail.

If intraluminal secretions do not vary and the nasal airway is considered noncompliant,* its patency is a function of vascular filling and the content of interstitial fluid within the mucosa. Open endothelial cell junctions have been recognized in capillaries and minute venules of the nasal vasculature, as well as transcellular fenestrae [17] and porous basement membranes [17,18], all of which

*Except for a limited portion near the mucocutaneous junction that acts as a Starling resistor and effects changes primarily during rapid inspiration [16].

should promote rapid fluid shifts. This arrangement also subserves the rapid intravascular uptake typical of mucosally applied agents [19]. As diagramed in Fig. 1, the nasal vasculature has several "levels" or components, each of which may respond distinctively to humoral and neural control. A system of arterioles has been recognized, running parallel to and just below the mucosal surface in humans and other mammals. These ("resistance") vessels probably are concerned most directly with heat and moisture exchange. In addition, they supply subepithelial and periglandular capillary plexuses, which foster absorption of water-soluble gases and solute. Deeper in the mucosa is a ("capacitance") system of thin-walled venous sinusoids ("lakes") and draining venules, capable of marked volume changes, and constituting an erectile tissue [10]. Connecting capillaries also link conventional arterial and venous segments; controlling sphincters, as well as arteriovenous shunts [18], may modify their function.

2. Autonomic Influences on Vascular Response

While the state of the venous sinusoids is a principal determinant of nasal patency, the contributions of additional vascular segments are uncertain, and current views of human physiology borrow generously from neural control studies in other species. In the cat, it is clear that total mucosal blood flow falls with sympathetic [20] and rises with parasympathetic stimulation [21] as nasal patency increases and diminishes, respectively. Although associated tone changes in capacitance and resistance vessels are qualitatively similar in the feline model, they may differ in

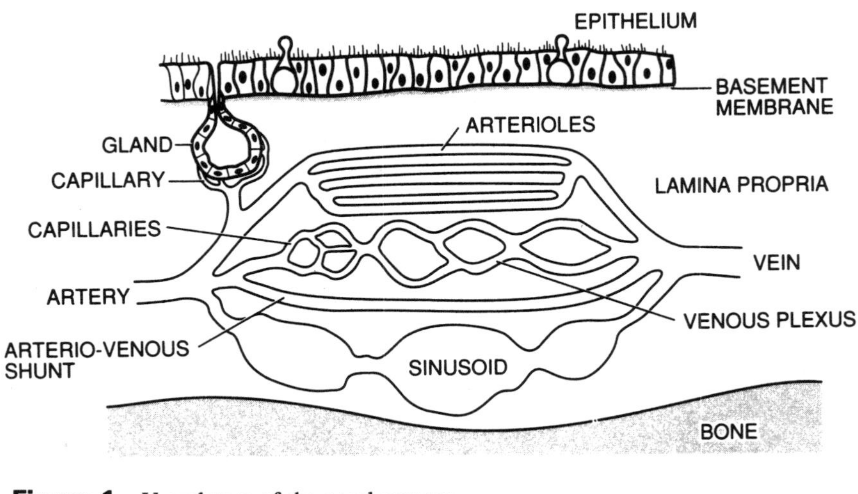

Figure 1 Vasculature of the nasal mucosa.

degree, depending on stimuli. Responses in nonhuman species to plasma levels of vasoactive agents also are documented [22,23], and it is possible that sensory nerve fibers accompanying blood vessels may subserve local axon reflexes involving neuropeptide effects on vascular elements.

Overall, human nasal patency also rises with sympathetic and falls with cholinergic influences; however, the segmental vascular changes responsible are not clear, and important interspecies differences may exist. For example, obstructive nasal responses to β-adrenergic agonists have seemed more evident in humans [24] than in cats [25]. In addition, atropine is said not to block the feline nasal vascular engorgement induced by direct parasympathetic stimulation [21].* In human volunteers, however, topical atropine has inhibited the increases in nasal airway resistance (NAR) induced by a methacholine aerosol [24]. Furthermore, we have observed locally applied atropine to decrease baseline NAR in some persons, suggesting inhibition of resting parasympathetic tone.

3. Environmental Determinants of Airway Response

A variety of "incidental" factors easily provoke nasal vascular responses, causing objective changes in airway patency, as well as in mucosal temperature, color, and heat flux; augmented secretion from tubular glands often is associated, presumably as a parasympathetic effect [26]. Strategies for challenging the upper airway and assessing its response must confront this exquisite reactivity if serous artifacts in data are to be minimized. Heightened nasal responsiveness to index stimuli, resulting in exaggerated drops in airway conductance (often with sneezing and hypersecretion), has been found with active inflammatory conditions—especially allergic rhinitis. Connell [27] described a decreasing dose threshold for nasal obstructive responses to (defatted) whole ragweed pollen challenges that was evident with sequential exposures. Similar findings with aqueous pollen extracts have been reported recently [28] (although preceding exposures to NH_3 gas did not increase subjects' nasal responses to ragweed in the same way). This "priming" effect [27] may persist for a month or more following natural pollen seasons [28] and apparently can augment nasal responsiveness to unrelated (normally subclinical) inhalant allergens [27] and probably to certain mediators of inflammation [29,30]. However, priming is not induced by challenging test subjects with histamine or methacholine.

Nasal patency decreases predictably with recumbency [31,32], probably reflecting passive vascular engorgement, as well as with excessive pressure applied (as by an over-tight mask) so as to encircle the nose [33]. Measurable nasal obstruction also may be induced by cooling the trunk and extremities [32,34], and both this and the effect of recumbency are accentuated in active allergic rhinitis [31,32]. Additional stimuli, including axillary pressure, have appeared to influ-

*The hypersecretion that results *is* effectively blocked by atropine.

ence nasal patency by reflex mechanisms. Prominent sneezing and hypersecretion following even modest tactile stimulation of the nasal mucosa are familiar events; in our experience, a decrease in nasal patency usually results as well. Apparently similar reflex responses may accompany painful disturbance of the vibrissae, nasal vestibule, upper lip, and intraoral structures. In addition, obstructive nasal changes have followed ocular stimulation, by corneal touch or strong retinal illumination, in some subjects [26,35].

The nasal response(s) to diminishing or increasing nasal ventilation have received little systematic study, although decreased patency is thought to occur following laryngectomy and tracheostomy, which abolishes nasal aeration [36]. Increased airway resistance also has been observed to follow short-term suspension of nasal breathing (by applying tape across the nares) with unimpaired oral respiration [32]. Furthermore, when deprived of nasal aeration, subjects with coexisting allergic rhinitis showed greater obstructive responses than normal subjects [32].

Inglestedt [37] has related these changes to the air-conditioning functions of the nose, emphasizing that the slitlike nasal cavities serve as relatively high-capacity, regenerative heat and water exchangers. This author observed a threefold increase in nasal flow resistance when expired air was excluded from the nasal passages for 5 min and ascribed this to interruption of normal heat and moisture transfer. In contrast to these observations, periods of complete breath holding generally present increased nasal patency [38] (unless effects of an associated Valsalva maneuver predominate). This response seems to result from the hypercapnia and hypoxia that develop during voluntary apnea and may be mediated by autonomic mechanisms, as shown in animal models [39]. Studies of human subjects confirm increases in nasal patency when $FICO_2$ is elevated but suggest that a direct vascular effect of hypercapnia is responsible [40,41]. The characteristic responses to nasal hyperventilation remain to be clarified. During strenuous overbreathing, an "exercise effect" (leading, predictably, to greater nasal patency [43,43]) might be expected. Since introduction of a passive flow at the nares or posterior choanae has been a feature of some measurement techniques [43,44], possible effects of this maneuver, alone, deserve study.

4. Central Coordination of Nasal Response

Induced Effects that Cross the Midline. Stimuli applied to a single nasal chamber or to facial structures on one side affect the corresponding nasal airway primarily; however, contralateral responses also are observed. In animals, bilateral nasal vascular responses follow stimulation of one cervical sympathetic chain [45], although the ipsilateral airway shows the greater change. Comparable human data are lacking; however, bilateral rhinorrhea has been observed following noxious stimulation of one eye [35] or nostril [46]. Related artifacts deserve concern, especially in anterior rhinomanometric procedures (see below, "Anterior

Rhinomanometry"), in which, reciprocally, each airway is gently instrumented to facilitate measurements on the opposite side.

The "Nasal Cycle." Reciprocal patency changes that occur spontaneously and sequentially in the paired nasal airways are well documented [47]. A spontaneous "nasal cycle" showing peak changes every 1½–6 h is displayed by three-fourths to four-fifths of subjects [47], although nasal inflammation and exogenous vasoactive agents may suspend these variations [45–50]. Central control is assumed to coordinate right- and left-sided airway changes so that total nasal resistance remains unchanged. Neither the mechanism for sensing nor that for coordinated autoregulation of nasal patency is understood, although cycling may be effaced also by stellate ganglion block [51,52]. Measurement techniques based on total nasal patency should be unaffected by these reciprocal airway changes. However, when sequential data are based on a single airway, phasic variations in that airway are a potential source of error.

III. THE ASSESSMENT OF NASAL AIRWAY RESPONSE

A. The Problem in Perspective

Although the parameters of nasal response are finite, methods used to asses them differ substantially among laboratories. This procedural disarray has grown during more than 50 years of nasal investigations and exists despite efforts to compare and standardize useful techniques [53–57]. Subjective assessments of pruritus (of nose, eyes, and pharynx), postnasal discharge, sneezing, and nasal stuffiness have been scored [58] to provide tractable data in extended efficacy studies of immunotherapy and drugs. However, the short-term format of challenge in clinic or laboratory requires more precisely measurable, "rapid-response" indicators.

It is often forgotten that the structurally complex nasal vasculature, with its capacity for rapid fluid exchange and somewhat arcane control system, afford a tenuous basis, at best, for inferring the minute (patho-) physiology of mucosal events. Deductions of blood flow, blood volume, differential "vascular tone," etc., from clinical variables such as mucosal color and temperature or even measured airway patency, while tempting, are subject to serious error. Similarly, hopeful generalizations based on "turgescence" and "ischemia" are best avoided in favor of more objective (though still indirect) indices of tissue change.* Precise measurements of secretory and segmental vascular activity have been employed in invasive animal studies but remain to be adapted to clinical investigations. While probably not ideal, test approaches based largely on flow-resistive properties of the nasal airways currently provide the most clinically useful parameters of

*Even with available quantitative methods, however (e.g., nasal patency parameters), subjective changes may be reported after challenge without recording of measurable change (and vice versa).

mucosal response. To apply these methods, it must be appreciated that measurement approaches favored by the pulmonary physiologist may prove unusable or require profound modification when applied to the nose.

B. Nasal Ventilation as a Measurable Function

1. Characteristics of Nasal Ventilation

In normal tidal breathing, the nasal airways act, essentially, as rigid conduits in which flow-resistive forces are opposed by a "transnasal" or driving pressure gradient (ΔP). Compliance, as such, is restricted (effectively) to a short segment, just central to each nasal vestibule, which acts as a Starling resistor [16], narrowing progressively as air velocity rises. This flow-resistive effect probably is best developed during inspiration, when negative intranasal pressures prevail, although, with forced breathing, it may be partially opposed by active flaring of the nasal alae. Reported excesses of inspiratory ΔP (compared with expiration) associated with an index flow $\dot{V}$ [59,60] may reflect phasic variation in the caliber of this segment, which abuts on the narrow "ostium internum," close to the mucocutaneous junction.

By comparison with the tracheobronchial airways, the nasal passages are remarkably tortuous and limited in mean cross-sectional area, imparting substantial angular accelerations to moving air. These qualities of the channel promote local eddies and mandate high flow velocities, which, in turn, determine that much nasal airflow is turbulent [55,60], even with quiet tidal breathing. Furthermore, the extent of turbulence must increase as patency diminishes or as increasingly high flow rates are achieved, even by subjects without notable nasal obstruction.

2. The Nasal Flow–Pressure Relationship

At normally prevailing rates of flow, the well-developed turbulence of nasal air streams contrasts with largely laminar regimes present in subglottic airways [60], seriously complicating the interpretation of nasal ventilatory parameters. With a variable combination of laminar and turbulent flow present, the nasal flow–pressure relationship is not linear (as in pure laminar flow) but describes a flattened S-shaped figure with a quasilinear central segment (see Fig. 2). Efforts to describe this relationship mathematically have been numerous and have generated no agreement on preferred approaches [54,55,57]. It is clear that neither an "Ohm's law analogue" (i.e., pressure = resistance × flow) typical of laminar flow nor a model supposing complete turbulence (i.e., pressure = resistance × flow^2) provides a realistic basis for most analyses. A "compromise" relationship (i.e., pressure = resistance $\text{flow}^{1.7}$) has theoretical advantages [55] and limited empirical support [61] but is not fully accepted by most workers. The formulation

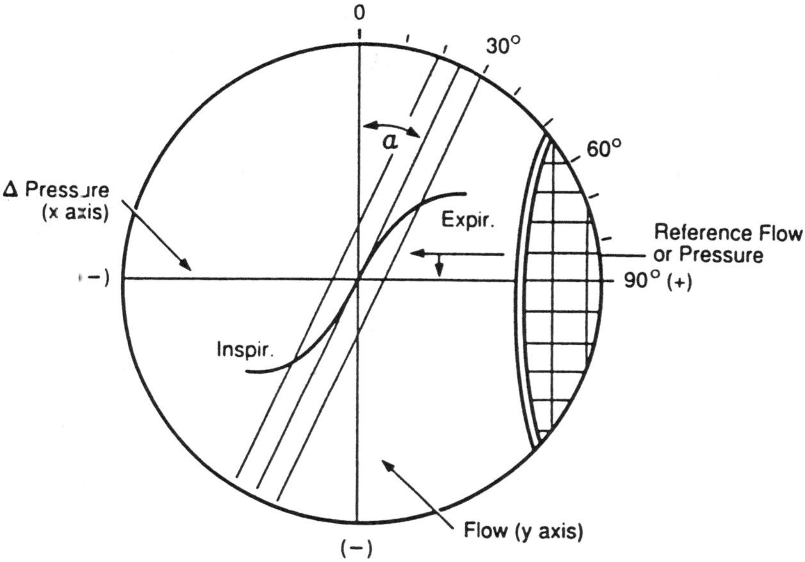

Figure 2 Nasal flow–pressure relationship.

proposed many years ago by Rohrer and discussed by Hamilton [55] still seems best to characterize the nasal pressure–flow (ΔP–$\dot{V}$ relationship):

$$P = K_1\dot{V}^2 = K_2\dot{V} + K_3 \tag{1}$$

In this equation, the constants K_1 and K_2 express the flow-resistive properties of a given nasal airway at any condition of patency.* Values of these constants change as nasal conductance is varied. Although it is possible to derive the values of constants K_1 and K_2 (see below, "Anterior Rhinomanometry") and to follow their changes, they have not been translated into a widely favored parameter of nasal patency.

3. Consequences of Turbulent Nasal Flow

Figure 2 emphasizes that the relationship of driving pressure (ΔP) and flow ($\dot{V}$) changes throughout the nasal respiratory cycle. As a result, measurements of nasal

*The term K_3 usually approximates 0 unless nasal obstruction is intense or respiration is rapid so that changes in flow direction must be made forcefully. Under these conditions, the complete nasal flow–pressure curve will display more or less hysteresis (i.e., a pressure deflection at 0 flow). It is probably that the value of term K_3 in the Rohrer equation and the degree of hysteresis are related and jointly reflect the work needed to overcome inertial forces during acceleration of airway gas.

ΔP alone (without the associated flow rate) or of submaximal $\dot{V}$ alone (without driving pressure) are virtually meaningless in gauging obstruction. The resistance of the nasal airway is essentially the pressure drop associated with a specific rate of flow and, operationally, is expressed as the slope of the nasal pressure–flow curve at the flow point considered. With low flows, in both inspiration and expiration, the ΔP–$\dot{V}$ relationship approaches linearity (reflecting a prominently laminar regime), but it becomes progressively curved at higher (more fully turbulent) flow levels. Nasal airway resistance thus varies through much of the respiratory cycle, its rise tending to accelerate as progressively higher flow rates are achieved. Comparison of NAR data (e.g., before and after challenge) therefore should relate to a single flow rate or other suitable reference point.*

Because nasal flow comprises turbulent and laminar components that vary with individual airway configuration and air velocities, as well as overall conductance, efforts [53,62] to deduce an "effective airway cross-sectional area" from nasal ventilatory measurements have shown limited value. Consequently, most recently active workers have sought indicators of nasal patency by direct analyses or by "processing" of nasal ΔP–$\dot{V}$ curves. However, it has been difficult to establish criteria for the relative significance of changes in resistance data, especially when subjects' baseline NAR values differ substantially. Consider, for example, (1) a challenge protocol in which a doubling of NAR (at a reference flow) is the predetermined minimal "positive" response to challenge, (2) a completely normal subject (A) with substantially laminar nasal flow, and (3) an entered subject (B) with preexisting mucosal edema producing turbulence virtually throughout nasal ventilation. The addition of an arbitrary "unit" of obstruction to each subject's airway will cause a greater proportional rise in NAR for the latter subject (B), whose ΔP–$\dot{V}$ relationship is nonlinear under baseline conditions and must become increasingly so as patency falls further. If the resulting NAR rise just exceeds 10% for B, subject A's response will fall well below this level of increment (as predictable from A's more quasilinear ΔP–$\dot{V}$ relationship). Thus, despite comparable decrements in patency, one (i.e., B) will be judged a "responder" and one (A) will not. This problem is of lesser concern in studies of subglottic airways, for which the ΔP–$\dot{V}$ relationship normally is linear up to flows of 2 L/s [60]. In the nose, however, the baseline level of patency can readily influence the magnitude of measured responses to incremental (or decreased) obstruction. The risk of design errors involving this effect is especially great where groups (e.g., normal subjects and subjects with symptomatic rhinitis) differing clinically and in mean nasal patency are studied for nasal response to a challenge or other intervention. For comparative purposes, sets of subjects should have similar (and preferably high)

*Since obstruction may limit attainable flow rates, a reference pressure point has been used empirically by many workers.

nasal conductivity. Individual responses to challenge are best studied during periods of minimal nasal obstruction, and for sequential studies, similar values for baseline NAR (coefficient of variation perhaps $<35\%$) are preferable in related test sessions. Deviations from these preferred conditions should be recognized, prospectively, as sources of concern and potential design defects. Efforts to reduce the impact of an exponential nasal ΔP–$\dot{V}$ relationship have included choosing a low flow range* for measurement [63] and a preference for experimental subjects with normal nasal patency, who also have shown minimal responses to "control" challenge. The use of nasal respiratory work as a variable, as suggested by Cole and co-workers [64], may provide a measurable relationship that is more extensively linear.

C. Specific Indicators of Nasal Airway Response

1. Preliminary Precautions

The diversity of measurement techniques advanced for nasal investigations is so broad, and their practical utility so variable, that any comprehensive catalog would have limited value. Instead, we will focus on a subset of methods judged useful by many current workers. Approaches that defy standardization are inadequate for challenge work and have been omitted. Where possible, related methods are described together as practical alternatives. The reader must recognize that too many published descriptions of nasal measurement approaches are technically incomplete and that few comparisons of proposed methods have been reported.

2. Methods Providing Nonventilatory Parameters

Attempts to use subjective assessments of nasal "obstruction" and pruritus systematically as indicators of nasal response to acute challenge have been disappointing. However, Mygind and co-workers have introduced a "sneeze-drip" variable [65] to quantitate equally homely events. In this approach, spontaneous sneezes are tallied simply following nasal challenge. With the subjects' neck flexed fully, nasal secretions are allowed to run from the nostrils, and the number of "drips" collected in a defined period (often 10–15 min) is also counted. By summing sneezes and drips, a quantitative index of response is derived. Since drip number will also vary with secretion viscosity and the topography of the nares (including the number and disposition of vibrissae), total secretion volume [66,67] (or weight [68]) might be preferable. In any case, the method presupposes rather florid nasal reactions, such as those provoked by "bolus" challenge with potent

*The low flow range is more readily treated as a laminar (and linear) region in which arithmetical changes are realistic. However, data based on low flows are probably less sensitive indicators of changes in patency than are variables based on higher attainable flows (and values of ΔP).

pollen extracts. The documentation of more subtle changes or of intense obstructive responses with minimal coryza would require other parameters.

Alternative indicators of nasal blood flow have been adapted for short-term studies in the human only recently. Thermography [69], reflecting mucosal heat flux, provides a correlate of at least one component of nasal blood flow (especially that in subepithelial arterioles); however, the high cost and complexity of required equipment seriously limit its use. The potential value of plethysmography [70], photoelectric plethysmography [71], and thermoelectric conductivity measurements [34] as indicators of "rapid" nasal response appears limited, on the basis of reported applications. Although substantially invasive, the clearance of xenon 133 following local injection has provided a useful indicator of nasal mucosal blood flow, applicable to challenge studies [72]. Widely available sensing equipment is used to monitor washout of the radionuclide. By contrast, laser-Doppler velocimetry requires specialized and costly hardware but provides an essentially noninvasive indicator for continuous monitoring of blood flow—primarily that in superficial mucosal arterioles—with the subject in a head-up position [73]. Comparisons between these methods suggest that they measure different but complementary microvascular functions [74]. Short-period changes in mucosal width at a constant reference point, measured with an operating microscope, provides a further, recently described, parameter [75].

Nasal responses to both allergens and nonimmunological stimuli often release phlogogenic mediator substances, derived from the mucosa, into nasal secretions [76]. Methods to recover and assay these in small volumes have been used recently to dissect pathogenic mechanisms of response following challenge. Fluid may be collected by continuous aspiration, e.g., using a fenestrated 8-French catheter lying along the nasal floor [66]; more commonly, repetitive nasal washings using approximately 5 ml of a physiological salt solution have been assayed. The latter approach is facilitated by first instilling an α-adrenergic agonist to increase and stabilize the nasal cavity volume and requires only brief breath holding and glottic closure by subjects [77]. Washings have been assayed for preformed mast cell products (e.g., histamine and TAME-esterase activity) as well as newly synthesized factors including a range of arachidonic acid metabolites and 2-lyso-PAF-acether [78]. Variations in kinin activity also have been documented [79]. In addition, assay of albumin in aspirate/washings provides an estimate of the relative contributions to the recovered fluid of transudation from plasma and glandular secretion [80]. Cell traffic through the nasal mucosa and airway secretions often changes in response to challenge, with a time scale measured in hours or days. Since nasal washings can provide only luminal, nonadherent cells, superficial scrapings, often obtained with a small plastic curette (Rhinoprobe, Synbiotics, San Diego, California), or direct biopsy is often favored. Particular interest has surrounded the cytology of the "late" response to allergens, which is dominated by neutrophils and eosinophils as well as small (absolute) increases in mucosal basophils, which still are increased manyfold over populations in the prechallenge state [79]. Several research groups have independently reported increased metachromatically staining cells in the allergen-challenged noses of sensitive atopic subjects, describing these as mast cells, basophils [81–83], or both. The full significance of these cells as contributors to the "late" response and, notably, to the exaggerated reactivity ("priming") that follows merits further study.

It is now evident that impaired eustachian tube function follows supraliminal upper airway challenge, dysfunction often continuing after the acute rhinitis response subsides [84,85]. Defective tubal patency causing reduced middle ear aeration can be demonstrated [85] in a primate model and in atopic subjects receiving intranasal allergen or histamine. In evaluating such dysfunction, tympanometry, using an electroacoustic impedance device, has been widely accepted. By contrast, recently demonstrated changes in sinus mucosal width following intranasal allergen challenge have yet to be used systematically as an indicator of tissue response [86].

3. Methods Providing Ventilatory Parameters

Peak Expiratory Flow Rate (Nasal). Taylor and associates proposed recording the peak rate of nasal expiratory flow ($PEFR_N$) as a parameter of airway patency [87]. To accomplish this, the subject makes a maximally rapid forced expiration through the nose following a full inspiratory effort. The lips are firmly pressed together during this maneuver, and the nose is enclosed in a nasal mask connected to a Wright peak flow meter. The highest of six readings has been proposed as peak flow (nasal) at a point in time. Care is needed to prevent undue pressure on the nose or its surrounding venous outflow. The $PEFR_N$ values achieved by apparently well persons have varied from less than 250 to over 600 L/min, but most normal adult values cluster in the range from 380 to 550 L/min [87]. In addition to nasal patency, $PEFR_N$ values reflect a subject's ventilatory capability, including lower airway conductance, efficiency of the thoracic bellows, and expiratory vigor. These sources of bias, often grouped as "effort," mandate use of a "blockage index" (BI) proposed by Taylor and associates and calculated as follows [87]:

$$BI = \frac{\text{Peak flow (oral)} - \text{Peak flow (nasal)}}{\text{Peak flow (oral)}} \tag{2}$$

Values for BI rise as nasal patency diminishes and generally are below 0.4 in ostensibly normal persons.

The $PEFR_N$ is easily recorded with simple components that are portable and require no power source. Subject cooperation is easily enlisted; however, since forced nasal expiration (without a handkerchief) is unfamiliar (and often somewhat intimidating), subject training is surprisingly important. In addition, middle ear discomfort (or fear of it) often prompts an inconsistent expiratory effort. These problems may be limiting when appreciable nasal secretions occur or other factors obstruct the nasal airway.

As expected, there is a strong positive correlation between baseline values of BI and nasal airway resistance [87,88] (see below), with the latter determined at submaximal flow rates.* This association is most evident in data from relatively unobstructed noses, decreasing when nasal patency falls. Airway resistance has appeared to be a more sensitive indicator of response in limited comparisons by the author and his colleagues. However, the $PEFR_N$ and BI may be useful where clear-cut change is provoked in nasal airway caliber [88].

Nasal Airway Resistance and Related Parameters. A variety of methods estimate NAR, which realistically expresses the relationship between air flow and the associated pressure drop across the nasal airway. For both conceptual and tactical purposes, NAR may be visualized as the slope of the curve relating flow $\dot{V}$ to pressure differential between the nasopharynx and the nares (transnasal pressure drop [ΔP]). As previously discussed and shown in Fig. 2, this relationship (and the slope of the curve representing it) changes throughout the respiratory cycle as more or less laminar and turbulent flow regimes predominate. Resistance is expressed as pressure differential/unit of flow—usually centimeters of H_2O per liter per second in North America, while investigators aboard have proposed a "standard international unit" [89] with dimensions of pascals† per square centimeter per second. Theoretically, any practically attainable level of flow may be chosen as a standard reference point for NAR measurements. However, valid comparisons among subjects or for sequential NAR values in one subject are possible only if data are based on a single, consistently used flow rate. It is desirable also to make measurements consistently in the inspiratory or expiratory phase of the respiratory cycle, since the ΔP–$\dot{V}$ relationship often is demonstrably phase-variable. Our experience suggests that expiration, especially its latter portion,‡ is the most stable and artifact-free component of nasal respiration in successive cycles. However, others have used inspiratory measurements exclusively, with apparent success in achieving study objectives.

Two basic approaches to the acquisition of ΔP–$\dot{V}$ data are widely employed: anterior and posterior rhinomanometry. Of the several differences between these methods, the most fundamental is in the means of sensing pharyngeal pressure.

Posterior Rhinomanometry. Posterior rhinomanometry (Fig. 3) employs a flexible tube, held between the pursed lips and supported on the midline of the tongue, that is open to the pharynx as a pressure tap. Flow is sensed by a clinical

*The correlation between nasal peak flow and airway resistance is negative and equally significant.

†A Pascal is a microunit of pressure approximating 0.01 cm H_2O (1 cm H_2O = 98 pascals).

‡When the ΔP-$\dot{V}$ curve has negligible hysteresis, the first and second halves of expiration are, of course, superimposed.

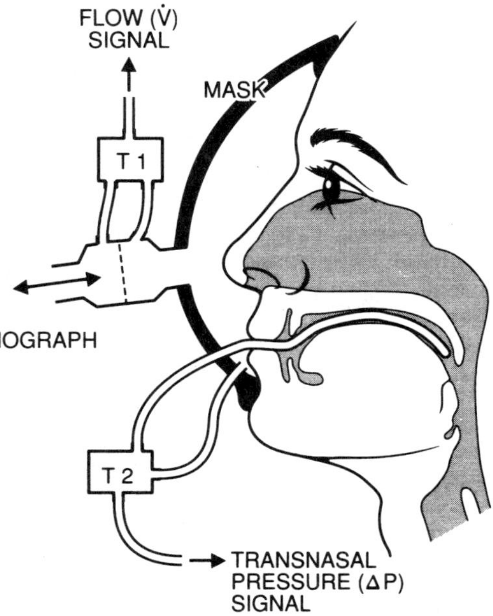

Figure 3 Posterior rhinomanometry.

pneumotachygraph (preferably with a linear output to 100 L/min) carried by a mask that encloses either the nose and mouth or the nose alone. Although this approach is used generally to study the total nasal airway as an integrated unit, modifications allowing study of the right and left channels separately are feasible [90,91]. In either case, bidirectional pressure transducers receive output from the pneumotachygraph(s). Similarly, pressure taps from oropharynx and mask* are connected to a separate transducer that generates a signal proportional to their difference (= transnasal pressure [ΔP]). Transducer outputs are amplified and may be recorded separately as time-related tracings on strip charges. Alternatively, $\dot{V}$ and ΔP are readily displayed on the precalibrated axes of an oscilloscope or an X-Y plotter. These signals also may be converted to quantities such as respiratory work by interposing suitable microprocessors, and data may be stored on magnetic tape for later review.

Posterior rhinomanometric methods require an airtight mask application without significant compression of the facial venous channels that drain intranasal

*Some investigators have substituted atmospheric for mask pressure, as a measure of expediency; however, these two quantities *do* differ, especially when respiratory effort is increased.

vessels. If these precautions are observed, both masks that exclude the mouth and larger types, enclosing the entire face, may be useful. In general, we have found models with a flexible, "knife-edge" margin, such as the Wright aviation mask or (scuba) units designed for underwater use, especially adaptable for nasal testing purposes.

Posterior rhinomanometry offers a potentially sensitive indicator of upper airway patency without instrumentation of the nasal passages. However, satisfactory recordings are not obtained from the oropharyngeal pressure tap, despite every reasonable effort, in about 15% of our subjects; failure rates as high as 40–50% have been claimed [92], although most experience matches our own, even in studies that include children. At times, a previously absent pressure signal is obtained after advancing (or, rarely, retracting) the tube a few millimeters. In any case, once the catheter is positioned satisfactorily, its length should be maintained throughout any set of studies on one subject. Persistent difficulty in securing a ΔP signal often is dissipated simply by allowing an unstressed opportunity for the subject to gain confidence and become familiar with the apparatus. Efforts to roll the lips inward and drop the tongue to the floor of the mouth during deep, slow nasal breathing also promote the necessary relaxation of oropharyngeal structures. If a continuous chart or oscilloscopic image is available, it often can provide useful feedback to a subject striving to produce the desired (S-shaped) ΔP–$\dot{V}$ curve. Secondary failures are rare following establishment of a consistent pharyngeal pressure signal and should suggest lateral deflection of the tube or blockage of its lumen by (removable*) secretions. Equipment for rhinomanometry may be assembled from widely used components. In addition, a test module (the Mercury nasal Resistance Meter, NR series), has been available from Mercury Electronics (Glasgow, Scotland) for some time. The device apparently has found increasing acceptance among British [93] and European [94] workers and has been adapted to permit testing of almost all adults and many children, including some preschoolers [95]. Additional commercial devices, generally for anterior rhinometry, are being introduced.

Anterior Rhinomanometry. The desire to avoid use of an oropharyngeal tube has prompted increasing interest in the variation of anterior rhinomanometry (Fig. 4). With this approach, posterior pharyngeal pressure is estimated by inserting a tap into one nostril while flow through the opposite airway is directed through a small pneumotachygraph. Both flow and pressure sensors require smooth-surface adaptors (often termed "nasal olives") affording an airtight fit with minimal airway distortion and mucosal stimulation. Alternatively, the nostril providing a pressure signal may be sealed with tape or a cast made of dental impression

*Commercial pipe cleaners are especially useful for this purpose during a single test session. Suitable precautions to preclude transfer of secretions among successive subjects are, of course, mandatory.

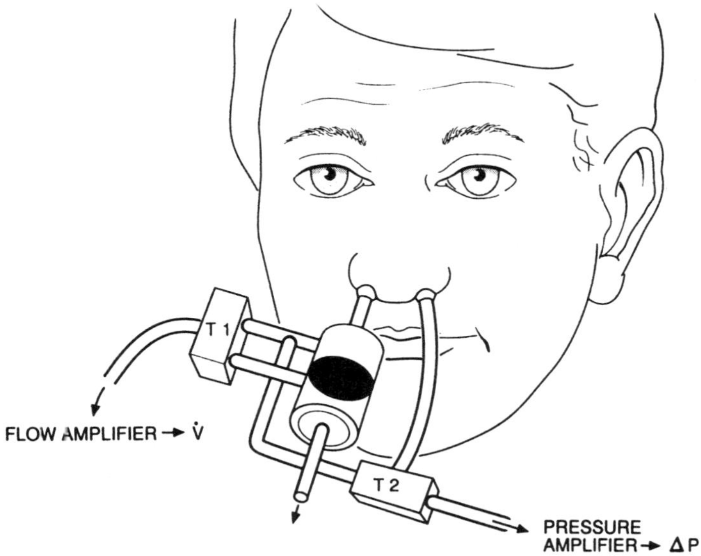

Figure 4 Anterior rhinomanometry.

material [96]. Since flow is suspended in one airway during any measurement, the two sides must be studied individually, with placement of the flow and pressure sensors alternated. Calculation of a resistance parameter for the entire nasal airway (R_N) is then possible using values (R_R and R_L, respectively) from the right and left nares:

$$\frac{1}{R_N} = \frac{1}{R_R} + \frac{1}{R_L} \tag{3}$$

and

$$R_N = \frac{R_R \times R_L}{R_R + R_L} \tag{4}$$

Less often, the responses of only one passage are studied sequentially, although the risk of error due to reciprocal spontaneous airway changes discourages this approach.

Anterior rhinomanometry can also provide flow and pressure readings from almost all adult subjects and many children [97]. However, this approach does involve tactical problems that are easily overlooked. Airtight sealing of adaptors in the nostrils is an evident necessity but difficult to achieve without stimulating or deforming the airway. The "nasal olives" used must be of low internal resistance and similarly positioned in sequential tests to avoid variable deformity of the narrow nasal valve [57,98] or random stimulation of mucosal sensory receptors. Although a variety of shapes and sizes are needed to approach ideal conditions, too often a single adaptor is used for all subjects, with the tactic hope that errors will be tractable. These concerns seem more critical, under many test conditions, than the questionable adequacy of an anterior nasal tap in reflecting conditions deeper in the airway. Pharyngeal pressure can be sensed across the nasal airway, although its transmission appears to vary with airway geometry and secretion volume. Rhinomanometric values by posterior and anterior approaches do appear to differ [92,99], despite reports to the contrary [100,101]. When compared in single subjects, the anterior mode has shown greater scatter and less consistency of data points [99]. Statistically, however, values obtained by anterior and posterior methods generally vary in parallel [101].

Body Plethysmography. Additional approaches to NAR measurement have been described by individual laboratories, with limited comparisons reported [98,101]. Particular interest has surrounded estimation of nasal patency using the body plethysmograph. The nose normally contributes at least half of total respiratory resistance (R_T) during nasal respiration [60] and provides a progressively larger fraction as upper airway obstruction increases. Accordingly, NAR has been determined plethysmographically as the difference between the respective values for R_T measured during oral and nasal breathing [99,102–104]. This approach makes the reasonable assumption that the R_T values compared are related to a single, specific rate of flow. In limited comparisons, NAR data obtained plethysmographically and by posterior rhinometry have shown close accord and parallel variations [99]. Laboratories experienced in body-box applications, including head-out models, may find this approach quite useful in challenge procedures that produce well-marked nasal change.

Approaches to the Analysis of Nasal Flow-pressure Data. Data derived from "anterior" or "posterior" measurements may be interrelated in several ways to produce indices of nasal patency. Perhaps the most technically simple approach is to record $\dot{V}$ and ΔP on adjacent chart strips. Since the tracings that result share a time axis, a perpendicular to this axis will intersect temporally related values, permitting calculation of an "Ohm's law analogue" of resistance, i.e., $\Delta P/\dot{V} = R$. Changes in this parameter, measured at a defined rate of flow and respiratory phase (e.g., end-expiration), reflect nasal patency more or less clearly.

The use of nasal airway conductance (= 1/NAR) as a parameter of response has been described by Dvoracek et al. [105], who favored this variable over other indicators of nasal patency. In their approach, conductance (liters per second/cm H_2O) was determined at an inspiratory ΔP of 0.390 cm H_2O. Because flow rates readily transmitted by unobstructed noses may be unattainable when congestion supervenes (e.g., after a "positive" challenge), the relation of measurements to an index ΔP rather than a reference flow has been proposed [55]. While this approach has theoretical defects, it has unquestioned practical advantages. Accordingly, resistance values now are widely related to a consistent pressure point, and this strategy has been embraced by an international working group on the standardization of rhinometry [89]; commonly favored pressures have been in the range from 1.0 to 3.0 cm H_2O (roughly 100–300 pascals), with 1.5 cm H_2O a frequent consensus point. Regardless of the reference value chosen, it should be recognized that, in any single breath, resistance parameters do change as pressure and flow vary; hence, the need for a "benchmark" or reference value.

Since the ΔP–$\dot{V}$ relationship may be visualized directly as an oscilloscopic image, many workers have favored this approach. Direct readings of points or slopes are possible with a conventional screen—especially if rhythmic breathing allows superimposition of successive images. However, use of an image-retentive screen or an oscilloscope camera (providing "Polaroid-type" prints) facilitates accurate measurements; alternatively, an X-Y plotter may be used. In practice, ΔP and $\dot{V}$ transducer outputs are electronically amplified and processed to allow projection on X/Y axes, usually with $\dot{V}$ as the Y axis. The transducers and screen deflections are calibrated regularly using an in-line rotameter for flow and a water manometer (in a Y-connection) as a pressure monitor; these standard indicators generally are removed at other times. Calibration is, of course, effected at the "gain" and "sensitivity" levels employed for clinical measurement.

Several apparently successful approaches to analysis of the S-shaped oscilloscopic image have been summarily described [54,55,57,89,98,106,107]. Probably the most widely popular approach is the "point" measurement of ΔP at a chosen index flow rate or of $\dot{V}$ at a defined ΔP. Others, including ourselves, have regarded the slope of the ΔP–$\dot{V}$ curve, at any flow level, as a more valid representation of the relevant NAR. Estimates of slope are facilitated by superimposing a moveable overlay, ruled with parallel lines, over the fluorescent ΔP–$\dot{V}$ image (Fig. 2).

Nasal airway resistance data for normal subjects, reported by several groups, are difficult to compare because of differences in technique and analysis among laboratories. In general, however, at flows less than 0.5 L/s, mean values cluster below 1.6 cm H_2O/L/s [59,63,106,108,109]. A mean of 1.05 ± 0.37 (range 0.35–1.85) has been obtained in 40 adults, aged 18–48 years, studied in our own laboratory [63], with a trend toward higher values during winter. Others have noted an age-associated decrease in NAR among adults without symptoms or signs of upper airway disease, although a progressive NAR rise during childhood also has been reported [97,110]. A subjective sense of obstruction has been reported as an increasingly consistent feature with total NAR > 3.0 cm H_2O/L/s (or 7.0 on one side) [111]; however, a true threshold for this perception is not suggested.

The index flow rate or reference pressure point should be one requiring little effort initially, and also attainable by most subjects even after development of moderate nasal stuffiness; in general, 0.5 L/s or flows below this have been employed. The relative merits of readings based on very low reference flows (where a quasilinear $\Delta P-\dot{V}$ association obtains) or on higher values (e.g., 0.3–0.5 L/s) at which turbulence determines a $\Delta P \sim \dot{V}^2$ or $\sim\dot{V}^{1.7}$ relationship is unclear; both ranges seem to have been usable in specific circumstances.

As previously emphasized, the absolute change in calculated resistance for any airway lumen event will depend (because of the exponential $\Delta P-\dot{V}$ relationship) on the initial level of patency as well as on the reference point for measurement. In practice, a doubling or 100% rise in NAR requires a substantial drop in patency at low reference flows but will occur with relatively lesser obstructive changes in a high-flow measurement range. Similarly, since flow and pressure are related nonlinearly, at any reference value, initially "stuffy" noses more easily display large NAR changes than relatively patent ones for a unit change in luminal size.

These sources of bias scarcely need concern the rhinologist seeking only to quantitate gross organic obstruction by making side-to-side comparisons [111–113] and perhaps assess the completeness of its relief postoperatively. By contrast, where nasal challenge quickly elicits relatively subtle and evanescent changes, care is needed to ensure sensitivity and minimize measurement errors. Experimental objectives often will limit or define the technical choices available to the investigator. Where feasible, we have preferred to use subjects for challenge with relatively low baseline NAR, i.e., <1.5 cm H_2O/L/s at lowest flows and < 4 cm H_2O/L/s at 0.5 L/s in (end-) expiration. Breathing rate and effort do not appear to bias NAR values related consistently to a reference level of pressure or flow. Normal subjects, comfortably seated at 20–22°C, show only modest spontaneous variations in patency if measured in this way during several hours under baseline conditions. For such persons, a doubling of NAR constitutes an "unexpected" airway event and a suitable end point for defining significant induced change. However, for liminal challenge stimuli, lesser NAR increments, denoting subtle airway changes, may (consistently) occur. Unless one were willing to sacrifice such responses as "falsely negative," the criteria of a "positive" challenge would require redefinition: i.e., (1) a 70% or greater NAR rise might serve more appropriately as "positive,"* or (2) measurements might be made at a higher reference flow (or pressure), with the change required to achieve "significance" chosen so as to be well beyond the expected normal limits of variation. When measured at that ventilatory point, minimal criteria for a "positive response" are less uniformly accepted and less easily defined in nasal than in bronchial provocation. Therefore, each testing facility should identify empirical norms for the

*In observations of 50 normal subjects, Hasegawa and co-workers [114] noted NAR differences of as much as 53% in values obtained 15 min apart. The *mean* change over this interval was, of course, substantially lower. These workers emphasized, however, that physiological variability could produce changes as great as 53% in this brief period.

response parameters it employs, establishing the expected range of variation under extended baseline conditions and after "control" challenge exposures.

An alternative approach to nasal patency testing has been the use of Rohrer constants, from Eq. 1 as variables. In this equation, K_1 and K_2 derive essentially from the resistance attributable to turbulent and laminar components of flow, respectively. These constants may be calculated, at any point in time, from measurements based on strip charts or an oscilloscopic image [115]; alternatively, they may be derivable automatically by the microprocessing of ΔP and $\dot{V}$ data. In practice, K_1 has received primary attention, and shorter versions of the Rohrer equation (e.g., $\Delta P = K_1\dot{V}^2$ or $P = K_1\dot{V}^{1.7}$) have been assumed [55,112]. This expedient is especially palatable if moderate to high flow rates are examined, respiration is not excessively rapid,* and nasal obstruction is moderate, at worst. At least one group has found K_1 to be a tractable variable when estimated, in inspiration, from 4–6 points on a ΔP–$\dot{V}$ curve [115]. In addition, they found a strong correlation between K_1, measured at 0.4 L/s, and NAR determined by rhinometry at the same flow; both variables were based on inspiratory recordings. In the same study, K_2 (the coefficient of the linear term) appeared to mirror nasal patency changes and NAR (also measured at 0.4 L/s) far less well than K_1. We, too, have observed a convincing correlation of calculated K_1 and measured NAR at 0.5 L/s in expiration. However, especially in view of the added steps generally required to derive K_1, it seems to offer no confirmed advantage over conventional rhinometric methodology.

An omnibus approach to analysis of the ΔP–$\dot{V}$ curve has been proposed by Broms and associates [107]. These workers use an oscilloscope precalibrated so as to permit superimposition of concentric circles, centered at the X-Y intersection. The circles pass through flows of ± 1.2 and 3 cm H_2O, respectively. At the intersections of the $\dot{V}$–ΔP curve with these circles, lines are drawn to the zero point, and the resulting angles made with the X(V) axis are determined. By combining the applicable (six) tangents, a parameter of NAR is derived, which samples all portions of the $\dot{V}$–ΔP cycle; automatic processing of the curve is feasible.

Microprocessing of ΔP and $\dot{V}$ data to give a continuous digital readout of NAR is technically feasible but apparently not widely employed. However, Cole and coworkers [64,90] have sampled ΔP and $\dot{V}$ outputs of posterior rhinometry every 20 ms with a microprocessor and derived direct readouts of nasal respiratory work (in joules per liter) and minute ventilation (liters per minute). They suggest that the graphic relationship between these quantities is broadly linear, with a slope characteristic of a subject's nasal patency at any given instant.

*To minimize inertial forces.

Some workers have employed "passive rhinometry," in which a constant flow of air is passed through an oropharyngeal tube and the pressure developed within the pharynx is measured, during mouth closure, as an index of nasal patency [43]. A related "anterior" approach [44,116] records the pressure developed when each nostril (or both together) passively receives a constant flow, with the lips parted. Both methods are simple in concept; however, many subjects cannot provide the complete glottic closure required. In addition, possible artifactual effects of passive aeration have not been systematically evaluated.

IV. NASAL CHALLENGE TECHNIQUES

A. The Problem in Perspective

A vast array of allergens, chemical irritants, autacoids, drugs, and physical factors have potential upper airway activity; yet remarkably few of these have been studied in the nose. Virtually any condition or agent that is suitable for bronchial provocation may be employed for nasal challenge. However, this section will focus primarily on methods for exposing the nasal airway to solutions or fluid extracts in aerosol form.

It must be appreciated that published (and personal) concepts of nasal reactivity are conditioned by the validity and sensitivity of the indicator systems used as well as the criteria for defining a response. Minor airway effects—for example, those due to a bland "control" aerosol—may be manifest when one technique is used but inapparent with less sensitive approaches. Such differences in the feasibility of ascertainment have led to many conflicts in the reported effects of nasal challenge using specific agents. Similarly, artifactual nasal effects of challenge and measurement maneuvers are easily overlooked if monitored by relatively insensitive methods.

While endorsing diverse nasal provocative methods, most workers concede (1) that in most cases, challenge should imitate ordinary "field" exposure, and (2) that finely metered delivery of most natural materials, under controlled conditions, is technically quite difficult. As a result, attention has been focused increasingly on the optimal delivery of solutions and extracts in aerosol form, creating unnaturally brief, intense exposures.

Kirkman's development of hay fever after sniffing sweet vernal grass pollen, in 1835, was perhaps the earliest recorded nasal challenge [117]. Decades later, Blackley tested responses to pollen by conjunctival, nasal, and parabuccal instillation [118]. Thereafter, nasal challenge was employed diagnostically by scattered clinicians both before and after the emergence of skin test procedures. These early efforts centered on the sniffing or dropping of dry pollens into the nose, usually from a toothpick, with subjective appraisal of clinical response. Subsequent workers have used inhalation of intact pollens from stirred dry suspension

[119,120] and continuously generated test chamber aerosols [121]; others (rarely) have injected allergen eluates into the nasal mucosa [122]. Aschan and Drettner [123] challenged the noses of allergic subjects with intact pollens or pollen extract aerosols, as well as histamine solution, and assessed the resulting changes by simultaneous measurements of nasal flow and pressure drop. The effects of H_1-blocking antihistaminics, phenylephrine, and immunotherapy on these responses were assessed similarly by these workers. Subsequent reports have confirmed the value of objective response parameters and of challenge with fluid-phase materials, delivered by various means. The cohesiveness of native pollen grains (especially those of ragweeds) has made their dispersion for direct airway challenge generally unfeasible.* Suspension of grains of powdered lactose has allowed their dispersion from a punctured capsule in a "Spinhaler" (Fisons Laboratories) [125]. Defatted grains were employed by Connell in an apparatus designed for challenge by active inhalation [119]. Although the pollen dose administered was not precisely measurable, a particle counter might be interposed to indicate levels of such a monodisperse aerosol.

B. Delivery Systems for Fluid-Phase Materials

1. Challenge with Directly Applied (Nonaerosol) Materials

Fluid-phase challenge materials have been delivered to the nose as aerosols, in fluid-soaked, felted media [126,127], and as droplets from a syringe [65,128], pipette [129], glass applicator [130], or dropper [115]. In choosing among these, primary concerns have been the mucosal distribution of introduced materials and the relative risks of eliciting factitious nasal vascular responses. Decreased nasal patency has followed introduction of even bland fluids (e.g., phosphate-buffered saline) by each method [24]; however, the use of saturated cotton pledgets and pipettes (especially when positioned through a nasal speculum) generally has caused greater responses than aerosols. Partially offsetting this concern is the predictable delivery of challenge material to a defined mucosal area that is afforded by saturated media. Applications of thin, fluid-soaked paper disks [127] to the mucosa may share this advantage while inciting less unwanted response. Okuda [131] has used paper disks 3 mm in diameter containing, for example, histamine, house dust extract, or saline to appraise the value of four mucosal sites: forward end of the inferior turbinate, middle of the agger nasi, nasal septum, and center of the middle turbinate. Changes were graded by clinical criteria but did suggest the inferior turbinate as the most reactive single location, followed by the agger nasi. However, maximum reactivity was observed when several sites—

*The use of a modified industrial dust feed device [124] to maintain stable levels of native short-ragweed pollen in a test chamber may be regarded as a qualified exception. However, this success was achieved with the "averaging influence" of a relatively large mixing volume.

involving both the right and left airways—were challenged. This approach provides control of the time and extent of mucosal contact at a cost of limited nasal manipulation, and it may have potential value where highly reactive substances are tested. Instillation of fluid by micropipette (usually 100 μl) offers precision in placement, but deposited droplets often coalesce and drain to the nares or nasopharynx.

A recently described nasal "pool" device may allow challenge of the mucosa and collection of nasal secretion/transudation by bulk fluid transfer. The anatomical level challenged may be roughly controlled, although the method precludes all approaches but assay of the collected washings for assessment of response [132].

2. Aerosol Challenge

Aerosolized fluids seem to afford satisfactory mucosal challenge with fewest technical artifacts and are favored by many current workers, although the number of proponents of Okuda's approach is increasing [133]. Despite their wide use in bronchial challenge, aerosols require special concerns in the upper airway. Since the volume of the nasal cavities is so limited, the timing of the challenge aerosol's introduction, with respect to inspiration, will critically affect its depth and pattern of deposition. The optimal extent (and duration) of contact of any test agent with the mucosa remains controversial. However, the injection of aerosol during breath holding will favor a shallow pattern of nasal deposition, which most workers would agree to avoid.

Particle size influences the probability of nasal trapping, with larger introduced units retained most efficiently. By contrast, relatively minute aerosols, e.g., the 2- to 3-μm droplets produced by many nebulizers, are captured less well by the nose, much passing to the subglottic airways. Accordingly, for nasal work, atomizers and other sources of relatively coarse aerosols have been preferred over devices with fine particle outputs. Materials that escape nasal trapping not only compromise challenge strength but also pose a risk of unwanted effects at lower respiratory levels. Many reports describing ipsilateral bronchial narrowing and/or changes in pulmonary aeration with nasal stimulation [103,134,135] suggest the existence of functional connections between respiratory levels. However, the direct passage of challenge materials to subglottic airways may underlie certain bronchial reactions following nasal challenge.

Published data permit very limited comparisons among aerosol delivery systems with respect to discharge volume and patterns of intranasal distribution. In general, the reproducibility of output has been distinctly less with hand-activated units than with those driven by a compressor or gas cylinder. For example, single-discharge volumes resulting from repetitive activations, by a hand bulb, of a DeVilbiss #251 atomizer have varied by at least ± 30%. This variability was three times that seen when the same unit was driven by an electronically timed (solenoid-controlled) compressor [63].

Deposition of dyed aerosol in a cadaver nasal model (without phasic air flow) generally was oriented around the long axis of the orifice adapter [136]. Two activations—with discharge directed both high and low in the nose—produced the broadest area of deposition. In this static model, freon-propelled and compressor-generated aerosols generally caused the deepest penetration. A broader and more shallow area of mucosal contact occurred with a "plastic bottle nebulizer," and the intensity of its manual compression was paralleled by the discharge volume and breadth of deposition. An atomized pump delivered an almost constant volume of 0.14 ml, which was well dispersed over the nasal lining. By contrast, "drip" bottles produced only limited areas of droplet accumulation.

We have studied the nasal deposition and clearance of phosphate-buffered saline (PBS) tagged with technetium 99m pertechnitate in adult volunteers [137]. The atomizers compared each delivered 0.10 ± 0.01 g of fluid per 0.10-s activation when pulsed with a flow of 11.5 L/min at 7 psi. Although intrasubject variation was evident, clearance of deposited radioactivity was greatest with a DeVilbiss #251 atomizer discharge and slower with models 144 and 127, as well as "Rhinilar" sprayer and a hand-activated spray bottle delivering comparable volumes. Slowed clearance was seen when aerosol impaction favored the vibrissae and nasal vestibule, with relatively less initial deposition deeper in the nasal airway.* The #251 atomizer produced delivery levels that correlated well with radioactivity instilled directly using a micropipette. Furthermore, clearance was substantially more rapid when a "sniffing" inhalation accompanied challenge than when the breath was held during aerosol delivery. However, even with this maneuver, deposition was largely in the anterior third of the nose, an experience also reported with a "hand-operated" nasal spray pump [138].

The volume of challenge material instilled has usually varied between 0.1 and 0.4 ml, although workers who employ micropipettes commonly use larger amounts to strengthen the provocative stimulus. Dalle and Melon, for example, have described applying 0.6 ml (total) as 0.1 ml applied to the septum, inferior, and middle turbinates bilaterally [139]. Such volumes also may elicit more prominent nonspecific (e.g., PBS-induced) responses than are desired. We have noted significantly greater NAR rises when subjects were challenged by intranasal aerosol with 0.4 ml volumes (0.2 ml/nostril) than with doses of half this amount [63]. Nasal patency changes were evident during the 15 min after challenge and were documented by posterior rhinomanometric testing at intervals of 1–2 min.

The diluent best suited to nasal testing is the one that, alone, empirically causes the least nasal response after direct mucosal challenge; however, most workers have found either 0.9% saline or PBS (pH 7.4) to be a preferred vehicle for

*Washing the nasal mucosa at 1 and 18 min produced the same total clearance, confirming that the technetium 99m pertechnitate did not enter or bind to mucosal elements.

provocative materials. The effects of added antimicrobial agents and protein stabilizers (e.g., dilute human serum albumin) largely remain undefined.*

Nasal challenge aerosols normally are administered at "room temperature," although, admittedly, the fluid may lose or gain heat during aerosolization and airway passage. Challenges with PBS administered by DeVilbiss #251 atomizer from a reservoir maintained at 37°C, caused slightly greater ($p > 0.05$) NAR rises than unheated fluid [63]. Warming of nasal provocative aerosols, therefore, cannot be recommended at present.

Nasal airway resistance will be found to increase transiently following even the most ideal challenge procedure with a diluent "control" in most, if not all, normal persons. The extent of this "nonspecific" reactivity must be considered both in subject selection and in defining the level of change that will be judged "significant." The rise above baseline values of NAR, measured at 10–15 min following a single (0.1 ml/nostril) PBS challenge, has averaged 25.5%, 26%, and 20.5%, respectively, in three subject groups [24,120,140]. Despite this concordance, intrasubject differences are definite, and individuals show some variability in response to a standardized PBS exposure on different days [24]. Therefore, as least one diluent challenge should be carried out on each day that a subject is tested. Most workers recognize this need and have incorporated into their testing protocols controls of one or more types, including sham challenges [63,109,114,119, 129,141] and challenge with irrelevant allergens [10,128,139,142,143] or "placebo" materials [106,119,139,144–146], as well as challenge of clinically defined control groups [147–149].

Since provocative protocols often demand repetitive exposure to a test substance, the nasal response to serial "control" challenges is of major importance. Accordingly, we have followed resistance values in subjects challenged six times, at 15-min intervals, with 0.1-ml portions of PBS per nostril. While half of the subjects' NAR values were increased to 50% or more over baseline, in only 15% did a doubling of resistance occur [24]. When this procedure was repeated on two or more occasions with single subjects, variability was clear-cut and occasionally marked. A positive correlation between such temporal differences in response to serial PBS challenge and baseline NAR values on the corresponding days of testing has been suggested [47] but requires confirmation. In any case, repeated nasal challenge in a format analogous to bronchial provocation appears feasible. Generous use of pretesting with control materials will enhance the significance of the data gathered and help identify subjects with aberrant reactivity to liminal stimuli.

That some nasal reaction should follow exposure to minute amounts of a bland

---

*However, we have noted apparently greater rises in NAR following nasal aerosols of PBS containing 0.4% phenol than with phenol-free PBS.

aerosol is not surprising, considering the function of the nose as guardian of the airway. The responses induced appear within minutes and presumably are mediated reflexly, in part through autonomic pathways. This view is supported by observations of the almost total suppression of PBS-induced changes in NAR 15 min following intranasal aerosolization of atropine [24]. Nasal airway resistance values following PBS challenge generally have returned to near-baseline levels in 15 min, while responses to allergens and other stimuli may persist longer. These patterns have prompted us to focus special attention on measurements made after 15 min and to conduct serial challenges at intervals only slightly longer. However, follow-up schedules are difficult to formulate, especially in view of the late or protracted responses reported after strong antigen challenge [79]. Dvoracek et al. [105] described immediately occurring obstructive responses that often persisted for 4 h after ragweed pollen extract. Pelikan [150] and Taylor [151] have reported similar reactions, beginning 2–6 h after challenge and lasting 12–24 h, as putative type III phenomena. Even longer delayed responses, evolving over 24–50 h, have been described [150]. Following repetitive allergen challenges, Taylor [106] has reported groups of subjects with increasing NAR responses, others with lessened reactivity NAR responses and, in some, a composite of the two.

C. The Author's Procedure for Nasal Provocative Testing

The following paragraphs describe nasal challenge with aerosols as performed in the Allergy Division at the University of Michigan Hospitals in Ann Arbor. While empirically useful, the method represents one stage in a process of accommodation to diverse problems rather than an ultimate product of technical evolution.

Testing is carried out in an evenly lit room with temperature (preferably 70–72°F) and relative humidity (preferably 20–40%) recorded. Adventitious factors such as drafts from equipment fans, odors (e.g., from heated lubricants or electronic components), and contamination by dust or arthropods are excluded as fully as possible.

Nasal airway resistance is measured by posterior rhinomanometry, using a Scott aviation mask (#801450-19), although several standard diving masks also have been adaptable for this purpose. A clinical pneumotachygraph is fitted to an anterior orifice of the mask, and its pressure ports are connected to a Hewlett-Packard #270 transducer. A plastic catheter of at least 3-mm interior diameter passes through the anteroinferior portion of the mask for use as a pharyngeal tap. Its external end and a segment of tubing that opens within the mask are connected to a second #270 transducer that provides a ΔP signal. Transducer outputs are processed by Hewlett-Packard flow and pressure amplifiers and preamplifiers and projected on precalibrated axes of an image-retentive oscilloscope. A ruled overlay is used to estimate the slope of the ΔP–$\dot{V}$ curve just above zero flow or at 0.3 l/s^{-1} in expiration; the resulting angle is expressed directly as "resistance" in centimeters of H_2O per liter per second. Because NAR testing intervals last only seconds, the mask is not strapped to the head, but rather is applied with minimum, firm, bimanual pressure by the subject while breathing with slightly supranormal depth and a rate of 20/min or below.

Subjects are seated comfortably in an upright position, unless another attitude is required. At least 30 min are allowed for acclimatization to conditions in the testing area. However, when the subject has passed through unusual extremes of temperature, humidity, air movement, or irritant exposure, longer periods are allowed for equilibration. Since diurnal variations in nasal patency and/or reactivity may occur [140], related studies on different test days are scheduled at similar times and with a constant relationship of testing to preceding meals.

Challenge is effected with the system of components represented in Fig. 5. Aerosol is produced by a DeVilbiss 251 atomizer modified to take small fluid volumes by insertion into the reservoir of the lower 45-mm segment of a test tube of 12-mm interior diameter. The atomizer is driven by compressed air adjusted to 7 psi with a needle valve, while a solenoid adjusts the flow pulses to a constant duration of 0.1 s. This sequence of components is a modification of the (French-Rosenthal) "dosimeter" developed at the Good Samaritan Hospital in Baltimore [152]. With the subjects' neck in slight hyperextension, aerosol is introduced while he or she makes a gentle inspiratory effort. The orifice of the atomizer is positioned 1–2 mm within the nasal verge, and the right and left airways are challenged individually in rapid succession.

Baseline NAR is determined, after acclimatization, at 5-min intervals. When values from each of three consecutive determinations are consistent (i.e., differ from their mean by less than 10%), aerosol testing may begin. As a preliminary to other exposures, an initial PBS challenge, using 0.1 ml into each nostril, is done routinely. Thereafter, a defined schedule of NAR determinations is followed; i.e., every min for the first 5 min after challenge, then every 2 min for the next 10 min. The resulting 10 values are averaged, and special attention is paid to the 15-min determination, which should approximate closely the pre-PBS value. If NAR has not returned to the baseline level at 15 min or if an intervening value has exceeded baseline by $> 30\%$, further testing of the subject on that day is deferred. Subjects who demonstrate responses to PBS of lesser degree and duration are suitable for further provocation. Challenges are followed by NAR determinations using the schedule described for PBS,* with testing every 5 min if continued after the first 15 min. Where progressively higher concentrations of a single agent are used for challenge, 15- to 20-min intervals generally separate the individual, incremental steps. However, a qualitatively different material (e.g., a control aerosol or

---

*We have maintained the option of excluding one single value from each set that exceeds all others by $>30\%$.

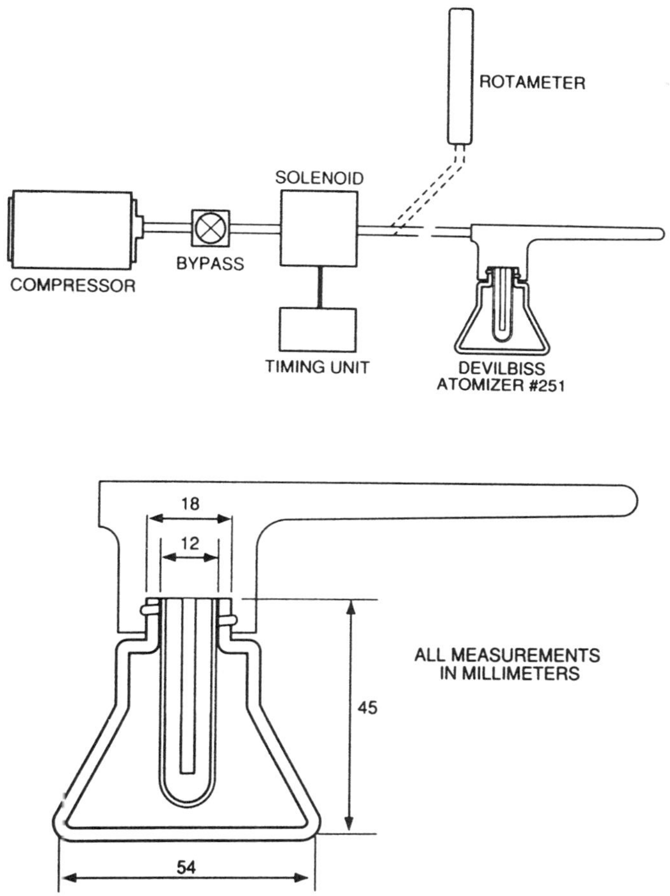

Figure 5 Nasal aerosol challenge system components.

blocking agent) usually is not introduced until NAR has returned to the baseline level established for that session. The significance of challenge-induced patency responses is judged ultimately by comparison with the effects of control exposure on the individual or on an appropriate subject group. Practically, however, in our subjects, a doubling of NAR is not provoked by aqueous vehicles suitable for allergens and many drugs. Therefore, changes of this magnitude (i.e., +100%) can be required as a standard of "significant change" unless NAR responses are found empirically to cluster below this level. As experience is gained with a specific challenge protocol, the limits of the NAR effect induced by both the "active" and the "control" agents employed should become progressively clear.

Nasal obstructive responses that follow testing with allergens, autacoids, and autonomic agonists generally are brief, making routine administration of decongestants unnecessary. However, "late" responses have been described following allergen aerosols [79,105,150,151], and resurgent "hay fever" occasionally has appeared many hours after intensive challenge, especially with native pollens. Subjects should recognize this possibility and may be provided with a topical agent (e.g., phenylephrine or tetrahydrazoline) for use as needed.*

V. EXPERIENCES WITH SPECIFIC NASAL CHALLENGE PROCEDURES

Although nasal testing has been reported extensively, efforts to synthesize this experience must confront the wide diversity of methods employed, many relying on "clinical" indicators of response. Since attention will be confined to work using quantifiable parameters as indicator systems, the following summary makes no pretense of completeness. Rather, it will indicate the scope of recorded efforts in nasal provocation and attempt to promote initial access to a diffuse and often unfamiliar literature.

A. Challenge with Allergens

Many investigators have used nasal challenge with allergens to explore immunological aspects of rhinitis and as a diagnostic correlate in clinical care. Increasing concentrations have been administrated and nasal patency sequentially followed in a format recalling that for bronchial provocation. As also with lower airway testing, the resulting data are difficult to interpret for diagnostic purposes, since the experimental challenge differs so completely, in strength and duration, from conditions of "field" exposure. Correlations between results of nasal testing and other criteria used for allergen-specific clinical diagnosis have varied from excellent to poor. Several workers, including Bernstein and Safferman [129], have noted a definite concordance of skin test reactions, nasal challenge results, and allergen-specific in vitro histamine release data. However, patients with positive skin and negative mucosal tests have also been evident in this and other test series [142]. Schumacher and Pain noted an overall concordance of skin and nasal test results [140] but no correlation between skin reaction size and the dose of intranasal allergen required to double NAR. Similarly, in this report, nasal

*Subjects with even mild reactive airway disease, challenged nasally with allergen, may present immediate or late *bronchospastic* responses. If asthmatic subjects are not excluded, resources to reverse such reactions must be available.

sensitivity appeared unrelated to clinical symptom severity or to serum IgE level; however, others have claimed correlation among these variables when using, especially, pollen extracts [127,139]. Malmberg et al. found nasal challenges more often positive than conjunctival tests performed simultaneously [152]. Yet these authors also reported on absence of rhinomanometric change in some subjects with strongly suggestive histories and/or inflammatory changes on specific nasal challenge.

Our own experience confirms that "negative" nasal tests are obtained commonly in persons with skin reactivity to the same allergen, especially when the corresponding natural exposure does not evoke symptoms. Of greater concern is the occurrence of decreased nasal patency after brief, "bolus" laboratory challenge in subjects who manifest no spontaneous clinical response to the eliciting allergen when it is encountered naturally. This seeming paradox requires only a potent aerosol, a subject with strong corresponding skin (or radioallergosorbent test) reactivity, and a sensitive indicator of nasal change. While such a reactivity pattern is not the rule, its potential occurrence demands that clinical interpretations of nasal provocative data be made with due caution. Chances for error are especially high when extracts rated at concentrations of 1:500 (weight/volume) or higher concentrations are employed. Above 1:100 we have noted an unacceptable level of nonspecific reactivity, especially with certain house dust and fungus extracts. Lacking widely endorsed guidelines, many workers begin nasal testing with extract 10 times more dilute than the lowest strength producing an intradermal titration end point for the subject. We regard a 1:10,000 or 1:5,000 aerosol as a reasonable starting point for skin test–negative persons. Concentration steps should progress regularly, and we have commonly preferred approximately threefold sequential increments (i.e., 1:10,000, 1:3,000, 1:1,000), although other series have been used with apparent success.

Except for isolated studies involving controlled exposure to intact pollens, most reports of nasal allergen challenge have been based on aerosolized extracts. Pollens tested have included types acknowledged widely as clinically important (i.e., grasses [65,106,123,128,139,140,142,144,148,153], ragweed [30,105, 120], birch [128,152], and Japanese cedar [146], as well as less familiar types (e.g., Rumex [142]) for which challenge results could aid an evaluation of significance. Apparently successful nasal provocative studies have also used extracts of green algae [129]; dog [152], cat [152], and human "danders" [148]; mites [148]; house dust [127,139,146,148]; and fungi [123].

Attention often has been limited to nasal responses following challenge by 5–30 min [154]. However, especially with pollens and mite, late obstructive responses are well recognized either alone or following initial brief NAR rises. Sequential exposures to pollen allergens have led to the concept of "priming" [27,28,141,155], which seem swell established, although others have described exceptional NAR responses that diminish with repeated specific allergen challenge

[143]. As yet, no syntheses have reconciled these disparate findings or suggested a coherent basis for the hyperresponsiveness often observed following significant allergen exposure. Tissue changes typical of "late phase" nasal responses may be a prerequisite for the expression(s) of priming; however, isolated allergen-induced early responses have apparently induced hyperreactivity (to aerosolized histamine) [156]. Nasal histopathology following allergen challenge has received only modest attention despite the relative simplicity of mucosal punch biopsy. After instillation of 2000–6000 timothy pollen grains by micropipette, Wihl and Mygind [154] noted clinical hay fever but no light or scanning electron microscope changes in biopsies 30 min after challenge. However, following four sequential daily ragweed pollen challenges, Connell [155] described marked histiocytosis and an infiltrate of foamy cells, reticular elements, and eosinophils, as well as basement membrane defects, with loss of ground substance.

Nasal washings (and brush "biopsies") provide a reflection of the proinflammatory events occurring in the mucosa following direct antigen (allergen) challenge [157,158]. While studies based on pelletized cells are not strictly quantitative, they clearly confirm an increase in activated eosinophils in challenged airways within 2 h; neutrophil abundance is associated, but peaks later [157]. Rising numbers of metachromatically staining cells—probably basophils—also are seen in the hours following challenge of sensitive subjects. Except for a secondary influx of eosinophils, the late nasal response has not yet been associated with discrete changes in inflammatory cell populations [158].

Nasal washing supernatants have been assayed for a variety of cell- and serum-derived soluble mediators of inflammation following allergen challenge. Preformed mast cell components such as histamine TAME-esterase and tryptase, as well as newly synthesized prostaglandin D_2 (PGD_2), appear rapidly as acute changes develop [79,159]; several components (but not PGD_2) show secondary peaks during late-phase reactions [79]. Nasal responses to allergen also include kininogen influx and kinin generation [160] as well as the appearance of eosinophil-derived macromolecules [158].

Lysine acetylsalicylate has been increasingly used, intranasally, as a relatively safe test for aspirin reactivity in predisposed asthmatics [161]. Especially in subjects with resulting coryza, nasal washings have shown elevations in histamine and leukotriene C_4 [161,162], without consistent changes in a cyclooxygenase product (PGE_2) [162], following this agent and oral aspirin.

B. Evaluations of Antiallergic Interventions

Allergen challenges, commonly in the form of pollen extracts, also have been exploited to evaluate therapeutic interventions in nasal disease. The usefulness of nasal provocation in choosing candidates for immunotherapy has been proposed [148] but has won few adherents. With a provocation-induced model, cromolyn has been shown to control allergic rhinitis changes [128,145,146] as it mitigates nasal symptoms during natural hay fever [145]. Similarly, NAR rises provoked by pollen extract have been partially blocked by fenoterol (a β_2-adrenergic agonist) [144,163]. In related efforts, objective indices of NAR have been used to document the favorable effects on perennial rhinitis of beclomethasone [115] and diminution of changes in subjects with allergic rhinitis challenged with antigen [79,164]. Evaluations of classic injection treatment [88,123,165] as well as intranasal immunotherapy [166] also have used rhinomanometric parameters. Studies, usually of simpler design, have also demonstrated the NAR-reducing properties of phenylephrine [123,167–169], pseudoephedrine [168,169,171], ephedrine [169,173], phenylpropanolamine [169,172], and desoxyephedrine [175], as well as Contac [176] and other widely used proprietary agents [177]. In addition, the effectiveness of certain commercial preparations for allergic rhinitis has been supported by correlations of symptom scores, "pollen counts," and NAR measurements [178]. Using direct nasal allergen testing, before and after controlled immunotherapy trials, active treatment has reduced the cellular responses and levels of mediators released in actively treated subjects [160].

C. Challenge with Neurohumors and Proinflammatory Agents

Direct challenge of the nasal mucosa with pharmacological agents (including autacoids) has helped clarify mechanisms of normal and disturbed upper airway physiology. In both healthy subjects and those with rhinitis, aerosols of histamine [115,123,126,148,171,172,179,180] or methacholine [126,179,181,182] provoke increases in NAR of relatively short duration, the latter agent, especially, also promoting nasal secretion volume. Borum [149] has attempted to correlate individual responses to methacholine with rhinitis severity and the overall effects of treatment; however, support for the validity of this approach is limited. Furthermore, reactivity to these agents has not differed notably among normal, allergic rhinitis, and vasomotor rhinitis groups studied by McLean et al. [147,179]. Repeated challenges with histamine also have not resulted in heightened reactivity to this agent [30,179]. Rhinitis symptoms and pharyngeal discomfort have followed nasal challenge with bradykinin [182]. However, the sneezing, pruritus, and substance P production observed after aerosolized serotinin have uncertain clinical relevance [183].

The modest nasal obstructive responses provoked by aerosols of isoproterenol can be blocked by topical propranolol, implying the presence of β-adrenergic receptors in human nasal vasculature. Analogous effects have been documented with other β-adrenoceptor stimulants [184,185] in both normal subjects and asymptomatic hay fever patients. Similarly, inhibition of methacholine effect on NAR by prior aerosolized atropine is easily demonstrated [179,185]. Atropine also attenuates the increased NAR induced by PBS [24], suggesting that this response also is mediated reflexly. The nasal obstruction of spontaneous pollinosis has been partially ameliorated by aerosols of atropine, chlorpheniramine, and phenylephrine [147]. However, only the last-named agent significantly increases nasal patency in normal subjects.

Polymyxin B, a direct histamine liberator that raises NAR, has been used to "probe nasal mast cell reactivity" and to compare this function in normal, allergic rhinitis, and vasomotor rhinitis groups [147]. Symptomatic hay fever subjects have shown the greatest responses to polymyxin B, but still can respond with further histamine-provoked rises in NAR following this agent.

Effects of arachidonic acid derivatives on the upper airway have been investigated extensively in other species but less so in humans. In limited trials, PGF_2 was thought to have no effect on NAR after administration as a nasal aerosol [186] and not to increase patency [182]. By contrast, E series prostaglandins diminished NAR in certain subjects ("responders") but produced no change in others ("nonresponders") [186,187]. The effect of PGD_2 has been marked increases in NAR among subjects with and without nasal allergy [182].

Considerable interest surrounds the observation of occasional subjects with sharp increases in NAR (but no mast cell–derived mediator release or cellular influx following nasal exposure to distilled water [78]. However, little aerodynamic change occurred in 10 swimmers following immersion in chlorinated fresh water [188]. In the laboratory, hyperosmolar solutions introduced into the nose have resulted in fluid shifts into the lumen and the evolution of mast cell–derived mediators, assayable in nasal washings [189]. Hyperosmolarity of the luminal surface fluid was postulated as a determinant of mediator release in a subset of subjects also specifically reporting nasal symptoms on exposure to cold, dry air [190]. When challenged with air at −3 to −10°C, these subjects experience recognizable symptoms, and increased tonicity of mucosal fluid has been documented.

D. Additional Agents and Interventions

Objective indicators of nasal patency have been adapted to studies of diverse factors and their possible upper-airway effects. Manipulable models have been developed, for example, on the basis of the transient nasal obstruction produced by SO_2 or NH_3. Water-soluble gases such as these are readily delivered to the nasal mucosa by relatively simple apparatus. The increase in NAR produced by NH_3 has been blocked by topical atropine but not by chlorpheniramine aerosol administered locally [191]. Nasal airway resistance values have been reported to increase during breathing of helium–air mixtures [192], although the factors responsible for this change are not obvious. Hypercapnia, induced by increasing $FICO_2$, strikingly decreases NAR [36,38], while oxygen-enriched mixtures have not caused measurable patency changes [38]. The effects of other atmospheric components on the nose remain speculative, although in limited studies, the inhalation of carbon black has not affected nasal patency [193].

Besides increasing NAR [15], inhaled SO_2 has been observed to decrease nasal mucus velocity, although these functions appear to vary independently. Saketkhoo et al. have described increased mucociliary clearance following ingestion of hot water and chicken soup with no associated change in NAR after 5 or 30 min [109]. Mucus velocity has been shown to increase with aerobic exercise even as the expected decrease [194] in NAR develops. By contrast, physically interrupting nasal air flow has been reported to slow mucociliary transport [195], and in undisturbed subjects, baseline nasal air conductance and saccharine transit times were correlated.

The value of NAR and related parameters in selecting patients for corrective dentofacial or nasal procedures and following them postoperatively has led to an extensive literature; in it, the studies of Warren et al. [197,198], Sorenson et al. [199], and McCaffrey and Kern [111] are especially notable. Effects of stellate ganglion block [51] and vidian nerve resection [200] on nasal patency also have been documented by comparing NAR measurements before and after these procedures.

VI. CONCLUSION

Nasal provocative testing is a useful investigative modality that can provide information unavailable by other means. Like other biomedical techniques, this approach demands reproducible methods and an objective evaluation of results, if data are to have value. Unfortunately, both the physical and physiological characteristics of the nose contribute procedural problems that are scarcely present in the lower airways. Remedial approaches to these difficulties have been multiple and, without exception, imperfect. Looking forward, the need to identify testing problems and to design techniques that recognize these perils remains paramount. In addition, progress will require critical (and occasionally tiresome) comparisons of available methods in accord with aerodynamic and neurovascular realities. The possibility that nasal models [201] based on postmortem material may facilitate hypothesis testing is intriguing.

While the importance of these development is unmistakable, so also are the technical resources now at hand. The reader should recognize that valid (but not necessarily uniform) methods of nasal testing have emerged, and that their use is providing an increasingly coherent picture of upper airway function. In this setting of proven feasibility, nasal challenge techniques can offer a direct approach to questions fundamental to allergy, rhinology, chest medicine, and environmental hygiene. At present, few areas would seem to provide more latitude or better prospects for fruitful clinical inquiry.

REFERENCES

1. Stenius-Aarniala, B. S. M., Malmberg, C. H. O., and Halopainen, E. E. A., Relationship between the results of bronchial, nasal and conjunctival provocation tests in patients with asthma, *Clin. Allergy*, *8*, 403 (1978).
2. Hilding, A. C., Phagocytosis, mucous flow and ciliary action, *Arch. Environ. Health*, *6*, 61 (1963).
3. Asmundsson, T., and Kilburn, K. H., Mechanisms of respiratory tract clearance in *Sputum* (M. J. Dulfano, ed.), Charles C. Thomas, Springfield, Illinois, 1973.
4. Andersen, I., Lundqvist, G., Jensen, D., et al., Human response to 78-hour exposure to dry air, *Arch. Environ. Health*, *28*, 31 (1974).
5. Papaioanou, H. A., Naylor, B., and McLean, J. A., Ciliocytophoria in nasal secretions; relationship to infection and atopic disease, *J. Allergy*, *44*, 167 (1969).
6. Mygind, N., *Nasal Allergy*, 2nd Ed., Blackwell Scientific Publishers, Oxford, 1979.
7. Hoorn, B., Organ cultures of ciliated epithelium for the study of respiratory viruses, *Acta Pathol. Microbiol. Scand.*, (Suppl) 183 (1966).
8. Torjussen, W., and Solberg, A., Histological findings in the nasal mucosa of nickel workers, *Acta Oto-Laryngol. (Stockh.)*, *82*, 266 (1976).
9. Andersen, I., Lundqvist, G., and Proctor, D., Human nasal mucosal function in a controlled climate, *Arch. Environ. Health*, *23*, 408 (1971).
10. Negus, V., *The Comparative Anatomy and Physiology of the Nose and Paranasal Sinuses*, Livingstone, Edinburgh and London, 1958.
11. May, K. R., and Clifford, R., The impaction of aerosol particles on cylinders, spheres, ribbons, and discs, *Ann. Occup. Hyg.*, *10*, 83 (1967).
12. Muir, D., *Clinical Aspects of Inhaled Particles*, Heinemann, London, 1972.
13. Douek, E. *The Sense of Smell and its Abnormalities*, Livingstone, Edinburgh, 1974.
14. Proctor, D., and Wagner, H., Jr., Mucociliary particle clearance in the human nose, in *Inhaled Particles and Vapours, II* (C. Davies, ed.), Pergamon Press, Oxford, 1966.
15. Speizer, F., and Frank, N., A comparison of changes in pulmonary flow resistance in healthy volunteers acutely exposed to SO_2 by mouth and by nose, *Br. J. Indust. Med.*, *23*, 75 (1966).
16. Bridger, G. P., and Proctor, D. F., Maximum nasal inspiratory flow and nasal resistance, *Ann. Otol. Rhinol. Laryngol.*, *79*, 481 (1970).
17. Watanabe, K., and Watanabe, I., The ultrastructural characteristics of the capillary walls in human nasal mucosa, *Rhinology*, *18*, 183 (1980).
18. Cauna, N., Electron microscopy of the nasal vascular bed and its nerve supply, *Ann. Otol. Rhinol. Laryngol.*, *79*, 443 (1970).
19. Kontou-Karakitsos, K., Salvaggio, J. E., and Mathews, K. P., Comparative nasal absorption of allergens in nonatopic subjects, *J. Allergy Clin. Immunol.*, *55*, 241 (1975).
20. Anggard, A., and Edwall, L., The effects of sympathetic nerve stimulation on the tracer disappearance rate and local blood content of the nasal mucosa of the cat, *Acta Oto-Laryngol. (Stockh.)*, *77*, 131 (1974).

21. Anggard, A., The effects of parasympathetic nerve stimulation on the microcirculation and secretion in the nasal mucosa of the cat, *Acta Oto-Laryngol. (Stockh.)*, *78*, 98 (1974).
22. Malm, L., Responses of resistance and capacitance vessels in feline nasal mucosa to vasoactive agents, *Acta Oto-Laryngol. (Stockh.)*, *78*, 90 (1974).
23. Jackson, R. T., Pharmacologic responsiveness of the nasal mucosa, *Ann. Otol. Rhinol. Laryngol.*, *79*, 461 (1970).
24. McLean, J. A., Mathews, K. P., Ciarkowski, A. A., et al., The effects of topical saline and isoproterenol on nasal airway resistance, *J. Allergy Clin. Immunol.*, *58*, 563 (1976).
25. Malm, L., Beta-adrenergic receptors in the vessels of the cat nasal mucosa, *Acta Oto-Laryngol. (Stockh.)*, *78*, 242 (1974).
26. Taylor, M., The nasal vasomotor reaction, *Otolaryngol. Clin. North Am.*, *6*, 645 (1973).
27. Connell, J. T., Quantitative intranasal pollen challenges III, the priming effect in allergic rhinitis, *J. Allergy*, *43*, 33 (1969).
28. Bacon, J. R., McLean, J. A., Mathews, K. P., et al. Priming of the nasal mucosa by ragweed extract or by an irritant (ammonia), *J. Allergy Clin. Immunol.*, *67*, 111 (1981).
29. Gerth Van Wijk, R., and Dieges, P. H., Comparison of nasal responsiveness to histamine, methacholine and phentolamine in allergic rhinitis patients and controls, *Clin. Allergy*, *17*, 563 (1987).
30. Walden, S. M., Proud, D., Lichtenstein, L. M., et al., Antigen-provoked increase in histamine reactivity, *Am. Rev. Respir. Dis.*, *144*, 642 (1991).
31. Hasegawa, M., and Saito, Y., Postural variation in nasal resistance and symptomatology in allergic rhinitis, *Acta Oto-Laryngol. (Stockh.)*, *88*, 264 (1979).
32. Solomon, W. R., Comparative effects of transient body surface cooling, recumbency and induced obstruction in allergic rhinitis and control subjects, *J. Allergy*, *37*, 216 (1966).
33. Kortekangas, A. E., Effect of testing technique on nasal pressure variation, *Acta Oto-Laryngol. (Stockh.)*, *75*, 249 (1973).
34. Drettner, B., Vascular reactions of the human nasal mucosa on exposure to cold, *Acta Oto-Laryngol. (Stockh.)*, (suppl) 166 (1961).
35. Solomon, W. R., Ocular mechanisms producing reflex nasal obstruction (abstr.), *J. Allergy*, *39*, 108 (1967).
36. Dixon, F. W., Hoerr, N. L., and McCall, J. W., The nasal mucosa in laryngectomized patients, *Ann. Otol. Rhinol. Laryngol.*, *58*, 535 (1949).
37. Ingelstedt, S., Humidifying capacity of the nose, *Ann. Otol. Rhinol. Laryngol.*, *79*, 475 (1970).
38. Hasegawa, M., and Kern, E. B., The effect of breath holding, hyperventilation, and exercise on nasal resistance, *Rhinology*, *16*, 243 (1978).
39. McCaffrey, T. V., and Kern, E. B., Response of nasal airway resistance to hypercapnia and hypoxia in the dog, *Acta Oto-Laryngol. (Stockh.)*, *87*, 545 (1979).
40. McCaffrey, T. V., and Kern, E. B., Response to nasal airway resistance to hypercapnia and hypoxemia, *Ann. Otol. Rhinol. Laryngol.*, *88*, 247 (1979).

41. Takagi, Y., Proctor, D. F., Salman, S., et al., Effects of cold air and carbon dioxide on nasal air flow resistance, *Ann. Otol. Rhinol. Laryngol.*, *80*, 736 (1971).
42. Dallimore, N. S., and Eccles, R., Changes in human nasal resistance associated with exercise, hyperventilation and rebreathing, *Acta Oto-Laryngol. (Stockh.)*, *84*, 416 (1977).
43. Richerson, H. B., and Seebohm, P. M., Nasal airway response to exercise, *J. Allergy*, *41*, 269 (1968).
44. Van Dishoeck, E. A., and van Dishoeck, H. E. A., Nasal resistance measurement without breathing, *Rhinology*, *8*, 37 (1970).
45. Wilson, H., and Yates, M. S., Bilateral nasal vascular responses to unilateral sympathetic stimulation, *Acta Oto-Laryngol. (Stockh.)*, *85*, 105 (1978).
46. Malmberg, H., Binder, E., and Fraki, J., Nasal reactions elicited by unilateral allergen challenge, *Acta Oto-Laryngol. (Stockh.)*, *107*, 446 (1989).
47. Hasegawa, M., and Kern, E. B., The human nasal cycle, *Mayo Clin. Proc.*, *52*, 28 (1977).
48. Eccles, R., Cyclic changes in human nasal resistance to air flow, *J. Physiol.*, *272*, 75P (1977).
49. Sternstein, H. J., Quantitative effects of physical and chemical agents on erectile tissue response in the nose, *Arch. Otolaryngol.*, *78*, 232 (1974).
50. Stoksted, P., The physiological cycle of the nose under normal and pathologic conditions, *Acta Oto-Laryngol. (Stockh.)*, *42*, 175 (1952).
51. Stoksted, P., and Thomsen, K. A., Changes in the nasal cycle under stellate ganglion block, *Acta Oto-Laryngol. (Stockh.)*, *109* (suppl), 176 (1953–4).
52. Keuning, J., On the nasal cycle, *Int. Rhinol.*, *6*, 99 (1968).
53. Foxen, E. H., Miles Preston, T. D., and Lack, J. A., The assessment of nasal airflow: a review of past and present methods, *J. Laryngol. Otol.*, *85*, 811 (1971).
54. Kern, E. B., Standardization of rhinomanometry, *Rhinology*, *15*, 115 (1977).
55. Hamilton, L. H., Nasal airway resistance: its measurement and regulation, *Physiologist*, *22*, 43 (1979).
56. Kortekangas, A. E., Problems in the standardization of rhinomanometry, *Allergy*, *35*, 255 (1980).
57. Cole, P., and Havas, T. E., Resistance to respiratory airflow of the nasal passages: comparisons between different common methods of calculation, *Rhinology*, *24*, 163 (1986).
58. Lichtenstein, L. M., Norman, P. S., and Winkenwerder, W. L., Clinical and *in vitro* studies on the role of immunotherapy in ragweed hay fever, *Am. J. Med.*, *44*, 514 (1968).
59. Salman, S. D., Proctor, D. F., Swift, D. L., et al., Nasal resistance: description of a method and effect of temperature and humidity changes, *Ann. Otol. Rhinol. Laryngol.*, *80*, 736 (1971).
60. Ferris, B. G., Jr., Mead, J., and Opie, L. N., Partitioning of respiratory flow resistance in man, *J. Appl. Physiol.*, *19*, 653 (1964).
61. Solomon, W. R., and Stohrer, A. W., Considerations in the measurement of nasal patency, *Ann. Otol. Rhinol. Laryngol.*, *74*, 978 (1965).
62. Reeves, H. M., Wright, W. K., and Novakovic, M., Quantitative measurement of nasal-airway resistance, *Arch. Otolaryngol.*, *92*, 573 (1970).

63. McLean, J. A., Ciarkowski, A. A., Solomon, W. R., et al., An improved technique for nasal inhalation challenge tests, *J. Allergy Clin. Immunol.*, *57*, 153 (1976).
64. Cole, P., Fastag, O., and Niinimaa, V., Computer-aided rhinometry: a research rhinometer for clinical trial, *Acta Oto-Laryngol. (Stockh.)*, *90*, 139 (1980).
65. Mygind, N., and Thomsen, J., ICI74,917: a new anti-allergic drug, administered by pressurized aerosol, *Acta Allergol.*, *30*, 298 (1975).
66. Druce, H. M., Wright, R. H., Kossoff, D., et al., Cholinergic nasal hyperreactivity in atopic subjects, *J. Allergy Clin. Immunol.*, *76*, 445 (1985).
67. Yagi, N., Hamada, E., and Ichikawa, R., The validity of the thread test for evaluating nasal secretion in nasal allergy, *Acta Oto-Laryngol.*, *103*, 312 (1987).
68. Knowles, G. K., Townsend, P., and Turner-Warwick, M., A standardized filter paper technique for assessing nasal secretory activity, *Clin. Allergy*, *11*, 287 (1981).
69. Phipatanakul, C., and Slavin, R. G., Use of thermography in clinical allergy, *J. Allergy Clin. Immunol.*, *50*, 264 (1972).
70. Drettner, B., and Aust, R., Plethysmographic studies of the blood flow in the mucosa of the human maxillary sinus, *Acta Oto-Laryngol. (Stockh.)*, *78*, 259 (1974).
71. Davis, D. L., and Hertzman, A. B., The analysis of vascular reactions in the nasal mucosa with the photoelectric plethysmograph, *Ann. Otol. Rhinol. Laryngol.*, *66*, 522 (1957).
72. Holmberg, K., Bake, B., and Pipkorn, U., Nasal mucosal blood flow after intranasal allergen challenge, *J. Allergy Clin. Immunol.*, *81*, 541 (1988).
73. Druce, H. M., Bonner, R. F., Patow, C., et al., Response of nasal blood flow to neurohormones as measured by laser-Doppler velocimetry, *J. Appl. Physiol.*, *54*, 1276 (1984).
74. Olsson, P., A comparison between the ^{133}Xe washout and laser Doppler techniques for estimation of nasal mucosal blood flow in humans, *Acta Oto-Laryngol. (Stockh.)*, *102*, 106 (1986).
75. Hallen, H., and Juto, J.-E., Nasal mucosa reaction. A model for mucosal reaction during challenge, *Rhinology*, *30*, 129 (1992).
76. Proud, D., Kagey-Sobotka, A., Naclerio, R. M., et al., Pharmacology of upper airways challenge, *Int. Arch. Allergy Appl. Immunol.*, *82*, 493 (1987).
77. Naclerio, R. M., Meijer, H. L., Kagey-Sobotka, A., et al., Mediator release after nasal airway challenge with allergen, *Am. Rev. Respir. Dis.*, *128*, 597 (1983).
78. Meslier, N., Braunstein, G., Lacronique, J., et al., Local cellular and humoral responses to antigenic and distilled water challenge in subjects with allergic rhinitis, *Am. Rev. Respir. Dis.*, *137*, 617 (1988).
79. Lichtenstein, L. M., The nasal late-phase response: an *in vivo* model, *Hosp. Pract.*, *23*, 119 (1988).
80. Konno, A., Terada, N., Okamoto, Y., et al., The role of chemical mediators and mucosal hyperreactivity in nasal hypersecretion in nasal allergy, *J. Allergy Clin. Immunol.*, *79*, 620 (1987).
81. Friedman, M. M., and Kaliner, M., In situ degranulation of human nasal mucosal mast cells: ultrastructural features and cell-cell associations, *J. Allergy Clin. Immunol.*, *76*, 70 (1985).
82. Okuda, M., Ohtsuka, H., and Kawabori, S., Studies of nasal surface basophilic cells, *Ann. Allergy*, *54*, 69 (1985).

83. Otsuka, H., Denburg, J. A., Befus, A. D., et al., Effect of beclomethasone dipropionate on nasal metachromatic cell subpopulations, *Clin. Allergy*, *16*, 589 (1986).
84. Doyle, W. J., Friedman, R., Fireman, P., et al., Eustachian tube obstruction after provocative nasal antigen challenge, *Acta Oto-Laryngol.*, *110*, 508 (1984).
85. Skoner, D. P., Doyle, W. J., and Fireman, P., Eustachian tube obstruction (ETO) after histamine nasal provocation: a double-blind dose-response study, *J. Allergy Clin. Immunol.*, *79*, 27 (1987).
86. Pelikan, Z., and Pelikan-Filipek, M., Role of nasal allergy in chronic maxillary sinusitis—diagnostic value of nasal challenge with allergen, *J. Allergy Clin. Immunol.*, *86*, 484 (1990).
87. Taylor, G., MacNeil, A. R., and Freed, D. L. J., Assessing degree of nasal patency by measuring peak expiratory flow rate through the nose, *J. Allergy Clin. Immunol.*, *52*, 193 (1973).
88. Frostad, A. B., Reproducibility of the nasal provocation test and of measuring peak expiratory flow rate through the nose, *Allergy*, *35*, 253 (1980).
89. Clement, P. A. R., Committee report on standardization of rhinomanometry, *Rhinology*, *22*, 151 (1984).
90. Cole, P., Niinimaa, V., Mintz, S., et al., Work of nasal breathing: measurement of each nostril independently, *Acta Oto-Laryngol. (Stockh.)*, *88*, 148 (1979).
91. Marshall, R., A nasal mask for posterior rhinometry of each side of the nose separately, *Rhinology*, *18*, 43 (1980).
92. Kortekangas, A. E., Significance of anterior and posterior technique in rhinometry, *Acta Oto-Laryngol. (Stockh.)*, *73*, 218 (1972).
93. Mackay, I. S., Measurement of nasal airflow and resistance, *J. Roy. Soc. Med.*, *72*, 852 (1979).
94. Mygind, N., Measurement of nasal airway resistance: is it only for article writers? *Clin. Otolaryngol.*, *5*, 161 (1980).
95. Solow, B., and Greve, E., Rhinomanometric recording in children, *Rhinology*, *18*, 31 (1980).
96. Babatola, F. D. O., and Eccles, R., A new technique using a nasal cast for anterior rhinomanometry, *Rhinology*, *25*, 109 (1987).
97. Saito, A., and Nishihata, S., Nasal airway resistance in children, *Rhinology*, *19*, 149 (1981).
98. Haight, J. S. J., and Cole, P., Site and function of the nasal valve, *Laryngoscope*, *93*, 49 (1983).
99. Nolte, E., and Luder-Luhr, I., Comparing measurements of nasal resistance by body plethysmography and by rhinomanometry, *Respiration*, *30*, 31 (1973).
100. Pelikan, Z., Feenstra, L., and Barree, G. O. F., Response of the nasal mucosa to allergen challenge measured by two different methods of rhinomanometry, *Ann. Allergy*, *38*, 263 (1977).
101. Jones, A. S., Lancer, J. M., Stevens, J. C., et al., Rhinomanometry: do the anterior and posterior methods give equivalent results?, *Clin. Otolaryngol.*, *12*, 109 (1987).
102. Butler, J., Work of breathing through the nose, *Clin. Sci.*, *19*, 55 (1960).
103. Ogura, J. H., and Harvey, J. E., Nasopulmonary mechanics: experimental evidence

of the influence of the upper airway upon the lower, *Acta Oto-Laryngol. (Stockh.)*, *71*, 123 (1971).

104. Cole, P., and Havas, T., Nasal resistance to respiratory airflow: a plethysmographic alternative to the face mask, *Rhinology*, *25*, 159 (1987).

105. Dvoracek, J. E., Solley, G. O., Gleich, G. J., et al., Induction of prolonged inflammation in nasal mucosa by insufflation of ragweed pollen extract, *J. Allergy Clin. Immunol.*, *63*, 210 (1979).

106. Taylor, G., and Shivalkar, P. R., Changes in nasal airways resistance on antigenic challenge in allergic rhinitis, *Clin. Allergy*, *1*, 63 (1971).

107. Broms, P., Jonson, B., and Lamm, C. J., A universal way to evaluate the curve in rhinomanometry, *Acta Oto-Laryngol. (Stockh.)*, *360* (suppl), 22 (1979).

108. Ingelstedt, S., Jonson, B., and Rundcrantz, H., A clinical method for determination of nasal airway resistance, *Acta Oto-Laryngol. (Stockh.)*, *68*, 189 (1969).

109. Saketkhoo, K., Janaszkiewicz, A., and Sackner, M. A., Effects of drinking hot water, cold water and chicken soup on nasal mucous velocity and nasal airflow resistance, *Chest*, *74*, 408 (1978).

110. Masing, H., Rhinomanometry, different techniques and results, *Acta Otorhinolaryngol. Belg.*, *33*, 566 (1979).

111. McCaffrey, T. V., and Kern, E. B., Clinical evaluation of nasal obstruction, *Arch. Otolaryngol.*, *105*, 542 (1979).

112. Eichler, J., and Lenz, H., Comparison of different coefficients and units in rhinomanometry, *Rhinology*, *23*, 149 (1985).

113. Postema, C. A., Huygen, P. L. M., Lecluse, R. G. M., et al., The lateralization percentage as a measure of nasal flow asymmetry in active anterior rhinomanometry, *Clin. Otolaryngol.*, *5*, 165 (1980).

114. Hasegawa, M., Kern, E. B., and O'Brien, P. C., Dynamic changes in nasal resistance, *Ann. Otol. Rhinol. Laryngol.*, *88*, 66 (1979).

115. Cockcroft, O. W., MacCormack, D. W., Tarlo, S. M., et al., Nasal airway inspiratory resistance, *Am. Rev. Respir. Dis.*, *119*, 921 (1979).

116. Syabbalo, N. C., Bundgaard, A., Entholm, P., et al., Measurement and regulation of nasal airflow resistance in man, *Rhinology*, *24*, 87 (1986).

117. Halpern, S. R., Holman, J., and Whittaker, C., The correlation between skin and respiratory mucous membrane tests with molds in allergic rhinitis, *Ann. Allergy*, *19*, 1407 (1961).

118. Blackley, C. H., *Experimental Researches on the Causes and Nature of Catarrhus Aestivus (Hay Fever or Hay Asthma)*, Balliere, Tindall and Cox, London, 1873.

119. Connell, J. T., Qualitative intranasal pollen challenge. I. Apparatus, design and technique, *J. Allergy*, *39*, 358 (1967).

120. Guercio, J. P., Birch, S., Fernandez, R. J., et al., Deposition of ragweed pollen and extract on nasal mucosa of patients with allergic rhinitis: effect on nasal air flow resistance and nasal mucus velocity, *J. Allergy Clin. Immunol.*, *66*, 61 (1980).

121. Solomon, W. R., Experimental ragweed pollinosis induced during normal respiration in a test chamber: initial observations (abstr.), *J. Allergy*, *43*, 181 (1969).

122. Dean, L., Linton, L., and Linton, C., An intramucosal test for hypersensitivity in allergic rhinitis, *Ann. Otol. Rhinol. Laryngol.*, *44*, 317 (1935).

123. Aschan, G., and Drettner, B., Nasal obstruction at provocation experiments in patients with hay fever, *Acta Oto-Laryngol. (Stockh.)*, *140* (suppl), 91 (1958).
124. Solomon, W. R., Modifications of the Wright dust feed mechanism permitting stable dispersion of native ragweed pollen, *J. Allergy Clin. Immunol.*, *57*, 177 (1976).
125. Bousquet, J., Lebel, B., Dhivert, H., et al., Nasal challenge with pollen grains, skin-prick tests and specific IgE in patients with grass pollen allergy, *Clin. Allergy*, *17*, 529 (1987).
126. Grobler, N. J., *Reactivity of the Nasal Mucosa (A Clinical and Epidemiological Study)*, Drukker J. Van Denderen, Groningen, the Netherlands, 1966.
127. Halopainen, E., Tarkianen, and Malmberg, H., Nasal challenge, *Rhinology*, *14*, 181 (1976).
128. Haahtela, T., Comparison among HC20-511 (ketotifen), clemastine, DSCG and beclomethasone diproprionate in nasal challenge, *Ann. Allergy*, *41*, 345 (1978).
129. Bernstein, I. L., and Safferman, R., Clinical sensitivity to green algae demonstrated by nasal challenge and *in vitro* tests of immediate hypersensitivity, *J. Allergy Clin. Immunol.*, *51*, 22 (1973).
130. Munzel, M., and Behbehani, A., The diagnostic value of intranasal tests in allergic rhinopathy, *Rhinology*, *14*, 37 (1976).
131. Okuda, M., Basic study of nasal provocative test. First report: side, site of the nose, size of site and allergen amount, *Arch. Otorhinolaryngol. (NY)*, *214*, 241 (1977).
132. Greiff, L., Pipkorn, V., Aikner, V., et al., The "nasal pool" device applies controlled concentrations of solutes on human nasal airway mucosa and samples its surface exudations/secretions, *Clin. Exp. Allergy*, *20*, 253 (1990).
133. Flowers, B. K., Proud, D., Kagey-Sobotka, A., et al., Localized antigen challenge of the nasal mucosa, *Arch. Otolaryngol. Head Neck Surg.*, *116*, 1407 (1990).
134. Drettner, B., Pathophysiological relationship between the upper and lower airways, *Ann. Otol. Rhinol. Laryngol.*, *79*, 499 (1970).
135. Sercer, A., Uber die Beeinflussung der Bronchien von der Nase aus, *Arch. Ohr Nas. Kehlkopfheilk.*, *161*, 264 (1952).
136. Mygind, N., and Vesterhauge, S., Aerosol distribution in the nose, *Rhinology*, *16*, 1 (1978).
137. McLean, J. A., Bacon, J. R., Mathews, K. P., et al., Distribution and clearance of radioactive aerosol on the nasal mucosa, *Rhinology*, *22*, 65 (1984).
138. Newman, S. P., Moren, F., and Clarke, S. W., Deposition pattern from a nasal pump spray, *Rhinology*, *25*, 77 (1987).
139. Dalle, J., and Melon, J., Skin tests, IgE, RAST and nasal provocation tests, *Acta Oto-Rhino-Laryngol. Belg.*, *33*, 572 (1979).
140. Schumacher, M. J., and Pain, M. C. F., Nasal challenge testing in grass pollen hay fever, *J. Allergy Clin. Immunol.*, *64*, 202 (1974).
141. Connell, J. T., Quantitative intranasal pollen challenge. II. Effect of daily pollen exposure, and placebo challenge on the nasal mucosa, *J. Allergy*, *41*, 123 (1968).
142. Solomon, W. R., An appraisal of Rumex as an aeroallergen, *J. Allergy*, *44*, 25 (1969).
143. Taylor, G., and Shivalker, P. R., Local nasal desensitization in allergic rhinitis, *Clin. Allergy*, *2*, 125 (1972).

144. Borum, P., and Mygind, N., Inhibition of the immediate allergic reaction in the nose by the beta-2 adrenostimulant fenoterol, *J. Allergy Clin. Immunol.*, *66*, 25 (1980).
145. Makol, G. J., Pinnas, J. L., and Chen, T. M., The effect of cromolyn upon nasal airway resistance in active rhinitis patients (abstr.), *J. Allergy Clin. Immunol.*, *63*, 210 (1979).
146. Hasegawa, M., Saito, Y., and Watanabe, K., The effect of sodium cromoglycate on antigen induced nasal reaction in allergic rhinitis as measured by rhinomanometry and symptomatology, *Clin. Allergy*, *6*, 359 (1976).
147. McLean, J. A., Mathews, K. P., Brayton, P. R., et al., Intranasal effects of pharmacologic agents in hay fever and in vasomotor rhinitis (abstr.), *J. Allergy Clin. Immunol.*, *61*, 191 (1978).
148. Clement, P. A. R., van Dishoek, E. A. V., van de Wal, R. J., et al., The nose provocation and passive anterior rhinomanometry (PAR), *Acta Onto-Rhino-Laryngol. Belg.*, *32*, 56 (1978).
149. Borum, P., Nasal methacholine challenge; a test for the measurement of nasal reactivity, *J. Allergy Clin. Immunol.*, *63*, 253 (1979).
150. Pelikan, Z., Late and delayed responses of the nasal mucosa to allergen challenge, *Ann. Allergy*, *41*, 37 (1978).
151. Taylor, G., and Shivalker, P. R., "Arthus-type" reactivity in the nasal airways and skin in pollen sensitive subjects, *Clin. Allergy*, *1*, 407 (1971)
152. Malmberg, H., Holopainen, E., and Stenius-Aarniala, B., Relationship between nasal and conjunctival tests in patients with allergic rhinitis, *Clin. Allergy*, *8*, 397 (1978).
153. Rosenthal, R., The emerging role of bronchoprovocation, *J. Allergy Clin. Immunol.*, *64* (pt. 2), 562 (1979).
154. Wihl, J. A., and Mygind, N., Studies on the allergen-challenged human nasal mucosa, *Acta Oto-Laryngol. (Stockh.)*, *84*, 281 (1977).
155. Connell, J. T., Quantitative pollen challenge VI: the priming effect and its relationship to histopathologic changes in nasal biopsies (abstr.), *J. Allergy*, *41*, 101 (1968).
156. Van Wijk, R., Zijlstra, F., van Toorenenbergen, A. W., et al., Isolated early response after nasal allergen challenge is sufficient to induce nasal hyperreactivity, *Ann. Allergy*, *69*, 43 (1992).
157. Pelikan, Z., and Pelikan-Filipek, M., Cytologic changes in the nasal secretions during the immediate nasal response, *J. Allergy Clin. Immunol.*, *82*, 1103 (1988).
158. Klementsson, H., Andersson, M., Baumgarten, C. R., et al., Changes in non-specific nasal reactivity and eosinophil influx and activation after allergen challenge, *Clin. Exp. Allergy*, *20*, 539 (1990).
159. Proud, D., Bailey, G. S., Naclerio, R. M., et al., Tryptase and histamine as markers to evaluate mast cell activation during the responses to nasal challenge with allergen, cold, dry air, and hyperosmolar solutions, *J. Allergy Clin. Immunol.*, *89*, 1098 (1992).
160. Iliopoulos, O., Proud, D., Adkinson, N. F., Jr., et al., Effects of immunotherapy on the early, late, and rechallenge reaction to provocation with allergen; changes in inflammatory mediators and cells, *J. Allergy Clin. Immunol.*, *87*, 855 (1991).
161. Ortolani, C., Mirone, C., Fontana, A., et al., Study of mediators of anaphylaxis in nasal wash fluids after aspirin and sodium metabisulfite nasal provocation in intolerant rhinitic patients, *Ann. Allergy*, *59*, 106 (1987).

162. Ferreri, N. R., Howland, W. C., Stevenson, D. D., et al., Release of leukotrienes, prostaglandins, and histamine into nasal secretions of aspirin-sensitive asthmatics during reaction to aspirin, *Am. Rev. Respir. Dis.*, *137*, 847 (1988).
163. Schumacher, M. J., Effect of a β-adrenergic agonist, fenoterol, on nasal sensitivity to allergen, *J. Allergy Clin. Immunol.*, *66*, 33 (1980)
164. Vilsvik, J. S., Jenssen, A. O., and Walstad, R., The effect of beclomethosone dipropionate aerosol on allergen induced nasal stenosis, *Clin. Allergy*, *5*, 291 (1975).
165. Irander, K., Olofsson, J., and Aschan, G., Hyposensitization in allergic seasonal rhinitis as evaluated by rhinomanometry, *Acta Oto-Laryngol. (Stockh.)*, *360* (suppl), 24 (1979).
166. Mathews, K. P., Bayne, N. K., Banas, J. M., et al., Controlled studies of intranasal immunotherapy for ragweed pollenosis, *Int. Arch. Allergy Appl. Immunol.*, *66*, 218 (1981).
167. Cohen, B. M., Nasal resistance in decongestant spray trials, *Clin. Pharmacol. Ther.*, *13*, 137 (1972).
168. Roth, P. R., Cantekin, E. I., Bluestone, C. D., et al., Nasal decongestant activity of pseudoephedrine, *Ann. Otol. Rhinol. Laryngol.*, *85*, 235 (1977).
169. McLaurin, J. W., Shipman, W. F., and Rosedale, R., Oral decongestants. A double blind comparison study of effectiveness of four sympathomimetic drugs; objective and subjective, *Laryngoscope*, *71*, 54 (1961).
170. Loth, S., and Bende, M., The effect of topical phenylpropanolamine on nasal secretion and nasal airway resistance after histamine challenge in man, *Clin. Otolaryngol.*, *10*, 15 (1985).
171. Mascia, A. V., Objective assessment of nasal airway in children: an evaluation of decongestant therapy, *Ann. Allergy*, *26*, 470 (1968).
172. Bagg, L. R., Empey, D. W., Hughes, D. T. D., et al., The determination of the optimal oral dose of pseudoephedrine for nasal decongestion using nasal histamine challenge and anterior rhinomanometry, *Br. J. Clin. Pharmacol.*, *7*, 426P (1979).
173. Britton, M. G., Empey, D. W., John, G. C., et al., Histamine challenge and anterior nasal rhinomanometry: their use in the assessment of pseudoephedrine and triprolidine as nasal decongestants in subjects with hay fever, *Br. J. Clin. Pharmacol.*, *6*, 57 (1978).
174. Sternstein, H. J., Efficacy of vasoconstrictor agents in the obstructed nose, *Arch. Otolaryngol.*, *36*, 713 (1942).
175. Butler, D. B., and Ivy, A. C., Effects of nasal inhalers on erectile tissues of the nose: quantitative studies, *Arch. Otolaryngol.*, *38*, 309 (1943).
176. Cohen, B. M., Physiologic/clinical comparisons of a sustained-release decongestant combination, its components and placebo in patients with allergic rhinitis, *J. Asthma Res.*, *13*, 7 (1975).
177. Dressler, W. E., Myers, T., London, S. J., et al., A system of rhinomanometry in the clinical evaluation of nasal decongestants, *Ann. Otol. Rhinol. Laryngol.*, *86*, 310 (1977).
178. Connell, J. T., A novel method to assess antihistamine and decongestant efficacy, *Ann. Allergy*, *42*, 278 (1979).
179. McLean, J. A., Mathews K. P., Solomon, W. R., et al., Effect of histamine and

methacholine on nasal airway resistance in atopic and nonatropic subjects, *J. Allergy Clin. Immunol.*, *59*, 165 (1977).

179a. Majchel, A. M., Proud, D., Freidhoff, L., et al., The nasal response to histamine challenge: effect of the pollen season and immunotherapy, *J. Allergy Clin. Immunol.*, *90*, 85 (1992).

180. Skoner, D., Doyle, W. J., Boehm, S., et al., Effect of terfenadine on nasal, eustachian tube, and pulmonary function after provocative intranasal histamine challenge, *Ann. Allergy*, *67*, 619 (1991).

181. Watase, T., and Okuda, M., The effects of autonomotropic drugs on allergic nasal mucosa, *Rhinology*, *24*, 181 (1986).

182. Doyle, W. J., Boehm, S., and Skoner, D. P., Physiological responses to intranasal dose–response challenges with histamine, methacholine, bradykinin and prostaglandin in adult volunteers with and without nasal allergy, *J. Allergy Clin. Immunol.*, *86*, 924 (1990).

183. Tonnesen, P., Schaffalitzky de Muckadell, O. B., and Mygind, N., Nasal challenge with serotonin in asymptomatic hay fever patients, *Allergy*, *42*, 447 (1987).

184. Svensson, G., Heguardt, B., and Lofkrist, T., Effects of topical use of β-adrenoceptor stimulants on nasal mucosa: rhinomanometric evaluations in experiments with terbutaline and KWD 2131. I. Normal persons and hay fever patients in asymptomatic period, *Acta Oto-Laryngol. (Stockh.)*, *90*, 297 (1980).

185. Svensson, G., Effects of topical use of β-adrenoreceptor stimulants on nasal mucosa. Rhinomanometric evaluations in experiments with terbutaline and DWD 2131. II. Nasal provocation tests with hay fever patients in asymptomatic period, *Acta Oto-Laryngol. (Stockh.)*, *90*, 130 (1980).

186. Anggard, A., The effect of prostaglandins on nasal airway resistance in man, *Ann. Otol. Rhinol. Laryngol.*, *78*, 657 (1969).

187. Jackson, R. T., Prostaglandin E_1 as a nasal constrictor in normal human volunteers, *Curr. Ther. Res.*, *12*, 711 (1970).

188. Small, M., and Murray, J. A. M., Nasal changes following immersion in chlorinated water, *Rhinology*, *25*, 153 (1987).

189. Sibler, G. Proud, D., Warner, J., et al., *In vivo* release of inflammatory mediators by hyperosmolar solutions, *Am. Rev. Respir. Dis.*, *137*, 606 (1988).

190. Togias, A. G., Proud, D., Lichtenstein, L. M., et al., The osmolality of nasal secretions increases when inflammatory mediators are released to response to inhalation of cold, dry air, *Am. Rev. Respir. Dis.*, *137*, 625 (1988).

191. McLean, J. A., Mathews, K. P., Solomon, W. R., et al., Effect of ammonia on nasal resistance in atopic and nonatopic subjects, *Ann. Otol. Rhinol. Laryngol.*, *88*, 228 (1979).

192. Cockcroft, D. W., Hargreave, F. E., and Pengelly, L. D., The effect of helium on nasal resistance and nasal flow, *Am. Rev. Respir. Dis.*, *120*, 697 (1979).

193. Andersen, I., Lundquist, G. R., Proctor, D. F., et al., Human response to controlled levels of inert dust, *Am. Rev. Respir. Dis.*, *119*, 619 (1979).

194. Saketkhoo, K., Kaplan, I., and Sackner, M. A., Effect of exercise on nasal mucous velocity and nasal air flow resistance in normal subjects, *J. Appl. Physiol.*, *46*, 369 (1979).

195. Deitmer, T., and Erwig, H., The influence of nasal obstruction on mucociliary transport, *Rhinology*, *24*, 159 (1986).
196. Doyle, W. J., and van Cauwenberge, P. B., Relationship between nasal patency and clearance, *Rhinology*, *25*, 167 (1987).
197. Watson, R. W., Warren, D. W., and Fischer, N. D., Nasal resistance, skeletal classification, and mouth breathing in orodontic patients, *Am. J. Orodont.*, *54*, 367 (1968).
198. Warren, D. W., Aerodynamic studies of upper airway; implications for growth, breathing and speech, in *Naso-Respiratory Function and Craniofacial Growth* (J. A. McNamara, Jr., ed.), Center for Human Growth and Development, University of Michigan, Ann Arbor, Michigan, 1979.
199. Sorenson, H., Solow, B., and Greve, E., Assessment of the nasopharyngeal airway, *Acta Oto-Laryngol. (Stockh.)*, *89*, 227 (1980).
200. Konna, A., and Togawa, K., Role for vidian nerve in nasal allergy, *Ann. Otol. Rhinol. Laryngol.*, *88*, 258 (1979).
201. Hornung, D. E., Leopold, D. A., Youngentob, S. L., et al., Airflow patterns in a human nasal model, *Arch. Otolaryngol. Head Neck Surg.*, *113*, 169 (1987).

25

Conjunctival Challenge

Michael B. Raizman

Tufts University School of Medicine
Boston, Massachusetts

I. INTRODUCTION

Provocative conjunctival challenge was first described in the medical literature over a century ago, yet for many years it had little use. Forstot has nicely outlined the history of the eye test, noting its replacement by skin testing in most situations [1]. Friedlaender has also summarized work with conjunctival provocative testing as a model of human disease [2]. Conjunctival challenge is now reemerging as a valuable clinical and research tool with the growing recognition of the role of hypersensitivity reactions in multiple clinically relevant ocular diseases. More sophisticated methods of evaluating conjunctival responses have prompted better research applications. The role of conjunctival challenge in the setting of systemic allergy remains unclear. At present, the primary application of conjunctival challenge is in the assessment of the efficacy of pharmacological agents for the treatment of allergic conjunctivitis. This chapter will focus on conjunctival challenge mechanics, evaluation, and applications, concentrating on the most recent important studies in this growing field. Recent refinements in these procedures hold the promise of increasing their utility to ophthalmologists and expanding their relevance to allergists as well.

II. CONJUNCTIVAL ANATOMY AND PATHOLOGICAL RESPONSES

The conjunctiva is a mucous membrane that covers both the surface of the globe (bulbar conjunctiva) and as the posterior or inner surface of the upper and lower eyelids (palpebral conjunctiva). These divisions are important, since the responses of each can vary. The superior palpebral conjunctiva is closely adherent to the underlying eyelid, providing little room for edema, while the abundant substantia propria elsewhere allows for the pathological response of chemosis. The superior palpebral conjunctiva also has a tendency to formation of papillae and rarely develops follicles; the converse is true for the bulbar and inferior palpebral conjunctiva. All portions of the human conjunctiva contain mast cells in high numbers. These are restricted to the substantia propria in normal persons, entering the epithelium only in pathological situations.

In conjunctival challenge evaluation, interest in focused primarily on the inferior fornix, where the inferior palpebral conjunctiva and bulbar conjunctiva merge. Because the anatomy of this region provides a natural reservoir, it is this location that most commonly receives the antigen. It has the added benefit of easy visibility during evaluation of the response.

The ocular tear film is composed not only of lacrimal gland products but of contributions from the conjunctiva as well. This is important, since it allows tear evaluation to complement other clinical observations during the response to provocative challenge. The normal tear volume is about 7 μl, but the tear film

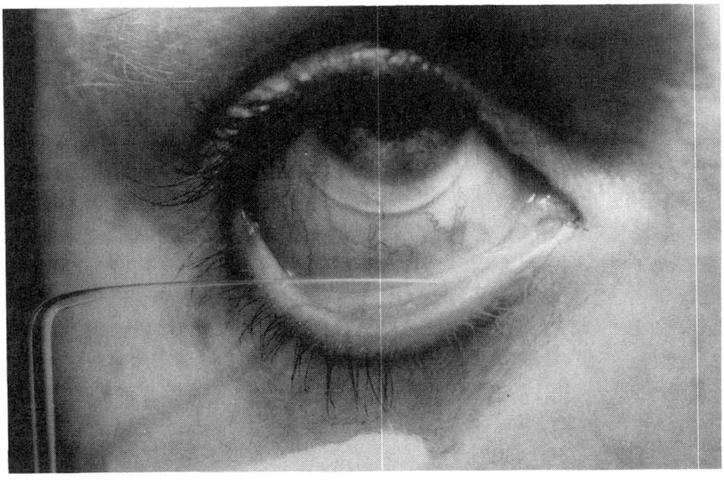

Figure 1 A heated and pulled capillary tube may be used to remove tears from the inferior fornix. (Note the high-water-content soft contact lens that is used to deliver antigen.)

accommodates up to 10–12 μl of fluid. Tear samples of 2 μl are easy to obtain (Fig. 1); application of challenge solutions ideally should not exceed 10 μl.

III. CONJUNCTIVAL CHALLENGE TECHNIQUES AND EVALUATION OF RESPONSES

The conjunctiva may be challenged with dry allergens or solutions. Dry materials are placed in the inferior conjunctival fornix with a spatula or wooden applicator. Solutions are easily applied with a calibrated micropipette into the inferior fornix (Fig. 2). The lacrimal puncta may be occluded during testing with solutions, to prevent rapid efflux and inconsistent test doses (Fig. 3). When a testing end point is reached, the conjunctiva may be rinsed with sterile normal saline solution to dilute the antigen. As a rule, the conjunctival test doses required are 1000–10,000 times greater than those used for skin testing.

A technique I have used in the laboratory and clinic involves challenge with high-water-content contact lenses that are soaked in the desired solution and then applied to the cornea. This provides a depot of test substance with slow release into the tear film, which may be left in place for extended periods if desired. I have found this especially useful for testing ocular medications and contact lens–related products (Fig. 1).

The subjective response to challenge may be graded by an adequately informed test subject. Useful subjective parameters include itching, tearing, and general irritation. Objective measurements may include grading of bulbar and inferior palpebral conjunctival hyperemia and edema (Fig. 4a–d), lower eyelid edema,

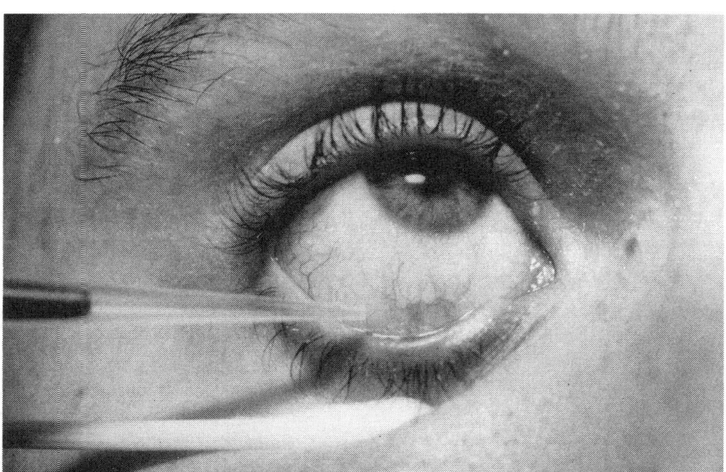

Figure 2 A micropipette may be used to instill test solutions.

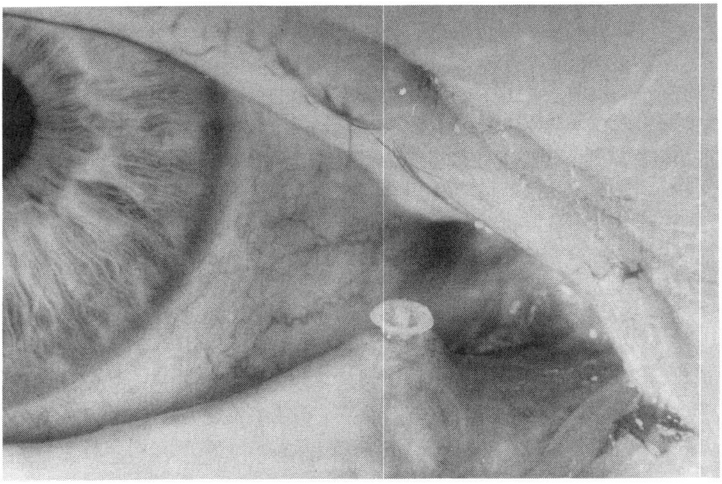

Figure 3 A silicone punctal plug occludes the inferior lacrimal punctum. Alternatively, collagen plugs that dissolve slowly can be used.

mucus discharge, tear volume, tear composition (including osmolarity, protein content, immunoglobulin composition, and cytokine concentrations), tear cytology, and surface cytology obtained from conjunctival scrapings. Tear samples may be easily obtained with a capillary tube (Fig. 1) or on a Schirmer filter paper strip placed at the lateral third of the lower eyelid margin. Friedlaender has described

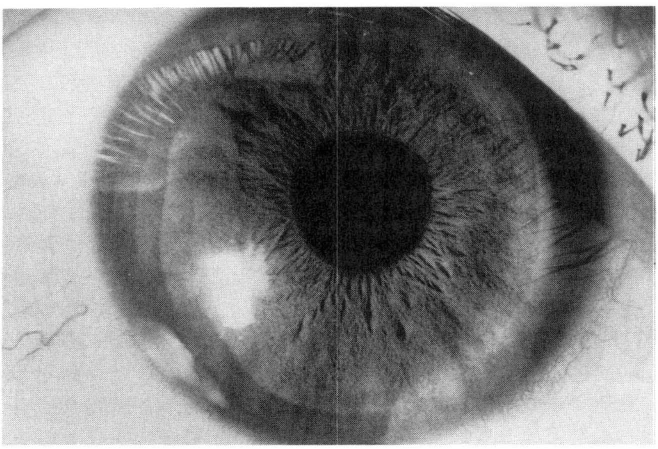

(a)

Figure 4 (**a**) Minimal bulbar conjunctival hyperemia; (**b**) mild bulbar conjunctival hyperemia; (**c**) moderate bulbar conjunctival hyperemia; (**d**) severe bulbar conjunctival hyperemia.

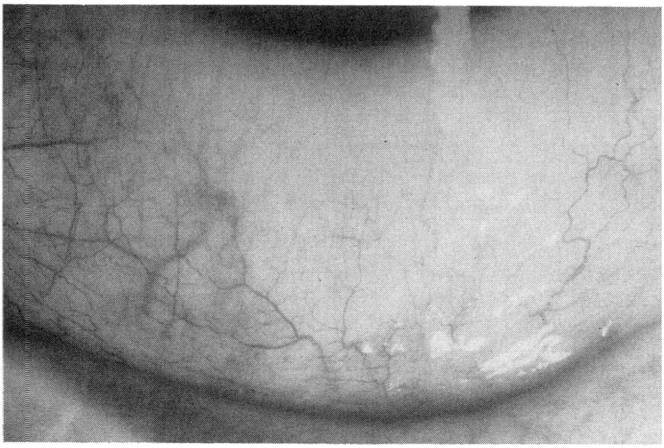
(b)

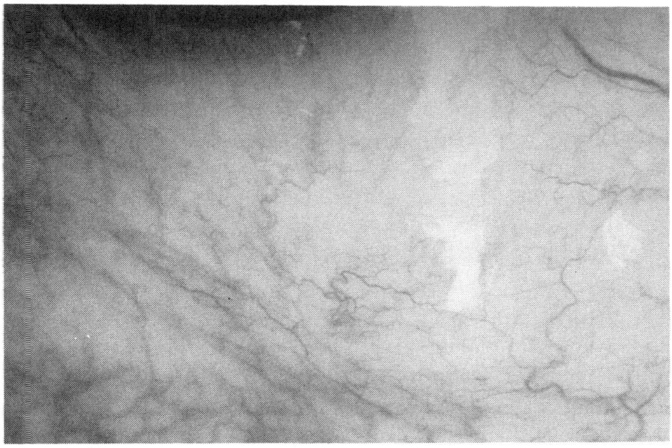
(c)

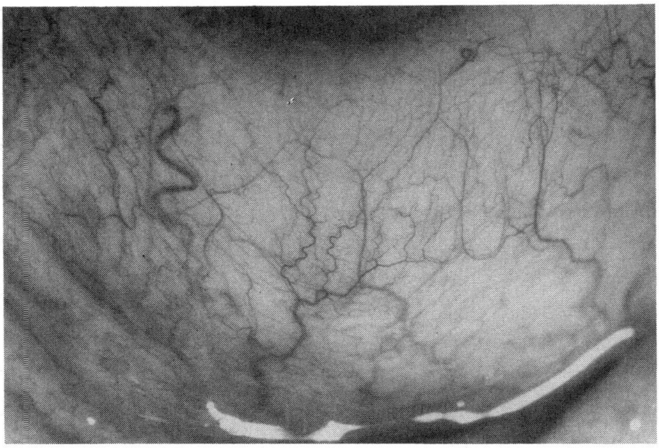
(d)

the measurement of surface conjunctival temperature as an objective way to quantify inflammation [2].

In animal research, the options are expanded. Conjunctival vasopermeability may be measured in vivo. Biopsy is a useful tool for evaluating edema quantitatively and, more important, for evaluating other histopathological responses. Much attention has focused on ocular mast cells in this regard.

In evaluating clinical responses, especially hyperemia and edema, I find photography to be an invaluable tool. Photographs should be taken before challenge and at multiple time points to provide unbiased documentation of responses. These may be evaluated respectively in a masked fashion and allow useful comparative studies.

Abelson et al. described a simple but useful method of testing therapeutic agents designed to alter the ocular response to airborne allergens [3]. Volunteers are challenged on the conjunctiva with a common allergen such as ragweed or cat dander at increasing doses until a positive response is obtained. They are retested several days later. A defined response to a specific quantity of allergen may be determined for each subject. The therapeutic medication may then be given, followed by ocular challenge. If a therapeutic eyedrop is under investigation, one eye may serve as a control and receive a placebo drop in addition to the antigen challenge. The initial screening allows control that is usually lacking in such studies.

IV. ANIMAL AND HUMAN RESEARCH APPLICATIONS

Practical animal models have allowed the investigation of immediate hypersensitivity responses to conjunctival challenge, including conjunctival mast cell participation, inflammatory cell infiltration, leukotriene production, and pharmacological modification of the responses. Preliminary studies suggest that a late-phase component of the conjunctival response may be demonstrable in animals. Late-phase responses in the human eye after conjunctival challenge have not been well described. It is not clear whether this reflects the absence of late-phase responses in the eye or the difficulty in detecting such responses with current techniques.

Recently, Woodward and Ledgard have described a technique for measuring alterations in conjunctival vasopermeability to local challenge in the guinea pig [4]. Radiolabeled erythrocytes and albumin are injected into sensitized animals 15 min before conjunctival challenge. After challenge, eyes are enucleated and conjunctiva is isolated, dried, and counted. Peripheral blood is obtained, and the tissue content of transudated albumin may be calculated. By comparison with the unchallenged eye, alterations in vasopermeability may be calculated.

Using this technique, Woodward and colleagues have added to our limited knowledge of the role of leukotrienes and histamine in the conjunctival response. The vasopermeability model allowed the demonstration that exogenously administered leukotriene E (LTE) and LTD, and to a lesser extent LTC, were able to increase vascular leakage, while LTB had no effect. The response to LTD was stereospecific: the naturally occurring 5S, 6R isomer was 1000 times more potent than the 5R, 6S isomer in eliciting this response [5,6].

This model was also used to demonstrate the primacy of the H_1 receptor in mediating conjunctival responses to histamine [7]. Further, in an ovalbumin-sensitized guinea pig, LT inhibitors were found to have an additive effect with antihistamines in inhibiting vascular leakage. Studies such as these should allow a more careful elucidation of ocular responses.

Human studies of physiological responses after conjunctival challenge have been more limited. Bisgaard et al. described the production of leukotrienes C_4, D_4, and E_4 in skin and tears after provocative tests using high-performance liquid chromatography [8,9]. Several investigators have focused on the production of histamine and the efficacy of topical antihistamines. Stegman and Miller described the measurement of tear protein in response to topical allergen as measured by refractometry [10], but this technique has not found widespread use. Moller et al. also measured leukotrienes in the tears after challenge with birch pollen [11].

TAME-esterases and kinins have been measured in nasal secretions [12] and, more recently, in human tears after conjunctival provocation [2], but the significance of these mediators and the value of their measurement has not been explored sufficiently.

V. CLINICAL APPLICATIONS

Provocative conjunctival challenge fell out of favor as other, more accessible means of challenge were described. It appears that only a few ophthalmologists still use the test for diagnostic purposes. The major diagnostic applications include the evaluation of adverse responses to topical ocular medications and to contact lenses and their associated products.

Many patients are sensitized to the components of a large number of ocular medications. Moreover, some patients, especially those with glaucoma, infectious diseases, or recent ocular surgery, are using several eye medications concurrently. When an adverse reaction develops, it is often best to determine the offending agent by conjunctival challenge rather than simply eliminating or changing drugs at random.

A similar problem arises in contact lens wearers. Most use several solutions in the care of their lenses. Provocative challenge may define the guilty component of their lens care regimen. The problem in this population is not trivial. Though many wear contact lenses for cosmetic purposes, a large number require lenses for therapeutic reasons or to correct aphakia.

Thimerosal is notorious for producing adverse ocular responses. It was once a common preservative in contact lens care products and other eye medications, but growing recognition of its deleterious effects prompted its removal from many of these. Mondino and co-workers [13,14] and Wilson et al. [15] used conjunctival challenge in association with skin testing to implicate thimerosal in cases of contact lens–induced keratitis and conjunctivitis.

Conjunctival challenge may have some advantage over other challenge sites in patients whose allergic involvement is primarily ocular, although the evidence for this is anecdotal. Unsubstantiated clinical evidence also suggests that conjunctival testing may help clarify equivocal tests at other sites. More extensive laboratory research in recent years and a greater understanding of the basic mechanisms of conjunctival inflammation suggest that provocative conjunctival challenge will find an increasing role in the clinic.

REFERENCES

1. Forstot, S. L., Conjunctival challenge, in *Provocative Challenge Procedures: Bronchial, Oral, Nasal, and Exercise* (S. L. Spector, ed.), CRC Press, Boca Raton, Florida, 1983.
2. Friedlaender, M. H., Conjunctival provocative tests: a model of human ocular allergy, *Trans. Am. Ophthalmol. Soc.*, *87*, 577–597 (1989).
3. Abelson, M. B., Chambers, W. A., and Smith, L. M., Conjunctival allergen challenge: a clinical approach to studying allergic conjunctivitis, *Arch. Ophthalmol.*, *108*, 84–88 (1990).
4. Woodward, D. F., and Ledgard, S. E., Effect of LTD_4 on conjunctival vasopermeability and blood-aqueous barrier integrity, *Invest. Ophthalmol. Vis. Sci.*, *26*, 481 (1985).
5. Woodward, D. F., and Ledgard, S. E., Comparison of leukotrienes as conjunctival microvascular permeability factors, *Ophthalm. Res.*, *17*, 318 (1985).
6. Gary, R. K., Woodward, D. F., Nieves, A. L., et al., Characterization of the conjunctival vasopermeability response to leukotrienes and their involvement in immediate hypersensitivity, *Invest. Ophthalmol. Vis. Sci.*, *29*, 119 (1988).
7. Woodward, D. F., Ledgard, S. E., Nieves, A. L., et al., Conjunctival immediate hypersensitivity: re-evaluation of histamine involvement in the vasopermeability response, *Invest. Ophthalmol. Vis. Sci.*, *27*, 57 (1986).
8. Bisgaard, H., Ford-Hutchinson, A. W., Charleson, S., et al., Detection of leukotriene C_4 immunoreactivity in tear fluid from subjects challenged with specific antigens, *Prostaglandins*, *27*, 369–374 (1984).
9. Bisgaard, H., Ford-Hutchinson, A. W., Charleson, S., et al., Production of leukotrienes in human skin and conjunctival mucosa after specific allergen challenge, *Allergy*, *40*, 417 (1985).
10. Stegman, R., and Miller, D., A human model of allergic conjunctivitis, *Arch. Ophthalmol.*, *93*, 1354 (1975).
11. Moller, C., Bjorksten, B., Nilsson, G., et al., The precision of the conjunctival provocation test, *Allergy*, *39*, 37–41 (1984).
12. Naclerio, R. M., Proud, D., Togias, A. C., et al., Inflammatory mediators in late antigen-induced rhinitis, *N. Engl. J. Med.*, *313*, 65–70 (1985).

13. Mondino, B. J., and Groden, L. R., Conjunctival hyperemia and corneal infiltrates with clinically disinfected soft contact lenses, *Arch. Ophthalmol.*, *98*, 1767 (1980).
14. Mondino, B. J., Salamon, S. M., and Zaidman, G. W., Allergic and toxic reactions in soft contact lens wearers, *Surv. Ophthalmol.*, *26*, 337 (1982).
15. Wilson, L. A., McNatt, J., and Reitschell, R., Delayed hypersensitivity to thimerosol in soft contact lens wearers, *Ophthalmology*, *88*, 804 (1981).

BIBLIOGRAPHY

Abelson, M. B., and Allansmith, M. R., Histamine and the eye, in *Immunology and Immunopathology of the Eye* (A. M. Silverstein and G. R. O'Connor, eds.), Mason Publishers, New York, 1979, p. 362.

Abelson, M. B., Allansmith, M. R., and Friedlaender, M. H., Effects of topically applied ocular decongestant and antihistamine, *Am. J. Ophthalmol.*, *90*, 254 (1980).

Abelson, M. B., and Udell, I. J., H_2-receptors in the human ocular surface, *Arch. Ophthalmol.*, *99*, 302 (1981).

Abelson, M. B., Yamamoto, G. K., and Allansmith, M. R., Effects of ocular decongestants, *Arch. Ophthalmol.*, *98*, 865 (1980).

Allansmith, M. R., Baird, R. S., and Bloch, K. J., Degranulation of ocular mast cells in rats undergoing systemic anaphylaxis, *Invest. Ophthalmol. Vis. Sci.*, *19*, 1521 (1980).

Bonini, S., Trocme, S. D., Barney, N. P., Brash, N. P., Block, K. J., and Allansmith, M. R., Late-phase reaction and tear cytology in the rat ocular anaphylaxis model, *Curr. Eye Res.*, *28*, 1970 (1987).

Dwyer, R. S., Turk, J. L., and Darougar, S., Immediate hypersensitivity in the guinea pig conjunctiva: characterization of the IgE and IgG1 antibodies involved, *Int. Arch. Allergy*, *46*, 910 (1974).

Hall, J. M., Pribnow, J. F., Meisler, D., et al., Immediate hypersensitivity in the guinea pig conjunctiva: intravitreal and topical sensitization, *Invest. Ophthalmol. Vis. Sci.*, *25*, 212 (1984).

Iso, T., Nakajima, N., Suda, H., et al., Passive anaphylaxis in rat conjunctiva and topical effects of antiallergic agents, *Ophthalm. Res.*, *12*, 9 (1980).

Khatami, M., Donnelly, J. J., John, T., et al., Vernal conjunctivitis: model studies in guinea pigs immunized topically with fluoresceinyl ovalbumin, *Arch. Ophthalmol.*, *102*, 1683 (1984).

Trocme, S. D., Bonini, S., Trocme, M. C., et al., A hapten model of topically induced ocular anaphylaxis in the rat, *Invest. Ophthalmol. Vis. Sci.*, *28*, 264 (1987).

Udell, I. J., and Abelson, M. B., Animal and human ocular surface response to a topical nonimmune mast-cell degranulating agent (compound 48/80), *Am. J. Ophthalmol.*, *91*, 226 (1981).

26

Clinical Application of Immediate Skin Testing

Harold S. Nelson

National Jewish Center for Immunology and Respiratory Medicine Denver, Colorado

I. INTRODUCTION

The immediate wheal and flare skin test has been the diagnostic method of choice for demonstration of immediate hypersensitivity since the days of Charles Blackley [1]. Studies addressing variables that affect the immediate skin test have appeared periodically in the literature for the last 60 years. In the last two decades, in part because of the development of in vitro tests for the diagnosis of immediate hypersensitivity, there has been a reexamination of the reliability of the immediate skin test [2]. Many of the variables affecting immediate skin tests have undergone careful study. If the resulting information is incorporated into the process of allergy skin testing, the results can be made as accurate as the clinical or research situation demands.

II. METHODS OF SKIN TESTING

Skin testing for the diagnosis of immediate hypersensitivity is performed by one of two methods, prick or intradermal (Table 1). The former method involves making a break in the epidermis that allows extract to diffuse passively into the superficial dermis. The break may be made with an upward motion, with downward pressure, or as a linear abrasion, and with a variety of instruments that will be discussed later. The intradermal test involves injection of the extract into the superficial layers of the dermis using a syringe and needle.

Table 1 Comparison of Prick and Intradermal Tests

Advantages, prick	Advantages, intradermal
Safer	More sensitive (1,000–30,000 fold)
Technically less demanding	More reproducible
Rapid	
Little discomfort	
Many allergens in one session	
Extracts stable (50% glycerin)	
Positive and negative easily distinguishable	
Positive test correlates better with clinical symptoms	
Steeper dose–response curve	

Source: Refs. 3 and 4.

Given wheal and flare reactions of equivalent size, systemic reactions appear to be less frequent with prick than with intradermal testing [5]. The difference probably relates to an effect of the depth to which the extract is introduced by the two methods on its rate of absorption into the systemic circulation.

Because of the ease with which prick tests can be performed and because they can be safely performed on the back, it is possible to test with many allergens in one session.

Allergy extracts are most stable when they are most concentrated [6]. Furthermore, 50% glycerin, which greatly increases the stability of extracts, can be employed for prick testing [6], while even 6% glycerin will cause a high incidence of false-positive reactions on intradermal testing [7].

Prick testing offers a potential advantage in interpretation over intradermal testing. With the less traumatic devices, nonspecific irritant reactions seldom occur. Using conventional techniques, Barbee et al. reported only six measurable wheals in 3101 consecutive saline controls [8]. When the diluent control is completely negative, no allowance is necessary in interpretation of positive reactions, and even an isolated erythematous reaction is suggestive of the presence of specific immunoglobulin E (IgE) for that antigen [5], although only wheals measuring 3 mm and greater are accepted as unequivocal evidence of a positive reaction [9]. However, the introduction of more traumatic devices for performing prick skin tests, as will be discussed later, has potentially eliminated this advantage of prick skin testing.

As will be discussed later, the prick test is said to correlate better than the intradermal test with the occurrence of clinical symptoms [10]. This clearly depends on the relative concentration of the extracts employed with the two methods. If intradermal testing is performed with extracts 1,000–30,000 times more dilute, the clinical relevance of a positive test will be same as for a prick test

[9]. However, if intracutaneous tests are performed, as they often are, with extracts only 25 to 50 times as dilute as those employed for prick testing, they will begin to yield frequent positive reactions in patients with no history suggestive of allergic disease [7].

The individual intradermal skin test is more reproducible than the individual prick test [11]. Malling obtained a coefficient of variation (CV; standard deviation/mean test size) of 29% for prick testing and of 17% for intradermal testing [12]. In titrated skin testing, however, he found that the greater reproducibility of intracutaneous testing was offset by a shallower dose–response slope. The log area of the reaction with prick testing increased twofold for each log increase in concentration, while the log area of the intracutaneous test (either wheal or flare) increased by only 1.7-fold ($p < 0.01$). Malling concluded that the steeper slope of the dose–response curve, in addition to the other advantages of the prick test enumerated above, made it preferable to the intracutaneous method for quantitative testing.

A. Techniques of Intradermal Testing

Intracutaneous testing is usually performed with a 1.0-ml disposable syringe and 25- or 26-gauge needles. The needle is introduced superficially into the dermis until the bevel is entirely within the skin. Then a volume of 0.01–0.02 ml is injected, raising a small bleb. To improve accuracy of delivery, a 0.1-ml syringe with a 30-gauge needle has been recommended and found to give greater reproducibility [13]. An alternative recommendation to increase reproducibility is injection of 0.05 ml of extract [2], but this has the disadvantage of being more painful and may result in more fluid leakage, reducing accuracy [14].

B. Techniques of Prick Skin Testing

The term "prick skin testing" is generically employed for techniques separately termed scratch, puncture, and prick. In the scratch test method, a superficial abrasion is made with a knife, needle, or other instrument. Extract is applied to the site. In the puncture test, the extract is first placed on the skin and a superficial break in the epidermis is made by downward pressure through the drop. In the prick test, a drop of extract is placed on the skin and a sharp instrument is passed thorough the drop at anywhere from a 20° to an 80° angle, just catching the skin. The instrument is then lifted, creating a small break in the epidermis. The extract appears to enter the dermis at the time of pricking through a small resulting channel, since it has been shown that immediate blotting of the liquid does not reduce the size of the reaction [15]. Studies comparing the prick and scratch methods have generally favored the former. The prick test has proved to be more sensitive [16,17], less variable [18,19], faster, less painful, and less likely to produce small scars [5]. A potential advantage of performing the prick test with an upward motion instead of downward pressure is that it can then be performed reliably in patients with dermatographism, since, with proper technique, there is not sufficient downward pressure to the skin to cause a wheal and flare at the site of the negative control.

The advantages of the prick method of testing have led to its more extensive use and to a proliferation of devices designed to break the integrity of the epidermis. The commonly employed instruments for prick testing include several types of hollow and solid-bore needle, blood-drawing lancets, lancets specifically designed for skin testing [20,21], the Morrow-Brown needle [22], the Multi-Test [22], and the DermaPIK. Skin test lancets have a 1-mm tip and shoulders that prevent further penetration into the skin. The Morrow-Brown needle is a plastic cylinder with a 1-mm tapered print, also with shoulders to prevent further penetration. The Multi-Test has eight clusters of plastic prongs, each with nine separate plastic points, the whole contained on a rigid frame, the distance between adjacent prongs being 2 cm.

A number of investigators have compared the performance of these prick skin test devices. One advantage of the individual lancets and the Morrow-Brown needle is said to be less dependence on the technician's experience [23]. In general, the Morrow-Brown needle produces a smaller reaction [24] and a larger number of false-negative reactions [23]. In direct comparison with the Morrow-Brown needle, the skin test lancet has been reported to produce less variable results [23]. The Multi-Test has received both favorable [22,25–27] and unfavorable [28–31] evaluations regarding its reliability.

The differences between the various prick skin test devices is perhaps best understood if they are viewed as varying in the degree of trauma that they impart to the skin. Those that produce the least trauma also produce the smallest reactions with allergen but, correspondingly, are less apt to produce positive reactions at the site of negative control. The least traumatic devices are also the least painful and are accepted better by the patients. Finally, if the trauma to the skin is insufficient, false-negative tests can result because of failure to penetrate the epidermis. From available studies it is apparent that the least traumatic of the commonly employed devices is the Morrow-Brown needle. Most skin test lancets and needles, whether employed with upward or downward pressure, are intermediate in the degree of trauma they produce. The blood-drawing lancet, the Multi-Test, and the DermaPIK are the most traumatic of the commercially available devices. It is important to know the characteristics of the device employed, since the more traumatic it is, the larger is the reaction that may occur at a negative site as a result of trauma alone, and the greater the size of reaction that is required for confidence that it truly is an allergic reaction [32]. The values for 95% confidence that a wheal exceeds the possible reaction at a saline control site are 0 mm for the Hollister-Steir lancetter; 2.5 mm for the ALK lancet; 3.5 mm for the ALO bifurcated needle employed with either upward or downward motion; 4.5 mm for the Multi-Test; and 5.0 m DermaPIK [32].

A disposable hypodermic needle may also be employed for prick testing [33]. With a hollow needle, as well as with the Morrow-Brown needle, blood-drawing lancet, skin test lancet, Multi-Test, and DermaPIK, the device must be discarded after each antigen to prevent carryover of extract from one site to the next. With solid-bore needles the device may be wiped and reused for all tests in a single subject. However, wiping must be performed after each prick with a wet, not dry, sponge (H. S. Nelson, unpublished), and, in addition, with the bifurcated needle swishing in liquid before wiping may be advisable to prevent carryover of extract in the narrow groove between the two points [28].

III. SKIN TEST AGENTS

The agents employed for immediate skin testing consist of allergenic extracts, nonimmunological mast cell mediator–releasing agents, histamine, and negative controls. The reliability of skin testing is in part dependent on the quality of the allergenic extracts employed. Following their development in the 1970s, in vitro tests were applied to assess the potency of the allergy extracts then available, with the disturbing finding that extracts with similar labeled potency could vary by as much as 1000-fold in their biological activity [34–36]. This problem has been corrected, to some extent, by the introduction of standardized extracts for a variety of inhalants (see Table 2).

Still to be addressed is standardization and, perhaps more important, stabilization of food extracts. Some food extracts, especially fruits, lose potency within days of preparation [37]. A markedly greater number of positive skin tests were reported with such foods as shrimp, clam, fish, peas, peanuts, potatoes, tomatoes, cabbage and bananas when frozen food was used, as compared with commercial extracts [38]. A study comparing fresh foods with commercial extracts reported that prick skin tests were much more frequently positive with fresh extracts of apple, cherry, orange, peach, pear, tomato, and hazelnut, while the commercial extracts gave as many or more positive reactions with banana, pea, peanut, potato, and walnut [39].

It has been suggested that extract mixes might be employed for initial screening for sensitivity [40]. However, when compared with positive reactions on individual tests, various mixes failed to detect 11–33% of reactions by prick and 4–29% of reactions by intradermal testing.

Table 2 Advantages of Standardized Extracts

1. Less variation between manufacturers and lots.
2. Development of meaningful schedules for diagnosis and treatment.
3. Ability to compare skin tests between patients and over time.
4. Greater safety with high-dose immunotherapy.

Nonimmunological releasers of mast cell mediators have been employed for skin testing. Commonly employed are opiates, either codeine (50 mg/ml by prick) [41] or morphine sulfate (0.1 mg/ml intradermally) [5]. A nonopiate mast cell mediator–releasing agent, compound 48/80, is employed in approximately the same concentrations as histamine [42]. The report that the dose–response slopes for allergen, nonimmunological mediator releasers, and histamine are parallel [43] and the observation that they are similar suppressed by antihistamine [44] bring into question what advantage these agent have over histamine as a positive control. One potential disadvantage of histamine as a control is that the wheal and flare reaction with histamine peaks in 8–10 min, while that with allergen peaks in 12–17 min, requiring two readings for scientific accuracy [13].

Histamine hydrochloride or phosphate has been employed for some time as a positive control. In the United States, the phosphate salt is usually employed, and the potency is expressed as the content of histamine base. The usual concentrations employed are 0.1 mg/ml (0.275 mg/ml histamine phosphate) as a control for intradermal testing and 1 mg/ml (2.75 mg/ml histamine phosphate) for prick testing [5]. If larger wheals are desired, or if titrated histamine testing is to be employed, the concentration can be 10 mg/ml histamine base (27.5 mg/ml histamine phosphate). In a recent study of devices for prick testing, 10 mg/ml histamine base produced mean wheal areas of 27–40 mm^2 with the six devices tested [28].

In northern Europe, histamine is used as a standard for extract potency, as well as a positive control [29,45]. The histamine equivalent potency (HEP) in skin testing was originally based on 1 mg/ml histamine hydrochloride (0.63 mg/ml histamine base) [29]. It was found that this gave a rather small reaction, and, subsequently, substitution of 10 mg/ml histamine hydrochloride (6.3 mg/ml histamine base) was recommended [46,47]. In one study [46], the comparative size and reproducibility of tests with 1 mg/ml and 10 mg/ml histamine hydrochloride were as follows: for 1 mg/ml, diameter 4.5 mm, area 16 mm^2, CV 27%; for 10 mg/ml, diameter 7.0 mm, area 38 mm^2, CV 17%.

IV. QUANTITATION OF IMMEDIATE SKIN TESTS

Skin testing may be used for diagnosis, to compare two or more extracts, to measure change over time as a result of either drug treatment or allergy immunotherapy.

For diagnostic purposes, it is customary in the United States to perform tests with only a single concentration of extract, although it has been recommended that duplicate prick skin tests be performed [9]. The results may then be expressed in several ways. A semiquantitative grading system may be used. As an example, that employed at the University of Michigan [5] is given, with modifications, in Table 3.

Table 3 A Semi-quantitative Grading System

	Prick skin tests	Intradermal skin tests	
		Control < 2 mm	Control ≥ 2 mm
Negative	No reaction or no different from control	No different from control	No different from control
1+	Erythema <21 mm	3- to 4-mm wheal with erythema, or erythema larger than 21-mm	Wheal 1½–2 times control with erythema, or erythema > 21-mm
2+	Erythema >20 mm	4- to 8-mm wheal without pseudopods	Wheal 2–3 times control
3+	Wheal ≥ 3 mm with surrounding erythema	Wheal > 8 mm without pseudopods	Wheal > 3 times control
4+	Wheal with pseudopods and surrounding erythema	Wheal with pseudopods	Wheal with pseudopods

Source: Ref. 5.

The Northern (Scandinavian) Society for Allergology recommended that a semiquantitative grading system be used, in which the size of the allergen-induced wheal was compared with that produced by a histamine control [45]. In their original recommendations, the control was to be 1 mg/ml of histamine hydrochloride (0.63 mg/ml histamine base). Reactions to allergen producing a wheal similar in size to that produced by histamine were to be graded 3+, those twice that size 4+, and those half that size 2+, and those between the negative control and 2+ in size were to be graded 1+. Among the arguments in favor of such a grading system is that it would compensate for difference due to technicians and instruments [29]. Furthermore, significant variation in skin reactivity to histamine has been reported [48], and in a large population the prevalence of six positive skin tests increased from 15% to 60% with a four 10-fold difference in the threshold of skin reactivity to histamine. Among the arguments against using a histamine standard are that it introduces another biological variable, that the histamine test must be read at 8–10 min whereas the allergen skin reactions peak at 12–17 min, and that it is unnecessary, since the variation in reactivity of subjects to histamine is not great [13]. In a study of skin reactivity to standardized dog extract, the use of a 3+ grade by the histamine reference system resulted in a sensitivity of 0.917, a specificity of 0.932, and a better correlation with RAST and provocation tests than was obtained with wheals not corrected for the size of the histamine reaction [49]. The overall efficiency of the 3+ histamine reference was 0.926, compared with 0.886 for the uncorrected 3-mm wheal. It might be added that end-point titration did not give better results than the histamine reference value, despite added complexity. Its overall efficiency was only 0.905. There is not agreement on the usefulness of correcting for the size of the histamine reaction. Vohlonen and co-workers examined reproducibility of the skin prick test performed in 20 subjects by four nurses. They found greatest reproducibility when uncorrected wheals were expressed by area. Reproducibility decreased when the wheals were corrected for the size of the histamine control or corrected for diluent control [50].

Alternatively the results of skin tests may be expressed by measuring the largest diameter, the mean diameter, or the area. Only the wheal may be employed [51], only the flare [51], or a combination of the two [52]. It has been shown that area is somewhat more reproducible than the product of the two diameters [51]. Progressively less precise, but still good, are average of the two diameters and measurement of the largest diameter [51]. Further improvement in accuracy is achieved by enlarging smaller wheals before measuring [28,51,53].

When the wheal is measured, it is not uncommon to disregard the size of the erythema and to accept as positive only prick skin tests with wheals 3 mm in diameter or larger. The 3-mm wheal diameter as the threshold for significance is also supported by several recent studies [9,49,54]. Sampson compared prick skin testing with double-blind food challenges in children with eczema [54]. He found that the 3-mm wheal diameter performed as well as or better than other criteria such as other wheal diameters, measuring wheal and flare, calculating allergen wheal/histamine wheal ratios, or recording the presence of pseudopods. Vanto compared the sensitivity and specificity of various prick test parameters in 202 children, of whom 84 were judged allergic to dogs when tested with a standardized dog extract. He found that a 3-mm wheal diameter performed better than any other wheal size, with a sensitivity of 0.976 and a specificity of 0.822 [49]. All these studies were performed with devices that impart limited trauma to the skin. With the more traumatic devices that have been introduced, such as the Multi-Test and DermaPIK, different standards for positive reactions must be set, since wheals larger than 3 mm are regularly produced at the saline control sites with these devices.

In scientific studies, a greater degree of precision than that provided by the single-dilution test is often desired. It is usually recommended that this be achieved by performing skin tests with serial three- to 10-fold dilutions of extract [55,56], and, for further accuracy, that prick skin tests be performed in duplicate or even quadruplicate [9].

It is believed that the dose-response of the skin is best expressed by the log of the dose and the log of the reaction [9]. Furthermore, it is believed to be linear only over a limited range [52,57], so that for quantitative studies, reactions with diameters larger than 17 mm and smaller than 4 mm should be avoided.

A number of methods have been employed to quantitate the results of skin testing for scientific studies, including end-point titration, sum of the wheals or sum of the flares, mean size of wheals produced by several concentrations, calculation of a linear regression from the results of tests with several dilutions (parallel-line comparisons), determination of the concentration giving a wheal of the same size as a given concentration of histamine [45], and calculation of an index of the wheal and flare produced by each concentration [58]. This index is calculated by the formula: index = (L + W) flare + 3.7 + 11.5 log (L + W) wheal, where L equals length and W equals width.

The end-point titration is usually performed down to a dilution giving a reaction of a certain minimum size. For the prick test, this is usually a 3-mm diameter, while for the intradermal test, a 10-mm wheal with a least 21-mm erythema [2] or a 5-mm wheal with at least 10-mm erythema [59] has been employed. When the latter criteria were applied to a comparison of two extracts using half-log increments, CVs of 6–9% were obtained [59].

A parallel-line skin test assay (PLSTA) has been recommended by the FDA Bureau of Biologics as the primary method by which allergen extract potency is to be estimated [60]. This method is preferred because the confidence intervals of the flare reactions are narrower (54–186%) than those for wheals [27–367%), because of the 5.5-fold steeper slope of the dose–response curve for erythema than for whealing [60]. This method involves

1. Determination of the dilution of each extract giving a reaction just above end point
2. Injection of each extract in quantities of 0.05 ml intradermally into the skin of the back in four serial threefold dilutions in triplicate
3. Measurement of the largest and midpoint orthogonal diameters of the flare of each reaction and summing of the triplicates
4. Determination that each slope has an *r* value of at least 0.85 and a slope of more than 10mm/log dilution, with the greatest sum of erythema being no more than 120 mm
5. Determination that the two slopes are parallel ($p > 0.01$) and calculation of a common slope
6. Determination of the relative potency by the distance between two parallel lines

There are a number of problems with the PLSTA [61], including the complexity of performing the study, the discomfort for the patient caused by multiple injections of 0.05 ml into the skin of the back, the frequency with which data have to be rejected as not meeting the listed criteria (5 of 21 sets of subject date in one report [61]), and, finally, the risk (in the same study of 2 of 21 subjects experienced systemic reactions following performance of PLSTAs). Malling has proposed a similar parallel-line assay employing prick skin testing [46]. Malling compared parallel assays employing prick and intradermal skin tests. He found the slope of the wheal and flare of the intradermal test to be similar, and less steep than that of the prick test wheal. He used criteria similar to those of the Bureau of Biologics, i.e., slope with a correlation coefficient of at least 0.90 and CV not greater than

40%. Given these criteria, he found the steeper slope of the prick test wheals compensated for the lesser reproducibility of individual prick test results.

Workers at Johns Hopkins University have suggested an alternative method termed "midpoint skin titration." Given two intradermal skin tests, one with a wheal < 7 mm, the other with a wheal > 7 mm, it is possible to interpolate for a dose producing a wheal of 7-mm diameter (ID-7). They found this measurement much more sensitive than the intradermal end-point titration in detecting significant changes in skin test reactivity induced by immunotherapy [62].

V. VARIABLES IN ALLERGY SKIN TESTING

The size of the immediate skin test reaction is a function of the amount of antigen that is injected into the skin, the amount of specific IgE present, the number of mast cells, the releasibility of the mast cells to the antigen used, and the reactivity of the patient's skin to the mediators released, particularly histamine. The reactivity to histamine has been shown to vary with age, with the region of the body used for testing, perhaps with the time of day, and certainly in response to medication that the patient may have ingested.

A. Age

In large population studies, there is a definite variation with age in the incidence of positive skin reactions [8]. In part, this is due to the level IgE, which rises during childhood, peaks during the second decade, then falls progressively with increasing age [63]. In addition to this variation in immediate hypersensitivity, however, there is an age-related variation in the reactivity of the skin to histamine. Infants have been shown to occasionally be nonreactive to 10 mg/ml of histamine hydrochloride up to 1 month of age and to 1 mg/ml up to 4 months of age [41]. Apart from these occasional nonreactors, there is significantly less reactivity overall in infants and young children than in adults [41]. Children from birth to 3 years had histamine reactions with 61% of the diameter of adult reactions [64]. At the other extreme, there is also a decrease in skin reactivity to histamine with advancing age [65]. The decline begins after age 50, and by age 71–85 years, the level of reactivity measured in wheal diameter had declined to 73% of the young adult level [64]. The overall effect of the age-related changes in specific IgE and skin reactivity to histamine is additive [63]. Thus, the incidence of positive skin tests rises throughout infancy and childhood, peaks in the first half of the third decade, declines slowly to age 50, and then rapidly declines with advancing age [8]. The percentage of subjects showing any positive skin reaction in a general-population sample in Tucson, Arizona, increased from 22% among the 3- to 4-year-olds to 52% in the first half of the third decade, and fell to 16% after age 75 [8].

B. Area of the Body

There are differences in the reactivity of different parts of the body to histamine, which are reflected in the response to antigens as well. The back has been reported to be more reactive to histamine than the forearm, where the area of reactions was half as large [66]. The responsiveness of the back both to histamine and to allergens shows a highly significant gradient. Reactions are smallest on the upper third and largest on the lower third, the diameter of reactions in the latter areas vs. the former averaging 124% for histamine and 142% for allergen [32]. With regard to the forearms, several studies have demonstrated that the more distal portions and the radial sides are less reactive than the more proximal and ulnar aspects [57,67]. Although statistically significant, these differences may not be detectable in ordinary clinical practice [68].

C. Time of Day

As with many body functions and responses, the reactivity of the skin to histamine has been reported to have a circadian rhythm. In a study in which the size of reactions was measured every 4 h through a 24-h days, significantly less reactivity to histamine and allergen was found at 7:00 h, while reactivity peaked between 19:00 and 23:00 h. The peak-to-trough ratio was reported to be 2.9 for whealing and 3.5 for erythema [69]. The authors suggested, on the basis of their study, that testing early in the day might yield false-negative reactions. A subsequent study, however, compared reactivity to ragweed in 20 children and 20 adults at 8:00 and 16:00 h, the usual range for allergy skin testing in clinical practice [70]. The investigators found only a minor variation in reactivity, and furthermore, the variation present was in the direction opposite to that suggested by the previous report, with reactions larger in the morning than in the afternoon to a statistically significant but clinically insignificant degree [70]. This report has been confirmed by a study in which skin testing was performed in 21 subjects twice at mean times of 9:45 a.m. and 7:46 p.m. These investigators also found that the histamine response was significantly larger in the morning, while there was no significant difference between morning and evening in the mean size of the reactions or in the number of positive prick skin test reactions to allergen [71]. Thus, within the usual range of clinical practice, the time of skin testing is probably not important.

D. Suppression by Medication

Some medications clearly can suppress skin tests. Most notable are the H_1 histamine antagonists. They have been shown to have a prolonged suppressive effect, the duration of which generally corresponds to the maximal suppression attained while subjects are taking the drugs. Thus, in the study of Cook et al., maximum skin test suppression with five drugs varied from 31% to 63%, and significant suppression persisted with the same order of potency for mean periods of 1.9–4.3 days [72]. The prolonged persistence of skin test suppression relates to the long half-life that many of these drugs possess in adults [73]. The tricyclic antidepressants also possess potent antihistaminic properties and can produce suppression of skin tests lasting at least as long as that produced by conventional antihistamines [74]. An exception to the general rule for the duration of suppression of skin reactivity by antihistamines is astemizole, which significantly suppressed prick skin test reactions to allergen for over 2 months, and to histamine for over 4 months (H. S. Nelson, unpublished data). H_2 histamine antagonists can also be demonstrated to have a small (10–15%) but significant suppressive effect [75], which can furthermore be shown to be additive to the H_1 effect [76].

In assessing the possibility of suppression by antihistamines, it is helpful to know that the immediate reactions to histamine and to mediators released from mast cells are depressed to the same degree by antihistamines [44]. Therefore, the histamine skin test can be used as an adequate control for testing for possible suppression in patients who may recently have ingested a drug with antihistaminic properties.

Apart from drugs employed for their histamine antagonism, the drugs commonly used in patients with allergies do not significantly suppress the skin reaction to histamine or to allergen. These include theophylline and β-adrenergic bronchodilators [77]. Short courses of corticosteroids in moderate doses, such as 24 mg methylprednisolone daily for 1 week, did not have a suppressive effect on immediate skin tests [78]. However, 25 subjects receiving long-term corticosteroid therapy reacted significantly less to codeine skin tests than did 25 control subjects (mean diameter 9.5 mm vs. 14 mm). There was no difference in the skin reactivity to histamine [79]. Chronic local application of potent steroid ointment will also suppress the skin test response because of reduction in skin mast cells and histamine content [80].

VI. RELIABILITY OF IMMEDIATE SKIN TESTING

A. Reproducibility

It is generally accepted that the carefully performed intradermal skin test is more reproducible than the epicutaneous test [11]. However, there are factors that can lessen the reproducibility of the intradermal test, such as variation in the volume injected, leakage of fluid out along the needle tract (most common with volumes greater than 0.04 ml), and variation in the depth of injection [81]. For prick skin testing, significant variation of wheal size among different technicians has been reported [28,34].

Recent interest in the prick test has resulted in a careful assessment of its reproducibility. It has become clear that the CV is greater for smaller reactions.

Coefficients of variation for wheals with an area less than 15 mm^2 were reported to be 30–60%, while for wheals greater than 15 mm^2 they were 20–30% [41], and in another study, the CVs of wheal areas on the back were only 10–20% for wheals with an area greater than 50 mm^2 [82]. Malling reported CVs less than 40% over the range of prick test wheal areas from 5 to 150 mm^2 [12]. He found that very large reactions (> 150 mm^2) resulted in a lower reproducibility (perhaps because of the irregular occurrence of pseudopods).

B. Positive Skin Tests in Nonallergic Subjects

Investigators have determined the prevalence of positive immediate skin tests in nonallergic subjects. Lindblad and Farr performed intradermal skin testing with concentrated extracts in 100 "wheeze-free, sneeze-free" subjects [7]. Employing pollen extracts at concentrations of 10,000 PNU/ml, they found a 28–35% prevalence of positive reactions (wheal ⩾ 5 mm); many of these positive reactions were transferable by Prausnitz–Küstner testing. At concentrations of 1000 PNU/ml, the prevalence of positive skin test reactions to pollen extracts decreased to 2–8%, while at 100 PNU/ml, there were no positive reactions to pollen. The prevalence of positive test reactions to house dust extract, which was only one-tenth as concentrated as the pollens, was 50%, 19%, and 4% for serial tenfold dilutions.

Adinoff and co-workers performed prick skin tests with 13 standardized extracts in 200 subjects [83]. Fifty had a personal history of asthma or rhinitis; 90% of them had at least one positive skin test. Fifty others had no such personal history, but had a close family member with a history of asthma or rhinitis; 46% had at least one positive prick skin test. One hundred subjects had neither a personal nor a family history of asthma or rhinitis, yet 29% had at least one positive prick skin test.

C. "True" False-Positive Skin Tests

False-positive skin tests may occur as a result of placement of the tests too close to a large positive reaction. Although some investigators recommend placement of prick skin tests at distances as little as 2 cm [84,85], there are strong arguments for placement of skin tests, either prick or intradermal, at least 5 cm apart [13,85,86]. Even with placement at recommended distances, false-positive reactions are sometimes observed: for example, when a histamine control was placed below venom skin tests on the upper arm [87]. Five of 50 patients tested in this manner with 0.001 μg/ml of various Hymenoptera venoms developed false-positive reactions at one or more of the test sites. A 9% incidence of false-positive reactions to intradermal testing with bee venom was reported when the tests were placed 4–5 cm distal to a histamine control. These authors recommended 6-cm spacing between intradermal tests [85]. It has been suggested that this decreased threshold, which can result in false-positive reactions to both allergen and saline, is mediated through the axon reflex [13]. Whatever the mechanism, it is important to consider any positive skin test reaction suspect if it is within or near the flare of a nearby positive reaction, and to repeat it at another site.

D. False-Negative Skin Tests

False-negative skin tests can be due to the quality of the extract, fluctuations in the subject's sensitivity, or suppression by medication, can follow a systemic reaction to the allergen used, and can perhaps be due to the presence of "localized allergy."

Allergy extracts of the same stated strength have been demonstrated to vary greatly in potency [34–36]. This problem has been overcome for at least some antigens by the introduction of extracts standardized by a Bureau of Biologics standard. Even for those extracts for which a standard exists, there is still a problem of deterioration after reconstitution [6,55]. For this reason it has been recommended that dilute extracts be prepared weekly and refrigerated between uses. Further stabilization of dilute extracts, as for use in intradermal testing, can be achieved by addition of 0.03% human serum albumin [6,88]. Deterioration of extract potency over the shelf life of an extract is usually not a problem with prick testing if the extracts are reconstituted in 50% glycerin [6]. In the case of extracts of some fruits, seafoods, and vegetables [37–39], deterioration occurs even in concentrated glycerinated extracts, and the use of frozen or fresh extracts may yield a higher incidence of positive reactions.

With exposures that are seasonal, the level of specific IgE in the serum may vary throughout the year, peaking shortly after the season and then declining until the next seasonal exposure. This has been reported to occur to a sufficient degree that subjects with a low level of reactivity may have negative skin tests in the months just before the season [89].

The suppressive effects of medications are discussed above.

It has been reported that skin tests may be falsely negative for several days after a systemic reaction to an antigen such as Hymenoptera venom or penicillin [90]. An interval of 2 weeks between the reaction and skin testing should be ample to allow return of full reactivity.

It has been suggested that some clinically sensitive subjects may have positive reactions to challenge of the target organ but negative reactions to skin testing. Huggins and Brostoff identified a group of patients they believed were sensitive to house dust mite, who had positive reactions to nasal challenge but negative prick skin tests and negative serum RASTs to house dust mite [91]. Huggins and Brostoff demonstrated that these patients had specific IgE in their nasal secretions, like patients with positive skin tests and unlike subjects with no history of mite sensitivity. Two articles have confirmed the occurrence of positive RASTs on nasal secretions in the presence of negative prick skin tests and negative RASTs on serum. However, neither study established the clinical relevance of the allergens in question [92,93].

VII. CORRELATION WITH IN VITRO TESTING

The results of skin testing correlate with those of in vitro measurement of specific IgE [2]. Generally, prick tests are somewhat more sensitive than in vitro tests, and intradermal tests, with the usually employed concentrations, are considerably more sensitive. When, in a large population survey in Tucson, Arizona, any prick test with a wheal of 1 mm or larger was considered positive, positive prick tests were associated with a positive RAST 78.5% of the time [94]. A negative prick skin test was accompanied by a negative RAST 97.5% of the time. Given a negative prick test, a positive intradermal test (wheal 5 mm or larger) was accompanied by a positive RAST in two of 12 cases, while a negative intradermal test was invariably accompanied by a negative RAST (38/38). Vanto, employing a standardized dog extract, found that 95% of prick tests with a mean wheal diameter of 3 mm or more were accompanied by a positive RAST, while no RASTs of grade 3 or 4 were found in patients with negative prick skin tests [49].

When the results of the various tests for specific IgE were compared with the occurrence of symptoms of allergic rhinitis during natural exposure, it was concluded that RAST, leukocyte histamine release, and titrated skin tests were comparable in predicting allergic rhinitis, the choice being dictated by relative expense and convenience [2]. Bousquet et al., on the other hand, found that nasal provocation and titrated prick skin tests to grass pollen performed following rush immunotherapy correlated significantly with symptoms during the subsequent grass pollen season, but did not correlate with RAST titers [56].

VIII. CORRELATION WITH BRONCHIAL CHALLENGE

Unlike the RAST, with which the skin test shows a strong correlation, there is a relatively poor correlation between skin testing and bronchial allergen challenge. The reason for this poor correlation is the presence of a second variable, nonspecific bronchial hyperresponsiveness as measured by histamine or methacholine challenge. The correlation between skin testing and bronchial allergen challenge can be improved considerably by incorporating the threshold of nonspecific bronchial responsiveness [95]. The validity of this retrospectively derived association was confirmed prospectively by Cockcroft and co-workers [96], who showed that the early airway response to allergen could be predicted within an eightfold range by a formula employing skin test reactivity and bronchial sensitivity to histamine. This degree of prediction was better than the reproducibility of bronchial allergen challenge achieved by some investigators.

IX. DIAGNOSTIC VALUE OF IMMEDIATE SKIN TESTING

A. Correlation with Clinical Disease

Skin testing is merely a bioassay indicating the presence of sensitivity; it is never "diagnostic" of the presence of clinical disease. The results must be correlated with the patient's history and known exposures to determine their significance. In doing so, it is helpful to think of the specificity, sensitivity, and efficiency of the skin test in relation to the historical diagnosis (Table 4).

It is clear from the data presented earlier (see above, "Positive Skin Tests in Nonallergic Subjects") that to interpret immediate skin tests properly, it is necessary to have some idea of the degree of reactivity that is encountered with a given concentration of extract in an asymptomatic population. It is also important to correlate degree of skin test reactivity with the likelihood of occurrence of symptoms in an allergic population. This latter has been more often examined in the case of skin tests to food, rather than inhalants. The reason is, perhaps, that oral challenges with food more closely mimic natural exposure than do most bronchial or nasal challenges, in which the form and concentration of allergen employed often have little relationship to natural exposures.

B. Food Testing

The predictive value of skin testing to food has been examined in a number of populations, predominantly in children. Hill skin-tested 100 asthmatic children to a variety of foods, then conducted open challenges whenever the significance of a food's giving a positive skin test was in doubt [97]. Of 218 foods that were positive by scratch testing, 20% were believed to cause asthma and 8% to cause other allergic symptoms, and 72% were tolerated without symptoms. However, Hill questioned the value of routine skin testing to foods, since most often foods that caused asthma had already been identified by the mothers. More rigorous double-blind testing was conducted by Bock et al. [98]. They found that all positive food challenges in children over 3 years of age occurred with foods

Table 4 Sensitivity, Specificity, Positive Predictive Value, and Efficiency of the Skin Test

Sensitivity: True positive as a percent of patients with the disease (TP/TP + FN)
Specificity: True negative as a percent of patients without disease (TN/TN + FP)
Positive predictive value: Patients with disease as a percent of test positive individuals (TP/TP + FP).
Efficiency: Tested individuals correctly classified by the test as a percent of total tested (TP + TN/all subjects tested).

TP = true positive; TN = true negative; FP = false positive; FN = false negative.

that had produced at least a 3-mm wheal on prick skin testing with commercial extracts [99].

Divergent results have been reported for the value of skin testing to foods in children with eczema and migraine headaches. In children with eczema, Sampson found positive prick tests to 34 of 40 foods that produced symptoms on double-blind challenge [54]. The sensitivity and specificity of prick skin testing were superior to those of the RAST whether a 2+ or a 3+ RAST reaction was accepted as significant. Egger et al., on the other hand, in a study of food allergy as a cause of migraine headaches in children [100], found a poor correlation between the results of prick skin tests and positive challenges to foods.

C. Inhalant Testing

Few studies of provocation testing with inhalant allergens relate the degree of skin test reactivity to the occurrence of symptoms on natural exposure. Norman et al. compared patient sensitivity by titrated intradermal skin testing with the occurrence of symptoms in placebo-treated patients observed during the ragweed pollen season [2]. All subjects had responded to an advertisement for persons with late summer allergic rhinitis symptoms, yet in many subjects the symptoms did not correlate with the ragweed pollen counts. The investigators found that 16 of 23 subjects with positive intradermal skin tests (10-mm wheal with 20-mm erythema) to ragweed extract at a concentration of <1 PNU/ml (0.0027 μg *Amb a I*) had symptoms correlating with ragweed pollen counts, while only 2 of 14 with threshold skin tests to concentrations of 1 PNU/ml or greater had symptoms that correlated. Brown examined the prevalence of positive intradermal skin tests to concentrations of 1:1000 weight/volume (w/v) of 14 inhalant allergens common in Tucson, Arizona [94]. Among subjects with a negative prick skin test to the same allergen, positive intradermal skin tests were recorded in 39.3% of "allergic" and 49.2% of "nonallergic" subjects. The authors suggested caution in the interpretation of positive intradermal skin tests with extracts of 1:1,000 w/v in subjects with negative prick skin tests to the same allergen.

Bousquet et al. have demonstrated, in at least one study, a highly significant correlation (Rs = .84) between postimmunotherapy prick skin test end point to grass extract and the number of days with symptoms during the subsequent grass pollen season [101].

Vanto employed a combination of history, RAST, and bronchial or conjunctival provocation to determine clinical sensitivity to dog [49]. He then calculated the sensitivity and specificity of prick skin testing in establishing the diagnosis. When wheal sizes were compared, a prick skin test with a 3-mm wheal was found to have the best combination of sensitivity (0.976) and specificity (0.822). When a prick skin test wheal equal in size to the histamine control was employed, it improved the overall accuracy to a sensitivity of 0.917 and a specificity of 0.932. Adinoff et al., on the other hand, found that either a wheal of 3 mm or greater or erythema of 10 mm or greater had 0.90 sensitivity and specificity in subjects giving a history of symptoms on exposure to cats [83]. Adjusting the size of a positive reaction to the size of the histamine control reduced both sensitivity (0.82) and specificity (0.88).

X. PREDICTIVE VALUE

A study of the predictive value of a positive skin test in an asymptomatic population was conducted by Hagy and Settipane [102,103]. They obtained an allergy history and performed a battery of scratch skin tests in 1836 freshmen during registration at Brown and Pembroke colleges. On follow-up after 3 and 7 years, they compared the occurrence of positive prick skin tests among freshmen to the subsequent development of allergic rhinitis. After 3 years, 1.7% of those with initially negative skin tests and 18.2% of those with positive skin tests had developed symptoms of hay fever [102]. After 7 years, the prevalence of symptoms of hay fever in the two groups was 7.7% and 32%, respectively [103].

XI. OTHER CONSIDERATIONS

A. Late Cutaneous Reactions

The occurrence of progressive erythema and induration, peaking 4–6 h following the immediate skin reaction, has been of increasing interest. These reactions can be triggered by mast cell mediators released by a variety of mechanisms including allergen, anti-IgE, and nonimmunological mast cell degranulating agents, but not by histamine alone [104]. There appears to be a threshold size of the immediate reaction below which the late-phase reaction does not occur [104]. Beyond that size, there is a rough correlation between the size of the immediate reaction and the size of the resulting late-phase reaction not only in the same individual [104], but also in unselected patents [105].

The late-phase cutaneous reaction is affected differently from the immediate reaction by medication employed in the treatment of allergy an asthma. Only corticosteroids produce major, consistent suppression of the cutaneous late-phase reaction [106].

B. Delayed Reaction to Immediate Skin Tests

Green et al. examined 292 patients 48 h following the performance of intradermal skin testing with extracts of 1000 PNU/ml concentration [107]. They found that overall, 6% of intradermal skin tests were followed by a delayed reaction, which occurred after 13% of positive immediate skin tests and 5% of negative immediate skin tests. The allergens that most commonly gave rise to late reactions were

Helminthosporium (13%), feathers (11%), ragweed (9%), and *Alternaria* (8%). All others gave rise to late reactions less than 6% of the time.

C. Effect of Immunotherapy on Immediate Skin Tests

It has been appreciated since the original report of allergy immunotherapy by Noon [108] that there is a rapid decrease in sensitivity of target organs with the initiation of allergy immunotherapy. This finding has been confirmed by modern laboratory assays [109,110]. Parallel decreases in cutaneous and bronchial sensitivity to the administered allergen have been documented [111,112]. The mechanism for the suppression of skin reactivity by immunotherapy has not been established; however, it is not due to decreased IgE, which is often higher at the time the decreased tissue sensitivity is demonstrated than it is before initiation of immunotherapy. It has been suggested that decreased generation of histamine-releasing factors may be responsible [113]. It has been shown that this decrease in skin and bronchial reactivity occurred concomitantly with a decrease in symptoms on natural exposure to cat [111]. It appears that the late-phase cutaneous reaction is reduced, as well, by immunotherapy [114].

REFERENCES

1. Taylor, G., and Walker, J., Charles Harrison Blackley (1820–1900), *Clin. Allergy*, *3*, 103 (1973).
2. Norman, P. S., Lichtenstein, L. M., and Ishizaka, K., Diagnostic tests in ragweed hay fever: comparison of direct skin tests, IgE antibody measurements, and basophil histamine release, *J. Allergy Clin. Immunol.*, *52*, 210 (1973).
3. Nelson, H. S., Diagnostic procedures in allergy: I. Allergy skin testing, *Ann. Allergy*, *51*, 411 (1983).
4. Nierop, G., Voorhorst, R., and Temmerman-van de Vijver, R. L., Atopic skin tests reevaluated. X. Comparison of a perfected technique of intracutaneous skin testing and the prick test performed with a modified Morrow-Brown needle, *Ann. Allergy*, *46*, 105 (1981).
5. Vanselow, N. A., Skin testing and other diagnostic procedures, in *A Manual of Clinical Allergy*, 2nd Ed. (J. M. Sheldon, R. G. Lovell, and K. P. Matthews, ed.), W. B. Saunders, Philadelphia, 1967, p. 55.
6. Nelson, H. S., The effect of preservatives and conditions of storage on the potency of allergy extracts, *J. Allergy Clin. Immunol.*, *67*, 64 (1981).
7. Lindblad, J. H., and Farr, R. S., The incidence of positive intradermal reactions and demonstration of skin sensitizing antibody to extracts of ragweed and dust in humans without history of rhinitis or asthma, *J. Allergy*, *32*, 392 (1961).
8. Barbee, R. A., Lebowitz, M. D., Thompson, H. C., et al., Immediate skin test reactivity in a general population sample, *Ann. Intern. Med.*, *84*, 129 (1976).
9. Dreborg, S., ed., Skin tests used in type I allergy testing. Position paper. Sub-Committee on Skin Tests of the European Academy of Allergology and Clinical Immunology, *Allergy*, *44* (suppl 10), 1–59 (1989).

10. Reddy, P. M., Nagaya, H., Pascual, H. C., et al., Reappraisal of the intracutaneous tests in the diagnosis of reaginic allergy, *J. Allergy Clin. Immunol.*, *61*, 36 (1978).
11. Voorhorst, R., and van Krieken, H., Atopic skin test reevaluated. II. Variability in results of skin testing done in octuplicate, *Ann. Allergy*, *31*, 195 (1973).
12. Malling, H.-J., Diagnosis and immunotherapy of mould allergy. II. Reproducibility and relationship between skin sensitivity estimated by end-point titration and histamine equivalent reaction using skin prick test and intradermal test, *Allergy*, *40*, 354 (1985).
13. Voorhorst, R., Perfection of skin testing technique, *Allergy*, *35*, 247 (1980).
14. Voorhorst, R., and van Krieken, H., Atopic skin test reevaluated. I. Perfection of skin testing technique, *Ann. Allergy*, *31*, 137 (1973).
15. Ownby, D. R., and Anderson, J. A., An improved prick skin test procedure for young children, *J. Allergy Clin. Immunol.*, *69*, 533 (1982).
16. Indrajana, J. T., Spieksma, T., and Voorhorst, R., Comparative study of the intracutaneous, scratch and prick tests in allergy, *Ann. Allergy*, *29*, 639 (1971).
17. Krouse, H. A., and Klaustermeyer, W. B., Immediate hypersensitivity skin testing: a comparison of scratch, prick and intradermal techniques, *Immunol. Allergy Pract.*, *2*, 13 (1980).
18. Imber, W. E., Allergic skin testing, *J. Allergy Clin. Immunol.*, *60*, 47 (1979).
19. James, J. M., and Simons, F. E. R., Allergy skin testing, *Can. Med. Assoc. J.*, *120*, 330 (1979).
20. Malling, H.-J., Anderson, C. E., Boas, M. D., Holgersen, F., Munch, E. P., and Weeke, B., The allergy pricker, *Allergy*, *37*, 563 (1982).
21. Osterballe, O., and Weeke, B., A new lancet for skin prick testing, *Allergy*, *34*, 175 (1979).
22. Menardo, J. L., Bousquet, J., and Michel, F. B., Comparison of three prick test methods with the intradermal test and the RAST in the diagnosis of mite allergy, *Ann. Allergy*, *48*, 235 (1982).
23. Basomba, A., Sastre, A., Pelaez, A., et al., Standardization of the prick test: a comparative study of three methods, *Allergy*, *40*, 395 (1985).
24. Perrin, L. F., Dechamp, C. H., Deviller, P., et al., Reproducibility of skin tests: a comparative study of the Pepys prick test and the Morrow-Brown needle and their correlation with the serum IgE level, *Clin. Allergy*, *14*, 581 (1984).
25. Murphree, J. T., and Kniker, W. T., Correlation of immediate skin test responses to antigens introduced by Multi-Test and intracutaneous routes, *Ann. Allergy*, *41*, 279 (1979).
26. Mahan, C., Spector, S. L., Siegel, S. C., et al., Multi-Test versus Morrow-Brown needle, *J. Allergy Clin. Immunol.*, *86*, 275 (1990).
27. Garibaldi, E., and Slavin, R. G., Positive Multi-Test reactions do not cause false positive reactions at adjacent sites, *Ann. Allergy*, *65*, 481 (1990).
28. Adinoff, A. D., McCall, L. L., Rosloniec, D. M., et al. Comparison of six epicutaneous devices in the performance of immediate hypersensitivity skin testing, *J. Allergy Clin. Immunol.*, *84*, 168 (1989).
29. Aas, K., Some variables in skin prick testing, *Allergy*, *35*, 250 (1980).

30. Guerin, B., Lelievre, D., Pellegrin, A., et al., Tests for allergy to housedust, *Clin. Allergy*, *14*, 319 (1984).
31. Huber, B., and Berdel, D., A comparison of the Multi-Test with the prick test and Multi-Test 2, *Clin. Allergy*, *13*, 467 (1983).
32. Nelson, H. S., Rosloniec, D. M., McCall, L. L., and Ikle, D., Comparative performance of five commercial prick skin test devices (submitted for publication).
33. Pepys, J., Skin tests in diagnosis, in *Clinical Aspects of Immunology*, 2nd Ed. (P. G. H. Gell and R. R. A. Coombs, ed.), F. A. Davis, Philadelphia, 1968, p. 189–220.
34. Baer, H., Maloney, C. J., Norman, P. S., et al., The potency and group I antigen content of six commercially prepared grass pollen extracts, *J. Allergy Clin. Immunol.*, *157*, 64 (1974).
35. Yunginger, J. W., Jones, R. T., and Gleich, G. J., Studies on Alternaria antigens: II. Measurement of the relative potency of commercial Alternaria extracts by the direct RAST and by RAST inhibition, *J. Allergy Clin. Immunol.*, *58*, 405 (1976).
36. Gleich, G. J., Larson, J. B., Jones, R. T., et al., Measurement of the potency of allergy extracts by their inhibitory capacities in the radioallergosorbent test, *J. Allergy Clin. Immunol.*, *53*, 158 (1974).
37. Tuft, L., and Blumstein, G. I., Studies in food allergy. II. Sensitization to fresh fruits: clinical and experimental observations, *J. Allergy*, *13*, 574 (1942).
38. Ancona, G. R., and Schumacher, I. C., The use of raw foods as skin testing material in allergic disorders, *Calif. Med.*, *73*, 473 (1950).
39. Ortolani, C., Ispano, M., Pasttorello, E. A., et al., Comparison of results of skin prick tests (with fresh foods and commercial food extracts) and RAST in 100 patients with oral allergy syndrome, *J. Allergy Clin. Immunol.*, *83*, 683 (1989).
40. Sugar, M. S., and Lawlor, G. J., Jr., Reliability of skin testing with allergen mixes, *Immunol. Allergy Pract.*, *8*, 169 (1986).
41. Menardo, J. L., Bousquet, J., Rodiere, M., et al., Skin reactivity in infancy, *J. Allergy Clin. Immunol.*, *75*, 646 (1985).
42. Voorhorst, R., and van der Hooft-van Asbeck, M. C., Atopic skin test re-evaluated. VI. Skin reactions to compound 48/80 and histamine in patients with atopic and non-atopic chronic respiratory complaints and in normal volunteers, *Ann. Allergy*, *42*, 185 (1979).
43. Dreborg, S., Holgersson, M., Nilsson, G., and Zetterstrom, O., Dose response relationship of allergen, histamine, and histamine releasers in skin prick test and the precision of the method, *Allergy*, *42*, 117 (1987).
44. Taylor, R. J., Long, W. F., and Nelson, H. S., The development of subsensitivity to chlorpheniramine, *J. Allergy Clin. Immunol.*, *76*, 103 (1985).
45. Standardization of diagnostic work in allergy, *Acta Allergol.*, *29*, 239 (1974).
46. Malling, H.-J., Skin prick testing and the use of histamine references, *Allergy*, *39*, 596 (1984).
47. Taudorf, E., Malling, H-J., Laursen, L. C., et al., Reproducibility of histamine prick skin test: inter- and intravariation using histamine dihydrochloride 1, 5, and 10 mg/ml, *Allergy*, *40*, 344 (1985).
48. Stuckey, M. S., Witt, C. S., Schmitt, L. H., et al., Histamine sensitivity influences reactivity in allergens, *J. Allergy Clin. Immunol.*, *75*, 373 (1985).

49. Vanto, T., Efficiency of different skin prick testing methods in the diagnosis of allergy to dog, *Ann. Allergy*, *49*, 340 (1982).
50. Vohlonen, I., Terho, E. O., Koivikko, A., et al., Reproducibility of the skin prick test, *Allergy*, *44*, 525 (1989).
51. Ownby, D. R., Computerized measurement of allergen-induced skin reactions, *J. Allergy Clin. Immunol.*, *69*, 536 (1982).
52. Voorhorst, R. T., and van Krieken, H., Atopic skin test reevaluated. III. The wheal:flare ratio, the long dose-response curve, and the bioassay of allergen extracts, *Ann. Allergy*, *34*, 77 (1975).
53. Sussman, G. L., Harvey, R. P., and Schocket, A. L., Evaluation of skin test response using two techniques of measurement, *Ann. Allergy*, *48*, 75 (1982).
54. Sampson, H. A., Role of immediate food hypersensitivity in the pathogenesis of atopic dermatitis, *J. Allergy Clin. Immunol.*, *71*, 473 (1983).
55. Van Metre, T. E., Jr., Adkinson, N. F., Jr., Kagey-Sobotka, A., et al., How should we use skin testing to quantify IgE sensitivity? *J. Allergy Clin. Immunol.*, *86*, 583 (1990).
56. Bousquet, J., Lebel, B., Dhivert, H., et al., Nasal challenge with pollen grains, skin-prick tests and specific IgE in patients with grass pollen allergy, *Clin. Allergy*, *17*, 529 (1987).
57. Becker, E. L., and Rappaport, B. Z., Quantitative studies in skin testing. II. The form of the dose-response curve utilizing a quantitative response, *J. Allergy*, *19*, 317 (1948).
58. Voorhorst, R., van der Hooft-van Asbeck, M.C ., van Krieken, H., et al.: Atopic skin test reevaluated. V. The wheal-flare ratio of skin reactions to extracts of grass pollen, *Dermatophagoides pteronyssinus* and to histamine and compound 48/80, *Ann. Allergy*, *42*, 183 (1979).
59. Grammer, L. L., Silvestri, L., Suszki, I. M., et al., Evaluation and standardization of polymerized ragweed extracts by chromatography, radioimmunoassay inhibition, and end point cutaneous titration, *J. Allergy Clin. Immunol.*, *72*, 160 (1983).
60. Turkeltaub, P. C., Rastogi, S. C., Baer, H., et al., A standardized quantitative skin-test assay of allergen potency and stability: studies on the allergen dose–response curve and effect of wheal, erythema and patient selection on assay results, *J. Allergy Clin. Immunol.*, *70*, 343 (1982).
61. Dolen, W. K., Miller, B. T., Ledoux, R. L., et al., Comparison of parallel line skin test assay (PLST) and ELISA inhibition (EI) methods for determination of relative potency of polymerized grass and ragweed antigen extracts, *J. Allergy Clin. Immunol.*, *81*, 489 (1988).
62. Van Metre, T. E., Jr., Adkinson, N. F., Jr., Kagey-Sobotka, A., et al., Immunotherapy decreases skin sensitivity to ragweed extract: demonstration by midpoint skin test titration, *J. Allergy Clin. Immunol.*, *86*, 587 (1990).
63. Barbee, R. A., Brown, W. G., Kaltenborn, W., et al., Allergen skin-test reactivity in a community population sample: correlation with age, histamine skin reactions, and total serum immunoglobulin E, *J. Allergy Clin. Immunol.*, *68*, 15 (1981).
64. Skassa-Brociek, W., Manderscheid, J.-C., Michel, F.-B., et al., Skin test reactivity to histamine from infancy to old age, *J. Allergy Clin. Immunol.*, *80*, 711 (1987).
65. Halonen, M., Barbee, R. A., Lebowitz, M. D., et al., An epidemiologic study of the

interrelationships of total serum immunoglobulin E, allergy skin test reactivity, and eosinophilia, *J. Allergy Clin. Immunol.*, *69*, 221 (1982).
66. Alexander, H. L., and McConnell, F. S., The variability of skin reactions in allergy, *J. Allergy*, *2*, 23 (1930).
67. Swain, H. H., and Becker, E. L., Quantitative studies in skin testing. V. The whealing reactions of histamine and ragweed pollen extract, *J. Allergy*, *23*, 441 (1952).
68. Clarke, C. W., Mitchell, J., Nunn, A. J., et al., Reproducibility of prick skin tests to five common allergens, *Clin. Allergy*, *12*, 1 (1982).
69. Lee, R. E., Smolensky, M. H., Leach, C. S., et al., Circadian rhythms in the cutaneous reactivity to histamine and selected antigens, including phase relationship to urinary cortisol excretion, *Ann. Allergy*, *38*, 231 (1977).
70. Vichyanond, P., and Nelson, H. S., Circadian variation of skin reactivity and allergy skin tests, *J. Allergy Clin. Immunol.*, *83*, 1101 (1989).
71. Paquet, F., Boulet, L.-P., Bedard, G., et al., Influence of time of administration on allergic skin prick tests response, *Ann. Allergy*, *67*, 163 (1991).
72. Cook, T. J., MacQueen, P. M., Wittig, H. J., et al., Degree and duration of skin test suppression and side effects with antihistamines, *J. Allergy Clin. Immunol.*, *51*, 71 (1973).
73. Bantz, E. W., Dolen, W. K., Chadwick, E. W., et al., Chronic chlorpheniramine therapy: subsensitivity, drug metabolism and compliance, *Ann. Allergy*, *59*, 341 (1987).
74. Rao, K. S., Menon, P. K., Hilman, B. C., et al., Duration of the suppressive effect of tricyclic antidepressants on histamine-induced wheal-and-flare reactions in human skin, *J. Allergy Clin. Immunol.*, *82*, 752 (1988).
75. Miller, J., and Nelson, H. S., Suppression of immediate skin tests by ranitidine, *J. Allergy Clin. Immunol.*, *84*, 895 (1989).
76. Harvey, R. P., and Schocket, A. L., The effect of H_1 and H_2 blockade on cutaneous histamine response in man, *J. Allergy Clin. Immunol.*, *65*, 136 (1980).
77. Abramowitz, P. W., Perez, M. M., Johnson, C. E., et al., Effect of theophylline, terbutaline, and their combination on the immediate hypersensitivity skin test reaction, *J. Allergy Clin. Immunol.*, *66*, 123 (1980).
78. Slott, R. I., and Zweiman, B., A controlled study of the effect of corticosteroids on immediate skin test reactivity, *J. Allergy Clin. Immunol.*, *54*, 229 (1974).
79. Olson, R., Karpink, M. H., Shelanski, S., et al., Skin reactivity to codeine and histamine during prolonged corticosteroid therapy, *J. Allergy Clin. Immunol.*, *86*, 153 (1990).
80. Pipkorn, U., Hammarlung, A., and Enerbaeck, L., Prolonged treatment with topical corticosteroids results in an inhibition of the allergen-induced weal-and-flare response and a reduction in skin mast cell numbers and histamine content, *Clin. Exp. Allergy*, *19*, 19 (1989).
81. Rappaport, B. Z., and Becker, E. L., Quantitative studies in skin testing IV. The volume–response relationship, *J. Allergy*, *20*, 358 (1949).
82. Stanworth, D. R., and Kuhns, W. S., Quantitative studies on the assay of human skin sensitizing antibodies (reagins). I. An examination of factors affecting the accuracy of the Prausnitz-Kustner (P-K) test, *Immunology*, *8*, 323 (1965).
83. Adinoff, A. D., Rosloniec, D. M., McCall, L. L., et al., Immediate skin test

reactivity to Food and Drug Administration–approved standardized extracts, *J. Allergy Clin. Immunol.*, *86*, 766 (1990).

84. Chanal, I., Horst, M., Segalen, C., et al., Comparison between modified skin prick test with standardized allergen extracts and Phazet, *J. Allergy Clin. Immunol.*, *82*, 878 (1988).
85. Koller, K. Y., Pirker, C., Jarisch, R., et al., Influence of the histamine control on skin reactivity in skin testing, *Allergy*, *47*, 58 (1992).
86. Terho, E. O., Husman, K., Kivekas, J., et al., Histamine control affects the weal produced by the adjacent diluent control in skin prick tests, *Allergy*, *44*, 30 (1989).
87. Tipton, W. R., Influence of histamine controls on skin tests with Hymenoptera venom, *Ann. Allergy*, *44*, 204 (1980).
88. Norman, P. S., and Marsh, D. G., Human serum albumen and Tween 80 as stabilizers of allergen solutions, *J. Allergy Clin. Immunol.*, *62*, 314 (1978).
89. Haahtela, T., and Jokela, H., Influence of the pollen season on immediate skin test reactivity to common allergens, *Allergy*, *35*, 15 (1980).
90. McLean, J. A., Management of hypersensitivity to stinging insects, in *A Manual of Clinical Allergy*, 2nd Ed. (J. M. Sheldon, R. G. Lovell, and K. P. Mathews, eds.), W. B. Saunders, Philadelphia, 1967, p. 315.
91. Huggins, K. G. S., and Brostoff, J., Local production of specific IgE antibodies in allergic rhinitis patients with negative skin tests, *Lancet*, *ii*, 148 (1975).
92. Small, P., Barrett, D., Frenkiel, S., et al., Measurement of antigen specific IgE in nasal secretions of patients with perennial rhinitis, *Ann. Allergy*, *55*, 68 (1985).
93. Miadonna, A., Leggieri, E., Tedeschi, A., et al., Clinical significance of specific IgE determination on nasal secretion, *Clin. Allergy*, *13*, 155 (1983).
94. Brown, W. E., Halonen, M. J., Kaltenborn, W. T., et al., The relationship of respiratory allergy, skin test reactivity, and serum IgE in a community population sample, *J. Allergy Clin. Immunol.*, *63*, 328 (1979).
95. Killian, D., Cockcroft, D. W., Hargreave, F. E., et al., Factors in allergen-induced asthma: relevance of the intensity of the airways allergen reaction and nonspecific bronchial reactivity, *Clin. Allergy*, *6*, 219 (1976).
96. Cockcroft, D. W., Murdock, K. Y., Kirby, J., et al., Prediction of airway responsiveness to allergen from skin sensitivity to allergen and airway responsiveness to histamine, *Am. Rev. Respir. Dis.*, *135*, 264 (1987).
97. Hill, L. W., Food sensitivity in 100 asthmatic children, *N. Engl. J. Med.*, *238*, 657 (1948).
98. Bock, S. A., Lee, W.-Y., Remigio, L. K., et al., Appraisal of skin tests with food extracts for diagnosis of food hypersensitivity, *Clin. Allergy*, *8*, 559 (1978).
99. Bock, S. A., Lee, W.-Y.., Remigio, L. K., et al., Studies of hypersensitivity reactions to foods in infants and children, *J. Allergy Clin. Immunol.*, *62*, 327 (1978).
100. Egger, J., Carter, C. M., Wilson, J., et al., Is migraine food allergy? A double-blind controlled trial of oligoantigenic diet treatment, *Lancet*, *ii*, 865 (1983).
101. Bousquet, J., Maasch, H., Martinot, B., et al., Double-blind, placebo-controlled immunotherapy with six grass-pollen allergoids. II. Comparison between parameters assessing the efficacy of immunotherapy, *J. Allergy Clin. Immunol.*, *82*, 439 (1988).
102. Hagy, G. W., and Settipane, G. A., Prognosis of positive allergy skin tests in an

asymptomatic population: a three-year follow-up of college students, *J. Allergy*, *48*, 200 (1971).

103. Hagy, G. W., and Settipane, G. A., Risk factors for developing asthma and allergic rhinitis: a 7-year follow-up of college students, *J. Allergy Clin. Immunol.*, *58*, 330 (1976).
104. DeShazo, R. D., Levinson, A. I., Dvorak, H. F., et al., The late phase skin reaction: evidence for activation of the coagulation system in an IgE dependent reaction in man, *J. Immunol.*, *122*, 692 (1979).
105. Agarwal, K., and Zetterstrom, O., Diagnostic significance of late cutaneous allergic responses and their correlation with radioallergosorbent test, *Clin. Allergy*, *12*, 489 (1982).
106. DeShazo, R. D., Levinson, A. I., and Dvorak, H. F., The late phase skin reaction: paradigm or epiphenomenon? *Ann. Allergy*, *51*, 166 (1983).
107. Green, G. R., Zweiman, B., Beerman, H., et al., Delayed skin reactions to inhalant antigens, *J. Allergy*, *40*, 224 (1967).
108. Noon, L., Prophylactic inoculation against hay fever, *Lancet*, *i*, 1572 (1911).
109. Dantzler, B. S., Tipton, W. R., Nelson, H. S., et al., Tissue threshold changes during the first months of immunotherapy, *Ann. Allergy*, *45*, 213 (1980).
110. Tipton, W. R., and Nelson, H. S., Experience with daily immunotherapy in 59 adult allergic patients, *J. Allergy Clin. Immunol.*, *69*, 194 (1982).
111. Ohman, J. L., Jr., Findlay, S. R., and Leiterman, K. M., Immunotherapy in cat-induced asthma: double-blind trial with evaluation of in vivo and in vitro response, *J. Allergy Clin. Immunol.*, *74*, 230 (1984).
112. Bousquet, J., Calvayrac, P. O., Guerin, B., et al., Immunotherapy with a standardized *Dermatophagoides pteronyssinus* extract. I. In vivo and in vitro parameters after a short course of treatment, *J. Allergy Clin. Immunol.*, *76*, 734 (1985).
113. Kuna, P., Alam, R., Kuzminska, B., et al., The effect of preseasonal immunotherapy on the production of histamine-releasing factor (HRF) by mononuclear cells from patients with seasonal asthma: results of a double-blind, placebo-controlled, randomized study, *J. Allergy Clin. Immunol.*, *83*, 816 (1989).
114. Pienkowski, M. M., Norman, P. S., and Lichtenstein, L. M., Suppression of late-phase skin reactions by immunotherapy with ragweed extract, *J. Allergy Clin. Immunol.*, *76*, 729 (1985).

27

Delayed Hypersensitivity, Cell-Mediated Immunity, and Anergy

Charles H. Kirkpatrick

*University of Colorado Health Sciences Center
Denver, Colorado*

I. INTRODUCTION

The cell-mediated components of the immune response are responsible for regulation of the intensity of responses by T lymphocytes and B lymphocytes, for production of interleukins and interferons that serve as growth factors and activators of defense mechanisms by effector cells such as T cells and macrophages, and for lysis of virus-infected cells and tumor cells. A number of clinical conditions such as contact allergic reactions, graft-versus-host disease, rejection of allografts, delayed hypersensitivity, and granuloma formation are expressions of cell-mediated immunity. It is also the component of the immune system that provides protective immunity against infections with mycobacteria, many fungi, and certain parasites and viruses, such as herpesviruses. Anergy is a condition in which a patient or experimental animal is unable to express delayed hypersensitivity or other cell-mediated responses. Anergy may be global, when the subject is unable to respond to any antigen, or limited, when the subject is unable to respond to antigens of one infectious agent. For example, some patients with chronic candidiasis are unable to develop cell-mediated immune responses to *Candida* antigens but are able to respond normally to other antigens.

This chapter will review the mechanisms of expression of cell-mediated immune responses and the consequences of deficient function of this portion of the immune system. Selected topics concerning correction of deficient cell-mediated immunity and induction of anergy in clinical situations will be discussed.

II. HISTORICAL CONSIDERATIONS

Perhaps the first studies of cell mediated immune responses involved experimental tuberculosis. In the late 1800s, Robert Koch [1] reported that mycobacterium-infected guinea pigs developed marked local inflammatory responses when tubercle bacilli or the culture fluids in which the mycobacteria had been grown were injected into the skin. In some experiments the inflammatory reactions killed the mycobacteria. The active material in the culture fluids became known as "old tuberculin," and for years it was used as a diagnostic reagent for detection of clinical tuberculosis.

The work of Zinsser [2] described features of delayed-type hypersensitivity that distinguished it from other forms of immunological inflammation. He reported that the reactions required several hours to become fully expressed and several days to subside. He also noted that this form of hypersensitivity could not be transferred to nonimmune recipients with the serum of immune donors. This feature of delayed-type hypersensitivity was confirmed by Dienes and Mallory in 1932 [3].

The "cellular" nature of contact allergic reactions and delayed hypersensitivity was established in guinea pigs by Landsteiner and Chase in the early 1940s [4,5]. The first report described transfer of contact sensitivity to picryl chloride with peritoneal exudate cells from sensitized donors [4]. The later paper [5] showed that delayed hypersensitivity to tuberculin could be transferred by the same procedure. In 1949, Lawrence [6] reported that peripheral blood leukocytes from tuberculin-sensitive human donors would transfer tuberculin reactivity to unsensitized human recipients.

The roles of cell-mediated immune responses in immunobiology have been defined in the past three decades. Mitchison, in 1954, described the role of specifically reactive lymphocytes in rejection of transplanted tumor cells [7]. The significance of cell-mediated immunity in the pathogenesis of certain infectious diseases was defined. Lurie [8–10] reported that macrophages from rabbits with tuberculosis had greater microbicidal activity than macrophages of control rabbits. It was also found that depletion of macrophages by in vivo irradiation abolished the ability to express delayed hypersensitivity, but the response could be restored by administration of peritoneal exudate cells or bone marrow cells [11].

By the mid-1960s, the importance of antigen-responsive lymphocytes in macrophage activation and cellular immunity had been established [12–14]. This led to experiments providing evidence that most of the cells in the inflammatory lesions of cell-mediated immune reactions were not specifically reactive against the test antigen. When radiolabeled lymphoid cells from sensitized donors were transferred to unsensitized recipients and delayed hypersensitivity reactions were elicited, only a few of the labeled donor cells were found in the lesions [15,16]. This suggested that there must be mechanisms for recruitment of many recipient cells into the inflammatory sites. The first in vitro studies that provided evidence for an amplification process in cellular immunity were reported by George and Vaughn in 1962 [17]. Ultimately, it was learned that antigen-reactive cells respond to antigenic stimulation by secreting factors known as lymphokines [18], and that these factors, through a variety of activities, are responsible for the inflammatory lesions and antimicrobial activities of cell-mediated immunity. The molecular nature of many of these factors, including interleukins, colony-stimulating factors, and interferons, has been defined, and their receptors have been identified. In mice, there is evidence that products of mast cells are also important for expression of delayed hypersensitivity [19].

III. PATHOGENESIS OF CELL-MEDIATED IMMUNITY

We now know that helper T cells, the cells that produce most of the lymphokines, can be divided into at least two subpopulations on the basis of their patterns of lymphokine production [20]. TH_1 cells produce interleukin-2, interferon-γ, lymphotoxin, interleukin-3 (IL-3), granulocyte-macrophage colony-stimulating factor (GM-CSF), and tumor necrosis factor (TNF). These lymphokines are essential for macrophage activation and expression of delayed-type hypersensitivity. The second subpopulation of helper T cells (TH_2 cells) produces IL-3, IL-4, IL-5, and IL-6, and these factors are essential for optimal functions of B lymphocytes, including antibody secretion and isotype switching to immunoglobulin G (IgG) and IgE production. Interleukin-5 is an important growth factor for eosinophils. Recent studies provide support for the presence of similar T-helper subpopulations in humans [21,22].

Activation of T-helper cells requires antigens that are processed by antigen-presenting cells and presented to the specific T lymphocyte receptor in association with class II molecules of the major histocompatibility complex (MHC). These T cells also bear CD4 molecules.

The second major population of T lymphocytes is composed of cells that have "suppressive" effects on immune responses, and cells that have cytolytic activity. These cells bear CD8 molecules. Cytolytic T lymphocytes are activated by endogenous antigens that are presented by a process that is restricted by class I MHC molecules.

IV. EVALUATION OF CELL-MEDIATED IMMUNITY

A. Delayed Hypersensitivity

The classic method for evaluating cell-mediated immunity in vivo involves injection of a small volume (usually 0.1 ml) of standardized antigen intradermally. A positive response is characterized by a field of induration at the injection site. In assessment of immune competence, diameters of induration of 0.5 cm or greater are scored as positive. In epidemiological surveys for tuberculosis, indurations of 1.0 cm or greater in response to intermediate-strength purified protein derivative (PPD) are scored as positive. Positive delayed hypersensitivity reactions are usually accompanied by erythema, but only the field of induration should be scored in quantitating the response.

In evaluation of immunocompetence, one should employ antigens to which most persons should be reactive. These include antigens that are used for childhood immunizations (diphtheria toxoid, tetanus toxoid, mumps skin test antigen) or antigens from ubiquitous microorganisms (streptococcal proteins, *Candida albicans*, *Trichophyton* sp.). The place of residence of the patient may increase the probability of sensitization to regional antigens such as histoplasmin, blastomycin, or coccidioidin.

Clinical studies have described the frequency of delayed-type hypersensitivity responses in patient populations. Gordon and associates [23] studied responsiveness to tetanus toxoid, *C. albicans*, streptokinase–streptodornase (SK/SD), *Trichophyton* sp., tuberculin (PPD), and coccidioidin in 81 adult volunteers aged 19–100 years (mean age 52 years). Positive responses to *C. albicans*, SK/SD, and tetanus toxoid were observed in 92%, 51%, and 49%, respectively (Table 1). None of their patients was anergic, and none of their subjects reacted to the glycerol-saline diluent. A positive skin test produced a field of induration of 25 mm^2 or greater. If one assumes that the fields of induration were circular, diameters of

Table 1 Delayed Hypersensitivity in Human Subjects[a]

	Percent Responders	
Test antigen	Gordon et al.	Palmer and Reed
Candida albicans	92	63
SK/SD	51	NT
Tetanus	49	NT
Trichophyton	42	62
PPD	30	33
Coccidioidin	10	12
Histoplasmin	NT	25
Mumps	NT	67

[a]These data are from publications by Gordon et al. [23] and Palmer and Reed [24]. The doses and sources of test antigens are summarized in Table 2.

SK/SD = streptokinase–streptodornase (Varidase, Lederle); NT = not tested; PPD = purified protein derivative.

approximately 5.6 mm were scored as positive. Only the delayed-type response to tetanus toxoid was age-related; positive responses were noted in only 27% of subjects over 70 years of age.

They concluded that screening for anergy could be done with *C. albicans*, 1:1000, and tetanus toxoid, 2 LfU/ml.

Palmer and Reed [24] studied delayed hypersensitivity responses by patients in the Albuquerque, New Mexico, Veterans Administration Hospital. All consenting subjects (n = 752) in the medial, surgical, orthopedic, neurosurgical, and intensive care wards were studied, irrespective of their diagnosis. The antigens used were similar to the panel described by Gordon et al. [23], except that there were instances in which the suppliers differed (Table 2). The age of their

Table 2 Dosages and Sources of Skin Test Antigens for Evaluating Delayed Hypersensitivity[a]

Antigen/dose	Gordon et al.	Palmer & Reed
Candida albicans		
1:100[b]	Pittsburgh VAH	NT
1:1000	Pittsburgh VAH	NT
1:500	NT	Hollister-Stier
SK/SD[c]		
50 U/ml	Lederle	NT
5 U/ml	Lederle	NT
Tetanus toxoid		
10 LfU/ml[b]	Merrill	NT
2 LfU/ml	Merrill	NT
Trichophyton		
1:100[b]	Pittsburgh VAH	NT
1:1000	Pittsburgh VAH	NT
1:500	NT	Hollister-Stier
PPD		
5 TU[b]	Connaught or Parke-Davis	CDC
Coccidioidin		
1:100[b]	Cutter or Iatric Corp.	Cutter
Histoplasmin	NT	Parke-Davis
Mumps	NT	Eli Lilly

[a]Antigens and concentrations as reported by Gordon et al. [23] and Palmer and Reed [24].
[b]Recommended concentration.
[c]SK/SD, marketed as Varidase, is no longer available.
Pittsburgh VAH = Pittsburgh Veterans Administration Hospital; NT = not tested; SK/SD = streptokinase–streptodornase; PPD = purified protein derivative; CDC = Centers of Disease Control.

population ranged from 18 to 85 years, and the median age was in the "fifth decade." Both erythema and induration were measured, but they noted that scoring erythema alone did not increase the number of positive reactors. The percentages of responders with indurations of 5 mm or greater are presented in Table 1. Fifty-seven (7.6%) of their patients did not respond to any test antigen. Most of the appropriate antigens are commercially available. Our institution uses Dermatophyton "O," 1:100 (Hollister-Stier), *fluid* tetanus toxoid (Wyeth-Ayerst) diluted to 10 LfU/ml, mumps skin test antigen (Eli Lilly), Trichophyton 1:40 (Hollister-Stier), and PPD 5TU (Parke-Davis). Other antigens such as histoplasmin and spherulin (coccidioidin) are used if the patient has resided in endemic areas. In special situations there may be an interest in studying the ability of a patient to *develop* delayed hypersensitivity. In this case a nonenvironmental antigen or "neoantigen" is used. Examples are the hemocyanin from the keyhole limpet (KLH) or the contact sensitizer 1-chloro-2,4-dinitrobenzene (CDNB). Sensitization to KLH is done by injecting 100 μg of the antigen intradermally. Sensitization to CDNB is done by dissolving 500 or 1000 μg of the material in acetone and applying it to a small area (approximately 5.0 cm^2) of the skin. In Chapter 28 in this volume, Drs. Lauerma and Maibach discuss the significance of various skin sites in contact allergy. Delayed hypersensitivity or contact allergy should be demonstrable about 10 days after sensitization. Delayed hypersensitivity to KLH is demonstrated by intradermal injection of 0.1 ml of a solution containing 1.0 or 10.0 μg KLH/ml. Contact allergy to CDNB is demonstrated by a spontaneous recurrence of inflammation at the site of application of the sensitizer or by application of 50 μg of CDNB in acetone to a different skin site. An inflammatory response develops in 48–72 h.

B. Lymphocyte Transformation

Antigen-responsive T lymphocytes respond to antigen in vitro by proliferation and increased DNA synthesis. In most laboratories, the radioactive label is tritiated thymidine and is added after the cells have been in culture for 5 or 6 days. The cells are harvested 4–16 h later, and the incorporated radioactivity is measured [25]. The results are calculated by comparing counts per minute (CPM) by the antigen-stimulated cells to the CPM by unstimulated cells. Some laboratories express results as CPM by stimulated cells minus CPM by unstimulated cells ($CPM_{stim} - CPM_{control}$). Others use a ratio of stimulated CPM to resting CPM ($CPM_{stim}/CPM_{control}$); a value of 3.0 or greater usually indicates a positive response. Since thymidine incorporation is related to doubling of the DNA, it has been argued that the values should be expressed as the logarithm of the CPM [26].

Lymphocyte transformation is the most widely used in vitro assay for cell-mediated immunity.

C. Lymphokine Production

Lymphokines are the effector molecules that produce the biological effects of cell-mediated immune reactions. Production of lymphokines by antigen-activated cells has been an important technique for defining cellular defects in certain immunodeficiency syndromes [27,28]. Currently available bioassays and immunoassays allow quantitation of interleukins, interferons, and growth factors that are produced by T cells in response to antigens. In situ hybridization techniques allow identification of individual cells that have produced the mRNA for selected lymphokines as a consequence of activation by antigens.

D. T Cell–Mediated Cytotoxicity

A consequence of activation of CD8+ T lymphocytes by antigens that are produced within the test animal or patient is production of T cells that are specifically cytotoxic for antigen-bearing cells. Examples of "internally" produced antigens are proteins produced during viral infections, antigens expressed by tumor cells, and alloantigens on transplanted cells. These antigens are presented to MHC class I–bearing CD8+ T cells. The interaction between these "killer" cells and the target cells is specific for the antigen against which the T cells are reactive and is restricted to targets that have the same MHC I determinants as the T cells.

Lytic injury to the target cell is quantitated by first labeling the target cells with a radioisotope such as ^{51}Cr and determining the percentage of the radiolabel that is released from the cells after incubation with the cytolytic T cells. While the test is specific and sensitive, it is rarely used in clinical medicine.

V. DISORDERS WITH IMPAIRED CELL-MEDIATED IMMUNITY

It is not the purpose of this chapter to provide a comprehensive discussion of immunodeficiency syndromes. However, most disorders in which development, maturation, or function of the T lymphocytes is abnormal are accompanied by impaired expression of cell-mediated immunity. This was first recognized in infants with severe combined immunodeficiency (SCID) and infants who were born without a thymus gland. These patients fail to thrive and have repeated infections with opportunistic organisms such as *Pneumocystis carinii* and *C. albicans*. Correction of the underlying defect with transplantation of bone marrow [29] or thymus tissue [30,31] has been accompanied, in some patients, by restoration of cell-mediated immunity and improved health. An especially exciting recent development in this field concerns infants who lack the enzyme adenosine deaminase and have a form of SCID. Transfection of their blood lymphocytes with the gene for adenosine deaminase has corrected the metabolic defect in their lymphoid cells and has been accompanied by restoration of immunocompetence [32].

Application of the techniques of molecular biology to the study of immunodeficiency patients has revealed a number of site-specific defects that cause impaired functions of T lymphocytes. The abnormalities vary and include impaired gene transcription and lymphokine production, impaired transduction of signals from T cell receptors to cellular G proteins, and impaired production of single chains of the CD3 complex, with subnormal expression of T cell receptors [reviewed in Ref. 28]. The end results are similar, although the magnitude of the defect differs from patient to patient. Identification of these "experiments of nature" greatly enhances our understanding of the biochemical events that occur as a consequence of the interaction of T cell receptors with antigens and eventuate in T cell activation and immune responses.

It is also recognized that diseases or treatments may modify immunocompetence. Immune deficiency and infections with opportunistic microorganisms are common in recipients of high doses of corticosteroids or cytoreductive therapy and in recipients of irradiation therapy [33]. In addition, there are a number of diseases such as Hodgkin's disease [34], certain lymphomas [34], uremia [35], and chronic infectious diseases [36–39] in which there is loss of cell-mediated immunity. The defect may be global, with inability to respond to any antigens in a test panel, or more selective, with impaired responses to some antigens and normal responses to others.

The induration in delayed hypersensitivity responses is due to deposition of fibrin and entrapment of water within the lesions [40]. Thus, patients who are deficient in fibrinogen or subjects who are anticoagulated cannot express palpable delayed hypersensitivity reactions even though they have cellular infiltration at the site [40–42].

The epidemic of human immunodeficiency virus (HIV) infection has demonstrated that a variety of mechanisms may lead to immunodeficiency and susceptibility to infections with opportunistic organisms. The most dramatic laboratory finding in HIV-infected patients is the profound depletion of CD4+ helper T cells [43], but HIV-infected patients have many abnormalities of T cell function, including impaired production of IL-2 and interferon-γ, impaired expression of IL-2 receptors by lymphocytes, and autoantibodies against their own T cells and B cells [44]. A curious finding in HIV infections has been that only a few T cells appear to be infected with HIV even in the presence of marked dysfunction of the T cell system. Recent studies may explain this. Infection of CD4+ cells with HIV or even crosslinking the CD4 molecules with gp120 from HIV renders the cells susceptible to killing by apoptosis [45–47]. This mechanism of cell death is important in normal differentiation, but it appears also to have a role in abnormal cell death and in susceptibility of T lymphocytes to corticosteroids.

VI. MODULATION OF CELL-MEDIATED IMMUNITY

Delayed hypersensitivity, lymphocyte transformation, and lymphokine production are cell-mediated immune responses that are naturally acquired during infection with many microorganisms including mycobacteria, many fungi, and certain viruses and parasites. These responses are also induced by immunization with certain vaccines, such as mumps vaccine and diphtheria and tetanus toxoids.

One of the first demonstrations of induced alteration of delayed hypersensitivity is known as the Chase–Sulzberger phenomenon [48,49]. Intravenous administration or feeding of simple chemicals or haptens prevented induction of delayed hypersensitivity in spite of subsequent sensitizations. The suppressive effect is antigen-specific and is mediated by T lymphocytes [50]. Two stages of suppression have been identified. "Afferent" suppression results from failure to develop T cells (TH_1) that express delayed hypersensitivity; T cells from these animals will not transfer delayed hypersensitivity to nonimmune syngeneic recipients. Animals with "efferent" suppression have T cells that are capable of expressing delayed hypersensitivity, but their function is suppressed by the host.

Of clinical importance are disorders in which infections or products of infectious organisms either directly or indirectly produce immunosuppression. Some patients with the recent diagnosis of tuberculosis have suppressed cell-mediated immunity. In vitro studies have shown that the impaired responses are due to a peripheral blood leukocyte that adheres to plastic and is radiation-resistant [51]. Other reports have identified these cells as monocytes/macrophages [52], and Kleinhenz et al. [37] have reported that in vitro addition of mycobacterial arabinogalactan stimulates production of prostaglandins by monocytes.

Impaired cell-mediated immune responses have been reported in patients with chronic coccidioidomycosis [36], cutaneous leishmaniasis [38], chronic infections with "atypical" mycobacteria such as *M. avium-intracellulare* (MAI) [39], and Hodgkin's disease [53].

A role for prostaglandins as mediators of immunosuppression is strongly suggested and is supported by the finding that addition of indomethacin to the cell cultures and treatment of immunosuppressed patients with indomethacin may produce improvements and even normalization of cell-mediated immune responses [39,53]. As shown in Fig. 1, in HIV-negative patients with chronic pulmonary infections with MAI, treatment with 25 mg t.i.d. of indomethacin was accompanied by expression of delayed-type hypersensitivity to PPD and normalization of T cell proliferation responses to PPD. T cell responses to the mitogen phytohemagglutinin also improved but did not become normal (Fig. 2). The suppressive factor that was present in the serum disappeared during indomethacin treatment [54]. A recent report described a patient with disseminated MAI and a defect in monocyte bactericidal activity who had clinical and bactericidal im-

Skin Tests

Patients	PRE	POST
1	2	15
2	0	10
3	0	13
4	0	15

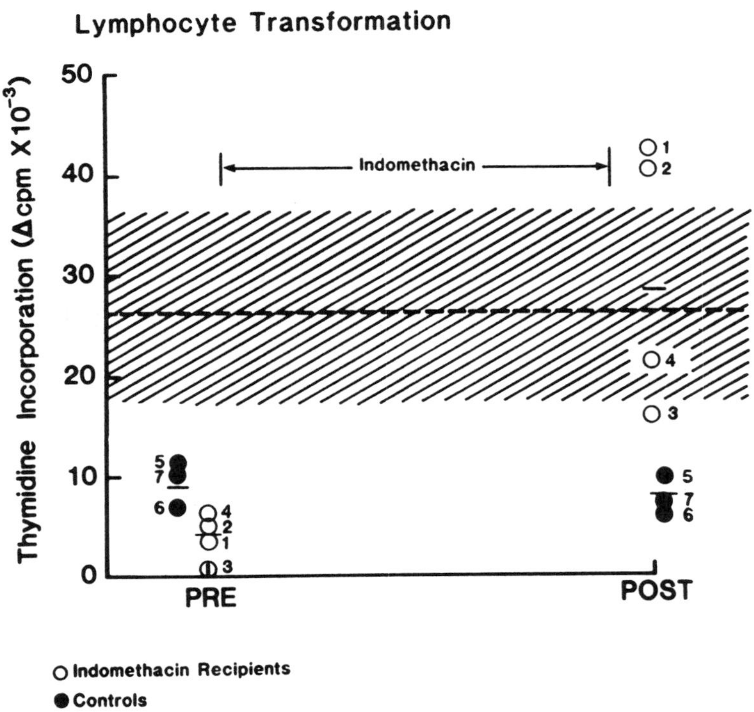

Figure 1 Effect of indomethacin on cell-mediated immune responses to purified protein derivative (PPD) by patients with pulmonary disease due to *Mycobacterium avium-intracellulare*. Indomethacin-treated patients are designated by open circles and control patients are designated by solid circles. All patients were receiving multidrug therapy; none was HIV-infected. Indomethacin was given orally, 25 mg t.i.d.

Note that all four indomethacin-treated patients acquired the ability to express delayed hypersensitivity to PPD (5 tuberculin units), and their peripheral blood lymphocytes showed normal proliferation responses to PPD (10 μg/ml). The hatched areas indicate the normal range for PPD-positive subjects. (From Ref. 39.)

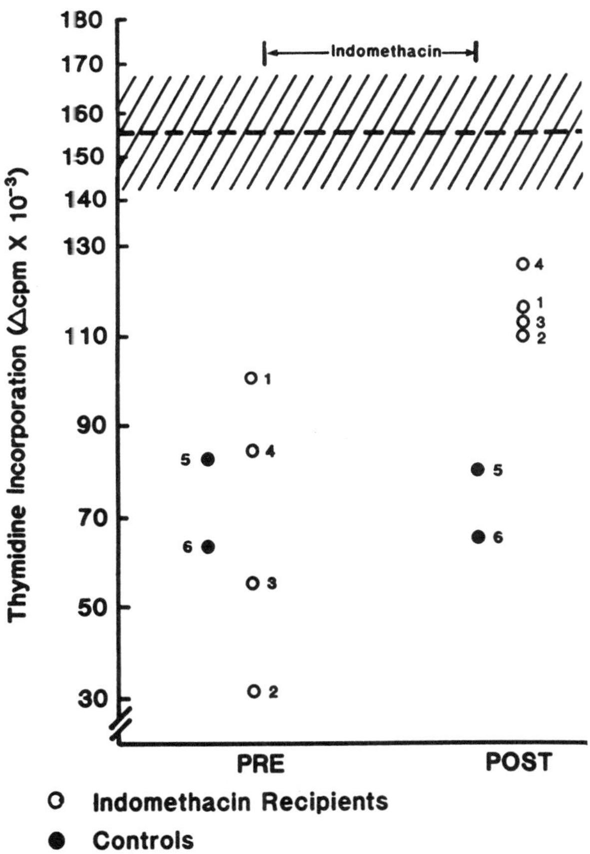

Figure 2 Effect of indomethacin on T cell proliferation responses to phytohemagglutinin. Indomethacin-treated patients are designated by open circles and control patients are designated by solid circles. Note that all indomethacin-treated patients had improved responses by phytohemagglutinin (0.33 μg/ml). The response by normal subjects is indicated by the hatched area. (From Ref. 39.)

provement during indomethacin treatment [55]. Preliminary data indicate that the improvements in cell-mediated immunity may be the result of increased production of cytokines by antigen-activated T-cells (D. E. Edwards and C. H. Kirkpatrick, unpublished).

There are other examples of clinical use of immunomodulators. Cimetidine therapy has improved cell-mediated immunity and produced clinical benefits in members of a family with chronic mucocutaneous candidiasis [56]. Parenteral treatment with interferon-γ has produced reversal-like reactions in the skin of patients with lepromatous leprosy [57]. Interleukin-2 has been studied as an agent for improving immunocompetence in patients with AIDS, but with little success [58]. However, interferon-α has been effective treatment for Kaposi's sarcoma in these patients [59].

Transfer factors have the potential for wide application in treatment of certain chronic infectious diseases. While many of the case reports of immunotherapy with transfer factors are anecdotal and involve patients in whom transfer factors were used as the last attempt to achieve clinical remissions, impressive results have been recorded. Especially noteworthy are the results in patients with chronic or recurrent infections with herpes simplex virus [60]. This clinical trial resulted in improvement of all 11 patients, six of whom had complete remissions. An important component of the study was the crossover design, in which some patients were changed to a similar preparation from a donor who lacked cell-mediated immunity to herpes simplex virus. These patients relapsed, but responded when they were returned to treatment with the transfer factor from the herpes-immune donor.

Patients with chronic mucocutaneous candidiasis have had reconstitution of immune responses [25] and clinical responses to treatment with *Candida*-specific transfer factor [61]. The best results were obtained if the patients were put in remission with systemic antifungal therapy and then given *Candida*-specific transfer factor to correct the immunological defect. None of these patients relapsed, while relapses were common in the patients who received a transfer factor–like material from a donor who lacked cell-mediated immunity to *Candida*.

The effects of transfer factors on immune responses are summarized in Fig. 3. In this study, the transfer factor donor had delayed hypersensitivity to streptococcal antigens (Varidase), *C. albicans*, and mumps, but not to PPD. Before treatment the recipient was anergic (unable to express any delayed-type responses), and her T cells did not respond to antigens by increased proliferation or lymphokine production. Transfer factor therapy corrected the deficient delayed hypersensitivity and lymphokine production; there was no change in the T cell proliferation response.

After a few months the effect of the transfer factor was lost, but it could be restored by additional treatments.

Recently, McMeeking et al. [63] have reported successful treatment of intestinal cryptosporidiosis in patients with AIDS. All but one of the patients responded to material from a coccidia-immune donor, but six of seven patients failed to respond to the placebo preparation.

An especially interesting study with a transfer factor was reported by Steele and associates [63]. They used a herpes zoster–specific transfer factor to protect children with acute leukemia from chickenpox. Only one patient in the treatment

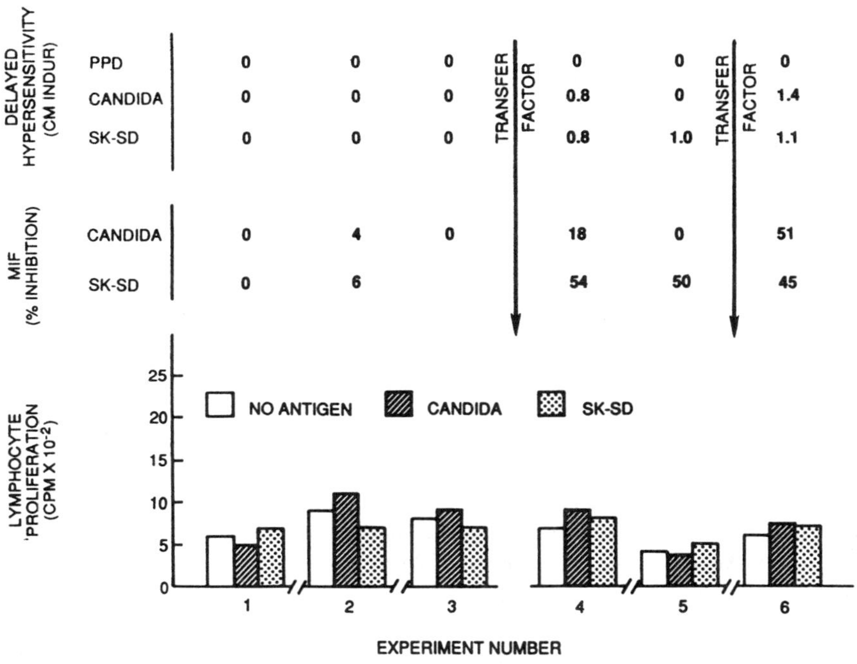

Figure 3 Effects of transfer factors on cell-mediated immune responses. The patient was a 27-year-old white women with chronic mucocutaneous candidiasis. She was anergic and her lymphocytes did not respond to in vitro activation with *Candida* or streptococcal antigens (SK-SD) by secreting lymphokines (MIF) or by increased proliferation. Administration of a transfer factor from a donor who had cell-mediated immune responses to *Candida* and SK-SD, but not to purified protein derivative (PPD), resulted in expression of delayed hypersensitivity and lymphokine production to *Candida* and SK-SD, but not PPD. The effect of the *Candida*-specific transfer factor was lost after a few months, but was restored when the transfer factor treatment was repeated.

group (n = 16) developed clinical chickenpox during the duration of the study, but 13 of the 15 patients in the control group developed chickenpox, and three patients had systemic infections. This result suggests that transfer factors may be useful for prevention of certain infectious diseases for which vaccines are not available.

Progress has been made in definition of the properties and activities of transfer factors (Table 3). The effects are antigen-specific and are primarily related to expression of cell-mediated immunity. A recent report describes purification of murine transfer factors with different specificities to apparent homogeneity [64].

Table 3 Properties of Transfer Factors

Antigen-specific
Proteinaceous
Molecular weight $\simeq$ 5000 Da
Produced by T cells
Transfer ability to express cell-mediated immunity
React with antigen

VII. INDUCTION OF ANERGY IN CLINICAL SITUATIONS

Autoimmune diseases are the result of immunological inflammatory responses to self-antigens. Normally, autoreactive T cells are eliminated in the thymus [65], or their functions may be suppressed in the peripheral lymphoid system. While autoimmunity may be simply described as an abnormality of immunoregulation and a breakdown in self-tolerance, many immunological abnormalities have been identified in various autoimmune diseases. These include activated lymphoid cells in the inflammatory lesions, autoantibody production, expression of MHC molecules or self-antigens by the target organ, and loss of normal suppressor mechanisms.

Currently, induction of tolerance or anergy against autoantigens is being investigated as a method for treatment of certain autoimmune diseases. Remarkable success has been achieved in certain animal models, and a clinical trial is under way in patients with multiple sclerosis.

Specific immunotherapy is possible because several antigens that serve as the targets of autoimmunity have been identified. These include myelin basic protein and proteolipid protein in multiple sclerosis, thyroperoxidase in Grave's disease, S-antigen in retinitis, and the acetylcholine receptor in myasthenia gravis. Oral administration of myelin basic protein can suppress development of experimental autoimmune encephalitis (EAE) and can slow the clinical course or even induce remissions in animals with early EAE [66]. The suppressive effect is mediated by CD8+ T cells that secrete transforming growth factor-β in response to activation by the antigen [67].

A second strategy involves immunization of the test animals with the portions of the variable regions of the T cell receptors that are involved in recognition of the alloantigen [68,69]. T cell vaccination induces anti-idiotypic responses against antigen-recognition units of T cell receptor and has also been effective in prevention and treatment of experimental autoimmune encephalitis [70,72]. T cells from vaccinated rats transfer protection against EAE to recipients [71] (Table 4). Administration to sensitized mice of peptides from myelin basic protein in Freund's incomplete adjuvant may prevent progression of the disease [72]. This effect also appears to be mediated by CD8+ T cells [73].

Table 4 Protection Against Experimental Autoimmune Encephalitis (EAE) by Vβ8-Specific T Cells

No. of Cells	Recipients with EAE
None	5/5
1×10^7	0/3
3×10^7	0/5

Source: Data from Ref. 71.

VIII. SUMMARY AND CONCLUSIONS

The cell-mediated immune system is essential for immunological resistance to infections with mycobacteria, certain fungi, and many parasites and viruses, such as the herpesviruses. Failure of this system to function normally can render patients susceptible to infections with opportunistic microorganisms. This is dramatically illustrated by patients with HIV infections, but has been known for years in patients with certain malignant diseases and patients who receive immunosuppressive treatments.

Delayed hypersensitivity is a means for assessing the integrity of cell-mediated immunity in vivo. To express delayed hypersensitivity, the patient must have antigen-presenting cells that are capable of processing and presenting the test antigen to CD4+ T cells, T cells that express the appropriate receptor for the antigen and are capable of transducing the signal to the cytoplasmic environment, normal secretion of the appropriate cytokines, and tissues that respond to the inflammatory stimuli from the cytokines. Thus the entire arc of a cell-mediated immune response may be examined by testing for delayed hypersensitivity.

Understanding of the mechanisms for altering cell-mediated immune responses is now being applied to clinical medicine. Correction of immunological defects has improved resistance of patients to a number of opportunistic infections. Induction of anergy, either to the autoantigen or to the T cell receptor that recognizes the antigen, may provide a novel approach to control of certain autoimmune diseases.

REFERENCES

1. Koch, R., Weitere Mittheilungen über ein Heilmittel gegen Tuberculose, *Dtsch. Med. Wochenschr.*, *16*, 1029–1032 (1890).
2. Zinsser, H., Studies on the tuberculin reaction and on specific hypersensitivities in bacterial infection, *J. Exp. Med.*, *34*, 495–524 (1921).
3. Dienes, L., and Mallory, T. B., Histological studies of hypersensitivity reactions. The

contrast between the histological responses in the tuberculin (allergic) type and the anaphylactic type of skin reactions, *Am. J. Pathol.*, *8*, 689–710 (1932).
4. Landsteiner, K., and Chase, M. W., Experiments on transfer of cutaneous sensitivity to simple chemical compounds, *Proc. Soc. Exp. Biol. Med.*, *49*, 688–690 (1942).
5. Chase, M. W., The cellular transfer of cutaneous hypersensitivity to tuberculin, *Proc. Soc. Exp. Biol. Med.*, *59*, 134–135 (1945).
6. Lawrence, H. S., The cellular transfer of cutaneous hypersensitivity to tuberculin in man, *Proc. Soc. Exp. Biol. Med.*, *71*, 516–522 (1949).
7. Mitchison, N. A., Passive transfer of transplantation immunity, *Proc. Roy. Soc. Lond. (Series B—Biol. Sci.)*, *142*, 72–87 (1954).
8. Lurie, M. B., Physiological properties of mononuclear phagocytes derived from normal and from tuberculous rabbits, *Arch. Pathol.*, *25*, 253–254 (1938).
9. Lurie, M. B., Studies on the mechanism of immunity in tuberculosis. The mobilization of mononuclear phagocytes in normal and immunized animals and their relative capacities for division and phagocytosis, *J. Exp. Med.*, *69*, 579–606 (1939).
10. Lurie, M. B., Studies on the mechanism of immunity in tuberculosis. The fate of tubercle bacilli ingested by mononuclear phagocytes derived from normal and immunized animals, *J. Exp. Med.*, *75*, 247–268 (1942).
11. Volkman, A., and Collins, F. M., The restorative effect of peritoneal macrophages on delayed hypersensitivity following ionizing irradiation, *Cell. Immunol.*, *2*, 552–566 (1971).
12. Mackaness, G. B., Cellular resistance to infection, *J. Exp. Med.*, *116*, 381–406 (1962).
13. Simon, H. B., and Sheagren, J. N., Cellular immunity in vitro. I. Immunologically mediated enhancement of macrophage bactericidal capacity, *J. Exp. Med.*, *133*, 1377–1389 (1971).
14. Nathan, C. F., Karnovsky, M. L., and David, J. R., Alterations of macrophage functions by mediators from lymphocytes, *J. Exp. Med.*, *133*, 1356–1376 (1971).
15. Najarian, J. S., and Feldman, J. D., Specificity of passively transferred delayed hypersensitivity, *J. Exp. Med.*, *118*, 341–352 (1963).
16. McCluskey, R. T., Benacerraf, B., and McCluskey, J. W., Studies on the specificity of the cellular infiltrate in delayed hypersensitivity reactions, *J. Immunol.*, *90*, 466–477 (1963).
17. George, M., and Vaughn, J. H., In vitro cell migration as a model for delayed hypersensitivity, *Proc. Soc. Exp. Biol. Med.*, *111*, 514–521 (1962).
18. Dumonde, D. C., Wolstencroft, R. A., Panayi, G. S., et al., Lymphokines: non-antibody mediators of cellular immunity generated by lymphocyte activation, *Nature*, *224*, 38–42 (1969).
19. Van Loveren, H., Meade, R., and Askenase, P. W., An early component of delayed-type hypersensitivity mediated by T-cells and mast cells, *J. Exp. Med.*, *157*, 1604–1617 (1963).
20. Mossman, T. R., and Coffman, R. L., TH_1 and TH_2 cells: different patterns of lymphokine secretion lead to different functional properties, *Annu. Rev. Immunol.*, *7*, 145–173 (1989).
21. Wierenga, E. A., Snoek, M., de Groot, C., et al., Evidence for compartmentalization of CD4+ T lymphocytes in atopic patients, *J. Immunol.*, *144*, 4561–4656 (1990).

22. Del Prete, G. F., De Carli, M., Mastromauro, C., et al., Purified protein derivative of *Mycobacterium tuberculosis* and excretory–secretory antigen(s) of *Toxocara canis* expand in vitro human T cells with stable and opposite (type 1 T helper and type 2 T helper) profiles of cytokine production, *J. Clin. Invest.*, *88*, 346–350 (1991).
23. Gordon, E. H., Krouse, H. A., Kinney, J. L., et al., Delayed cutaneous hypersensitivity in normals: choice of antigens and comparison to in vitro assays of cell mediated immunity, *J. Allergy Clin. Immunol.*, *72*, 487–494 (1983).
24. Palmer, D. L., and Reed, W. P., Delayed hypersensitivity skin testing. I. Response rates in a hospitalized population, *J. Infect. Dis.*, *130*, 132–137 (1974).
25. Kirkpatrick, C. H., Lymphocyte transformation test, in *Encyclopedia of Immunology* (I. M. Roitt and P. J. Delves, eds.), Academic Press, London, 1992, pp. 1005–1008.
26. Alling, D. W., and Kahan, B. D., Growth rates of mixed leukocyte cultures, *Transplantation*, *8*, 1–8 (1969).
27. Kirkpatrick, C. H., Rich, R. R., and Smith, T. K., Effects of transfer factor on lymphocyte function in anergic patients, *J. Clin. Invest.*, *51*, 2948–2958 (1972).
28. Arnaiz-Villena, A., Timon, M., Rodriguez-Gallego, C., et al., Human T-cell activation deficiencies, *Immunol. Today*, *13*, 259–265 (1992).
29. Fischer, A., Landais, P., Friedrich, W., et al., European experience of bone marrow transplantation for severe combined immunodeficiency, *Lancet*, *336*, 850–854 (1990).
30. Kirkpatrick, C. H., Ottesen, E. A., Smith, T. K., et al., Reconstitution of defective cellular immunity with fetal thymus and dialysable transfer factor. Long term studies in a patient with chronic mucocutaneous candidiasis, *Clin. Exp. Immunol.*, *23*, 414–428 (1976).
31. Stiehm, E. R., Immunodeficiency disorders: general considerations, in *Immunologic Disorders in Infants and Children* (E. R. Stiehm, ed.), W.B. Saunders, Philadelphia, 1989, pp. 157–195.
32. Blaese, R. M., and Culver, K. W., Gene therapy for primary immunodeficiency disease, *Immunodefic. Rev.*, *3*, 329–349 (1992).
33. Bodey, G. P., Candidiasis in cancer patients, *Am. J. Med.*, *77*, 13–19 (1984).
34. Sokal, J. E., and Primikirios, N., The delayed skin test response in Hodgkin's disease and lymphosarcoma. Effect of disease activity, *Cancer*, *14*, 597–607 (1961).
35. Wilson, W. E. C., Kirkpatrick, C. H., and Talmage, D. W., Suppression of immunologic responses in uremia, *Ann. Intern. Med.*, *62*, 1–14 (1965).
36. Catanzaro, A., Suppressor cells in coccidioidomycosis, *Cell. Immunol.*, *64*, 235–245 (1981).
37. Kleinhenz, M. E., Ellner, J. J., Spagnuolo, P. J., et al., Suppression of lymphocyte responses by tuberculous plasma and mycobacterial arabinogalactan, *J. Clin. Invest.*, *68*, 153–162 (1981).
38. Petersen, E. A., Neva, F. A., Oster, C. N., et al., Specific inhibition of lymphocyte proliferation responses by adherent suppressor cells in diffuse cutaneous leishmaniasis, *N. Engl. J. Med.*, *306*, 387–392 (1982).
39. Mason, U. G., and Kirkpatrick, C. H., Modulation of immunologic responses in nontuberculous mycobacterial infections with indomethacin, *J. Clin. Immunol.*, *4*, 112–117 (1984).
40. Colvin, R. B., Mosesson, M. W., and Dvorak, H. W., Delayed type hypersensitivity

skin reactions in congenital afibrinogenemia lack fibrin deposition and induration, *J. Clin. Invest.*, *63*, 1302–1306 (1979).
41. Cohen, S., Benacerraf, B., McCluskey, R. T., et al., Effect of anticoagulants on delayed hypersensitivity reactions, *J. Immunol.*, *98*, 351–358 (1967).
42. Edwards, R. L., and Rickles, F. R., Delayed hypersensitivity in man: effects of systemic anticoagulation, *Science*, *200*, 541–543 (1978).
43. Dobozin, B. S., Judson, F. N., Cohen, D. L., et al., The relationship of abnormalities of cellular immunity to antibodies to HTLV-III in homosexual men, *Cell. Immunol.*, *98*, 156–171 (1986).
44. Siegel, F. P., Lopez, C., Fitzgerald, P. A., et al., Opportunistic infections in acquired immune deficiency syndrome result from synergistic defects of both the natural and adaptive components of cellular immunity, *J. Clin. Invest.*, *78*, 115–123 (1986).
45. Terai, C., Kornbluth, R. S., Pavza, C. D., et al., Apoptosis as a mechanism of cell death in cultured T lymphoblasts acutely infected with HIV-1, *J. Clin. Invest.*, *87*, 1710–1715 (1991).
46. Banda, N. K., Bernier, J., Kurahara, D. K., et al., Crosslinking CD4 by human immunodeficiency virus gp120 primes T cells for activation induced apoptosis, *J. Exp. Med.*, *176*, 1099–1106 (1992).
47. Ameisen, J. C., Programmed cell death and AIDS: from hypothesis to experiment, *Immunol. Today*, *13*, 388–391 (1992).
48. Chase, M. W., Inhibition of experimental drug allergy by prior feeding of the sensitizing agent, *Proc. Soc. Exp. Biol. Med.*, *61*, 257–259 (1946).
49. Sulzberger, M. B., Hypersensitiveness to neoarsphenamine in guinea pigs. I. Experiments in prevention and desensitization, *Arch. Derm. Syph.*, *20*, 669–697 (1929).
50. Asherson, G. L., Zembala, M., Perera, M. A. C. C., et al., Production of immunity and unresponsiveness in the mouse by feeding contact sensitizing agents and the role of suppressor cells in the Peyer's patches, mesenteric lymph nodes and other lymphoid tissues, *Cell. Immunol.*, *33*, 145–155 (1977).
51. Ellner, J. J., Suppressor adherent cells in human tuberculosis, *J. Immunol.*, *121*, 2573–2579 (1978).
52. Stobo, J. D., Immunosuppression in man: suppression in macrophages can be mediated by interactions with regulatory T-cells, *J. Immunol.*, *119*, 918–924 (1977).
53. DeShazo, R. D., Indomethacin-responsive mononuclear cell dysfunction in Hodgkin's disease, *Clin. Immunol. Immunopathol.*, *17*, 66–75 (1980).
54. Mason, U. G., Greenberg, L. E., Yen, S. S., et al. Indomethacin responsive mononuclear cell dysfunction in "atypical" mycobacteriosis, *Cell Immunol.*, *71*, 54–65 (1982).
55. Ridgway, D., Wolff, L. J., Wall, M., et al., Indomethacin-sensitive monocyte killing defect in a child with disseminated atypical mycobacterial disease, *J. Clin. Immunol.*, *11*, 357–362 (1991).
56. Jorizzo, J. L., Sams, W. M., Jr., Jegasothy, B. V., et al., Cimetidine as an immunomodulator: chronic mucocutaneous candidiasis as a model, *Ann. Intern. Med.*, *92*, 192–195 (1980).
57. Sampaio, E. P., Moreira, A. L., Sarno, E. N., et al., Prolonged treatment with recombinant interferon γ induces erythema nodosum leprosum in lepromatous leprosy patients, *J. Exp. Med.*, *175*, 1729–1737 (1992).

58. Fauci, A. S., Rosenberg, S. A., Sherwin, S. A., et al., Immunomodulators in clinical medicine, *Ann. Intern. Med.*, *106*, 421–433 (1987).
59. Walker, R. E., and Lane, H. C., Interferon-α in HIV infection, in *AIDS. Etiology, Diagnosis, Treatment and Prevention*, 3rd Ed. (V. T. De Vita, S. Hellman, and S. A. Rosenberg, eds.), J. B. Lippincott, Philadelphia, 1992, pp. 395–406.
60. Dwyer, J. M., The use of antigen specific transfer factor in the management of infections with herpes viruses, in *Immunobiology of Transfer Factor* (C. H. Kirkpatrick, D. R. Burger, and H. S. Lawrence, eds.), Academic Press, New York, 1983, pp. 233–243.
61. Kirkpatrick, C. H., and Greenberg, L. E., Treatment of chronic mucocutaneous candidiasis with transfer factor, in *Immune Regulators in Transfer Factor* (A. Kahn, C. H. Kirkpatrick, and N. O. Hill, eds.), Academic Press, New York, 1979, pp. 547–562.
62. McMeeking, A., Borkowsky, W., Klesius, P. H., et al., A controlled trial of bovine dialyzable leukocyte extract for cryptosporidiosis in patients with AIDS, *J. Infect. Dis.*, *161*, 108–112 (1990).
63. Steele, R. W., Myers, M. G., and Vincent, M. M., Transfer factor for the prevention of varicella-zoster infection in childhood leukemia, *N. Engl. J. Med.*, *303*, 355–359 (1980).
64. Rozzo, S. J., and Kirkpatrick, C. H., Purification of transfer factors, *Mol. Immunol.*, *29*, 167–182 (1992).
65. Kappler, J. W., Roehm, N., and Marrack, P., T cell tolerance by clonal elimination in the thymus, *Cell*, *49*, 273–280 (1987).
66. Brod, S. A., Al-Sabbagh, A., Sobel, R. A., et al., Suppression of experimental autoimmune encephalomyelitis by oral administration of myelin antigens. IV. Suppression of chronic relapsing disease in the Lewis rat and strain 13 guinea pig, *Ann. Neurol.*, *29*, 615–622 (1991).
67. Lider, O., Santos, L. M. B., Lee, C. S. Y., et al., Suppression of experimental allergic encephalitis by oral administration of myelin basic protein. II. Suppression of disease and in vitro immune responses is mediated by antigen-specific CD8+ T lymphocytes, *J. Immunol.*, *142*, 748–752 (1989).
68. Urban, J. L., Kumar, V., Kono, D. H., et al., Restricted use of T cell receptor V genes in murine autoimmune encephalitis raises possibilities for antibody therapy, *Cell*, *54*, 577–592 (1988).
69. Davies, T. F., Martin, A., Concepcion, E. S., et al., Evidence of limited variability of antigen receptors on intrathyroidal T-cells in autoimmune thyroid disease, *N. Engl. J. Med.*, *325*, 238–244 (1991).
70. Howell, M. D., Winters, S. T., Olee, T., et al., Vaccination against experimental allergic encephalitis with T cell receptor peptides, *Science*, *246*, 668–670 (1989).
71. Vandenbark, A. A., Hashim, G., and Offner, H., Immunization with a synthetic T cell receptor of V region peptide protects against experimental autoimmune encephalitis, *Nature*, *341*, 541–544 (1989).
72. Gaur, A., Wiers, B., Liu, A., et al., Amelioration of autoimmune encephalitis by myelin basic protein synthetic peptide-induced anergy, *Science*, *258*, 1491–1494 (1992).
73. Gaur, A., Haspel, R., Mayer, J. P., et al., Requirement for CD8+ cells in T cell receptor peptide-induced clonal unresponsiveness, *Science*, *259*, 91–94 (1993).

28

Provocative Tests in Dermatology

Antti I. Lauerma and Howard I. Maibach

University of California School of Medicine
San Francisco, California

I. INTRODUCTION

Provocative in vivo skin tests are used in dermatology to detect and define the possible exogenous chemical agent that causes a skin disorder. Such chemical agents often cause skin disorders by hypersensitivity mechanisms, which can thus be diagnosed by a provocative test. The anatomical advantage of studying skin disorders is that the skin is the foremost frontier of human body and therefore easily accessible for testing. Although it has been shown that differences in the reactivity of different skin sites exist, many causative agents may be tested locally on one skin site, thus exposing only limited areas of skin to the diagnostic procedures. Such procedures include patch, intradermal, prick, scratch, scratch–chamber, open, rub, photo, and photopatch tests. In cases of some generalized skin reactions, however, systemic exposure to the external agent may be necessary for diagnosis.

The value of provocative tests is identification of the causative agent, which enables restarting of those medications not responsible for the eruption. This chapter will briefly describe the in vivo provocation test methods used for making diagnoses of skin disorders. The skin disorders in which such tests are useful include drug eruptions, contact dermatitis and immediate contact reactions, and possibly subjective irritation (Table 1).

Table 1 Skin Disorders Diagnosable Through Provocative Testing

Disorder	Mechanism[a]	Provocation
Drug eruption	Type I	Prick test
		Scratch test
		Intradermal test
		Systemic challenge
	Type II	Patch test
		Systemic challenge
	Type III	Intradermal test
		Systemic challenge
	Type IV	Patch test
		Systemic challenge
	Nonimmunological	Systemic challenge
Allergic contact dermatitis	Type IV	Patch test
		Intradermal test
		Open test
Immediate contact reaction	Type I	Prick test
		Scratch test
		Scratch–chamber test
		Rub test
		Open test
	Nonimmunological	Rub test
		Open test
Subjective irritation	Unknown	Lactic acid test

[a]Types I–IV: Coombs–Gell classification.

II. DRUG ERUPTIONS

Drug eruptions are a heterogeneous class of adverse skin reactions due to ingestion or injection of therapeutic drugs. The drug eruptions should ideally be diagnosed through systemic rechallenge, because many factors (e.g., systemic drug metabolism) may contribute to the process, and skin tests therefore are not as reliable. Because systemic challenge is not always easy to perform, skin tests may, however, precede such challenges, according to reaction type. If skin tests do not provide information about the causative agent and a medication needs to be restarted, the next step is a controlled drug rechallenge, preferably in a hospital environment [1].

The choice of provocation protocols depends on the type of reaction involved. Although much work has been directed toward classifying drug eruptions and elucidating their mechanisms, they are still not well understood. Many of them are presumably mediated by immunological mechanisms, but there are also *nonimmunological drug eruptions*, idiosyncrasies, in genetically predisposed persons.

In cases of nonimmunological drug eruptions, skin tests are usually negative, and systemic provocations are often negative (Tables 2 and 3). Immunological drug eruptions may be classified into the four reaction types according to Coombs and Gell [2].

Anaphylactic (*Coombs–Gell type I*) reactions include *anaphylaxis*, *urticaria*, and *angioneurotic edema*. They are usually mediated by immunoglobulin E (IgE) antibodies. Penicillin is one well-known causative agent for type I reactions. Prick (Table 4) and scratch (Table 5) tests are used in diagnosis of type I reactions and are a relatively safe way of detecting the causative agent. Intradermal tests (Table 6) may also be used in such cases, although a much larger amount of the antigen is introduced into the body, which makes systemic reactions more likely. Also, in vitro tests such as the radioallergosorbent test (RAST) are used in diagnosis [2]. Because type I reactions are potentially life-threatening, systemic challenges (Tables 2 and 3) [1], if done, should be performed with extreme care, starting with very low doses, under hospital conditions. Physician should always be readily available, and the patient should be monitored frequently.

Cytotoxic (*type II*) reactions are mediated by cytotoxic mechanisms; quinine and quinidine are examples of causative agents. Patch tests (Table 7) may be attempted before systemic challenges (Tables 2 and 3) [1], for example, in the case of *thrombocytopenic purpura* caused by carbromal or bromisovalum [2].

Immune complex–mediated (*type III*) reactions include *Arthus* and *vasculitic* reactions. Type III reactions are mediated by immunoglobulins, complement, and the antigen itself, which form complexes. For example, sulfa preparations, pyrazolones, and hydantoin derivatives have caused vascular purpura via type III mechanisms. Intradermal tests (Table 6) may be tried for diagnosis before systemic challenges (Tables 2 and 3) [2].

Delayed hypersensitivity (*type IV*) reactions are cell-mediated immune reactions involving the antigen, antigen-presenting cells, and T lymphocytes. Drug

Table 2 Systemic Challenge: Protocol[a]

The patient should be monitored under hospital conditions throughout the study.
Especially if the initial drug eruption was strong, challenge should be started at a low dose, i.e., no more than one-tenth of the initial dose.
A dose of suspected drug is given in the morning. Patient's skin, temperature, pulse, and other signs are followed at 1 h intervals for 10 h and recorded.
If no reactions appear during 24 h, the challenge is repeated at higher dose (e.g., one-third of the dose) the next morning.
If no reactions appear on days 1 and 2, then on the third morning a full therapeutic dose is given as third challenge.
If necessary, different drug challenges may be repeated every 24 h.

[a]See Kauppinen and Alanko [1] for detailed instructions.

Table 3 Systemic Challenge: Precautions[a]

Challenge is not advisable if the patient has had
Toxic epidermal necrolysis
Stevens–Johnson syndrome and/or erythema multiforme
Systemic lupus erythematosus–like reaction
Extreme care should be exercised if the patient has had
Anaphylaxis
Urticaria
Any other immediate-type reaction

[a]See Kauppinen and Alanko [1] for detailed instructions.

Table 4 Prick Test

Materials:	(1) Allergens in vehicles. (2) Vehicle (negative control). (3) Histamine in 0.9% NaCl (positive control). (4) Prick lancets.
Method:	One drop of each test allergen, vehicle, and histamine control is applied to the volar aspects of forearms. The test site is pierced with a lancet to introduce the allergen into the skin.
Reading time:	15–30 min.
Interpretation:	An edematous reaction (wheal) of at least 3 mm in diameter and at least half the size of the histamine control is considered positive, in the absence of such reaction in the vehicle control.
Precautions:	General anaphylaxis not very likely, because of the small amount of allergen introduced, but a physician should always be available for such occurrences. The patient should not leave the premises during the first 30 min after the test.

Table 5 Scratch Test

Materials:	(1) Allergens in vehicles. (2) Vehicle (negative control). (3) Histamine in 0.9% NaCl (positive control). (4) Needles.
Method:	A drop of each test allergen, vehicle, and histamine control is applied to the volar aspects of forearms or back, and needles are used to scratch the skin slightly at these sites.
Reading time:	Up to 30 min.
Interpretation:	Difficult because of unstandardized procedure. Edematous reaction at least as wide as the histamine control is considered positive in the absence of such reaction in the vehicle control.
Precautions:	As with prick test.

Table 6 Intradermal Test

Materials:	(1) Allergens in isotonic solution vehicles. (2) Solution vehicle (negative control). (3) Tuberculin (1 cc) syringes and needles.
Method:	0.05–0.1 ml of allergen solution and vehicle solution is applied intradermally to the skin of the volar aspects of the forearms or back.
Reading time:	30 min., 24 h, and 48 h.
Interpretation:	Erythematous and edematous reaction at 30 min is suggestive of immediate type (type I) allergy in the absence of such a reaction in the vehicle control. Arthus reaction with polymorphonuclear leukocyte infiltration appearing in 2–4 h, which may progress into necrosis in hours or days, suggests cytotoxic (type III) reaction. Erythema and edema of at least 5 mm in diameter at 48 h indicates delayed-type hypersensitivity (type IV), for example contact allergy.
Precautions:	The risk of general anaphylaxis is higher than in prick or scratch tests because of larger amount of allergen introduced; therefore, a physician should always be available for such occurrences. The risk is greater in asthmatic patients. The patient should not leave the premises during the first 30 min after the test.

Table 7 Patch Test

Materials:	(1) Allergens in vehicle (e.g., petrolatum, ethanol, water). (2) Vehicles. (3) Aluminum chambers (Finn Chamber), Scanpor tape, and filter papers (for solutions). OR: (1) Ready-made patch test series (TRUE test).
Method:	Patches on tape or ready-made patch test series are applied on intact skin of the back. Filter papers are used for solutions. 17 μl of allergen in vehicle is used for each patch. Ready-made patch series are applied as is on similar skin sites. The patches are removed after 48 h.
Reading time:	48 h, and 96 h.
Interpretation:	Erythema and edema or more is positive. Distinguishing between allergic and irritant reaction is important. If the reaction is spreading across the boundaries of the patch site, the reaction is likely to be allergic. If the reaction peaks at 48 h and starts to fade rapidly after that, it may be irritant.
Precautions:	Intense skin reactions possible; these can be treated with topical glucocorticosteroids. Active sensitization possible.

Table 8 Photo Test

Materials:	Ultraviolet (UV) radiation source.
Method:	Minimal erythema dose (MED) of UVA or UVB is measured (1) while the subject is taking the suspected medication and (2) after discontinuing the same medication.
Interpretation:	If MED is much lower while the subject is taking the medication, this suggests a photosensitive reaction to the drug.

reactions of this type are often *maculopapular* or *eczematous*, although *photoallergic* reactions and *fixed drug eruptions* are also presumably mediated by type IV mechanisms. Other type IV reactions include some cases of *erythroderma*, *exfoliative dermatitis*, *lichenoid* and *vesicobullous eruptions*, *erythema exudavitum multiforme*, and *toxic epidermal necrolysis*. Type IV reactions may be detected by patch tests with the causative agent (Table 7) [2]. In the case of a fixed drug eruption, in which the reaction reoccurs in the same skin site every time the drug is ingested, the patch test should be done in that particular skin site for a positive result [3]. For photosensitivity reactions, photo (Table 8) or photopatch tests (Table 9) should be done [4]. A negative patch test does not rule out the possibility that the tested drug may be causative. This is because patch testing involves potential limitations, such as insufficient penetration. In this case a systemic provocation (Tables 2 and 3) should be done [1].

III. CONTACT DERMATITIS

Contact dermatitis is commonly divided into irritant contact dermatitis and allergic contact dermatitis. *Irritant contact dermatitis*, the more common of the

Table 9 Photopatch Test

Materials:	(1) Ultraviolet (UV) radiation source. (2) Patch test materials (see Table 8).
Method:	Two sets of patch tests are applied for 48 h. After removal, one set is irradiated with UV at a dose below minimal erythema dose (MED) (5 J/cm^2 or 50% of MED, whichever is smaller), and the other set is protected from UV dose.
Reading time:	72–96 h.
Interpretation:	Reaction only at irradiated site suggests photoallergy. Reaction at both sites suggests contact allergy. Reaction at both sites and a much stronger reaction at the irradiated site suggests both contact allergy and photoallergy.

two, is initiated by *nonimmunological* toxic mechanisms and is not diagnosable through provocative testing, while allergic contact dermatitis is. In *allergic contact dermatitis* the patient becomes topically sensitized to a low-molecular-weight hapten and in subsequent topical contact develops an eczematous skin reaction, which is mediated by *delayed hypersensitivity (type IV)* mechanisms. Allergic contact dermatitis is tested with patch tests (Table 7), intradermal tests (Table 6) or open tests (Table 10).

Of these three methods, patch testing is the most common and standardized. The problems involved in patch testing are insufficient penetration of the allergenic compound, which may result in false-negative results, and irritation from the test compound, which may cause a false-positive result. Also, patch testing may cause a worsening of eczema in other skin sites (excited skin syndrome) or active sensitization to patch compounds [5].

Two methods for patch testing exist, the Finn Chamber and TRUE Test methods. Both have been shown to be rather reliable, especially when stronger reactions (contact allergies) are investigated [6]. The TRUE Test is somewhat easier to handle, as it is ready to use. However, the Finn Chamber method provides more flexibility for the dermatologist and the allergist to test substances not in routine patch test use. Regardless of the test method, the most important factor in successful patch testing is the experience and skill of the interpretator.

A standard patch test series is shown in Table 11. It is the standard series of the International Contact Dermatitis Research Group and the European Environmental and Contact Dermatitis Research Group [7]. A standard patch test series has been compiled to represent the most commonly encountered contact allergens, and it is meant to act as a screening tray. Its content is subject to change due to research findings about contact allergy [7]. A multitude of other patch test series are available when the causative agents of the individual patient's contact dermatitis

Table 10 Open Test (Repeated Open Application Test)

Materials:	(1) Allergen in vehicle (petrolatum, ethanol, water). (2) Vehicle. (3) Cotton-tipped applicators or other devices to spread the preparations.
Method:	Patient applies allergen and vehicle on antecubital fossa (outpatient) or shoulder regions of upper back, two times a day, for 7 days or until a positive reaction appears.
Reading time:	Patient reports whether positive reaction appears. At 7 days the patient returns for reading of the test site.
Interpretation:	Erythema and edema or more is positive.
Precautions:	Active sensitization possible.

Table 11 Standard Patch Test Series

Potassium dichromate	0.5% pet.
Neomycin sulfate	20.0% pet.
Thiuram mix	1.0% pet.
p-Phenylenediamine free base	1.0% pet.
Cobalt chloride	1.0% pet
Benzocaine	5.0% pet.
Formaldehyde	1.0% aq.
Colophony	20.0% pet
Quinoline mix	6.0% pet.
Balsam of Peru	25.0% pet.
PPD–black rubber mix	0.6% pet.
Wool alcohols (lanolin)	30.0% pet.
Mercapto mix	2.0% pet.
Epoxy resin	1.0% pet.
Paraben mix	15.0% pet.
p-tert-Butylphenol–formaldehyde resin	1.0% pet.
Fragrance mix	8.0% pet.
Ethylenediamine dihydrochloride	1.0% pet.
Quaternium 15	1.0% pet.
Nickel sulfate	5.0% pet.
Kathon C6	0.01% aq.
Mercaptobenzothiazole	2.0% pet.
Primin	0.01% pet.

pet. = petrolatum vehicle; aq. = aqueous vehicle.

are known better; these include, for example, patch test series for preservatives, rubber chemicals, topical drugs, and cloth chemicals. There are also special series to investigate occupational contact allergies in, for example, dental personnel or hairdressers.

Patch tests should be applied on the back for 48 h and be read after removal. A second reading 24–48 h after patch removal is necessary, as irritant reactions, which are often easily misinterpreted as allergic, often tend to fade during the third and fourth days, while allergic reactions tend to persist. Additionally, with some allergens, such as corticosteroids and neomycin, late reactions may occur, possibly because of poor percutaneous penetration. Therefore, a third reading approximately 1 week after patch application may be advisable, although this may be difficult to do routinely in practice.

Intradermal testing (Table 6) has recently been shown to be of value in diagnosing hydrocortisone contact allergy [8]. Open tests or repeated open application tests (Table 10) are not as sensitive as patch or intradermal tests, possibly because of insufficient penetration of the compound under unoccluded conditions [9,10].

IV. CONTACT URTICARIA SYNDROME: IMMEDIATE CONTACT REACTIONS

Contact urticaria syndrome includes a group of skin reactions, i.e., immediate contact reactions, that appear usually within 1 hr of skin contact with the causative agent. Immediate skin reactions are divided into immunological (IgE-mediated) and nonimmunological immediate contact reactions. The symptoms range from mere itching and tingling to local wheal and flare. In cases of intense sensitivity, a generalized urticaria, systemic symptoms, and even anaphylaxis (contact urticaria syndrome) may occur [11].

Immunological immediate contact reactions are usually urticarial, although they may range from mere tingling in the skin to a generalized anaphylactic reaction in the whole body. Immunological immediate reactions are Coombs–Gell type I reactions mediated mainly via allergen-specific IgE bound to skin mast cells. Coupling of membrane-bound IgE by allergen causes mast cells to liberate histamine, which with other inflammatory mediators makes skin vessels permeable, and edema (urticaria) results. The sensitization in IgE-mediated contact urticaria may occur through skin or possibly the respiratory or gastrointestinal tract. Exposure through skin is the most likely route in latex allergy. The provocative in vivo methods usually performed first are prick test (Table 4), scratch test (Table 5), and scratch–chamber test (Table 12). However, the test methods simulating the clinical contact situation more realistically are the rub test (Table 13) and open application test (Table 14). A previously affected skin site is more sensitive to immunological skin reactions than a nonaffected site. In addition to in vivo methods, the diagnosis of immunological immediate contact reactions can be done with RAST, which detects antigen-specific IgE molecules from the patient's serum [11].

Table 12 Scratch–Chamber Test

Materials:	(1) Scratch test materials (see Table 5). (2) Chambers.
Method:	As with scratch test, but scratch sites are covered with aluminum chambers for 15 min.
Reading time:	30 min.
Interpretation:	See Table 5.
Precautions:	As with prick and scratch tests.

Table 13 Rub Test

Materials:	(1) Allergen in vehicle (petrolatum, ethanol, water). (2) Vehicle. (3) Cotton-tip applicators or other devices to spread the preparations.
Method:	Allergen and vehicle are rubbed to skin.
Reading time:	Up to 1 h.
Interpretation:	Urticarial reaction is positive.
Precautions:	See Table 4.

Nonimmunological immediate contact reactions range from erythema to urticaria and occur in persons not sensitized to the compounds [11]. Nonimmunological contact reactions are probably more common than immunological contact reactions. They are possibly due to the causative agent's ability to release inflammatory mediators, such as histamine, prostaglandins, and leukotrienes, from skin cells, without the participation of IgE molecules. Agents capable of causing nonimmunological contact reactions are numerous; the most potent and best-studied agents are benzoic acid, sorbic acid, cinnamic aldehyde, and nicotinic acid esters. Provocative skin tests for diagnosis of nonimmunological contact urticaria include the rub test (Table 13) and open test (Table 14). In nonimmunological contact reactions, the reactions appear within 45–60 min after application, while in immunological reactions they should appear in 15–20 min [12].

V. SUBJECTIVE IRRITATION

Although *subjective irritation* or "sensitive skin" is not yet well characterized, there is evidence for a group of such persons, known as "stingers" [13]. The lactic acid test (Table 15) has been used experimentally to distinguish between "stingers," who more often have subjective irritation, and "nonstingers" [14].

Table 14 Open Application Test for Immediate Contact Reactions

Materials:	(1) Allergen in vehicle (petrolatum, ethanol, water). (2) Vehicle. (3) Cotton-tipped applicators or other devices to spread the preparations.
Method:	As with rub test, but preparations are merely applied, not rubbed, on top of skin.
Reading time:	See Table 13.
Interpretation:	See Table 13.
Precautions:	See Table 4.

Table 15 Lactic Acid Test

Materials:	(1) Facial sauna. (2) 5% lactic acid in water. (3) Vehicle (water). (4) Soap, paper towels, cotton-tipped applicators.
Method:	Facial area below eyes is cleansed with soap, paper towels, and water, rinsed with water, and patted dry. Face is exposed to sauna heat for 15 min. Moisture of face is blotted away. Lactic acid in water is rubbed on one side of face (cheek) and water on other. Face is exposed to sauna again.
Reading time:	2 and 5 min after second sauna exposure.
Interpretation:	Any subjective sensation is graded by patient: 0 = none; 1 = slight; 2 = moderate; 3 = severe. If cumulative score of two time points is 3 or more, patient is "stinger."
Precautions:	Irritation may occur.

REFERENCES

1. Kauppinen K. and Alanko, K., Oral provocation: uses, *Semin. Dermatol.*, *8*, 187–191 (1989).
2. Bruynzeel, D. P., and Ketel, W. G. V., Patch testing in drug eruptions, *Semin. Dermatol.*, *8*, 196–203 (1989).
3. Alanko, K., Stubb, S., and Reitamo, S., Topical provocation of fixed drug eruption, *Br. J. Dermatol.*, *116*, 561–567 (1987).
4. Rosen, C., Photo-induced drug eruptions, *Semin. Dermatol.*, *8*, 149–157 (1989).
5. Fischer, T., and Maibach, H., Improved, but not perfect, patch testing, *Am. J. Cont. Derm.*, *1*, 73–90 (1990).
6. Ruhnek-Forsbeck, M., Fischer, T., Meding, B., Petterson, L., Stenberg, B., Strand, A., Sundberg, K., Svensson, L., Wahlberg, J. E., Widström, L., Wrangsjö, K., and Billberg, K., Comparative multi-center study with TRUE Test and Finn Chamber patch test methods in eight Swedish hospitals, *Acta Dermatol. Venereol. (Stockh.)*, *58*, 123–128 (1988).
7. Andersen, K., Burrows, D., and White, I. R., Allergens from the standard series, in *Textbook of Contact Dermatitis* (R. J. G. Rycroft, T. Menne, P. J. Frosch, and C. Benezra, eds.), Springer-Verlag, Berlin, 1991, pp. 416–456.
8. Wilkinson, S. M., Cartwright, P. H., and English, J. S. C., Hydrocortisone: an important cutaneous allergen, *Lancet*, *337*, 761–762 (1991).
9. Hannuksela, M., and Salo, H., The repeated open application test (ROAT), *Cont. Derm.*, *14*, 221–227 (1986).
10. Hannuksela, M., Sensitivity of various skin sites in the repeated open application test, *Am. J. Cont. Derm.*, *2*, 102–104 (1991).
11. Lahti, A., and Maibach, H. I., Contact urticaria syndrome, in *Dermatology* (S. L. Moschella and H. J. Hurley, eds.), Philadelphia, W. B. Saunders, 1992, pp. 433–440.

12. Gollhausen, R., and Kligman, A. M., Human assay for identifying substances which induce non-allergic contact urticaria: the NICU-test, *Cont. Derm.*, *13*, 98–106 (1985).
13. Maibach, H. I., Lammintausta, K., Berardesca, E., and Freeman, S., Tendency to irritation: sensitive skin, *J. Am. Acad. Dermatol.*, *21*, 833–835 (1989).
14. Lammintausta, K., Maibach, H. I., and Wilson, D., Mechanisms of subjective (sensory) irritation. Propensity to non-immunologic contact urticaria and objective irritation in stingers, *Dermatosen*, *36*, 45–49 (1988).

29

Drug Desensitization

John A. Anderson

Henry Ford Hospital
Detroit, Michigan

I. INTRODUCTION

Treatment of a patient with an adverse reaction to a drug or a biological agent should include (1) discontinuation of the medication or agent, wherever possible; (2) prompt management of the adverse clinical signs and symptoms; (3) substitution of another drug or agent, if necessary; and (4) consideration of drug challenge or drug desensitization when the alternative drug or agent is not appropriate [1]. Usually, substitution can be made among a variety of medications. In some cases, however, this is not so, and the most appropriate medication or agent is the one to which the patient had a reaction.

II. INCREMENTAL DRUG CHALLENGE

In cases where the history of the drug-related reaction is vague, the reaction is not life threatening, and there is no objective test, other than challenge, to confirm the association, then a drug challenge under controlled conditions may be considered. Such a challenge has been termed "test dosing" by Patterson and colleagues [2,3]. This procedure has been reserved for cases in which the history is suggestive of an allergic or allergic-like reaction to a drug or biological agent but the likelihood of a serious reaction is low and, therefore, the risk of rechallenge with the drug is also low [3]. The term "test dosing" should probably be replaced by the term "incremental drug challenge (under controlled conditions)" [4]. The former term can be confused with a previously common, but dangerous, clinical practice of routinely giving a small dose of medication before a large one to a patient suspected of having had a previous reaction to that agent (e.g., conventional radiocontrast medium reactions). Incremental drug challenge should not be confused with drug desensitization [3,4]. The procedures for these challenges have not been standardized or subjected to critical review. An exception is the procedure for challenge with a local anesthetic. Detailed protocols for such challenges are available [1,2,4,5]. Most of these current protocols are based on the 1979 experience of deShazo and Nelson, who evaluated 90 patients with an alleged history of an adverse reaction to a local anesthetic [6]. Table 1 represents a local anesthetic challenge protocol in which IgE, immediate-reacting skin testing is first done, followed by serial, incremental challenges at 15-min intervals. DeSwarte has suggested creating individual protocols like this local anesthetic protocol with other drugs when specific challenges are indicated [4]. If that is done, however, the investigators should understand the following:

1. The need for initial drug skin testing, especially for medication reactions that do not involve any proven or suspected IgE reaction, is questionable.
2. The starting dose for a specific drug challenge is arbitrary.
3. The route of administration for the drug or agent depends on the medication and the availability of suitable dosage forms.

Table 1 Skin Testing and Provocative Challenge for Local Anesthetics

Route	Dilution	Dose
Prick skin test[a]	Undiluted	1.0 drop
ID skin test	1:100	0.02 ml
SQ challenge[b]	1:100	0.1 ml
	1:10	0.1 ml
	Full strength	0.1 ml
	Full strength	0.5 ml
	Full strength	1.0 ml
	(Full strength)	(2.0 ml)[c]

[a]Skin test with a battery of local anesthetic types (free of epinephrine/parabens).
[b]Challenge with single type of local anesthetic (negative on skin test) sequentially at 15-min intervals, as recommended by deShazo and Nelson [6].
[c]As recommended by Patterson et al. [2].
ID = intradermal; SQ = subcutaneous.
Source: Ref. 1.

4. The interval of challenge may vary depending on the half-life of the drug.
5. The incremental challenge dosage of the drug or agent is arbitrary.
6. The final top or "safe" dose and the cumulative dose also are arbitrary, but it probably is safe to use the equivalent of one usual therapeutic drug dose in a 24-h period.

Certainly, any incremental drug challenge, even in a patient whose suspected reaction has been mild, must be taken seriously and be done under some control, even in an office setting. The patient should be observed for at least 2 h after such a challenge, and the equipment and personnel should be available to manage potential serious side effects such as anaphylaxis or an anaphylactoid reaction, even though such a serious reaction is unlikely.

III. DESENSITIZATION WITH A DRUG OR BIOLOGICAL AGENT

In cases where the history of a reaction to a specific drug or biological agent is definite, the reaction is serious and perhaps life-threatening, and, finally, there is no appropriate substitute drug or agent, then the procedure of desensitization may be considered. Desensitization is defined as the process of eliminating the natural or acquired reactivity or sensitivity to an external stimulus [7]. In its broadest sense, desensitization denotes reducing the degree of reaction to a drug or biological agent by repeated and increased exposure to that drug or agent [8].

The process of desensitization has been used to manage patients who react to drugs such as the β-lactam antibiotics [9], insulin [5] and to biological agents such as horse serum in vaccine containing antivenom or antilymphocyte globulin (ALG) [10]. In these situations, an IgE immunological mechanism has been clearly identified as being responsible for the anaphylactic reaction in the patient. Drug desensitization has been successfully used to manage a cystic fibrosis patient who reacted to an aminoglycoside antibiotic (tobramycin) and a leukemic patient who reacted to cytarabine—both of whom were suspected of reacting on the basis of an IgE mechanism [11,12]. DeSwarte has called this process "immunological desensitization" [4].

Desensitization has also been applied to the management of patients who have reacted to other drugs, such as aspirin [13,14], trimethoprim/sulfamethoxazole (TMP-SMX) [15], sulfasalazine (SSZ) [16], sulfadiazine (SDZ), allopurinol [17], vancomycin [18], and pentamidine [19]. In each of these latter situations, the rhinitis/asthma, rash, or fever reaction has been recognized as involving other (and usually unknown) mechanisms. Desensitization to these latter medications has been referred to by DeSwarte as the process of acquiring "clinical tolerance" to the agent in question [4]. Other authors simply describe this process as non-immunological desensitization.

The exact pathophysiological or immunological process by which the state of desensitization occurs with most of these medications is unclear. In the case of insulin desensitization, serum insulin-specific IgE antibodies have been shown to decrease rapidly, and insulin IgE skin tests that were positive before desensitization become negative on repeat testing after desensitization [20,21]. Lieberman has stated that this situation is an example of IgE neutralization or "true drug desensitization" [5].

Following penicillin desensitization in a penicillin-allergic patient, repeat penicillin skin testing may be negative. However, the level of circulating IgE antipenicillin antibodies usually does not change [22]. Also, any change in penicillin allergen–specific IgG "blocking" antibody levels does not correlate with the acquisition of the "desensitized state." Evidence is against mast cell mediator "depletion" as an explanation for the development of the desensitized state during penicillin desensitization. The most attractive hypothesis to explain immunological (IgE) desensitization is a progressive decrease of mast cell or basophil mediator release on a cellular level [23]. However, one study has shown that in vitro basophil histamine release to penicillin antigens appears to be unaffected during desensitization by penicillin [24].

The best-studied nonimmunological desensitization process is that of aspirin desensitization in an aspirin-sensitive patient who has rhinitis and asthma. The desensitization state in this case is an extension of a refractory period that occurs after an asthmatic reaction with aspirin challenge. This was first recognized in a single patient in 1922 by Widal et al. and confirmed in another patient by Zeiss and Lockey in 1976 [8]. This refractory state has been found to last as little as 2 days and as much as 5–7 days following the induction of asthma by aspirin challenge [13]. This observation led to studies of aspirin-sensitive patients in which it was found possible to desensitize those who had aspirin-induced rhinitis or asthma, but not those with urticaria, for long periods of time, with demonstrable decreases in their primary clinical condition [14].

The exact mechanism by which aspirin desensitization occurs is unknown, but the following hypotheses have been proposed: (1) mast cell degranulation (as a result of depletion of mast cell mediators); (2) direct drug-related inhibition of mast cell activity; (3) tachyphylaxis of bronchial smooth muscle receptors; (4) inhibition of leukotriene generation or metabolism [13]. None of these hypotheses have ever been proved.

In both types of desensitization (IgE-mediated immunological reactions, and other, nonimmunological drug reactions), once the procedure is over, the patient reverts to the predesensitized or sensitive state—and is at risk for another anaphylactic or anaphylactoid reaction if exposed again to the medication in question. Long-term desensitization, for chronic conditions, is also possible with either type desensitization. In the case of penicillin allergy, the state of "desensitization" has been maintained at a therapeutic drug dose for as long as 10 weeks, provided the medication is given no less often than every 12 h [9]. Once a diabetic who had reacted to insulin has been desensitized to it, this state can be maintained indefinitely, as long as insulin is administered daily [5]. A state of desensitization has been maintained with aspirin in aspirin-sensitive asthmatics for as long as 8 years, provided the medication is taken regularly within 2-day intervals [14]. Long-term desensitization has been maintained with SSZ in patients with Crohn's disease and with TMP-SMX in patients with AIDS receiving prophylactic therapy for *Pneumocystis carinii* infection [15,16,19].

IV. TEN PRINCIPLES CONCERNING THE DESENSITIZATION PROCEDURE

1. *The need for desensitization must be clearly established.* This includes ascertaining that the patient is reactive to a specific drug or biological agent and that the sensitivity is severe and potentially life-threatening (e.g., anaphylaxis or anaphylactoid reaction). It also includes establishing that there is no suitable alternative medication available to treat the condition in question.

2. *The adverse reaction to the medication should be one that is expected to be modified by the desensitization procedure*. In most cases, this is established in the literature relating to the specific adverse drug reaction. Cutaneous reactions as a group are the most common manifestation of drug reactions. In the case of erythema multiforme or the febrile mucocutaneous syndromes (Stevens–Johnson syndrome or Lyell's syndrome [toxic epidermal necrolysis]) reexposure to an associated drug may cause a severe exacerbation. Therefore, desensitization to such a medication is inappropriate [1,4]. In the case of adverse reactions to radiocontrast media, desensitization is ineffectual and is not recommended for the management of patients with a previous history of reaction [1,4,5].

3. *Informed consent must be obtained from the patient, parent, or caretaker before the desensitization procedure begins.*

4. *For acute desensitization, the patient should be in the hospital, preferably in an intensive care unit setting* [1,4]. In the case of a prolonged desensitization procedure that takes weeks to complete, if the adverse reactions are not expected to be immediate (e.g., extended oral SSD or TMP-SMX), this may not be necessary or practical beyond the initial few days of the procedure.

5. *The patient's cardiac, pulmonary, renal, and metabolic state should be as stable as possible.*

6. *Concurrent medication that may exacerbate anaphylaxis or anaphylactoid reactions (e.g., β-adrenergic blocking agents) or mask an adverse event during the desensitization procedure (e.g., antihistamines, sympathomimetics, or corticosteroids), should be withheld before the desensitization procedure* [4]. However, these latter medications (antihistamines, sympathomimetics, and corticosteroids) may be needed to treat an adverse reaction should one occur during the procedure.

7. *Acute desensitization procedures should be done under optimal controlled*

conditions. This usually includes the available of adequately trained personnel and experience with the management of anaphylaxis or anaphylactoid reactions, as well as an intravenous access and cardiovascular and pulmonary monitoring of vital signs as appropriate. Usually, desensitizations are better performed as elective procedures on weekdays and during the daylight hours, when the availability of personnel and adequate equipment and supplies is probably better in most institutions than at other times of the day or week.

8. *Published protocols of desensitization procedures for drugs and biological agents should be considered only as guidelines* [1]. Often, these protocols are based on limited information, and the specific starting, incremental, and final doses, as well as the timing of administration of the drug, must be adjusted according to the individual patient's circumstances (e.g., specific patient sensitivity).

9. *Adverse reactions during and after the desensitization procedure should be expected*. In penicillin desensitization procedures, reactions occur in about one-third of cases, regardless of the route of administration (oral vs. parental) [4,25–28]. Adverse reactions must be treated as they occur, and the initial desensitization schedule of dosing must be appropriately adjusted. The next dose following the treatment of an adverse event should be lower than the dose that caused the reaction [1]. Any patient who is desensitized must be carefully observed for 48–72 h following the completion of the desensitization procedure, in case a late reaction should occur [4]. Acute desensitization to an agent does not necessarily block the late onset of reactions such as serum sickness or nephritis, which may occur because of another mechanism [1,9,26,27,29].

10. *Following completion of the desensitization procedure and discontinuation of the drug or biological agent, the patient will quickly revert to his previous, sensitized state* [1,4,9,13].

V. SPECIFIC DRUG DESENSITIZATION PROTOCOLS

A. β-Lactam Antibiotics

Tables 2 (oral route) and 3 (intravenous [IV] route) represent protocols for the administration of β-lactam antibiotics during a desensitization procedure. These protocols are based on studies of penicillin-allergic patients who have been successfully desensitized to penicillin [9,25–27]. These approaches can also be applied to other β-lactam antibiotics such as the semisynthetic penicillins and cephalosporins [28]. The oral route, which is preferred by many, is convenient for the patient able to take oral medications, and although reactions such as pruritus and urticaria occur, they are usually mild and can be easily managed [4,9,29].

The method of oral desensitization as depicted in Table 2 is based on studies using similar protocols in 43 penicillin-allergic subjects aged 17–72 years, by

Table 2 β-Lactam Oral Desensitization Protocol

Dose no.	Stock drug conc.[a] (mg/ml)	Amount (ml)	Drug dose (mg)	Cumulative drug (mg)
1[b]	0.5 mg/ml	0.05	0.025	0.025
2		0.10	0.05	0.075
3		0.20	0.10	0.175
4		0.40	0.20	0.375
5		0.80	0.40	0.775
6	5.0 mg/ml	0.15	0.75	1.525
7		0.30	1.50	3.025
8		0.60	3.00	6.025
9		1.20	6.00	12.025
10		2.40	12.00	24.025
11	50 mg/ml	0.50	25.00	49.025
12		1.20	60.00	109.025
13		2.50	125.00	234.025
14		5.00	250.00	484.025

[a]Dilutions using pediatric syrup 250 mg/5 ml
[b]Oral dose approximately doubled every 15–30 minutes; modified from Sullivan et al. [25] and Wendel et al. [26].
Source: Ref. 1.

Table 3 β-Lactam Intravenous Desensitization Protocol

Dose no.	Stock drug conc.[a] (mg/ml)	Amount per 50 mg (mg/ml)[a]	Cumulative drug (mg)
1[b]	0.004	0.00008	0.004
2	0.020	0.0004	0.024
3	0.1	0.002	0.124
4	0.6	0.012	0.724
5	3.0	0.06	3.724
6[c]	15.0	0.3	18.724
7	30.0	0.6	48.724
8	62.0	1.2	110.724
9	125.0	2.5	235.724
10	250.0	5.0	485.724

[a]Mix 1 ml of stock drug solution in 50 ml D5/0.2% saline. Infuse each dose within 20–45 min. Dilution volume may vary with age/weight. Modified from Borish et al. [27].
[b]Doses 1–5 represent fivefold dilutions
[c]Doses 6–10 represent twofold dilutions
Source: Ref. 1.

Sullivan et al. and Wendel et al. [25,26]. It is similar to desensitization protocols using oral β-lactam antibiotics that are published and recommended elsewhere [4,30].

The β-lactam antibiotic oral desensitization protocol described in Table 2 represents a generally conservative approach in which the starting dose is one step (twofold) less than is usually recommended [4,25,26,30]. The starting dose of 0.025 mg is calculated to be less than a standard 0.125-mg intradermal skin test that might be responsible for a local (positive) skin test reaction (0.02 ml of a 10,000-unit or 6.25 mg/ml penicillin test solution) [1]. This starting dose is more than the amount of a penicillin test solution that is thought to be introduced into the epidermis during a usual epicutaneous allergy skin test, such as a prick or puncture test (3.3×10^{-6} ml) [31]. Thus, in an exquisitely sensitive (allergic) subject, the starting dose in the protocol depicted in Table 2 may have to be modified even further [1,32].

The protocol in Table 2 represents a serial twofold solution or doubling increase adjusted every 15–30 min. This also represents a conservative approach, as most investigators and other authorities advocate strict every-15-minute dosing, on the basis of patient experience [4,25,26,30]. All authorities recommend altering the dosing schedule should the patient react during the desensitization procedure. Following restabilization of the patient with treatment for the reaction, the remaining desensitization protocol should be adjusted. The next subsequent desensitization dose should be lower than the dose that produced the reaction [1]. The top desensitization dose is up to the clinician treating the patient. The protocol represented in Table 2 tops out at a single dose of 250 mg and a cumulative dose of approximately 500 mg. This represents 25–33% of a usual total 24-h daily dose of antibiotic and a single dose that is typically given every 6 or 8 h for an adult patient [1]. In other situations, when patients require higher doses of β-lactam antibiotics, the protocol can be extended, following the same pattern of regular dosing and administration [4,32].

For patients who require parenteral administration of antibiotics, both the subcutaneous and the IV route can be used in desensitization protocols. Saxon and colleagues have described a subcutaneous desensitization procedure for penicillin-allergic patients beginning with either the dose that produces a positive intradermal skin test with the usual penicillin testing solution (0.125 mg; see description under oral desensitization procedure), or a smaller dose [32]. In sensitive subjects, Saxon and colleagues recommended finding the epicutaneous penicillin skin test dose that produces only a small test reaction (wheal less than 4 mm), on the basis of testing with tenfold dilutions of the original test concentration that produced a positive test. Once the "nonreactive" dose is determined, a tenfold increase of this dose is then used as an intradermal test (0.02 ml), and subsequently, the dose is doubled every 15 min, with the antibiotic being administered subcutaneously [32].

Many investigators prefer the intravenous route for β-lactam antibiotic desensitization, since if offers a more precise control of the rate and concentration of drug administered than either the subcutaneous route or the oral route [4,27]. The protocol represented in Table 3 is an intravenous desensitization schedule adapted from the studies of Borish et al., in which 12 β-lactam antibiotic–allergic subjects (age 9 months to 64 years) were successfully desensitized on 15 occasions [27]. A similar IV β-lactam protocol was used by Moss et al. in 15 patients (aged 12–37 years) [28].

In both of these study situations, the procedure for desensitization was based on the IV administration of stock solutions made up from serial dilutions of the dose of antibiotic usually given every 4–6 h on a treatment basis (17–25% of total daily requirement) [27,28]. That represented 500 mg in the study of Borish et al. and 50 mg/kg in the study of Moss et al. [27,28]. Serial tenfold dilutions are then mae up so that the beginning IV solution is 10^{-6} of the therapeutic dose [27,28].

The IV desensitization protocol in Table 3 is adjusted to represent a more gradual desensitization that begins with a drug dose approximating the usual skin test reaction levels (see oral desensitization procedure). Thus, there is a similarity between the oral and IV protocols depicted in Tables 2 and 3. Typically, the stock IV drug solution is administered in 50 ml 5% dextrose/10.2% saline over a 20- to 45-min period [27,28]. The desensitization mixtures are placed either in separate IV bags or in the burette. The exact rate of administration will depend on the patient and the possibility of an allergic reaction to the administered antibiotic. The fluid volume for each drug increment may have to be adjusted for the age and weight of the patient [1].

As with oral antibiotic desensitization, the top desensitizing dose will vary with the needs of the patient. In the studies of Borish et al. and Moss et al., higher IV end drug concentrations were safely given than indicated in the desensitization protocol depicted in Table 3 [27,28]. This protocol, like the oral protocol in Table 2, should be adjusted to fit the specific clinical need by following the same general principles. Again, should an allergic reaction occur during the IV infusion, the dosing should be stopped and resumed only after stabilization of the patient at a lower drug concentration.

Table 4 lists the reported adverse reactions to β-lactam antibiotic desensitization. Before 1980, the overall reaction rate in 43 desensitization procedures from 13 reports was 56%. This included four instances of systemic anaphylaxis (9%), in which two fatalities resulted [33,34]. Since 1980, the overall reaction rate in 115 desensitization procedures in 101 patients was reported to be 30%, of which 21% were acute cutaneous reactions (pruritus, urticaria), 2% were anaphylaxis, which resulted in unsuccessful desensitization in one patient, and 8% were late reactions such as late onset urticaria, serum sickness, and nephritis.

Most reports of penicillin desensitization published since 1980 have involved the use of the oral route. Although the systemic route for drug desensitization seems more risky, on the basis of experience before 1980, the limited experience

Table 4 Adverse Reactions to β-Lactam Antibiotics with Desensitization

Route of administration	Patients	Reactions (%) Cutaneous (%)	Anaphylaxis (%)	Late (%)	Total (%)
Before 1980					
SQ, IM, IV[a] 13 reports [25,27,33,34]	43	13 (30)	4[b] (9)	7 (16)	24 (56)
After 1980					
Oral, 4 reports [9,15,23,25]	74	19 (26)	1 (1)	7 (10)	27 (36)
IV,[a] 2 reports [27,28]	26	5 (19)	1[c] (4)	0	6 (23)

[a]SQ = Subcutaneous; IM = intramuscular; IV = intravenous.
[b]Two deaths.
[c]One unsuccessful desensitization.

of two separate investigators using the IV route is at least comparable in safety to the results obtained with the oral route. However, no direct comparison of these two routes of desensitization has been made in a controlled fashion and reported in the contemporary literature.

B. Insulin

Generalized urticaria and other systemic reactions indicative of anaphylaxis to insulin administration usually are the result of interruption of regular insulin replacement therapy in a diabetic patient [1]. Systemic symptoms usually occur within 12 days of resumption of insulin replacement therapy, following progressively larger local dermal reactions at the site of subcutaneous insulin injections [4,5].

Patients with systemic reactions to insulin should be hospitalized. If the patient is seen within 24–48 h of the reaction, and the signs and symptoms of anaphylaxis are mild (usually cutaneous only), the patient's usual insulin dose can be reduced to approximately one-third and then gradually increased by 2–5 units per injection until the previous dose or diabetic control is achieved [4,5].

If 48 or more hours have elapsed, or the systemic signs and symptoms of anaphylaxis are more severe, then it is appropriate to desensitize the patient to insulin. This procedure begins with allergy skin testing to various insulins from both animal and human sources to find the least antigenic insulin for the individual patient. Typically, patients are least reactive (by skin test) to recombinant DNA human insulin. Table 5 shows a typical insulin desensitization protocol for a patient who can be safely controlled over several days [1]. This protocol is similar to other insulin desensitization schedules published in the literature [2,4,5]. More rapid insulin desensitization may be necessary if diabetic ketoacidosis is present. Insulin desensitization may be accomplished with dosage adjustments as rapid as every 15–30 min, as with β-lactam antibiotic desensitization, which follows the same principles of immunological desensitization in a patient with an IgE sensitization. The same precautions should be followed in the desensitization procedure for insulin allergy in a diabetic patient as for penicillin allergy and β-lactam antibiotic desensitization, with regard to anticipation of an adverse reaction and possible protocol adjustments. In addition, in insulin desensitization, the staff should be prepared to treat rapid changes in blood glucose levels, including hypoglycemia.

Once the maintenance insulin dose has been achieved, the patient can usually be kept at therapeutic dosing of insulin indefinitely. Thus, the "desensitized state" continues as long as insulin replacement therapy is given daily.

Table 5 Insulin Desensitization

Day	Time	Route[a]	Type[b]	Units[c]
1	AM	ID	Reg	0.00001
	Noon	ID	Reg	0.0001
	PM	ID	Reg	0.001
2	AM	ID	Reg	0.01
	Noon	ID	Reg	0.1
	PM	ID	Reg	1.0
3	AM	ID	Reg	2.0
	Noon	SQ	Reg	4.0
	PM	SQ	Reg	8.0
4	AM	SQ	Reg	12.0
	Noon	SQ	Reg	16.0
5	AM	SQ	NPH/Lente	20.0
6	AM	SQ	NPH/Lente	25.0
7 and on	AM	SQ	NPH/Lente	Increase 5 U/d until reaching therapeutic level

[a]ID = intradermal; SQ = subcutaneous

[b]Reg = regular crystalline zinc insulin; NPH/Lente = long-acting insulin.

[c]The starting dose may be modified by the patient's insulin sensitivity, based on skin testing, 24–48 h after start of severe reaction.

Soruce: Ref. 1.

C. Horse Serum–Derived (Equine) Antivenin

In the rare case in which a patient requires a lifesaving antiserum such as antivenin for snakebite, the possibility of allergy to horses must be considered before the biological agent is administered. A patient who has had previous allergic symptoms on exposure to horses (asthma, hay fever, or urticaria) can be assumed also to be allergic to blood products from the horse. The existence of allergy can be confirmed by allergy skin testing to either horse extract or to a 1:10 weight/volume dilution of the specific biological product (e.g., antivenin), using a 0.02 intradermal test dose.

If the patient is allergic and has a positive skin test to the biological agent, the clinician should follow the directions of the package insert of the biological product regarding a desensitization procedure. Table 6 represents a protocol based on published information in the *Physician's Desk Reference* and a Wyeth Laborato-

Table 6 Snake Antivenin (Horse Serum) Skin Test, Desensitization, Treatment (℞)[a]

Route	Dilution	Dose (ml)	Cumulative dose (ml)
ID skin tests	1:100	0.02	—
	1:10	0.02	—
SC desensitization	1:100	0.1	0.001
		0.2	0.003
		0.5	0.008
	1:10	0.1	0.018
		0.2	0.038
		0.5	0.088
IM℞	FS	0.1	0.188
		0.2	0.388
		0.4	0.788
		0.8	1.588
		1.6	3.2
		3.2	6.4
		6.4	12.8
Minimum ℞[b]	FS	12.8	25.6
Minimum to moderate ℞	FS	25.6	51.2
Moderate to severe ℞	FS	50	101.2
Severe ℞	FS	50	151.2

[a]Following positive skin tests, advances in doses every 15 min. From *Physician's Desk Reference*, 47th Ed., 1993, pp. 2541–2543.

[b]Envenomation: minimum-involvement ℞; moderate-involvement ℞; severe-involvement ℞.

ID = intradermal; SC = subcutaneous; IM = intramuscular; FS = full strength.

ries package insert concerning the use of snake antivenin from an equine source [35]. If the patient is known to be severely reactive to horse or horse serum, a more conservative desensitization schedule should be individually established. The basic principles used in other immunological desensitizations, as with β-lactam antibiotics or insulin, would also apply to desensitization using horse serum–containing vaccines.

The top doses listed in the protocol in Table 6 relate to the amount of antivenin that is necessary to treat a patient who is mildly, moderately, or severely afflicted by snakebite.

If a reaction to horse serum–derived antivenin occurs during the desensitization procedure, it must be managed promptly. The next dose of antivenin should not be given before 30 min, according to the published reports, and preferably should be lower than the dose of antivenom provoking the reaction [1].

Once the patient has tolerated 0.5 ml of a full-strength subcutaneous administration of antivenin, it is advised that the patient be given either progressive intramuscular doses or IV antivenom at a 1:1 to 1:10 dilution in sodium chloride injection (USP) or 5% dextrose injection (USP). Antivenin treatment will usually require a minimum of 20 ml (two 10-ml vials) and a maximum of 150 ml or more (15 or more vials), depending on the severity of the snakebite reaction [35].

In the allergic patient who requires desensitization with horse serum antivenin or other horse serum–derived biological products, anaphylaxis should be anticipated throughout the procedure, including skin testing, subcutaneous desensitization, and IV antivenin treatment. Furthermore, serum sickness reactions are common with horse serum administration and are not blocked by acute desensitization.

D. Aspirin

The usual recommendation for the aspirin-intolerant patient is strict avoidance of aspirin and nonsteroidal anti-inflammatory drugs (NSAIDs) [1]. Aspirin desensitization has been performed successfully in many patients with chronic rhinitis and asthma, but not with aspirin-induced urticaria [8]. This includes 25 aspirin-sensitive asthmatics in a 7-month, randomized, placebo-controlled, double-blind, crossover, extended trial [36]. There are follow-up reports of 107 patients who either were desensitized with aspirin for as long as 8 years (35 patients), were told to avoid aspirin (42 patients), or finally, were desensitized for a mean of 2 years and then discontinued the drug because of side effects, avoiding aspirin thereafter (30 patients) [14]. Statistical evaluation of these three groups demonstrated more improvement in both rhinitis and aspirin symptoms in the patient continuously maintained in the "aspirin-desensitized state."

According to Manning and Stevenson, all aspirin-sensitive asthmatic patients are capable of undergoing desensitization [8]. Usually, patients are first sequentially challenged with serial oral doses of aspirin under controlled conditions (see protocol, Table 7). The end point for a positive challenge in the studies of Stevenson et al. is either a drop of 20% or more in pulmonary function (forced expired volume in 1 second [FEV_1]) or early signs of hay fever–like symptoms such as rhinorrhea, ocular injection, or periorbital edema.

Typically, oral aspirin challenges are done on an inpatient basis, over a 3-day period, using a single blind method (Table 7) [8]. Following three negative placebo doses on day 1 at 8 a.m., 11 a.m., and 2 p.m., progressive doses of oral aspirin are given at the same time intervals on days 2 and 3. The beginning aspirin doses range from 3 to 30 mg and progress to 60 mg, 100 mg, 150 mg, 325 mg, and 650 mg—unless the patient reacts.

In 30 patients challenged in the above manner, cumulative provocative doses of aspirin ranged from 33 to 1083 mg [13]. Declines in FEV_1 ranged from 25% to 65%. Nasal symptoms were provoked in 28 of 30 patients. Eleven of 30 patients (37%) reacted to doses of aspirin of 150 mg or less. Twelve of 30 patients (40%) reacted to doses between 180 and 450 mg. Seven patients (23%) reacted to aspirin doses of 500 mg or more.

Aspirin desensitization is accomplished by reinstituting the oral dose of aspirin that initiated a positive challenge, on the following day, once the patient is stabilized. If no reaction occurs, the next higher dose of aspirin is given, as used in the challenge protocol (Table 7). A maximum of three desensitization doses are given per day. Should the patient react again, at any of the desensitizing doses, subsequent challenge is suspended for the rest of the day. The following day, once the patient is stabilized, rechallenge and desensitization is repeated again using the last dose of aspirin that was responsible for the previous reaction. This procedure is repeated until the patient has been shown to tolerate 650 mg of aspirin without any reaction. At this point, the patient is considered desensitized [8]. This "desensitized state" can then be maintained, long-term, by maintaining the aspirin doses at 650 mg every 12 h [14].

Table 7 Single-Blind 3-Day Oral Aspirin Challenge and Desensitization[a]

Time	Day 1	Day 2	Day 3
8:00 a.m.	Placebo	Aspirin, 3 or 30 mg	Aspirin, 150 mg
11:00 a.m.	Placebo	Aspirin, 60 mg	Aspirin, 325 mg
2:00 a.m.	Placebo	Aspirin, 100 mg	Aspirin, 650 mg

[a]Individualized by the physician with respect to both incremental increases in aspirin dosage and timing of administration.
Source: Ref. 8.

E. Sulfonamide Antimicrobial Drugs

The risk of an adverse reaction to sulfonamide drugs, particularly a macular/papular rash, urticaria, and, in AIDS patients, fever, is substantial [37,38]. This class of antimicrobial agents is a frequently associated with medication reactions of the febrile mucocutaneous syndrome type such as Stevens–Johnson syndrome and Lyell's syndrome (toxic epidermal necrolysis). However, the occurrence of severe, life-threatening reactions to the sulfonamide drugs, such as systemic anaphylaxis or Lyell's syndrome, is uncommon [39].

Of particular importance are reactions to TMP-SMX. The incidence of cutaneous reactions to these drugs in the general population is estimated to be 3% [38]. This drug reaction rate increases to 12% among immunosuppressed patients who are HIV-seronegative and is estimated to be 29–70% among patients who have AIDS. This is of particular concern because TMP-SMX is the principal medication for both treatment of and prophylaxis against *Pneumocystis carinii* pneumonia (PCP), a common result of immunodeficiency in AIDS patients [39,40].

In AIDS patients who have mild to moderate reactions to TMP-SMX, such as rash or fever, further treatment with this medication is often still advisable [39]. In a study involving 21 AIDS patients who reacted to IV TMP-SMX when treated for PCP, only four (20%) reacted a second time when this medication was subsequently given by mouth for prophylactic control of recurrent infection [41]. In a controlled trial of 310 adult AIDS patients who had recently recovered from PCP following TMP-SMX treatment, 154 were randomly placed on the same drug and the rest on another medication as prophylaxis [40]. Of these patients receiving prophylactic TMP-SMX, there was little difference in the percentage of patients who tolerated this medication when readministered based on whether they had a previous mild or moderate reaction to TMP-SMX (68% vs. 74%). Furthermore, the severity of the subsequent reaction was approximately the same based on the necessity to switch to another prophylactic treatment (8 of 25 with a history of previous TMP-SMX reaction [32%] vs. 33 of 129 without a history of a previous TMP-SMX reaction [26%]) [40]. It is for this reason that some authorities feel that for AIDS patients requiring PCP prophylaxis who have had a reaction to TMP-SMX that was mild to moderate, repeat administration of the drug is advisable and does not necessitate either incremental challenge or desensitization [38,39].

On the other hand, when patients have initially had febrile mucocutaneous reactions to TMP-SMX, such as the Stevens–Johnson syndrome, repeat administration of the drug has almost always resulted in a more severe reaction [38]. It is this type of reaction that has resulted in discontinuation of the drug in up to 14% of cases [38]. Development of febrile mucocutaneous reactions precludes drug desensitization, for when this has been tried, the result has usually been a more severe reaction upon rechallenge.

Sulfadiazine has been used to treat central nervous system toxoplasmosis in

AIDS patients. Reaction rates of 10–40% have been reported [38]. Sulfasalazine (SSZ) has been used to manage ulcerative colitis. Rash and fever have been reported as side effects in 1–5% of patients [16].

Desensitization to the sulfonamide antimicrobial agents may appropriately be considered if there is no suitable alternative treatment in life-threatening conditions such as PCP or CNS toxoplasmosis in AIDS patients or for patients with ulcerative colitis. Case reports of successful desensitization using TMP-SMX, SDZ, and SSZ have been published [15,16,38,41–44].

Desensitization to the sulfonamide drugs is usually an extended procedure taking place over many days, up to 1 month. Table 8 represents a TMP-SMX desensitization protocol adjusted from the report of Smith et al. [15]. With this protocol, it takes approximately 2 weeks to reach a tolerated dose of medication comparable to a single usual dose of TMP-SMX, or a "desensitized state."

Table 9 represents an extended oral SSZ desensitization protocol adapted from Purdy et al., who successfully desensitized 12 of 13 patients with inflammatory bowel disease [16]. With this protocol, it takes at least 25 days to reach a tolerated drug dose comparable to a single usual dose of SSZ. It should be noted, however,

Table 8 Extended Oral Trimethoprim–Sulfamethoxazole Desensitization[a]

Day	Sulfamethoxazole (mg/ml or tablet)	Drug dose per day
1	2 mg/ml	1 mg
2	2 mg/ml	2 mg
3	2 mg/ml	4 mg
4	2 mg/ml	8 mg
5	2 mg/ml	10 mg
6	2 mg/ml	16 mg
7	40 mg/ml	24 mg
8	40 mg/ml	40 mg
9	40 mg/ml	80 mg
10	40 mg/ml	100 mg
11	40 mg/ml	120 mg
12	40 mg/ml	160 mg
13	40 mg/ml	200 mg
14	40 mg/ml	300 mg
15	80 mg trimethoprim/400 mg sulfamethoxazole (tablet)	400 mg (1 tab./day)
16–22		800 mg (2 tab./day)
23+		1600 mg (4 tab./day)

[a]Modified from Smith et al. [16].
Source: Ref. 1.

Table 9 Extended Oral Sulfasalazine Desensitization[a]

Day	Sulfasalazine mg/ml suspension or tablet	Drug dose per day
1	1 mg/ml	1 mg
2	1 mg/ml	2 mg
3	1 mg/ml	4 mg
4	1 mg/ml	8 mg
5–11	1 mg/ml	10 mg (each day)
12	20 mg/ml	20 mg
13	20 mg/ml	40 mg
14	20 mg/ml	80 mg
15–21	20 mg/ml	100 mg (each day)
22	20 mg/ml	200 mg
23	20 mg/ml	400 mg
24	20 mg/ml	800 mg
25–31	500 mg/ml	1000 mg (2 tab./day)
32+	500 mg/ml	2000 mg (4 tab./day)

[a]Modified from Purdy et al. [15].
Source: Ref. 1.

that in the 12 patients treated by Purdy et al., it usually took 32 days to reach a minimum therapeutic dose of 2 g SSZ/day, and in 3 of 12 patients (25%) it took 2–7 months to achieve this treatment dose.

Similar desensitization procedures have been reported for SDZ used to treat cerebral toxoplasmosis in AIDS patients, in which oral medication was slowly increased over days [38,43]. Although Bell et al. performed the desensitizing procedure under concurrent corticosteroid therapy, the use of corticosteroids or antihistamines is not advised, as they could mask a treatable reaction during the desensitization procedure [38,43]. These drugs should be reserved for use if a reaction occurs.

Desensitization procedures with sulfonamide medications still carry a significant risk of a serious reaction during or after the procedure—and may not be successful. An anaphylactoid reaction with severe hypotension induced by oral TMP-SMX during a desensitization procedure using a protocol for such a procedure published by Finegold was reported by Scher et al. [42,45]. Of 13 patients who were placed on a desensitization protocol with SSZ by Purdy et al., five (38%) developed an allergic-like reaction (pruritus or rash), which was severe enough in one patient to cause discontinuation of the procedure [16].

Carr et al. [38] reported upon 27 patients desensitized to SDZ on 33 occasions. In five patients (19%), an allergic-like reaction prompted discontinuation of the procedure. Greenberger and Patterson [19] have reported on 2 patients with AIDS who developed a reaction to sulfonamide medication. One patient was rapidly desensitized using an oral SDZ protocol with dosing every 4 h. This patient developed a rash at 10 days. A rapid desensitization with TMP-SMX was attempted in the second patient with IV dosing every 20 min. This procedure was discontinued after two attempts because of high fever and rash at 3 h after beginning the IV TMP-SMX infusion.

F. Desensitization Using Other Drugs

Reports of successful desensitization with drugs other than the β-lactam antibiotics, insulin, vaccines containing horse serum, aspirin, and sulfonamide antibiotics are few in number. Table 10 lists individual reports relating to desensitization procedures using allopurinol in gout, cytarabine in leukemia, pentamidine in AIDS, tobramycin in cystic fibrosis, and vancomycin in AIDS. The original reaction to these medications that prompted consideration for desensitization was usually allergic-like [1]. The exact mechanism of these reactions is usually unknown, but it probably is not an IgE mechanism, although this was suspected in the reports on cytarabine and vancomycin. Patterson has stated that the "use of allopurinol in patients with a history of drug reaction . . . is a dangerous procedure. The expected reaction is delayed and thus the onset of symptoms of a drug reaction may follow a dose by 2–4 days" [2]. Webster and Panush, however, have reported on a single patient with chronic tophaceous gout who developed a pruritic maculopapular rash with allopurinol [17]. Having failed to respond to other medication, the patient was successfully desensitized with slowly increasing

Table 10 Reports of Successful Drug Desensitizations Based on Very Limited Experience

Drug	Reaction (disease)	Starting dose	Increment	Interval	Final
Allopurinol [17]	Rash (gout)	0.008 mg	1.5–2 ×	p.o. 1 × every day × 30 days	300,000 mg
Cytarabine [12]	Anaphylaxis (leukemia)	10 ml of 0.002% sol.	10 ×	IV every 30 min.	200 mg in 500 ml
Pentamidine [19]	Rash and anaphylactoid reactions (AIDS)	0.00016 mg	10 × to 0.16 mg in 2 ml	IV for 2 min every 15 min	200 mg in 250 ml over 2 h
Tobramycin [11]	Anaphylaxis (cystic fibrosis)	0.001 mg	2 ×	IV every 30 min.	16 mg
Vancomycin [18]	"Red-man" syndrome (AIDS)	0.5 mg in 500 ml	10 ×	5 h/day for 6 days	500 mg

oral doses, advancing daily over a 1-month period. Other similar individual case reports of allopurinol desensitization can be found in the published literature, but the experience is limited.

Successful intravenous desensitization with the pyrimidine nucleoside cytarabine was performed in a single leukemic patient [12]. Evidence for an IgE-type reaction was reported on the basis of a positive intradermal skin test and the ability to passively transfer cutaneous hypersensitivity in guinea pigs using a 4-h passive cutaneous anaphylaxis (PCA) test. No allergic-like reaction occurred during the desensitization procedure, but the patient died 5 days later of sepsis.

Pentamidine has been used as an alternative medication for the treatment of PCP (especially when the patient has reacted to TMP-SMX). Although allergic-like reactions to pentamidine are usually reported to be less frequent than with the use of TMP-SMX, one prospective study demonstrated a rate of adverse reactions to pentamidine of approximately 15% [38]. Intravenous administration of pentamidine during the treatment of PCP in AIDS patients has been associated with profound and fatal hypotension [39]. The aerosolized route has been used as an alternative in prophylactic treatment attempting to protect against primary or recurrent PCP. Bronchoconstriction has been reported to occur in 30–40% of cases, but it can be treated without discontinuation of the drug with concomitant inhaled β_2-adrenergic medications such as albuterol [39].

Greenberger and Patterson described two patients with AIDS and PCP who were successfully desensitized with an IV pentamidine desensitization protocol [19]. These patients either had a rash or wheezed repeatedly with pentamidine medication. Immediate or late allergic-like reaction occurred during the IV pentamidine desensitization procedure, but both patients were observed only for a short time, since they died in 2 days and in 4 days [19].

Earl and Sullivan described a 15-year-old patient with cystic fibrosis who developed urticaria in reaction to the aminoglycoside antibiotic tobramycin [11]. This patient was successfully desensitized to this antibiotic by the IV route but could not be desensitized to penicillin, to which she was also allergic. Evidence for an IgE mechanism in tobramycin reaction was reported. An intradermal immediate-reacting skin test to this antibiotic was slightly positive, with a reaction greater than that to a similar skin test in four control subjects. The size of the skin test reaction lessened somewhat after the desensitization procedure.

Lin et al. reported upon a desensitization procedure of a single AIDS patient who developed the "red-man (or red-neck) syndrome" while being treated with vancomycin for methicillin-resistant septicemia [18]. An IgE etiology in this patient was suspected on the basis of an immediate-reacting skin test to vancomycin before the desensitization procedure and a decrease in size after desensitization and 5 weeks of full therapeutic dosing of this medication. In most cases of this type of reaction (red-man or red-neck), direct mast cell mediator release rather than allergy is the proposed mechanism [1].

VI. SUMMARY

Drug desensitization can be a useful procedure in some carefully selected patients who have had an allergic or an allergic-like reaction to an agent but require the drug because their illness is serious and no suitable substitute is available. Most information exists on desensitization procedures involving immunological IgE reactions, especially those involving β-lactam antibiotics (e.g., penicillin) and insulin. Desensitization has also proved helpful in the case of some nonimmunological anaphylactoid reactions, such as those to aspirin and sulfonamide-containing antimicrobial agents. Drug desensitization has not been proved helpful for anaphylactoid reactions to radiocontrast media. Desensitization has been proved to be unsuccessful and dangerous when attempted for reactions of the febrile mucocutaneous type (e.g., Stevens–Johnson syndrome and Lyell's syndrome).

Important considerations in the use of the drug desensitization procedure, as well as protocols for drug administration available in the recently published U.S. literature, have been presented in this chapter. Attention has been given to risk factors that must be considered before utilizing this therapeutic approach.

The potential risk to the patient must always be weighed against the possible benefit. If drug desensitization is attempted, the procedure must be done under controlled conditions by knowledgeable physicians and support staff. Adverse reactions to the drug desensitization procedure should be expected in at least one-third of the cases.

Finally, although protocols for drug desensitization have been published, those attempting to perform this procedure should use these protocols only as guidelines, since they are based on limited information and usually have to be altered for each patient desensitized.

REFERENCES

1. Anderson, J. A., Allergic reactions to drugs and biologic agents, *JAMA*, *268*, 2845–2857 (1992).
2. Patterson, R., DeSwarte, R. D., Greenberger, P. A., and Grammer, L. C., Drug allergy and protocols for management of drug allergies, *NER Allergy Proc.*, *7*, 325–342 (1986).
3. Patterson, R., Diagnosis and treatment of drug allergy, *J. Allergy Clin. Immunol.*, *81*, 380–384 (1985).
4. DeSwarte, R. D., Drug allergy, in *Allergic Diseases—Diagnosis and Management*, 4th Ed. (R. Patterson, L. C. Grammar, P. A. Greenberger, and C. R. Zeiss, eds.), J. B. Lippincott, Philadelphia, 1993; pp. 395–552.
5. Lieberman, P., Difficult allergic drug reactions, *Immunol. Allergy Clin. North Am.*, *11*, 213–231 (1991).
6. DeShazo, R. D., and Nelson, H. S., An approach to the patient with a history of local

anesthetic hypersensitivity: experience with 90 patients, *J. Allergy Clin. Immunol.*, *63*, 387–394 (1979).
7. *Random House Dictionary of the English Language*, unabridged edition, Random House, New York, 1986.
8. Manning, M. E., and Stevenson, D. D., Pseudoallergic drug reactions. Aspirin, nonsteroidal anti-inflammatory drugs, dyes, additives, and preservatives, *Immunol. Allergy Clin. North Am.*, *11*, 659–678 (1991).
9. Stark, B., Earl, H., Gross, G., Lumry, W. R., Goodman, E. L., and Sullivan, T. J., Acute and chronic desensitization of penicillin allergic patients using oral penicillin, *J. Allergy Clin. Immunol.*, *79*, 523–532 (1987).
10. Wedner, H. J., Drug allergy prevention and treatment, *Immunol. Allergy Clin. North Am.*, *11*, 679–694 (1991).
11. Earl, H. S., and Sullivan, T. J., Acute desensitization of a patient with cystic fibrosis allergic to both beta-lactam and aminoglycoside antibiotics, *J. Allergy Clin. Immunol.*, *79*, 477–483 (1987).
12. Rassiga, A. L., Schwartz, H. J., Forman, W. B., and Crum, .E D., Cytarabine-induced anaphylaxis, *Arch. Intern. Med.*, *140*, 425–426 (1980).
13. Pleskow, W. W., Stevenson, D. D., Mathison, D. A., Simon, R. A., Shatz, M., and Zeiger, R. S., Aspirin desensitization in aspirin sensitive asthmatic patients: clinical manifestation and characterization of the refractory period, *J. Allergy Clin. Immunol.*, *69*, 11–19 (1982).
14. Sweet, J. M., Stevenson, D. D., Simon, R. A., and Mathison, D. A., Long-term effects of aspirin desensitization—treatment for aspirin-sensitive rhinosinusitis-asthma, *J. Allergy Clin. Immunol.*, *85*, 59–65 (1990).
15. Purdy, B. H., Phillips, D. R., and Summers, R. W., Desensitization for sulfasalazine skin rash, *Ann. Intern. Med.*, *100*, 512–514 (1984).
16. Smith, R. M., Iwamoto, G. K., Richerson, H. B., and Flaherty, J. P., Trimethoprim-sulfamethoxazole desensitization in the acquired immunodeficiency syndrome (letter), *Ann. Intern. Med.*, *106*, 335 (1987).
17. Webster, E., and Panush, R. S., Allopurinol hypersensitivity in a patient with severe, chronic, tophaceous gout, *Arthritis Rheum.*, *28*, 707–709 (1985).
18. Lin, R. Y., Desensitization in the management of vancomycin hypersensitivity, *Arch. Intern. Med.*, *150*, 2197–2198 (1990).
19. Greenberger, P. A., and Patterson, R., Management of drug allergy in patients with acquired immunodeficiency syndrome, *J. Allergy Clin. Immunol.*, *79*, 484–488 (1987).
20. Patterson, R., Mellies, C. J., and Roberts, M., Immunologic reactions against insulin: IgE anti-insulin, insulin allergy and combined IgE and IgG immunologic insulin resistance, *J. Allergy Clin. Immunol.*, *110*, 1135 (1973).
21. Lamkin, N., Lieberman, P., Hashimoto, K., et al., Allergic reactions to insulin. Allergy grand rounds, *J. Allergy Clin. Immunol.*, *58*, 213 (1976).
22. Naclerio, R., Mizrahi, E. A., and Adkinson, N. F., Immunologic observations during desensitization and maintenance of clinical tolerance to penicillin, *J. Allergy Clin. Immunol.*, *71*, 294 (1983).
23. Sullivan, T. J., Antigen specific desensitization of patients allergic to penicillin, *J. Allergy Clin. Immunol.*, *69*, 500–508 (19820.

24. Pienkowski, M. M., Kazmier, J., and Adkinson, N. F., Basophil histamine release remains unaffected by clinical desensitization to penicillin, *J. Allergy Clin. Immunol.*, *82*, 171–178 (1988).
25. Sullivan, T. J., Yecies, L. D., Shatz, G. S., Parker, C. W., and Wedner, H. J., Desensitization of patients allergic to penicillin using orally administered β-lactam antibiotics, *J. Allergy Clin. Immunol.*, *69*, 275–282 (1982).
26. Wendel, G. D., Stark, B. J., Jamison, R. B., Molina, R. D., and Sullivan, T. J., Penicillin allergy and desensitization in serious infections during pregnancy, *N. Engl. J. Med.*, *312*, 1229–1232 (1985).
27. Borish, L., Tamir, R., and Rosenwasser, I. J., Intravenous desensitization to beta-lactam antibiotics, *J. Allergy Clin. Immunol.*, *80*, 314–319 (1987).
28. Moss, R. B., Babin, S., Hsu, Y. P., Blessing-Moore, J., and Lewiston, N. J., Allergy to semisynthetic penicillins in cystic fibrosis, *J. Pediatr.*, *104*, 460–466 (1984).
29. Lin, R. Y., A perspective on penicillin allergy, *Arch. Intern. Med.*, *152*, 930–937 (1991).
30. Morbidity and Mortality Weekly Report, Centers for Disease Control, Atlanta, Georgia, Sept. 1, 1988; pp. 14–15.
31. Bousquet, J., *In-vivo* methods for study of allergy: skin test techniques and interpretation in allergy, in *Allergy Principles and Practice*, 3rd Ed. (E. Middleton, Jr., C. Reed, E. Ellis, N. F. Adkinson, Jr., and J. Yunginger, eds.), CV Mosby, St. Louis, 1988, pp. 422–425.
32. Saxon, A., Beall, G. N., Rohr, A. S., and Adelman, D. C., Immediate hypersensitivity reactions to beta-lactam antibiotics, *Ann. Intern. Med.*, *107*, 204–215 (1987).
33. Grieco, M. H., Drubin, M. R., Robinson, J. L., and Schwartz, M. J., Penicillin hypersensitivity in patients with bacterial endocarditis, *Ann. Intern. Med.*, *60*, 203 (1964).
34. Graybill, J. R., Sande, M. A., Reinarz, J. A., and Shapiro, S. R., Controlled penicillin anaphylaxis leading to desensitization, *South. Med. J.*, *67*, 62 (1974).
35. Antivenin (Crotalidae) polyvalent (equine origin), Wyeth Laboratories, Division of American Home Products Corp., Philadelphia, package insert and *Physician's Desk Reference* 47th Ed., 1993, pp. 2541–2543.
36. Stevenson, D. D., Pleskow, W. W., Simon, R. A., Mathison, D. A., Lumry, W. R., Schatz, M., and Zeiger, R. S., Aspirin-sensitive rhinosinusitis asthma: a double-blind crossover study of treatment of aspirin, *J. Allergy Clin. Immunol.*, *73*, 500–507 (1984).
37. Bigby, M., Jick, S., Jick, H., and Arndt, K., Drug-induced cutaneous reactions: a report from the Boston Collaborative Drug surveillance program on 15,438 consecutive inpatients, 1975 to 1983, *JAMA*, *256*, 3358–3363 (1986).
38. Carr, A., Cooper, D., and Penny, R., Allergic manifestations of human immunodeficiency virus (HIV) infection, *J. Clin. Immunol.*, *11*, 55–64 (1991).
39. Masur, H., Prevention and treatment of pneumocystis pneumonia, *N. Engl. J. Med.*, *327*, 1853–1860 (1992).
40. Hardy, W. D., Feinberg, J., Finkelstein, D. M., et al., A controlled trial of trimethoprim-sulfamethoxazole or aerosolized pentamidine for secondary prophylaxis of *Pneumocystis carinii* pneumonia in patients with acquired immunodefi-

ciency syndrome. AIDS Clinical Trials Group Protocol 021, *N. Engl. J. Med.*, *327*, 1842–1848 (1992).

41. Shafer, R. W., Seitzman, P. A., and Tapper, M. L., Successful prophylaxis of *Pneumocystis carinii* pneumonia with trimethoprim-sulfamethoxazole in AIDS patients with previous allergic reactions, *J. AIDS*, *2*, 389–393 (1989).
42. Finegold, I., Oral desensitization to trimethoprim-sulfamethoxazole in a patient with acquired immunodeficiency syndrome, *J. Allergy Clin. Immunol.*, *78*, 905–908 (1986).
43. Bell, E. T., Sulphadiazine desensitization in AIDS patients (letter), *Lancet*, *i*, 163 (1985).
44. Holdsworth, C. D., Sulphasalazine desensitization (letter), *Br. Med. J.*, *282*, 110 (1981).
45. Sher, M. R., Suchar, C., and Lockey, R. F., Anaphylactic shock induced by oral desensitization to trimethoprim/sulfamethoxazole (TMP-SMX) (abstr.), *J. Allergy Clin. Immunol.*, *77*, 133A (1986).

Index

About the Editor

SHELDON L. SPECTOR is a Clinical Professor in the Department of Medicine at the University of California Los Angeles School of Medicine. The coauthor, editor, or coeditor of five books and the author or coauthor of over 190 professional papers and some 90 abstracts, he is a Fellow of the American College of Physicians, the American College of Chest Physicians, the American Academy of Allergy and Immunology, and the American College of Allergy and Immunology, and a member of the American Society of Internal Medicine and the American Thoracic Society, among other organizations, and he serves on the editorial boards of several journals, including the *Journal of Asthma* (Marcel Dekker, Inc.). Dr. Spector received the M.D. degree (1964) from Wayne State University, Detroit, Michigan. He is certified by the American Board of Internal Medicine and the American Board of Allergy and Immunology.